Antimicrobial Resistance

in Bacteria from Livestock and Companion Animals

Antimicrobial Resistance

in Bacteria from Livestock and Companion Animals

EDITORS

Stefan Schwarz
Freie Universität Berlin, Berlin, Germany

Lina Maria Cavaco
Statens Serum Institute, Copenhagen, Denmark

Jianzhong Shen
China Agricultural University, Beijing, China

with Frank Møller Aarestrup

ASM
PRESS

Washington, DC

Library of Congress Cataloging-in-Publication Data

Names: Schwarz, Stefan (Professor of veterinary medicine), editor. | Cavaco, Lina Maria, editor. | Shen, Jianzhong (Professor of agricultural science), editor. | Aarestrup, Frank M., 1966- editor.
Title: Antimicrobial resistance in bacteria from livestock and companion animals / editors: Stefan Schwarz, Lina Maria Cavaco, and Jianzhong Shen, with Frank M?ller Aarestrup.
Description: Washington, DC : ASM Press, [2018] | Includes index.
Identifiers: LCCN 2018025722 (print) | LCCN 2018027927 (ebook) | ISBN 9781555819804 (ebook) | ISBN 9781555819798 | ISBN 9781555819798q (hard cover)
Subjects: LCSH: Drug resistance in microorganisms. | Antibiotics in veterinary medicine.
Classification: LCC QR177 (ebook) | LCC QR177 .A58565 2018 (print) | DDC 616.9/041--dc23
LC record available at https://lccn.loc.gov/2018025722

10 9 8 7 6 5 4 3 2 1

Address editorial correspondence to
ASM Press, 1752 N St., N.W.,
Washington, DC 20036-2904, USA

Send orders to ASM Press, P.O. Box 605, Herndon, VA 20172, USA
Phone: 800-546-2416; 703-661-1593
Fax: 703-661-1501
E-mail: books@asmusa.org
Online: http://www.asmscience.org

We would like to thank our families for their support and to all our corresponding and contributing authors who shared their expertise, time, and effort in producing this book.

Contents

Contributors

SAM ABRAHAM
School of Veterinary and Life Sciences
Murdoch University
Murdoch, Western Australia
Australia

BEN ADLER
School of Biomedical Sciences
Monash University
Clayton, Victoria
Australia

CARLA ANDREA ALONSO
Biochemistry and Molecular Biology Unit
University of La Rioja
Logroño, La Rioja
Spain

MUNA F. ANJUM
Department of Bacteriology,
Animal and Plant Health Agency
Addlestone, Surrey
United Kingdom

MIKE APLEY
Clinical Sciences
College of Veterinary Medicine
Kansas State University
Manhattan, KS 66506

MARIE ARCHAMBAULT
Département de Pathologie et Microbiologie
Faculté de Médecine Vétérinaire
Université de Montréal
Saint-Hyacinthe, Québec
Canada

CRISTINA ARROYO
UCD School of Agriculture and Food Science
University College Dublin
Dublin
Ireland

LI BAI
Key Laboratory of Food Safety Risk Assessment of Ministry of Health
China National Center for Food Safety Risk Assessment
Beijing
China

LONDA J. BERGHAUS
Department of Large Animal Medicine,
College of Veterinary Medicine,
University of Georgia,
Athens, GA

JANINE T. BOSSÉ
Section of Pediatrics,
Department of Medicine
Imperial College London
London
United Kingdom

PATRICK BUTAYE
Department of Biomedical Sciences
Ross University School of Veterinary Sciences
Basseterre
Saint Kitts and Nevis
And
Department of Pathology, Bacteriology and Poultry Diseases
Ghent University, Faculty of Veterinary Medicine
Merelbeke
Belgium

BOUDEWIJN CATRY
Scientific Institute of Public Health
Brussels
Belgium

LINA MARIA CAVACO
Department for Bacteria, Parasites and Fungi, Infectious Disease Preparedness
Statens Serum Institute
Copenhagen
Denmark
and
Department for Cellular and Molecular Medicine
Faculty of Health and Medical Sciences
University of Copenhagen
Copenhagen
Denmark

PETER J. COLLIGNON
Infectious Diseases and Microbiology
Canberra Hospital
Garran, Australian Capital Territory
Australia
and
Medical School
Australian National University
Acton, Australian Capital Territory
Australia

TERESA M. COQUE
Department of Microbiology
Ramón y Cajal University Hospital
Ramón y Cajal Health Research Institute (IRYCIS)
Madrid
Spain

SALLY J. CUTLER
School of Health, Sport & Bioscience
University of East London
London
United Kingdom

ROSA DEL CAMPO
Department of Microbiology
Ramón y Cajal University Hospital
Ramón y Cajal Health Research Institute (IRYCIS)
Madrid
Spain
and
Red Española de Investigación en Patología Infecciosa (REIPI)

ANA SOFIA R. DUARTE
Unit for Genomic Epidemiology
National Food Institute
Technical University of Denmark
Lyngby
Denmark

JORDI TORREN EDO
European Medicines Agency
London
United Kingdom
and
Facultat de Veterinària
Universitat Autònoma de Barcelona (UAB)
Cerdanyola del Vallès
Spain

SÉAMUS FANNING
UCD-Centre for Food Safety
University College Dublin
Dublin
Ireland

ANDREA T. FEßLER
Institute of Microbiology and Epizootics
Department of Veterinary Medicine
Freie Universität Berlin
Berlin
Germany

EDWARD M. FOX
CSIRO Agriculture and Food
Werribee, Victoria
Australia

ANNE V. GAUTIER-BOUCHARDON
Mycoplasmology, Bacteriology and Antimicrobial Resistance Unit
Anses Ploufragan
France

STEEVE GIGUÈRE (DECEASED)
Department of Large Animal Medicine,
College of Veterinary Medicine,
University of Georgia,
Athens, GA 30605

LUCA GUARDABASSI
Department of Veterinary and Animal Sciences
Faculty of Health and Medical Sciences,
University of Copenhagen,
Frederiksberg
Denmark

MARISA HAENNI
Unité Antibiorésistance et Virulence Bactériennes (AVB)
Université Claude Bernard Lyon 1
and
French agency for food environmental and occupational health & safety (Anses)
Lyon
France

TINE HALD
Unit for Genomic Epidemiology
National Food Institute
Technical University of Denmark
Lyngby
Denmark

HENRIK HASMAN
Reference Laboratory for Antimicrobial Resistance,
Department for Bacteria, Parasites and Fungi, Infectious Disease Preparedness,
Statens Serum Institute,
Copenhagen
Denmark

HEATHER HARBOTTLE
US Food and Drug Administration
Center for Veterinary Medicine
Division of Human Food Safety
Rockville, MD 20855

TAO HE
Institute of Food Safety and Nutrition
Jiangsu Academy of Agricultural Sciences
Jiangsu
China

HELEN JUKES
Veterinary Medicines Directorate
Addlestone
United Kingdom

KRISTINA KADLEC
Institute of Farm Animal Genetics
Friedrich-Loeffler-Institut
Neustadt-Mariensee,
Germany

NICOLAS KIEFFER
Emerging Antibiotic Resistance Unit
Medical and Molecular Microbiology
Department of Medicine
University of Fribourg
Fribourg
Switzerland
and
French INSERM European Unit
University of Fribourg (LEA-IAME)
Fribourg
Switzerland
and
National Reference Center for Emerging Antibiotic Resistance (NARA)
Switzerland

LOTHAR KREIENBROCK
Institute for Biometry, Epidemiology and Information Processing
WHO Collaborating Center for Research and Training at the Human-Animal-
Environment Interface
University of Veterinary Medicine Hannover
Hannover
Germany

RICARDO LEÓN-SAMPEDRO
Department of Microbiology
Ramón y Cajal University Hospital
Ramón y Cajal Health Research Institute (IRYCIS)
Madrid
Spain
and
Centro de Investigación Biomédica en Red de Epidemiología y Salud Pública
(CIBER-ESP)
Madrid
Spain

FENGQIN LI
Key Laboratory of Food Safety Risk Assessment of Ministry of Health
China National Center for Food Safety Risk Assessment
Beijing
China

DAVID H. LLOYD
Department of Clinical Sciences and Services
Royal Veterinary College
Hatfield, Hertfordshire
United Kingdom

IGOR LONCARIC
Institute of Microbiology
University of Veterinary Medicine
Vienna
Austria

BRIAN V. LUBBERS
Kansas State Veterinary Diagnostic Laboratory
Kansas State University
Manhattan, KS 66506

AGNESE LUPO
Unité Antibiorésistance et Virulence Bactériennes (AVB)
Université Claude Bernard Lyon 1
and
French agency for food environmental and occupational health & safety (Anses)
Lyon
France

LAURA LUQUE-SASTRE
UCD-Centre for Food Safety
UCD Centre for Molecular Innovation and Drug Discovery (Science Centre South)
University College Dublin
Dublin
Ireland

JEAN-YVES MADEC
Unité Antibiorésistance et Virulence Bactériennes (AVB)
Université Claude Bernard Lyon 1
and
French agency for food environmental and occupational health & safety (Anses)
Lyon
France

JEAN-YVES MAILLARD
Cardiff School of Pharmacy and Pharmaceutical Sciences,
Cardiff University
Cardiff
United Kingdom

PATRICK F. MCDERMOTT
Office of Research
Center for Veterinary Medicine,
US Food & Drug Administration
Laurel, MD 20708

SYLVIA MCDEVITT
Biology Department
Skidmore College
Saratoga Springs, NY 12866

SCOTT A. MCEWEN
Department of Population Medicine
Ontario Veterinary College
University of Guelph
Guelph, ON
Canada

BARRY J. MCMAHON
UCD School of Agriculture and Food Science
University College Dublin
Dublin
Ireland

GEOVANA B. MICHAEL
Institute of Microbiology and Epizootics
Department of Veterinary Medicine
Freie Universität Berlin
Berlin
Germany

RON A. MILLER
US Food and Drug Administration
Center for Veterinary Medicine
Division of Human Food Safety
Rockville, MD 20855

ARSHNEE MOODLEY
Department of Veterinary and Animal Sciences
Faculty of Health and Medical Sciences,
University of Copenhagen,
Frederiksberg
Denmark

THI LOAN ANH NGUYEN
Department of Animal Sciences and Aquatic Ecology
Ghent University
Ghent
Belgium

PATRICE NORDMANN
Emerging Antibiotic Resistance Unit
Medical and Molecular Microbiology
Department of Medicine
University of Fribourg
Fribourg
Switzerland
and
French INSERM European Unit
University of Fribourg (LEA-IAME)
Fribourg
Switzerland
and
National Reference Center for Emerging Antibiotic Resistance (NARA)
Switzerland

JOHN ELMERDAHL OLSEN
Department of Veterinary and Animal Sciences
Faculty of Health and Medical Sciences,
University of Copenhagen,
Frederiksberg
Denmark

STEPHEN W. PAGE
Advanced Veterinary Therapeutics
Newtown, New South Wales
Australia

SARA M. PIRES
Division of Diet, Disease Prevention and Toxicology
National Food Institute
Technical University of Denmark
Lyngby
Denmark

LAURENT POIREL
Emerging Antibiotic Resistance Unit
Medical and Molecular Microbiology
Department of Medicine
University of Fribourg
Fribourg
Switzerland
and
French INSERM European Unit
University of Fribourg (LEA-IAME)
Fribourg
Switzerland
and
National Reference Center for Emerging Antibiotic Resistance (NARA)
Switzerland

CONSTANÇA F. POMBA
Faculty of Veterinary Medicine
University of Lisbon
Lisbon
Portugal
and
Antimicrobial and Biocide Resistance Laboratory,
Centre for Interdisciplinary Research in Animal Health (CIISA)
Lisbon
Portugal

JOHN F. PRESCOTT
Department of Pathobiology
Ontario Veterinary College
University of Guelph
Guelph, ON
Canada

CHRISTOPHER RENSING
Institute of Environmental Microbiology
College of Resource and Environment
Fujian Agriculture and Forestry University
Fuzhou, Fujian
China

MARILYN C. ROBERTS
Department of Environmental and Occupational Health Sciences
University of Washington
Seattle, WA 98195

JOSEPH E. RUBIN
Department of Veterinary Microbiology
Western College of Veterinary Medicine
University of Saskatchewan
Saskatoon, Saskatchewan,
Canada

LAURA RUIZ-RIPA
Biochemistry and Molecular Biology Unit
University of La Rioja
Logroño, La Rioja
Spain

CHUANCHUEN RUNGTIP
Department of Veterinary Public Health
University of Chulalongkorn
Bangkok
Thailand

ANNE-KATHRIN SCHINK
Institute of Microbiology and Epizootics
Department of Veterinary Medicine
Freie Universität Berlin
Berlin
Germany

STEFAN SCHWARZ
Institute of Microbiology and Epizootics
Department of Veterinary Medicine
Freie Universität Berlin
Berlin,
Germany

JIANZHONG SHEN
Beijing Advanced Innovation Center for Food Nutrition and Human Health
College of Veterinary Medicine
China Agricultural University
Beijing
China

ZHANGQI SHEN
Beijing Advanced Innovation Center for Food Nutrition and Human Health
College of Veterinary Medicine
China Agricultural University
Beijing
China

SHABBIR SIMJEE
Elanco Animal Health
Basingstoke
Hampshire
United Kingdom

MICHAEL T. SWEENEY
Veterinary Medicine Research and Development
Zoetis, Inc.
Kalamazoo, MI 49007

HEATHER TATE
Office of Research
Center for Veterinary Medicine,
US Food & Drug Administration
Laurel, MD 20709

CARMEN TORRES
Biochemistry and Molecular Biology Unit
University of La Rioja
Logroño, La Rioja
Spain

PIERRE-LOUIS TOUTAIN
Ecole Nationale Vétérinaire de Toulouse Université de Toulouse
Toulouse
France
And
Department of Veterinary Basic Sciences Royal Veterinary College
London, United Kingdom

DARREN J. TROTT
Australian Centre for Antimicrobial Resistance Ecology
School of Animal and Veterinary Sciences
The University of Adelaide
Roseworthy, South Australia
Australia

ENGELINE VAN DUIJKEREN
Centre for Infectious Disease Control
National Institute for Public Health and the Environment (RIVM)
Bilthoven
The Netherlands

DAISY VANROMPA
Department of Animal Sciences and Aquatic Ecology
Faculty of Bioscience Engineering
Ghent University
Ghent
Belgium

YANG WANG
Beijing Advanced Innovation Center for Food Nutrition and Human Health
College of Veterinary Medicine
China Agricultural University
Beijing
China

JEFFREY L. WATTS
Veterinary Medicine Research and Development
Zoetis, Inc.
Kalamazoo, MI 49007

SCOTT WEESE
Department of Pathobiology
Ontario Veterinary College
University of Guelph
Guelph, ON,
Canada

NICOLE WERNER
Institute for Biometry, Epidemiology and Information Processing
WHO Collaborating Center for Research and Training at the Human-Animal-
Environment Interface
University of Veterinary Medicine Hannover
Hannover
Germany

JENNIFER WILLINGHAM-LANE
Department of Large Animal Medicine,
College of Veterinary Medicine,
University of Georgia,
Athens, GA 30605

CONGMING WU
Beijing Advanced Innovation Center for Food Nutrition and Human Health
College of Veterinary Medicine
China Agricultural University
Beijing
China

EA ZANKARI
Unit for Genomic Epidemiology
National Food Institute
Technical University of Denmark
Lyngby
Denmark

QIJING ZHANG
Department of Veterinary Microbiology and Preventive Medicine
College of Veterinary Medicine
Iowa State University
Ames, IA 50011

SHAOHUA ZHAO
Office of Research
Center for Veterinary Medicine,
US Food & Drug Administration
Laurel, MD 20710

Foreword

I am honored to be asked to write a preface for the collection of articles that comprise *Antimicrobial Resistance in Bacteria from Livestock and Companion Animals*. The authors are all leaders in the field and have provided comprehensive summaries of their knowledge in all aspects of the use of antibiotics and development of resistance in animal health.

It is regrettable that it has taken 50 years to recognize that this worldwide plague of misuse and resistance development cannot be reversed. Given recent publications, the extent of antibiotic use in commercial fish farming in Southeast Asia reminds us that there are still many hurdles to be overcome if we want to control the misuse of antibiotics in humans.

Finding new antimicrobials has always been difficult, and it is to be hoped that modern molecular biology and its constant technical improvements will save the day and provide humans with reliable agents for disease treatment without the inevitability of drug resistance. Improving knowledge of the science of low-molecular-weight microbial compounds will perhaps, in time, teach us how to use antibiotics for human use. Antimicrobial discovery must continue apace such that a source of reliable agents will always be available, whether for human or animal health.

This compendium of interesting and focused articles is valuable, and it promises to provide expert advice on all aspects of antimicrobial resistance and ways of controlling it. Remember that in the 1950s antibiotics were miracles, but they have become menaces! It is up to us to focus on intelligent use of small molecules as cures and to finally eliminate infectious diseases in humans.

Julian Davies
University of British Columbia
Vancouver, British Columbia, Canada

Preface

Antimicrobial agents are indispensable for the treatment of bacterial infections not only in humans, but also in animals. In veterinary medicine, no new classes of antimicrobial agents are expected to be licensed in the coming years. In fact, virtually all antimicrobial agents that have been approved during the past 2 decades for veterinary applications are derivatives of already approved antimicrobial agents. Given this situation, it is most important to use the currently available antimicrobial agents as wisely as possible to preserve their efficacy for the future. To this end, it is important to better educate all those people who prescribe antimicrobial agents in human and veterinary medicine about antimicrobial resistance, resistant bacteria, management practices, and measures to prevent infections as well as prudent use of antimicrobial agents. On one hand, it is important to refresh continuously the knowledge on the aforementioned topics, and on the other hand, it is necessary to raise awareness on antimicrobial resistance of bacteria from livestock and companion animals so that measures to counteract resistance development will be implemented.

This book, *Antimicrobial Resistance of Bacteria from Livestock and Companion Animals*, is intended to become a valuable reference for persons who treat, research, or monitor resistance in bacteria of animal origin. The first book of this kind—*Antimicrobial Resistance in Bacteria of Animal Origin*, edited by Frank M. Aarestrup—was published in 2006 by ASM Press. More than a decade later, we felt that it was time to compile a new book for ASM Press that would include the wealth of data on antimicrobial resistance in bacteria from animals that has been published in the meantime.

The new book is composed of 31 individual chapters, some of which have been updated and expanded from the 2006 book by including in part new authors and coauthors. Other chapters have been included for the first time and represent a valuable addition to this book.

The first six chapters introduce the reader to general aspects of antimicrobial resistance. Chapters 1 to 3 describe the history and current use of antimicrobial drugs in veterinary medicine; the particularities of antimicrobial susceptibility testing of bacteria from animals and veterinary-specific breakpoints to evaluate the results; and new and molecular methods for the detection of antimicrobial resistance (including MALDI-TOF mass spectrometry, next-generation sequencing, and DNA microarrays), respectively. Chapter 4 provides a comprehensive overview of the multiple mechanisms by which bacteria become resistant to antimicrobial agents, while chapters 5 and 6 give important information on resistance to metals used in livestock production and bacterial resistance to biocides. Both metals and biocides represent important substances that can coselect for antimicrobial resistance in bacteria.

The next 18 chapters provide the latest information on antimicrobial resistance in specific groups of bacteria that represent important obligate or facultative pathogens in livestock and companion animals. In comparison to the book published in 2006, separate chapters describing antimicrobial resistance in staphylococci (inclu ding the livestock-associated methicillin-resistant *Staphylococcus aureus* and methicillin-resistant *Staphylococcus pseudintermedius*, which have gained much public health attention during the past decade) and streptococci have been included. Moreover, new chapters on antimicrobial resistance in *Listeria* spp., *Rhodococcus equi*, *Bordetella bronchiseptica*, *Stenotrophomonas* spp., *Pseudomonas* spp., *Acinetobacter* spp., *Trueperella pyogenes*, *Arcanobacterium* spp., and *Corynebacterium* spp. were added. In addition, chapters were included that deal with antimicrobial resistance in *Chlamydia*, *Chlamydophila*, *Rickettsia*, *Coxiella*, and other intracellular pathogens, as well as *Leptospira*, *Brucella*, and other rarely investigated veterinary and zoonotic pathogens. The remaining chapters on antimicrobial resistance in *Enterococcus*, nontyphoidal salmonellae, *Escherichia coli*, *Campylobacter* spp., *Pasteurellaceae*, and fish pathogens as well as *Clostridium* spp., *Brachyspira* spp., and other anaerobes were completely revised and expanded.

The final seven chapters provide insight into antimicrobial resistance with a One Health perspective, licensing and approval of antimicrobial agents for use in animals, and methods and applications for monitoring of antimicrobial drug usage in animals and provide an overview of principles and practices of monitoring antimicrobial resistance in bacteria from animal origin. In addition, single chapters describe risk assessment and source attribution models, the optimization of treatment of animals to avoid resistance selection, and last but not least, antimicrobial stewardship in veterinary medicine.

All in all, this book provides a comprehensive and up-to-date overview of the various aspects associated with antimicrobial resistance. The information provided in this book will be useful to all people interested in this topic, including veterinary practitioners, students, researchers, industry, and decision-makers. To compile all this information, we recruited the very best experts worldwide in antimicrobial resistance of livestock and companion animals to write the corresponding chapters. We are deeply indebted to the 84 authors and coauthors from institutions in 16 countries, including Australia, Austria, Belgium, Canada, China, Denmark, France, Germany, Ireland, Portugal, St. Kitts and Nevis, Spain, Switzerland, Thailand, the United Kingdom, and the United States, who rendered this book a truly international collaboration product. This book would not have been possible without their invaluable input and participation. We also thank our many colleagues who reviewed the various chapters. We also thank ASM Press, not only for the opportunity to compile this book, but also for being patient with us during this process.

Stefan Schwarz
Lina M. Cavaco
Jianzhong Shen

About the Authors

Prof. Dr. Med. Vet. Stefan Schwarz is Director of the Institute of Microbiology and Epizootics at the Department of Veterinary Medicine of the Freie Universität Berlin Germany. Previously, he worked for 24 years for governmental research institutions in Germany, such as the Friedrich-Loeffler-Institut (Federal Institute for Animal Health) and the Federal Agricultural Research Center. Prof. Schwarz is also a visiting professor at the College of Veterinary Medicine at China Agricultural University in Beijing.

His research group is involved in the analysis of the molecular genetics of antimicrobial resistance, antimicrobial susceptibility testing methods, and monitoring of antimicrobial resistance. He has published more than 400 papers in international peer-reviewed journals and has received several research awards. Prof. Schwarz acts as editor of or serves on the editorial board of six international journals. A cat lover, he spends his free time taking care of abandoned cats at a small animal shelter in Berlin.

Lina M. Cavaco, PhD, is Portuguese but was born in Germany in 1976 and began her education there. When she moved to Portugal in 1984 and spent part of her childhood in a small town in the south of Portugal, she became attracted to the country life and the veterinary profession. Dr. Cavaco received a degree in Veterinary Science from the Veterinary Faculty of the University of Lisbon (formerly the Technical University) in 2000 and began research into the diagnosis of bacterial diseases in domestic and zoo species at the bacteriology section of the University of Lisbon, where she obtained an MSc degree in Veterinary Public Health.

At the end of 2005, Dr. Cavaco moved to Denmark to start studies on the mechanisms and selection of antimicrobial resistance at Copenhagen University and obtained her PhD degree in September 2008. From October 2008 to May

2017, she worked at the Technical University of Denmark, focusing her research on antimicrobial resistance mechanisms and selection of resistance to antimicrobials and metals in Enterobacteriaceae and MRSA while also teaching undergraduates and performing proficiency testing and training. This peaked her interest in online education, and she developed and launched a massive open online course (MOOC) on antimicrobial resistance methods and participated in the preparation of another MOOC on whole-genome sequencing, both of which are accessible to a global audience.

Dr. Cavaco has been at the Statens Serum Institute and Copenhagen University since June 2017, where her primary research is focused on new antimicrobial candidate compounds and studies assessing efficacy for treatment of infections with multiresistant bacteria.

Prof. Jianzhong Shen is a member of the Chinese Academy of Engineering and Dean of the College of Veterinary Medicine at China Agriculture University (CAU). He received his bachelors, masters, and doctoral degrees from CAU and has been working at CAU for 30 years, since 1988. He has actively served as a committee member for multiple national organizations and scientific communities, including the Veterinary Drug Evaluation Commission of the Ministry of Agriculture of China, the Veterinary Drug Residue Commission of China, the Feed Additive Evaluation Commission of the Ministry of Agriculture of China, and the Chinese Association of Animal Science and Veterinary Medicine.

Dr. Shen's research focuses on the development of detection methods for veterinary drug residues as well as on the emergence, transmission, and molecular mechanisms of antibiotic resistance in bacteria of animal origin. In the past decade, he has published more than 200 peer-reviewed papers in international journals and received more than 40 patents. He has also received several major Chinese national awards, including the National Technology Invention Award (2015), the National Agriculture Science and Technology Award (2013), the National Agricultural Scientific Research Talent award (2012), and the National Excellent Scientific and Technological Workers award (2010).

Antimicrobial Resistance in Bacteria from Livestock and Companion Animals
Edited by Frank Møller Aarestrup, Stefan Schwarz, Jianzhong Shen, and Lina Cavaco
© 2018 American Society for Microbiology, Washington, DC
doi:10.1128/microbiolspec.ARBA-0002-2017

History and Current Use of Antimicrobial Drugs in Veterinary Medicine

1

John F. Prescott[1]

INTRODUCTION

The introduction of antimicrobial drugs into agriculture and veterinary medicine shortly after the Second World War caused a revolution in the treatment of many diseases of animals. In the "wonder drug era" of the late 1940s and early 1950s, the effective treatment of many infections that were previously considered incurable astonished veterinarians, such that some even feared for their livelihoods. Not all use of antimicrobial drugs in food animals is yet under veterinary prescription globally, despite repeated recommendations by the World Health Organization and other responsible organizations, so that the term "veterinary medicine" is used here rather generically to suggest use in animals rather than just use by veterinarians.

A broad overview of key features of the history of antimicrobial drug use in animals is given in Table 1, which traces developments from the preantibiotic era to the present day, where there are arguable fears that we are moving into the "postantibiotic" era but which may better be described as the antimicrobial stewardship era. Much of this overview will focus on antimicrobial use in food animals, the subject of an earlier review that partly focused on the public health aspects of the use of antimicrobials in food animals (1), but will include important aspects of use in companion animals.

The table illustrates many important features in the history of the use of antimicrobials in animals: (i) The development of resistance to antimicrobial drugs followed soon after their introduction. (ii) Resistance was usually dealt with by the development of new classes of antimicrobials by the isolation from nature of novel antibiotics within a particular class or by development of synthetic analogs of an existing class. (iii) The antimi-

crobial drugs used in animals were the same as those in human medicine, although a number of them that were rejected by human medicine because of toxicity problems (e.g., bacitracin) became growth-promoting feed antimicrobials in food animals. At least one of these drugs (colistin) is now being reclaimed for systemic use in humans. (iv) Antimicrobials were used in agriculture in feed as growth promoters, or for subtherapeutic purposes, almost as soon as they were discovered. (v) The majority of antimicrobial drugs used in animals (and shared with human medicine) belong to a small number of major classes, and only one major new class of antimicrobial drugs (fluoroquinolones; pleuromutilins are an exception, but have very restricted use) has been introduced for food animal use in the past 30 years. (vi) Significant antimicrobial contamination in carcasses or selected tissues was detected in the 1970s and 1980s, leading either to the banning of potentially toxic (e.g., carcinogenic or idiosyncratic effects) drugs or to rigorous, ongoing programs of detection in carcasses after slaughter. This was the major focus of regulations of use in food animals in those decades, and there is still confusion in some quarters about the difference between residues and resistance. (vii) The public health impacts resulting from the development of resistance, and especially because of transmissible resistance, have been a major battleground between agriculture and medicine for nearly 50 years. (viii) The resistance crisis in human medicine has led to unprecedented concern at the highest political levels globally about the threat of resistance to humanity, to an unprecedented focus on stewardship, and to major ongoing reduction and ongoing changes in agricultural use of antibiotics, at least in the developed world. (ix)

[1]Department of Pathobiology, University of Guelph, Guelph, Ontario N1G 2W1, Canada.

Table 1 Historical time line of important events and trends in the use of antimicrobial drugs in animals, with emphasis on food animals

Timeline	Feature of period	Antimicrobial drug development	Important events
1925–1935	Antiseptic era	Discovery of sulfonamides	Discovery of penicillin, first beta-lactam, by Alexander Fleming
1936–1940	Antiseptic, sulfonamide period	Penicillin efficacy shown in humans	Sulfonamides introduced into food animal use
1941–1945	Dawn of "wonder drug" era	Streptomycin, first aminoglycoside, discovered	Second World War is impetus for antimicrobial drug discovery for treatment of war wounds
1946–1950	"Wonder drug" era	Discovery bacitracin, chloramphenicol, neomycin, polymyxin, streptogramins, tetracycline antibiotics, all natural products of microorganisms, usually fungi	Penicillin, streptomycin released from military use for civilian population and animal use; widespread use in animals by 1950, largely empirical; far more wonder than science
1951–1955	"Wonder drug" era	Discovery of erythromycin, first macrolide; introduction of neomycin, aminoglycoside, for topical or intestinal infections in animals Introductions of nitrofurans into clinical use, especially for intestinal infections	Tetracyclines, chloramphenicol used therapeutically in animals; widespread, largely empirical, use Intramammary use of antibiotics for mastitis treatment widespread Discovery of and extensive use of antibiotics for growth promotion in food animals, pioneered in the USA
1956–1960	"Wonder drug" era	Discovery of vancomycin, first glycopeptide Tylosin, novel macrolide Virginiamycin, streptogramin, used as growth promoters	More science and less wonder, but drug dosage still largely empirical Early studies of drug excretion in Denmark
1961–1965	Emerging resistance period	Methicillin and other penicillinase-resistant penicillins Introduction of spiramycin, a macrolide, into animal use Gentamicin, antipseudomonal aminoglycoside	Discovery of transmissible, plasmid- or "R" factor-based, multiple drug resistance in *Enterobacteriaceae* Studies of drug residues and withdrawal periods in animals
1966–1970	New drug analog period	Cephalothin, first-generation cephalosporin Ampicillin, first broad-spectrum penicillin, used in food and companion animals, example of a successful synthetic alteration of side chains of basic beta-lactam ring to expand activity Amikacin, for gentamicin-resistant infections Flavomycin introduced as growth promoter	New drug analogs successfully address resistance problem Transmissible, multiple-drug resistant, serious *Salmonella* infections, transmission from calves to human in UK Because of transmissible resistance, Swann Report in UK removes drugs important in human medicine as feed antibiotics, allows their veterinary prescription-only use therapeutically in food animals
1971–1975	New drug analog period	Carbenicillin, antipseudomonal penicillin Other first-generation cephalosporins introduced Trimethoprim-sulfonamide combination	New drug analogs successfully address resistance problem FDA report (1972) suggests stopping feed use of subtherapeutic penicillin, tetracyclines; not implemented
1976–1980	Tissue drug residue problems in food animals; early pharmacokinetic period	Cexotin, first extended-spectrum (second-generation) cephalosporin Moxalactam, unusual beta-lactam Introduction in Europe of avoparcin, glycopeptide, for growth promotion in food animals	Chloramphenicol use in food animals banned in USA and Denmark because of potential human toxicity through residues, followed by other countries Transmissible, multiple-drug resistant, *Salmonella typhimurium* phage type 204

(Continued)

Table 1 *(Continued)*

Timeline	Feature of period	Antimicrobial drug development	Important events
			spreads from calves to humans
			Journal of Veterinary Pharmacology and Therapeutics started, to improve drug use in animals
			Focus on pharmacokinetics and drug metabolism in food animals by J.D. Baggot (Ireland, USA), L.E. Davis (USA), P. Nielsen and F. Rasmussen (Denmark)
1981–1985	Pharmacokinetic, drug dosage prediction period	Cefotaxime, antipseudomonal cephalosporin, and other third-generation cephalosporins Broad-beta-lactamase inhibitors combined with aminopenicillins, e.g., sulbactam-ampicillin used in food animals Imipenem-cilastatin, unusual broad-spectrum beta-lactam	Antimicrobial drug dosage prediction based on pioneering pharmacokinetic approach in food animals developed by Ziv in Israel, Hjerpe in USA, and others Changes in sulfamethazine use in swine to address residue issue Ban on nitrofuran and nitroimidazole drugs for food animals in USA because of mutagenicity
1986–1990	Increasing resistance problems in humans: MRSA emerges	Quinolones, fluoroquinolones introduced into human medicine Ceftiofur, a second- to third-generation cephalosporin, introduced for food animals	Development of Food Animal Residue Avoidance Database (FARAD) in USA Moratorium on sulfamethazine use in dairy cows in USA Moratorium on most use of aminoglycosides in food animals in USA because of kidney residues
1991–1995	Increasing resistance problems in humans: VREs emerge	Azithromycin and other improved macrolides introduced into human medicine Tilmicosin (macrolide), tiamulin (pleuromutilin), florfenicol (nontoxic introduced for food animal selected use Fluoroquinolones introduced for selected use in food animals in Europe	First fluoroquinolone, enrofloxacin, introduced into food animal (poultry) use in USA, with severe restrictions; includes resistance monitoring through National Antimicrobial Resistance Monitoring System that integrates food animal and medical data National Council on Clinical Laboratory Standards (NCCLS) in USA establishes veterinary subcommittee to develop susceptibility testing methods and interpretations Animal Medicines Use Clarification Act in USA allows veterinary prescription extra-label use of certain approved drugs
1996–2000	Resistance crisis in medicine; now includes penicillin-resistant *Streptococcus pneumoniae*	Oral, third-generation cephalosporins in human medicine may partially drive resistance crisis Effective antivirals introduced into human medicine Fluoroquinolone introduced for treatment of acute pneumonia in cattle in USA	VRE emergence linked to avoparcin use in food animals in Europe; ban of avoparcin and four other growth promoters in Europe WHO (1998) recommends withdrawal of growth-promoting antimicrobials if significant for human medicine Global emergence of multidrug-resistant *S. typhimurium* DT104 Japanese Veterinary Antimicrobial Resistance Monitoring Program started NCCLS guidelines for veterinary bacterial susceptibility testing published Center for Veterinary Medicine of FDA proposes "an approach for establishing thresholds in association with the use of antimicrobial drugs in food-producing animals" (Framework document)

(Continued)

Table 1   *(Continued)*

Timeline	Feature of period	Antimicrobial drug development	Important events
2001–2005	Resistance crisis in medicine continues, expands	No new antimicrobial drugs introduced for food animals	FDA Center for Veterinary Medicine proposes withdrawal of fluoroquinolones in poultry because of resistance in *Campylobacter* WHO Global Strategy for Containment of Antimicrobial Resistance calls for prescription-only use of antimicrobials in food animals, national usage and resistance monitoring, phasing out of growth promoters if drugs important for humans Withdrawal of fluoroquinolones for use in poultry in USA because of emerging resistance in *C. jejuni* Spread of multidrug resistance including cephalosporinase (CMY2) genes among certain *Salmonella* serovars. Development of prudent use guidelines by practitioner specialty groups at national levels
2005–2010	Resistance crisis in medicine continues; MRSA and MRSP emerge in animals, spread partly by people	No new antimicrobial drugs introduced for food animals Voluntary ban on use of ceftiofur in pigs in Denmark, and on use of ceftiofur in chickens in Canada	Resistance crisis in medicine focuses intense effort on improved infection and antimicrobial drug use control by physicians; some benefits observed Veterinary "prudent" or "judicious" use approaches increasingly replaced by emerging concept of stewardship Global spread of food animal-associated MRSA, driven by zinc oxide use in food animals Voluntary ban on ceftiofur use in Danish pigs followed by marked reduction in extended-spectrum cephalosporinase *E. coli* excretion MRSA emerges in Dutch animal workers; Holland proposes 50% reduction in antibiotic use in food animals within 5 years MRSP emerges in dogs, clonal spread in Europe and North America
2011–2016	Resistance crisis in medicine reaches highest political levels United Nations affirms global collective action	Avilamycin introduced as first-in-class, animal-use-only, orthosomycin antibiotic to prevent mortality due to necrotic enteritis of broilers under veterinary prescription; first "new" antimicrobial drug for food animals in 10 years	Transatlantic Task Force on Antimicrobial Resistance to cooperate between USA and European Union on resistance Innumerable calls for global solutions to antibiotic resistance WHO Options for Action promotes development of national action plans incorporating human and animal health sectors Human medicine antibiotic resistance threats identified by microorganism level in USA, most unrelated to animal use Consumer demands for "antibiotic-free" animal production; McDonald's Corporation adopts antimicrobial stewardship requirements for sourcing meat G7 agrees to address the resistance crisis O'Neill Report in UK's final recommendations includes reducing unnecessary use in agricul-

(Continued)

Table 1 *(Continued)*

Timeline	Feature of period	Antimicrobial drug development	Important events
			...ture as one of 10 planks to fight resistance
			Plasmid-mediated colistin resistance gene *mcr1* related to agricultural use in animals and humans identified in China, shown to be globally widespread
			United Nations High-Level Meeting on the antimicrobial resistance threat unprecedented meeting
2017–	Stewardship era	Intense activity to find alternatives to antibiotics or "animal only" antibiotics for food animals	Political will to address the resistance crisis continues in place
			Anticipated enhancement of surveillance, stewardship, and innovation as global response to antimicrobial resistance crisis
			Innovation in numerous fields relating to use of antibiotics anticipated
			Increasing adoption of a "One Health" approach to resistance may remove some of the conflict between agriculture and human medicine
			The story continues

The science and practices supporting optimal antimicrobial drug use in animals and in humans has developed relatively slowly and is not complete.

DISCOVERY OF ANTIBIOTICS AND EARLY USAGE

Antimicrobial drugs were introduced for animal (and human) use with a minimum of controlled experimental studies, so that from the start of their use there were frequent calls to move from the wonder to the science. As in human medicine, much of the early dosage used was empirical and based on inadequately controlled small-scale trials (2, 3), so that there was a "confusing hodge-podge of widely divergent optimum dose-ranges for the many livestock diseases allegedly amenable to the activity of penicillin" (4). In the United States such empiricism led to a licensed dosage of penicillin G in cattle that was clearly inadequate. It took four or five decades before the licensed drug dosage was more scientifically determined, based on quantitative understanding of the interaction of drug with the target microorganism (dosage, pharmacokinetic and pharmacodynamic parameters, *in vitro* susceptibility) as well as clinical data (Table 1). Clinical evaluation is still an important component used in the licensing of antimicrobial drugs, in part because the predictive science is imperfect.

In retrospect, for drugs whose use "has advanced the practice of medicine farther than any other single factor of any of the previous centuries" (5), the time taken to establish the science of the clinical use of antimicrobial drugs seems astonishing. As human medicine's poor cousin, veterinary medicine lagged in the development of the science of optimal antimicrobial drug use, but the lag was only relative since the same delay was clearly visible in human medicine. In general, the science and practice of antimicrobial usage in animals has largely paralleled that in human medicine, in the same way that most antimicrobial drugs used were the same or were in the same drug class. There have been, however, a number of features unique to animal agriculture, as discussed below.

In most countries, approval by the appropriate regulatory authority must be obtained before an antimicrobial drug can be legally sold, and this depends on extensive testing to ensure safety and efficacy, as well as, in the case of food animals, studies of safety for people consuming their products. Registration requirements for veterinary medical products have been largely harmonized internationally under the International Cooperation on Harmonization of Technical Requirements of Veterinary Medicinal products (VICH) of the World Organization for Animal Health, membership of which includes the European Union and the United States. A harmonized VICH guideline, GL 27, defines the data requirements for risk of transfer of resistant bacteria or resistance determinants from foods of animal origin to humans. These data are assessed in terms of exposure of food-borne pathogens and commensal bacteria, and the "qualitative probability" that human exposure to resistant bacteria results in adverse human consequences. As part of this assessment, many countries are attempting to stratify the stringency of regulatory requirements by how important a drug is to public health, also discussed below. This is a highly contentious issue, since most antimicrobial drugs can, under various criteria, be claimed as "critically important." A more useful and a more rational approach, which could be adopted in both human and veterinary medicine, is categorization into "lines" based in part on culture and susceptibility results (Table 2) (6). This approach has the advantage of simplicity (for example, labels on bottles could indicate the category) and would enhance the use of laboratory diagnosis. Research is needed into whether such a categorization scheme would be accepted in the animal (and human) health world, including the barriers to acceptance and what it would take to implement such a system so that it would be widely accepted.

The regulation of antimicrobial drug use in animals is a complex process that has jurisdictional differences. Regulation is more stringent for use of these drugs in food animals, although "off- or extra-label" use (use of the product in any manner not specified on the label) is often approved under specific circumstances and constraints. Use of antimicrobial drugs in companion animals is subject to less stringent regulation, and there is likely more off-label use in companion animals (as there is in human medicine).

Although the situation is changing, there has been historically no formal interest by regulatory authorities in postapproval use (or periodic relicencing) of antimicrobial drugs in animals. Some of the label claims for some antimicrobial drugs list approval for use in bacteria that have had their names changed several times since approval or for diseases that have subsequently been shown to be caused by other agents, so that reading the labels can be like reading a outdated veterinary microbiology textbook from the 1960s. The postapproval monitoring of resistance in *Campylobacter jejuni* following the introduction of fluoroquinolones for use in broiler chickens in the United States, and the subsequent withdrawal of fluoroquinolones from use in poultry in the United States is, however, a well-known example of postapproval monitoring of the approved use of a drug.

PRACTICES IN ANTIMICROBIAL DRUG USAGE UNIQUE TO ANIMAL HUSBANDRY

The greatest differences in usage of antimicrobial drugs between animal husbandry and human medicine were, and in many countries still are, in the use in agriculture of antimicrobials for growth promotion and for long-term disease prophylaxis, although the situation is changing relatively rapidly. This has occurred particularly in countries where livestock, notably chickens and pigs, are reared intensively.

Table 2 Suggested categorization of antimicrobial drugs for veterinary use (6)

Class	Definition	Examples
First-line (primary)	Initial treatment of known or suspected bacterial infection in absence of culture and susceptibility results These drugs may commonly be used in human medicine but are usually considered less important for treating serious human (and animal) infections or raise less concern about development of resistance	Penicillin, most cephalosporins, trimethoprim-sulfonamides, tetracyclines
Second-line (secondary)	Used when culture and susceptibility testing, plus patient or infection factors, indicate that no first-line drugs are reasonable choices Drugs in this class may be more important for treatment of serious human (and animal) infections, or there may be particular concern about development of infection	Fluoroquinolones, third and later generation cephalosporins
Third-line (tertiary)	Used in serious, life-threatening infections, with the support of culture and susceptibility results, when no first-line or second-line drugs are indicated Not for use in food animals	Carbapenems
Restricted, voluntarily prohibited	Used only in life-threatening infections when culture and susceptibility testing indicate no other options Not for use in food animals Additional requirements may be indicated, or use may be voluntarily prohibited	Vancomycin

The growth-promotional benefits of adding low concentrations of many antibacterial drugs to feed was recognized almost as soon as antibiotics were introduced. The enhancement of growth rates and improved efficiency of use of feed were noted when pigs and poultry were fed the fungal waste derived from antibiotic production, originally intended as a source of vitamins and protein, but mostly as an efficient way to use the waste. The effect was originally attributed to the presence of vitamin B_{12} ("animal protein factor") in the mycelial mass, but with time it was recognized to be a direct effect of residual antibiotic. Interestingly, how antimicrobial drugs improve growth rate and efficiency of utilization is still unknown, although it is thought to be through an inhibitory or metabolic effect of some kind on the Gram-positive intestinal microflora. Curiously, until about the mid-1950s, low prolonged oral dosage of tetracycline was even used to improve the growth of underweight human infants and children, but this practice was dropped because of both resistance and discoloration of teeth. In animals, the growth-promotional and disease-prophylactic benefits appear to have remained constant over the years (7), supporting the idea that these effects result from metabolic rather than antibacterial activities. As the use of antibiotics as growth promoters in intensively reared livestock becomes illegal in much of the world, alternative approaches to manipulation of the microbiome may replace their growth-promoting effects.

Not only have antimicrobial drugs been used for growth promotion, but some drugs were and in some countries still are administered in feed for prolonged periods at somewhat higher concentrations, the "subtherapeutic levels" (defined in the United States as less than 200 g per ton of feed), which are lower concentrations than those approved for therapeutic purposes. The historical origin of subtherapeutic usage and indeed the meaning of this term are obscure, but it seems to have both beneficial growth-promotional and disease-prophylactic effects, particularly against pathogens that do not readily develop or acquire resistance. Drugs such as tetracyclines are administered "subtherapeutically" for many defined, licensed purposes at a range of concentrations varying with the drug, the food-animal species, and the purpose. Such usage, which can often be prolonged and thus inconsistent with important general principles of antimicrobial drug dosage (6), has been particularly widespread in the swine industry in countries in which the drugs are still allowed for this purpose (8). The practice is coming under increased scrutiny and will likely also be banned and replaced by short-term antimicrobial prophylaxis or short-term treatment targeted to specific pathogens. As noted earlier, a number of antimicrobial drugs (such as the streptogramins) that were too toxic for parenteral use in humans were relegated to growth-promotional and disease-prophylactic use in food animals.

Another practice that has historically been far more common in food animal use than in human medicine has been short-term mass medication with therapeutic concentrations of drugs immediately before an outbreak of disease can be anticipated, or immediately at the onset of disease in a population (9). This type of prophylaxis has been commonly practiced in beef feedlot and swine medicine and is most akin to the prophylactic use of antimicrobial drugs to prevent *Haemophilus* or *Neisseria* meningitis in humans. Prophylactic use of intramammary antimicrobial drugs to prevent development of new infections and to treat existing infections has become a standard practice in dairy cows in the two months before calving and re-entering the milking herd ("dry cow treatment"), with no apparent adverse effect on resistance development, perhaps in part because the very high concentrations of drugs achieved in the udder result in rapid killing of the target bacteria. Blanket use of dry cow treatment is also coming under scrutiny and is being replaced by use only when udders are known to be infected and likely to carry an infection over to the next lactation.

USE OF ANTIMICROBIAL DRUGS IN ANIMALS

Food Animals

Data on the quantities and types of antimicrobial used in food animals are increasingly available in highly developed countries, with countries such as Denmark and Sweden leading the way. A global assessment of trends in antimicrobial use in food animals recognized the relative lack of reliable quantitative data globally but forecasted a marked increase as livestock production practices intensified in middle- and low-income countries (10). In Europe, the Danish Integrated Antimicrobial Monitoring and Research Program (DANMAP), started in 1995, is a ground-breaking and very high-quality program that monitors both resistance in selected food-animal indicator organisms and pathogens and usage of antimicrobials in human and animal medicine. DANMAP can accurately record national antimicrobial use in animals to the kilogram level. In Sweden, the Swedish Veterinary Antibiotic Resistance Monitoring organization has had a similar program since 2000 and has integrated this with Swedish Antibiotic Utilization and Resistance in Human Medicine since 2011. In the United States, the National Antimicrobial Resistance Monitoring System has monitored resistance in food-animal indicator organisms and select human and animal pathogens nationally, but has not monitored use, since 1996. In Canada, the Canadian Integrated Program for Antimicrobial Resistance Surveillance has a similar program but has struggled for national jurisdictional reasons to obtain accurate food animal use data. In Europe, the European Medicines Agency collects data on antimicrobial use in animals from member countries (European Surveillance on Veterinary Antimicrobial Consumption).

These data have great value in "benchmarking" comparisons between antimicrobial use in food animals between different countries, which can vary widely, but there is uncertainty about the best way to compare antimicrobial use between different species (e.g., milligram/population corrected unit, animal daily dose) and about the validity of some of the comparisons based on sales data, differences in dosages, and differences in animal demographics including weight estimates (11, 12). This is discussed further in chapter 28. The importance of benchmarking cannot be underestimated as a driver for reducing antimicrobial use in food animals at the farm and the veterinarian level, as illustrated by the use of the "yellow" card system in Denmark and the experience of the value of benchmarking in Holland in its 50% reduction of use in food animals between 2007 and 2012 (13, 14). Reduction in use in food animals is associated with reduction of resistance in indicator bacteria (15), and a correlation between antimicrobial use in animals and resistance in indicator bacteria is well established (16). A robust approach to benchmarking has been developed (17).

The documentation of antimicrobial drug use in food animals nationally and internationally is a rapidly growing, fast moving, and evolving field that can only be briefly touched on here but is reviewed in detail in chapter 28. As promoted by the World Health Organization and others, surveillance and documentation of use, and of the impacts of reduction in use in animals, is an essential element in addressing the resistance crisis and improving how antimicrobials are used in animals.

There are now numerous studies of the antimicrobial-prescribing habits of veterinarians and factors influencing those habits (18, 19) which can be expected to continue as veterinary medicine embraces antimicrobial stewardship.

Companion Animals
The use of antimicrobials in companion animals essentially mirrors their use in human medicine, a discus-

sion of which is far beyond the scope of this chapter. Only in recent years have antimicrobial use practices in companion animals come under scrutiny, both as sources of important emerging resistance issues (such as methicillin-resistant *Staphylococcus aureus* [MRSA] and *Staphylococcus pseudintermedius* [MRSP]) (20) and as potential sources for multidrug-resistant pathogens for humans. The rapid emergence and clonal spread of methicillin-resistant *S. pseudintermedius* has been a "wake-up call" for companion animal practice (20–22). Untreatable multidrug-resistant hospital-associated infections are now being encountered in companion animals. Studies of the use of antimicrobials in primary care companion animal veterinary practice have been characterized by their small sample size and labor-intensive nature. However, studies are now being reported that involve analysis of mega-data on usage obtained from shared practice software to obtain that involving large numbers of animals (e.g., one million dogs) (23). However, documentation of usage alone is not particularly useful since it may not be appropriate to the infections being treated. For example, in Canada, one study found that there was overuse of cefovecin and of fluoroquinolones for the treatment of cat and dog diseases for which antibiotics were either not indicated or for which first-line antimicrobials were appropriate (24). The potential value of companion animal usage data obtained electronically is that, as has been shown for food animals, it can be used for benchmarking purposes as part of a broader approach to improved antimicrobial stewardship.

PUBLIC HEALTH ASPECTS OF ANTIMICROBIAL DRUG USE IN ANIMALS

Food Animals
The effect of antimicrobial drug use in food animals on the development of resistance in bacteria that can cause disease in humans has been the subject of prolonged, acrimonious, and ongoing debate. The major and most accessible reviews of this issue are summarized in Table 3, which shows that the intensity of the criticism of agricultural usage of antimicrobial drugs intensified from the mid-1990s and has now reached a crescendo, paralleling the antimicrobial resistance crisis in human medicine (Table 1).

The first major review of the effect of antimicrobial drug use on resistance in human and animal pathogens was carried out in the United Kingdom under the chairmanship of M.M. Swann. The impetus for the review was a combination of recognition of the increasing im-

Table 3 Historical time line of major reports and their conclusions or recommendations relating to the public health aspects of antimicrobial drug use in food animals

Date	Report/country	Major conclusions or recommendations
1962	Netherthorpe Committee *UK, Joint Committee, Agricultural and Medical Research Councils*	Recognized economic benefit of antimicrobials as growth promoters, saw no reason to discontinue However, continue to examine situation and substitute penicillin and tetracycline use if alternative nontherapeutic growth promoters become available
1969	Committee on Antibiotic Uses in Animal Husbandry and Veterinary Medicine; The Swann Report *UK, Report to Parliament*	Restriction of use of antimicrobials into prescription-only therapeutic use and nonprescription feed additives Growth-promotional and subtherapeutic use of drugs important in human medicine were banned
1972	The Use of Antibiotics in Animal Feeds *USA, FDA Task Force*	Use of antimicrobial drugs in food animals may promote resistance in *Salmonella*; manufacturers to show this is not a problem Sufficient evidence to stop use of penicillin and chlortetracycline as growth promoters
1979	Drugs in Livestock Feed *USA, Office of Technology Assessment*	Stop use of penicillin and tetracyclines as growth promoters, even though this would have short-term economic cost
1980	The Effects on Human Health of Subtherapeutic Use of Antimicrobials in Animals *USA, National Research Council*	Could not conclude from data available that there was a direct relationship between subtherapeutic drug use in animal feed and human health Insufficient data from UK that implementation of Swann report had reduce postulated hazards to human health
1981	Antibiotics in Animal Feeds *USA, Council for Agricultural Sciences and Technology*	Irrational to ban subtherapeutic dosage without also banning therapeutic use Cost of a ban on feed antimicrobials: about $3.5 billion
1989	Human Health Risks with the Subtherapeutic Use of Penicillin or Tetracyclines in Animal Feed *USA, Institute of Medicine*	Unable to find substantial direct evidence of definite human health hazard in the use of subtherapeutic concentrations of penicillins and tetracyclines in animal feeds
1995	Impacts of Antibiotic-Resistant Bacteria *USA, Office of Technology Assessment*	Need to collect more data to resolve the issue of the effect of feed antimicrobials in animals on human health A further report will not resolve the issue
1997	Antimicrobial Feed Additives *Sweden, Ministry of Agriculture, Commission on Antimicrobial Feed Additives*	As part of negotiations leading to European Union membership, Sweden, which had banned use of antimicrobial growth promoters in 1985, re-reviewed benefits of antibacterial feed additives and again concluded that benefits did not outweigh the risks
	The Medical Impact of the Use of Antimicrobials in Food Animals *WHO*	Stop using antimicrobials for growth promotion or subtherapeutic purposes in animals if used in human therapeutics or if they select for cross-resistance to antimicrobials used in human medicine
1998	A Review of Antimicrobial Resistance in the Food Chain *UK, Ministry of Agriculture, Fisheries, and Food*	Resistance in animal pathogens and commensal bacteria is selected for by antimicrobial drug use, can reach people through food chain, may cause disease or colonize people, can transfer resistance to human pathogens, *Campylobacter* and *Salmonella*, and certain antimicrobials are especially problematic
1999	The Use of Drugs in Food Animals: Benefits and Risks *USA, Committee on Drug Use in Food Animals: Panel on Animal Health, Food Safety and Public Health, National Research Council and Institute of Medicine*	Use of drugs in food animals does not appear to constitute an immediate public health concern; additional data may alter conclusion, but data are lacking Recommended integrated national databases to support rational, visible, science-driven decision-making and policy development for regulatory approval and use of antimicrobials in food animals Estimated cost of ban on nontherapeutic use in animals: between $5 and 10 per person per year in USA
2000	The Use of Antibiotics in Food-Producing Animals: Antibiotic-Resistant Bacteria in Animals and Humans	Stop using growth promoters if same drugs important in human medicine

(Continued)

Table 3 *(Continued)*

Date	Report/country	Major conclusions or recommendations
	Australia: Joint Expert Advisory Committee on Antibiotic Resistance	All antimicrobials for animals prescription only Predetermine "resistance thresholds" for animal antimicrobials that trigger investigation or mitigation Develop a comprehensive and integrated resistance surveillance system Monitor antimicrobial usage Find alternatives to antimicrobials for food animals
2001	Risk Assessment on the Human Health Impact of Fluoroquinolone Resistant *Campylobacter* Associated with the Consumption of Chicken *USA, Center for Veterinary Medicine*	Risk assessment by highly detailed mathematical model with numerous explicit assumptions suggested that in 1998 mean estimate of 8,678 U.S. citizens had fluoroquinolone-resistant *Campylobacter* illnesses acquired from chicken and received fluoroquinolones for treatment
2002	The Need to Improve Antimicrobial Use in Agriculture: Ecological and Human Health Consequences *USA, Alliance for the Prudent Use of Antibiotics. Clinical Infectious Diseases 34; Supplement 3*	Elimination of nontherapeutic use of antimicrobials in food animals will lower burden of antimicrobial resistance in the environment, with benefits to human and animal health
	Uses of Antimicrobials in Food Animals in Canada: Impact on Resistance and Human Health *Canada, Health Canada Advisory Committee on Animal Uses of Antimicrobials and Impact on Resistance and Human Health*	Make all antimicrobials for disease control prescription only Develop extra-label policy Control an importation of drugs "loop-hole" Stringently reassess growth-promotional use of drugs Develop national surveillance of resistance and use
	Food Safety and Pig Production in Denmark. Controls on antibiotics, veterinary medicines and *Salmonella* Verner Wheelock Associates Limited; Danish Bacon and Meat Council	Control of antimicrobial-resistant bacteria by banning antimicrobial growth promoters, and *Salmonella* control programs, has made Denmark a model and given the Danish pig industry competitive economic advantage
2003	Joint FAO/OIE/WHO Expert Workshop on Non-Human Antimicrobial Usage and Antimicrobial Resistance: Scientific Assessment *WHO*	Clear evidence of adverse human health consequences due to resistant organisms resulting from nonhuman usage Surveillance of usage and resistance important to identify problems and choose interventions Magnitude of impact accompanied by considerable uncertainty
	Impacts of Antimicrobial Growth Promotion Termination in Denmark *WHO*	Review of the "Danish experiment" of terminating use of growth promoters on efficiency of food animal production, animal health, food safety, and consumer prices concluded that there have been no serious negative effects Very beneficial in reducing total quantity of antimicrobials used and reducing antimicrobial resistance in important food animal reservoirs
2004	Second Joint FAO/OIE/WHO Expert Panel on Non-Human Antimicrobial Usage and Antimicrobial Resistance: Management Options *WHO*	Establish national surveillance programs on use and resistance; follow WHO/OIE guidelines on responsible use; implement strategies to prevent transmission through food etc.
	Antibiotic Resistance: Federal Agencies Need to better Focus Efforts to Reduce Risk to Humans from Antibiotic Use in Animals *U.S. General Accounting Office*	Expedite risk assessments in animals of antibiotics critically important to humans; develop plan to assess and mitigate risk
2008	Antimicrobial Resistance from Food Animals. *World Health Organization*	Continues to press for multiple approaches to improve antimicrobial use in food animals, prescription only, integrated use and resistance surveillance, identify barriers to implementation of international guidelines, etc.
	Putting Meat on the Table: Industrial Farm Animal Production in America	Phase out nontherapeutic antimicrobial use in food animals, restrict use to veterinary oversight and prescription, require

(Continued)

Table 3 *(Continued)*

Date	Report/country	Major conclusions or recommendations
	USA, Pew Commission on Industrial Farm Animal Production	reporting of annual sales, review previously approved antibiotics for animals etc.
		General approach very critical of modern intensive agriculture
2009	The American Veterinary Medical Association Response to the Final Report of the Pew Commission on Industrial Farm Animal Production *American Veterinary Medical Association (AVMA)*	Described Pew Report as having some value but "dangerous and uninformed" and "shocking"
		The Pew Report and the AVMA response highlights the highly conflictive nature of the debate in the USA
2010–2014	No major reports during this period but numerous scientific papers investigating development and spread of livestock-associated MRSA, spread of extended-spectrum β-lactamase-producing *E. coli* or *Salmonella* in food animals treated with ceftiofur, and possible or definite spread to humans	
	Many examples during this period of small groups of engaged academics reviewing the issue in different forums and making recommendations	
2015	Antimicrobials in Agriculture and the Environment: Reducing Unnecessary Use and Waste *UK, Review on Antimicrobial Resistance: O'Neill Report*	Scale of antimicrobial use in global agriculture is massive
		A review of the evidence supports a link between antimicrobial use in animals and resistance in human pathogens
		Proposed global targets for antimicrobial use in animals, restrictions on use of certain antimicrobials, and improved surveillance
2016	Tackling Drug-Resistant Infections Globally: Final Report and Recommendations. *UK, Review on Antimicrobial Resistance: O'Neill Report*	Influential economist's view of the present and future scale and costs, call for urgent global action
		Highlights agricultural area as one of 10 major recommendations

portance of (i) the phenomenon of "infectious," transferable, drug resistance associated in part with the pioneering work of the distinguished British veterinary microbiologist H. Williams Smith, (ii) the emergence and dissemination in calves in Britain of multidrug-resistant *Salmonella enterica* serotype Typhimurium and its spread to humans, and (iii) experiences around this time of a difficult-to-control epidemic of chloramphenicol-resistant *S. enterica* serovar Typhi in Central America. Chloramphenicol was then the drug of last resort for typhoid fever in humans (25). The 1969 Swann Report to the British government gave a careful analysis of how different usage of antimicrobial drugs in animals might lead to selection of resistant bacteria and resistance plasmids and how such resistant bacteria, or their transmissible resistance traits, could lead to difficult to treat infections in humans. The major recommendations of the committee were as follows: (i) "Feed" antimicrobial drugs could only be used for growth promotion without prescription if they had little or no implication as therapeutic agents in humans, would not impair the value of prescribed drugs, and produced an economic benefit. Since penicillin and tetracyclines did not meet these criteria, they were withdrawn from growth-promotional use and could only be used therapeutically by veterinary prescription. (ii) The "therapeutic" antimicrobials (those other than growth-promotional antimicrobials) tylosin, sulfonamides, and nitrofurans

should no longer be used without veterinary prescription. The spirit of the Swann report was to restrict the use of therapeutically effective antibiotics to only therapeutic use on a veterinary prescription basis. Withdrawal of penicillin and tetracyclines for growth-promotional and subtherapeutic purposes was, however, soon followed by their substitution by bacitracin, flavomycin, nitrovin, and virginiamycin for similar purposes.

It was perhaps unfortunate that little effort was made in Britain following the Swann report to improve the scientific base of understanding of the effect of antimicrobial drug use in animals on human health, or to document the effect of implementation of the report. Nevertheless, the sustained work of A.H. Linton (26) and that of his colleagues led to important conceptual understanding of the routes of movement of resistant bacteria between animals and humans, and the factors which enhanced the movement, although the scale of the movement still has considerable uncertainty (Fig. 1).

In the United States, the response to the issues raised in the Swann report was largely unenthusiastic and critical (Table 3). Resistance to Swann's recommendations was based on the estimates of the considerable economic contribution that growth-promoting and subtherapeutic (feed) antimicrobial drugs made to agriculture in comparison to what was criticized as the inadequate evidence, the dubious and slender risk, and the "special case pleading" on which the recommendations of the

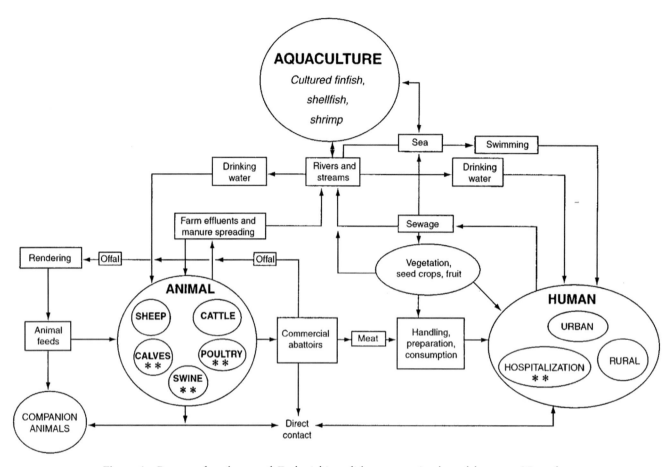

Figure 1 Routes of exchange of *Escherichia coli* between animals and humans. Note the areas where antimicrobial drug selection for resistance is most likely. The size of the circles or boxes does not indicate the extent of the scale of the movement. After Linton (26), modified by R. Irwin; reproduced with permission.

Swann report were regarded as based. The strong lobby of antimicrobial drug manufacturers and the absence in the United States of a national health system (i.e., the patient pays for illness, whereas in Europe it is the nation that bears the cost) may have helped to fuel the criticism. The data were regarded as inadequate to make clear judgements, but the scale of the problem was also thought to be minor. For example, the 1989 Institute of Medicine study (Table 3) suggested that use of subtherapeutic or growth-promoting drugs might contribute to perhaps 26 human deaths a year from antimicrobial-resistant *Salmonella*. For perspective, these numbers would have compared to about 40,000 automobile accident and 10,000 gunshot fatalities in the United States in the same year.

Despite the inconclusive nature of many of the reports in the United States in the period between 1972 and 1995, the issue refused to die. There were periodic highly publicized reports throughout this period of serious human illness caused by *Salmonella* carrying resistance genes thought to be acquired from subtherapeutic, or even therapeutic, use of antimicrobials in animals. One of several examples was that of Spika and others (27) of chloramphenicol-resistant *S. enterica* serotype Newport traced from hamburger meat to dairy farms. Such reports led to apparently carefully orchestrated media and even major science journal frenzies about the discovery of the "smoking gun," with consequent fervent denials by the animal antimicrobial drug industry. Given the existing well-established understanding of the epidemiology of the movement of resistant intestinal bacteria (Fig. 1), these periodic frenzies seemed at the time both astonishing and somehow hysterical. The periodic surges in public interest, however, produced no political will in the United States to re-examine the problem.

The reason for the extensive re-examination of the issue from the mid-1990s was related to several factors. The most important of these was the antimicrobial resistance crisis in medicine, in which for the first time resistant bacteria moved "out of the hospital and into the community." The very serious nature of the crisis led to a re-examination within the human medicine community of all aspects of antimicrobial use and even to the apparent rediscovery of the importance of basic infection control procedures such as hand-washing. The antimicrobial resistance crisis in medicine again focused the medical establishment on agricultural usage of antimicrobials, in some cases almost to the extent of using it as the scapegoat for the crisis in medicine.

Improvements in understanding of the microbiology of infectious diseases acquired from animals were less important, but also critical, forces in the re-examination of antimicrobial usage in agriculture. For example, at the time of the Swann report, *C. jejuni* was not recognized as a human pathogen, although it subsequently became identified as the most common cause of bacterial gastroenteritis in humans. The emergence of fluoroquinolone resistance in *C. jejuni* of poultry origin in the United States because of the use of fluoroquinolones to treat *Escherichia coli* infections in chickens (28) subsequently led to the ban of all use of this class of drug in chickens in the United States (Table 3). A subsequent risk analysis in the United States suggested that 8,678 citizens treated for this illness with fluoroquinolones had fluoroquinolone-resistant *C. jejuni* illness acquired from chickens (Table 3), a huge number compared to the "26 possible deaths because of resistant *Salmonella*" identified in the 1989 Institute of Medicine report.

Similarly, at the time of the Swann report, vancomycin-resistant enterococci (VREs) were also unknown, although subsequently, enterococcal infections emerged as major nosocomial, largely hospital-acquired, infections in humans, with vancomycin as the "drug of last resort" in such infections. Acquisition of transmissible vancomycin-resistance genes by these hospital-associated bacteria made them essentially untreatable, again raising the specter of the postantibiotic era (Table 1). Work by Aarestrup and his colleagues in Denmark was important in identifying avoparcin, a glycopeptide antimicrobial related to vancomycin, as selecting for the massive presence of VREs in the intestine of poultry and swine fed this drug as a growth promoter (29). For the first time, there was convincing large-scale evidence that eliminating the use of antimicrobial drugs in food animals could dramatically reverse the rise of resistant bacteria in these animals (30). Convincing molecular genetic typing evidence showed that VREs from animals colonized humans (31) and, most dramatically, the marked decline in human intestinal colonization by VREs in Europe following the withdrawal of avoparcin as a growth promo-

ter (32) suggested that the scale of the movement of resistant intestinal bacteria from animals to humans, which had always been a matter of great uncertainty, was far larger than generally suspected previously. Molecular genetic typing and whole-genome sequencing of resistance genes and gene regions were unavailable at the time of the Swann Report but were subsequently used extensively to characterize the relatedness (and therefore sometimes the source) of both bacteria and their resistance genes obtained from animals and humans.

More recent application of whole-genome sequencing to antimicrobial-resistant extrapathogenic *E. coli* from human urinary tract infections and comparison to isolates from healthy chickens clearly indicates that some resistant human isolates derive from chickens (33). Recognition of the likelihood of such a previously unsuspected "insidious epidemic" suggests that the scale and importance of the movement of resistant bacteria and their genes into the human population may be far greater than suspected. One group suggested that cephalosporin use in poultry was responsible for about 1,500 human deaths annually in Europe (34). A voluntary ban on ceftiofur use in Danish swine production was shown to effectively reduce extended-spectrum cephalosporinase-producing *E. coli* in slaughter pigs (35). It seems likely that similar bans, voluntary or involuntary, may be adopted in different jurisdictions in agriculture. The World Health Organization ranking of antimicrobials according to their importance in human medicine (36) remains an important issue for animal use, since the World Health Organization classification of "critically important" includes drugs such as penicillin, and essentially all antibiotics are classified as important, highly important, or critically important. Further discussion, which will likely focus on "highest-priority critically-important antimicrobials" (36), is clearly required as one of the steps in addressing the global resistance crisis.

It is highly ironic that the recent emergence and global dissemination of MRSA in livestock, particularly of clonal complex 398 associated with swine, and the emergence and dissemination of livestock-associated MRSA infections in humans (37, 38) has been linked to the use of zinc oxide in the feed of intensively reared livestock (39). Following the European ban on antimicrobial growth promoters, zinc oxide was introduced as an alternative to to prevent enteric infections in young animals.

Companion Animals

There has been no systematic study of the effect of antimicrobial drug use in companion animals (meaning, particularly, dogs and cats) and transfer of resistant bacteria or their genes to humans. As a generalization, resistance to antimicrobials is growing among bacteria that cause infection in pets, such as *S. aureus*, *S. pseudintermedius*, and *E. coli* (40), and such bacteria can be transmitted between pets, owners, and veterinary staff both directly and indirectly. Practicing veterinarians are far more likely than controls to be nasally colonized by *S. aureus* (41). Companion animals have been documented to act as reservoirs of some of the high-risk multidrug-resistant clones of *Enterobacteriaceae* (42–44), some of which are likely to be acquired from their human owners. Infection with such resistant bacteria may be amplified by antimicrobial use in veterinary clinics or hospitals and subsequently spread back to animal owners in the dance of infection (Fig. 1).

THE EMERGING CONCEPT AND PRACTICE OF ANTIMICROBIAL STEWARDSHIP IN VETERINARY MEDICINE

As the science of antimicrobial resistance moves onto the political stage, the past 2 years have seen dramatic changes in the global response to the antimicrobial resistance crisis, culminating most recently in the September 2016 United Nations High-Level Meeting and the commitment of members to address the issue in a multifaceted way. This follows earlier similar commitment by members of the G7 and numerous important analyses of how to address the crisis (45, 46) (Table 1). In the United States, there has been game-changing commitment (Guidance 213, Guidance for Industry 233) to remove antibiotics from use as growth promoters and to bring all antibiotics used in feed or water of food animals under veterinary oversight. Canada has followed suit. Another major change has been adoption of a "One Health" approach to resistance (reviewed in chapter 26), an approach that involves multidisciplinary and multi jurisdictional approaches to very complex problems involving people, animals, and the environment (47). An evolving concept and practice, a One Health approach may reduce some of the conflict between the use of antimicrobials in human and veterinary medicine by focusing efforts and energy on resolving resistance issues in a collaborative rather than blaming manner.

Antimicrobial resistance is a multifaceted problem with all the complexities of climate change, to which it is highly analogous. It has multiple causes, with no single actor or factor that can be blamed, has the well-established ability to be self-sustaining, and has the potential to be catastrophic. No single intervention will address the problem, but the combination of multiple interventions and approaches has the potential to have a cumulative impact that will help in its control. A stewardship approach which integrates so much of what we now know about effective antimicrobial use (6), and about infection generally, is the best approach for first-line veterinary practitioners to address the resistance crisis. "Antimicrobial stewardship," reviewed in chapter 32, is the term increasingly used in medicine to describe the multifaceted approaches required to sustain the efficacy of antibiotics and minimize the emergence of resistance. The concept and practice of antimicrobial stewardship continues to evolve in human and veterinary medicine, but it is an approach that takes an active, dynamic process of continuous improvement encapsulated in the idea of good stewardship practice (GSP) (6, 48). Only a GSP mind-set will ensure the long-term sustainability of antimicrobial drugs. Antimicrobial stewardship and GSP involve coordinated approaches and interventions designed to promote, improve, monitor, and evaluate the judicious use of antimicrobials to preserve their future effectiveness and promote and protect human and animal health. This involves a "5R" approach of responsibility, reduction, refinement, replacement, and review (49). Critically, a GSP approach to stewardship also could be evaluated quantitatively as a standard of veterinary practice.

The question for the future is how to preserve existing and develop new drugs in the face of bacterial pathogens, some of which appear to have become particularly adept at developing or acquiring resistance over the past 60 years. Using some of the tools available as we enter the "golden age of microbiology" to improve the way we diagnose infections and develop new, likely targeted, antimicrobials is promising (50). However, as noted by one writer in respect to resistant bacterial infections in companion animal practice (40), resolving the issue of multidrug-resistant endemic bacterial infections will not be through development of new antibiotics if current hygiene practices remain and if we don't undertake good stewardship practices to preserve our existing drugs.

With respect to the changing relationship to antimicrobial drugs in human and veterinary medicine that the resistance crisis has produced, there's a sense that humanity is perhaps in the intermission after the first act of a three-act play, and we're still trying to determine if the play is a comedy or a tragedy. It currently feels like both. There's a huge amount to be done.

Citation. Prescott JF. 2017. History and current use of antimicrobial drugs in veterinary medicine. Microbiol Spectrum 5(6):ARBA-0002-2017.

References

1. Prescott JF. 2006. History of antimicrobial usage in agriculture: an overview, p 19–27. *In* Aarestrup FM (ed), *Antimicrobial Resistance in Bacteria of Animal Origin.* ASM Press, Washington, DC.

2. Little RB, Bryan CS, Petersen WE, Plastridge WN, Schalm OW. 1946. INTRAMAMMARY therapy of bovine mastitis. *J Am Vet Med Assoc* 108:127–135.

3. Roberts SJ. 1953. Antibiotic therapy in large animals, p 39–48. *Conference Proceedings, Am Vet Med Assoc.*

4. Collins JH. 1948. The present status of penicillin in veterinary medicine. *J Am Vet Med Assoc* 113:330–333.

5. Hussar AE, Holley HW. 1954. *Antibiotics and Antibiotic Therapy.* MacMillan, New York, NY.

6. Weese JS, Page S, Prescott JF. Antimicrobial stewardship in animals, p 117–132. *In* Giguère S, Prescott JF, Dowling PM (ed), *Antimicrobial Therapy in Veterinary Medicine*, 5th ed. Wiley Blackwell, Ames, IA.

7. Shryock T, Page S. 2013. Performance uses of antimicrobial agents and non-antimicorbial alternatives, p 379–394. *In* Giguère S, Prescott JF, Dowling PM (ed), *Antimicrobial Therapy in Veterinary Medicine*, 5th ed. Wiley Blackwell, Ames, IA.

8. Burch DGS. 2013. Antimicrobial drug use in swine, p 553–568. *In* Giguère S, Prescott JF, Dowling PM (ed), *Antimicrobial Therapy in Veterinary Medicine*, 5th ed. Wiley Blackwell, Ames, IA.

9. Apley MD, Coetzee JF. 2013. Antimicrobial drug use in cattle, p 495–518. *In* Giguère S, Prescott JF, Dowling PM (ed), *Antimicrobial Therapy in Veterinary Medicine*, 5th ed. Wiley Blackwell, Ames, IA.

10. Van Boeckel TP, Brower C, Gilbert M, Grenfell BT, Levin SA, Robinson TP, Teillant A, Laxminarayan R. 2015. Global trends in antimicrobial use in food animals. *Proc Natl Acad Sci USA* 112:5649–5654.

11. Grave K, Torren-Edo J, Muller A, Greko C, Moulin G, Mackay D, Fuchs K, Laurier L, Iliev D, Pokludova L, Genakritis M, Jacobsen E, Kurvits K, Kivilahti-Mantyla K, Wallmann J, Kovacs J, Lenharthsson JM, Beechinor JG, Perrella A, Mičule G, Zymantaite U, Meijering A, Prokopiak D, Ponte MH, Svetlin A, Hederova J, Madero CM, Girma K, Eckford S, ESVAC Group. 2014. Variations in the sales and sales patterns of veterinary antimicrobial agents in 25 European countries. *J Antimicrob Chemother* 69:2284–2291.

12. Dupont N, Fertner M, Sonne Kristensen C, Toft N, Stege H. 2016. Reporting the national antimicrobial consumption in Danish pigs: influence of assigned daily dosage values and population measurement. *Acta Vet Scan* 58:27.

13. Speksnijder DC, Mevius DJ, Bruschke CJM, Wagenaar JA. 2015. Reduction of veterinary antimicrobial use in the Netherlands. The Dutch success model. *Zoonoses Public Health* 62(Suppl 1):79–87.

14. Speksnijder DC, Jaarsma DAC, Verheij TJM, Wagenaar JA. 2015. Attitudes and perceptions of Dutch veterinarians on their role in the reduction of antimicrobial use in farm animals. *Prev Vet Med* 121:365–373.

15. Dorado-Garcia A, Mevius D, Jacobs JJ, Van Geijlswijk M, Mouton JW, Wagenaar J, Heederik DJ. 2016. Quantitative assessment of antimicrobial resistance in livestock during the course of a nationwide antimicrobial use reduction in the Netherlands. *J Antimicrob Chemother* 71:3607–3619.

16. Chantziaras I, Boyen F, Callens B, Dewulf J. 2014. Correlation between veterinary antimicrobial use and antimicrobial resistance in food-producing animals: a report on seven countries. *J Antimicrob Chemother* 69:827–834.

17. Bos MEH, Mevius DJ, Wagenaar JA, van Geijlswijk IM, Mouton JW, Heederik DJJ, Netherlands Veterinary Medicines Authority (SDa). 2015. Antimicrobial prescription patterns of veterinarians: introduction of a benchmarking approach. *J Antimicrob Chemother* 70:2423–2425.

18. De Briyne N, Atkinson J, Pokludová L, Borriello SP, Price S. 2013. Factors influencing antibiotic prescribing habits and use of sensitivity testing amongst veterinarians in Europe. *Vet Rec* 173:475.

19. De Briyne N, Atkinson J, Pokludová L, Borriello SP. 2014. Antibiotics used most commonly to treat animals in Europe. *Vet Rec* 175:325.

20. Lloyd DH. 2012. Multi-resistant *Staphylococcus pseudintermedius*: a wake-up call in our approach to bacterial infection. *J Small Anim Pract* 53:145–146.

21. Perreten V, Kadlec K, Schwarz S, Grönlund Andersson U, Finn M, Greko C, Moodley A, Kania SA, Frank LA, Bemis DA, Franco A, Iurescia M, Battisti A, Duim B, Wagenaar JA, van Duijkeren E, Weese JS, Fitzgerald JR, Rossano A, Guardabassi L. 2010. Clonal spread of methicillin-resistant *Staphylococcus pseudintermedius* in Europe and North America: an international multicentre study. *J Antimicrob Chemother* 65:1145–1154.

22. McCarthy AJ, Harrison EM, Stanczak-Mrozek K, Leggett B, Waller A, Holmes MA, Lloyd DH, Lindsay JA, Loeffler A. 2015. Genomic insights into the rapid emergence and evolution of MDR in *Staphylococcus pseudintermedius*. *J Antimicrob Chemother* 70:997–1007.

23. Buckland EL, O'Neill D, Summers J, Mateus A, Church D, Redmond L, Brodbelt D. 2016. Characterisation of antimicrobial usage in cats and dogs attending UK primary care companion animal veterinary practices. *Vet Rec* 179:489.

24. Murphy CP, Reid-Smith RJ, Boerlin P, Weese JS, Prescott JF, Janecko N, McEwen SA. 2012. Out-patient antimicrobial drug use in dogs and cats for new disease events from community companion animal practices in Ontario. *Can Vet J* 53:291–298.

25. Randall CJ. 1969. The Swann Committee. *Vet Rec* 85:616–621.

26. Linton AH. 1977. Antibiotic resistance: the present situation reviewed. *Vet Rec* 100:354–360.

27. Spika JS, Waterman SH, Hoo GW, St Louis ME, Pacer RE, James SM, Bissett ML, Mayer LW, Chiu JY, Hall B, Greene K, Potter ME, Cohen ML, Blake P. 1987. Chloramphenicol-resistant *Salmonella newport* traced through hamburger to dairy farms. A major persisting source of human salmonellosis in California. *N Engl J Med* 316:565–570.

28. Smith KE, Besser JM, Hedberg CW, Leano FT, Bender JB, Wicklund JH, Johnson BP, Moore KA, Osterholm MT, Investigation Team. 1999. Quinolone-resistant *Campylobacter jejuni* infections in Minnesota, 1992–1998. *N Engl J Med* 340:1525–1532.

29. Bager F, Madsen M, Christensen J, Aarestrup FM. 1997. Avoparcin used as a growth promoter is associated with the occurrence of vancomycin-resistant *Enterococcus faecium* on Danish poultry and pig farms. *Prev Vet Med* 31:95–112.

30. Aarestrup FM, Seyfarth AM, Emborg HD, Pedersen K, Hendriksen RS, Bager F. 2001. Effect of abolishment of the use of antimicrobial agents for growth promotion on occurrence of antimicrobial resistance in fecal enterococci from food animals in Denmark. *Antimicrob Agents Chemother* 45:2054–2059.

31. Jensen LB, Hammerum AM, Poulsen RL, Westh H. 1999. Vancomycin-resistant *Enterococcus faecium* strains with highly similar pulsed-field gel electrophoresis patterns containing similar Tn*1546*-like elements isolated from a hospitalized patient and pigs in Denmark. *Antimicrob Agents Chemother* 43:724–725.

32. Klare I, Badstübner D, Konstabel C, Böhme G, Claus H, Witte W. 1999. Decreased incidence of VanA-type vancomycin-resistant enterococci isolated from poultry meat and from fecal samples of humans in the community after discontinuation of avoparcin usage in animal husbandry. *Microb Drug Resist* 5:45–52.

33. Nordstrom L, Liu CM, Price LB. 2013. Foodborne urinary tract infections: a new paradigm for antimicrobial-resistant foodborne illness. *Front Microbiol* 4:29.

34. Collignon P, Aarestrup FM, Irwin R, McEwen S. 2013. Human deaths and third-generation cephalosporin use in poultry, Europe. *Emerg Infect Dis* 19:1339–1340.

35. Agersø Y, Aarestrup FM. 2013. Voluntary ban on cephalosporin use in Danish pig production has effectively reduced extended-spectrum cephalosporinase-producing *Escherichia coli* in slaughter pigs. *J Antimicrob Chemother* 68:569–572.

36. Collignon PC, Conly JM, Andremont A, McEwen SA, Aidara-Kane A, Agerso Y, Andremont A, Collignon P, Conly J, Dang Ninh T, Donado-Godoy P, Fedorka-Cray P, Fernandez H, Galas M, Irwin R, Karp B, Matar G, McDermott P, McEwen S, Mitema E, Reid-Smith R, Scott HM, Singh R, DeWaal CS, Stelling J, Toleman M, Watanabe H, Woo GJ, World Health Organization Advisory Group, Bogotá Meeting on Integrated Surveillance of Antimicrobial Resistance (WHO-AGISAR). 2016. World Health Organization ranking of antimicrobials according to their importance in human medicine: A critical step for developing risk management strategies to control antimicrobial resistance from food animals. *Clin Infect Dis* 63:1087–1093.

37. Smith TC, Pearson N. 2011. The emergence of *Staphylococcus aureus* ST398. *Vector Borne Zoonotic Dis* 11:327–339.

38. Cuny C, Wieler LH, Witte W. 2015. Livestock-associated MRSA: the impact on humans. *Antibiotics (Basel)* 4:521–543.

39. Cavaco LM, Hasman H, Aarestrup FM, Wagenaar JA, Graveland H, Veldman K, Mevius D, Fetsch A, Tenhagen B-A, Concepcion Porrero M, Dominguez L, Granier SA, Jouy E, Butaye P, Kaszanyitzky E, Dán A, Zmudzki J, Battisti A, Franco A, Schwarz S, Gutierrez M, Weese JS, Cui S, Pomba C, Members of MRSA-CG. 2011. Zinc resistance of *Staphylococcus aureus* of animal origin is strongly associated with methicillin resistance. *Vet Microbiol* 150:344–348.

40. Lloyd DH. 2007. Reservoirs of antimicrobial resistance in pet animals. *Clin Infect Dis* 45(Suppl 2):S148–S152.

41. Jordan D, Simon J, Fury S, Moss S, Giffard P, Maiwald M, Southwell P, Barton MD, Axon JE, Morris SG, Trott DJ. 2011. Carriage of methicillin-resistant *Staphylococcus aureus* by veterinarians in Australia. *Aust Vet J* 89:152–159.

42. Ewers C, Bethe A, Stamm I, Grobbel M, Kopp PA, Guerra B, Stubbe M, Doi Y, Zong Z, Kola A, Schaufler K, Semmler T, Fruth A, Wieler LH, Guenther S. 2014. CTX-M-15-D-ST648 *Escherichia coli* from companion animals and horses: another pandemic clone combining multiresistance and extraintestinal virulence? *J Antimicrob Chemother* 69:1224–1230.

43. Ewers C, Stamm I, Pfeifer Y, Wieler LH, Kopp PA, Schönning K, Prenger-Berninghoff E, Scheufen S, Stolle I, Günther S, Bethe A. 2014. Clonal spread of highly successful ST15-CTX-M-15 *Klebsiella pneumoniae* in companion animals and horses. *J Antimicrob Chemother* 69:2676–2680.

44. Abraham S, Wong HS, Turnidge J, Johnson JR, Trott DJ. 2014. Carbapenemase-producing bacteria in companion animals: a public health concern on the horizon. *J Antimicrob Chemother* 69:1155–1157.

45. O'Neill J. 2016. *Tackling Drug Resistant Infections Globally: Final Report and Recommendations.* The Review on Antimicrobial Resistance. https://amr-review.org/sites/default/files/160518_Final%20paper_with%20cover.pdf44.

46. Laxminarayan R, Duse A, Wattal C, Zaidi AKM, Wertheim HF, Sumpradit N, Vlieghe E, Hara GL, Gould IM, Goossens H, Greko C, So AD, Bigdeli M, Tomson G, Woodhouse W, Ombaka E, Peralta AQ, Qamar FN, Mir F, Kariuki S, Bhutta ZA, Coates A, Bergstrom R, Wright GD, Brown ED, Cars O. 2013. Antibiotic resistance-the need for global solutions. *Lancet Infect Dis* 13:1057–1098.

47. Robinson TP, Bu DP, Carrique-Mas J, Fèvre EM, Gilbert M, Grace D, Hay SI, Jiwakanon J, Kakkar M, Kariuki S, Laxminarayan R, Lubroth J, Magnusson U, Thi Ngoc P, Van Boeckel TP, Woolhouse MEJ. 2016. Antibiotic resistance is the quintessential One Health issue. *Trans R Soc Trop Med Hyg* 110:377–380.

48. Guardabassi L, Prescott JF. 2015. Antimicrobial stewardship in small animal veterinary practice: from theory to practice. *Vet Clin North Am Small Anim Pract* 45:361–376, vii.

49. Page S, Prescott J, Weese S. 2014. The 5Rs approach to antimicrobial stewardship. *Vet Rec* 175:207–208.

50. Prescott JF. 2014. The resistance *tsunami*, antimicrobial stewardship, and the golden age of microbiology. *Vet Microbiol* 171:273–278.

Antimicrobial Resistance in Bacteria from Livestock and Companion Animals
Edited by Frank Møller Aarestrup, Stefan Schwarz, Jianzhong Shen, and Lina Cavaco
© 2018 American Society for Microbiology, Washington, DC
doi:10.1128/microbiolspec.ARBA-0001-2017

Antimicrobial Susceptibility Testing of Bacteria of Veterinary Origin

2

Jeffrey L. Watts[1], Michael T. Sweeney[1], and Brian V. Lubbers[2]

INTRODUCTION

The emergence of multidrug-resistant bacteria in both human and veterinary medicine over the past decade has limited the therapeutic choices available to clinicians (1–4). This has, in turn, led to increased pressure on the veterinary community to reduce the overall use of antimicrobial agents, with an emphasis on those deemed critically important for use in human health (4–6). Thus, selection of the most appropriate agent for treatment is essential in preserving the future utility of the currently available agents in both human and veterinary medicine while also ensuring animal welfare. Antimicrobial susceptibility tests (ASTs) can provide essential information to guide the veterinarian in selecting the most appropriate agent and are considered an essential component of responsible use and antimicrobial stewardship programs (2, 7).

The foundational characteristics of ASTs are as follows: (i) a standardized, reproducible test methodology; (ii) quality control (QC) guidelines to ensure day-to-day and interlaboratory assay performance; and (iii) an established relationship between the test outcome and the clinical outcome following treatment (8–12). While standardized test methods have been available in human medicine since the 1960s, the development of rigorous AST methods for use in veterinary medicine was not undertaken until the early 1990s (9, 13). This is not surprising given the variety of host species (companions, food animals, and exotics) and the differences in the application of test results. AST results for a pathogen from a canine, for example, will be used to select treatment for the individual animal, while the same information for a swine isolate may be used to devise therapy for the entire herd. This diversity in host animals and the application of test results has made the development of ASTs that provide accurate, reproducible, clinically relevant results for veterinary pathogens daunting, but substantial progress has been made over the past 2 decades.

Historical Perspective

The use of ASTs in veterinary medicine closely paralleled the development of ASTs in human medicine (as reviewed in reference 7). Because the AST methods for human pathogens such as *Staphylococcus aureus* or *Escherichia coli* could be readily applied to the same organisms isolated from animal diseases with equivalent values, the use of these methods for testing veterinary isolates was a logical extension of the human AST methodologies. However, the use of these methods for the more fastidious veterinary pathogens, as well as the use of human interpretive criteria, was problematic. For example, four different media were recommended by various authors for susceptibility testing of *Histophilus somni* ("*Haemophilus somnus*"), and five different media were recommended for testing of *Actinobacillus pleuropneumoniae* (as reviewed in reference 7, 13). This not only made comparison of AST results from different laboratories difficult, but no single medium would reliably support the growth of all strains. Moreover, the only interpretive criteria available for categorizing isolates as susceptible or resistant were those developed for use with human pathogens, and veterinary laboratories routinely used these breakpoints for similar animal pathogens regardless of the host species. By the early 1980s, it had become apparent that the use of human interpretive criteria did not reliably predict clinical outcomes when applied to veterinary pathogens and antimicrobial agents. This led some authors to question the use of AST methods

[1]Veterinary Medicine Research and Development, Zoetis, Inc., Kalamazoo, MI 49009; [2]Kansas State Veterinary Diagnostic Laboratory, Manhattan, KS 66506.

in veterinary medicine, while other investigators attempted to develop veterinary-specific interpretive criteria (as reviewed in references 7, 14). It was apparent by the late 1980s that there was a need for the development of veterinary-specific AST methods and interpretive criteria.

In 1993, the Clinical and Laboratory Standards Institute (CLSI, formerly the National Committee for Clinical Laboratory Standards [NCCLS]) formed the Subcommittee on Veterinary Antimicrobial Susceptibility Testing (V-AST) with the task of developing veterinary-specific AST standards (9). This group decided that rather than attempt to address all uses of antimicrobial agents in veterinary medicine (such as growth promotion, prophylaxis, and extra-label usage), it would limit its efforts to therapeutic uses for systemic diseases. This allowed the V-AST to use experience gained from human pathogens for the development of veterinary-specific methods and interpretive criteria. The group also decided it would limit the development of interpretive criteria to the approved indication and pathogens for specific agents. At the time, this eliminated the problems associated with establishing interpretive criteria for extra-label antimicrobial uses and allowed the development of host/pathogen/antimicrobial-specific interpretive criteria (9, 13); however, this has become increasingly difficult recently as the V-AST has attempted to create international standards and guidelines because approved indications vary considerably by jurisdiction.

By 1999, the V-AST had published the first standard for the performance of ASTs with veterinary pathogens, M31 (now VET01), as well as the first guideline on the data requirements for interpretive criteria development, M37 (now VET02) (9, 10, 13). The first version of VET01 included a standardized test method for *H. somni* and *A. pleuropneumoniae* that utilized a common test medium, veterinary fastidious medium, as well as QC organisms for use when testing these organisms (9, 13). The document also included the first publication of veterinary-specific interpretive criteria for several veterinary-use-only antimicrobial agents such as ceftiofur and tilmicosin. The current version adds a standardized method for testing of *Campylobacter* spp. as well as veterinary-specific interpretive criteria for antimicrobial agents in each of the major antimicrobial classes (9). In addition to the sponsor-supported interpretive criteria, the V-AST formed a working group in 1998 to address the development of interpretive criteria for older, generic agents. Since its inception, the Generic Working Group has developed host-pathogen-specific interpretive criteria for several

generic compounds such as tetracycline and penicillin. The FDA-approved antimicrobial agents in the United States with veterinary-specific interpretive criteria are listed in the CLSI VET01 document. VET01 is the accepted worldwide standard for susceptibility testing of veterinary pathogens and is used by laboratories accredited by the American Association of Veterinary Laboratory Diagnosticians (9). Additionally, the V-AST has developed standards for the antimicrobial susceptibility testing of pathogens that cause diseases of fish and other aquatic animals and has developed guidelines for laboratories to use when testing infrequently encountered or unusual organisms (15, 16).

At present, there are only a few groups other than the CLSI that are developing standards for antimicrobial susceptibility testing of veterinary pathogens. In 1996, the European Society for Clinical Microbiology and Infectious Diseases established the European Committee on Antimicrobial Susceptibility Testing (EUCAST) to harmonize antimicrobial breakpoints across Europe (17, 18). Since its inception, EUCAST has addressed susceptibility testing of human pathogens, and clinical breakpoints have been harmonized for a large number of agents (19, 20). In 2014, EUCAST expanded into the antimicrobial susceptibility testing of veterinary pathogens with the formation of the VETCAST group (http://www.eucast.org/ast_of_veterinary_pathogens/). The VETCAST group has defined its responsibility for developing veterinary-specific testing and clinical breakpoints for new and generic agents exclusively in Europe. At present, VETCAST is developing its standards and operating processes for antimicrobial susceptibility testing of veterinary pathogens. Additionally, veterinary-specific methods and interpretive criteria have been developed for the calibrated dichotomous sensitivity method widely used in Australia (21).

AST METHODS

Antimicrobial susceptibility testing is performed when the antimicrobial susceptibility of a bacterial pathogen cannot be determined solely from its identification or if bacterial resistance is suspected due to poor clinical response (9). Bacterial pathogens from infected animals are normally cultured from clinical specimens (such as skin or lung tissue) using selective or nonselective growth media. However, only potential pathogens, not contaminants or normal bacterial flora, are selected for antimicrobial susceptibility testing, and the identification of any isolated bacterial pathogen may be determined using biochemical and/or automated methods. It is highly recommended that isolation and identification procedures be performed prior to *in vitro* antimicrobial susceptibility testing.

Veterinary diagnostic laboratories can select from several methodologies for antimicrobial susceptibility testing of veterinary pathogens, with most laboratories using the agar disk diffusion (ADD) method or the broth microdilution MIC method or both (10). To ensure the generation of accurate, reproducible results, laboratories should adhere to a standard, well-defined method that includes the appropriate QC information. The purpose of an AST method is not to mimic *in vivo* conditions but to provide reproducible results that can be correlated to clinical outcome. In the United States, the majority of veterinary laboratories use either a CLSI reference method or a commercial method that adheres to this standard (9, 12). The method a laboratory selects depends on a variety of factors, including the cost per test, the availability of appropriate antimicrobial agents (since veterinary-specific agents are not available in all test systems), and the volume of samples to be handled by the laboratory. In general, smaller laboratories with relatively low test volumes tend to prefer the ADD method, and larger laboratories prefer the more semiautomated MIC methods.

ADD Method

The ADD method remains a flexible, low-cost means of conducting antimicrobial susceptibility testing and is widely used in many veterinary laboratories. In general, appropriate agar plates are inoculated with a standardized concentration of a pure bacterial culture, to which antimicrobial-impregnated paper disks are then added to the test plate. The outcome of the assay is a "zone of inhibition," and although results are read to the nearest millimeter, the final results are reported categorically as susceptible, intermediate, or resistant to the antimicrobial agent of interest. If ADD test results are to be reliable, the methodology must be standardized and controlled as originally described (22), from which interpretive criteria (susceptible, intermediate, resistant) have been developed. Care must be taken when reading zones with hazy endpoints or the presence of small colonies within the larger defined zone of inhibition. Advantages of the ADD test include its lower material cost per test compared to other susceptibility test methods, flexibility in antimicrobial selection, and ease of setting up the assay. Disadvantages may include inherent test and user variabilities such as inoculum size used, measuring of zones, labor requirements, and stability of disks. Guidelines for proper media preparation and storage, as well as proper storage of antimicrobial susceptibility disks, are available for veterinary laboratories (9). The ADD zone diameters inversely correlate (larger zone is correlated to a lower MIC) with MIC values from a standard dilution test (usually from a broth microdilution method), and the CLSI provides the most up-to-date zone diameter (and MIC) interpretive criteria for clinical breakpoints (10).

Numerous veterinary-specific antimicrobial agents are commercially available in antimicrobial-impregnated disks used with the ADD method (9). However, certain veterinary-specific agents or infrequently tested disks may only be available from the pharmaceutical manufacturer. Additionally, smaller veterinary laboratories may have difficulties in standardizing the inoculum used in this method, but commercial systems are available for this purpose.

MIC Methods

A variety of MIC methods ranging from the agar dilution method to a commercially available gradient strip method, as well as semiautomated broth microdilution methods, are available for veterinary laboratories (9, 10). Both broth and agar dilution techniques can be used to quantitatively determine the *in vitro* activity of an antimicrobial agent against a bacterial culture of interest. In general, a standardized inoculum of a pure culture of the isolate of interest is added to a series of tubes, agar plates, or wells that contain a broth or agar medium with increasing concentrations of an antimicrobial agent based on a log2 scale (for example, 0.5 g/ml, 1.0 g/ml, 2.0 g/ml, etc.). Commercial microdilution systems are available that may contain dried or frozen antimicrobial agents in a dilution series, and appropriate QC tests should be performed for any method that is used. The MIC method provides a value that is expressed in micrograms per milliliter and allows categorization of the organism as susceptible, intermediate, or resistant based on available clinical breakpoints.

The techniques described are primarily for testing commonly isolated pathogens that grow well after overnight incubation when using Mueller-Hinton broth. However, Mueller-Hinton broth is not adequate to support the growth of many fastidious pathogens encountered in veterinary medicine. Media that are supplemented with additional growth factors such as yeast or lysed blood may adequately support growth of certain fastidious organisms. When an appropriate medium has been identified for use, QC procedures and interpretive criteria need to be established for testing that organism. Standardized methods for testing the more-fastidious organisms such as anaerobes and *Campylobacter* spp. have been developed for the MIC methodology (9, 10).

The MIC method is preferred for use in surveillance or epidemiological programs because it allows the calculation of quantitative summary statistics. Of the various MIC formats, the broth microdilution method is the most widely used. However, the primary disadvantage of the available systems is inflexibility in antimicrobial selection and dilution test ranges unless the laboratory is willing to bear the cost of custom panels. The number of dilutions tested in the MIC method may vary from laboratory to laboratory depending on the final use of the results. Laboratories involved in surveillance programs usually prefer to test a smaller number of antimicrobial agents over an extended number of drug dilutions, while many diagnostic laboratories choose to use a "clinical breakpoint" panel. These breakpoint panels allow the laboratory to test a larger number of compounds with more limited dilution ranges spanning the interpretive criteria or clinical breakpoint values for each antimicrobial agent. Care should be taken in selecting a breakpoint panel that has in-range values for at least one QC strain to allow for validation of test results.

Antimicrobial Combination (Checkerboard) Test Methods

Laboratories may want to understand the activity of antibiotic combinations on pathogens in specific situations, especially where a multidrug-resistant phenotype is exhibited by the pathogen. Although not considered a standardized technique, the checkerboard assay is an *in vitro* method that may be used to evaluate synergy, indifference, or antagonism between two antimicrobial agents when they are combined. Antimicrobial combinations are considered to be synergistic if the effect of the antimicrobial combination is greater than the effect of either agent alone or greater than the sum of the effects of the individual agents. Indifference is defined as a drug combination that has an effect equal to the effect of either agent alone, and antagonism is defined as a combination that has an effect less than the effect of either agent alone (23). In the checkerboard assay, one antimicrobial agent is added vertically at 2-fold dilutions to a 96-well plate while another agent is added horizontally to produce a "checkerboard" of various combined drug concentrations (Fig. 1). The outcome of the checkerboard assay is the fractional inhibitory concentration (FIC). FIC values are determined by identifying the MIC values for each drug alone, as well as the lowest MIC of the drugs in combination (Fig. 1). FICs can be determined by the following formula:

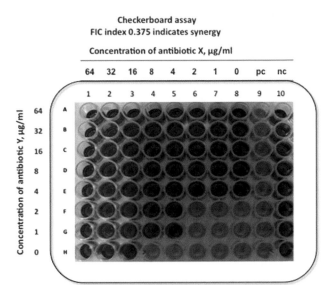

Figure 1 Example of a checkerboard plate setup that shows a synergistic reaction between two combined antibiotics (http://www.ibg.kit.edu/nmr/548.php).

$$\text{(MIC of drug X in combination/}$$
$$\text{MIC of drug X alone)}$$
$$+ \text{(MIC of drug Y in combination/}$$
$$\text{MIC of drug Y alone)}$$

An FIC value that is ≤0.5 is considered to be synergistic, while values of >4.0 would be considered antagonistic (23).

Although checkerboard assays are laborious and time-consuming, this method is valuable in understanding the potential effect of two drugs when administered closely together to help avoid interference from either drug (24). Additionally, this method is helpful when determining if synergistic activity of combination therapy would be expected in the therapy of drug-resistant pathogens. Synergism and antagonism may be drug-pathogen specific, so test results should be considered case by case, and it should be noted that most tests will result in indifference instead of synergism or antagonism for the majority of drug-pathogen combinations. Any evidence of synergy or antagonism based on the checkerboard method should be confirmed by time-kill studies with the combined agents, followed by animal and clinical studies to establish whether combination therapy is a truly effective option for treatment.

QC and Test Standardization

Regardless of the susceptibility test method that is selected, the routine administration of QC testing is an essential component of AST. The routine testing of QC strains allows the veterinary laboratory to verify that personnel, incubation conditions, test media, and antimicrobial agents are performing at an acceptable, standardized level. Numerous QC strains have been defined by various standards organizations for use in their systems (17, 25, 26). Any QC ranges should be developed using a multilaboratory study that examines both inter- and intralaboratory reproducibility such as those defined by the CLSI (9, 10) or by using an external quality assurance system (25). The overall performance of the susceptibility test system should be monitored using those ranges listed by testing the appropriate control strains each day (or week) the test is performed. The interval at which QC strains are tested varies among laboratories. While inclusion of QC strains on each day of testing is preferred, this may be too costly and time-consuming for smaller veterinary laboratories, and these laboratories may choose to run these QC strains on a weekly basis or less often. A procedure for conversion from daily to weekly QC testing is described in document VET01 (9).

REPORTING OF AST RESULTS

The overall goal of AST is to assist the clinician with antimicrobial selection; therefore, a primary responsibility of the veterinary laboratory is to select the most appropriate agents for routine testing and reporting. Reporting AST results for veterinary pathogens is more complicated than for human pathogens due to the differences in approved antimicrobial agents and approved interpretive criteria for the various animal host species. For this reason, most veterinary laboratories have predefined panels of compounds specifically used for testing pathogens from specific hosts or specific disease indications. This may include a specific panel for testing bovine/porcine pathogens, a bovine mastitis panel, an equine panel, or a companion animal (canine/feline) panel. In addition to species-specific drug panels, there are separate Gram-negative and Gram-positive panels for both diagnostic and surveillance purposes.

The veterinary laboratory should not report specific antibacterial agents in certain host animals, and the reporting of agents that do not have specific approvals in a host species (termed "extra-label use" in the United States) should only be done with extreme care after consultation with a veterinarian. Extra-label use is defined as an antimicrobial agent used in any manner not specifically listed on the drug packaging and may include use in a different animal species; for treatment of a different disease; at a different dose, route, or frequency of administration; or with a different withdrawal time (27). For example, federal regulations in the United States prohibit the extra-label use of chloramphenicol, fluoroquinolones and glycopeptides in food-producing animals, and AST results for these agents should not be reported when a clear extra-label use situation exists (28). However, the individual laboratory must make decisions to report antimicrobial results for certain antimicrobials, such as aminoglycosides in cattle. This antimicrobial is not strictly prohibited from use in cattle and may be used at the discretion of a practicing veterinarian; however, this use requires a significantly extended withdrawal time, and bovine practitioners in the United States have therefore adopted a voluntary "no use" policy (29). Similar types of regulations exist for regions outside of the United States, and in some countries the restrictions on extra-label use are even more stringent. Antimicrobial products in the European Union with formularies and drug classes that are deemed critically important for human health may therefore be ranked accordingly for first-line, second-line, or third-line use in animals and should be reported accordingly by diagnostic laboratories in those jurisdictions.

Preference in reporting should be given to those agents with veterinary-specific interpretive criteria for the host-pathogen combination being tested, because these are the most clinically relevant values (Table 1). The use of clinical breakpoints developed for a specific disease in one host species for categorizing isolates from another host species as susceptible or resistant may not accurately predict clinical outcome and should be minimized whenever possible. If agents are to be reported using interpretive criteria developed for other animal species or humans, then this should be indicated to the veterinarian. For example, if a *Pasteurella multocida* isolate from a case of bovine respiratory disease is tested against tetracyclines, it is inappropriate to report this isolate as susceptible based on swine breakpoints for this drug-pathogen combination; rather, it should be reported based on the interpretive criteria for the bovine breakpoint. In this example, a *P. multocida* isolate with a MIC of 2 g/ml would be considered resistant for swine respiratory disease but susceptible for bovine respiratory disease. While each laboratory bears the responsibility for developing specific reporting cascades for the various host animals and pathogens to be tested, most veterinary microbiology laboratories use the information provided in Table 1 of CLSI document VET01 as a guideline for selecting antimicrobial agents that could be considered for routine testing (9). It is preferred to test and report those antimicrobial agents that have veterinary-specific interpretive criteria (called

Table 1 Summary of antimicrobial agents with veterinary-specific interpretive criteria[a]

Antimicrobial agent	Host species with approved interpretive criteria
Amikacin	Dogs, horses
Amoxicillin-clavulanate	Dogs, cats
Ampicillin	Dogs, horses, swine
Cephalothin	Dogs
Cefazolin	Dogs, horses
Cefpodoxime	Dogs
Ceftiofur	Horses, swine cattle, bovine mastitis
Chloramphenicol	Dogs
Clindamycin	Dogs
Danofloxacin	Cattle
Difloxacin	Dogs
Doxycycline	Dogs
Enrofloxacin	Dogs, cats, cattle, chickens, turkeys
Florfenicol	Swine, cattle
Gamithromycin	Cattle
Gentamicin	Dogs, horses
Marbofloxacin	Dogs, cats
Orbifloxacin	Dogs, cats
Penicillin	Dogs, horses, swine, cattle
Penicillin-novobiocin	Bovine mastitis
Pirlimycin	Bovine mastitis
Pradofloxacin	Dogs, cats
Spectinomycin	Cattle
Tetracycline	Dogs, swine, cattle
Tilmicosin	Swine, cattle
Tiamulin	Swine
Tildipirosin	Swine, cattle
Tulathromycin	Swine, cattle

[a]From reference 10.

group A agents) over those antimicrobial agents that use human interpretive criteria (group B) since the relationship from human to veterinary application has not been demonstrated. Antimicrobial agents that have neither veterinary-specific nor human-specific CLSI-approved interpretive criteria (group C) should be selectively reported due to differences in dosage and pharmacokinetics, and those agents listed in group D should be selectively tested and selectively reported. Reporting in this manner allows the clinician to evaluate the clinical relevance (or lack thereof) of the test results.

Cumulative AST Data

The preferred method for reporting cumulative MIC results is to report all data in a frequency distribution table or graph, because this allows the user to understand the activity of a specific agent against a given population of target organisms. Only a single bacterial species should be used to understand the activity of a particular antibiotic, and the laboratory should not combine distributions from different bacterial species. When large numbers of antibacterial agents and pathogens need to be reported in a succinct manner, summary statistics are often the most practical method for reporting MIC data (4). The most common summary statistics would include total number of isolates, MIC_{50} (the MIC at which 50% of the isolates are inhibited), MIC_{90} (the MIC at which 90% of the isolates are inhibited), and the MIC test range. These are based on populations of bacterial isolates and are not the concentration of antimicrobial that inhibits 50% or 90% of the growth from a single culture. A minimum of 10 isolates, but ideally at least 50 isolates, should be used and tested to calculate MIC_{50}, MIC_{90}, and MIC range values from the population of isolates used. Only on-scale dilution values should be reported, and the MIC_{50} and MIC_{90} values may be indicated when MIC distribution data are presented (http://aac.asm.org/site/misc/ifora.xhtml). If data for a single interpretive category are to be summarized, the percent susceptible is preferred because it avoids the issue of handling the intermediate and resistant categories. Additional analyses can be performed, but direct comparison of MIC data across antimicrobial classes should not be done due to potential differences in the relative *in vitro* activity of these two classes on a per-weight basis and differences in the dosing and pharmacokinetics of the two antimicrobials. For example, if ceftiofur has an MIC_{90} of ≤0.06 g/ml for *Mannheimia haemolytica*, compared to an MIC_{90} of 16.0 g/ml for tulathromycin, the efficacy of these two compounds may still be comparable (because both values are below the susceptible breakpoints for each drug) when used to treat bovine respiratory disease. When summary comparisons between antimicrobials are made, it is more appropriate to use the percent-susceptible data.

Class Testing

Veterinary diagnostic laboratories may report AST results for a particular antimicrobial agent within an antibiotic class to predict the susceptibility of other agents within the same class, and this is often referred to as "class testing." The CLSI has recommended the use of certain antimicrobial agents to predict antimicrobial susceptibility to multiple agents within the same class as a means of increasing testing efficiencies in diagnostic laboratories (9). For example, ampicillin, tetracycline, and clindamycin are routinely tested as the representatives for their respective antimicrobial classes. In contrast, there are significant differences in the activity of other antimicrobial agents within a class in which class testing cannot be performed. Such is the case when using the veterinary macrolide tilmicosin as the class representative for tulathromycin and other veterinary macrolides. In this example, no information is available that supports the use of tilmicosin as the class representative for other veterinary macrolides since veterinary macrolides have different substituted ring structures, as well as different *in vitro* and *in vivo* properties with regard to MIC activity, dosage regimen, and pharmacokinetics. Additionally, there is evidence that the presence of different macrolide resistance genes has a differential effect on the MICs of drugs in this class (30). Therefore, any susceptibility results for tilmicosin to predict the activity and potential treatment outcome for tulathromycin, gamithromycin, or tildipirosin is strongly discouraged due to the unique attributes of each antibiotic.

ESTABLISHMENT OF VETERINARY-SPECIFIC INTERPRETIVE CRITERIA

The methodology for establishing veterinary interpretive criteria can be found in the most current version of CLSI document VET02 (10). In establishing veterinary-specific interpretive criteria, the CLSI V-AST committee evaluates a tripartite database: MIC distribution data, pharmacokinetic/pharmacodynamic (PK/PD) data, and clinical outcome data (10).

MIC Distribution Data

In general, bacteria that possess a genetic resistance element will have increased MICs relative to bacteria without that same resistance mechanism. By plotting a MIC distribution (histogram) for a single bacterial species-antimicrobial combination, the bacterial population can be divided into two groups: (i) bacteria with low MIC values for that antimicrobial that likely do not possess a resistance mechanism, also known as the wild-type population, and (ii) bacteria with high MIC values indicating the presence of an antimicrobial resistance mechanism, the non-wild-type population. The terms "low MIC values" and "high MIC values" are not absolute values but are relative and based on the specific bacteria-antimicrobial combination. For example, a low MIC for a population of *M. haemolytica* isolates to danofloxacin would be ≤0.25 g/ml, while a low MIC for the same population of isolates to tulathromycin would be ≤16 g/ml.

For some antimicrobial-pathogen combinations, a bimodal MIC distribution may not exist, and determination of a distinct non-wild-type population is not possible. This is most often found in cases where specific resistance mechanisms are rare in that particular bacterial species. In these cases, the CLSI and V-AST may only delineate a "susceptible" category. If a laboratory isolate test result is "nonsusceptible," the identity of the organism and antimicrobial susceptibility should be reconfirmed. For example, ampicillin has only a "susceptible" category for β-hemolytic streptococci, as does danofloxacin for *M. haemolytica* and *P. multocida*, although in the latter case, the "intermediate" and "resistant" categories were recently added based on new data demonstrating a resistant subpopulation (31).

It is also worth noting that in some instances, rather than a clear distinction between wild-type and non-wild-type populations, a particular resistance mechanism will cause small incremental increases in the MIC, leading to a less distinct division of the population.

Because the MIC distribution data (and the subsequent interpretive criteria on which it is built) are based on a specific pathogen-antimicrobial combination, attempts to extrapolate interpretive criteria to a different pathogen or antimicrobial should not be done for reasons further discussed below.

PK/PD Data

Evaluating only the *in vitro* microbiological response to an antimicrobial ignores the role of the animal host, so interpretive criteria must also consider some of the animal host factors that impact disease outcome. Considering that the total effect of an antimicrobial in treating an infection is a reflection of how the antimicrobial is absorbed by the animal following administration, distributed to the site of infection, metabolized (this can increase or decrease the antimicrobial's activity) by the animal, and finally eliminated from the animal, it seems intuitive that pharmacokinetics would be part of establishing veterinary interpretive criteria. The effect of the antimicrobial on the bacterial pathogen is the pharmacodynamic response of interest (Table 2). Together, the host animal contribution to the change in drug exposure and the bacterial response over time becomes the PK/PD relationship and is generally categorized as either the time that antimicrobial concentrations in the plasma are greater than the MIC of the infecting pathogen ($fT > MIC$), the ratio of the total antimicrobial exposure (expressed as the area under the drug plasma concentration curve) to the MIC of the infecting pathogen ($fAUC/MIC$), or the ratio of peak drug plasma concentrations to the MIC of the infecting pathogen ($fCmax/MIC$). The PK/PD index associated with veterinary antimicrobial classes can be found in Table 3 (32–40).

Table 2 Definitions of pharmacodynamic parameters

Time above MIC ($fT > MIC$)
Antimicrobial activity is based on the time that the active (non-protein bound) concentration of the drug is above the MIC of the infecting bacterium.
Area under the curve to MIC ratio ($fAUC/MIC$)
Activity for antimicrobials associated with this PK/PD index is based on the total exposure, as measured by the area under the drug plasma concentration curve (pharmacokinetic profile) of active (non-protein bound) antimicrobial in relation to the MIC of the infecting bacterium.
Peak plasma concentration to MIC ratio (Cmax/MIC)
Some antimicrobials have activity based on the ratio of the peak plasma concentration of active (non-protein bound) antimicrobial to the MIC of the infecting bacterium.

During the breakpoint development process, a statistical process known as Monte Carlo simulation is used to capture the variation in host animal pharmacokinetics (41). In doing so, an interpretive category is based not on the average plasma concentrations of an antimicrobial for that animal species, but rather on the concentrations that will likely be achieved by 90% of animals in the population treated with that particular antimicrobial dosing regimen.

Clinical Outcome Data

The third and final piece of data used to establish veterinary interpretive criteria comes from clinical studies in which animals affected with the particular disease and infecting pathogen are treated with the specific antimicrobial and dosing regimen. Clinical outcomes are compared to the MIC distribution of isolates from that study. Generally, clinical response will be good at low MIC values (again, low is relative to the antimicrobial-pathogen combination) and will decrease as MIC values increase. Clinical outcome data in support of interpretive criteria are usually based on a small number of animals (and isolates); therefore, these data generally become supportive in nature to the more robust microbiological distribution and PK/PD data. As with microbiological distribution and PK/PD data, clinical outcome data similarly constrain the ability to extrapolate interpretive criteria to other situations, for example, other disease conditions, caused by other pathogens, in different host species (classes), treated with different dosing regimens.

Table 3 Mechanism of action and associated pharmacokinetic/pharmacodynamics (PK/PD) indices of antimicrobial agents used in veterinary medicine

Antimicrobial class	Representative antimicrobials	Mechanism of action	PK/PD index associated with activity	Reference for PK/PD
Macrolides/azalides/ lincosamides/ketolides	Erythromycin, clarithromycin Azithromycin Clindamycin Telithromycin	Protein synthesis inhibitor	AUC/MIC	37
Beta-lactams	Penicillins, cephalosporins, carbapenems	Cell wall synthesis inhibitor	Time > MIC	38
Glycopeptides	Vancomycin	Cell wall synthesis inhibitor	Time > MIC, Cmax/MIC	39
Fluoroquinolones	Enrofloxacin, danofloxacin, marbofloxacin, pradofloxacin	DNA replication/transcription inhibitor	AUC/MIC Cmax/MIC	40 36
Aminoglycosides	Gentamicin, amikacin, neomycin, spectinomycin	Protein synthesis inhibitor	Cmax/MIC	41
Tetracyclines	Oxytetracycline, chlortetracycline, doxycycline, minocycline	Protein synthesis inhibitor	Time > MIC	42
Phenicols	Florfenicol, chloramphenicol	Protein synthesis inhibitor		
Trimethoprim		Folic acid synthesis inhibitor		
Sulfonamides	Sulfadimethoxine, sulfamethazine	Folic acid synthesis inhibitor		
Oxazolidinones	Linezolid Novobiocin	Protein synthesis inhibitor Exact mechanism unknown; proposed mechanisms include: Cell wall synthesis inhibitor Nucleic acid synthesis inhibitor Protein synthesis inhibitor	AUC/MIC	43

Re-Evaluation of Clinical Breakpoints

Over time, breakpoints may need to be revised due to the emergence of new bacterial resistance mechanisms and subsequent changes in clinical response rates. In human medicine, case reports/case series documenting clinical failures and description of the resistance mechanism may initiate revision of a clinical breakpoint; however, there is no formal timeline in place for re-evaluation of veterinary breakpoints (42–44). In veterinary medicine, breakpoint revision could be considered by the CLSI V-AST upon presentation of microbiological, PK/PD, and clinical cutoff data; however, there seems to be a significant communication gap between clinicians, diagnostic laboratories, and the V-AST subcommittee that would signal the need for breakpoint revision. Closing this gap should be considered a priority if breakpoints are to maintain their clinical relevance.

ROLE OF AST FOR CLINICAL OUTCOME

The role of AST in managing patients was best summarized by Doern et al. (45) with the statement "Susceptibility testing is not done in a vacuum." Microbiology laboratories often go to great lengths to ensure standardization and repeatability of the methods they use. While this is an extremely important aspect of AST, laboratories need to recognize that the utility of AST for the clinician is predicated on two important factors: the test must be timely enough to be clinically useful, and the test must have predictive value. Provided that these criteria are met, AST becomes a powerful tool in the judicious selection of antimicrobial therapy.

Testing Timing

Broth dilution and disk diffusion susceptibility testing of most veterinary pathogens requires a minimum of 36 hours from specimen submission to AST result: approximately 18 hours of incubation for the initial culture and 18 hours to perform the actual AST. Specimen transport, mixed cultures, and contaminant growth and slow-growing organisms can add significantly to the testing turnaround time. Direct susceptibility testing of clinical specimens has been reported to reduce turnaround time and in studies evaluating its use for urine and blood culture was nearly equivalent to the standardized method; however, because this is a nonstandard method, results should be reported as preliminary and confirmed with the standard method (46). The primary disadvantage to direct testing of clinical specimens is that the purity of the culture and bacterial inoculum cannot be controlled. Testing bacterial inocula above 5 × 10⁵ CFU/ml has been reported to lead to an increase

in MIC values (47, 48), which could lead to a false-resistant test result and lead the clinician to rule out the use of an appropriate antimicrobial, perhaps encouraging the use of a more advanced or more toxic antimicrobial, while testing a lower bacterial inoculum could lead to a false-susceptible result and the use of an antimicrobial that would be clinically inappropriate for that infection. Alternative AST methods with the potential to reduce the turnaround time associated with testing are currently being investigated. A brief discussion of these methods can be found at the end of this chapter under "Future Directions and Trends."

Correlation of AST Results with Clinical Outcome

While cost and turnaround time certainly influence the decision to pursue diagnostic testing, the primary benefit, or limitation, of culture and susceptibility testing rests on the predictive ability of the test. The "90-60 rule" has been used to summarize the predictive value of AST: infections due to susceptible isolates will respond approximately 90% of the time, while infections due to resistant isolates will respond approximately 60% of the time (49). The actual evidence for and against the predictive value of AST is quite sparse and often contradictory. The predictive value of AST for predicting therapeutic outcomes for mastitis in dairy cows was reviewed by Constable and Morin (50), who "do not currently recommend the use of susceptibility testing to guide treatment decisions for individual cows," despite reporting several studies that did, indeed, demonstrate statistically significant associations between AST and therapeutic outcomes. Conversely, a review by Barlow (51), which evaluated many of the same references as the review by Constable and Morin, reported that many of these studies had limited statistical power due to high rates of spontaneous bacteriological cure and low proportions of resistant isolates. The Barlow review highlighted the need for "unbiased randomized clinical trials with sufficient sample size" to evaluate the correlation between AST and clinical outcomes for mastitis therapy.

In a publication by McClary et al. (52), the authors also did not demonstrate a correlation between AST and bovine respiratory disease treatment response. However, as with the mastitis studies, this study also reported a low proportion of resistant isolates (6/745 for *M. haemolytica*; 16/231 for *P. multocida*). Additionally, in this study, the authors used bacterial isolates obtained by deep nasopharyngeal swab to measure the pretreatment MIC values. This may have impacted the correlation of AST result to clinical outcome, because it has been demonstrated in several studies that bacterial pathogens from the upper respiratory tract may be different from those cultured from the lower respiratory tract of bovine respiratory disease-affected calves (53–55).

Reports from the human medical experience are also not definitive. Studies have been reported that demonstrate clear statistical associations between AST result and clinical outcome (56–58). Some reports have highlighted situations where the categorical interpretation (susceptible, intermediate, resistant) does not accurately predict clinical outcome, but an association between increasing MIC values and worsening of patient outcomes occurs; many of these papers call for revision of the established breakpoints (42, 59–61). Other studies fail to demonstrate any relationship at all between the *in vitro* result and the patient outcome (62, 63).

It is important for readers to understand that all veterinary-specific breakpoints have been evaluated for correlation to clinical outcome through the breakpoint development process. Through an expert consensus process, over 90 antimicrobial, pathogen, and host species combinations have been approved to provide guidance to clinical decision-making.

While even staunch proponents of AST will readily admit that an *in vitro* test cannot fully account for all the variables within an individual animal that will ultimately impact clinical outcome, the clinician needs to know, "Is there value in the test?". Our contention is that AST has value in the antimicrobial selection process. Therefore, what are the factors/considerations that potentially increase or decrease the relationship between the *in vitro* result and the clinical outcome?

Factors Impacting the Relationship Between *In Vitro* Result and Clinical Outcomes

Laboratory factors
Assuming that a standardized susceptibility test method is being utilized, one of the most important factors that can potentially affect the *in vitro-in vivo* relationship is selecting the right isolate, that is, the isolate responsible for clinical disease, for susceptibility testing. Both the clinician collecting the specimen and the laboratory microbiologist can have a profound impact on selecting the right isolate. The veterinary clinician has the responsibility to submit samples that limit normal flora/contaminant growth and are representative of the disease process in that individual or group of animals. For example, selecting the right isolate for AST when an *E. coli* isolate is recovered from a cystocentesis sample from a canine patient showing clinical signs of a urinary tract infection that then grows in pure culture

in the laboratory would be a relatively straightforward process. The selection of the right isolate becomes less clear if the *E. coli* is recovered from a mixed culture and the sample was collected by free catch in a patient showing signs of polyuria. In the latter case, the *E. coli* could be a primary urinary tract infection pathogen, or it could be a contaminant that results in antimicrobial treatment when none was indicated and misdiagnosis of the underlying disease condition.

In the laboratory, the microbiologist will generally select a single CFU from the original culture to perform AST. The degree to which this impacts the *in vitro-in vivo* relationship is generally dependent on the degree to which there are mixed-strain infections (64).

Extrapolating breakpoints
Clinical interpretive categories are designed to predict the contribution of the antimicrobial to therapeutic success (or failure) (65). This correlation is imperfect, at best, at the individual patient level but does allow the clinician to evaluate the relative odds for success in a population of patients (66, 67). Because a clinical interpretive criterion is designed for a specific bacterial species-antimicrobial-host species-disease process-dosing regimen combination, extrapolation of any of those factors would potentially affect the predictive value of the test result. While in most situations this would seem intuitive, i.e., a clinical interpretive category for *S. aureus* may or may not apply to *M. haemolytica*, oftentimes, the clinician may not be aware of which host species-disease process-dosing regimen was used to determine the "S"/"I"/"R" on the report. Clinical microbiology laboratories should be encouraged to make this more transparent on reports.

Host factors
An *in vitro* AST will not account for all of the factors that ultimately lead to clinical outcome in a patient. The test is not intended to mimic the disease process in an animal, but rather to provide a result that can provide the clinician with an expectation of the biology of the specific pathogen and what the drug can (or cannot) contribute to clinical outcome. In cases where the immune function contributes significantly to disease outcome, the predictive value of AST will be reduced.

ROLE OF SURVEILLANCE AND ANTIMICROBIAL STEWARDSHIP
Surveillance is defined as the continuous collection of data to understand the prevalence of antimicrobial-resistant bacteria, while monitoring is defined as the

routine measurement and analysis of antimicrobial susceptibility testing information to detect trends (60, 68, 69). Data generated from surveillance and monitoring studies can be used to detect the emergence of antimicrobial-resistant phenotypes, to understand any trends for reduced susceptibility to a certain antimicrobial agent, to determine mechanisms of resistance in bacteria, and to provide information for prudent use recommendations. Surveillance and monitoring programs are one component in providing an overall framework or plan of action for antimicrobial stewardship and the judicious use of antibacterial agents.

Numerous government and industry-sponsored veterinary surveillance programs already exist, and particular thought should given to designing and implementing a veterinary surveillance program. Components related to sampling strategies such as deciding on active or passive surveillance, which animal species to sample, which bacterial organisms from what body sites should be selected, and the species of bacteria to be collected (animal bacterial target pathogens, zoonotic, and/or commensal bacteria), as well as the maximum number of isolates per geographical location or disease outbreak, are just a few key considerations to help address the defined objective of any long-term surveillance study. Additionally, selecting the most appropriate antimicrobial agents for testing, the type of AST method used, the standardized testing method and appropriate QC, and reporting and analysis of data should be well thought out prior to program initiation (70).

The proper design and methodology of any surveillance program helps to address the biggest challenge for cross-comparison of surveillance studies, which is harmonization. Therefore, comparing surveillance data across programs may be difficult since each surveillance study may not be measuring the same parameter. This is especially true for surveillance programs that use epidemiological cutoff values (ECVs) rather than clinical breakpoints or breakpoints from different host species to determine bacterial resistance (65). CLSI document VET05 offers guidance on areas in which harmonization can be achieved in veterinary antimicrobial surveillance programs (65).

Judicious antimicrobial use is the attempt to both maximize therapeutic efficacy and minimize the selection of resistant microorganisms (71), and antimicrobial stewardship is defined as a coordinated program that promotes the appropriate use of antimicrobials, improves patient outcomes, reduces microbial resistance, and decreases the spread of infections caused by multidrug-resistant organisms (http://www.apic.org/Professional-Practice/Practice-Resources/Antimicrobial-Stewardship). As concern about antimicrobial resistance in human and veterinary pathogens has increased, so has the number of surveillance and monitoring activities in government, academic, and industry settings which have led to improved judicious use and stewardship of antimicrobial agents. The most recent example in the United States centers on The President's Council of Advisors on Science and Technology (PCAST), which released a report in 2014 recommending steps the federal government can take to combat antibiotic resistance. The PCAST report includes action steps for human health care, animal agriculture, drug development, and surveillance, with the goal of preventing infections, improving surveillance, encouraging appropriate use of antibiotics in people and animals, and developing new antimicrobial drugs (https://obamawhitehouse.archives.gov/sites/default/files/microsites/ostp/PCAST/pcast_carb_report_sept2014.pdf).

EPIDEMIOLOGIC CUT-OFF VALUES

Veterinary diagnosticians and practitioners will be most familiar with using standardized AST methods and clinical breakpoints to guide the treatment of individual veterinary patients. However, another important use of AST is in the area of antimicrobial resistance surveillance. While the testing methodology is exactly the same for both clinical diagnostics and antimicrobial resistance surveillance, the overall goal and intended use of test results are slightly different. Where the goal of clinical diagnostics is to predict therapeutic outcome in a patient (or group of patients in production settings) and the test result is an interpretive category, the goal of surveillance is to detect new and emerging antimicrobial resistance mechanisms within a population of bacteria as soon as possible, and the test result is an epidemiological cutoff value, also known as an ECV or ECOFF. As such, clinical breakpoints and ECVs should not be used interchangeably (72). ECVs are determined through evaluation of the distribution of MICs, very similar to the process of evaluating MIC distributions to establish a clinical interpretive criteria (73, 74). However, ECVs only separate the microbial populations into wild-type and non-wild-type categories based on the presence or absence of resistance mechanisms. Thus, ECVs do not consider PK/PD data or clinical outcome data and are often set lower than the "susceptible" clinical interpretive criteria, again, to facilitate detection of emerging antimicrobial resistance within a population of bacterial isolates as early as possible. A comparison of ECVs and clinical breakpoints is provided in Fig. 2.

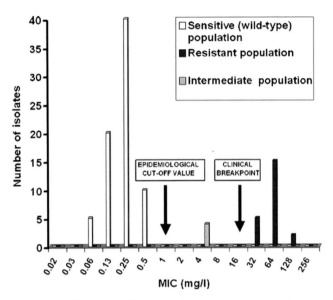

Figure 2 Illustrated differences between an epidemiological cutoff value and a clinical breakpoint (67).

FUTURE DIRECTIONS AND TRENDS

Much progress has been made in the past decade in the development of veterinary-specific testing methods and interpretive criteria. Test methods for additional veterinary pathogens including mycoplasma species commonly encountered in veterinary medicine, such as *Mycobacterium bovis*, need to be developed. A test method for susceptibility testing of *Haemophilus parasuis* has been published recently (73). The development of veterinary-specific interpretive criteria for older, generic agents has increased greatly over the past 10 years, but much work still remains in which additional clinical breakpoints for these older drugs are often used in veterinary surveillance and monitoring programs. At present, standardized methods for susceptibility testing of *Campylobacter* spp. and *Arcobacter butzleri* have been developed, but no interpretive criteria for these organisms or other enteric pathogens are available (75). The standardization of test methods for *Campylobacter* spp. has been particularly beneficial to monitoring programs such as the National Antimicrobial Resistance Monitoring System. Additionally, the relevance of AST results to antimicrobial agents used in control (prophylaxis) or growth promotion has not been established. The continued development of veterinary-specific interpretive criteria will play an increasingly important role in the prudent use of antimicrobial agents, and the pharmaceutical industry must be encouraged to participate in this process. While much of the interpretive criteria to date have been developed by CLSI for agents approved in the United States, this work needs to be ex-

panded to include agents approved in Europe and elsewhere. As other organizations such as EUCAST and the World Organisation for Animal Health begin to address veterinary AST methods and interpretive criteria, the need for collaboration and harmonization among the various standards organizations will become critical.

Alternative test methodologies to traditional phenotypic AST have been evaluated with the primary goal of increasing the speed at which test results are delivered to the clinician, and these have been discussed in detail elsewhere (76). Those methodologies that are currently used in a limited capacity or hold the most potential for future adoption are PCR, matrix-assisted laser desorption ionization–time of flight (MALDI-TOF), and next-generation sequencing. The utility and limitations of these three methods are briefly discussed here. Currently, PCR testing is being used primarily as an adjunct method to phenotypic susceptibility testing. In this manner, PCR is used to confirm the presence of a specific resistance gene, such as the *mecA* gene that confers resistance to beta-lactamase stable penicillins in *S. aureus*. As a primary testing method, PCR can be performed more rapidly than MIC or disk diffusion testing because it does not require overnight incubation. Use of PCR can decrease the turnaround time for clinicians compared to traditional AST methods (77). However, the primary limitations of PCR are that the "target" gene must be known—a challenging proposition for new, emerging, or rare resistance mechanisms—and the presence of a gene may not accurately predict activity of the genetic element.

MALDI-TOF mass spectrometry has also been recently evaluated as a method to improve the turnaround time associated with bacterial identification. There are three primary methods for determining antimicrobial susceptibility using MALDI-TOF. When bacterial isolates are incubated in the presence of the antimicrobial, MALDI-TOF can be used to measure antimicrobial breakdown products from bacterial enzyme hydrolysis (78). MALDI-TOF has also been used in combination with a PCR amplification step to detect resistance elements and to measure the protein spectral changes that occur with antimicrobial exposure, although the latter use has primarily focused on fungi (79, 80). While the use of MALDI-TOF as an AST method requires further comparison to current reference methods, the technology holds promise since many laboratories currently have the instrumentation because they are using this equipment for bacterial identification.

Yet another technology that is being evaluated for antimicrobial susceptibility testing is whole-genome sequencing (WGS). Its role is more limited at this time, but it has the potential to be transformative for the veterinary diagnostic laboratory, especially for susceptibility testing of bacterial species that are difficult to culture. One challenge for WGS will be its cost compared to phenotypic testing, which is relatively inexpensive. However, the cost of WGS seems to decrease yearly as the technology advances and becomes easier to perform. Additionally, speed, accuracy, and resolution are improving, thereby potentially allowing this technology to compete with conventional techniques. A specific undertaking for WGS will be its ability to equal the sensitivity and robustness of phenotypic susceptibility testing due to the currently incomplete database information that links genotype to phenotype (81). If WGS can provide accurate results that are faster than the 18 to 24 hours required for standard disk or broth susceptibility testing, it could supplement phenotypic testing, which would still be necessary to detect any novel mechanisms of resistance, but could be used to quickly identify resistance for certain antibiotics where known drug-resistance genes are present before results from the currently used phenotypic AST methods become available (82). Other possible applications for WGS may include detecting multidrug-resistant veterinary and zoonotic pathogens as well as serving as a useful tool in the monitoring and spread of bacterial pathogens in epidemiological studies (76, 77).

Though not related to technologies, but rather to the need for improved responsible use of anti-infectives, another component of antimicrobial stewardship that will receive more attention in the future is the monitoring of actual antimicrobial usage. Because the need for harmonization in surveillance and monitoring programs continues to be challenging, there will also be a need for harmonization when recording and reporting on antimicrobial usage to more accurately understand the overall sales and consumption of antimicrobial agents in veterinary medicine and the associations between antimicrobial consumption, use, and resistance at the individual patient/herd level.

Citation. Watts JL, Sweeney MT, Lubbers BV. 2018. Antimicrobial susceptibility testing of bacteria of veterinary origin. Microbiol Spectrum 6(2): ARBA-0001-2017.

References

1. Michael GB, Freitag C, Wendlandt S, Eidam C, Feßler AT, Lopes GV, Kadlec K, Schwarz S. 2015. Emerging issues in antimicrobial resistance of bacteria from food-producing animals. *Future Microbiol* **10**:427–443.

2. Guardabassi L, Prescott JF. 2015. Antimicrobial stewardship in small animal veterinary practice: from theory to practice. *Vet Clin North Am Small Anim Pract* **45**:361–376, vii.

3. DeDonder KD, Harhay DM, Apley MD, Lubbers BV, Clawson ML, Schuller G, Harhay GP, White BJ, Larson RL, Capik SF, Riviere JE, Kalbfleisch T, Tessman RK. 2016. Observations on macrolide resistance and susceptibility testing performance in field isolates collected from clinical bovine respiratory disease cases. *Vet Microbiol* **192**:186–193.

4. Levy SB. 2001. Antibiotic resistance: consequences of inaction. *Clin Infect Dis* **33**(Suppl 3):S124–S129.

5. Phillips I, Casewell M, Cox T, De Groot B, Friis C, Jones R, Nightingale C, Preston R, Waddell J. 2004. Does the use of antibiotics in food animals pose a risk to human health? A critical review of published data. *J Antimicrob Chemother* **53**:28–52.

6. Seyfarth AM, Wegener HC, Frimodt-Møller N. 1997. Antimicrobial resistance in *Salmonella enterica* subsp. *enterica* serovar typhimurium from humans and production animals. *J Antimicrob Chemother* **40**:67–75.

7. Watts JL, Yancey RJ Jr. 1994. Identification of veterinary pathogens by use of commercial identification systems and new trends in antimicrobial susceptibility testing of veterinary pathogens. *Clin Microbiol Rev* **7**:346–356.

8. Ferraro MJ. 2001. Should we reevaluate antibiotic breakpoints? *Clin Infect Dis* **33**(Suppl 3):S227–S229.

9. Clinical and Laboratory Standards Institute (CLSI). 2013. Performance standards for antimicrobial disk and dilution susceptibility tests for bacteria isolated from animals; approved standard—4th ed. CLSI document VET01-A4. CLSI, Wayne, PA.

10. Clinical and Laboratory Standards Institute (CLSI). 2013. Development of *in vitro* susceptibility testing criteria and QC parameters for veterinary antimicrobial agents; approved guideline—3rd ed. CLSI document VET02-A3. CLSI, Wayne, PA.

11. Clinical and Laboratory Standards Institute (CLSI). 2015. Performance standards for antimicrobial disk and dilution susceptibility tests for bacteria isolated from animals—3rd ed. CLSI supplement VET01S. CLSI, Wayne, PA.

12. Turnidge JD, Ferraro MJ, Jorgensen JH. 2003. Susceptibility test methods: general considerations, p 1102–1107. *In* Murray PR, Baron EJ, Jorgensen JH, Pfaller MA, Yolken RH (ed), *Manual of Clinical Microbiology*, 8th ed. ASM Press, Washington, DC.

13. National Committee on Clinical Laboratory Standards. 2002. Performance standards for antimicrobial disk and dilution susceptibility tests for bacteria isolated from animals; approved standard—2nd ed. NCCLS document M31-A2, NCCLS, Wayne, PA.

14. Woolcock JB, Mutimer MD. 1983. Antibiotic susceptibility testing: caeci caecos ducentes? *Vet Rec* **113**:125–128.

15. Clinical and Laboratory Standards Institute (CLSI). 2013. Methods for broth dilution susceptibility testing of bacteria isolated from aquatic animals—2nd ed. CLSI document VET04-A2. CLSI, Wayne, PA.

16. Clinical and Laboratory Standards Institute (CLSI). 2017. Methods for Antimicrobial Susceptibility Testing of Infrequently Isolated or Fastidious Bacteria Isolated

from Animals - 1st ed. CLSI Supplement VET06. CLSI, Wayne PA.

17. European Committee for Antimicrobial Susceptibility Testing (EUCAST) of the European Society of Clinical Microbiology and Infectious Dieases (ESCMID). 2000. EUCAST definitive document E.DEF 3.1, June 2000: determination of minimum inhibitory concentrations (MICs) of antibacterial agents by agar dilution. *Clin Microbiol Infect* 6:509–515.

18. European Committee for Antimicrobial Susceptibility Testing (EUCAST) of the European Society of Clinical Microbiology and Infectious Diseases (ESCMID). 2000. EUCAST definitive document E.DEF 2.1, August 2000: determination of antimicrobial susceptibility test breakpoints. *Clin Microbiol Infect* 6:570–572.

19. Kahlmeter G, Brown DFJ, Goldstein FW, MacGowan AP, Mouton JW, Osterlund A, Rodloff A, Steinbakk M, Urbaskova P, Vatopoulos A. 2003. European harmonization of MIC breakpoints for antimicrobial susceptibility testing of bacteria. *J Antimicrob Chemother* 52:145–148.

20. Kahlmeter G, Brown D. 2004. Harmonisation of European breakpoints: can it be achieved. *Clin Microbiol Newsl* 26:187–192.

21. Bell SM, Gatus BJ, Pham JN, Rafferty DL. 2002. Antibiotic susceptibility testing by the CDS method. The Antibiotic Reference Laboratory, Department of Microbiology, The Prince of Wales Hospital, New South Wales, Australia.

22. Clinical and Laboratory Standards Institute (CLSI). 2014. Analysis and presentation of cumulative antimicrobial susceptibility test data; approved guideline—4th ed. CLSI document M39-A4. CLSI, Wayne, PA.

23. Sweeney MT, Zurenko GE. 2003. *In vitro* activities of linezolid combined with other antimicrobial agents against staphylococci, enterococci, pneumococci, and selected Gram-negative organisms. *Antimicrob Agents Chemother* 47:1902–1906.

24. Sweeney MT, Brumbaugh GW, Watts JL. 2008. *In vitro* activities of tulathromycin and ceftiofur combined with other antimicrobial agents using bovine *Pasteurella multocida* and *Mannheimia haemolytica* isolates. *Vet Therap* 9:212–222.

25. Aarestrup F. 2004. *Antibiotic Resistance in Bacteria of Animal Origin II: External Quality Assurance Systems*. Danish Inst. Food Vet. Res., Copenhagen, Denmark.

26. Andrews JM, BSAC Working Party on Susceptibility Testing. 2001. BSAC standardized disk susceptibility test method. *J Antimicrob Chemother* 48(suppl 1):S43–S57.

27. AVMF. Animal Medicinal Drug Use Clarification Act (AMDUCA). https://www.avma.org/KB/Resources/Reference/Pages/AMDUCA.aspx.

28. U.S. GPO. 2018. Electronic Code of Federal Regulations. http://www.ecfr.gov/cgi-bin/text-idx?SID=054808d261de27898e02fb175b7c9ff9&node=21:6.0.1.1.16&rgn=div5#21:6.0.1.1.16.2.1.2.

29. AVMA. AVMA policies. https://www.avma.org/KB/Policies/Pages/default.aspx.

30. Michael GB, Eidam C, Kadlec K, Meyer K, Sweeney MT, Murray RW, Watts JL, Schwarz S. 2012. Increased MICs of gamithromycin and tildipirosin in the presence of the genes erm(42) and msr(E)-mph(E) for bovine *Pasteurella multocida* and *Mannheimia haemolytica*. *J Antimicrob Chemother* 67:1555–1557.

31. Sweeney MT, Papich MG, Watts JL. 2017. New interpretive criteria for danofloxacin antibacterial susceptibility testing against Mannheimia haemolytica and Pasteurella multocida associated with bovine respiratory disease. *J. Vet. Diagn. Invest.* 29:224–227.

32. Forrest A, Nix DE, Ballow CH, Goss TF, Birmingham MC, Schentag JJ. 1993. Pharmacodynamics of intravenous ciprofloxacin in seriously ill patients. *Antimicrob Agents Chemother* 37:1073–1081.

33. Drusano GL, Johnson DE, Rosen M, Standiford HC. 1993. Pharmacodynamics of a fluoroquinolone antimicrobial agent in a neutropenic rat model of *Pseudomonas* sepsis. *Antimicrob Agents Chemother* 37:483–490.

34. Ambrose PG, Bhavnani SM, Rubino CM, Louie A, Gumbo T, Forrest A, Drusano GL. 2007. Pharmacokinetics-pharmacodynamics of antimicrobial therapy: it's not just for mice anymore. *Clin Infect Dis* 44:79–86.

35. Turnidge JD. 1998. The pharmacodynamics of beta-lactams. *Clin Infect Dis* 27:10–22.

36. Knudsen JD, Fuursted K, Espersen F, Frimodt-Møller N. 1997. Activities of vancomycin and teicoplanin against penicillin-resistant pneumococci *in vitro* and *in vivo* and correlation to pharmacokinetic parameters in the mouse peritonitis model. *Antimicrob Agents Chemother* 41:1910–1915.

37. Forrest A, Nix DE, Ballow CH, Goss TF, Birmingham MC, Schentag JJ. 1993. Pharmacodynamics of intravenous ciprofloxacin in seriously ill patients. *Antimicrob Agents Chemother* 37:1073–1081.

38. Blaser J, Stone BB, Groner MC, Zinner SH. 1987. Comparative study with enoxacin and netilmicin in a pharmacodynamic model to determine importance of ratio of antibiotic peak concentration to MIC for bactericidal activity and emergence of resistance. *Antimicrob Agents Chemother* 31:1054–1060.

39. van Ogtrop ML, Andes D, Stamstad TJ, Conklin B, Weiss WJ, Craig WA, Vesga O. 2000. *In vivo* pharmacodynamic activities of two glycylcyclines (GAR-936 and WAY 152,288) against various Gram-positive and Gram-negative bacteria. *Antimicrob Agents Chemother* 44:943–949.

40. Andes D, van Ogtrop ML, Peng J, Craig WA. 2002. *In vivo* pharmacodynamics of a new oxazolidinone (linezolid). *Antimicrob Agents Chemother* 46:3484–3489.

41. Rey JF, Laffont CM, Croubels S, De Backer P, Zemirline C, Bousquet E, Guyonnet J, Ferran AA, Bousquet-Melou A, Toutain PL. 2014. Use of Monte Carlo simulation to determine pharmacodynamic cutoffs of amoxicillin to establish a breakpoint for antimicrobial susceptibility testing in pigs. *Am J Vet Res* 75:124–131.

42. Shukla BS, Shelburne S, Reyes K, Kamboj M, Lewis JD, Rincon SL, Reyes J, Carvajal LP, Panesso D, Sifri CD, Zervos MJ, Pamer EG, Tran TT, Adachi J, Munita JM, Hasbun R, Arias CA. 2015. Influence of minimum inhib-

itory concentration in clinical outcomes of *Enterococcus faecium* bacteremia treated with daptomycin: is it time to change the breakpoint? *Clin Infect Dis.* 62:1514–1520.

43. Turnidge J, Paterson DL. 2007. Setting and revising antibacterial susceptibility breakpoints. *Clin Microbiol Rev* 20:391–408.

44. Turnidge JD, Subcommittee on Antimicrobial Susceptibility Testing of the Clinical and Laboratory Standards Institute. 2011. Cefazolin and *Enterobacteriaceae*: rationale for revised susceptibility testing breakpoints. *Clin Infect Dis* 52:917–924.

45. Doern GV, Brecher SM. 2011. The clinical predictive value (or lack thereof) of the results of *in vitro* antimicrobial susceptibility tests. *J Clin Microbiol* 49(Supplement):S11–S14.

46. Breteler KBK, Rentenaar RJ, Verkaart G, Sturm PDJ. 2011. Performance and clinical significance of direct antimicrobial susceptibility testing on urine from hospitalized patients. *Scand J Infect Dis* 43:771–776.

47. Egervärn M, Lindmark H, Roos S, Huys G, Lindgren S. 2007. Effects of inoculum size and incubation time on broth microdilution susceptibility testing of lactic acid bacteria. *Antimicrob Agents Chemother* 51:394–396.

48. Udekwu KI, Parrish N, Ankomah P, Baquero F, Levin BR. 2009. Functional relationship between bacterial cell density and the efficacy of antibiotics. *J Antimicrob Chemother* 63:745–757.

49. Rex JH, Pfaller MA. 2002. Has antifungal susceptibility testing come of age? *Clin Infect Dis* 35:982–989.

50. Constable PD, Morin DE. 2003. Treatment of clinical mastitis. Using antimicrobial susceptibility profiles for treatment decisions. *Vet Clin North Am Food Anim Pract* 19:139–155.

51. Barlow J. 2011. Mastitis therapy and antimicrobial susceptibility: a multispecies review with a focus on antibiotic treatment of mastitis in dairy cattle. *J Mammary Gland Biol Neoplasia* 16:383–407.

52. McClary DG, Loneragan GH, Shryock TR, Carter BL, Guthrie CA, Corbin MJ, Mechor GD. 2011. Relationship of *in vitro* minimum inhibitory concentrations of tilmicosin against *Mannheimia haemolytica* and *Pasteurella multocida* and *in vivo* tilmicosin treatment outcome among calves with signs of bovine respiratory disease. *J Am Vet Med Assoc* 239:129–135.

53. Allen JW, Viel L, Bateman KG, Rosendal S, Shewen PE, Physick-Sheard P. 1991. The microbial flora of the respiratory tract in feedlot calves: associations between nasopharyngeal and bronchoalveolar lavage cultures. *Can J Vet Res* 55:341–346.

54. DeRosa DC, Mechor GD, Staats JJ, Chengappa MM, Shryock TR. 2000. Comparison of *Pasteurella* spp. simultaneously isolated from nasal and transtracheal swabs from cattle with clinical signs of bovine respiratory disease. *J Clin Microbiol* 38:327–332.

55. Godinho KS, Sarasola P, Renoult E, Tilt N, Keane S, Windsor GD, Rowan TG, Sunderland SJ. 2007. Use of deep nasopharyngeal swabs as a predictive diagnostic method for natural respiratory infections in calves. *Vet Rec* 160:22–25.

56. Nguyen MH, Yu VL, Morris AJ, McDermott L, Wagener MW, Harrell L, Snydman DR. 2000. Antimicrobial resistance and clinical outcome of *Bacteroides* bacteremia: findings of a multicenter prospective observational trial. *Clin Infect Dis* 30:870–876.

57. Bastos ML, Hussain H, Weyer K, Garcia-Garcia L, Leimane V, Leung CC, Narita M, Penã JM, Ponce-de-Leon A, Seung KJ, Shean K, Sifuentes-Osornio J, Van der Walt M, Van der Werf TS, Yew WW, Menzies D, Collaborative Group for Meta-analysis of Individual Patient Data in MDR-TB. 2014. Treatment outcomes of patients with multidrug-resistant and extensively drug-resistant tuberculosis according to drug susceptibility testing to first- and second-line drugs: an individual patient data meta-analysis. *Clin Infect Dis* 59:1364–1374.

58. López-Góngora S, Puig I, Calvet X, Villoria A, Baylina M, Muñoz N, Sanchez-Delgado J, Suarez D, García-Hernando V, Gisbert JP. 2015. Systematic review and meta-analysis: susceptibility-guided versus empirical antibiotic treatment for *Helicobacter pylori* infection. *J Antimicrob Chemother* 70:2447–2455.

59. Sakoulas G, Moise-Broder PA, Schentag J, Forrest A, Moellering RC Jr, Eliopoulos GM. 2004. Relationship of MIC and bactericidal activity to efficacy of vancomycin for treatment of methicillin-resistant *Staphylococcus aureus* bacteremia. *J Clin Microbiol* 42:2398–2402.

60. Mavros MN, Tansarli GS, Vardakas KZ, Rafailidis PI, Karageorgopoulos DE, Falagas ME. 2012. Impact of vancomycin minimum inhibitory concentration on clinical outcomes of patients with vancomycin-susceptible *Staphylococcus aureus* infections: a meta-analysis and meta-regression. *Int J Antimicrob Agents* 40:496–509.

61. Silley P, Simjee S, Schwarz S. 2012. Surveillance and monitoring of antimicrobial resistance and antibiotic consumption in humans and animals. *Rev Sci Tech* 31:105–120.

62. Venugopal AA, Riederer K, Patel SM, Szpunar S, Jahamy H, Valenti S, Shemes SP, Khatib R, Johnson LB. 2012. Lack of association of outcomes with treatment duration and microbiologic susceptibility data in *Clostridium difficile* infections in a non-NAP1/BI/027 setting. *Scand J Infect Dis* 44:243–249.

63. Smith AL, Fiel SB, Mayer-Hamblett N, Ramsey B, Burns JL. 2003. Susceptibility testing of *Pseudomonas aeruginosa* isolates and clinical response to parenteral antibiotic administration: lack of association in cystic fibrosis. *Chest* 123:1495–1502.

64. Zetola NM, Modongo C, Moonan PK, Ncube R, Matlhagela K, Sepako E, Collman RG, Bisson GP. 2014. Clinical outcomes among persons with pulmonary tuberculosis caused by *Mycobacterium tuberculosis* isolates with phenotypic heterogeneity in results of drug-susceptibility tests. *J Infect Dis* 209:1754–1763.

65. Silley P. 2012. Susceptibility testing methods, resistance and breakpoints: what do these terms really mean? *Rev Sci Tech* 31:33–41.

66. Giguère S, Lee E, Williams E, Cohen ND, Chaffin MK, Halbert N, Martens RJ, Franklin RP, Clark CC, Slovis NM. 2010. Determination of the prevalence of antimicrobial resistance to macrolide antimicrobials or rifampin

in *Rhodococcus equi* isolates and treatment outcome in foals infected with antimicrobial-resistant isolates of *R equi*. *J Am Vet Med Assoc* **237**:74–81.

67. Cosgrove SE, Sakoulas G, Perencevich EN, Schwaber MJ, Karchmer AW, Carmeli Y. 2003. Comparison of mortality associated with methicillin-resistant and methicillin-susceptible *Staphylococcus aureus* bacteremia: a meta-analysis. *Clin Infect Dis* **36**:53–59.

68. Hunter PA, Reeves DS. 2002. The current status of surveillance of resistance to antimicrobial agents: report on a meeting. *J Antimicrob Chemother* **49**:17–23.

69. Franklin A, Acar J, Anthony F, Gupta R, Nicholls T, Tamura Y, Thompson S, Threlfall EJ, Vose D, van Vuuren M, White DG, Wegener HC, Costarrica ML, Office International des Epizooties Ad hoc Group. 2001. Antimicrobial resistance: harmonisation of national antimicrobial resistance monitoring and surveillance programmes in animals and in animal-derived food. *Rev Sci Tech* **20**:859–870.

70. Clinical and Laboratory Standards Institute (CLSI). 2011. Generation, presentation, and application of antimicrobial susceptibility test data for bacteria of animal origin; a report. CLSI document VET05-R. CLSI, Wayne, PA.

71. U.S. Food and Drug Administration. Judicious use of antimicrobials. http://www.fda.gov/AnimalVeterinary/SafetyHealth/AntimicrobialResistance/JudiciousUseof Antimicrobials/.

72. Schwarz S, Silley P, Simjee S, Woodford N, van Duijkeren E, Johnson AP, Gaastra W. 2010. Editorial: assessing the antimicrobial susceptibility of bacteria obtained from animals. *J Antimicrob Chemother* **65**:601–604.

73. Prüller S, Turni C, Blackall PJ, Beyerbach M, Klein G, Kreienbrock L, Strutzberg-Minder K, Kaspar H, Meemken D, Kehrenberg C. 2016. Towards a standardized method for broth microdilution susceptibility testing of *Haemophilus parasuis*. *J Clin Microbiol* **55**:264–273.

74. Miller RA, Reimschuessel R. 2006. Epidemiologic cutoff values for antimicrobial agents against *Aeromonas salmonicida* isolates determined by frequency distributions of minimal inhibitory concentration and diameter of zone of inhibition data. *Am J Vet Res* **67**:1837–1843.

75. Riesenberg A, Frömke C, Stingl K, Feßler AT, Gölz G, Glocker E-O, Kreienbrock L, Klarmann D, Werckenthin C, Schwarz S. 2017. Antimicrobial susceptibility testing of *Arcobacter butzleri*: development and application of a new protocol for broth microdilution. *J Antimicrob Chemother* **72**:2769–2774.

76. van Belkum A, Dunne WM Jr. 2013. Next-generation antimicrobial susceptibility testing. *J Clin Microbiol* **51**:2018–2024.

77. Waldeisen JR, Wang T, Debkishore M, Lee LP. 2011. A real-time PCR antibiogram for drug-resistant sepsis. *PLoS One* **6**:e28528. http://journals.plos.org/plosone/article?id=10.1371/journal.pone.0028528

78. Hooff GP, van Kampen JJA, Meesters RJW, van Belkum A, Goessens WHF, Luider TM. 2012. Characterization of β-lactamase enzyme activity in bacterial lysates using MALDI-mass spectrometry. *J Proteome Res* **11**:79–84.

79. Marinach C, Alanio A, Palous M, Kwasek S, Fekkar A, Brossas J-Y, Brun S, Snounou G, Hennequin C, Sangland D, Datry A, Golmard J-L, Mazier D. 2009. MALDI-TOF MS-based drug susceptibility testing of pathogens: the example of *Candida albicans* and fluconazole. *Proteomics* **9**:4627–4631.

80. De Carolis E, Vella A, Florio AR, Posteraro P, Perlin DS, Sanguinetti M, Posteraro B. 2012. Use of matrix-assisted laser desorption ionization-time of flight mass spectrometry for caspofungin susceptibility testing of *Candida* and *Aspergillus* species. *J Clin Microbiol* **50**:2479–2483.

81. Köser CU, Ellington MJ, Cartwright EJP, Gillespie SH, Brown NM, Farrington M, Holden MTG, Dougan G, Bentley SD, Parkhill J, Peacock SJ. 2012. Routine use of microbial whole genome sequencing in diagnostic and public health microbiology. *PLoS Pathog* **8**:e1002824.

82. Punina NV, Makridakis NM, Remnev MA, Topunov AF. 2015. Whole-genome sequencing targets drug-resistant bacterial infections. *Hum Genomics* **9**:19.

Antimicrobial Resistance in Bacteria from Livestock and Companion Animals
Edited by Frank Møller Aarestrup, Stefan Schwarz, Jianzhong Shen, and Lina Cavaco
© 2018 American Society for Microbiology, Washington, DC
doi:10.1128/microbiolspec.ARBA-0011-2017

Molecular Methods for Detection of Antimicrobial Resistance

3

Muna F. Anjum[1], Ea Zankari[2], and Henrik Hasman[2,3]

INTRODUCTION

Molecular characterization of the genetic mechanism(s) underlying a given phenotypic result, obtained by traditional antimicrobial sensitivity testing, is now an integral part of many clinical investigations in relation to bacterial infections, whether in humans or animals. In some cases, when phenotypic results are too time-consuming, nonconclusive, or unavailable, molecular analysis can be used to investigate the presence of a given gene or point mutation and thereby give direct support to ensure that an optimal treatment or control strategy is undertaken in a timely manner. In addition, molecular characterization is frequently used as an indirect method to aid in epidemiological investigations following an outbreak, when phenotypic data is not sufficiently detailed to control possible outbreaks involving resistant bacteria. Finally, molecular characterization of antimicrobial resistance (AMR) determinants is also used for local, national, or even global surveillance of AMR. Currently, the European Food Safety Authority (EFSA) and the European Center for Disease Control (ECDC) are involved in monitoring and coordinating surveillance of AMR in important zoonotic bacteria from food animals and humans, and systems such as the European Antimicrobial Resistance Surveillance System (EARSS) have helped generate data regarding the prevalence of AMR in many European countries. However, most of the data are based on phenotypic characterization of isolates, although genotypic detection of AMR genes is also being increasingly performed by member states.

Discussing phenotypic detection of AMR in bacteria is not meaningful unless the purpose of the analysis is defined. In relation to treatment of clinical infections, parameters such as sites of infection, clinical manifestation, and toxic concentration of the antimicrobial agent used need to be considered to define a relevant clinical breakpoint, which distinguishes between treatable (sensitive), potentially treatable (intermediate resistant), and nontreatable (resistant) infections. Alternatively, the epidemiological cutoff, or ECOFF, can be used to differentiate between the wild type, fully susceptible populations of bacteria, and bacteria with reduced susceptibility due to an acquired resistance mechanism.

Acquired resistance to antimicrobial agents is correlated with a multitude of molecular mechanisms depending on the organism and the antimicrobial agent involved. These mechanisms include very different genetic events such as constitutive or inducible expression of (acquired) resistance genes, upregulated expression of resistance genes because of mutations in the promoter/regulator region, and insertion of strong active promoters as part of, e.g., insertion elements upstream of the resistance gene, mutations in housekeeping genes acting as targets for antimicrobial agents, and loss-of-function mutations in regulatory elements or specific porins (1). In addition, bacteria can be intrinsically resistant to certain types or even whole classes of antimicrobial agents when these are given in therapeutic concentrations. For example, enterococci are inherently resistant to cephalosporins, partly due to low binding affinity of the penicillin binding protein 5, which is involved in cell wall synthesis in this organism (2). Common causes of intrinsic resistance are lack of (or low affinity to) the target for the antimicrobial agent, an inability of the drug to access the target, expression of chromosomally located resistance genes encoding enzymes, and the presence of multidrug efflux pumps (3).

[1]Department of Bacteriology, Animal and Plant Health Agency, Surrey, United Kingdom; [2]National Food Institute, Technical University of Denmark, Lyngby, Denmark; [3]Reference Laboratory for Antimicrobial Resistance and Staphylococci, Staten Serum Institut, Copenhagen, Denmark.

Because of the large diversity of possible mechanisms involved in reduced antimicrobial susceptibility, it is not a trivial task to transform all of these mechanisms or genes into sequence-based detection algorithms if genotypic methods are eventually to substitute for phenotypic methods, especially because new genes or allelic variants of current resistance mechanisms are continuously being discovered. In the case of intrinsic resistance, *a priori* knowledge of a given organism is required to predict if it is intrinsically resistant to certain antimicrobials, which makes translation of sequence-based data into predicted susceptibility even more complicated. For example, anaerobic bacteria are intrinsically resistant to aminoglycosides, while *Helicobacter pylori* is intrinsically resistant to metronidazole and *Pseudomonas aeruginosa* shows natural resistance to sulfonamides and trimethoprims (4–6). Conversely, some genetic resistance mechanisms are inherently difficult to detect by classical *in vitro* phenotypic methods and can therefore remain undetected, even though they can lead to treatment failure *in vivo*, thereby increasing the importance of detecting these mechanisms by molecular methods. This is evident for Gram-negative pathogens carrying the bla_{OXA-48} gene, often conferring only a minor reduction in their susceptibility to carbapenems (7), and some clonal lineages of methicillin-resistant *Staphylococcus aureus* (MRSA), where heterologous expression of the *mecA* gene can lead to inconclusive interpretation of the organism's susceptibility to beta-lactams (8).

Despite the varied challenges posed by genotypic detection of mechanisms leading to reduced susceptibility to different antimicrobial agents, molecular methods are being used extensively by both research and reference laboratories. Some of the methods employed, such as PCR and hybridization techniques, have been used for decades, while new methods such as whole-genome sequencing (WGS) and matrix-assisted laser desorption ionization–time of flight mass spectrometry (MALDI-TOF MS) are just emerging. The most commonly used modern molecular methods in relation to detection of determinants involved in conferring reduced susceptibility to antimicrobial agents are discussed in this article. The main advantages and disadvantages of using the different genotypic methods for detecting AMR will be described individually below; a more elaborate discussion of these methods has been published recently (9).

PCR

PCR is a technique that was developed in the 1980s by Kary Mullis (10) and has revolutionized molecular biology, enabling rapid and exponential amplification of target DNA sequences using a forward and reverse PCR primer and an enzyme known as DNA polymerase in the presence of deoxyribonucleotides. Conventional PCR comprises three steps: (i) denaturing of the double-stranded DNA at 95°C, (ii) annealing of the PCR primers at 50 to 60°C, and (iii) extension of the DNA at 72°C. PCR is used routinely in microbiology laboratories for detecting any genes that may be present within bacteria, as long as a DNA sequence is available for the whole or partial gene which can be used to design the PCR primers. The PCR-amplified gene product can be visualized by running agarose gels and staining DNA with ethidium bromide or other fluorescent DNA-chelating dyes. The whole process, including amplification and visualization, can take between 4 and 5 h.

Since the development of PCR, there have been several advances, which include real-time PCR (RT-PCR) and isothermal amplifications, e.g., loop-mediated isothermal amplification (LAMP) and recombinase polymerase amplification (RPA). The main difference between conventional PCR and RT-PCR is that in the latter, amplification of the target DNA sequence is monitored in real time as it occurs, rather than at the end, due to the presence of fluorescent dyes in the reaction, and thus is also known as quantitative PCR (qPCR). Therefore, in RT-PCR, agarose gel electrophoresis is not required; this can save considerable time and is safer, because the use of ethidium bromide, which is a carcinogen, is not required. RT-PCR can use either (i) nonspecific dyes that intercalate with any double-stranded DNA or (ii) sequence-specific DNA probes consisting of oligonucleotides that are labeled with a fluorescent reporter which permits detection only after hybridization of the probe with its complementary sequence (11). Isothermal PCR techniques such as LAMP and RPA, in contrast, differ from conventional or RT-PCR in that the whole process is performed at a constant temperature and does not require ramping up and down of temperatures. For LAMP, the temperature is around 65°C, while it is around 40°C for RPA; up to six different primers are used for LAMP, whereas RPA uses two primers (12, 13). The presence of intercalating dyes in the reaction allows fluorescent detection of target DNA amplification in real time using a real time PCR machine, which can be considerably faster than PCR or RT-PCR. However, LAMP and RPA PCR amplification can also occur using a simple water bath or heating element and be measured by photometry for turbidity, which makes both methods amenable for point-of-care applications and use in low-resource settings (14).

Multiplex PCR, in which several target DNA fragments are amplified simultaneously, can be performed using either conventional or RT-PCR. The application of PCR for monitoring multiple AMR genes in bacteria has become easier with the use of multiplexing, and this technique is widely used today, where appropriate, to replace PCR and RT-PCR applications to amplify single genes. In a multiplex PCR assay, several resistance genes can be detected simultaneously with different primers included in the assay mix. The products must be of different sizes and can be visualized either by gel electrophoresis, if from conventional PCR, or by addition of different dyes for RT-PCR. Multiplex PCRs are often designed to detect different genes, all relating to the same resistance phenotype such as detection of the most prevalent beta-lactamases present in Gram-negative bacteria which are involved in resistance to cephalosporins (15) or carbapenems (16, 17). Therefore, by screening for these genes simultaneously, considerable time and effort can be saved in detecting the possible mechanism(s) responsible for the resistance phenotype.

The robustness of any PCR strategy relies on multiple factors such as optimal primer design, GC content of the target template, and presence of inhibitory molecules in the sample. The primers require close to 100% identity to the target DNA and are thus sensitive to the presence of single nucleotide polymorphisms within the binding sequence, especially at the 3′ end of the primer, where elongation initiates. It is therefore important to select primers in binding areas with low or no nucleotide variation. To ensure the robustness of new PCR assays, a thorough validation process should always be performed to evaluate the specificity (number of false-positive results) and sensitivity (number of false-negative results) of the assay. Designing primers is relatively easy, but to ensure that these primers have both a high specificity and high sensitivity is not a trivial task, because this requires access to a diverse sequencing dataset representing the variation expected to be present in the test material. If multiplexing is also required, software programs can be employed to help in defining relevant sets of primer pairs (18). Finally, both a positive and a negative control are required every time a PCR assay is performed, to ensure that the sensitivity and specificity are maintained each time the assay is performed.

Conventional PCR assays are well suited to detect the presence or absence of (resistance) genes but are less suited for detection of point mutations within target genes, unless subsequent Sanger sequencing is performed to detect these mutations. RT-PCR can detect single point mutations in a given gene if sequence-specific DNA probes targeting the mutation area are used. However, an advantage that conventional PCR has over RT-PCR is that the latter can only be used to detect the presence of short fragments of DNA, optimally up to 150 bp, whereas conventional PCR can easily detect much larger fragments.

AMR Gene Detection

The use of PCR to detect the presence of AMR genes in a bacterial isolate or even in samples from different environments is commonplace. Due to the ease of designing conventional PCR primers, there are a plethora of PCRs that have been used to detect the presence of different AMR genes from bacteria, in both aerobes and anaerobes. A highly cited paper in this area is by Schwartz et al. (19), who discuss PCR used to monitor for the presence of *vanA* (encoding vancomycin resistance), *mecA* (encoding methicillin resistance), and *ampC* (encoding ampicillin resistance) in wastewater systems and water biofilms. The authors found the *vanA* gene in both wastewater and drinking water biofilms, with the *vanA* gene being found in the latter in the absence of enterococci. While *mecA* was only detected in hospital wastewater, *ampC* was the most widespread and was present in wastewater, surface water, and drinking water biofilms. Another paper is one by Lévesque et al. (20), which describes PCR mapping used to determine AMR genes and the order in which they were present in integron cassettes. In 1995, when this paper was published, integrons were a new type of mobile element, and this work was quite novel. A comprehensive, although not exhaustive, list of primers to detect AMR genes is available at the website of the European Reference Laboratory for Antimicrobial Resistance (EURL AMR) in bacteria from animals and food (http://www.eurl-ar.eu/data/images/faq/primerliste %20til%20web_07.11.2013.pdf).

Conventional PCR has also been used to detect resistance genes in bacteria during infection to antibiotics used in first-line therapy such as those associated with extended-spectrum beta-lactamase (ESBL) resistance (21–23). These PCR assays are often performed in addition to antimicrobial susceptibility testing of the isolates because PCR results can be obtained more quickly, enabling control measures or accurate treatment. More recently, both PCR and RT-PCR have been used widely across Europe and for rapid large-scale epidemiological surveillance of archived bacterial isolates to look for the presence of the plasmid-mediated *mcr-1* and *mcr-2* genes harboring plasmid-mediated resistance to antibiotics of last resort such as colistin, which has attracted much interest since its detection and reporting in 2015 (24–31). As demonstrated by the colistin outbreak, the use of RT-PCRs as a rapid, easy, and cheap method for targeting AMR gene detection during outbreak response remains unrivalled by any other technology (28).

Examples of the application of multiplex PCR for detecting AMR genes in clinical samples include studies by Strommenger et al. (32) and Chung et al. (33), in which the resistance present in multidrug-resistant *S. aureus* was determined by conventional PCR or in which a multiplex RT-PCR was employed to detect the presence of *mecA* and species-specific genes. Another example is a multiplex PCR which is used routinely for surveillance in reference laboratories to detect some of the most prevalent ESBL genes: *bla*TEM, *bla*SHV, *bla*CTX-M, and *bla*OXA (34). Using this multiplex PCR, Randall et al. (35) determined the prevalence of ESBL-producing *Escherichia coli* strains present in pigs at slaughter in the United Kingdom in 2013 to be 23.4%. They also showed that *bla*CTX-M was the most common ESBL type present in these isolates; Sanger sequencing of the PCR product showed *CTX-M-1* to be the most prevalent variant to be carried by these isolates, although some *CTX-M-15* were also detected.

LAMP assays for the detection of resistance include several assays which have been developed for detecting genes encoding resistance to antibiotics for first-line therapeutics or antibiotics of last resort. Examples include LAMP assays developed for the detection of ESBLs, AmpC genes, and carbapenemases in bacteria purified from both humans and animals (12, 36). Due to the rapidity of LAMP assays and the ease of conducting them at a constant temperature, several LAMP assays have been developed (*bla*VIM, *bla*NDM, *bla*KPC, *OXA-48* family, *CTX-M-1* family, and *CTX-M-9* family) to detect carbapenemase and ESBL-producing *Enterobacteriaceae* using the eazyplex SuperBug CRE system (Amplex Biosystems GmbH, Giessen, Germany) (36). As with PCR, LAMP assays can be used to look for the presence of ESBL genes in a bacterial community rather than in single isolates. For example, Kirchner et al. (37) have used LAMP assays to determine the presence of *bla*CTX-M genes in lysates made from the mix of bacteria present in overnight enrichment broths prepared from neck flap and cecal samples from poultry carcasses collected at an abattoir. The results showed that just less than a third of the ceca from poultry carcasses were contaminated with bacteria harboring the *bla*CTX-M gene, but this figure was much higher in skin flaps (>60%), probably due to cross-contamination.

DNA MICROARRAY TECHNOLOGY

DNA microarrays are genomic tools which have been used successfully in the past decade to assess bacterial genomic diversity by detecting the presence or absence of genes in a test organism in comparison to a reference strain or genes. The DNA microarray technology was initially based on glass slides that were spotted with thousands of specific DNA probes based on genes present in one reference strain for which a whole-genome sequence was available. As more isolates of a particular species or genus were whole-genome sequenced, the numbers of probes present on the microarray slide increased substantially to represent accessory genes not present in the reference strain that were part of the "pan-genome." Comparative genomic hybridizations were performed whereby test and reference isolate DNA were fluorescently labeled and hybridized to a microarray slide (38). The presence or absence of genes in the test isolate, in comparison to a reference, was determined by analyzing the hybridization results. This method enabled comparison of the genomic diversity in a relatively large number of test isolates (tens to hundreds) for which WGS was not available. Examples include *E. coli* and *Salmonella*, for which a large number of studies were performed looking at AMRs (39–41).

However, the use of glass slides and fluorescent dyes made the process expensive and time-consuming. Furthermore, there were several advancements in the technology. Although a number of different technologies were available and are reviewed in more detail elsewhere, especially in the context of AMR (42), in this section we will concentrate on that available from Alere Technologies. The Alere microarrays had several advantages that made them suitable for use in routine diagnostic laboratories, which may receive hundreds of samples. Advantages included adaptation of the microarray slide containing DNA probes to a simpler platform such as the bottom of an Eppendorf test tube or a 96-well plate, the use of horseradish peroxidase instead of expensive fluorescent dyes, simple protocols which enable large numbers of test sample DNA to be processed more rapidly and economically, and no requirement for dual hybridization including test and reference. However, disadvantages included the numbers of DNA probes that could be printed in comparison to the full microarray glass slide, which were a few hundred instead of several thousand. In addition, this platform is not suitable for detecting gene expression, but only gene presence and absence, due to inclusion of a preamplification step during labeling of the test DNA prior to hybridization.

AMR Detection Using Microarrays

Several groups have used the Alere microarrays to investigate AMR and virulence genes that may be present on mobile genetic elements such as plasmids and transposons and can be coselected. Characterization of enteric pathogens and commensals such as field and clinical isolates of both human and animal origin is important in understanding the dissemination these genes by zoonotic bacteria that may ultimately affect human health and therapeutics. This application was first developed by the Animal and Plant Health Agency (formerly the Veterinary Laboratories Agency) in collaboration with Alere through Identibac for determining virulence genes present in *E. coli* to distinguish between pathogenic and commensal *E. coli* (43), but later it was applied for detecting AMR genes in *E. coli* and *Salmonella* from food animals, as well as from human clinical isolates in several studies (44–50). Examples of the use of these microarrays include the characterization of animal isolates collected through surveillance studies, which revealed that AMR genes in *Salmonella* and *E. coli* may be present on different mobile genetic elements such as plasmids and *Salmonella* genomic island 1 (48, 51).

The Identibac microarrays have been used to determine the presence of AMR genes in both aerobic and anaerobic Gram-negative bacteria isolated from healthy human feces in two longitudinal studies performed with a cohort of healthy human subjects in the United Kingdom and Sweden over 1 year following a course of antibiotic treatment, as part of a European Commission 7th Framework Program project called Antiresdev (45, 52–54). Analysis of isolates from feces purified pre-antibiotic treatment indicated widespread presence of AMR genes in healthy individuals aged between 20 and 60, from both the Swedish and United Kingdom groups, with certain AMR isolates persisting over time. Following treatment, an effect was seen in individuals treated only with amoxicillin, in which a temporary increase in the number of isolates harboring the beta-lactamase gene *bla*TEM was seen in the treated group but not in the placebo group. No other antibiotic had such a profound effect (45, 53). Examination of anaerobic gut microbiota for mobile genetic elements associated with aerobes, to determine if the former acts as an AMR "sink," indicated that these genes were uncommon in anaerobes and that only the *sul* gene, encoding resistance to sulfonamide, was present in *Bacteroides*; however, the genetic element which may be associated with the *sul* gene could not be determined (54). It would be of interest to perform a similar type of study on farms, to determine if certain

AMR bacteria and genes persist on farms over time and the possible risk to food safety associated with such persistence.

Another application of the Identibac AMR microarrays has been to look at the resistome of the microbiota, i.e., the AMR gene content present in the whole microbial population rather than in individual isolates, using human DNA. In a study by Card et al. (55), the resistomes present in the oral and fecal microbiota of humans from five countries were compared using the microarray. The results showed the prevalence of AMR genes associated with anaerobic bacteria such as *tetX* and *ermB*, as well as *bla*TEM and *sul2*, which are common in aerobic bacteria, present in the majority of samples. Interestingly, a functionally based screening approach which was also undertaken by the authors to determine the genetic context of the AMR genes such as *bla*TEM and *sul2* that were detected in the microbiota only recovered chromosomal genes. This is probably because AMR genes such as *bla*TEM and *sul2* are present in sufficient abundance to be detected by microarray, which employs a linear multiplex amplification process, but are nevertheless not present in high enough abundance to be present in the bacterial artificial chromosome functional libraries that were prepared. It was therefore indicated that microarrays may be more suited to detect AMR genes present on mobile genetic elements which may be present in low copy numbers than a functional genomic approach, although microarrays may be less sensitive than next-generation sequencing methods, in which the depth of sequencing can be very high (see "Whole Genome Sequence Analysis to Detect AMR"). Although in the above study the human oral and fecal microbiota was used, this technique can be applied to any sample, including from farm animals and the environment.

Other microarrays that have been described for determining AMR include those based on glass slides, which for example, have been applied for the characterization of virulence and AMR genes present in *Salmonella* strains of human clinical relevance (56). There are also arrays in which AMR genes associated with both Gram-positive and Gram-negative bacteria are present. One such array was developed for diagnostic and surveillance activities and was used to test *S. aureus* isolates recovered from milk samples from dairy farms in Quebec, Canada (57). Other organizations, including Alere, have also developed microarrays for detection of virulence and AMR in *S. aureus* isolates recovered from hospital, community, and farm settings (58–64). These arrays are still widely used in both human and veterinary settings.

WGS ANALYSIS TO DETECT AMR

Like PCR and microarrays, WGS has the potential to detect genetic determinants (genes and mutations) conferring AMR (65, 66). The main advantage of using WGS for this purpose is the ability to cover many different targets at the same time and to subtype specific gene variants. The current WGS technology and methodology for analysis offers similar results as well as some of the same shortcomings as PCR (followed by Sanger sequencing of amplicons) and microarrays, which will be described and discussed in detail below. However, as opposed to microarrays, WGS also offers the possibility to rapidly add new target sequences to the analysis database as well as the ability to perform fast *in silico* reanalysis on already sequenced isolates (26).

Current Technologies and Bioinformatic Tools

Sequencing platforms

WGS data are generated on highly sophisticated sequencing platforms, which produce large amounts of sequence data compared to the traditional Sanger sequencing technology. Today, the most common platforms for high-throughput sequencing of bacterial genomes are Illumina and Ion Torrent machines, which perform what has been called second-generation or next-generation sequencing (as opposed to traditional Sanger sequencing). Common to these machines is that the output consists of relatively short reads (100 to 400 bp, depending on the technology), which in most cases are shorter than the genes conferring resistance to antimicrobial agents. Also, the rate of randomly occurring, as well as methodology-based, sequencing errors on single reads originating from the next-generation sequencing technology is relatively high compared to errors encountered with traditional Sanger sequencing. To overcome this problem, a huge surplus (termed *x-fold coverage*) of short-read data is produced for each genome and used for error correction by majority calling. This surplus of (overlapping) short-read data can be either mapped onto known references (reference assembly) or used to build larger fragments (*de novo* assembly) of sequence data (so-called *contigs*), which are combined to constitute the draft genome of the isolate (67–69).

An important prerequisite to detect the presence of any relevant gene, including genes conferring resistance to antimicrobial agents, is that the quality and quantity of short reads are large enough to ensure that a given gene is being correctly detected by downstream analysis to avoid false-negative results. Due to the potentially high sensitivity of the analysis methods used for WGS, another important consideration is to ensure that the WGS data do not contain any traces of contaminant DNA, because this can lead to false-positive results. Unfortunately, low levels of DNA from intraspecies contamination can be very difficult to detect, and good laboratory practice when preparing the DNA and sequencing libraries, in combination with extensive use of appropriate negative controls, is often the best way to avoid, or at least minimize, contamination issues (70). When WGS data from an isolate are found free of contaminants and obtained with a sufficiently high quality and quantity to ensure that relevant genetic information is unlikely to be missing, they can then be used to search for genetic determinants related to AMR (67; http://www.phgfoundation.org/file/16848/).

Bioinformatic approaches for using WGS data to detect genetic determinants related to AMR

Extracting the relevant information to detect genetic determinants related to decreased antimicrobial susceptibility from WGS data is far from being a simple task. The main challenges are (i) to obtain comprehensive databases containing the relevant DNA or protein sequence targets and (ii) to apply appropriate bioinformatic methodologies to accurately extract the relevant information from WGS data based on these target databases. Target databases for WGS analysis are in principle not much different from primer lists directed toward certain PCR targets or DNA probes attached to microarrays as described in the sections above, even though WGS databases have the potential to contain more targets than most PCR or microarray systems. In many instances, a clear correlation between a specific resistance phenotype and a given (resistance) gene exists and has been well-characterized by another method, e.g., PCR or microarray, which makes it relatively easy to include these genes in a target database. However, the task of building a comprehensive database covering all possible genetic variations for a given AMR phenotype is far more complicated. As mentioned above, many genetic mechanisms can be accountable for the AMR phenotype, and a plethora of genetic mechanisms are responsible for resistance phenotypes to different antimicrobial agents. For many of these mechanisms it is difficult to generate simplified *in silico* decision rules for prediction of their corresponding resistance phenotype, especially because some bacterial species employ specialized mechanisms, which may not even be well-characterized or generally applicable beyond a given species (71). Therefore, many of the bioinformatic tools to detect genetic determinants conferring reduced antimicrobial susceptibility are based on target databases containing well-defined genes or specific single point mutations, where a strong correlation between the genetic determinant and a given phenotype exists and can be extracted from either published peer-reviewed articles or from pre-existing archives such as the Antibiotic Resistance Gene Database (ARDB) (https://ardb.cbcb.umd.edu/). A disadvantage of such target databases is that they are based on *a priori* data and are therefore not suitable for detecting completely new genes families, novel genes, or new point mutations. Also, a constant curation of the target database is required to maintain updates when new genes are published.

Because comprehensive knowledge of genetic determinants for AMRs varies among bacterial species, the sensitivity of gene-based target databases can be too low to be applied for WGS as a first-line decision tool for treatment due to the risk of false-negative results. To unveil the current status of employing WGS data for antimicrobial susceptibility testing, EUCAST recently initiated a consultation involving leading experts in the field (71; http://www.eucast.org/fileadmin/src/media/PDFs/EUCAST_files/Consultation/2016/EUCAST_WGS_report_consultation_20160511.pdf). Here, the applicability of WGS for this purpose was thoroughly evaluated in relation to the most common human pathogens, with the main conclusion being that the available published evidence does not currently support the use of WGS inferred susceptibility to guide clinical decision making. However, target databases can still be a valuable tool for local, regional, and global surveillance of AMR, because they offer unprecedented resolution of gene variants, which are difficult to obtain by phenotypic as well as most other genotypic methods. Finally, a WGS-based approach enables fast *in silico* reanalysis of existing data each time the database is updated to ensure backward screening for the presence of new genes or single nucleotide polymorphisms. This approach was successfully used to rapidly reanalyze existing WGS data from Denmark shortly after the first report of the emergence of a mobile colistin resistance gene from China, termed *mcr-1* (24). Here, the *mcr-1* gene was retrieved from GenBank as soon as it became available and was added to the ResFinder database, described below, which was used in combination with the CGE Bacterial Analysis Platform (72) to reanalyze 534 bacterial genomes from humans and 380 bacterial genomes from animal and food samples within 2 days after the release of *mcr-1*, thus enabling detection and reporting of *mcr-1* to the scientific community outside China within 3 weeks of the original publication (26).

The two most common bioinformatic approaches to detect the presence of relevant genes are so-called mapping analysis of raw sequencing reads and BLAST-based analysis of (*de novo* assembled) draft genome contigs against a reference target database (67). In general, the reference mapping approaches using raw reads are more sensitive than BLAST-based analysis of draft genomes when it comes to detecting AMR genes because *de novo* assembly is not required for reference mapping. The lower sensitivity of the BLAST-based approach is most likely to be caused by the inability of *de novo* assembler algorithms to assemble all reads into complete genes, either because the raw read coverage of the particular DNA segment containing the resistance gene is too low for full assembly or because several resistance genes with almost identical sequences are present in the isolate, which will cause most assemblers to split the sequence into separate DNA fragments, thus also splitting the resistance gene (73). Conversely, the higher sensitivity of the mapping algorithms is more prone to produce false-positive results from samples with undetected contamination, because the contaminating DNA may not always be assembled into full-length genes by the *de novo* assemblers and therefore may not be reported by the BLAST alignment, but the algorithm will still be able to map to the target genes, though potentially with lower coverage than correctly mapping reads.

Currently available bioinformatic tools to detect genetic determinants for AMR

The number of freely available bioinformatic tools for detecting genetic determinants for AMR in WGS data is constantly increasing. The tools are available as web services, as standalone programs to be downloaded on a local computer through a graphical user interface, or as command-line tools, which means that the user is required to download the program and run it command-line on a computer running a Unix-based operation system. A selection of the most commonly used, publicly availably tools will be presented below and summarized in Table 1. A more exhaustive list and in-depth presentation and discussion of bioinformatic tools for detecting molecular mechanisms conferring reduced susceptibility to antimicrobial agents has recently been published (74). In addition, some of the target databases, which these tools are using for detection, have been implemented into commercial software solutions such as the CLCbio Genomic Workbench from Qiagen (http://www.qiagen.com) and the Bionumerics Seven software from Applied Math (http://www.applied-maths.com). Below, only the noncommercial solutions

Table 1 Overview of different open-access bioinformatic tools for identification of antimicrobial resistance

Method	Method for gene detection	Database	Reference

ARG-ANNOT	Local BLAST program in Bio-Edit software. Program is downloaded and run on users computer does not work on MAC
	
	User selective settings, % identity
	
	Analyzes assembled data
	
	Analyze without Web interface
	
	User sort output results
	
	Possible to run with user-created database
		FASTA format
		Three databases:
		  Nucleotide sequences for acquired resistance gene database and corresponding protein database
		  Mutational gene database
		Do not state when/if the databases are updated
			(66)

CARD	Analyzes assembled data
	Two analysis tools; BLAST and RGI
	BLAST method
	  BLASTn, BLASTp, BLASTx, tBLASTn, tBLASTx
	  Against CARD protein or nucleotide database
	RGI (currently only analyze protein sequences)
	Uses BLAST and curated SNP matrices
	Possible to download:
	  RGI command-line tool to bulk analyze (Unix)
	  Heatmap
	  BLAST output (excel)
	  ORFs FASTA
		FASTA format
		Four nucleotide databases with corresponding protein databases
		  Resistance genes and mechanisms
		  rRNA mutation genes
		  Mutational genes
		  Wild type genes
		State on download page when database is updated
			(80, 81)

ResFinder	BLASTn
	User selective settings, % identity and % coverage
	Program sort output according to user selected thresholds, outputs only best matches.
	Possible to analyze assembled data or raw reads
	Possible to download:
	  Results as text
	  Results as tab separated file
	  FASTA with hit in genome
	  FASTA with found resistance genes
		FASTA format
		One database for each antimicrobial class with nucleotide sequences for acquired resistance genes
		Note file with phenotypic information on resistance genes
		State on homepage and download page when database is updated
			(65)

KmerResistance	Mapping using *K*-mers Analyses raw reads Calculates quality of the raw reads and uses this to set threshold for detected genes Predicts the species of the genome Possible to run as web-server or to download program and run command-line Possible to run with user-created database	Uses the ResFinder database	(73)
SRST2	Mapping using Bowtie2 Analyzes raw reads Threshold for detected genes has been set to 90% identity and 90% coverage Program is downloaded from GitHub and is a command-line tool (Unix) Possible to run with user-created database	Can only handle databases in FASTA format with a specific header format Choose between the ARG-ANNOT database or the ResFinder database, the databases is not regularly updated	(82)

RGI; Resistance Gene Identifier. ORF; Open Reading Frame. SNP; Single Nucleotide Polymorphism.

will be presented and discussed in more detail. However, the numbers and diversity of AMR tools are vast, with many government and research institutions using their own custom-made databases and analytical approaches, some of which may not be publicly available (27, 75–79).

ResFinder

ResFinder (65) is a web server composed of a BLAST-based alignment for detection of acquired AMR genes in assembled WGS data and a curated database in FASTA format containing the resistance genes. The BLAST output is sorted, so only the best hit within a given position in the data, with a 30-bp overlap allowance, is given as a result. This makes it possible to detect the same gene located in multiple positions of the genomic data. ResFinder allows user selection of the minimum percent identity and minimum percent length of the sequence alignment and reports only the best hit for each gene target which meets these parameters. The ideal percent identity and percent length to employ are dependent on the purpose as well as the quality and type of sequence data.

ResFinder allows upload of both preassembled genomes as well as raw data from various sequencing platforms; when raw WGS data is uploaded, it is assembled by Velvet before being analyzed by ResFinder. ResFinder has been included in a web service called the CGE Bacterial Analysis Platform to allow for automated bulk analysis (72).

Because ResFinder detects only acquired genes, it does not detect genetic elements such as chromosomal mutations and multidrug transporters, as well as intrinsic resistance genes. This makes ResFinder well suited for surveillance of AMR in relation to acquired mechanisms but less suited to be used as an alternative for phenotypic antimicrobial sensitivity testing in the clinic.

CARD

The Comprehensive Antibiotic Resistance Database (CARD) is a web service and has two analysis options: BLAST and RGI (Resistance Gene Identifier) (80, 81). The BLAST option performs standard BLAST searches on smaller sequences uploaded by the user (but not whole genomes) against the CARD reference sequences. The RGI supports two detection model types: (i) protein homolog models, which employ BLAST sequence similarity cutoffs to detect AMR genes, and (ii) protein variant models for detection of mutations conferring AMR. Currently, the RGI only analyzes protein sequences, and if assembled contigs are submitted to the tool, the RGI first predicts open reading frames and

then analyzes the predicted protein sequences. The RGI is also developed as a command-line tool for bulk analysis of many genomes simultaneously.

ARG-ANNOT

Antibiotic Resistance Gene-Annotation (ARG-ANNOT) (66) uses a local BLAST algorithm in conjunction with the BioEdit software (http://www.mbio.ncsu.edu/BioEdit/bioedit.html), which allows the user to analyze sequences on a local computer without Internet access once the software is installed. Unfortunately, BioEdit does not currently run on Mac OS environments. ARG-ANNOT provides the user with three databases in FASTA format with phenotypic information in the FASTA header, acquired AMR genes with nucleotide or protein sequences, and a mutational gene database. Currently, the ARG-ANNOT system does not detect mutations automatically but outputs the sequence that matches the reference genes so the user is manually able to search from possible mutations. It is also possible for the user to make a custom-made database for specific analysis through ARG-ANNOT.

KmerResistance

KmerResistance (73) is a mapping tool and is available both as a web server and as a command-line tool. KmerResistance performs mapping against the ResFinder gene database by examining the number of co-occurring k-mers between the raw sequence data and the database. A k-mer is a subsequence of the length k.

To detect possible resistance gene contaminants, a novel quality validation estimation of the data has been added to minimize false-positive results. This is done by predicting the bacterial species from the genome data, which gives an estimate of both coverage and depth of the data, and thereby the quality of the data. With this quality measure of the data, the exponential survival function is used to measure the quality of detected genes. Only genes above the quality threshold set by the exponential survival function are given as output, under the assumption that hits to genes with a significantly lower k-mer coverage than the k-mer hits to the chromosome originate from contamination as described above.

SRST2

Short Read Sequence Typing for Bacterial Pathogens (SRST2) (82) is a command-line tool based on the mapping tool Bowtie2 (83). SRST2 maps raw sequence reads directly against an input database of preference, for example, resistance genes. SRST2 also enables further analysis of the identified genes, such as mutations compared to reference sequence. The authors have set the threshold of SRST2 to 90% identity and 90% coverage.

In addition to the above-mentioned programs, other programs and methods for detecting AMR genes, not only for single isolates but also for metagenomic samples, are available online for free download, most of them as command-line tools. In the future, comparison of results obtained using the same WGS data set but different programs or tools will be useful to understand the benefits and possible shortcomings of each and to determine whether under certain circumstances some tools will provide more accurate results than others.

Detection of antimicrobial determinants in complex samples

The tools mentioned above are best suited for the detection of AMR determinants in WGS data from single (pure) isolates, even though they may to some extent also be applicable for complex samples containing whole bacterial communities. However, more dedicated tools for the analysis of DNA samples originating from whole bacterial communities (often called the microbiome) do exist, even though they are still in their infancy. Such microbiome DNA samples are often referred to as whole-community metagenomic samples and should not be confused with traditional metagenomic samples, in which only species-relevant targets such as 16S DNA, are sequenced and used to estimate species distributions in complex samples. The latter is now often referred to as microbial community profiling to avoid confusion with metagenomic sequence analysis. These methods will be able to cover not only bacteria and AMR, but also other pathogens such as viruses, fungi, and parasites. Additionally, part of the sample can also be tested for chemicals/residues in parallel, thus increasing the amount of information about the sample. Analysis of whole-community metagenomic samples can be useful especially for AMR surveillance, but other applications such as rapid investigation of clinical samples have also been demonstrated (84–86). As a proof-of-concept for whole-community metagenomics in AMR surveillance, shotgun Illumina sequencing of toilet waste from 18 international airplane flights arriving at Copenhagen Airport, Denmark, was performed and mapped against the ResFinder database using the online tool MGmapper (https://cge.cbs.dtu.dk/services/MGmapper/), which builds on a combination of the Burrows-Wheeler Aligner (BWA) algorithm and SAMtools software packages (87, 88). An average of 0.06% of the reads from the samples were assigned to (known) resistance genes, with genes encoding resistance to tetracycline and macrolide and beta-lactam resistance genes as the most abundant in the samples (89).

An initial challenge is to ensure that a representative sampling is performed and then to ensure that the DNA purification method is able to extract DNA from all species present at an equal ratio, especially if the downstream analysis includes quantification and comparison of (resistance) gene distributions for AMR surveillance. Knudsen and Bergmark recently evaluated eight commercial kits for extracting DNA from three microbiome sample types and found large variation in species composition obtained between the different kits (90). This makes it virtually impossible to compare microbiome data across studies unless the same methodology has been used. DNA extracted from whole-community metagenomic samples covers not only species-related information but all available DNA information present in the sample, including that originating from the host, the environment, and bacteria of interest (74).

The amount and variation of DNA can be extremely high in extractions from whole-community samples, and it is often economically unrealistic to sequence more than a subsample of this, even on the large-capacity second-generation sequencing platforms. However, even if samples are sequenced at high depth it can become time-consuming to process the data generated due to computational requirements. Therefore, it is rare to obtain all available sequence information present in the sample, which makes it difficult to perform *de novo* assembly prior to analysis for determinants related to reduced susceptibility to antimicrobial agents. Hence, detection of AMR determinants in DNA from complex communities often relies on mapping of raw sequencing reads to gene databases using mapping approaches similar to those mentioned above and is therefore dependent on the quality of these databases. Furthermore, genes such as AMR genes may be harbored by organisms that are of low prevalence in the microbiota and may be difficult to detect unless DNA extracted from metagenomics samples is sequenced to a high depth, which currently may not be economically viable beyond specific purposes such as research. However, as next-generation sequencing technologies advance, there is no doubt that these difficulties will be overcome.

MALDI-TOF MS IN RELATION TO AMR

MALDI-TOF MS is a powerful analytical tool which has only recently been introduced in many clinical laboratories. In short, MALDI-TOF MS is a technique used to analyze biomolecules such as DNA, carbohydrates, proteins, and peptides by their ability to become ionized and enter gas phase and then measuring their time of flight. Here, the mass/charge (m/z) ratio of the resulting molecular fragments is analyzed to produce a molecular signature. Analysis can be made directly on biological samples of single organisms in standardized or complex matrices including blood and urine, and each spectrum can then be compared to commercial databases containing, e.g., species-specific spectral information, which has proved useful especially for species identification of microorganisms (91). Furthermore, MALDI-TOF MS offers the possibility to detect specific proteins or enzymes as well as smaller biomolecules such as antimicrobial agents and their degradation products (92). The main explanation for the rapid implementation of MALDI-TOF MS in clinical microbiology is probably its ability to generate rapid and relatively reliable results with a high throughput at a low cost. However, considerable cost is required to purchase and maintain the equipment, as is the case with most instrumentation, but once the equipment is acquired, processing each sample is relatively inexpensive. The practical applications of MALDI-TOF MS in relation to detecting AMR can generally be divided into one of three categories, described in detail below.

Species Identification and Targeted Antimicrobial Treatment

One of the most common applications of MALDI-TOF MS in the clinical microbial laboratory is to perform organism (bacterial species) identification. Application of this method is typically based on the detection of highly abundant proteins in a mass range between 2 and 20 kDa by computing their m/z values (91, 93). The same level of information can be obtained as from classical culture-based species identification methods, but with MALDI-TOF MS, where results are generated much more rapidly than by culture, hours or even days can be saved in initiating the correct treatment. This can have a direct impact on the clinical outcome as shown by Kumar et al., where the survival rate of septic shock patients decreased by 7.6% for each hour of delay in antimicrobial administration, for the first 6 hours (94). Therefore, an obvious benefit of rapid organism identification using MALDI-TOF MS is to utilize this information to perform targeted antimicrobial treatment based on *a priori* knowledge of expected treatment outcomes for each bacterial pathogen or to conduct proper antimicrobial stewardship if no pathogen can be detected in a given sample (95, 96).

Direct Detection of AMR Determinants

A large proportion of AMR determinants are proteins, so it is in principle possible to detect these, or proteo-

lytic fragments of these, directly in the molecular signature from the MALDI-TOF MS, thus providing an on-the-fly resistance profile (97). An initial requirement for this detection is that the resistance genes are actually expressed, which can be an issue in relation to the inducible resistance systems. Initial attempts, however, have not found support for this approach. A study by Schaumann et al., analyzing mass spectra from protein extracts of ESBL-producing and non-ESBL-producing bacteria at the m/z range of 2,000 to 20,000, failed to obtain reliable discrimination between the two populations (98). An alternative approach is to collect spectra from uninduced and induced (by a given antimicrobial agent) cultures and then to perform spectral analysis of these to identify induced peaks in the data (99). A substantial obstacle for both of these methods is that many thousands of resistance protein variants exist, thus making it very difficult to develop specific databases covering all variants, which would need considerable effort and have to be done over time. In addition, signal shielding from nonresistance protein can occur, thus masking the relevant protein signals. This can to some extent be minimized if spectra from protein extracts rather than complete cell extracts are studied and by focusing on a small subset of resistance protein groups such as enzymes involved in resistance to critically important antimicrobial agents such as third-generation cephalosporins and carbapenems (100).

Detection of Antimicrobial Biomolecules and their Degradation Products

Because direct detection of resistance proteins by MALDI-TOF MS has not yet proven to be feasible to implement at the clinical laboratory, an alternative approach, in which the specific antimicrobial biomolecules and their degradation products resulting from the enzymatic activity are detected by MALDI-TOF MS, has been suggested (100). This approach is targeted to specific enzyme-drug combinations and is again mostly relevant in relation to the subgroup of critically important drugs, which are known to be subjected to enzymatic degradation. Therefore, most studies have examined the feasibility of this approach in relation to carbapenem resistance, as a result of carbapenemase activity, and have shown very high sensitivity and specificity (101, 102). However, one drawback of this approach in the clinical laboratory is that detection of carbapenems such as imipenem and meropenem, and their enzymatic degradation products, relies on a preincubation step to allow time for the degradation process to occur. Another drawback is that the analysis has to be performed at a shorter m/z range (0 to 700 m/z) than that used for species identification because these molecules are relatively small (103). Implementation at a clinical laboratory as a routine analysis is therefore impeded by the need to reset the MALDI-TOF MS machine several times daily or by investing in two identical machines: one for each purpose (Dennis S. Hansen, unpublished data). A final drawback is the lack of enzymatic inactivation for several of the clinically important antimicrobial agents such as methicillin-resistant *S. aureus* and vancomycin-resistant enterococci, which renders this approach impossible.

DISCUSSION

This article has demonstrated that molecular methods for characterizing AMR genes are not only important because they provide insight to the possible mechanism of resistance, but are also increasingly becoming commonplace. For example, methods such as PCR are routinely used by laboratories worldwide both for surveillance and for research and are still irreplaceable in terms of cost and throughput compared with other molecular methods. However, methods such as WGS, which are increasingly being used for molecular characterization of AMR determinants and provide a more comprehensive picture of all AMR genes that may be present in an isolate, could supersede PCR in the future if the cost of WGS continues to fall and if analytical processes are further simplified. WGS provides an advantage over methods such as microarray because once isolates are sequenced, the data are in theory available in perpetuity and can be interrogated infinitely with new genes or data sets. In comparison, microarrays, once performed using a set of genes, cannot be interrogated again for new genes. Designing and printing new primers and probes for genes *in silico* to update microarrays is not an inconsiderable bioinformatic effort. Any new probe and primer not only have to be specific for that gene, but they also cannot cross-react with any other, and they have to have melting temperatures similar to all other existing probes present on the microarray. In addition, the cost of printing new arrays with new primers and probes often means that these additions are performed as batch updates, so *ad hoc* immediate response to new outbreaks, such as the global *mcr-1* outbreak response, is difficult to perform.

However, the rise of WGS and its application in routine AMR surveillance poses the problem of implementation and harmonization of this methodology globally. With some resource-limited countries still struggling to implement simple molecular methods such as PCR in routine surveillance activities, it is unlikely that they will acquire the funds or infrastructure required to perform WGS and ensuing bioinformatic analysis of the data. This will probably affect mitigation and control of AMR, because AMR is a global issue, with new variants likely to arise in different areas of the world but being able to disseminate worldwide due to international trade of food and animals and extensive human travel.

However, with the introduction of WGS, researchers and primary investigators can now have an unprecedented resolution of sequence information, which shifts the workload from running the assay to analyzing the WGS data. Also, for PCR, RT-PCR, and microarrays, results are in most cases either negative or positive, depending on a given cutoff criterion. For instance, a PCR product with the expected size is interpreted as a positive result, even though it may not be 100% identical at the nucleotide level to the result from the positive control. When analyzing WGS data, if nucleotide variations in the genes of interest are reported, the investigator has to decide (or prove) if the phenotype associated with the reference gene is also applicable to the new variant present in the WGS data. For surveillance and infection control purposes, this may not be of primary concern, but if WGS results are used to guide clinical treatment, matters may be different and require further work to gain experimental proof.

Detection of genetic determinants conferring reduced susceptibility to antimicrobial agents requires application of validated analytical methods and target databases for these genotypic-phenotypic correlations to be fully useful. Combining the right bioinformatic and biological competences often requires interdisciplinary collaboration, where construction of the software algorithms and target databases are thoroughly documented and validated by the use of well-documented test sets. Furthermore, it is important to ensure that all genetic mechanisms are correctly and comprehensively assigned to particular resistance phenotypes, which are then added to target databases. This is a complex task which requires in-depth knowledge of AMR genes and includes periodic updating and curation of the databases. In addition, a common nomenclature for genes belonging to the same family, and for reporting the results from various analytical tools, is needed if not only WGS data, but also results of WGS data analysis, are to be shared beyond the local setting. Finally, appropriate quality assurance testing protocols to test the quality of all steps of WGS and WGS analysis will need to be developed and implemented routinely in the future. This is an important criterion to ensure that WGS and data interpretation performed from different laboratories are comparable. Similar quality assurance testing protocols have been implemented for a number of phenotypic and molecular tests of isolates by reference laboratories across Europe, e.g., antimicrobial susceptibility testing for *Enterobacteriaceae* and variable-number tandem repeat testing for *Salmonella*.

Another important point for consideration of the use of genotypic data for detecting resistance, as discussed by Anjum (9), is that new variants may be overlooked by PCR, microarrays, and WGS, because these detect the presence of genes using primers, probes, and sequences based on prior knowledge. Therefore, as demonstrated by the *mcr-1* gene (24), resistance to even critical antibiotics may be overlooked if only molecular methods are used. Therefore, it is important to continue to perform both methods in reference laboratories, but care must be taken in correlating genotypic and phenotypic data, as already mentioned, because there may be redundancy, i.e., more than one gene or genetic mechanism that can result in the same phenotype. For instance, continuing with the colistin example, Anjum et al. (27) showed that colistin-resistant *E. coli* and *Salmonella* isolates could harbor both the *mcr-1* gene and single nucleotide polymorphisms in several chromosomal genes associated with colistin resistance that would account for the colistin-resistance phenotype seen in these isolates. Until recently, when only chromosomal changes were known to be associated with colistin resistance, detection of single nucleotide polymorphism variants in relevant chromosomal genes was sufficient to declare colistin resistance to be present in *Enterobacteriaceae*; researchers did not look further. Because these chromosomal mutations are rarely transferable in nature, it was therefore deemed safe to use colistin for animal husbandry. However, identification of a transferable plasmid-borne colistin-resistance gene which has been shown to be prevalent worldwide has been a game changer. It has resulted in the recommendation for limited use of colistin in animal husbandry by competent authorities such as the European Medicines Agency (http://www.ema.europa.eu/docs/en_GB/document_library/Scientific_guideline/2016/05/WC500207233.pdf). The impact and risk of the presence of the *mcr-1* transferable plasmid in *Enterobacteriaceae* is still being assessed in many countries, including in China, where it was first detected and may have been present for longer than previously known (104).

MALDI-TOF MS is a relatively new method which holds promise and could become more commonplace in the future for AMR characterization, but this requires further exploration and validation of data. An important point for consideration when using this method is the upfront cost of buying MALDI-TOF MS equipment solely for AMR diagnostics, which at current prices may not be cost-effective. It may, however, be cost-effective for use in laboratories where the machine is already available for other purposes. For example, MALDI-TOF MS is used routinely in hospitals and other reference laboratory settings in many countries for rapid identification of bacteria isolated from clinical specimens. If any AMR are present in these isolates that could also be accurately characterized using MALDI-TOF, then it would no doubt aid both rapid clinical diagnosis and treatment of bacterial infections. MALDI-TOF also has the added advantage that it is a "phenotypic" method so in principle should be able to detect new and variant forms of proteins or enzymes that may be responsible for AMRs attributed to bacterial isolates.

This article has undertaken to review some of the most common and popular molecular methods that have been or are currently used by researchers and reference laboratories working with AMR. This review is not an exhaustive list of all approaches available but aims to provide readers, especially those new to the field, with some ideas and examples of work being implemented in this area, and some of the possible pitfalls. Because the field of AMR is an area of growing importance, it is expected that other molecular methods, which are not included in this review, may come to prominence in the future. Microbial community profiling and metagenomic sequence analyses are some of the rapidly developing methods which will probably be used for AMR gene detection in the future, although based on current popularity and convenience, the use of PCR and single-isolate WGS seems irreplaceable.

Citation. Anjum MF, Zankari E, Hasman H. 2017. Molecular methods for detection of antimicrobial resistance. Microbiol Spectrum 5(6):ARBA-0011-2017.

References

1. Chan KG. 2016. Whole-genome sequencing in the prediction of antimicrobial resistance. *Expert Rev Anti Infect Ther* **14:**617–619.

2. Hollenbeck BL, Rice LB. 2012. Intrinsic and acquired resistance mechanisms in *Enterococcus*. *Virulence* **3:** 421–433.

3. Cox G, Wright GD. 2013. Intrinsic antibiotic resistance: mechanisms, origins, challenges and solutions. *Int J Med Microbiol* **303:**287–292.

4. Schlessinger D. 1988. Failure of aminoglycoside antibiotics to kill anaerobic, low-pH, and resistant cultures. *Clin Microbiol Rev* **1:**54–59.

5. Goodwin A, Kersulyte D, Sisson G, Veldhuyzen van Zanten SJ, Berg DE, Hoffman PS. 1998. Metronidazole

resistance in *Helicobacter pylori* is due to null mutations in a gene (*rdxA*) that encodes an oxygen-insensitive NADPH nitroreductase. *Mol Microbiol* 28:383–393.

6. Huovinen P. 2001. Resistance to trimethoprim-sulfamethoxazole. *Clin Infect Dis* 32:1608–1614.

7. Poirel L, Potron A, Nordmann P. 2012. OXA-48-like carbapenemases: the phantom menace. *J Antimicrob Chemother* 67:1597–1606.

8. Boyce JM, Medeiros AA, Papa EF, O'Gara CJ. 1990. Induction of beta-lactamase and methicillin resistance in unusual strains of methicillin-resistant *Staphylococcus aureus*. *J Antimicrob Chemother* 25:73–81.

9. Anjum MF. 2015. Screening methods for the detection of antimicrobial resistance genes present in bacterial isolates and the microbiota. *Future Microbiol* 10:317–320.

10. Saiki RK, Gelfand DH, Stoffel S, Scharf SJ, Higuchi R, Horn GT, Mullis KB, Erlich HA. 1988. Primer-directed enzymatic amplification of DNA with a thermostable DNA polymerase. *Science* 239:487–491.

11. Arya M, Shergill IS, Williamson M, Gommersall L, Arya N, Patel HR. 2005. Basic principles of real-time quantitative PCR. *Expert Rev Mol Diagn* 5:209–219.

12. Anjum MF, Lemma F, Cork DJ, Meunier D, Murphy N, North SE, Woodford N, Haines J, Randall LP. 2013. Isolation and detection of extended spectrum β-lactamase (ESBL)-producing enterobacteriaceae from meat using chromogenic agars and isothermal loop-mediated amplification (LAMP) assays. *J Food Sci* 78: M1892–M1898.

13. Glais L, Jacquot E. 2015. Detection and characterization of viral species/subspecies using isothermal recombinase polymerase amplification (RPA) assays. *Methods Mol Biol* 1302:207–225.

14. Abdullahi UF, Naim R, Taib WRW, Saleh A, Muazu A, Aliyu S, Baig AA. 2015. Loop-mediated isothermal amplification (LAMP), an innovation in gene amplification: bridging the gap in molecular diagnostics; a review. *Indian J Sci Technol* 8:1–12.

15. Dallenne C, Da Costa A, Decré D, Favier C, Arlet G. 2010. Development of a set of multiplex PCR assays for the detection of genes encoding important beta-lactamases in *Enterobacteriaceae*. *J Antimicrob Chemother* 65:490–495.

16. Solanki R, Vanjari L, Subramanian S, B A, E N, Lakshmi V. 2014. Comparative evaluation of multiplex PCR and routine laboratory phenotypic methods for detection of carbapenemases among Gram negative bacilli. *J Clin Diagn Res* 8:DC23–DC26.

17. Poirel L, Walsh TR, Cuvillier V, Nordmann P. 2011. Multiplex PCR for detection of acquired carbapenemase genes. *Diagn Microbiol Infect Dis* 70:119–123.

18. Shen Z, Qu W, Wang W, Lu Y, Wu Y, Li Z, Hang X, Wang X, Zhao D, Zhang C. 2010. MPprimer: a program for reliable multiplex PCR primer design. *BMC Bioinformatics* 11:143.

19. Schwartz T, Kohnen W, Jansen B, Obst U. 2003. Detection of antibiotic-resistant bacteria and their resistance genes in wastewater, surface water, and drinking water biofilms. *FEMS Microbiol Ecol* 43:325–335.

20. Lévesque C, Piché L, Larose C, Roy PH. 1995. PCR mapping of integrons reveals several novel combinations of resistance genes. *Antimicrob Agents Chemother* 39:185–191.

21. Chagas TP, Alves RM, Vallim DC, Seki LM, Campos LC, Asensi MD. 2011. Diversity of genotypes in CTX-M-producing *Klebsiella pneumoniae* isolated in different hospitals in Brazil. *Braz J Infect Dis* 15:420–425.

22. Hasman H, Mevius D, Veldman K, Olesen I, Aarestrup FM. 2005. beta-Lactamases among extended-spectrum beta-lactamase (ESBL)-resistant *Salmonella* from poultry, poultry products and human patients in The Netherlands. *J Antimicrob Chemother* 56:115–121.

23. Mulvey MR, Bryce E, Boyd DA, Ofner-Agostini M, Land AM, Simor AE, Paton S. 2005. Molecular characterization of cefoxitin-resistant *Escherichia coli* from Canadian hospitals. *Antimicrob Agents Chemother* 49: 358–365.

24. Liu YY, Wang Y, Walsh TR, Yi LX, Zhang R, Spencer J, Doi Y, Tian G, Dong B, Huang X, Yu LF, Gu D, Ren H, Chen X, Lv L, He D, Zhou H, Liang Z, Liu JH, Shen J. 2016. Emergence of plasmid-mediated colistin resistance mechanism MCR-1 in animals and human beings in China: a microbiological and molecular biological study. *Lancet Infect Dis* 16:161–168.

25. Haenni M, Poirel L, Kieffer N, Châtre P, Saras E, Métayer V, Dumoulin R, Nordmann P, Madec JY. 2016. Co-occurrence of extended spectrum β lactamase and MCR-1 encoding genes on plasmids. *Lancet Infect Dis* 16:281–282.

26. Hasman H, Hammerum AM, Hansen F, Hendriksen RS, Olesen B, Agersø Y, Zankari E, Leekitcharoenphon P, Stegger M, Kaas RS, Cavaco LM, Hansen DS, Aarestrup FM, Skov RL. 2015. Detection of *mcr-1* encoding plasmid-mediated colistin-resistant *Escherichia coli* isolates from human bloodstream infection and imported chicken meat, Denmark 2015. *Euro Surveill* 20:20.

27. Anjum MF, Duggett NA, AbuOun M, Randall L, Nunez-Garcia J, Ellis RJ, Rogers J, Horton R, Brena C, Williamson S, Martelli F, Davies R, Teale C. 2016. Colistin resistance in *Salmonella* and *Escherichia coli* isolates from a pig farm in Great Britain. *J Antimicrob Chemother* 71:2306–2313.

28. Duggett NA, Sayers E, AbuOun M, Ellis RJ, Nunez-Garcia J, Randall L, Horton R, Rogers J, Martelli F, Smith RP, Brena C, Williamson S, Kirchner M, Davies R, Crook D, Evans S, Teale C, Anjum MF. 2017. Occurrence and characterization of *mcr-1*-harbouring *Escherichia coli* isolated from pigs in Great Britain from 2013 to 2015. *J Antimicrob Chemother* 72:691–695.

29. Nijhuis RH, Veldman KT, Schelfaut J, Van Essen-Zandbergen A, Wessels E, Claas EC, Gooskens J. 2016. Detection of the plasmid-mediated colistin-resistance gene *mcr-1* in clinical isolates and stool specimens obtained from hospitalized patients using a newly developed real-time PCR assay. *J Antimicrob Chemother* 71: 2344–2346.

30. Veldman K, van Essen-Zandbergen A, Rapallini M, Wit B, Heymans R, van Pelt W, Mevius D. 2016. Location

of colistin resistance gene *mcr-1* in *Enterobacteriaceae* from livestock and meat. *J Antimicrob Chemother* 71: 2340–2342.

31. Figueiredo R, Card RM, Nunez J, Pomba C, Mendonça N, Anjum MF, Da Silva GJ. 2016. Detection of an *mcr-1*-encoding plasmid mediating colistin resistance in *Salmonella enterica* from retail meat in Portugal. *J Antimicrob Chemother* 71:2338–2340.

32. Strommenger B, Kettlitz C, Werner G, Witte W. 2003. Multiplex PCR assay for simultaneous detection of nine clinically relevant antibiotic resistance genes in *Staphylococcus aureus*. *J Clin Microbiol* 41:4089–4094.

33. Chung Y, Kim TS, Min YG, Hong YJ, Park JS, Hwang SM, Song KH, Kim ES, Park KU. 2016. Usefulness of multiplex real-time PCR for simultaneous pathogen detection and resistance profiling of staphylococcal bacteremia. 2016:6913860.

34. Fang H, Ataker F, Hedin G, Dornbusch K. 2008. Molecular epidemiology of extended-spectrum beta-lactamases among *Escherichia coli* isolates collected in a Swedish hospital and its associated health care facilities from 2001 to 2006. *J Clin Microbiol* 46:707–712.

35. Randall LP, Lemma F, Rogers JP, Cheney TE, Powell LF, Teale CJ. 2014. Prevalence of extended-spectrum-β-lactamase-producing *Escherichia coli* from pigs at slaughter in the UK in 2013. *J Antimicrob Chemother* 69:2947–2950.

36. García-Fernández S, Morosini MI, Marco F, Gijón D, Vergara A, Vila J, Ruiz-Garbajosa P, Cantón R. 2015. Evaluation of the eazyplex SuperBug CRE system for rapid detection of carbapenemases and ESBLs in clinical *Enterobacteriaceae* isolates recovered at two Spanish hospitals. *J Antimicrob Chemother* 70:1047–1050.

37. Kirchner M, Lemma F, Randall L, Anjum MF. 2017. Loop-mediated isothermal amplification (LAMP) for extended spectrum β-lactamase gene detection in poultry carcase. *Vet Rec* 181:119.

38. Carter B, Wu G, Woodward MJ, Anjum MF. 2008. A process for analysis of microarray comparative genomics hybridisation studies for bacterial genomes. *BMC Genomics* 9:53.

39. Yu X, Susa M, Knabbe C, Schmid RD, Bachmann TT. 2004. Development and validation of a diagnostic DNA microarray to detect quinolone-resistant *Escherichia coli* among clinical isolates. *J Clin Microbiol* 42:4083–4091.

40. Barl T, Dobrindt U, Yu X, Katcoff DJ, Sompolinsky D, Bonacorsi S, Hacker J, Bachmann TT. 2008. Genotyping DNA chip for the simultaneous assessment of antibiotic resistance and pathogenic potential of extraintestinal pathogenic *Escherichia coli*. *Int J Antimicrob Agents* 32:272–277.

41. Call DR, Bakko MK, Krug MJ, Roberts MC. 2003. Identifying antimicrobial resistance genes with DNA microarrays. *Antimicrob Agents Chemother* 47:3290–3295.

42. Aarts HJM, Guerra B, Malorny B. 2006. Molecular methods for detection of antimicrobial resistance, p 37–48. *In* Aarestrup FM (ed), *Antimicrobial Resistance in Bacteria of Animal Origin*. ASM Press, Washington, DC.

43. Anjum MF, Mafura M, Slickers P, Ballmer K, Kuhnert P, Woodward MJ, Ehricht R. 2007. Pathotyping *Escherichia coli* by using miniaturized DNA microarrays. *Appl Environ Microbiol* 73:5692–5697.

44. Card R, Zhang J, Das P, Cook C, Woodford N, Anjum MF. 2013. Evaluation of an expanded microarray for detecting antibiotic resistance genes in a broad range of Gram-negative bacterial pathogens. *Antimicrob Agents Chemother* 57:458–465.

45. Card RM, Mafura M, Hunt T, Kirchner M, Weile J, Rashid MU, Weintraub A, Nord CE, Anjum MF. 2015. Impact of ciprofloxacin and clindamycin administration on Gram-negative bacteria isolated from healthy volunteers and characterization of the resistance genes they harbor. *Antimicrob Agents Chemother* 59:4410–4416.

46. Mendonça N, Figueiredo R, Mendes C, Card RM, Anjum MF, da Silva GJ. 2016. Microarray evaluation of antimicrobial resistance and virulence of *Escherichia coli* isolates from Portuguese poultry. *Antibiotics (Basel)* 5:5.

47. Szmolka A, Fortini D, Villa L, Carattoli A, Anjum MF, Nagy B. 2011. First report on IncN plasmid-mediated quinolone resistance gene qnrS1 in porcine *Escherichia coli* in Europe. *Microb Drug Resist* 17:567–573.

48. Batchelor M, Hopkins KL, Liebana E, Slickers P, Ehricht R, Mafura M, Aarestrup F, Mevius D, Clifton-Hadley FA, Woodward MJ, Davies RH, Threlfall EJ, Anjum MF. 2008. Development of a miniaturised microarray-based assay for the rapid identification of antimicrobial resistance genes in Gram-negative bacteria. *Int J Antimicrob Agents* 31:440–451.

49. Szmolka A, Anjum MF, La Ragione RM, Kaszanyitzky EJ, Nagy B. 2012. Microarray based comparative genotyping of gentamicin resistant *Escherichia coli* strains from food animals and humans. *Vet Microbiol* 156:110–118.

50. Olowe OA, Choudhary S, Schierack P, Wieler LH, Makanjuola OB, Olayemi AB, Anjum M. 2013. Pathotyping bla CTX-M *Escherichia coli* from Nigeria. *Eur J Microbiol Immunol (Bp)* 3:120–125.

51. Anjum MF, Choudhary S, Morrison V, Snow LC, Mafura M, Slickers P, Ehricht R, Woodward MJ. 2011. Identifying antimicrobial resistance genes of human clinical relevance within *Salmonella* isolated from food animals in Great Britain. *J Antimicrob Chemother* 66:550–559.

52. Kirchner M, Abuoun M, Mafura M, Bagnall M, Hunt T, Thomas C, Weile J, Anjum MF. 2013. Cefotaxime resistant *Escherichia coli* collected from a healthy volunteer; characterisation and the effect of plasmid loss. *PLoS One* 8:e84142.

53. Kirchner M, Mafura M, Hunt T, Abu-Oun M, Nunez-Garcia J, Hu Y, Weile J, Coates A, Card R, Anjum MF. 2014. Antimicrobial resistance characteristics and fitness of Gram-negative fecal bacteria from volunteers treated with minocycline or amoxicillin. *Front Microbiol* 5:722.

54. Kirchner M, Mafura M, Hunt T, Card R, Anjum MF. 2013. Antibiotic resistance gene profiling of faecal and

oral anaerobes collected during an antibiotic challenge trial. *Anaerobe* **23**:20–22.

55. Card RM, Warburton PJ, MacLaren N, Mullany P, Allan E, Anjum MF. 2014. Application of microarray and functional-based screening methods for the detection of antimicrobial resistance genes in the microbiomes of healthy humans. *PLoS One* **9**:e86428.

56. Huehn S, La Ragione RM, Anjum M, Saunders M, Woodward MJ, Bunge C, Helmuth R, Hauser E, Guerra B, Beutlich J, Brisabois A, Peters T, Svensson L, Madajczak G, Litrup E, Imre A, Herrera-Leon S, Mevius D, Newell DG, Malorny B. 2010. Virulotyping and antimicrobial resistance typing of *Salmonella enterica* serovars relevant to human health in Europe. *Foodborne Pathog Dis* **7**:523–535.

57. Garneau P, Labrecque O, Maynard C, Messier S, Masson L, Archambault M, Harel J. 2010. Use of a bacterial antimicrobial resistance gene microarray for the identification of resistant *Staphylococcus aureus*. *Zoonoses Public Health* **57**(Suppl 1):94–99.

58. Perreten V, Kadlec K, Schwarz S, Grönlund Andersson U, Finn M, Greko C, Moodley A, Kania SA, Frank LA, Bemis DA, Franco A, Iurescia M, Battisti A, Duim B, Wagenaar JA, van Duijkeren E, Weese JS, Fitzgerald JR, Rossano A, Guardabassi L. 2010. Clonal spread of methicillin-resistant *Staphylococcus pseudintermedius* in Europe and North America: an international multicentre study. *J Antimicrob Chemother* **65**:1145–1154.

59. El-Adawy H, Ahmed M, Hotzel H, Monecke S, Schulz J, Hartung J, Ehricht R, Neubauer H, Hafez HM. 2016. Characterization of methicillin-resistant *Staphylococcus aureus* isolated from healthy turkeys and broilers using DNA microarrays. *Front Microbiol* **7**:2019.

60. McManus BA, Coleman DC, Deasy EC, Brennan GI, O'Connell B, Monecke S, Ehricht R, Leggett B, Leonard N, Shore AC. 2015. Comparative genotypes, staphylococcal cassette chromosome mec (SCCmec) genes and antimicrobial resistance amongst *Staphylococcus epidermidis* and *Staphylococcus haemolyticus* isolates from infections in humans and companion animals. *PLoS One* **10**:e0138079.

61. Nimmo GR, Steen JA, Monecke S, Ehricht R, Slickers P, Thomas JC, Appleton S, Goering RV, Robinson DA, Coombs GW. 2015. ST2249-MRSA-III: a second major recombinant methicillin-resistant *Staphylococcus aureus* clone causing healthcare infection in the 1970s. *Clin Microbiol Infect* **21**:444–450.

62. Schlotter K, Huber-Schlenstedt R, Gangl A, Hotzel H, Monecke S, Müller E, Reißig A, Proft S, Ehricht R. 2014. Multiple cases of methicillin-resistant CC130 *Staphylococcus aureus* harboring *mecC* in milk and swab samples from a Bavarian dairy herd. *J Dairy Sci* **97**:2782–2788.

63. Piccinini R, Tassi R, Daprà V, Pilla R, Fenner J, Carter B, Anjum MF. 2012. Study of *Staphylococcus aureus* collected at slaughter from dairy cows with chronic mastitis. *J Dairy Res* **79**:249–255.

64. Pilla R, Castiglioni V, Gelain ME, Scanziani E, Lorenzi V, Anjum M, Piccinini R. 2012. Long-term study of MRSA ST1, t127 mastitis in a dairy cow. *Vet Rec* **170**:312.

65. Zankari E, Hasman H, Cosentino S, Vestergaard M, Rasmussen S, Lund O, Aarestrup FM, Larsen MV. 2012. Identification of acquired antimicrobial resistance genes. *J Antimicrob Chemother* **67**:2640–2644.

66. Gupta SK, Padmanabhan BR, Diene SM, Lopez-Rojas R, Kempf M, Landraud L, Rolain JM. 2014. ARG-ANNOT, a new bioinformatic tool to discover antibiotic resistance genes in bacterial genomes. *Antimicrob Agents Chemother* **58**:212–220.

67. Kwong JC, McCallum N, Sintchenko V, Howden BP. 2015. Whole genome sequencing in clinical and public health microbiology. *Pathology* **47**:199–210.

68. Padmanabhan R, Mishra AK, Raoult D, Fournier PE. 2013. Genomics and metagenomics in medical microbiology. *J Microbiol Methods* **95**:415–424.

69. Edwards DJ, Holt KE. 2013. Beginner's guide to comparative bacterial genome analysis using next-generation sequence data. *Microb Inform Exp* **3**:2.

70. Gargis AS, Kalman L, Berry MW, Bick DP, Dimmock DP, Hambuch T, Lu F, Lyon E, Voelkerding KV, Zehnbauer BA, Agarwala R, Bennett SF, Chen B, Chin EL, Compton JG, Das S, Farkas DH, Ferber MJ, Funke BH, Furtado MR, Ganova-Raeva LM, Geigenmüller U, Gunselman SJ, Hegde MR, Johnson PL, Kasarskis A, Kulkarni S, Lenk T, Liu CS, Manion M, Manolio TA, Mardis ER, Merker JD, Rajeevan MS, Reese MG, Rehm HL, Simen BB, Yeakley JM, Zook JM, Lubin IM. 2012. Assuring the quality of next-generation sequencing in clinical laboratory practice. *Nat Biotechnol* **30**: 1033–1036.

71. Ellington MJ, Ekelund O, Aarestrup FM, Canton R, Doumith M, Giske C, Grundman H, Hasman H, Holden MT, Hopkins KL, Iredell J, Kahlmeter G, Köser CU, MacGowan A, Mevius D, Mulvey M, Naas T, Peto T, Rolain JM, Samuelsen Ø, Woodford N. 2017. The role of whole genome sequencing in antimicrobial susceptibility testing of bacteria: report from the EUCAST Subcommittee. *Clin Microbiol Infect* **23**:2–22.

72. Thomsen MC, Ahrenfeldt J, Cisneros JL, Jurtz V, Larsen MV, Hasman H, Aarestrup FM, Lund O. 2016. A bacterial analysis platform: an integrated system for analysing bacterial whole genome sequencing data for clinical diagnostics and surveillance. *PLoS One* **11**: e0157718.

73. Clausen PT, Zankari E, Aarestrup FM, Lund O. 2016. Benchmarking of methods for identification of antimicrobial resistance genes in bacterial whole genome data. *J Antimicrob Chemother* **71**:2484–2488.

74. McArthur AG, Tsang KK. 2017. Antimicrobial resistance surveillance in the genomic age. *Ann N Y Acad Sci* **1388**:78–91.

75. Sharma M, Nunez-Garcia J, Kearns AM, Doumith M, Butaye PR, Argudín MA, Lahuerta-Marin A, Pichon B, AbuOun M, Rogers J, Ellis RJ, Teale C, Anjum MF. 2016. Livestock-associated methicillin resistant *Staphylococcus aureus* (LA-MRSA) clonal complex (CC) 398 isolated from UK animals belong to European lineages. *Front Microbiol* **7**:1741.

76. Doumith M, Godbole G, Ashton P, Larkin L, Dallman T, Day M, Day M, Muller-Pebody B, Ellington MJ, de

Pinna E, Johnson AP, Hopkins KL, Woodford N. 2016. Detection of the plasmid-mediated *mcr-1* gene conferring colistin resistance in human and food isolates of *Salmonella enterica* and *Escherichia coli* in England and Wales. *J Antimicrob Chemother* 71:2300–2305.

77. Garvey MI, Pichon B, Bradley CW, Moiemen NS, Oppenheim B, Kearns AM. 2016. Improved understanding of an outbreak of meticillin-resistant *Staphylococcus aureus* in a regional burns centre via whole-genome sequencing. *J Hosp Infect* 94:401–404.

78. Stoesser N, Batty EM, Eyre DW, Morgan M, Wyllie DH, Del Ojo Elias C, Johnson JR, Walker AS, Peto TE, Crook DW. 2013. Predicting antimicrobial susceptibilities for *Escherichia coli* and *Klebsiella pneumoniae* isolates using whole genomic sequence data. *J Antimicrob Chemother* 68:2234–2244.

79. Bradley P, Gordon NC, Walker TM, Dunn L, Heys S, Huang B, Earle S, Pankhurst LJ, Anson L, de Cesare M, Piazza P, Votintseva AA, Golubchik T, Wilson DJ, Wyllie DH, Diel R, Niemann S, Feuerriegel S, Kohl TA, Ismail N, Omar SV, Smith EG, Buck D, McVean G, Walker AS, Peto TE, Crook DW, Iqbal Z. 2015. Rapid antibiotic-resistance predictions from genome sequence data for *Staphylococcus aureus* and *Mycobacterium tuberculosis*. *Nat Commun* 6:10063.

80. McArthur AG, Waglechner N, Nizam F, Yan A, Azad MA, Baylay AJ, Bhullar K, Canova MJ, De Pascale G, Ejim L, Kalan L, King AM, Koteva K, Morar M, Mulvey MR, O'Brien JS, Pawlowski AC, Piddock LJ, Spanogiannopoulos P, Sutherland AD, Tang I, Taylor PL, Thaker M, Wang W, Yan M, Yu T, Wright GD. 2013. The comprehensive antibiotic resistance database. *Antimicrob Agents Chemother* 57:3348–3357.

81. McArthur AG, Wright GD. 2015. Bioinformatics of antimicrobial resistance in the age of molecular epidemiology. *Curr Opin Microbiol* 27:45–50.

82. Inouye M, Dashnow H, Raven LA, Schultz MB, Pope BJ, Tomita T, Zobel J, Holt KE. 2014. SRST2: rapid genomic surveillance for public health and hospital microbiology labs. *Genome Med* 6:90.

83. Langmead B, Salzberg SL. 2012. Fast gapped-read alignment with Bowtie 2. *Nat Methods* 9:357–359.

84. Hasman H, Saputra D, Sicheritz-Ponten T, Lund O, Svendsen CA, Frimodt-Møller N, Aarestrup FM. 2014. Rapid whole-genome sequencing for detection and characterization of microorganisms directly from clinical samples. *J Clin Microbiol* 52:139–146.

85. Schmieder R, Edwards R. 2012. Insights into antibiotic resistance through metagenomic approaches. *Future Microbiol* 7:73–89.

86. Wang Z, Zhang XX, Huang K, Miao Y, Shi P, Liu B, Long C, Li A. 2013. Metagenomic profiling of antibiotic resistance genes and mobile genetic elements in a tannery wastewater treatment plant. *PLoS One* 8:e76079.

87. Li H, Durbin R. 2010. Fast and accurate long-read alignment with Burrows-Wheeler transform. *Bioinformatics* 26:589–595.

88. Li H, Handsaker B, Wysoker A, Fennell T, Ruan J, Homer N, Marth G, Abecasis G, Durbin R, 1000 Genome Project Data Processing Subgroup. 2009. The Sequence Alignment/Map format and SAMtools. *Bioinformatics* 25:2078–2079.

89. Nordahl Petersen T, Rasmussen S, Hasman H, Carøe C, Bælum J, Schultz AC, Bergmark L, Svendsen CA, Lund O, Sicheritz-Pontén T, Aarestrup FM. 2015. Metagenomic analysis of toilet waste from long distance flights; a step towards global surveillance of infectious diseases and antimicrobial resistance. *Sci Rep* 5:11444.

90. Knudsen BE, Bergmark L. 2016. Impact of sample type and DNA isolation procedure on genomic inference of microbiome composition. *mSystems* 1:e00095-16.

91. Murray PR. 2012. What is new in clinical microbiology-microbial identification by MALDI-TOF mass spectrometry: a paper from the 2011 William Beaumont Hospital Symposium on molecular pathology. *J Mol Diagn* 14:419–423.

92. Hrabák J, Chudáčková E, Papagiannitsis CC. 2014. Detection of carbapenemases in *Enterobacteriaceae*: a challenge for diagnostic microbiological laboratories. *Clin Microbiol Infect* 20:839–853.

93. Panda A, Kurapati S, Samantaray JC, Srinivasan A, Khalil S. 2014. MALDI-TOF mass spectrometry proteomic based identification of clinical bacterial isolates. *Indian J Med Res* 140:770–777.

94. Kumar A, Roberts D, Wood KE, Light B, Parrillo JE, Sharma S, Suppes R, Feinstein D, Zanotti S, Taiberg L, Gurka D, Kumar A, Cheang M. 2006. Duration of hypotension before initiation of effective antimicrobial therapy is the critical determinant of survival in human septic shock. *Crit Care Med* 34:1589–1596.

95. Frickmann H, Masanta WO, Zautner AE. 2014. Emerging rapid resistance testing methods for clinical microbiology laboratories and their potential impact on patient management. *BioMed Res Int* 2014:375681.

96. Bauer KA, Perez KK, Forrest GN, Goff DA. 2014. Review of rapid diagnostic tests used by antimicrobial stewardship programs. *Clin Infect Dis* 59(Suppl 3):S134–S145.

97. Kostrzewa M, Sparbier K, Maier T, Schubert S. 2013. MALDI-TOF MS: an upcoming tool for rapid detection of antibiotic resistance in microorganisms. *Proteomics Clin Appl* 7:767–778.

98. Schaumann R, Knoop N, Genzel GH, Losensky K, Rosenkranz C, Stîngu CS, Schellenberger W, Rodloff AC, Eschrich K. 2012. A step towards the discrimination of beta-lactamase-producing clinical isolates of *Enterobacteriaceae* and *Pseudomonas aeruginosa* by MALDI-TOF mass spectrometry. *Med Sci Monit* 18:MT71–MT77.

99. dos Santos KV, Diniz CG, Veloso LC, de Andrade HM, Giusta MS, Pires SF, Santos AV, Apolônio AC, de Carvalho MA, Farias LM. 2010. Proteomic analysis of *Escherichia coli* with experimentally induced resistance to piperacillin/tazobactam. *Res Microbiol* 161:268–275.

100. Hrabák J, Chudáckova E, Walková R. 2013. Matrix-assisted laser desorption ionization-time of flight (MALDI-TOF) mass spectrometry for detection of antibiotic resistance mechanisms: from research to routine diagnosis. *Clin Microbiol Rev* 26:103–114.

101. Burckhardt I, Zimmermann S. 2011. Using matrix-assisted laser desorption ionization-time of flight mass spectrometry to detect carbapenem resistance within 1 to 2.5 hours. *J Clin Microbiol* **49:**3321–3324.

102. Studentova V, Papagiannitsis CC, Izdebski R, Pfeifer Y, Chudackova E, Bergerova T, Gniadkowski M, Hrabak J. 2015. Detection of OXA-48-type carbapenemase-producing *Enterobacteriaceae* in diagnostic laboratories can be enhanced by addition of bicarbonates to cultivation media or reaction buffers. *Folia Microbiol (Praha)* **60:**119–129.

103. Chong PM, McCorrister SJ, Unger MS, Boyd DA, Mulvey MR, Westmacott GR. 2015. MALDI-TOF MS detection of carbapenemase activity in clinical isolates of *Enterobacteriaceae* spp., *Pseudomonas aeruginosa*, and *Acinetobacter baumannii* compared against the Carba-NP assay. *J Microbiol Methods* **111:**21–23.

104. Wang Y, Tian GB, Zhang R, Shen Y, Tyrrell JM, Huang X, Zhou H, Lei L, Li HY, Doi Y, Fang Y, Ren H, Zhong LL, Shen Z, Zeng KJ, Wang S, Liu JH, Wu C, Walsh TR, Shen J. 2017. Prevalence, risk factors, outcomes, and molecular epidemiology of mcr-1-positive *Enterobacteriaceae* in patients and healthy adults from China: an epidemiological and clinical study. *Lancet Infect Dis* **17:**390–399.

Antimicrobial Resistance in Bacteria from Livestock and Companion Animals
Edited by Frank Møller Aarestrup, Stefan Schwarz, Jianzhong Shen, and Lina Cavaco
© 2018 American Society for Microbiology, Washington, DC
doi:10.1128/microbiolspec.ARBA-0019-2017

Mechanisms of Bacterial Resistance to Antimicrobial Agents

4

Engeline van Duijkeren,[1] Anne-Kathrin Schink,[2] Marilyn C. Roberts,[3] Yang Wang,[4] and Stefan Schwarz[2]

INTRODUCTION

With regard to their structures and functions, antimicrobial agents represent a highly diverse group of low-molecular-weight substances which interfere with bacterial growth, resulting in either a timely limited growth inhibition (bacteriostatic effect) or the killing of the bacteria (bactericidal effect). For more than 60 years, antimicrobial agents have been used to control bacterial infections in humans, animals, and plants. Nowadays, antimicrobial agents are among the most frequently used therapeutics in human and veterinary medicine (1, 2). In the early days of antimicrobial chemotherapy, antimicrobial resistance was not considered as an important problem, since the numbers of resistant strains were low and a large number of new highly effective antimicrobial agents of different classes were detected. These early antimicrobial agents represented products of the metabolic pathways of soil bacteria (e.g., *Streptomyces*, *Bacillus*) or fungi (e.g., *Penicillium*, *Cephalosporium*, *Pleurotus*) (Table 1) and provided their producers with a selective advantage in the fight for resources and the colonization of ecological niches (3). This in turn forced the susceptible bacteria living in close contact with the antimicrobial producers to develop and/or refine mechanisms to circumvent the inhibitory effects of antimicrobial agents. As a consequence, the origins of bacterial resistance to antimicrobial agents can be assumed to be in a time long before the clinical use of these substances. With the elucidation of the chemical structure of the antimicrobial agents, which commonly followed soon after their detection, it was possible not only to produce an-

timicrobial agents synthetically in larger amounts at lower costs, but also to introduce modifications that altered the pharmacological properties of these substances and occasionally also extended their spectrum of activity.

The increased selective pressure imposed by the widespread use of antimicrobial agents since the 1950s has distinctly accelerated the development and the spread of bacterial resistance to antimicrobial agents. In most cases, it took not longer than three to five years after the introduction of an antimicrobial agent into clinical use until the first resistant target bacteria occurred (1). This is particularly true for broad-spectrum antimicrobial agents, such as tetracyclines, aminoglycosides, macrolides, and β-lactams, which have been used for multiple purposes in human and veterinary medicine, horticulture, and/or aquaculture. In contrast, this time span was extended to ≥15 years for narrow-spectrum agents, such as glycopeptides, which were used at distinctly lower quantities and only for specific applications. Multiple studies have also revealed that resistance to completely synthetic antimicrobial agents, such as sulfonamides, trimethoprim, fluoroquinolones, and oxazolidinones, can develop quickly (4–7). These observations underline the enormous flexibility of the bacteria to cope with less favorable environmental conditions by constantly exploring new ways to survive in the presence of antimicrobial agents.

This chapter summarizes the latest information on resistance mechanisms and the mobile elements involved. It is a completely revised and updated version of the chapter that was published in 2006 (8).

[1]Center for Infectious Disease Control, National Institute for Public Health and the Environment (RIVM), 3720 BA Bilthoven, The Netherlands; [2]Institute of Microbiology and Epizootics, Centre of Infection Medicine, Department of Veterinary Medicine, Freie Universität Berlin, 14163 Berlin, Germany; [3]Department of Environmental and Occupational Health Sciences, University of Washington, Seattle, WA 98195-7234; [4]Beijing Advanced Innovation Center for Food Nutrition and Human Health, College of Veterinary Medicine, China Agricultural University, Beijing, 100193, China.

Table 1 Origins of antimicrobial agents

Class	Antimicrobial agent	Producing organisms	Year(s) of isolation/ description
β-Lactam antibiotics	Natural penicillins	*Penicillium notatum, Penicillium chrysogenum*	1929, 1940
	Cephalosporin C	*Cephalosporium acremonium*	1945, 1953
	Imipenem	*Streptomyces cattleya*	1976
	Aztreonam	*Gluconobacter* spp., *Chromobacterium violaceum*	1981
Glycopeptides	Vancomycin	*Amycolatopsis orientalis*	mid-1950s
	Teicoplanin, avoparcin	*Amycolatopsis coloradensis* subsp. *labeda*	1975
Macrolides	Erythromycin	*Streptomyces erythreus*	1952
	Spiramycin	*Streptomyces ambofaciens*	1955
Lincosamides	Lincomycin	*Streptomyces lincolnensis*	1963
Streptogramins	Streptogramin A+B	*Streptomyces diastaticus*	1953
	Virginiamycin A+B	*Streptomyces virginiae*	1955
Tetracyclines	Chlortetracycline	*Streptomyces aureofaciens*	1948
	Oxytetracycline	*Streptomyces rimosus*	1950
Phenicols	Chloramphenicol	*Streptomyces venezuelae*	1947
Aminoglycosides	Streptomycin	*Streptomyces griseus*	1943
	Neomycin	*Streptomyces fradiae*	1949
	Kanamycin	*Streptomyces kanamyceticus*	1957
	Gentamicin	*Micromonospora purpura*	1963
	Tobramycin	*Streptomyces tenebrarius*	1967
Aminocyclitols	Spectinomycin	*Streptomyces spectabilis*	1961
Pleuromutilins	Pleuromutilin, Tiamulin	*Pleurotus* spp.; synthetic	1951, 1976
Polypeptide antibiotics	Polymyxin B	*Bacillus polymyxa (aerosporus)*	1947
	Polymyxin E (colistin)	*B. polymyxa* var. *colistinus*	1949
	Bacitracin	*Bacillus licheniformis*	1943
Epoxide antibiotics	Fosfomycin	*Streptomyces fradiae, Streptomyces wedmorensis, Pseudomonas syringae*	1969
Pseudomonic acid antibiotics	Mupirocin	*Pseudomonas fluorescens*	1971
Steroid antibiotics	Fusidic acid	*Fusidium coccineum*	1960
Streptothricins	Nourseothricin	*Streptomyces noursei*	1963
Sulfonamides	Prontosil, sulfamethoxazole, etc.	Synthetic	1935
Trimethoprim	Trimethoprim	Synthetic	1956
Quinolones	Nalidixic acid	Synthetic	1962
Fluoroquinolones	Flumequine, enrofloxacin, etc.	Synthetic	1973
Oxazolidinones	Linezolid	Synthetic	1987, 1996

RESISTANCE TO ANTIMICROBIAL AGENTS

Resistance to antimicrobial agents can be divided into two basic types, intrinsic resistance and acquired resistance (1, 3, 8, 9). Intrinsic resistance, also known as primary or innate resistance, describes a status of general insensitivity of bacteria to a specific antimicrobial agent or class of agents. This is commonly due to the lack or the inaccessibility of target structures for certain antimicrobial agents, e.g., resistance to β-lactam antibiotics and glycopeptides in cell wall-free bacteria, such as *Mycoplasma* spp., or vancomycin resistance in Gram-negative bacteria due to the inability of vancomycin to penetrate the outer membrane. It can also be due to the presence of export systems or the production of species-specific inactivating enzymes in certain bacteria, e.g., the

AcrAB-TolC system or the production of AmpC β-lactamase in certain *Enterobacteriaceae*. In addition, some bacteria, such as enterococci, can use exogenous folates and are thus not dependent on a functional folate synthesis pathway. As a consequence, they are intrinsically resistant to folate pathway inhibitors, such as trimethoprim and sulfonamides (9). Intrinsic resistance is a genus- or species-specific property of bacteria. In contrast, acquired resistance is a strain-specific property which can be due to the acquisition of foreign resistance genes or mutational modification of chromosomal target genes. Mutations that upregulate the expression of multidrug transporter systems may also fall into this category. Three different basic types of resistance mechanisms can be differentiated: (i) enzymatic inactivation by either disintegration or chemical modification of the antimicrobials (Table 2), (ii) reduced intracellular accumulation by decreased influx and/or increased efflux of antimicrobials (Table 3), and (iii) modification of the cellular target sites by mutation, chemical modification, or protection of the target sites, but also overexpression of sensitive targets or the replacement of sensitive target structures by alternative resistant ones (Table 4) (1, 3, 8, 9).

The following subsections illustrate that bacterial resistance to antimicrobial agents varies depending on the agents, the bacteria, and the resistance mechanism. Resistance to the same antimicrobial agent can be mediated by different mechanisms. In some cases, the same resistance gene/mechanism is found in a wide variety of bacteria, whereas in other cases, resistance genes or mechanisms appear to be limited to certain bacterial species or genera. The data presented in the following subsections do not focus exclusively on resistance genes and mechanisms so far detected in bacteria of animal origin but also include resistance genes and mechanisms identified in bacteria from humans. For the best possible overview of the mechanisms and genes accounting for resistance to a specific class of antimicrobial agents, all data are presented under the names of the classes of antimicrobial agents.

Resistance to -Lactam Antibiotics

A number of penicillins, alone or in combination with a β-lactamase inhibitor, as well as first- to fourth-generation cephalosporins, are licensed for use in veterinary medicine. No carbapenems or monobactams are currently approved for use in animals. Resistance to β-lactam antibiotics is mainly due to inactivation by β-lactamases (10) and decreased ability to bind to penicillin-binding proteins (PBPs) (11) in both Gram-positive and Gram-negative bacteria, but may also be based on decreased uptake of β-lactams due to perme-

Table 2 Examples of resistance to antimicrobials by **decreased intracellular drug accumulation** (modified from ref. 8)[a,b]

Resistance mechanism	Resistance gene(s)	Gene product	Resistance phenotype	Bacteria involved	Location of the resistance gene
efflux via specific exporters	mef(A)	10-TMS efflux system of the major facilitator superfamily	14-, 15-membered macrolides	Streptococcus, other Gram+ and Gram– bacteria	T, P, C
	tet(A-E, G, H, I, J, K, L, Z), tetA(P), tet(30)	12-, 14-TMS efflux system of the major facilitator superfamily	tetracyclines	various Gram+ and Gram– bacteria	P, T, C
	pp-flo, floR, floR$_V$	12 TMS efflux system of the major facilitator superfamily	chloramphenicol, florfenicol	Photobacterium, Vibrio, Salmonella, Escherichia, Klebsiella, Pasteurella	T, P, C
	cmlA	12 TMS efflux system of the major facilitator superfamily	chloramphenicol	Pseudomonas, Salmonella, E. coli	T, P, C
	fexA	14 TMS efflux system of the major facilitator superfamily	chloramphenicol, florfenicol	Staphylococcus	T, P, C
	fexB	14 TMS efflux system of the major facilitator superfamily	chloramphenicol, florfenicol	Enterococcus	P
efflux via multidrug transporters	emrE	4-TMS multidrug efflux protein	tetracyclines, nucleic acid binding compounds	E. coli	C
	blt, norA	12-TMS multidrug efflux protein of the major facilitator superfamily	chloramphenicol, fluoroquinolones, nucleic acid binding compounds	Bacillus, Staphylococcus	C
	mexB-mexA-oprM, acrA-acrB-tolC	multidrug efflux in combination with specific OMP's	chloramphenicol, β-lactams, macrolides, fluoroquinolones, tetracyclines, etc.	Pseudomonas, E. coli, Salmonella	C

[a]P = plasmid; T = transposon; GC = gene cassette; C = chromosomal DNA.
[b]TMS = transmembrane segments.

Table 3 Examples of resistance to antimicrobials by enzymatic inactivation[a]

Resistance mechanism	Resistance gene(s)	Gene product	Resistance phenotype	Bacteria involved	Location of the resistance gene[b]
Hydrolytic degradation	*bla*	β-lactamases	β-lactam antibiotics	Various Gram+, Gram–, aerobic, anaerobic bacteria	P, T, GC, C
	ere(A), *ere*(B)	esterases	macrolides	Gram+, Gram– bacteria	P, GC
	vgb(A), *vgb*(B)	lactone hydrolases	streptogramin B antibiotics	*Staphylococcus, Enterococcus*	P
Chemical modification	*aac, aad (ant), aph*	acetyl-, adenyl-, phosphotransferases	aminoglycosides	Gram+, Gram–, aerobic bacteria	T, GC, P, C
	aad (ant)	adenyltransferases	aminoglycosides/ aminocyclitols	Gram+, Gram–, aerobic bacteria	T, GC, P, C
	catA, catB	acetyltransferases	chloramphenicol	Gram+, Gram–, aerobic, anaerobic bacteria	P, T, GC, C
	vat(A-G)	acetyltransferases	streptogramin A antibiotics	*Bacteroides, Staphylococcus, Enterococcus, Lactobacillus, Yersinia*	P, C
	mph(A-G)	phosphotransferases	macrolides	Gram+, Gram– bacteria	P, T, C
	lnu(A-P)	nucleotidyltransferases	lincosamides	Gram+, Gram– bacteria	P
	tet(X), *tet*(37), *tet*(56)	oxidoreductases	tetracyclines	Gram– bacteria, unknown, *Legionella*	T, P

[a]Modified from reference 8.
[b]Abbreviations: P, plasmid; T, transposon; GC, gene cassette; C, chromosomal DNA.

ability barriers or increased efflux via multidrug transporter systems (12, 13). Inactivation via β-lactamases is most commonly seen, with a wide range of β-lactamases involved. The evolution of β-lactamases which differ distinctly in their substrate spectra is believed to have occurred in response to the selective pressure imposed by the various β-lactam antibiotics that have been introduced into clinical use during the past decades (14).

Enzymatic inactivation of β-lactam antibiotics is based on the cleavage of the amino bond in the β-lactam ring by β-lactamases (10, 15, 16). At present, more than 1,000 β-lactamases have been described, most of which are variants of known β-lactamases that differ in their substrate spectra or their enzyme stability. Two classification schemes are currently in use. The initial classification scheme was based on the similarities in the amino acid sequences and divided the β-lactamases into two molecular classes, A and B (17), which were later expanded to four molecular classes, A to D (18). The second functional classification of β-lactamases was updated in 2010 by Bush and Jacoby (18) and is done on the basis of their substrate spectra and their susceptibility to β-lactamase inhibitors such as clavulanic acid (18). This system subdivides the β-lactamases into three groups, 1 to 3, with group 1 currently comprising 2 subgroups, group 2 comprising 12 subgroups, and group 3 comprising 2 subgroups.

Group 1 β-lactamases (molecular class C), for example, AmpC, CMY, ACT, DHA, FOX, and MIR, are cephalosporinases that are more active on cephalosporins than benzylpenicillin and are usually not inhibited by clavulanic acid. They are widespread among Gram-negative bacteria. The *ampC* genes are commonly located on the chromosome but may also be found on plasmids. Some of these *ampC* genes are expressed inducibly; others are expressed constitutively (18). Point mutations in the promotor or attenuator region may increase β-lactamase production. Subgroup 1e enzymes are group 1 variants with greater activity against ceftazidime and other oxyimino-β-lactams as a result of amino acid substitutions, insertions, or deletions and include GC1 in *Enterobacter cloacae* and plasmid-mediated CMY-10, CMY-19, and CMY-37. They have been named extended-spectrum AmpC β-lactamases (18).

Group 2 β-lactamases (molecular classes A and D) represent diverse enzymes, most of which are sensitive to inhibition by clavulanic acid. Subgroup 2a (molecular class A) includes enzymes such as BlaZ from staphylococci, which can inactivate only penicillins. Subgroup 2b (molecular class A) comprises broad-spectrum β-lactamases, such as TEM-1, TEM-2, SHV-1, and ROB-1, which can hydrolize penicillins and broad-spectrum cephalosporins. Subgroup 2be represents extended-spectrum β-lactamases (ESBLs; e.g., variants of TEM and SHV families and CTX-M type enzymes), which can also inactivate oxyimino cephalosporins and monobactams. Subgroups 2a, 2b, and 2be enzymes are sensi-

Table 4 Examples of resistance to antimicrobials by **target modification** (modified from ref. 8)[a]

Resistance mechanism	Resistance gene(s)	Gene product	Resistance phenotype	Bacteria involved	Location of the resistance gene
methylation of the target site	erm	rRNA methylase	macrolides, lincosamides, streptogramin B compounds	various Gram+ bacteria, Escherichia, Bacteroides	P, T, C
protection of the target site	tet(M, O, P, Q, S, T)	ribosome protective proteins	tetracyclines	various Gram+ and Gram– bacteria	T, P, C
	vga(A)	ribosome protective ABC-F protein	lincosamides, pleuromutilins, streptogramin A-compounds	Staphylococcus,	P, T, C
	optrA	ribosome protective ABC-F protein	oxazolidinones, phenicols	Enterococcus, Staphylococcus	P, C
replacement of a sensitive target by an alternative drug-resistant target	sul1, sul2, sul3	sulfonamide-resistant dihydropteroate synthase	sulfonamides	various Gram– bacteria	P, I
	dfrA, dfrB, dfrD, dfrG, dfrK	trimethoprim-resistant dihydrofolate reductase	trimethoprim	various Gram+ and Gram– bacteria	P, GC, T, C
	mecA, mecC	penicillin-binding proteins with altered substrate specificity	penicillins, cephalosporins, carbapenems, monobactams	Staphylococcus	C
	vanA-E	alternative D-Ala-D-Lac or D-Ala-D-Ser peptidoglycan precursors	glycopeptides	Enterococcus, Staphylococcus	T, P, C
alteration of the LPS	mcr-1 to mcr-5	phosphoethanolamine transferase	colistin	Enterobacteriaceae	T, P, C
mutational modification of the target site	—	mutation in the gene coding for ribosomal protein S12	streptomycin	several Gram+ and Gram– bacteria	C
	—	mutation in the 16S rRNA	streptomycin	Mycobacterium	C
	—	mutation in the 23S rRNA	macrolides	Mycobacterium	C
	—	mutation in the 16S rRNA	tetracyclines	Propionibacterium	C
	—	mutations in the genes for DNA gyrase and topoisomerase	fluoroquinolones	various Gram+ and Gram– bacteria	C
	—	mutation in the gene for the ribosomal protein L3	tiamulin	E. coli	C
mutational modification of regulatory elements	—	mutations in the marRAB soxR or acrR genes	fluoroquinolones	E. coli	C

[a]P = plasmid; T = transposon; GC = gene cassette; C = chromosomal DNA, I = integron.

tive to inhibition by clavulanic acid. Due to their wide spectrum of activity, ESBLs are a serious cause of concern (19). Most currently known ESBLs belong to the TEM, SHV, CTX-M, or OXA families of β-lactamases. Less common ESBLs include BEL-1, BES-1, SFO-1, TLA-1, TLA-2, and members of the PER and VEB enzyme families. Details about the structure and function of these ESBLs, their location on mobile elements, their dissemination among bacteria of different species and genera, and information on ESBL detection methods can be found in several reviews (19–21). Moreover,

a continuosly updated database which lists the known ESBLs and inhibitor-resistant β-lactamases including TEM, SHV, OXA, CTX-M, CMY, IMP, and VIM types can be found at https://www.ncbi.nlm.nih.gov/pathogens/beta-lactamase-data-resources/. The enzymes of subgroup 2br (molecular class A) are also broad-spectrum β-lactamases, such as TEM-30, TEM-31, and SHV-10, which however, are not inhibited by clavulanic acid. Analysis of the β-lactamases of subgroups 2b, 2be, and 2br—in particular, those of the TEM and SHV types—revealed the presence of mutations which either extended the substrate spectrum or affected the enzyme stability (10, 14, 19). TEM enzymes that exhibit an extended spectrum and increased resistance to clavulanic acid inhibition are organized in subgroup 2ber and are called complex mutant TEM (CMT); these include TEM-50 (CMT-1) and TEM-158 (CMT-9) (18). Subgroup 2c (molecular class A) includes inhibitor-sensitive carbenicillinases such as CARB-3, PSE-1, and RTG, whereas the extended-spectrum carbenicillinase RTG-4 in subgroup 2ce shows enhanced activity against cefepime and cefpirome. The β-lactamases of subgroup 2d (molecular class D) (e.g., OXA-type enzymes) exhibit variable sensitivity to inhibitors and can hydrolyze oxacillin or cloxacillin. The extended spectrum of the enzymes in subgroup 2de (e.g., OXA-11 and OXA-15) is defined by their ability to hydrolize oxacillin or cloxacillin as well as oxyimino β-lactams with a preference for ceftazidime. The subgroup 2df assembles OXA enzymes which are not inhibited by clavulanic acid and show carbapenem-hydrolyzing activities. The genes have been detected on plasmids and in the chromosome of Gram-negative bacteria (18). The β-lactamases of subgroups 2e and 2f represent cephalosporinases (e.g., CepA) or serine-carbapenemases (e.g., SME-1, IMI-1, KPC-2), which are sometimes inhibited by clavulanic acid (18).

While the β-lactamases of groups 1 and 2 have a serine residue in the catalytic center, the β-lactamases of group 3 (molecular class B) hydrolyze β-lactams by divalent cations (Zn^{2+}) and are referred to as metallo-β-lactamases (e.g., IMP-type, VIM-type, and NDM-type enzymes). Subgroup 3a consists of plasmid-encoded metallo-β-lactamases, which require two bound zinc ions for their activity. These enzymes can inactivate all β-lactams except monobactams and are insensitive to clavulanic acid but are inhibited by metal ion chelators such as EDTA. The metallo-β-lactamases in subgroup 3b preferentially hydrolyze carbapenems, especially if only one zinc-binding side is occupied (18). The location of many of the β-lactamase genes (bla) on either plasmids, transposons, or gene cassettes favors their dissemination (20–22).

Altered PBPs are often associated with resistance due to decreased binding of β-lactam antibiotics (11). PBPs are transpeptidases which play an important role in cell wall synthesis. They are present in most cell wall-containing bacteria, but they vary from species to species in number, size, amount, and affinity to β-lactam antibiotics (11). The acquisition of a novel PBP, such as the mecA-encoded PBP2a, which replaces the original β-lactam-sensitive PBP, is the cause of methicillin resistance in *Staphylococcus aureus*, *Staphylococcus pseudintermedius*, and coagulase-negative staphylococci

(23, 24). Methicillin-resistant staphylococci are resistant to virtually all β-lactam antibiotics except cefpirome. The *mecA* gene, which codes for the alternative PBP2a, is part of a genetic element, designated *Staphylococcus* cassette chromosome *mec* (SCC*mec*) (25). So far, 11 SCC*mec* types have been described (26). In 2011, a new *mecA* homologue, *mecC* (formerly called *mec*$_{LGA251}$), which is part of a distinct SCC*mec* type (SCC*mec* XI), was identified in methicillin-resistant *S. aureus* (MRSA) (27, 28). The majority of known MRSA-carrying *mecC* belong to clonal complex (CC) 130, but other CCs (CC425, CC1943, CC599, CC49) have also been found to harbor *mecC*. In addition, *mecC* is not restricted to *S. aureus* but has been found in several staphylococcal species including *Staphylococcus saprophyticus*, *Staphylococcus sciuri*, *Staphylococcus stepanovicii*, and *Staphylococcus xylosus* (29–31). In addition to PBP2a, the Fem proteins are involved in expression of methicillin resistance. The FemAB proteins contribute to the formation of the pentaglycine crossbridge, which is a unique staphylococcal cell wall component (32). Inactivation of *femAB* has been found to completely restore susceptibility to β-lactams and other antimicrobial agents in MRSA strains (33). PBPs with low affinity for β-lactams have also been detected in streptococci and enterococci (11). Homologous recombinations in the genes coding for PBPs 1a, 2a, and 2b are assumed to result in mosaic proteins with decreased affinity to β-lactams in *Streptococcus pneumoniae* and *Neisseria* spp.. PBPs, which have a low affinity to β-lactams, have been reported to be overproduced in resistant strains of *Enterococcus faecium* and *Enterococcus faecalis*. It is noteworthy that alterations in PBPs do not necessarily result in complete resistance to all β-lactams but can also lead to elevated MICs of selected β-lactam antibiotics (11).

Reduced uptake of β-lactams is due to decreased outer membrane permeability and/or the lack of certain outer membrane proteins, which serve as entries for β-lactams to the bacterial cell, and has been described in various *Enterobacteriaceae*, *Pseudomonas aeruginosa*, and other bacteria (34–36). In *Escherichia coli* and *Klebsiella pneumoniae*, β-lactam resistance can be based on the decreased expression or the structural alteration of the porins OmpF (37) and OmpK36 (38), by which β-lactams cross the outer membrane. In *P. aeruginosa*, resistance to imipenem has been shown to be based on the loss of the porin OprD (39).

Several multidrug transporters such as the MexAB/OprM and the MexCD/OprJ systems in *P. aeruginosa*, the SmeAB/SmeC system in *Stenotrophomonas maltophilia*, and the AcrAB/TolC system in *Salmonella enterica* and *E. coli* (40, 41) are known to mediate the export of β-lactam antibiotics.

Resistance to Tetracyclines

Among this family of antimicrobial agents, oxytetracycline, chlortetracycline, and tetracycline have been used in veterinary medicine since the 1950s. More recently, doxycycline has been approved for dogs, cats, and pigs. Up to now, minocycline and glycylcyclines have not been licensed for use in animals. Based on aggregated data from a survey on sales of veterinary antimicrobial agents in 25 European countries, the sales of tetracyclines accounted for 37% of the total sales of veterinary antimicrobial agents in 2011 (42). Thus, it is not surprising that tetracycline resistance has become widespread among bacteria of veterinary importance, including in aquaculture (43–45). Tetracycline resistance is usually due to the acquisition of new genes (46). There are 33 efflux genes, which code for energy-dependent efflux of tetracyclines, 12 ribosomal protection genes, which code for a protein that protects bacterial ribosomes, 13 genes which code for enzymes that modify and inactivate the tetracycline molecule, and 1 gene [*tet*(U)] which specifies tetracycline resistance by an unknown mechanism. The products of different *tet* genes share ≤79% amino acid identity (47). An updated database listing the currently known *tet* genes and their occurrence in various bacteria is available at http://faculty.washington.edu/marilynr/. This website is updated twice each year. New *tet* gene names are approved by Dr. Stuart B. Levy, Tufts University, Boston. Antibiotic resistance genes are not randomly distributed among bacteria. This has been well documented with the distribution of *tet* genes (47–50).

The energy-dependent efflux of tetracyclines is mediated by membrane-associated proteins which exchange a proton for a tetracycline-cation complex (46, 51). These tetracycline resistance efflux proteins are part of the major facilitator superfamily and share amino acid and protein structure similarities with other efflux proteins (12). Of the 33 efflux genes, 14 [*tet*(A) to *tet*(E), *tet*(G), *tet*(H), *tet*(J), *tet*(Y), *tet*(30), *tet*(31), *tet*(35), *tet*(41), *tet*(57)] are found only in Gram-negative genera. The remaining are found in both Gram-negative and Gram-positive genera or in bacteria of unknown source. The *tet*(B) gene has been identified in 33 Gram-negative genera, while the *tet*(L) gene has been identified in a total of 46 genera, including 24 Gram-negative and 22 Gram-positive genera (http://faculty.washington.edu/marilynr/). The Tn*10*-associated *tet*(B) gene codes for a unique efflux protein, which confers resistance to both tetracycline and minocycline but not to the new

glycylcyclines (46). All the 32 other efflux proteins confer resistance to tetracycline but not to minocycline or glycylcyclines. Laboratory-derived mutations in the *tet*(A), *tet*(B), *tet*(K), and *tet*(L) genes have led to glycylcycline resistance, suggesting that bacterial resistance to tigecycline may develop over time and with clinical use (46, 52, 53). The *tet* efflux genes code for an approximately 46-kDa membrane-bound efflux protein.

The tetracycline efflux proteins present in Gram-negative bacteria commonly exhibit 12 transmembrane segments (TMSs), and upstream of the structural gene and read in the opposite direction is a specific *tet* repressor gene. Induction of the structural gene is based on the binding of a tetracycline-Mg^{2+} complex to the *tet* repressor protein which, in the absence of tetracycline, blocks transcription of the *tet* structural gene (54). The *tet*(A) (*n* = 25), *tet*(B) (*n* = 33), *tet*(C) (*n* = 16), *tet*(D) (*n* = 22), *tet*(G) (*n* = 16), *tet*(H) (*n* = 12), and *tet*(L) (*n* = 22) genes are most widespread among Gram-negative bacteria of human and veterinary origin, while *tet*(D) and *tet*(E) are often associated with aquaculture environments and fish (44). Their location on either transposons, such as Tn*1721* [*tet*(A)] (55), Tn*10* [*tet*(B)] (56, 57), or Tn*5706* [*tet*(H)] (58), and plasmids facilitates their spread within the Gram-negative gene pool. The Gram-positive *tet*(K) and *tet*(L) efflux genes are not regulated by repressors and confer resistance to tetracyclines, but not to minocycline. They code for proteins with 14 TMSs and are regulated by translational attenuation, which requires the presence of tetracyclines as inducers for the translation of the *tet* gene transcripts (59). These genes are generally found on small transmissible plasmids, which on occasion become integrated into the chromosome and occasionally may undergo interplasmidic recombination with other resistance plasmids (54, 59–61).

The ribosomal protection genes code for cytoplasmic proteins which protect the ribosomes from the action of tetracycline both *in vitro* and *in vivo* and confer resistance to tetracycline, doxycycline, and minocycline (46, 62). These proteins have sequence similarity to the ribosomal elongation factors EF-G and EF-Tu and are grouped in the translation factor superfamily of GTPases (63). Their interaction with the ribosome causes an allosteric disruption of the primary tetracycline binding site(s), which then leads to the release of the tetracycline from the ribosome. This allows the ribosome to return to its functional normal posttranslocational conformational state, which was altered by the binding of tetracycline. A detailed review of the various experiments conducted to elucidate the mode of action of these proteins can be found in Connell et al. (63). The ribosomal protection genes are of Gram-positive origin and are found extensively among Gram-positive cocci. However, they have also been found in a number of Gram-negative genera. The first gene of this group, the *tet*(M) gene, has the widest host range of all *tet* genes, with 79 genera, of which 41 are Gram-positive and 38 are Gram-negative (http://faculty.washington.edu/marilynr/). This gene is located on conjugative transposons or integrative and conjugative elements, such as Tn*916* (64, 65). The other commonly found genes of both human and veterinary origin are *tet*(O) (20 Gram-positive, 18 Gram-negative genera), *tet*(Q) (eight Gram-positive, 11 Gram-negative genera), and *tet*(W) (11 Gram-positive, 22 Gram-negative genera). Recent work suggests that mutations within the *tet*(M) gene may confer increased resistance to tigecycline and thus may over time increase resistance to tigecycline in nature (52).

Enzymatic inactivation of tetracycline is mediated by 13 genes found in Gram-negative bacteria, nine of which [*tet*(47) to *tet*(55)] have recently been identified by soil functional metagenomic studies (66). The first inactivating gene described was the *tet*(X) gene (67) (which encodes an NADP-requiring oxidoreductase), which modifies and inactivates the tetracycline molecule in the presence of oxygen but was originally found only in a strict anaerobe, *Bacteroides*, where oxygen is excluded. The *tet*(X) gene has now been identified in 13 Gram-negative genera (http://faculty.washington.edu/marilynr/). This gene confers weak intrinsic resistance to tigecycline. The tigecycline activity can be improved by at least four different amino acid substitutions in the Tet(X) protein to obtain clinically relevant tigecycline resistance levels without loss of activity to other tetracyclines and was thought to be alarming for the future of tigecycline therapy (52). The gene *tet*(37) has been identified from the oral cavity of humans but is unrelated to the *tet*(X) or other genes in this class, and the function of the corresponding enzyme depends on oxygen (68). No bacterial host has been identified which carries *tet*(37). A third gene, *tet*(34), with similarities to the xanthine-guanine phosphoribosyl transferase gene of *Vibrio cholerae*, has also been identified in four Gram-negative genera (69). The recently described gene *tet*(56) has been identified in one Gram-negative genus (66), while the genes *tet*(47) to *tet*(55) have been isolated from grasslands and agricultural soils by functional genomics, where the genes were cloned into *E. coli* and shown to inactivate tetracycline (66). With this recent study, the number of new genes coding for inactivating enzymes from the environment

has greatly increased and may also be found in the future in bacteria of veterinary importance.

The *tet*(U) gene has been identified in the three Gram-positive genera: *Enterococcus*, *Staphylococcus*, and *Streptococcus*. However, it is still not clear if the gene confers tetracycline resistance in any of the bacteria it has been identified in.

A mutation in the 16S rRNA consisting of a single base exchange (1058G → 1058C) has been identified in tetracycline-resistant *Propionibacterium acnes* (70). Position 1058 is located in a region which plays an important role in the termination of peptide chain elongation as well as in the accuracy of translation.

Mutations which alter the permeability of the outer membrane porins and/or LPSs in the outer membrane can also affect resistance to tetracycline. A permeability barrier due to the reduced production of the OmpF porin, by which tetracyclines cross the outer membrane, has been described in *E. coli*. Mutations in the *marRAB* operon, which also regulates OmpF expression, may play a role in this type of tetracycline resistance (13).

Different types of multidrug transporters mediating resistance to tetracycline in addition to resistance to a number of structurally unrelated compounds have been described, for instance, in *E. coli* (EmrE), *S. enterica* (AcrAB/TolC), and *P. aeruginosa* (MexAB/OprM, MexCD/OprJ) (12, 40, 41).

Resistance to Macrolides, Lincosamides, and Streptogramins (MLS)

Several macrolide antibiotics, such as erythromycin, spiramycin, tylosin and tilmicosin, tulathromycin, gamithromycin, and tildipirosin, as well as lincosamide antibiotics, such as clindamycin, lincomycin, and pirlimycin, are approved for use in animals. Since the ban of growth promotors in the European Union, no streptogramin antibiotics are licensed for veterinary use in the European Union, but they may be used in other countries. The 16-membered macrolide antibiotics tylosin and spiramycin were previously used as feed additives for animal growth promotion but remain as therapeutics for veterinary use for the control of bacterial dysentery, respiratory disease, and mastitis. Erythromycin, the first macrolide, was introduced into clinical use over 60 years ago and has good activity against Gram-positive cocci and other Gram-positive bacteria and activity against some Gram-negative bacteria such as *Campylobacter* spp.. *Enterobacteriaceae* and *Pseudomonas* spp. have been considered to be innately nonsusceptible to erythromycin due to multidrug transporters which have 14-membered macrolides as substrates

(71). A number of Gram-negative aerobic, facultatively aerobic, and anaerobic genera carry a variety of acquired macrolide-lincosamide and/or streptogramin resistance genes (http://faculty.washington.edu/marilynr/). The data over the past 20 years clearly show that both Gram-positive and Gram-negative bacteria may become MLS resistant by acquisition of new genes normally associated with mobile elements. Acquired resistance mechanisms include specific efflux pumps, rRNA methylases that reduce binding of the antibiotic to the 50S subunit of the ribosome, or a variety of genes that inactivate the antibiotics (72–77). MLS antibiotics, though chemically distinct, are usually considered together because they share overlapping binding sites on the 50S ribosomal subunit, and a number of resistance genes confer resistance to more than one class of these antibiotics (72–74).

Target site modification occurs by rRNA methylases, which are encoded by *erm* genes. The *erm* genes were the first acquired genes that were identified to confer resistance to macrolides, lincosamides, and streptogramin B (MLS$_B$) antibiotics (74, 75). These genes are found in Gram-positive, Gram-negative, aerobic, and anaerobic genera. Currently, 43 rRNA methylases have been characterized. Each of these enzymes adds one or two methyl groups to a single adenine (A2058 in *E. coli*) in the 23S rRNA moiety which prevents binding of the antibiotic to the target site and thus confers MLS$_B$ resistance to the host bacterium (http://faculty.washington.edu/marilynr; 74–76). The *erm* genes may be expressed all the time (constitutively) or inducibly via translational attenuation (77). This means that the gene is turned on in the presence of low doses of specific antibiotics (74–77); the type of expression depends on a regulatory region upstream of the *erm* gene and on which the antibiotic is able to cause induction (75, 77). In staphylococci, erythromycin and other 14- and 15-membered macrolides are able to induce *erm* gene expression, whereas 16-membered macrolides, lincosamides, and streptogramin B antibiotics are considered noninducers (77). Laboratory selection of *S. aureus* produced mutants that had structural alterations in the translational attenuator region due to deletions, tandem duplications, point mutations, and the insertion of IS*256* (78–80). Similar mutations have also been detected in naturally occurring strains carrying the *erm* genes (81).

Efflux genes include 21 ATP transporters and 5 major facilitator superfamily transporters. These genes confer a variety of resistance patterns including resistance to carbomycin, erythromycin, lincomycin, oleandomycin, spiramycin, tylosin, streptogramin A, streptogramin B, and pleuromutilins, alone or in varying combinations (http://faculty.washington.edu/marilynr; 71–74, 82). Recent work by Sharkey et al. (83) suggests that Vga(A) and Lsa(A) are ABC-F proteins, which lack transmembrane domains, not confer resistance by active efflux, but instead mediate resistance through ribosome protection (83). Further work is needed to determine if other proteins in these classes represent the same mechanism of resistance. The *vga*(A) and *vga*(B) have G+C contents of 29 to 36% and their gene products share 59% identical amino acids. The *msr*(A) gene confers inducible resistance to 14- and 15-membered macrolides and streptogramin B (MS$_B$) and is found in staphylococci. The hydrophilic protein made from the *msr*(A) gene contains two ATP-binding motifs characteristic of the ABC proteins (74, 83, 84, 85). The *msr*(A) gene confers lower levels of erythromycin resistance than the rRNA methylases (86). There are two groups of major facilitator superfamily transporters: one group encompasses *lmr*(A) and *lmr*(B), which code for lincomycin-specific efflux pumps, and the second group includes *mef*(A), *mef*(B) and *mef*(C) genes, which code for specific efflux pumps for 14- and 15-membered macrolides. The *mef*(A) gene was first described in the 1990s from *Streptococcus* spp. (87), but more recently it has been shown to be present in old isolates of pathogenic *Neisseria* spp. (88) and is now found in 30 different genera. It was the most common acquired macrolide resistance gene in a collection of 176 randomly collected commensal Gram-negative bacteria (89). Downstream of the *mef*(A) gene is a gene for an ABC protein that has now been shown to independently confer macrolide resistance and has been named *msr*(D) (90). In contrast, the *mef*(B) gene is found in *Escherichia* spp. and the *mef*(C) gene in *Photobacterium* spp. and *Vibrio* spp..

The 28 inactivating enzymes identified so far encode three esterases, two lyases, 16 transferases, and seven phosphorylases (http://faculty.washington.edu/marilynr; 74, 82). The esterases [Ere(A), Ere(B), and Ere(D)] hydrolyze the lactone ring of the macrolides. The esterases have been found in both Gram-negative and Gram-positive bacteria, and their genes are often associated with plasmids, though the *ere*(A) gene has been associated with both class 1 and class 2 integrons (91). The lyase gene, *vgb*(A), has been identified in the genera *Enterococcus* and *Staphylococcus*, while the *vgb*(B) gene has been identified in *Staphylococcus*. These enzymes inactivate quinupristin by opening the lactone ring (92). The newest inactivating enzymes have been identified as transferases which confer resistance by adding an acetyl group to streptogramin A, thereby inactivating the antibiotic. Sixteen genes have been found in both Gram-positive and/or Gram-negative genera as described below (http://faculty.washington.edu/marilynr; 74, 82). The nine lincosamide nucleotidyltransferases [*lnu* genes] confer resistance to lincosamides but not to macrolides by modification and inactivation of the antibiotic. The *lnu*(A) gene has been identified in five Gram-positive genera, and the *lnu*(B) gene in four Gram-positive genera. The gene *lnu*(C) was identified in *Streptococcus* and *Haemophilus*. The gene *lnu*(E) was found in *Streptococcus* and *Enterococcus*, while *lnu*(F) was identified in *Aeromonas*, *Comamonas*, *Desulfobacterium*, *Escherichia*, *Leclercia*, *Morganella*, *Proteus*, and *Salmonella*. The gene *lnu*(D) is associated with *Streptococcus*, *lnu*(G) with *Enterococcus*, and *lnu*(H) with *Riemerella*. Furthermore, *lnu*(P) has been identified in *Clostridium*. Seven virginiamycin O-acetyltransferases (*vat* genes) have been identified, six of which are associated with mobile elements in *Enterococcus*, *Lactobacillus*, *Staphylococcus*, and/or *Bacteroides*. Each gene was found in only one or two of these genera. In contrast, *vat*(F) is chromosomally encoded in *Yersinia enterocolitica*.

There are seven enzymes, encoded by *mph* genes, which confer resistance by phosphorylation of erythromycin. The *mph*(A) gene is unqiue because it confers resistance to azithromycin, while *mph*(B) and *mph*(C) confer resistance to spiramycin (93). Six phosphorylases, encoded by the genes *mph*(A), *mph*(B), *mph*(D), *mph*(E), *mph*(F), and *mph*(G), have been found exclusively in Gram-negative species. To date, the gene *mph*(A) is found in 11 genera, while *mph*(D) and *mph*(E) are each found in six genera. The *mph*(B) gene is present in four genera, while *mph*(F) is found in *Pseudomonas*. The *mph*(G) gene has been found in the fish pathogens *Photobacterium* and *Vibrio* spp. The *mph*(C) gene, which was originally characterized in *Staphylococcus* spp., has now been identified in a clinical *S. maltophilia* isolate (http://faculty.washington.edu/marilynr/).

Usually, mutational changes that affect the 23S RNA, ribosomal proteins, and/or innate efflux pumps may lead to moderate changes in susceptibility (76, 82). Various mutations have been identified in the 23S rRNA (94). Originally, mutations at either the A2058 or A2059 position (*E. coli* numbering) were found in pathogens that had one or two copies of the 23S rRNA, such as *Mycobacterium* or *Helicobacter* (95). Resistance to tylosin, erythromycin, and clindamycin in *Brachyspira hyodysenteriae* was also associated with an A → T substitution at the nucleotide position homologous with position 2058 of the *E. coli* 23S rRNA gene (96). Variations at positions 2058 and 2059 in the 23S rRNA have also

been described in erythromycin-resistant *Streptococcus pyogenes*, *S. pneumoniae*, *Campylobacter coli*, *Campylobacter jejuni*, and *Haemophilus influenzae* (97, 98). An A → G substitution at position 2075 of the 23S rRNA was detected in *C. coli* from poultry and pigs which exhibited high-level erythromycin resistance (98). Mutations in ribosomal proteins L4 and/or L22 have been identified which confer elevated MICs of the newer agent telithromycin and/or of other members of the MLS group. Clinical Gram-positive bacteria have been found with the same mutations as mutants created in laboratories. Missense mutations, deletions, and/or insertions may alter the expression of innate pumps which then may alter resistance to the MLS antibiotics. A detailed discussion can be found in reference 71.

Resistance to Aminoglycosides and Aminocyclitols

Various aminoglycoside antibiotics, including gentamicin, kanamycin, amikacin, neomycin, (dihydro)streptomycin, paromomycin and framycetin, are licensed for use in both human and veterinary medicine. Among the aminocyclitol antibiotics, spectinomycin is approved for use in humans and animals, whereas apramycin is used exclusively in veterinary medicine. The main mechanism of resistance to aminoglycosides and aminocyclitols is enzymatic inactivation (99–102). In addition, reduction of the intracellular concentrations of aminoglycosides and modification of the molecular target can also result in resistance to aminoglycosides (103). Decreased intracellular concentration can result from either reduced drug uptake or from active efflux mechanisms. Chromosomal mutations conferring high-level resistance to streptomycin have also been described (13) and are the main resistance mechanism in mycobacteria.

Enzymatic inactivation of aminoglycosides and aminocyclitols is conferred by any of the three types of modifying enzymes: *N*-acetyltransferases (AACs), *O*-nucleotidyltransferases (also referred to as *O*-adenyltransferases [ANTs]), or *O*-phosphotransferases (APHs) (99–102). Acetyl-coenzyme A serves as a donor of acetyl groups in acetylation reactions at amino groups, while ATP is used for the adenylation and phosphorylation reactions at hydroxyl groups. For each of these three classes of aminoglycoside-modifying enzymes, numerous members are known which differ more or less extensively in their structure. Most modifying enzymes exhibit a narrow substrate spectrum. Several reviews have listed the known enzymes involved in modification of aminoglycosides/aminocyclitols and their molecular relationships (49, 99–102). However, new genes for aminoglycoside/aminocyclitol-inactivating enzymes or variants of already known ones are constantly being reported. Unfortunately, a continuously updated database for the currently known aminoglycoside/aminocyclitol-inactivating enzymes is not available. Another problem is the lack of an unambiguous nomenclature. There are at least two alternatively used designations for genes coding for the same modifying enzyme: one designation, for example, *aph(3″)-Ib*, refers to the type of modification (*aph*) and the position where the modification is introduced (*3″*) and lists the subtype of the gene (*Ib*); the other designation, for example, *strA*, is easier to handle, refers only to the corresponding resistance phenotype (*str* for streptomycin resistance), and indicates the subtype (A).

So far, four classes of AACs are known which acetylate the amino groups at positions 1, 3, 2′, and 6′ (99–103). To date, at least 80 AACs have been identified, most of which vary in their substrate spectra. The vast majority of the AAC enzymes were identified in Gram-negative bacteria. Combined resistance to apramycin and gentamicin is due to the enzyme AAC(3)-IV; the corresponding gene emerged after the introduction of apramycin into veterinary use. It was first detected in *E. coli* and *Salmonella* from animals (104) and was found later in *E. coli* from humans as well (105–107). A gene for a bifunctional enzyme, which displays acetyltransferase AAC(6′) and phosphotransferase APH (2″) activities, is usually found on Tn*4001*-like transposons, which are widely spread among staphylococci, streptococci, and enterococci (108–111).

To date, five classes of ANTs are categorized depending on the position of adenylation (6, 9, 4′, 2″, and 3″) on the aminoglycoside molecule (99–102). The ANT (2″) and ANT(3″) enzymes are more frequent among Gram-negative bacteria, whereas the ANT(4′), ANT (6), and ANT(9) enzymes are usually found in Gram-positive bacteria (101). The different ANT enzymes also vary considerably in their substrate spectra. Among the seven phosphotransferases [APH(2″), APH(3′), APH (3″), APH(4), APH(6), APH(7″), and APH(9)] which modify the aminoglycosides at positions 2″, 3′, 3″, 4, 6, 7″, and 9 (101), numerous variants have been identified which confer distinctly different resistance phenotypes. Most *aac*, *ant*, and *aph* genes are located on mobile genetic elements, such as plasmids, transposons, and gene cassettes (99–103, 112, 113).

The gene *apmA* codes for an acetyltransferase, which confers resistance to apramycin and decreased susceptibility to gentamicin. It has been detected on plasmids of variable sizes in MRSA ST398 (114–116). In staphylococci, spectinomycin resistance is mediated by the adenyltransferase genes *spc*, *spd*, and *spw* (117–121).

Multidrug efflux systems, such as MexXY in *P. aeruginosa* and AmrAB in *Burkholderia pseudomallei* (40), or the multidrug transporter AcrD in *E. coli* (122) can export aminoglycosides. The transporter MdfA from *E. coli* (123) has also been reported to mediate the efflux of the aminoglycosides kanamycin, neomycin, and hygromycin A.

Decreased uptake of aminoglycosides may be based on a mutation in lipopolysaccharide (LPS) phosphates or on a change in the charge of the LPS in *E. coli* and *P. aeruginosa*, respectively (124). Since the entry of aminoglycosides across the cytoplasmic membrane is mainly based on the electron transport system, anaerobic bacteria and facultative anaerobic bacteria exhibit relatively high insensitivity to aminoglycosides (13).

Methylation of the ribosomal target (16S rRNA) is responsible for high-level aminoglycoside resistance. It is also an emerging mechanism of great concern in clinically relevant Gram-negative bacteria. The first plasmid-mediated gene identified was the 16S rRNA methylase *armA* (125). To date, nine additional genes that encode methylases have been reported: *rmtA*, *rmtB*, *rmtC*, *rmtD*, *rtmD2*, *rmtE*, *rmtF*, *rmtG*, and *npmA* (126). The *rmt* genes confer resistance to gentamicin and amikacin, whereas *npmA* confers resistance to gentamicin, neomycin, amikacin, and apramycin, but not to streptomycin (127).

Mutations in the gene *rpsL* for the ribosomal protein S12 have been shown to result in high-level streptomycin resistance (128). Single base-pair substitutions at different positions in the gene *rrs*, which encodes 16S rRNA in mycobacteria, have been described to be involved in either streptomycin resistance (129) or resistance to amikacin, kanamycin, gentamicin, tobramycin, and neomycin, but not to streptomycin (130). In *Mycobacterium tuberculosis*, mutations in the gene *rpsL*, which encodes the ribosomal protein S12, can cause high-level streptomycin resistance. Overexpression of the acetyltransferase-encoding gene, *eis*, has mainly been associated with resistance to kanamycin. Mutations in the *gidB* gene, which encodes a 7-methylguanosine methyltransferase, are also associated with resistance to aminoglycosides in mycobacteria. It has been suggested that loss of function of this gene confers resistance (130).

Resistance to Sulfonamides and Trimethoprim

Various sulfonamides, trimethoprim, and combinations of sulfonamides and trimethoprim are licensed for use in humans and animals. There are no restrictions on the use of any of these compounds in food animals. Sulfonamides and trimethoprim are competitive inhibitors of different enzymatic steps in folate metabolism. In this regard, sulfonamides represent structural analogs of *p*-aminobenzoic acid and inhibit the enzyme dihydropteroic acid synthase (DHPS), whereas trimethoprim inhibits the enzyme dihydrofolate reductase (DHFR). Various mechanisms of intrinsic and acquired resistance to sulfonamides and trimethoprim have been described in bacteria (131–135).

Permeability barriers and efflux pumps play a relevant role by either preventing the influx or promoting the efflux of both compounds. Intrinsic resistance to both compounds in *P. aeruginosa* was initially thought to be based on outer membrane impermeability. However, the multidrug exporter system MexAB/OprM was found to be mainly responsible for resistance to sulfonamides and trimethoprim in *P. aeruginosa* (136). For other bacteria, such as *K. pneumoniae* and *Serratia marcescens*, impaired membrane permeability is still considered to play a role in sulfonamide and trimethoprim resistance (132, 133).

Naturally insensitive DHFR enzymes and folate auxotrophy play an important role in intrinsic resistance to sulfonamides and trimethoprim. DHFR enzymes which exhibit low affinity for trimethoprim and thus render their hosts intrinsically resistant to trimethoprim are known to occur in several bacterial genera including *Clostridium*, *Neisseria*, *Brucella*, *Bacteroides*, and *Moraxella* (13). Bacteria such as enterococci and lactobacilli which can utilize exogenous folates also show intrinsic resistance to trimethoprim and sulfonamides.

Mutational or recombinational changes in the target enzymes have been observed in a wide variety of bacteria. Mutations in the chromosomal *dhps* gene that lead to sulfonamide resistance by single amino acid substitutions can be generated under *in vitro* conditions but also occur *in vivo*. Such mutations have been identified in *E. coli*, *S. aureus*, *Staphylococcus haemolyticus*, *C. jejuni*, and *Helicobacter pylori* (132). In *S. pneumoniae*, two amino acid duplications which change the tertiary structure of the DHPS have been found to be responsible for sulfonamide resistance (137). Recombinational events between the naturally occurring gene coding for a susceptible DHPS and that of a horizontally acquired resistant DHPS are believed to account for sulfonamide resistance in *Neisseria meningitidis* (132). Trimethoprim resistance has also been shown to be due to a single amino acid substitution in the DHFR protein in *S. aureus* (138) and *S. pneumoniae* (139). Mutations in the promoter region of chromosomal *dhfr* genes have been described to occur in *E. coli* and resulted in overexpression of the trimethoprim-susceptible DHFR (132). Mutations in both the promoter region and the

dhfr gene have been identified in trimethoprim-resistant *H. influenzae* (140).

The replacement of sensitive enzymes by resistant enzymes usually causes high-level resistance (131–135). To date, three types of resistant DHPS enzymes encoded by the genes *sul1*, *sul2*, and *sul3* have been described to occur in Gram-negative bacteria (141–144). The gene *sul1* is part of class 1 integrons and thus is often associated with other resistance genes. As part of transposons, such as Tn*21*, and conjugative plasmids, it is spread into various Gram-negative species and genera (141, 143). The *sul2* gene often occurs together with the Tn*5393*-associated streptomycin resistance genes *strA-strB* on conjugative or nonconjugative plasmids (142, 143). The gene *sul3* was originally found on a conjugative plasmid from porcine *E. coli*, where it was flanked by copies of the insertion sequence IS*15/26* (144). Meanwhile, it has also been identified in *E. coli* from humans and animals other than pigs, as well as in *S. enterica* from animal and food sources (144–147).

More than 40 DHFR (*dfr*, formerly also referred to as *dhfr*) genes have been identified. The genes occurring in Gram-negative bacteria are subdivided on the basis of their structure into two major groups, *dfrA* and *dfrB* (148). The 33 *dfrA* genes code for DHFR enzymes of 152 to 189 amino acids (aa), whereas the eight *dfrB*-encoded DHFR enzymes consist of only 78 aa. The *dfrA* genes have been detected more frequently than the *dfrB* genes. Additionally, there are *dfr* gene groups in Gram-positive bacteria that currently consist of only one gene each. The gene *dfrG* codes for an enzyme of 165 aa and has been detected in the chromosome of *S. aureus* (149). In *S. haemolyticus* and *Listeria monocytogenes*, the gene *dfrD*, which codes for an enzyme of 162 aa, has been identified on plasmids (150, 151). The gene for the 163-aa DHFR DfrK was first detected on plasmids in *S. aureus* and linked to the *tet*(L) gene (152). Since then, *dfrK* has been found as part of transposon Tn*559* in the chromosomal DNA of staphylococci and enterococci (153, 154) and on small plasmids from *Staphylococcus hyicus* that confer only trimethoprim resistance (115). In staphylococci, the composite transposon Tn*4003* has been identified on various multiresistance plasmids. Tn*4003* is composed of a central *dfrA* gene (also known as *dfrS1*) bracketed by copies of the insertion sequence IS*257* (155).

Transferable trimethoprim resistance genes have been identified in a wide variety of Gram-negative bacteria; several of these genes are part of plasmids, transposons, or gene cassettes (112, 133, 135, 156) and thus are easily disseminated across species and genus borders.

Several studies showed the relationships between the *dfr* genes (133, 135, 156).

Resistance to Quinolones and Fluoroquinolones

Quinolones and fluoroquinolones are potent inhibitors of bacterial DNA replication. While early quinolones such as nalidixic acid and pipemidic acid have not been used in veterinary medicine, oxolinic acid and flumequine (the first fluorinated quinolone) have been used in food-producing animals, including fish, worldwide (1, 157). Since the first of the newer fluoroquinolones, enrofloxacin, was licensed for use in animals in the late 1980s (158), several other fluoroquinolones have been approved for veterinary use in recent years, including marbofloxacin, orbifloxacin, difloxacin, ibafloxacin, danofloxacin, and pradofloxacin. Two major mechanisms account for resistance to fluoroquinolones: mutations in the genes for DNA topoisomerases and decreased intracellular drug accumulation (159–163). In addition, plasmid-mediated (fluoro)quinolone resistance genes have been described in the past decade (163).

Mutational alteration of the target genes *gyrA* and *gyrB* (coding for the A and B subunits of the DNA gyrase) as well as *parC* and *parE* (coding for A and B subunits of the DNA topoisomerase IV) is frequently seen in (fluoro)quinolone-resistant bacteria. Both enzymes are tetramers consisting of two A and B units. The mutations in *gyrA* are commonly located within a region of ca. 130 bp which is referred to as the "quinolone resistance-determining region" (164). Mutations resulting in changes of Ser-83 (to Tyr, Phe, or Ala) and Asp-87 (to Gly, Asn, or Tyr) have been detected most frequently. In addition, double mutations at both positions and various other mutations have been described in Gram-positive and Gram-negative bacteria of human and veterinary importance (157, 160–162, 165). Stepwise mutations in *gyrA* and *parC* can result in an incremental increase in resistance to quinolones (157). Moreover, various mutations may also have different effects on resistance to the various fluoroquinolones (166). The complex interplay between individual mechanisms may also have different effects on fluoroquinolone resistance (167).

Multidrug efflux systems also conferring fluoroquinolone resistance have been identified in various Gram-positive and Gram-negative bacteria, such as *P. aeruginosa* (MexAB/OprM, MexCD/OprJ), *S. aureus* (NorA), *S. pneumoniae* (PmrA), *Bacillus subtilis* (Blt), *E. coli*, and *S. enterica* (AcrAB/TolC); for reviews see references 162, 168, and 169. Since the basal level of expression of these efflux systems is low, upregulation of their expression is required to confer resistance to

fluoroquinolones and other antimicrobials. In *E. coli* the level of production of the AcrAB-TolC efflux system is under the control of several regulatory genes, in particular the global regulatory systems *marRAB* and *soxRS*, but also *acrR* (168–171). Mutations in these regulatory systems may lead to overproduction of the AcrAB-TolC efflux pump and expression of the multidrug resistance phenotype (172, 173). Besides overproduction of the AcrAB-TolC efflux pump, it has been recently shown using macroarrays that *E. coli* strains constitutively expressing *marA* showed altered expression of more than 60 chromosomal genes (174).

Interplay between several resistance mechanisms may lead to high-level resistance to quinolones and to other antibiotics when multidrug efflux pumps and decreased outer membrane permeability are involved (167, 175). For *in vitro* selected quinolone-resistant *E. coli* mutants, it has been shown that first-step quinolone-resistant mutants acquire a *gyrA* mutation. Second-step mutants reproducibly acquire a multidrug resistance phenotype and show enhanced fluoroquinolone efflux. In some third-step mutants, fluoroquinolone efflux is further enhanced and additional topoisomerase mutations are acquired. In clinical *E. coli* isolates from humans and animals, the situation appears to be the same, where high-level fluoroquinolone resistance is reached when mutations at several chromosomal loci are acquired (167, 175). It is noteworthy that inactivation of the AcrAB efflux pump renders resistant *E. coli* strains, including those with target gene mutations, hypersusceptible to fluoroquinolones and certain other unrelated drugs (175). Thus, in the absence of the AcrAB efflux pump, gyrase mutations fail to produce clinically relevant levels of fluoroquinolone resistance (176). The same observation has been made for *P. aeruginosa*, in which deletion of the MexAB-OprM efflux pump, which is the homolog of the AcrAB-TolC efflux pump in this species, resulted in a significant decrease in resistance to fluoroquinolones even for strains carrying target gene mutations (177). In high-level fluoroquinolone-resistant *S. enterica* serovar Typhimurium DT204 strains, carrying multiple target gene mutations in *gyrA*, *gyrB*, and *parC*, inactivation of AcrB or TolC resulted in a 16- to 32-fold decrease of resistance levels to fluoroquinolones (178, 179).

Decreased drug uptake in Gram-negative bacteria is due to the *marRAB*-mediated downregulation of OmpF porin production. OmpF is an important porin for the entry of quinolones and fluoroquinolones into the bacterial cell (180, 181). Moreover, mutations in different gene loci (*cfxB*, *norB*, *nfxB*, *norC*, or *nalB*) are also associated with decreased permeability (182, 183).

Plasmid-mediated quinolone resistance mechanisms have been described in recent years in addition to the aforementioned chromosomal resistance mechanisms (184–186). These plasmid-mediated quinolone resistance mechanisms usually confer low-level (fluoro) quinolone resistance by (i) target protection, (ii) acetylation, and (iii) efflux pumps. The protection of the DNA gyrase is mediated by *qnr* genes. Six *qnr* gene families (*qnrA, qnrB, qnrC, qnrD, qnrS, qnrVC*) with multiple alleles per gene have been described and are organized in a database (www.lahey.org/qnrStudies). The *qnr* genes are associated with several mobile genetic elements and located on plasmids of varying sizes and different incompatibility groups (185, 186). The gene *aac(6′)-Ib-cr* codes for an aminoglycoside acetyltransferase, which is able to acetylate the amino nitrogen on the piperazinyl ring of quinolones such as ciprofloxacin and norfloxacin (185, 186). Efflux pumps are encoded by the genes *qepA* and *oqxAB*. The OqxAB efflux pump has a wide substrate specificity and is found not only on plasmids but also in the chromosomal DNA. These plasmid-mediated resistance genes have been found in several Gram-negative bacteria. The plasmid-located gene for an efflux pump *qacBIII* is able to confer decreased susceptibility to ciprofloxacin and norfloxacin in *S. aureus* and is the first plasmid-mediated quinolone resistance gene in Gram-positive bacteria (185, 186).

Resistance to Phenicols

Two members of the phenicols, chloramphenicol and its fluorinated derivative florfenicol, are currently approved for use in animals. The predominant mechanism of chloramphenicol resistance in Gram-positive and Gram-negative bacteria is enzymatic inactivation (187–189). In addition, efflux systems that mediate either resistance to only chloramphenicol or combined resistance to chloramphenicol and florfenicol have also been identified (188). Furthermore, permeability barriers and multidrug transporters play a role in certain Gram-negative bacteria (8, 12, 188, 190). Detailed reviews on the different genes and mechanisms accounting for bacterial resistance to chloramphenicol and florfenicol have been published (48, 188).

Enzymatic inactivation of chloramphenicol is commonly achieved by chloramphenicol acetyltransferases (CATs) which transfer acetyl groups from acetyl-CoA to the C3 position of the chloramphenicol molecule. Subsequent transfer of the acetyl group to the C1 position and transfer of a second acetyl group to C3 results in mono- or diacetylated chloramphenicol derivatives, both of which are unable to inhibit bacterial protein

biosynthesis (187–189). Two distinct types of CAT enzymes, which differ in their structures, are known: the classical CATs (type A) and a novel type of CAT (type B) (187, 188). All type A and type B CATs have a trimeric structure composed of three identical monomers. The *cat* gene codes for a CAT monomer, the size of which varies between 207 and 238 aa (type A CATs) and 209 and 212 aa (type B CATs) (188). Using the cutoff as set for the classification of tetracycline and MLS resistance genes (47, 74), 16 classes of *catA* determinants and at least another five classes of *catB* determinants can be differentiated (48). Among the *catA* genes, those formerly referred to as *catI, catII,* and *catIII* are most widespread among Gram-negative bacteria (48, 191–193). They are associated with either nonconjugative transposons such as Tn9 or plasmids. Expression of these *catA* genes is constitutive. Various *catA* genes, indistinguishable from or closely related to those present on the *S. aureus* plasmids pC221, pC223/pSCS7, and pC194 (48, 193–196), have been detected in coagulase-positive and -negative staphylococci, but also in members of the genera *Streptococcus, Bacillus,* and *Listeria,* respectively. Expression of these mostly plasmid-borne *catA* genes is inducible by chloramphenicol via translational attenuation (197), whereas the Tn4451-borne *catA* genes of *Clostridium* spp. are expressed constitutively (198). The *catB* genes—also referred to as *xat* (xenobiotic acetyltransferase) genes—differ distinctly from the *catA* genes but are related to acetyltransferase genes, such as *vat*(A-E), involved in streptogramin resistance (187). Some of the *catB* genes have been found exclusively on the chromosome of either *Agrobacterium tumefaciens, P. aeruginosa,* or *V. cholerae,* whereas others proved to be part of transposons (Tn2424, Tn840) or plasmid-borne integrons. Studies of the level of *catB*-mediated chloramphenicol resistance revealed a distinctly lower level of chloramphenicol resistance compared to that conferred by type A CATs (187).

In addition to inactivation via CATs, enzymatic inactivation of chloramphenicol can also occur by O-phosphorylation or by hydrolytic degradation to p-nitrophenylserinol (48). Since these mechanisms have so far only been seen in the chloramphenicol producer *Streptomyces venezuelae* and in a soil metagenome library, they are believed to play a role as self-defense mechanisms (48, 188).

A total of 11 classes of specific exporters which mediate either chloramphenicol or chloramphenicol/florfenicol resistance have been identified (48, 188). Among them, seven classes are represented by 10- to 12-TMS chloramphenicol exporters of soil bacteria of the genera *Streptomyces*, *Rhodococcus*, and *Coryne-bacterium* or of bacteria of unknown origin, whereas four classes of 12-TMS exporters were found among Gram-negative bacteria of medical importance (188, 199). Among these latter classes, one class represents the *cmlA* subgroup, and the others represent the *floR* subgroup. The gene *cmlA*, which codes for a chloramphenicol exporter, is a Tn*1696*-associated cassette-borne gene which, however, is inducibly expressed via translational attenuation (200). Genes related to *cmlA* are mainly found in *Enterobacteriaceae* and *Pseudomonas*. Genes related to *floR* have been identified in *Photobacterium*, *Vibrio*, *Klebsiella*, *E. coli*, and various *S. enterica* serovars and in *Pasteurella multocida* as part of the chromosomally located ICE*Pmu1* (48, 201–208). In *Vibrio* and *Salmonella*, the gene *floR* has been detected as part of chromosomal multiresistance gene clusters (207, 209), and in *E. coli*, as part of conjugative and nonconjugative multiresistance plasmids (201, 202). In *S. maltophilia* of porcine origin, a novel *floR* variant, *floR*$_V$, has been identified as part of a chromosomal genomic island (210). Another class of phenicol exporters is represented by FexA, the first specific chloramphenicol/florfenicol exporter of Gram-positive bacteria (211). The gene *fexA*, located on the transposon Tn*558* (212) from *Staphylococcus lentus*, codes for a 14-TMS exporter of the major facilitator superfamily and is expressed inducibly via translational attenuation. A second phenicol exporter, FexB, which exhibited 56.1% amino acid identity with the FexA protein, has been exclusively identified in enterococci (213).

Multidrug transporter systems that export chloramphenicol have been described to occur in several Gram-negative bacteria, including the systems MexAB/OprM and MexCD/OprJ in *P. aeruginosa*, AcrAB/TolC in *E. coli* and *S. enterica*, CeoAB/OpcM in *Burkholderia cepacia*, and ArpAB/ArpC and TtgAB/TtgC in *Pseudomonas putida* (40, 181).

Permeability barriers based on the reduced expression of the OmpF porin in *S. enterica* serovar Typhi or a major outer membrane protein in *H. influenzae* (188) have also been described to confer chloramphenicol resistance. The *mar* locus which is found in various *Enterobacteriaceae* can contribute to chloramphenicol resistance in two ways: on one hand, it can activate the AcrAB/TolC efflux system, leading to increased efflux of chloramphenicol, and on the other hand, MarA can activate the gene *micF*, whose transcripts represent an antisense RNA that effectively inhibits translation of *ompF* transcripts, which results in a decreased influx of chloramphenicol (180, 181).

Mutations in the major ribosomal protein clusters of *E. coli* and *B. subtilis*, but also mutations in the 23S rRNA of *E. coli*, have been described to mediate chloramphenicol resistance (214).

Resistance to Oxazolidinones

Oxazolidinones are a class of synthetic antibiotics that are highly active against Gram-positive bacteria. Currently, two oxazolidinones, linezolid and tedizolid, are exclusively approved for use in human medicine and are considered last-resort antimicrobial agents for the treatment of infections caused by MRSA, vancomycin-resistant enterococci, and penicillin-resistant *S. pneumoniae*.

Initially, point mutations within either the 23S rRNA and/or the genes coding for the ribosomal proteins L3 (*rplC*), L4 (*rplD*), and L22 (*rplV*) were recognized as the main mechanisms of reduced oxazolidinone susceptibility (215–217). Mutations in clinical staphylococcal and enterococcal isolates, including G2247T, T2500A, A2503G, T2504C, G2505A, and G2576T, usually were found in the vicinity of the peptidyltransferase center (217). Mutations in the gene *rplC*, including F147L and A157R, resulted in at least 2-fold increases of the oxazolidinone MICs of laboratory and clinical staphylococci (218). The mutations in the *rplD* gene, which resulted in amino acid exchanges K68N or K68Q, and the insertions $_{71}$GGR$_{72}$, $_{65}$WR$_{66}$, and $_{68}$KG$_{69}$ lead to oxazolidinone resistance in *S. pneumoniae* (219). Little is known about the effects of L22 mutations on linezolid resistance; whether the amino acid exchange A29V in L22 detected in two linezolid-resistant MRSA isolates is responsible for the linezolid resistance in these isolates remains to be investigated (220).

The gene *cfr* from *S. sciuri* was the first transferable oxazolidinone resistance gene (221). Initially described as a novel chloramphenicol/florfenicol resistance gene, the elucidation of the resistance mechanism revealed that *cfr* codes for an rRNA methylase, which confers resistance not only to phenicols but also to lincosamides, oxazolidinones, pleuromutilins, and streptogramin A by methylating the adenine residue at position 2503 in 23S rRNA, which is located in the overlapping ribosomal binding site of these antibiotics (222, 223). The gene *cfr* is mainly located on plasmids in staphylococci and has been distributed across species and genus boundaries. In recent years, it has been detected in both Gram-positive and Gram-negative genera, including *Bacillus*, *Enterococcus*, *Escherichia*, *Jeotgalicoccus*, *Macrococcus*, *Staphylococcus*, *Streptococcus*, and *Proteus* (48, 224, 225). Recently, variants of the *cfr* gene have been identified, including *cfr*(B) in *E. faecium* and

Clostridium difficile (226, 227) and *cfr*(C) in *Campylobacter* and *Clostridium* (228).

An ABC-F protein, which is able to mediate resistance to chloramphenicol and florfenicol as well as the oxazolidinones linezolid and tedizolid, is encoded by the gene *optrA*, which has been identified on a conjugative plasmid in *E. faecalis* (229). The insertion sequence IS*1216E* and the transposon Tn*558* have been identified in the *optrA* flanking regions on plasmids and on the chromosome of enterococci from humans, pigs, and chickens (230). Moreover, the gene *optrA* has also been detected on plasmids and in the chromosomal DNA of porcine *S. sciuri* (231, 232). Since then, this gene has been identified in genomes of clinical isolates of staphylococci, enterococci, and streptococci (233).

Resistance to Glycopeptides

Since the ban of the growth promotor avoparcin in 1996, no glycopeptide antibiotics are approved for use in animals. Glycopeptide antibiotics, such as vancomycin and teicoplanin, act by binding to the D-alanine-D-alanine termini of peptidoglycan precursors, thereby preventing transglycosylation and transpeptidation of the bacterial cell wall (234, 235).

Modification of the target site is the common mechanism of bacterial resistance to glycopeptides. So far, four D-Ala-D-Lac operons (*vanA*, *vanB*, *vanD*, and *vanM*) and five D-Ala-D-Ser operons (*vanC*, *vanE*, *vanG*, *vanL*, and *vanN*) have been described in enterococci (236). They differ in their levels of resistance to vancomycin and teicoplanin (235). In the D-Ala-D-Lac operons, the terminal dipeptide D-alanine-D-alanine is replaced by D-alanine-D-lactate, whereas in the D-Ala-D-Ser operons, it is replaced by D-alanine-D-serine. These replacements reduce the ability of glycopeptides to bind to the peptidoglycan precursors and result in the case of D-lactate in high-level and in the case of D-serine in low-level glycopeptide resistance.

The VanC operon is responsible for the intrinsic resistance of *Enterococcus gallinarum*, *Enterococcus casseliflavus*, and *Enterococcus flavescens* to glycopeptides (235). Similar to VanC, VanD and VanE, both from *E. faecalis*, have been reported not to be transferable (235). In contrast, the *vanA* and *vanB* operons are associated with transposons which can be located on conjugative and nonconjugative plasmids in enterococci. The VanA phenotype is associated with the nonconjugative transposon Tn*1546*, which contains a total of nine reading frames, five of which are essential for high-level glycopeptide resistance (237). Among these, the two genes *vanR* and *vanS* code for a response regulator protein and a sensor protein, respectively, involved in regulatory processes. Three genes are directly involved in resistance: *vanH*, *vanA*, and *vanX*. The gene *vanH* codes for a cytoplasmatic dehydrogenase that produces D-lactate from pyruvate, whereas the gene *vanX* codes for a D,D-dipeptidase which cleaves the D-alanine-D-alanine, and the gene *vanA* codes for a ligase that joins the remaining D-alanine with D-lactate. While glycopeptide resistance is often found in enterococci (238, 239), transfer studies showed that conjugative transfer of VanA-mediated vancomycin resistance from *E. faecalis* to *S. aureus* is possible under *in vitro* conditions (240). In 2002, the first patients infected with *vanA*-carrying high-level vancomycin-resistant *S. aureus* isolates were detected in the United States (241). Genes homologous to enterococcal glycopeptide resistance genes *vanA* and *vanB* have also been detected among members of the genera *Paenibacillus* and *Rhodococcus* (242). Moreover, a new glycopeptide resistance operon, *vanOHX*, has recently been identified in *Rhodococcus equi* (236).

Impaired membrane permeability renders Gram-negative bacteria intrinsically resistant to glycopeptides, large molecules which can cross the outer membrane only poorly, if at all (235).

Resistance to Pleuromutilins

The pleuromutilins tiamulin and valnemulin are mainly used in veterinary medicine for the control and specific therapy of gastrointestinal and respiratory tract infections in swine and to a lesser extent in poultry and rabbits. Retapamulin is used as an ointment to treat bacterial skin infections in humans. Products for systemic use in humans with infections caused by multidrug-resistant bacteria are currently being developed.

The main target bacteria in veterinary medicine are *B. hyodysenteriae*, *Brachyspira pilosicoli*, *Lawsonia intracellularis*, and *Mycoplasma* spp. Resistance derives from chromosomal mutations in the 23S rRNA and *rplC* genes or mobile resistance genes located on plasmids or transposons, such as the *cfr* genes and certain *vga*, *lsa*, and *sal* genes (243, 244). The mechanism of resistance varies among bacterial species.

In *B. hyodysenteriae*, reduced susceptibility to tiamulin has been associated with point mutations in the V domain of the 23S rRNA gene (positions 2032, 2055, 2447, 2499, 2504, and 2572 in *E. coli* numbering) and/or the ribosomal protein L3 gene (245, 246). Mutation at nucleotide position 2032 appears to be related to pleuromutilin resistance and to decreased susceptibility to lincosamides (246). Tiamulin resistance in *B. hyodysenteriae* develops in a stepwise manner both *in vitro* and *in vivo*, suggesting that multiple mutations are needed to achieve high levels of resistance. The MICs of valnemulin are generally a few dilution steps lower than those of tiamulin (247). To date, data on the resistance mechanisms of *B. pilosicoli* and *L. intracellularis* are lacking, and data on resistance mechanisms of mycoplasmata are limited. A single mutation of the 23S rRNA gene caused elevated tiamulin and valnemulin MICs in *Mycoplasma gallisepticum*, but combinations of two or three mutations were necessary to produce high levels of resistance to these drugs (248).

Resistance in staphylococci can be due to point mutations in the V domain of 23S rRNA or in the *rplC* gene, encoding the ribosomal protein L3 (249). Transferable resistance in staphylococci can be caused by *vga* genes, encoding ABC transporters or ABC-F proteins, resulting in resistance to pleuromutilins, streptogramin A, and lincosamides. There are several *vga* genes which confer pleuromutilin resistance in addition to lincosamide and streptogramin A resistance: *vga*(A) and its variants, *vga*(C), and *vga*(E) and its variant. All these genes have been found on plasmids and transposons of staphylococci (243). Transferable resistance to five classes of antimicrobials (phenicols, lincosamides, oxazolidinones, pleuromutilins, streptogramin A) in staphylococci is mediated by the gene *cfr*. The *sal*(A) gene from *S. sciuri*, also encoding a putative ABC-F protein, has been shown to mediate combined resistance to lincosamides, pleuromutilins, and streptogramin A antibiotics (244).

E. faecalis is intrinsically resistant to pleuromutilins, streptogramin A antibiotics, and lincosamides by the production of the ABC-F protein Lsa(A). In *E. faecium*, acquired resistance to the above-mentioned antimicrobials is mediated by the gene *eat*(A)$_V$ which may encode a putative ABC-F protein (83, 250). The enterococcal gene *lsa*(E), which may also code for a putative ABC-F protein (83), has been detected in methicillin-susceptible *S. aureus* and in MRSA of human and animal origin (251).

Resistance to Polypeptide Antibiotics

There are three polypeptide antibiotics that are used in human and/or veterinary medicine: bacitracin, polymyxin B, and colistin (polymyxin E). Bacitracin inhibits cell wall synthesis and is active against Gram-positive bacteria. It used to be used as a growth promoter (252). Since the ban of antimicrobial growth promoters in 2006 in the European Union, it is no longer approved for veterinary use as growth promotor in the EU. In China, colistin has also been banned from use as growth promoter in food animals, as of April 2017. However, it is used for that purpose in other countries, and it is still

approved for therapeutic purposes in the European Union and China. Polymyxin B and colistin (polymyxin E) disrupt the outer bacterial cell membrane of certain Gram-negative bacteria, such as most *Enterobacteriaceae*, *P. aeruginosa*, and *Acinetobacter baumannii*, whereas other Gram-negative bacteria, including *Proteus* spp., *Providencia* spp., *Morganella morganii*, *Serratia* spp., *Edwardsiella tarda*, and bacteria of the *B. cepacia* complex exhibit intrinsic resistance to these polypeptide antibiotics. Recently, colistin was included in the WHO list of critically important antibiotics (253). In human medicine, colistin is used as a last-line drug in the treatment of severe infections caused by multiresistant Gram-negative bacteria, whereas it is used in veterinary medicine for the treatment of enteric diseases, mainly in swine and poultry (254). So far, several mechanisms of resistance to polymyxins (polymyxin B and colistin) have been described (255). These include a variety of LPS modifications, such as modifications of lipid A with phosphoethanolamine and 4-amino-4-deoxy-L-arabinose, efflux pumps, the formation of capsules, and overexpression of the outer membrane protein OprH (255). Such resistance is chromosomally encoded, and hence spread entailed either *de novo* emergence or clonal expansion of resistant isolates.

The alteration of the LPS on its lipid A moiety is the primary mechanism of resistance to polycationic polymyxins. 4-Amino-4-deoxy-L-arabinose (L-Ara4N) or phosphoethanolamine is added to lipid A by enzymes such as ArnT and EptA, resulting in a decrease of the negative charge of the LPS, thereby lowering the affinity of the positively charged polymyxins to the outer membrane. The genes *arnT* (part of the operon *arnBCADTEF*) and *eptA*, which code for those enzymes, are controlled by chromosomally encoded two-component regulatory systems, such as PmrAB and PhoPQ. Mutations in the operons *pmrAB* and *phoPQ* may lead to an upregulation of *arnT* and *eptA* expression, resulting in polymyxin resistance. This has been described in *E. coli*, *K. pneumoniae*, *S. enterica*, and *P. aeruginosa* (255). Furthermore, mutations in the gene for the negative feedback regulator of PhoPQ, *mgrB*, can activate the *arnBCADTEF* operon in *K. pneumoniae* (256). Other genes coding for phosphoethanolamine transferases are *eptB* in *E. coli*, *eptC* in *C. jejuni*, and *lptA* in *N. meningitidis*. Those phosphoethanolamine transferases add phosphoethanolamine to different positions on lipid A. The main polymyxin resistance mechanism in *A. baumannii* is mutations in the genes of the PmrAB system and the resulting overexpression of *pmrC*, which codes for an EptaA-like phosphoethanolamine transferase. In

P. aeruginosa five two-component regulatory systems (PhoPQ, PmrAB, ParRS, CprRS, ColRS) have been identified, and mutations in the genes for those systems play a role in overexpression of the *arnBCADTEF-ugd* operon (256).

In addition, plasmid-mediated resistance to polymyxins was reported in 2016 (257). The gene *mcr-1* has been identified on a conjugative plasmid in *E. coli* of animal and human origin and codes for a phosphoethanolamine transferase. The *mcr-1* gene was first identified among isolates from China, but since then it has been detected in isolates of various *Enterobacteriaceae* from five continents (254). Furthermore, the gene *mcr-2* has been described in porcine and bovine *E. coli* isolates from Belgium (258). Most recently, another three *mcr* genes, designated *mcr-3* (259), *mcr-4* (260), and *mcr-5* (261), have been identified in *E. coli* and/or *S. enterica*. Several variants of *mcr-1* have been detected in *Enterobacteriaceae* (259), while *mcr-2* variants have been found in *Moraxella* spp. (262). Variants of the gene *mcr-3* have been identified in *Aeromonas* spp. (263, 264).

Polymyxin resistance due to the complete loss of LPS in *A. baumannii* is based on the inactivation of genes such as *lpxA*, *lpxC*, *lpxD*, and *lpsB*, the products of which are involved in LPS biosynthesis (265).

A variety of efflux pumps in several bacterial species have been described to be involved in polymyxin resistance in Gram-negative bacteria. Sensitive antimicrobial peptide proteins, encoded by the *sapABCDF* operon, and the resistance-nodulation-cell division transporter AcrAB-TolC seem to play a role in the susceptibility to polymyxins in *E. coli*, *S. enterica*, and *Proteus mirabilis* (266). The resistance-nodulation-cell division transporter VexB is involved in polymyxin resistance in *V. cholerae* (267). The efflux pump KpnEF, which has been described in isolates of *K. pneumoniae*, belongs to the small multidrug resistance protein family and is part of the Cpx regulon, which regulates capsule synthesis. Resistance to several antibiotics such as colistin, rifampicin, erythromycin, and ceftriaxone is influenced by KpnEF (267). Other efflux pumps of the small multidrug resistance protein family involved in polymyxin resistance have been identified in *B. subtilis* (EbrAB) and in *A. baumannii* (AbeS) (266).

Capsule formation is another mechanism of polymyxin resistance. Capsule polysaccharides limit the interaction of polymyxins with their target sites, thus playing an important role in polymyxin resistance, not only in intrinsically resistant bacteria such as *N. meningitidis* and *C. jejuni*, but also in *K. pneumoniae*, *E. coli*, and *P. aeruginosa* (268, 269). Moreover, anionic bacterial capsule polysaccharides have been shown to neutralize the bactericidal activity of cationic polypeptide antibiotics and antimicrobial peptides (269).

Overexpression of the outer membrane protein OprH contributes to polymyxin resistance in *P. aeruginosa*. OprH is a basic protein that binds to divalent cation-binding sites of LPSs, making these sites unavailable for polymyxins (270).

Resistance to Mupirocin

Mupirocin is a topical antibiotic used mainly for decolonization of MRSA and methicillin-susceptible *S. aureus* in patients and in health care personnel, but also for treatment of local skin and soft tissue infections caused by *S. aureus* and streptococci (271). It is not approved for veterinary use. Mupirocin prevents bacterial protein synthesis by inhibiting the bacterial isoleucyl-tRNA synthetase. Low-level resistance against mupirocin results from point mutations in the native isoleucyl-tRNA synthetase gene, whereas the acquisition of genes coding for alternative isoleucyl-tRNA synthetases leads to high-level resistance. The gene *mupA* (also referred to as *ileS2*) has been identified on conjugative plasmids (272–274), while the gene *mupB* has been found on nonconjugative plasmids in staphylococci (274, 275).

Resistance to Ansamycins

Certain ansamycins, such as rifampicin and rifamycin, are used in veterinary medicine for the treatment of infections of horses caused by *R. equi*. Rifampicin inhibits the bacterial RNA polymerase by interacting with the β-subunit, which is encoded by the gene *rpoB*. Resistance to rifampicin and related compounds is mainly due to point mutations that cause amino acid substitutions in at least one of three rifampicin resistance-determining regions within the *rpoB* gene. It is noteworthy that not all amino acid substitutions have the same effect. In *R. equi*, mutations at different positions within the *rpoB* gene have been shown to correlate with different rifampicin MIC values (276, 277). Mutations of *rpoB* have been described in several bacteria, such as *R. equi* (276, 277), *E. coli* (278), *Mycobacterium* spp. (279), *B. subtilis* (280), *S. aureus* (281), and *S. pseudintermedius* (282).

Furthermore, RNA polymerase binding proteins, such as RbpA in *Streptomyces coelicolor* and DnaA in *E. coli*, play a role in increased insensitivity to rifampicin (283).

Arr enzymes are ADP-ribosyltransferases, which are able to modify rifampicin by ADP-ribosylation and thus inactivate it. *M. smegmatis* carries the *arr* gene in its chromosomal DNA (284), homologues of which have been identified in the genomes of bacteria such as *S. maltophilia*, *Burkholderia cenocepacia*, and other environmental bacteria (284). The gene *arr-2* has been identified in chromosomal DNA and on various plasmids as part of class 1 integrons or composite transposons in Gram-negative bacteria such as *P. aeruginosa*, *K. pneumoniae*, and *E. coli* (283). An *arr-3* gene was detected in a class 1 integron of *Aeromonas hydrophila* from a koi carp (285).

Other modification mechanisms are glucosylation and phosphorylation in *Nocardia* spp. and phosphorylation in *Bacillus* spp. (283).

Resistance to Fosfomycin

Fosfomycin interferes with the peptidoglycan synthesis of bacteria by inhibiting the enzyme MurA. The irreversible inhibition is due to alkylation of the catalytic cysteine of MurA (286, 287). The exchange of cystein for asparagine is a target alteration, leading to intrinsic fosfomycin resistance in bacteria such as *M. tuberculosis*, *Chlamydia trachomatis*, and *Borrelia burgdorferi* (286, 287). Fosfomycin reaches its target site through GlpT, a glycerol-3-phosphate transporter, or via UhpT, a glucose-6-phosphate transporter. Both substrates induce the expression of their transporter, which is regulated by cAMP. Mutations in the genes coding for GlpT and UhpT or their regulators may lead to defective or inactive transporters, resulting in fosfomycin resistance (286, 287).

Enzymatic inactivation of fosfomycin can be achieved by several fosfomycin-modifying enzymes. The main enzymes described are three types of metalloenzymes (FosA, FosB, and FosX) and two kinases (FomA and FomB). FosA and FosB are thiol transferases, while FosX is a hydrolase. The metalloenzymes open the oxirane ring of fosfomycin and thus render it inactive. FosA enzymes are glutathione-*S*-transferases which use Mn^{2+} and K^+ as metal cofactors. They add glutathione to the oxirane ring, thereby opening the ring and inactivating fosfomycin (281). Various *fosA* genes have been identified on plasmids or in the chromosomal DNA of Gram-negative bacteria such as *S. marcescens*, *E. coli*, *K. pneumoniae*, *E. cloacae*, and *P. aeruginosa* (286, 287). They have been described as parts of transposons such as Tn*2921* or flanked by copies of IS26 on plasmid pFOS18 (288). The gene *fosC2*, which also codes for a glutathione-*S*-transferase, has been identified on a gene cassette in a class 1 integron on a conjugative plasmid in *E. coli* (289). Other *fos* genes have been described in numerous bacteria, including *fosC* in *Achromobacter denitrificans* and *fosK* in *Acinetobacter soli* (290).

FosB enzymes are bacillithiol-*S*-transferases that use Mg^{2+} as a cofactor. Several *fosB* gene variants have been detected in the chromosomal DNA of Gram-positive bacteria, such as *Staphylococcus epidermidis* (291), *B. subtilis*, *Bacillus anthracis*, and *S. aureus* (286, 287). The gene *fosB3* has been identified on a conjugative plasmid in *E. faecium* (292), while the genes *fosB1*, *fosB5*, and *fosB6* were located on small plasmids in *S. aureus* (293). The gene *fosD* is related to *fosB* and has been found in avian *Staphylococcus rostri* (294).

FosX enzymes are Mn^{2+}-dependent epoxide hydrolases, which use water to break the oxirane ring (286, 287). Variants of the gene *fosX* have been detected in the chromosomal DNA of *Clostridium botulinum*, *L. monocytogenes*, and *Brucella melitensis* (287). The gene *fosX*^{CC} was detected as part of a multidrug-resistance genomic island in *C. coli* (295).

FomA and FomB are kinases that originate from the fosfomycin producer *Streptomyces wedmorensis*. They sequentially add phosphates to the phosphonate moiety of fosfomycin by using Mg^{2+} as a cofactor (286). Most likely, these enzymes represent part of the self-defense system of the fosfomycin producer (286). Another such kinase, originally called FosC and found in another fosfomycin producer, *Pseudomonas syringae*, is an ortholog of FomA (296).

Resistance to Fusidic Acid

Fusidic acid is a steroidal compound which was isolated from *Fusidium coccineum*. It exhibits antimicrobial activitiy against Gram-positive bacteria, such as staphylococci and *Corynebacterium* spp., as well as the Gram-negative *Neisseria gonorrhoeae*, *N. meningitidis*, and *Moraxella catarrhalis* (297). Fusidic acid is mainly used topically to treat skin infections caused by staphylococci, but it can also be administered systemically. Fusidic acid binds to elongation factor G and thus prevents polypeptide chain elongation during protein synthesis (298). Elongation factor G is encoded by the gene *fusA*. Several mutations in the gene *fusA* that cause resistance to fusidic acid have been described in *S. aureus*, with L461K being the most prevalent (298). Protection of the target site and subsequent fusid acid resistance is conferred by the protein FusB, which prevents the interaction of fusidic acid with elongation factor G (299). The gene *fusB* has been identified on the widespread plasmid pUB101 in *S. aureus* (300). A *fusB*-related gene, *fusF*, has recently been identified in *Staphylococcus cohnii* (301). In contrast, the genes *fusC* and *fusD*, which also confer fusidic acid resistance by target protection, have been detected as part of a chimeric SCC*mec*IV-SCC$_{476}$ element in the chromosomal DNA of *S. aureus* (302) and in the chromosomal DNA of *S. saprophyticus* (303), respectively.

Resistance to Streptothricins

Streptothricins are antibiotics that consist of a streptolidine ring, a glucosamine, and a polylysine side chain. One of them, nourseothricin, was used as an antimicrobial feed additive in industrial animal farming in the former East Germany (304). Several *sat* genes have been identified which mediate streptothricin resistance by enzymatic inactivation via acetylation. In Gram-negative bacteria, particularly in *Enterobacteriaceae*, *sat* or *sat2* genes are usually located on gene cassettes in class 1 or class 2 integrons (305, 306). In staphylococci, the *sat4* gene is part of Tn*5405* and, as such, is commonly detected in staphylococci that also harbor *aphA3* and *aadE*. Furthermore, this gene has been detected in canine and feline *S. pseudintermedius* (307–309) and in MRSA of CC8 (ST254) from horses in Germany (310).

Resistance to Substances with Antimicrobial Activity Formerly Used as Growth Promoters

A number of substances with antimicrobial activity have been licensed as growth promoters for livestock. In the European Union, all growth promoters with antimicrobial activity were banned or withdrawn by 2006.

The mechanisms of resistance to the macrolides tylosin and spiramycin, the streptogramin virginiamycin, and the glycopeptide avoparcin were described in the sections "Resistance to Macrolides, Lincosamides, and Streptogramins (MLS)" and "Resistance to Glycopeptides." Hence, a brief summary of resistance to the remaining classes of growth promoters is given below. Two reviews (252, 311) are recommended for detailed insight into the various aspects of the use of growth promoters.

Bacitracin resistance was first described in the producer organism *Bacillus licheniformis*, in which an ABC transporter system, BcrABC, acts as a self-defense system by exporting the antibiotic from the producer cell (312). In *B. subtilis*, two independent but complementary-acting resistance mechanisms have been detected: an ABC transporter, YtsCD, that mediates the efflux of bacitracin, and a protein designated YwoA, which is believed to compete with bacitracin for the dephosphorylation of the C55-isoprenyl pyrophosphate (313). In *E. coli*, the gene *bacA*, which codes for an undecaprenyl pyrophosphate phosphatase, may account for bacitracin resistance (314). An ABC transporter, also termed BcrAB, that mediates bacitracin resistance was identified on a conjugative plasmid in *E. faecalis* (315).

Avilamycin resistance in the producer organism *Streptomyces viridochromogenes* Tü57 is based on the activity of an ABC transporter and two rRNA methyltransferases (316). In *E. faecalis* and *E. faecium*, resistance to avilamycin was initially described to be due to variations in the ribosomal protein L16 (317). Later, an rRNA methyltransferase, EmtA, which confers high-level resistance to avilamycin and evernimicin, was identified (318). Another two methylases—AviRa, which methylates 23S rRNA at the guanosine 2535 base, and AviRb, which methylates the uridine 2479 ribose—have been shown to confer avilamycin resistance (319). In addition, mutations at specific positions in the 23S rRNA also give rise to avilamycin resistance (320). Flavophospholipol (also known as flavomycin or bambermycin) has been reported to have a "plasmid-curing effect" on multiresistant *E. coli* under experimental conditions *in vitro* and *in vivo* (321). Cross-resistance to other antimicrobials has not been observed (252). Moreover, no genes or mutations conferring flavophospholipol resistance have been observed, to date.

Ionophores, such as salinomycin-Na and monensin-Na, are mainly used for the prevention of infections with parasites, such as *Eimeria* spp. (coccidiosis), *Plasmodium* spp., and *Giardia* spp. (252). Resistance or decreased susceptibility has been described in *S. hyicus*, coagulase-negative staphylococci from cattle and from *E. faecium* and *E. faecalis* from poultry and pigs. Genes or mutations accounting for acquired resistance to ionophores have not yet been described (252). Resistance to quinoxalines, such as carbadox and olaquindox, has been reported. An early study identified carbadox resistance to be associated with a conjugative multiresistance plasmid in *E. coli* (322). More than 20 years later, the genes *oqxA* and *oqxB*, which are responsible for olaqindox resistance, were cloned from a conjugative plasmid in *E. coli* (323). The corresponding gene products are homologous to several resistance-nodulation-cell-division family efflux systems and use TolC as the outer membrane component. Interestingly, the OqxAB-TolC system also mediates resistance to chloramphenicol and ethidium bromide (323).

CONCLUSION

The development of antimicrobial resistance—by either mutations, development of new resistance genes, or the acquisition of resistance genes already present in other bacteria—is a complex process that involves various mechanisms. Numerous resistance genes specifying different resistance mechanisms have been identified in various bacteria. The speed of resistance development differs with regard to the bacteria involved, the selective pressure imposed by the use of antimicrobial agents, and the availability and transferability of resistance genes in the gene pools accessible to the bacteria. These basic facts apply to resistance development in bacteria from humans as well as in bacteria from animals. The loss of acquired resistance properties is often a cumbersome process which is influenced mainly by selective pressure, but also by the colocation of the resistance genes on multiresistance plasmids or in the chromosomal DNA and the organization of the resistance genes in multiresistance gene clusters or integron structures. When organized in resistance gene clusters or integrons, loss of resistance genes may not be expected even in the absence of direct selective pressure. Because we know that the use of every antimicrobial substance can select for resistant bacteria, prudent use of antimicrobial agents is strongly recommended in both human and veterinary medicine, but particularly in food animal production to retain the efficacy of antimicrobial agents for the control of bacterial infections in animals.

Citation. van Duijkeren E, Schink A-K, Roberts MC, Wang Y, Schwarz S. 2017. Mechanisms of bacterial resistance to antimicrobial agents. Microbiol Spectrum 6(2):ARBA-0019-2017.

References

1. **Schwarz S, Chaslus-Dancla E.** 2001. Use of antimicrobials in veterinary medicine and mechanisms of resistance. *Vet Res* **32:**201–225.

2. **Schwarz S, Kehrenberg C, Walsh TR.** 2001. Use of antimicrobial agents in veterinary medicine and food animal production. *Int J Antimicrob Agents* **17:**431–437.

3. **Schwarz S, Noble WC.** 1999. Aspects of bacterial resistance to antimicrobial agents used in veterinary dermatological practice. *Vet Dermatol* **10:**163–176.

4. **Fiebelkorn KR, Crawford SA, Jorgensen JH.** 2005. Mutations in *folP* associated with elevated sulfonamide MICs for *Neisseria meningitidis* clinical isolates from five continents. *Antimicrob Agents Chemother* **49:**536–540.

5. **Datta N, Hedges RW.** 1972. Trimethoprim resistance conferred by W plasmids in *Enterobacteriaceae. J Gen Microbiol* **72:**349–355.

6. **Endtz HP, Ruijs GJ, van Klingeren B, Jansen WH, van der Reyden T, Mouton RP.** 1991. Quinolone resistance in campylobacter isolated from man and poultry following the introduction of fluoroquinolones in veterinary medicine. *J Antimicrob Chemother* **27:**199–208.

7. **Tsiodras S, Gold HS, Sakoulas G, Eliopoulos GM, Wennersten C, Venkataraman L, Moellering RC Jr, Ferraro MJ.** 2001. Linezolid resistance in a clinical isolate of *Staphylococcus aureus. Lancet* **358:**207–208.

8. **Schwarz S, Cloeckaert A, Roberts MC.** 2006. Mechanisms and spread of bacterial resistance to antimicrobial agents, p 73–98. *In* Aarestrup FM (ed), *Antimicrobial Resistance in Bacteria of Animal Origin.* ASM Press, Washington, DC.

9. **Schwarz S, Loeffler A, Kadlec K.** 2017. Bacterial resistance to antimicrobial agents and its impact on veterinary and human medicine. *Vet Dermatol* **28:**82–e19.

10. **Livermore DM.** 1995. β-Lactamases in laboratory and clinical resistance. *Clin Microbiol Rev* **8:**557–584.

11. **Georgopapadakou NH.** 1993. Penicillin-binding proteins and bacterial resistance to β-lactams. *Antimicrob Agents Chemother* **37:**2045–2053.

12. **Paulsen IT, Brown MH, Skurray RA.** 1996. Proton-dependent multidrug efflux systems. *Microbiol Rev* **60:**575–608.

13. **Quintiliani R Jr, Sahm DF, Courvalin P.** 1999. Mechanisms of resistance to antimicrobial agents, p 1505–1525. *In* Murray PR, Baron EJ, Pfaller MA, Tenover FC, Yolken RH (ed), *Manual of Clinical Microbiology,* 7th ed. ASM Press, Washington, DC.

14. **Petrosino J, Cantu C III, Palzkill T.** 1998. β-Lactamases: protein evolution in real time. *Trends Microbiol* **6:**323–327.

15. **Bush K.** 2001. New beta-lactamases in gram-negative bacteria: diversity and impact on the selection of antimicrobial therapy. *Clin Infect Dis* **32:**1085–1089.

16. **Bush K, Jacoby GA, Medeiros AA.** 1995. A functional classification scheme for β-lactamases and its correlation with molecular structure. *Antimicrob Agents Chemother* **39:**1211–1233.

17. **Ambler RP.** 1980. The structure of β-lactamases. *Philos Trans R Soc Lond B Biol Sci* **289:**321–331.

18. **Bush K, Jacoby GA.** 2010. Updated functional classification of beta-lactamases. *Antimicrob Agents Chemother* **54:**969–976.

19. **Bradford PA.** 2001. Extended-spectrum β-lactamases in the 21st century: characterization, epidemiology, and detection of this important resistance threat. *Clin Microbiol Rev* **14:**933–951.

20. **Bonnet R.** 2004. Growing group of extended-spectrum β-lactamases: the CTX-M enzymes. *Antimicrob Agents Chemother* **48:**1–14.

21. **Brolund A, Sandegren L.** 2016. Characterization of ESBL disseminating plasmids. *Infect Dis (Lond)* **48:**18–25.

22. **Weldhagen GF.** 2004. Integrons and β-lactamases: a novel perspective on resistance. *Int J Antimicrob Agents* **23:**556–562.

23. **Gilmore KS, Gilmore MS, Sahm DF.** 2002. Methicillin resistance in *Staphylococcus aureus,* p 331–354. *In* Lewis K, Salyers AA, Taber HW, Wax RG (ed), *Bacterial Resistance to Antimicrobials.* Marcel Dekker, New York, NY.

24. **Hackbarth CJ, Chambers HF.** 1989. Methicillin-resistant staphylococci: genetics and mechanisms of resistance. *Antimicrob Agents Chemother* **33:**991–994.

25. **Katayama Y, Ito T, Hiramatsu K.** 2000. A new class of genetic element, *Staphylococcus* cassette chromosome *mec,* encodes methicillin resistance in *Staphylococcus aureus. Antimicrob Agents Chemother* **44:**1549–1555.

26. http://www.sccmec.org/Pages/SCC_TypesEN.html

27. García-Álvarez L, Holden MT, Lindsay H, Webb CR, Brown DF, Curran MD, Walpole E, Brooks K, Pickard DJ, Teale C, Parkhill J, Bentley SD, Edwards GF, Girvan EK, Kearns AM, Pichon B, Hill RL, Larsen AR, Skov RL, Peacock SJ, Maskell DJ, Holmes MA. 2011. Meticillin-resistant *Staphylococcus aureus* with a novel *mecA* homologue in human and bovine populations in the UK and Denmark: a descriptive study. *Lancet Infect Dis* 11:595–603.

28. Shore AC, Deasy EC, Slickers P, Brennan G, O'Connell B, Monecke S, Ehricht R, Coleman DC. 2011. Detection of staphylococcal cassette chromosome *mec* type XI carrying highly divergent *mecA*, *mecI*, *mecR1*, *blaZ*, and *ccr* genes in human clinical isolates of clonal complex 130 methicillin-resistant *Staphylococcus aureus*. *Antimicrob Agents Chemother* 55:3765–3773.

29. Loncaric I, Kübber-Heiss A, Posautz A, Stalder GL, Hoffmann D, Rosengarten R, Walzer C. 2013. Characterization of methicillin-resistant *Staphylococcus* spp. carrying the *mecC* gene, isolated from wildlife. *J Antimicrob Chemother* 68:2222–2225.

30. Harrison EM, Paterson GK, Holden MT, Morgan FJ, Larsen AR, Petersen A, Leroy S, De Vliegher S, Perreten V, Fox LK, Lam TJ, Sampimon OC, Zadoks RN, Peacock SJ, Parkhill J, Holmes MA. 2013. A *Staphylococcus xylosus* isolate with a new *mecC* allotype. *Antimicrob Agents Chemother* 57:1524–1528.

31. Małyszko I, Schwarz S, Hauschild T. 2014. Detection of a new *mecC* allotype, *mecC2*, in methicillin-resistant *Staphylococcus saprophyticus*. *J Antimicrob Chemother* 69:2003–2005.

32. Ehlert K. 1999. Methicillin-resistance in *Staphylococcus aureus*: molecular basis, novel targets and antibiotic therapy. *Curr Pharm Des* 5:45–55.

33. Ling B, Berger-Bächi B. 1998. Increased overall antibiotic susceptibility in *Staphylococcus aureus femAB* null mutants. *Antimicrob Agents Chemother* 42:936–938.

34. Charrel RN, Pagès J-M, De Micco P, Mallea M. 1996. Prevalence of outer membrane porin alteration in β-lactam-antibiotic-resistant *Enterobacter aerogenes*. *Antimicrob Agents Chemother* 40:2854–2858.

35. Hopkins JM, Towner KJ. 1990. Enhanced resistance to cefotaxime and imipenem associated with outer membrane protein alterations in *Enterobacter aerogenes*. *J Antimicrob Chemother* 25:49–55.

36. Mitsuyama J, Hiruma R, Yamaguchi A, Sawai T. 1987. Identification of porins in outer membrane of *Proteus*, *Morganella*, and *Providencia* spp. and their role in outer membrane permeation of β-lactams. *Antimicrob Agents Chemother* 31:379–384.

37. Simonet V, Malléa M, Pagès J-M. 2000. Substitutions in the eyelet region disrupt cefepime diffusion through the *Escherichia coli* OmpF channel. *Antimicrob Agents Chemother* 44:311–315.

38. Martínez-Martínez L, Hernández-Allés S, Albertí S, Tomás JM, Benedi VJ, Jacoby GA. 1996. *In vivo* selection of porin-deficient mutants of *Klebsiella pneumoniae* with increased resistance to cefoxitin and expanded-spectrum-cephalosporins. *Antimicrob Agents Chemother* 40:342–348.

39. Wolter DJ, Hanson ND, Lister PD. 2004. Insertional inactivation of *oprD* in clinical isolates of *Pseudomonas aeruginosa* leading to carbapenem resistance. *FEMS Microbiol Lett* 236:137–143.

40. Poole K. 2002. Multidrug efflux pumps and antimicrobial resistance in *Pseudomonas aeruginosa* and related organisms, p 273–298. *In* Paulsen IT, Lewis K (ed), *Microbial Multidrug Efflux*. Horizon Scientific Press, Wymondham, United Kingdom.

41. Putman M, van Veen HW, Konings WN. 2000. Molecular properties of bacterial multidrug transporters. *Microbiol Mol Biol Rev* 64:672–693.

42. Grave K, Torren-Edo J, Muller A, Greko C, Moulin G, Mackay D, Fuchs K, Laurier L, Iliev D, Pokludova L, Genakritis M, Jacobsen E, Kurvits K, Kivilahti-Mantyla K, Wallmann J, Kovacs J, Lenharthsson JM, Beechinor JG, Perrella A, Mičule G, Zymantaite U, Meijering A, Prokopiak D, Ponte MH, Svetlin A, Hederova J, Madero CM, Girma K, Eckford S, ESVAC Group. 2014. Variations in the sales and sales patterns of veterinary antimicrobial agents in 25 European countries. *J Antimicrob Chemother* 69:2284–2291.

43. Casas C, Anderson EC, Ojo KK, Keith I, Whelan D, Rainnie D, Roberts MC. 2005. Characterization of pRAS1-like plasmids from atypical North American psychrophilic *Aeromonas salmonicida*. *FEMS Microbiol Lett* 242:59–63.

44. DePaola A, Roberts MC. 1995. Class D and E tetracycline resistance determinants in Gram-negative catfish pond bacteria. *Mol Cell Probes* 9:311–313.

45. Miranda CD, Kehrenberg C, Ulep C, Schwarz S, Roberts MC. 2003. Diversity of tetracycline resistance genes in bacteria from Chilean salmon farms. *Antimicrob Agents Chemother* 47:883–888.

46. Chopra I, Roberts M. 2001. Tetracycline antibiotics: mode of action, applications, molecular biology, and epidemiology of bacterial resistance. *Microbiol Mol Biol Rev* 65:232–260.

47. Levy SB, McMurry LM, Barbosa TM, Burdett V, Courvalin P, Hillen W, Roberts MC, Rood JI, Taylor DE. 1999. Nomenclature for new tetracycline resistance determinants. *Antimicrob Agents Chemother* 43:1523–1524.

48. Roberts MC, Schwarz S. 2016. Tetracycline and phenicol resistance genes and mechanisms: importance for agriculture, the environment, and humans. *J Environ Qual* 45:576–592.

49. Roberts MC, Schwarz S, Aarts HJ. 2012. Erratum: acquired antibiotic resistance genes: an overview. *Front Microbiol* 3:384.

50. Roberts MC, No D, Kuchmiy E, Miranda CD. 2015. Tetracycline resistance gene *tet*(39) identified in three new genera of bacteria isolated in 1999 from Chilean salmon farms. *J Antimicrob Chemother* 70:619–621.

51. Speer BS, Shoemaker NB, Salyers AA. 1992. Bacterial resistance to tetracycline: mechanisms, transfer, and clinical significance. *Clin Microbiol Rev* 5:387–399.

52. Linkevicius M, Sandegren L, Andersson DI. 2015. Potential of tetracycline resistance proteins to evolve tigecycline resistance. *Antimicrob Agents Chemother* **60**: 789–796.

53. Fiedler S, Bender JK, Klare I, Halbedel S, Grohmann E, Szewzyk U, Werner G. 2016. Tigecycline resistance in clinical isolates of *Enterococcus faecium* is mediated by an upregulation of plasmid-encoded tetracycline determinants *tet*(L) and *tet*(M). *J Antimicrob Chemother* **71**: 871–881.

54. Roberts MC. 1996. Tetracycline resistance determinants: mechanisms of action, regulation of expression, genetic mobility, and distribution. *FEMS Microbiol Rev* **19**: 1–24.

55. Allmeier H, Cresnar B, Greck M, Schmitt R. 1992. Complete nucleotide sequence of Tn*1721*: gene organization and a novel gene product with features of a chemotaxis protein. *Gene* **111**:11–20.

56. Chalmers R, Sewitz S, Lipkow K, Crellin P. 2000. Complete nucleotide sequence of Tn*10*. *J Bacteriol* **182**: 2970–2972.

57. Lawley TD, Burland V, Taylor DE. 2000. Analysis of the complete nucleotide sequence of the tetracycline-resistance transposon Tn*10*. *Plasmid* **43**:235–239.

58. Kehrenberg C, Werckenthin C, Schwarz S. 1998. Tn*5706*, a transposon-like element from *Pasteurella multocida* mediating tetracycline resistance. *Antimicrob Agents Chemother* **42**:2116–2118.

59. Projan SJ, Kornblum J, Moghazeh SL, Edelman I, Gennaro ML, Novick RP. 1985. Comparative sequence and functional analysis of pT181 and pC221, cognate plasmid replicons from *Staphylococcus aureus*. *Mol Gen Genet* **199**:452–464.

60. Schwarz S, Noble WC. 1994. Tetracycline resistance genes in staphylococci from the skin of pigs. *J Appl Bacteriol* **76**:320–326.

61. Werckenthin C, Schwarz S, Roberts MC. 1996. Integration of pT181-like tetracycline resistance plasmids into large staphylococcal plasmids involves IS*257*. *Antimicrob Agents Chemother* **40**:2542–2544.

62. Taylor DE, Chau A. 1996. Tetracycline resistance mediated by ribosomal protection. *Antimicrob Agents Chemother* **40**:1–5.

63. Connell SR, Tracz DM, Nierhaus KH, Taylor DE. 2003. Ribosomal protection proteins and their mechanism of tetracycline resistance. *Antimicrob Agents Chemother* **47**:3675–3681.

64. Flannagan SE, Zitzow LA, Su YA, Clewell DB. 1994. Nucleotide sequence of the 18-kb conjugative transposon Tn*916* from *Enterococcus faecalis*. *Plasmid* **32**: 350–354.

65. Salyers AA, Shoemaker NB, Stevens AM, Li L-Y. 1995. Conjugative transposons: an unusual and diverse set of integrated gene transfer elements. *Microbiol Rev* **59**: 579–590.

66. Forsberg KJ, Patel S, Wencewicz TA, Dantas G. 2015. The tetracycline destructases: A novel family of tetracycline-inactivating enzymes. *Chem Biol* **22**:888–897.

67. Speer BS, Bedzyk L, Salyers AA. 1991. Evidence that a novel tetracycline resistance gene found on two *Bacteroides* transposons encodes an NADP-requiring oxidoreductase. *J Bacteriol* **173**:176–183.

68. Diaz-Torres ML, McNab R, Spratt DA, Villedieu A, Hunt N, Wilson M, Mullany P. 2003. Novel tetracycline resistance determinant from the oral metagenome. *Antimicrob Agents Chemother* **47**:1430–1432.

69. Nonaka L, Suzuki S. 2002. New Mg^{2+}-dependent oxytetracycline resistance determinant tet 34 in *Vibrio* isolates from marine fish intestinal contents. *Antimicrob Agents Chemother* **46**:1550–1552.

70. Ross JI, Eady EA, Cove JH, Cunliffe WJ. 1998. 16S rRNA mutation associated with tetracycline resistance in a Gram-positive bacterium. *Antimicrob Agents Chemother* **42**:1702–1705.

71. Sutcliffe JA, Leclercq R. 2003. Mechanisms of resistance to macrolides, lincosamides and ketolides, p 281–317. *In* Schonfeld W, Kirst HA (ed), *Macrolide Antibiotics*. Birkhauser Verlag, Basel, Switzerland.

72. Schwarz S, Shen J, Kadlec K, Wang Y, Brenner Michael G, Feßler AT, Vester B. 2016. Lincosamides, streptogramins, phenicols, and pleuromutilins: mode of action and mechanisms of resistance. *Cold Spring Harb Perspect Med* **6**:a027037.

73. Fyfe C, Grossman TH, Kerstein K, Sutcliffe J. 2016. Resistance to macrolide antibiotics in public health pathogens. *Cold Spring Harb Perspect Med* **6**:a025395.

74. Roberts MC, Sutcliffe J, Courvalin P, Jensen LB, Rood J, Seppala H. 1999. Nomenclature for macrolide and macrolide-lincosamide-streptogramin B resistance determinants. *Antimicrob Agents Chemother* **43**:2823–2830.

75. Leclercq R, Courvalin P. 1991. Bacterial resistance to macrolide, lincosamide, and streptogramin antibiotics by target modification. *Antimicrob Agents Chemother* **35**:1267–1272.

76. Weisblum B. 1995. Erythromycin resistance by ribosome modification. *Antimicrob Agents Chemother* **39**: 577–585.

77. Weisblum B. 1995. Insights into erythromycin action from studies of its activity as inducer of resistance. *Antimicrob Agents Chemother* **39**:797–805.

78. Schmitz F-J, Petridou J, Jagusch H, Astfalk N, Scheuring S, Schwarz S. 2002. Molecular characterization of ketolide-resistant *erm*(A)-carrying *Staphylococcus aureus* isolates selected *in vitro* by telithromycin, ABT-773, quinupristin and clindamycin. *J Antimicrob Chemother* **49**:611–617.

79. Schmitz F-J, Petridou J, Astfalk N, Köhrer K, Scheuring S, Schwarz S. 2002. Molecular analysis of constitutively expressed *erm*(C) genes selected *in vitro* by incubation in the presence of the noninducers quinupristin, telithromycin, or ABT-773. *Microb Drug Resist* **8**:171–177.

80. Lüthje P, Schwarz S. 2007. Molecular analysis of constitutively expressed *erm*(C) genes selected *in vitro* in the presence of the non-inducers pirlimycin, spiramycin and tylosin. *J Antimicrob Chemother* **59**:97–101.

81. Werckenthin C, Schwarz S, Westh H. 1999. Structural alterations in the translational attenuator of constitutively

expressed ermC genes. *Antimicrob Agents Chemother* 43:1681–1685.

82. **Leclercq R, Courvalin P.** 1991. Intrinsic and unusual resistance to macrolide, lincosamide, and streptogramin antibiotics in bacteria. *Antimicrob Agents Chemother* 35:1273–1276.

83. **Sharkey LK, Edwards TA, O'Neill AJ.** 2016. ABC-F proteins mediate antibiotic resistance through ribosomal protection. *MBio* 7:e01975.

84. **Ross JI, Eady EA, Cove JH, Cunliffe WJ, Baumberg S, Wootton JC.** 1990. Inducible erythromycin resistance in staphylococci is encoded by a member of the ATP-binding transport super-gene family. *Mol Microbiol* 4:1207–1214.

85. **Reynolds E, Ross JI, Cove JH.** 2003. *Msr*(A) and related macrolide/streptogramin resistance determinants: incomplete transporters? *Int J Antimicrob Agents* 22:228–236.

86. **Lüthje P, Schwarz S.** 2006. Antimicrobial resistance of coagulase-negative staphylococci from bovine subclinical mastitis with particular reference to macrolide-lincosamide resistance phenotypes and genotypes. *J Antimicrob Chemother* 57:966–969.

87. **Clancy J, Petitpas J, Dib-Hajj F, Yuan W, Cronan M, Kamath AV, Bergeron J, Retsema JA.** 1996. Molecular cloning and functional analysis of a novel macrolide-resistance determinant, *mefA*, from *Streptococcus pyogenes. Mol Microbiol* 22:867–879.

88. **Cousin S Jr, Whittington WL, Roberts MC.** 2003. Acquired macrolide resistance genes in pathogenic *Neisseria* spp. isolated between 1940 and 1987. *Antimicrob Agents Chemother* 47:3877–3880.

89. **Ojo KK, Ulep C, Van Kirk N, Luis H, Bernardo M, Leitao J, Roberts MC.** 2004. The *mef*(A) gene predominates among seven macrolide resistant genes identified in 13 Gram-negative genera from healthy Portuguese children. *Antimicrob Agents Chemother* 48:3451–3456.

90. **Daly MM, Doktor S, Flamm R, Shortridge D.** 2004. Characterization and prevalence of MefA, MefE, and the associated *msr*(D) gene in *Streptococcus pneumoniae* clinical isolates. *J Clin Microbiol* 42:3570–3574.

91. **Plante I, Centrón D, Roy PH.** 2003. An integron cassette encoding erythromycin esterase, *ere*(A), from *Providencia stuartii. J Antimicrob Chemother* 51:787–790.

92. **Lipka M, Filipek R, Bochtler M.** 2008. Crystal structure and mechanism of the *Staphylococcus cohnii* virginiamycin B lyase (Vgb). *Biochemistry* 47:4257–4265.

93. **Chesneau O, Tsvetkova K, Courvalin P.** 2007. Resistance phenotypes conferred by macrolide phosphotransferases. *FEMS Microbiol Lett* 269:317–322.

94. **Vester B, Douthwaite S.** 2001. Macrolide resistance conferred by base substitutions in 23S rRNA. *Antimicrob Agents Chemother* 45:1–12.

95. **Meier A, Kirschner P, Springer B, Steingrube VA, Brown BA, Wallace RJ Jr, Böttger EC.** 1994. Identification of mutations in 23S rRNA gene of clarithromycin-resistant *Mycobacterium intracellulare. Antimicrob Agents Chemother* 38:381–384.

96. **Karlsson M, Fellström C, Heldtander MU, Johansson KE, Franklin A.** 1999. Genetic basis of macrolide and lincosamide resistance in *Brachyspira* (*Serpulina*) *hyodysenteriae. FEMS Microbiol Lett* 172:255–260.

97. **Haanperä M, Huovinen P, Jalava J.** 2005. Detection and quantification of macrolide resistance mutations at positions 2058 and 2059 of the 23S rRNA gene by pyrosequencing. *Antimicrob Agents Chemother* 49:457–460.

98. **Harrow SA, Gilpin BJ, Klena JD.** 2004. Characterization of erythromycin resistance in *Campylobacter coli* and *Campylobacter jejuni* isolated from pig offal in New Zealand. *J Appl Microbiol* 97:141–148.

99. **Mingeot-Leclercq M-P, Glupczynski Y, Tulkens PM.** 1999. Aminoglycosides: activity and resistance. *Antimicrob Agents Chemother* 43:727–737.

100. **Shaw KJ, Rather PN, Hare RS, Miller GH.** 1993. Molecular genetics of aminoglycoside resistance genes and familial relationships of the aminoglycoside-modifying enzymes. *Microbiol Rev* 57:138–163.

101. **Ramirez MS, Tolmasky ME.** 2010. Aminoglycoside modifying enzymes. *Drug Resist Updat* 13:151–171.

102. **Wright GD.** 1999. Aminoglycoside-modifying enzymes. *Curr Opin Microbiol* 2:499–503.

103. **Davies J, Wright GD.** 1997. Bacterial resistance to aminoglycoside antibiotics. *Trends Microbiol* 5:234–240.

104. **Hedges RW, Shannon KP.** 1984. Resistance to apramycin in *Escherichia coli* isolated from animals: detection of a novel aminoglycoside-modifying enzyme. *J Gen Microbiol* 130:473–482.

105. **Chaslus-Dancla E, Glupczynski Y, Gerbaud G, Lagorce M, Lafont JP, Courvalin P.** 1989. Detection of apramycin resistant *Enterobacteriaceae* in hospital isolates. *FEMS Microbiol Lett* 52:261–265.

106. **Chaslus-Dancla E, Pohl P, Meurisse M, Marin M, Lafont JP.** 1991. High genetic homology between plasmids of human and animal origins conferring resistance to the aminoglycosides gentamicin and apramycin. *Antimicrob Agents Chemother* 35:590–593.

107. **Johnson AP, Burns L, Woodford N, Threlfall EJ, Naidoo J, Cooke EM, George RC.** 1994. Gentamicin resistance in clinical isolates of *Escherichia coli* encoded by genes of veterinary origin. *J Med Microbiol* 40:221–226.

108. **Lyon BR, Skurray R.** 1987. Antimicrobial resistance of *Staphylococcus aureus*: genetic basis. *Microbiol Rev* 51:88–134.

109. **Rouch DA, Byrne ME, Kong YC, Skurray RA.** 1987. The *aacA-aphD* gentamicin and kanamycin resistance determinant of Tn4001 from *Staphylococcus aureus*: expression and nucleotide sequence analysis. *J Gen Microbiol* 133:3039–3052.

110. **Lange CC, Werckenthin C, Schwarz S.** 2003. Molecular analysis of the plasmid-borne *aacA/aphD* resistance gene region of coagulase-negative staphylococci from chickens. *J Antimicrob Chemother* 51:1397–1401.

111. **Leelaporn A, Yodkamol K, Waywa D, Pattanachaiwit S.** 2008. A novel structure of Tn4001-truncated element, type V, in clinical enterococcal isolates and multiplex PCR for detecting aminoglycoside resistance genes. *Int J Antimicrob Agents* 31:250–254.

112. Recchia GD, Hall RM. 1995. Gene cassettes: a new class of mobile element. *Microbiology* **141**:3015–3027.

113. Sandvang D, Aarestrup FM. 2000. Characterization of aminoglycoside resistance genes and class 1 integrons in porcine and bovine gentamicin-resistant *Escherichia coli*. *Microb Drug Resist* **6**:19–27.

114. Feßler AT, Kadlec K, Schwarz S. 2011. Novel apramycin resistance gene *apmA* in bovine and porcine methicillin-resistant *Staphylococcus aureus* ST398 isolates. *Antimicrob Agents Chemother* **55**:373–375.

115. Kadlec K, Feßler AT, Couto N, Pomba CF, Schwarz S. 2012. Unusual small plasmids carrying the novel resistance genes *dfrK* or *apmA* isolated from methicillin-resistant or -susceptible staphylococci. *J Antimicrob Chemother* **67**:2342–2345.

116. Feßler AT, Zhao Q, Schoenfelder S, Kadlec K, Brenner Michael G, Wang Y, Ziebuhr W, Shen J, Schwarz S. 2017. Complete sequence of a plasmid from a bovine methicillin-resistant *Staphylococcus aureus* harbouring a novel *ica*-like gene cluster in addition to antimicrobial and heavy metal resistance genes. *Vet Microbiol* **200**:95–100.

117. Murphy E. 1985. Nucleotide sequence of a spectinomycin adenyltransferase AAD(9) determinant from *Staphylococcus aureus* and its relationship to AAD(3″) (9). *Mol Gen Genet* **200**:33–39.

118. Wendlandt S, Li B, Lozano C, Ma Z, Torres C, Schwarz S. 2013. Identification of the novel spectinomycin resistance gene *spw* in methicillin-resistant and methicillin-susceptible *Staphylococcus aureus* of human and animal origin. *J Antimicrob Chemother* **68**:1679–1680.

119. Jamrozy DM, Coldham NG, Butaye P, Fielder MD. 2014. Identification of a novel plasmid-associated spectinomycin adenyltransferase gene *spd* in methicillin-resistant *Staphylococcus aureus* ST398 isolated from animal and human sources. *J Antimicrob Chemother* **69**:1193–1196.

120. Wendlandt S, Feßler AT, Kadlec K, van Duijkeren E, Schwarz S. 2014. Identification of the novel spectinomycin resistance gene *spd* in a different plasmid background among methicillin-resistant *Staphylococcus aureus* CC398 and methicillin-susceptible *S. aureus* ST433. *J Antimicrob Chemother* **69**:2000–2003.

121. Wendlandt S, Kadlec K, Schwarz S. 2015. Four novel plasmids from *Staphylococcus hyicus* and CoNS that carry a variant of the spectinomycin resistance gene *spd*. *J Antimicrob Chemother* **70**:948–949.

122. Rosenberg EY, Ma D, Nikaido H. 2000. AcrD of *Escherichia coli* is an aminoglycoside efflux pump. *J Bacteriol* **182**:1754–1756.

123. Edgar R, Bibi E. 1997. MdfA, an *Escherichia coli* multidrug resistance protein with an extraordinarily broad spectrum of drug recognition. *J Bacteriol* **179**:2274–2280.

124. Salyers AA, Whitt DD. 1994. *Bacterial Pathogenesis: a Molecular Approach*. ASM Press, Washington, DC.

125. Galimand M, Courvalin P, Lambert T. 2003. Plasmid-mediated high-level resistance to aminoglycosides in *Enterobacteriaceae* due to 16S rRNA methylation. *Antimicrob Agents Chemother* **47**:2565–2571.

126. Potron A, Poirel L, Nordmann P. 2015. Emerging broad-spectrum resistance in *Pseudomonas aeruginosa* and *Acinetobacter baumannii*: mechanisms and epidemiology. *Int J Antimicrob Agents* **45**:568–585.

127. Wachino J, Arakawa Y. 2012. Exogenously acquired 16S rRNA methyltransferases found in aminoglycoside-resistant pathogenic Gram-negative bacteria: an update. *Drug Resist Updat* **15**:133–148.

128. Meier A, Sander P, Schaper KJ, Scholz M, Böttger EC. 1996. Correlation of molecular resistance mechanisms and phenotypic resistance levels in streptomycin-resistant *Mycobacterium tuberculosis*. *Antimicrob Agents Chemother* **40**:2452–2454.

129. Prammananan T, Sander P, Brown BA, Frischkorn K, Onyi GO, Zhang Y, Böttger EC, Wallace RJ Jr. 1998. A single 16S ribosomal RNA substitution is responsible for resistance to amikacin and other 2-deoxystreptamine aminoglycosides in *Mycobacterium abscessus* and *Mycobacterium chelonae*. *J Infect Dis* **177**:1573–1581.

130. Cohen KA, Bishai WR, Pym AS. 2014. Molecular basis of drug resistance in *Mycobacterium tuberculosis*. *Microbiol Spectr* **2**:.

131. Elwell LP, Fling ME. 1989. Resistance to trimethoprim, p 249–290. *In* Bryan LE (ed), *Microbial Resistance to Drugs*. Springer Verlag, Berlin, Germany.

132. Huovinen P. 2001. Resistance to trimethoprim-sulfamethoxazole. *Clin Infect Dis* **32**:1608–1614.

133. Huovinen P, Sundström L, Swedberg G, Sköld O. 1995. Trimethoprim and sulfonamide resistance. *Antimicrob Agents Chemother* **39**:279–289.

134. Sköld O. 2000. Sulfonamide resistance: mechanisms and trends. *Drug Resist Updat* **3**:155–160.

135. Sköld O. 2001. Resistance to trimethoprim and sulfonamides. *Vet Res* **32**:261–273.

136. Köhler T, Kok M, Michea-Hamzehpour M, Plesiat P, Gotoh N, Nishino T, Curty LK, Pechere J-C. 1996. Multidrug efflux in intrinsic resistance to trimethoprim and sulfamethoxazole in *Pseudomonas aeruginosa*. *Antimicrob Agents Chemother* **40**:2288–2290.

137. Padayachee T, Klugman KP. 1999. Novel expansions of the gene encoding dihydropteroate synthase in trimethoprim-sulfamethoxazole-resistant *Streptococcus pneumoniae*. *Antimicrob Agents Chemother* **43**:2225–2230.

138. Dale GE, Broger C, D'Arcy A, Hartman PG, DeHoogt R, Jolidon S, Kompis I, Labhardt AM, Langen H, Locher H, Page MG, Stüber D, Then RL, Wipf B, Oefner C. 1997. A single amino acid substitution in *Staphylococcus aureus* dihydrofolate reductase determines trimethoprim resistance. *J Mol Biol* **266**:23–30.

139. Pikis A, Donkersloot JA, Rodriguez WJ, Keith JM. 1998. A conservative amino acid mutation in the chromosome-encoded dihydrofolate reductase confers trimethoprim resistance in *Streptococcus pneumoniae*. *J Infect Dis* **178**:700–706.

140. de Groot R, Sluijter M, de Bruyn A, Campos J, Goessens WHF, Smith AL, Hermans PWM. 1996. Genetic characterization of trimethoprim resistance in *Haemophilus influenzae*. *Antimicrob Agents Chemother* **40**:2131–2136.

141. Sundström L, Rådström P, Swedberg G, Sköld O. 1988. Site-specific recombination promotes linkage between trimethoprim- and sulfonamide resistance genes. Sequence characterization of *dhfrV* and *sulI* and a recombination active locus of Tn*21. Mol Gen Genet* 213: 191–201.

142. Rådström P, Swedberg G. 1988. RSF1010 and a conjugative plasmid contain *sulII*, one of two known genes for plasmid-borne sulfonamide resistance dihydropteroate synthase. *Antimicrob Agents Chemother* 32:1684–1692.

143. Swedberg G, Sköld O. 1980. Characterization of different plasmid-borne dihydropteroate synthases mediating bacterial resistance to sulfonamides. *J Bacteriol* 142: 1–7.

144. Perreten V, Boerlin P. 2003. A new sulfonamide resistance gene (*sul3*) in *Escherichia coli* is widespread in the pig population of Switzerland. *Antimicrob Agents Chemother* 47:1169–1172.

145. Grape M, Sundström L, Kronvall G. 2003. Sulphonamide resistance gene *sul3* found in *Escherichia coli* isolates from human sources. *J Antimicrob Chemother* 52:1022–1024.

146. Guerra B, Junker E, Helmuth R. 2004. Incidence of the recently described sulfonamide resistance gene *sul3* among German *Salmonella enterica* strains isolated from livestock and food. *Antimicrob Agents Chemother* 48:2712–2715.

147. Guerra B, Junker E, Schroeter A, Malorny B, Lehmann S, Helmuth R. 2003. Phenotypic and genotypic characterization of antimicrobial resistance in German *Escherichia coli* isolates from cattle, swine and poultry. *J Antimicrob Chemother* 52:489–492.

148. Pattishall KH, Acar J, Burchall JJ, Goldstein FW, Harvey RJ. 1977. Two distinct types of trimethoprim-resistant dihydrofolate reductase specified by R-plasmids of different compatibility groups. *J Biol Chem* 252:2319–2323.

149. Sekiguchi J, Tharavichitkul P, Miyoshi-Akiyama T, Chupia V, Fujino T, Araake M, Irie A, Morita K, Kuratsuji T, Kirikae T. 2005. Cloning and characterization of a novel trimethoprim-resistant dihydrofolate reductase from a nosocomial isolate of *Staphylococcus aureus* CM.S2 (IMCJ1454). *Antimicrob Agents Chemother* 49:3948–3951.

150. Dale GE, Langen H, Page MG, Then RL, Stüber D. 1995. Cloning and characterization of a novel, plasmid-encoded trimethoprim-resistant dihydrofolate reductase from *Staphylococcus haemolyticus* MUR313. *Antimicrob Agents Chemother* 39:1920–1924.

151. Charpentier E, Courvalin P. 1997. Emergence of the trimethoprim resistance gene *dfrD* in *Listeria monocytogenes* BM4293. *Antimicrob Agents Chemother* 41: 1134–1136.

152. Kadlec K, Schwarz S. 2009. Identification of a novel trimethoprim resistance gene, *dfrK*, in a methicillin-resistant *Staphylococcus aureus* ST398 strain and its physical linkage to the tetracycline resistance gene *tet* (L). *Antimicrob Agents Chemother* 53:776–778.

153. Kadlec K, Schwarz S. 2010. Identification of the novel *dfrK*-carrying transposon Tn*559* in a porcine methicillin-susceptible *Staphylococcus aureus* ST398 strain. *Antimicrob Agents Chemother* 54:3475–3477.

154. López M, Kadlec K, Schwarz S, Torres C. 2012. First detection of the staphylococcal trimethoprim resistance gene *dfrK* and the *dfrK*-carrying transposon Tn*559* in enterococci. *Microb Drug Resist* 18:13–18.

155. Rouch DA, Messerotti LJ, Loo LSL, Jackson CA, Skurray RA. 1989. Trimethoprim resistance transposon Tn*4003* from *Staphylococcus aureus* encodes genes for a dihydrofolate reductase and thymidylate synthetase flanked by three copies of IS*257. Mol Microbiol* 3:161–175.

156. Kehrenberg C, Schwarz S. 2005. *dfrA20*, a novel trimethoprim resistance gene from *Pasteurella multocida*. *Antimicrob Agents Chemother* 49:414–417.

157. Webber M, Piddock LJV. 2001. Quinolone resistance in *Escherichia coli*. *Vet Res* 32:275–284.

158. Bager F, Helmuth R. 2001. Epidemiology of quinolone resistance in *Salmonella*. *Vet Res* 32:285–290.

159. Drlica K, Zhao X. 1997. DNA gyrase, topoisomerase IV, and the 4-quinolones. *Microbiol Mol Biol Rev* 61: 377–392.

160. Everett MJ, Piddock LJV. 1998. Mechanisms of resistance to fluoroquinolones, p 259–296. *In* Kuhlmann J, Dalhoff A, Zeiler H-J (ed), *Quinolone Antibacterials*. Springer Verlag, Berlin, Germany.

161. Hooper DC. 1999. Mechanisms of fluoroquinolone resistance. *Drug Resist Updat* 2:38–55.

162. Ruiz J. 2003. Mechanisms of resistance to quinolones: target alterations, decreased accumulation and DNA gyrase protection. *J Antimicrob Chemother* 51:1109–1117.

163. Guan X, Xue X, Liu Y, Wang J, Wang Y, Wang J, Wang K, Jiang H, Zhang L, Yang B, Wang N, Pan L. 2013. Plasmid-mediated quinolone resistance: current knowledge and future perspectives. *J Int Med Res* 41:20–30.

164. Yoshida H, Bogaki M, Nakamura M, Nakamura S. 1990. Quinolone resistance-determining region in the DNA gyrase *gyrA* gene of *Escherichia coli*. *Antimicrob Agents Chemother* 34:1271–1272.

165. Cloeckaert A, Chaslus-Dancla E. 2001. Mechanisms of quinolone resistance in *Salmonella*. *Vet Res* 32:291–300.

166. Jones ME, Sahm DF, Martin N, Scheuring S, Heisig P, Thornsberry C, Köhrer K, Schmitz F-J. 2000. Prevalence of *gyrA*, *gyrB*, *parC*, and *parE* mutations in clinical isolates of *Streptococcus pneumoniae* with decreased susceptibilities to different fluoroquinolones and originating from worldwide surveillance studies during the 1997-1998 respiratory season. *Antimicrob Agents Chemother* 44:462–466.

167. Everett MJ, Jin YF, Ricci V, Piddock LJV. 1996. Contributions of individual mechanisms to fluoroquinolone resistance in 36 *Escherichia coli* strains isolated from humans and animals. *Antimicrob Agents Chemother* 40:2380–2386.

168. Poole K. 2000. Efflux-mediated resistance to fluoroquinolones in Gram-negative bacteria. *Antimicrob Agents Chemother* **44:**2233–2241.

169. Poole K. 2000. Efflux-mediated resistance to fluoroquinolones in Gram-positive bacteria and the mycobacteria. *Antimicrob Agents Chemother* **44:**2595–2599.

170. Alekshun MN, Levy SB. 1999. The *mar* regulon: multiple resistance to antibiotics and other toxic chemicals. *Trends Microbiol* **7:**410–413.

171. Okusu H, Ma D, Nikaido H. 1996. AcrAB efflux pump plays a major role in the antibiotic resistance phenotype of *Escherichia coli* multiple-antibiotic-resistance (Mar) mutants. *J Bacteriol* **178:**306–308.

172. Olliver A, Vallé M, Chaslus-Dancla E, Cloeckaert A. 2004. Role of an *acrR* mutation in multidrug resistance of *in vitro*-selected fluoroquinolone-resistant mutants of *Salmonella enterica* serovar Typhimurium. *FEMS Microbiol Lett* **238:**267–272.

173. Oethinger M, Podglajen I, Kern WV, Levy SB. 1998. Overexpression of the *marA* or *soxS* regulatory gene in clinical topoisomerase mutants of *Escherichia coli*. *Antimicrob Agents Chemother* **42:**2089–2094.

174. Barbosa TM, Levy SB. 2000. Differential expression of over 60 chromosomal genes in *Escherichia coli* by constitutive expression of MarA. *J Bacteriol* **182:**3467–3474.

175. Lee A, Mao W, Warren MS, Mistry A, Hoshino K, Okumura R, Ishida H, Lomovskaya O. 2000. Interplay between efflux pumps may provide either additive or multiplicative effects on drug resistance. *J Bacteriol* **182:**3142–3150.

176. Oethinger M, Kern WV, Jellen-Ritter AS, McMurry LM, Levy SB. 2000. Ineffectiveness of topoisomerase mutations in mediating clinically significant fluoroquinolone resistance in *Escherichia coli* in the absence of the AcrAB efflux pump. *Antimicrob Agents Chemother* **44:**10–13.

177. Lomovskaya O, Lee A, Hoshino K, Ishida H, Mistry A, Warren MS, Boyer E, Chamberland S, Lee VJ. 1999. Use of a genetic approach to evaluate the consequences of inhibition of efflux pumps in *Pseudomonas aeruginosa*. *Antimicrob Agents Chemother* **43:**1340–1346.

178. Baucheron S, Chaslus-Dancla E, Cloeckaert A. 2004. Role of TolC and *parC* mutation in high-level fluoroquinolone resistance in *Salmonella enterica* serotype Typhimurium DT204. *J Antimicrob Chemother* **53:**657–659.

179. Baucheron S, Imberechts H, Chaslus-Dancla E, Cloeckaert A. 2002. The AcrB multidrug transporter plays a major role in high-level fluoroquinolone resistance in *Salmonella enterica* serovar Typhimurium phage type DT204. *Microb Drug Resist* **8:**281–289.

180. Cohen SP, McMurry LM, Levy SB. 1988. *marA* locus causes decreased expression of OmpF porin in multiple-antibiotic-resistant (Mar) mutants of *Escherichia coli*. *J Bacteriol* **170:**5416–5422.

181. McMurry LM, George AM, Levy SB. 1994. Active efflux of chloramphenicol in susceptible *Escherichia coli* strains and in multiple-antibiotic-resistant (Mar) mutants. *Antimicrob Agents Chemother* **38:**542–546.

182. Hooper DC, Wolfson JS, Bozza MA, Ng EY. 1992. Genetics and regulation of outer membrane protein expression by quinolone resistance loci nfxB, nfxC, and cfxB. *Antimicrob Agents Chemother* **36:**1151–1154.

183. Juárez-Verdayes MA, Parra-Ortega B, Hernández-Rodríguez C, Betanzos-Cabrera G, Rodríguez-Martínez S, Cancino-Diaz ME, Cancino-Diaz JC. 2012. Identification and expression of *nor* efflux family genes in *Staphylococcus epidermidis* that act against gatifloxacin. *Microb Pathog* **52:**318–325.

184. Tran JH, Jacoby GA. 2002. Mechanism of plasmid-mediated quinolone resistance. *Proc Natl Acad Sci USA* **99:**5638–5642.

185. Jacoby GA, Strahilevitz J, Hooper DC. 2014. Plasmid-mediated quinolone resistance. *Microbiol Spectrum* **2:**PLAS-0006-2013

186. Rodríguez-Martínez JM, Machuca J, Cano ME, Calvo J, Martínez-Martínez L, Pascual A. 2016. Plasmid-mediated quinolone resistance: two decades on. *Drug Resist Updat* **29:**13–29.

187. Murray IA, Shaw WV. 1997. O-Acetyltransferases for chloramphenicol and other natural products. *Antimicrob Agents Chemother* **41:**1–6.

188. Schwarz S, Kehrenberg C, Doublet B, Cloeckaert A. 2004. Molecular basis of bacterial resistance to chloramphenicol and florfenicol. *FEMS Microbiol Rev* **28:**519–542.

189. Shaw WV. 1983. Chloramphenicol acetyltransferase: enzymology and molecular biology. *CRC Crit Rev Biochem* **14:**1–46.

190. Alekshun MN, Levy SB. 2000. Bacterial drug resistance: response to survival threats, p 323–366. *In* Storz G, Hengge-Aronis R (ed), *Bacterial Stress Responses*. ASM Press, Washington, DC.

191. Alton NK, Vapnek D. 1979. Nucleotide sequence analysis of the chloramphenicol resistance transposon Tn9. *Nature* **282:**864–869.

192. Murray IA, Hawkins AR, Keyte JW, Shaw WV. 1988. Nucleotide sequence analysis and overexpression of the gene encoding a type III chloramphenicol acetyltransferase. *Biochem J* **252:**173–179.

193. Murray IA, Martinez-Suarez JV, Close TJ, Shaw WV. 1990. Nucleotide sequences of genes encoding the type II chloramphenicol acetyltransferases of *Escherichia coli* and *Haemophilus influenzae*, which are sensitive to inhibition by thiol-reactive reagents. *Biochem J* **272:**505–510.

194. Brenner DG, Shaw WV. 1985. The use of synthetic oligonucleotides with universal templates for rapid DNA sequencing: results with staphylococcal replicon pC221. *EMBO J* **4:**561–568.

195. Horinouchi S, Weisblum B. 1982. Nucleotide sequence and functional map of pC194, a plasmid that specifies inducible chloramphenicol resistance. *J Bacteriol* **150:**815–825.

196. Schwarz S, Cardoso M. 1991. Nucleotide sequence and phylogeny of a chloramphenicol acetyltransferase encoded by the plasmid pSCS7 from *Staphylococcus aureus*. *Antimicrob Agents Chemother* **35:**1551–1556.

197. Lovett PS. 1990. Translational attenuation as the regulator of inducible *cat* genes. *J Bacteriol* **172:**1–6.

198. Bannam TL, Rood JI. 1991. Relationship between the *Clostridium perfringens catQ* gene product and chloramphenicol acetyltransferases from other bacteria. *Antimicrob Agents Chemother* **35:**471–476.

199. Lang KS, Anderson JM, Schwarz S, Williamson L, Handelsman J, Singer RS. 2010. Novel florfenicol and chloramphenicol resistance gene discovered in Alaskan soil by using functional metagenomics. *Appl Environ Microbiol* **76:**5321–5326.

200. Stokes HW, Hall RM. 1991. Sequence analysis of the inducible chloramphenicol resistance determinant in the Tn*1696* integron suggests regulation by translational attenuation. *Plasmid* **26:**10–19.

201. Cloeckaert A, Baucheron S, Chaslus-Dancla E. 2001. Nonenzymatic chloramphenicol resistance mediated by IncC plasmid R55 is encoded by a *floR* gene variant. *Antimicrob Agents Chemother* **45:**2381–2382.

202. Cloeckaert A, Baucheron S, Flaujac G, Schwarz S, Kehrenberg C, Martel JL, Chaslus-Dancla E. 2000. Plasmid-mediated florfenicol resistance encoded by the *floR* gene in *Escherichia coli* isolated from cattle. *Antimicrob Agents Chemother* **44:**2858–2860.

203. Hochhut B, Lotfi Y, Mazel D, Faruque SM, Woodgate R, Waldor MK. 2001. Molecular analysis of antibiotic resistance gene clusters in *Vibrio cholerae* O139 and O1 SXT constins. *Antimicrob Agents Chemother* **45:**2991–3000.

204. Kehrenberg C, Schwarz S. 2005. Plasmid-borne florfenicol resistance in *Pasteurella multocida*. *J Antimicrob Chemother* **55:**773–775.

205. Keyes K, Hudson C, Maurer JJ, Thayer S, White DG, Lee MD. 2000. Detection of florfenicol resistance genes in *Escherichia coli* isolated from sick chickens. *Antimicrob Agents Chemother* **44:**421–424.

206. Kim E, Aoki T. 1996. Sequence analysis of the florfenicol resistance gene encoded in the transferable R-plasmid of a fish pathogen, *Pasteurella piscicida*. *Microbiol Immunol* **40:**665–669.

207. White DG, Hudson C, Maurer JJ, Ayers S, Zhao S, Lee MD, Bolton L, Foley T, Sherwood J. 2000. Characterization of chloramphenicol and florfenicol resistance in *Escherichia coli* associated with bovine diarrhea. *J Clin Microbiol* **38:**4593–4598.

208. Michael GB, Kadlec K, Sweeney MT, Brzuszkiewicz E, Liesegang H, Daniel R, Murray RW, Watts JL, Schwarz S. 2012. ICE*Pmu1*, an integrative conjugative element (ICE) of *Pasteurella multocida*: analysis of the regions that comprise 12 antimicrobial resistance genes. *J Antimicrob Chemother* **67:**84–90.

209. Hall RM. 2010. *Salmonella* genomic islands and antibiotic resistance in *Salmonella enterica*. *Future Microbiol* **5:**1525–1538.

210. He T, Shen J, Schwarz S, Wu C, Wang Y. 2015. Characterization of a genomic island in *Stenotrophomonas maltophilia* that carries a novel *floR* gene variant. *J Antimicrob Chemother* **70:**1031–1036.

211. Kehrenberg C, Schwarz S. 2004. *fexA*, a novel *Staphylococcus lentus* gene encoding resistance to florfenicol and chloramphenicol. *Antimicrob Agents Chemother* **48:**615–618.

212. Kehrenberg C, Schwarz S. 2005. Florfenicol-chloramphenicol exporter gene *fexA* is part of the novel transposon Tn*558*. *Antimicrob Agents Chemother* **49:**813–815.

213. Liu H, Wang Y, Wu C, Schwarz S, Shen Z, Jeon B, Ding S, Zhang Q, Shen J. 2012. A novel phenicol exporter gene, *fexB*, found in enterococci of animal origin. *J Antimicrob Chemother* **67:**322–325.

214. Ettayebi M, Prasad SM, Morgan EA. 1985. Chloramphenicol-erythromycin resistance mutations in a 23S rRNA gene of *Escherichia coli*. *J Bacteriol* **162:**551–557.

215. Long KS, Vester B. 2012. Resistance to linezolid caused by modifications at its binding site on the ribosome. *Antimicrob Agents Chemother* **56:**603–612.

216. Mendes RE, Deshpande LM, Farrell DJ, Spanu T, Fadda G, Jones RN. 2010. Assessment of linezolid resistance mechanisms among *Staphylococcus epidermidis* causing bacteraemia in Rome, Italy. *J Antimicrob Chemother* **65:**2329–2335.

217. Shaw KJ, Barbachyn MR. 2011. The oxazolidinones: past, present, and future. *Ann N Y Acad Sci* **1241:**48–70.

218. Locke JB, Hilgers M, Shaw KJ. 2009. Mutations in ribosomal protein L3 are associated with oxazolidinone resistance in staphylococci of clinical origin. *Antimicrob Agents Chemother* **53:**5275–5278.

219. Wolter N, Smith AM, Farrell DJ, Schaffner W, Moore M, Whitney CG, Jorgensen JH, Klugman KP. 2005. Novel mechanism of resistance to oxazolidinones, macrolides, and chloramphenicol in ribosomal protein L4 of the pneumococcus. *Antimicrob Agents Chemother* **49:**3554–3557.

220. Shore AC, Lazaris A, Kinnevey PM, Brennan OM, Brennan GI, O'Connell B, Feßler AT, Schwarz S, Coleman DC. 2016. First report of *cfr*-carrying plasmids in the pandemic sequence type 22 methicillin-resistant *Staphylococcus aureus* staphylococcal cassette chromosome *mec* type IV clone. *Antimicrob Agents Chemother* **60:**3007–3015.

221. Schwarz S, Werckenthin C, Kehrenberg C. 2000. Identification of a plasmid-borne chloramphenicol-florfenicol resistance gene in *Staphylococcus sciuri*. *Antimicrob Agents Chemother* **44:**2530–2533.

222. Kehrenberg C, Schwarz S, Jacobsen L, Hansen LH, Vester B. 2005. A new mechanism for chloramphenicol, florfenicol and clindamycin resistance: methylation of 23S ribosomal RNA at A2503. *Mol Microbiol* **57:**1064–1073.

223. Long KS, Poehlsgaard J, Kehrenberg C, Schwarz S, Vester B. 2006. The Cfr rRNA methyltransferase

confers resistance to phenicols, lincosamides, oxazolidinones, pleuromutilins, and streptogramin A antibiotics. *Antimicrob Agents Chemother* **50**:2500–2505.

224. Shen J, Wang Y, Schwarz S. 2013. Presence and dissemination of the multiresistance gene *cfr* in Gram-positive and Gram-negative bacteria. *J Antimicrob Chemother* **68**:1697–1706.

225. Wang Y, Li D, Song L, Liu Y, He T, Liu H, Wu C, Schwarz S, Shen J. 2013. First report of the multiresistance gene *cfr* in *Streptococcus suis*. *Antimicrob Agents Chemother* **57**:4061–4063.

226. Hansen LH, Vester B. 2015. A *cfr*-like gene from *Clostridium difficile* confers multiple antibiotic resistance by the same mechanism as the *cfr* gene. *Antimicrob Agents Chemother* **59**:5841–5843.

227. Deshpande LM, Ashcraft DS, Kahn HP, Pankey G, Jones RN, Farrell DJ, Mendes RE. 2015. Detection of a new *cfr*-like gene, *cfr*(B), in *Enterococcus faecium* isolates recovered from human specimens in the United States as part of the SENTRY antimicrobial surveillance program. *Antimicrob Agents Chemother* **59**:6256–6261.

228. Tang Y, Dai L, Sahin O, Wu Z, Liu M, Zhang Q. 2017. Emergence of a plasmid-borne multidrug resistance gene *cfr*(C) in foodborne pathogen *Campylobacter*. *J Antimicrob Chemother* **72**:1581–1588.

229. Wang Y, Lv Y, Cai J, Schwarz S, Cui L, Hu Z, Zhang R, Li J, Zhao Q, He T, Wang D, Wang Z, Shen Y, Li Y, Feßler AT, Wu C, Yu H, Deng X, Xia X, Shen J. 2015. A novel gene, *optrA*, that confers transferable resistance to oxazolidinones and phenicols and its presence in *Enterococcus faecalis* and *Enterococcus faecium* of human and animal origin. *J Antimicrob Chemother* **70**:2182–2190.

230. He T, Shen Y, Schwarz S, Cai J, Lv Y, Li J, Feßler AT, Zhang R, Wu C, Shen J, Wang Y. 2016. Genetic environment of the transferable oxazolidinone/phenicol resistance gene *optrA* in *Enterococcus faecalis* isolates of human and animal origin. *J Antimicrob Chemother* **71**:1466–1473.

231. Li D, Wang Y, Schwarz S, Cai J, Fan R, Li J, Feßler AT, Zhang R, Wu C, Shen J. 2016. Co-location of the oxazolidinone resistance genes *optrA* and *cfr* on a multiresistance plasmid from *Staphylococcus sciuri*. *J Antimicrob Chemother* **71**:1474–1478.

232. Fan R, Li D, Wang Y, He T, Feßler AT, Schwarz S, Wu C. 2016. Presence of the *optrA* gene in methicillin-resistant *Staphylococcus sciuri* of porcine origin. *Antimicrob Agents Chemother* **60**:7200–7205.

233. Huang J, Chen L, Wu Z, Wang L. 2017. Retrospective analysis of genome sequences revealed the wide dissemination of *optrA* in Gram-positive bacteria. *J Antimicrob Chemother* **72**:614–616.

234. Arthur M, Reynolds P, Courvalin P. 1996. Glycopeptide resistance in enterococci. *Trends Microbiol* **4**:401–407.

235. Walsh C. 2003. *Antibiotics: Actions, Origins, Resistance.* ASM Press, Washington, DC.

236. Gudeta DD, Moodley A, Bortolaia V, Guardabassi L. 2014. *vanO*, a new glycopeptide resistance operon in

environmental *Rhodococcus equi* isolates. *Antimicrob Agents Chemother* **58**:1768–1770.

237. Arthur M, Molinas C, Depardieu F, Courvalin P. 1993. Characterization of Tn*1546*, a Tn*3*-related transposon conferring glycopeptide resistance by synthesis of depsipeptide peptidoglycan precursors in *Enterococcus faecium* BM4147. *J Bacteriol* **175**:117–127.

238. Aarestrup FM. 1995. Occurrence of glycopeptide resistance among *Enterococcus faecium* isolates from conventional and ecological poultry farms. *Microb Drug Resist* **1**:255–257.

239. Klare I, Heier H, Claus H, Reissbrodt R, Witte W. 1995. *vanA*-mediated high-level glycopeptide resistance in *Enterococcus faecium* from animal husbandry. *FEMS Microbiol Lett* **125**:165–171.

240. Noble WC, Virani Z, Cree RG. 1992. Co-transfer of vancomycin and other resistance genes from *Enterococcus faecalis* NCTC 12201 to *Staphylococcus aureus*. *FEMS Microbiol Lett* **72**:195–198.

241. Weigel LM, Clewell DB, Gill SR, Clark NC, McDougal LK, Flannagan SE, Kolonay JF, Shetty J, Killgore GE, Tenover FC. 2003. Genetic analysis of a high-level vancomycin-resistant isolate of *Staphylococcus aureus*. *Science* **302**:1569–1571.

242. Guardabassi L, Christensen H, Hasman H, Dalsgaard A. 2004. Members of the genera *Paenibacillus* and *Rhodococcus* harbor genes homologous to enterococcal glycopeptide resistance genes *vanA* and *vanB*. *Antimicrob Agents Chemother* **48**:4915–4918.

243. Wendlandt S, Shen J, Kadlec K, Wang Y, Li B, Zhang WJ, Feßler AT, Wu C, Schwarz S. 2015. Multidrug resistance genes in staphylococci from animals that confer resistance to critically and highly important antimicrobial agents in human medicine. *Trends Microbiol* **23**: 44–54.

244. Wendlandt S, Kadlec K, Feßler AT, Schwarz S. 2015. Identification of ABC transporter genes conferring combined pleuromutilin-lincosamide-streptogramin A resistance in bovine methicillin-resistant *Staphylococcus aureus* and coagulase-negative staphylococci. *Vet Microbiol* **177**:353–358.

245. Pringle M, Poehlsgaard J, Vester B, Long KS. 2004. Mutations in ribosomal protein L3 and 23S ribosomal RNA at the peptidyl transferase centre are associated with reduced susceptibility to tiamulin in *Brachyspira* spp. isolates. *Mol Microbiol* **54**:1295–1306.

246. Hidalgo Á, Carvajal A, Vester B, Pringle M, Naharro G, Rubio P. 2011. Trends towards lower antimicrobial susceptibility and characterization of acquired resistance among clinical isolates of *Brachyspira hyodysenteriae* in Spain. *Antimicrob Agents Chemother* **55**:3330–3337.

247. Pringle M, Landén A, Unnerstad HE, Molander B, Bengtsson B. 2012. Antimicrobial susceptibility of porcine *Brachyspira hyodysenteriae* and *Brachyspira pilosicoli* isolated in Sweden between 1990 and 2010. *Acta Vet Scand* **54**:54.

248. Li BB, Shen JZ, Cao XY, Wang Y, Dai L, Huang SY, Wu CM. 2010. Mutations in 23S rRNA gene associated with decreased susceptibility to tiamulin and

valnemulin in *Mycoplasma gallisepticum. FEMS Microbiol Lett* **308:**144–149.

249. van Duijkeren E, Greko C, Pringle M, Baptiste KE, Catry B, Jukes H, Moreno MA, Pomba MC, Pyörälä S, Rantala M, Ružauskas M, Sanders P, Teale C, Threlfall EJ, Torren-Edo J, Törneke K. 2014. Pleuromutilins: use in food-producing animals in the European Union, development of resistance and impact on human and animal health. *J Antimicrob Chemother* **69:**2022–2031.

250. Isnard C, Malbruny B, Leclercq R, Cattoir V. 2013. Genetic basis for *in vitro* and *in vivo* resistance to lincosamides, streptogramins A, and pleuromutilins (LS$_A$P phenotype) in *Enterococcus faecium. Antimicrob Agents Chemother* **57:**4463–4469.

251. Wendlandt S, Lozano C, Kadlec K, Gómez-Sanz E, Zarazaga M, Torres C, Schwarz S. 2013. The enterococcal ABC transporter gene *lsa*(E) confers combined resistance to lincosamides, pleuromutilins and streptogramin A antibiotics in methicillin-susceptible and methicillin-resistant *Staphylococcus aureus. J Antimicrob Chemother* **68:**473–475.

252. Butaye P, Devriese LA, Haesebrouck F. 2003. Antimicrobial growth promoters used in animal feed: effects of less well known antibiotics on gram-positive bacteria. *Clin Microbiol Rev* **16:**175–188.

253. WHO. 2017. Critically important antimicrobials for human medicine. 5th revision. http://who.int/food safety/publications/antimicrobials-fifth/en/.

254. Schwarz S, Johnson AP. 2016. Transferable resistance to colistin: a new but old threat. *J Antimicrob Chemother* **71:**2066–2070.

255. Olaitan AO, Morand S, Rolain JM. 2014. Mechanisms of polymyxin resistance: acquired and intrinsic resistance in bacteria. *Front Microbiol* **5:**643.

256. Jeannot K, Bolard A, Plésiat P. 2017. Resistance to polymyxins in Gram-negative organisms. *Int J Antimicrob Agents* **49:**526–535.

257. Liu YY, Wang Y, Walsh TR, Yi LX, Zhang R, Spencer J, Doi Y, Tian G, Dong B, Huang X, Yu LF, Gu D, Ren H, Chen X, Lv L, He D, Zhou H, Liang Z, Liu JH, Shen J. 2016. Emergence of plasmid-mediated colistin resistance mechanism MCR-1 in animals and human beings in China: a microbiological and molecular biological study. *Lancet Infect Dis* **16:**161–168.

258. Xavier BB, Lammens C, Ruhal R, Kumar-Singh S, Butaye P, Goossens H, Malhotra-Kumar S. 2016. Identification of a novel plasmid-mediated colistin-resistance gene, *mcr-2*, in *Escherichia coli*, Belgium, June 2016. *Euro Surveill* **21:**pii=30280. http://www.eurosurveillance.org/content/10.2807/1560-7917.ES.2016.21.27.30280.

259. Yin W, Li H, Shen Y, Liu Z, Wang S, Shen Z, Zhang R, Walsh TR, Shen J, Wang Y. 2017. Novel plasmid-mediated colistin resistance gene *mcr-3* in *Escherichia coli. MBio* **8:**e00543-17.

260. Carattoli A, Villa L, Feudi C, Curcio L, Orsini S, Luppi A, Pezzotti G, Magistrali CF. 2017. Novel plasmid-mediated colistin resistance *mcr-4* gene in *Salmonella* and *Escherichia coli*, Italy 2013, Spain and Belgium, 2015 to 2016. *Euro Surveill* **22:**30589. http://www.eurosurveillance.org/content/10.2807/1560-7917.ES.2017.22.31.30589.

261. Borowiak M, Fischer J, Hammerl JA, Hendriksen RS, Szabo I, Malorny B. 2017. Identification of a novel transposon-associated phosphoethanolamine transferase gene, *mcr-5*, conferring colistin resistance in d-tartrate fermenting *Salmonella enterica* subsp. *enterica* serovar Paratyphi B. *J Antimicrob Chemother* **72:**3317–3324.

262. AbuOun M, Stubberfield EJ, Duggett NA, Kirchner M, Dormer L, Nunez-Garcia J, Randall LP, Lemma F, Crook DW, Teale C, Smith RP, Anjum MF. 2017. *mcr-1* and *mcr-2* variant genes identified in *Moraxella* species isolated from pigs in Great Britain from 2014 to 2015. *J Antimicrob Chemother* **72:**2745–2749.

263. Ling Z, Yin W, Li H, Zhang Q, Wang X, Wang Z, Ke Y, Wang Y, Shen J. 2017. Chromosome-mediated *mcr-3* variants in *Aeromonas veronii* from chicken meat. *Antimicrob Agents Chemother* **61:**e01272-17. Epub ahead of print.

264. Eichhorn I, Feudi C, Wang Y, Kaspar H, Feßler AT, Lübke-Becker A, Michael GB, Shen J, Schwarz S. 2018. Identification of novel variants of the colistin resistance gene *mcr-3* in *Aeromonas* spp. from the national resistance monitoring program GERM-Vet and from diagnostic submissions. *J Antimicrob Chemother.*

265. Vila-Farrés X, Ferrer-Navarro M, Callarisa AE, Martí S, Espinal P, Gupta S, Rolain JM, Giralt E, Vila J. 2015. Loss of LPS is involved in the virulence and resistance to colistin of colistin-resistant *Acinetobacter nosocomialis* mutants selected *in vitro. J Antimicrob Chemother* **70:**2981–2986.

266. Baron S, Hadjadj L, Rolain JM, Olaitan AO. 2016. Molecular mechanisms of polymyxin resistance: knowns and unknowns. *Int J Antimicrob Agents* **48:**583–591.

267. Bina XR, Provenzano D, Nguyen N, Bina JE. 2008. *Vibrio cholerae* RND family efflux systems are required for antimicrobial resistance, optimal virulence factor production, and colonization of the infant mouse small intestine. *Infect Immun* **76:**3595–3605.

268. Campos MA, Vargas MA, Regueiro V, Llompart CM, Albertí S, Bengoechea JA. 2004. Capsule polysaccharide mediates bacterial resistance to antimicrobial peptides. *Infect Immun* **72:**7107–7114.

269. Llobet E, Tomás JM, Bengoechea JA. 2008. Capsule polysaccharide is a bacterial decoy for antimicrobial peptides. *Microbiology* **154:**3877–3886.

270. Young ML, Bains M, Bell A, Hancock RE. 1992. Role of *Pseudomonas aeruginosa* outer membrane protein OprH in polymyxin and gentamicin resistance: isolation of an OprH-deficient mutant by gene replacement techniques. *Antimicrob Agents Chemother* **36:**2566–2568.

271. Hetem DJ, Bonten MJ. 2013. Clinical relevance of mupirocin resistance in *Staphylococcus aureus. J Hosp Infect* **85:**249–256.

272. Hodgson JE, Curnock SP, Dyke KG, Morris R, Sylvester DR, Gross MS. 1994. Molecular characterization of the gene encoding high-level mupirocin resistance in *Staphylococcus aureus* J2870. *Antimicrob Agents Chemother* **38:**1205–1208.

273. Needham C, Rahman M, Dyke KG, Noble WC. 1994. An investigation of plasmids from *Staphylococcus aureus* that mediate resistance to mupirocin and tetracycline. *Microbiology* **140**:2577–2583.

274. Poovelikunnel T, Gethin G, Humphreys H. 2015. Mupirocin resistance: clinical implications and potential alternatives for the eradication of MRSA. *J Antimicrob Chemother* **70**:2681–2692.

275. Seah C, Alexander DC, Louie L, Simor A, Low DE, Longtin J, Melano RG. 2012. MupB, a new high-level mupirocin resistance mechanism in *Staphylococcus aureus*. *Antimicrob Agents Chemother* **56**:1916–1920.

276. Fines M, Pronost S, Maillard K, Taouji S, Leclercq R. 2001. Characterization of mutations in the *rpoB* gene associated with rifampin resistance in *Rhodococcus equi* isolated from foals. *J Clin Microbiol* **39**:2784–2787.

277. Riesenberg A, Feßler AT, Erol E, Prenger-Berninghoff E, Stamm I, Böse R, Heusinger A, Klarmann D, Werckenthin C, Schwarz S. 2014. MICs of 32 antimicrobial agents for *Rhodococcus equi* isolates of animal origin. *J Antimicrob Chemother* **69**:1045–1049.

278. Severinov K, Soushko M, Goldfarb A, Nikiforov V. 1993. Rifampicin region revisited. New rifampicin-resistant and streptolydigin-resistant mutants in the β subunit of *Escherichia coli* RNA polymerase. *J Biol Chem* **268**:14820–14825.

279. Telenti A, Imboden P, Marchesi F, Lowrie D, Cole S, Colston MJ, Matter L, Schopfer K, Bodmer T. 1993. Detection of rifampicin-resistance mutations in *Mycobacterium tuberculosis*. *Lancet* **341**:647–650.

280. Perkins AE, Nicholson WL. 2008. Uncovering new metabolic capabilities of *Bacillus subtilis* using phenotype profiling of rifampin-resistant *rpoB* mutants. *J Bacteriol* **190**:807–814.

281. Li J, Feßler AT, Jiang N, Fan R, Wang Y, Wu C, Shen J, Schwarz S. 2016. Molecular basis of rifampicin resistance in multiresistant porcine livestock-associated MRSA. *J Antimicrob Chemother* **71**:3313–3315.

282. Kadlec K, van Duijkeren E, Wagenaar JA, Schwarz S. 2011. Molecular basis of rifampicin resistance in methicillin-resistant *Staphylococcus pseudintermedius* isolates from dogs. *J Antimicrob Chemother* **66**:1236–1242.

283. Tupin A, Gualtieri M, Roquet-Banères F, Morichaud Z, Brodolin K, Leonetti JP. 2010. Resistance to rifampicin: at the crossroads between ecological, genomic and medical concerns. *Int J Antimicrob Agents* **35**:519–523.

284. Baysarowich J, Koteva K, Hughes DW, Ejim L, Griffiths E, Zhang K, Junop M, Wright GD. 2008. Rifamycin antibiotic resistance by ADP-ribosylation: structure and diversity of Arr. *Proc Natl Acad Sci USA* **105**:4886–4891.

285. Kadlec K, von Czapiewski E, Kaspar H, Wallmann J, Michael GB, Steinacker U, Schwarz S. 2011. Molecular basis of sulfonamide and trimethoprim resistance in fish-pathogenic *Aeromonas* isolates. *Appl Environ Microbiol* **77**:7147–7150.

286. Silver LL. 2017. Fosfomycin: mechanism and resistance. *Cold Spring Harb Perspect Med* **7**:a025262.

287. Castañeda-García A, Blázquez J, Rodríguez-Rojas A. 2013. Molecular mechanisms and clinical impact of acquired and intrinsic fosfomycin resistance. *Antibiotics (Basel)* **2**:217–236.

288. Jiang Y, Shen P, Wei Z, Liu L, He F, Shi K, Wang Y, Wang H, Yu Y. 2015. Dissemination of a clone carrying a *fosA3*-harbouring plasmid mediates high fosfomycin resistance rate of KPC-producing *Klebsiella pneumoniae* in China. *Int J Antimicrob Agents* **45**:66–70.

289. Wachino J, Yamane K, Suzuki S, Kimura K, Arakawa Y. 2010. Prevalence of fosfomycin resistance among CTX-M-producing *Escherichia coli* clinical isolates in Japan and identification of novel plasmid-mediated fosfomycin-modifying enzymes. *Antimicrob Agents Chemother* **54**:3061–3064.

290. Kitanaka H, Wachino J, Jin W, Yokoyama S, Sasano MA, Hori M, Yamada K, Kimura K, Arakawa Y. 2014. Novel integron-mediated fosfomycin resistance gene *fosK*. *Antimicrob Agents Chemother* **58**:4978–4979.

291. Zilhao R, Courvalin P. 1990. Nucleotide sequence of the *fosB* gene conferring fosfomycin resistance in *Staphylococcus epidermidis*. *FEMS Microbiol Lett* **56**:267–272.

292. Xu X, Chen C, Lin D, Guo Q, Hu F, Zhu D, Li G, Wang M. 2013. The fosfomycin resistance gene *fosB3* is located on a transferable, extrachromosomal circular intermediate in clinical *Enterococcus faecium* isolates. *PLoS One* **8**:e78106.

293. Fu Z, Liu Y, Chen C, Guo Y, Ma Y, Yang Y, Hu F, Xu X, Wang M. 2016. Characterization of fosfomycin resistance gene, *fosB*, in methicillin-resistant *Staphylococcus aureus* isolates. *PLoS One* **11**:e0154829.

294. He T, Wang Y, Schwarz S, Zhao Q, Shen J, Wu C. 2014. Genetic environment of the multi-resistance gene *cfr* in methicillin-resistant coagulase-negative staphylococci from chickens, ducks, and pigs in China. *Int J Med Microbiol* **304**:257–261.

295. Wang Y, Yao H, Deng F, Liu D, Zhang Y, Shen Z. 2015. Identification of a novel $fosX^{CC}$ gene conferring fosfomycin resistance in *Campylobacter*. *J Antimicrob Chemother* **70**:1261–1263.

296. Kim SY, Ju K-S, Metcalf WW, Evans BS, Kuzuyama T, van der Donk WA. 2012. Different biosynthetic pathways to fosfomycin in *Pseudomonas syringae* and *Streptomyces* species. *Antimicrob Agents Chemother* **56**:4175–4183.

297. Biedenbach DJ, Rhomberg PR, Mendes RE, Jones RN. 2010. Spectrum of activity, mutation rates, synergistic interactions, and the effects of pH and serum proteins for fusidic acid (CEM-102). *Diagn Microbiol Infect Dis* **66**:301–307.

298. Farrell DJ, Castanheira M, Chopra I. 2011. Characterization of global patterns and the genetics of fusidic acid resistance. *Clin Infect Dis* **52**(Suppl 7):S487–S492.

299. Lannergård J, Norström T, Hughes D. 2009. Genetic determinants of resistance to fusidic acid among clinical bacteremia isolates of *Staphylococcus aureus*. *Antimicrob Agents Chemother* **53**:2059–2065.

300. O'Brien FG, Price C, Grubb WB, Gustafson JE. 2002. Genetic characterization of the fusidic acid and cadmium

resistance determinants of *Staphylococcus aureus* plasmid pUB101. *J Antimicrob Chemother* 50:313–321.

301. Chen HJ, Hung WC, Lin YT, Tsai JC, Chiu HC, Hsueh PR, Teng LJ. 2015. A novel fusidic acid resistance determinant, *fusF*, in *Staphylococcus cohnii*. *J Antimicrob Chemother* 70:416–419.

302. Baines SL, Howden BP, Heffernan H, Stinear TP, Carter GP, Seemann T, Kwong JC, Ritchie SR, Williamson DA. 2016. Rapid emergence and evolution of *Staphylococcus aureus* clones harboring *fusC*-containing Staphylococcal Cassette Chromosome elements. *Antimicrob Agents Chemother* 60:2359–2365.

303. O'Neill AJ, McLaws F, Kahlmeter G, Henriksen AS, Chopra I. 2007. Genetic basis of resistance to fusidic acid in staphylococci. *Antimicrob Agents Chemother* 51:1737–1740.

304. Werner G, Hildebrandt B, Witte W. 2001. Aminoglycoside-streptothricin resistance gene cluster *aadE-sat4-aphA-3* disseminated among multiresistant isolates of *Enterococcus faecium*. *Antimicrob Agents Chemother* 45:3267–3269.

305. Kadlec K, Schwarz S. 2008. Analysis and distribution of class 1 and class 2 integrons and associated gene cassettes among *Escherichia coli* isolates from swine, horses, cats and dogs collected in the BfT-GermVet monitoring study. *J Antimicrob Chemother* 62:469–473.

306. Ahmed AM, Shimamoto T. 2004. A plasmid-encoded class 1 integron carrying *sat*, a putative phosphoserine phosphatase gene and *aadA2* from enterotoxigenic *Escherichia coli* O159 isolated in Japan. *FEMS Microbiol Lett* 235:243–248.

307. Boerlin P, Burnens AP, Frey J, Kuhnert P, Nicolet J. 2001. Molecular epidemiology and genetic linkage of macrolide and aminoglycoside resistance in *Staphylococcus intermedius* of canine origin. *Vet Microbiol* 79:155–169.

308. Kadlec K, Schwarz S, Perreten V, Andersson UG, Finn M, Greko C, Moodley A, Kania SA, Frank LA, Bemis DA, Franco A, Iurescia M, Battisti A, Duim B, Wagenaar JA, van Duijkeren E, Weese JS, Fitzgerald JR, Rossano A, Guardabassi L. 2010. Molecular analysis of methicillin-resistant *Staphylococcus pseudintermedius* of feline origin from different European countries and North America. *J Antimicrob Chemother* 65:1826–1828.

309. Perreten V, Kadlec K, Schwarz S, Grönlund Andersson U, Finn M, Greko C, Moodley A, Kania SA, Frank LA, Bemis DA, Franco A, Iurescia M, Battisti A, Duim B, Wagenaar JA, van Duijkeren E, Weese JS, Fitzgerald JR, Rossano A, Guardabassi L. 2010. Clonal spread of methicillin-resistant *Staphylococcus pseudintermedius* in Europe and North America: an international multicentre study. *J Antimicrob Chemother* 65:1145–1154.

310. Walther B, Monecke S, Ruscher C, Friedrich AW, Ehricht R, Slickers P, Soba A, Wleklinski CG, Wieler LH, Lübke-Becker A. 2009. Comparative molecular analysis substantiates zoonotic potential of equine methicillin-resistant *Staphylococcus aureus*. *J Clin Microbiol* 47:704–710.

311. Aarestrup FM. 2000. Occurrence, selection and spread of resistance to antimicrobial agents used for growth promotion for food animals in Denmark. *APMIS Suppl.* 101:1–8.

312. Podlesek Z, Comino A, Herzog-Velikonja B, Zgur-Bertok D, Komel R, Grabnar M. 1995. *Bacillus licheniformis* bacitracin-resistance ABC transporter: relationship to mammalian multidrug resistance. *Mol Microbiol* 16:969–976.

313. Bernard R, Joseph P, Guiseppi A, Chippaux M, Denizot F. 2003. YtsCD and YwoA, two independent systems that confer bacitracin resistance to *Bacillus subtilis*. *FEMS Microbiol Lett* 228:93–97.

314. El Ghachi M, Bouhss A, Blanot D, Mengin-Lecreulx D. 2004. The *bacA* gene of *Escherichia coli* encodes an undecaprenyl pyrophosphate phosphatase activity. *J Biol Chem* 279:30106–30113.

315. Manson JM, Keis S, Smith JM, Cook GM. 2004. Acquired bacitracin resistance in *Enterococcus faecalis* is mediated by an ABC transporter and a novel regulatory protein, BcrR. *Antimicrob Agents Chemother* 48:3743–3748.

316. Weitnauer G, Gaisser S, Trefzer A, Stockert S, Westrich L, Quiros LM, Mendez C, Salas JA, Bechthold A. 2001. An ATP-binding cassette transporter and two rRNA methyltransferases are involved in resistance to avilamycin in the producer organism *Streptomyces viridochromogenes* Tü57. *Antimicrob Agents Chemother* 45:690–695.

317. Aarestrup FM, Jensen LB. 2000. Presence of variations in ribosomal protein L16 corresponding to susceptibility of enterococci to oligosaccharides (avilamycin and evernimicin). *Antimicrob Agents Chemother* 44:3425–3427.

318. Mann PA, Xiong L, Mankin AS, Chau AS, Mendrick CA, Najarian DJ, Cramer CA, Loebenberg D, Coates E, Murgolo NJ, Aarestrup FM, Goering RV, Black TA, Hare RS, McNicholas PM. 2001. EmtA, a rRNA methyltransferase conferring high-level evernimicin resistance. *Mol Microbiol* 41:1349–1356.

319. Treede I, Jakobsen L, Kirpekar F, Vester B, Weitnauer G, Bechthold A, Douthwaite S. 2003. The avilamycin resistance determinants AviRa and AviRb methylate 23S rRNA at the guanosine 2535 base and the uridine 2479 ribose. *Mol Microbiol* 49:309–318.

320. Kofoed CB, Vester B. 2002. Interaction of avilamycin with ribosomes and resistance caused by mutations in 23S rRNA. *Antimicrob Agents Chemother* 46:3339–3342.

321. van den Bogaard AE, Hazen M, Hoyer M, Oostenbach P, Stobberingh EE. 2002. Effects of flavophospholipol on resistance in fecal *Escherichia coli* and enterococci of fattening pigs. *Antimicrob Agents Chemother* 46:110–118.

322. Ohmae K, Yonezawa S, Terakado N. 1981. R plasmid with carbadox resistance from *Escherichia coli* of porcine origin. *Antimicrob Agents Chemother* 19:86–90.

323. Hansen LH, Johannesen E, Burmølle M, Sørensen AH, Sørensen SJ. 2004. Plasmid-encoded multidrug efflux pump conferring resistance to olaquindox in *Escherichia coli*. *Antimicrob Agents Chemother* 48:3332–3337.

Antimicrobial Resistance in Bacteria from Livestock and Companion Animals
Edited by Frank Møller Aarestrup, Stefan Schwarz, Jianzhong Shen, and Lina Cavaco
© 2018 American Society for Microbiology, Washington, DC
doi:10.1128/microbiolspec.ARBA-0025-2017

Resistance to Metals Used in Agricultural Production

5

Christopher Rensing,[1] Arshnee Moodley,[2]
Lina M. Cavaco,[3] and Sylvia Franke McDevitt[4]

INTRODUCTION

Metal compounds are widely used in livestock production because they are necessary supplements and play a very important role as essential trace elements that are part of the nutritional requirements of most animal species. However, copper and zinc compounds are also added to feed in larger concentrations for achieving additional beneficial effects. Therefore, we will focus this chapter on copper and zinc; their use and indications; the concerns related to the selection of resistance, toxicity, and environmental pollution and policies; and the alternatives and new developments regarding their use. Compounds derived from the nonessential metal arsenic, such as roxarsone, which have been used in livestock for feed supplementation in some countries around the world, will not be discussed in great detail in this chapter.

USE OF METAL COMPOUNDS IN AGRICULTURAL PRODUCTION: REQUIREMENTS AND RECOMMENDATIONS

Copper

Copper is an essential trace element that is necessary for the human body because it has major functions regarding fetal growth and early postnatal development, hemoglobin synthesis, maturation of the connective tissues, proper nerve function and bone development, and inflammatory processes. Therefore, most animal species are required to have copper in their feed and exhibit copper deficiency symptoms if copper is insufficient. Copper is also expected to interact with other compounds in the feed (phytates, fiber fraction, zinc, iron, calcium, ascorbic acid, molybdenum, and sulfur), and therefore the concentrations added to feed are increased to ensure that the necessary amount is available for absorption by the target animal species. This is also dependent on the animal's intestinal tract, and these interactions influence the absorption, as extensively reviewed by Suttle (1).

An excess of copper can also be detrimental and lead to toxicity manifested as anemia and liver dysfunction. Release of copper from the liver may lead to vascular hemolysis and death. The toxicity of copper depends on speciation, with Cu(I) being more toxic then Cu(II). Certain animal species such as sheep and young calves are sensitive to excess copper (2). Copper might also exert a selection pressure on the gut microbiota and influence the composition of the gut flora. Furthermore, the use of therapeutic concentrations might select for resistance, which is addressed later in this chapter. Requirements for copper in animal feed depend on the target species, the age group and the feed composition (2).

Copper is contained in a number of plants and seeds in varying concentrations and may become concentrated with the use of copper compounds in agriculture, but the availability of copper in feed is not well known. For food-producing animals and small pet animals such as rabbits, the copper background levels in complete feeds are rather low and in the range of 5 (salmon feed) to 15 (rabbit feed) mg Cu/kg feed, and higher values are observed in feed for dairy cows, containing about 20 mg Cu/kg feed. Supplementation of animal feed is common practice, and the current limits for supplemen-

[1]Institute of Environmental Microbiology, College of Resource and Environment, Fujian Agriculture and Forestry University, Fuzhou, Fujian 350002, China; [2]Veterinary Clinical Microbiology, Department of Veterinary and Animal Sciences, Faculty of Health and Medical Sciences, University of Copenhagen, 1870 Frederiksberg, Denmark; [3]Department for Bacteria, Parasites, and Fungi, Infectious Disease Preparedness, Statens Serum Institut and Faculty of Health and Medical Sciences, University of Copenhagen, 2300 Copenhagen, Denmark; [4]Biology, Skidmore College, Saratoga Springs, NY 12866.

tation (3) were revised by the European Union in 2016 (Table 1) (4).

Copper additives

The list of copper compounds authorized for copper supplementation in feed is extensive and includes cupric acetate, monohydrate; basic cupric carbonate, monohydrate; cupric chloride, dihydrate; cupric methionate; cupric oxide; cupric sulfate, pentahydrate; cupric chelate of amino acid hydrate; copper lysine sulfate; cupric chelate of glycine hydrate; copper chelate of hydroxy analogue of methionine; dicopper chloride trihydroxide; and copper bislysinate. These authorized compounds fall under European Economic Community (EEC) number E4 (3). Most copper-containing compounds show bioavailability similar to copper sulfate for all animal species. However, cupric oxide and cupric carbonate (and cuprous iodide in poultry) showed a lower and more variable relative bioavailability (4).

Therapeutic use of copper

Copper may be prescribed for copper deficiency and is normally administered orally using premixes in feed, or it may be administrated using injectable solutions. Additionally, copper has antimicrobial properties, and copper sulfate may be used in footbaths as a fungicide for the control of foot-rot in cattle and sheep (5 to 10% solution) (5). Copper has also been used as a growth promoter, even though the efficacy of this practice has not been very well demonstrated. Growth promotion might depend on the feed antagonists present and relate to improved appetite or digestibility in pigs and poultry (1).

Zinc

Similar to copper, zinc is also an essential trace element and therefore is necessary to comply with the nutritional requirements of livestock. Zinc is part of 10% of all proteins and contributes to their tertiary structure and the function of enzymes, and therefore its role is essential in diverse organs and systems. For example, zinc is needed for glucose and lipid metabolism, cell proliferation, embryogenesis, and systems related to the nervous and immune systems.

Symptoms of zinc deficiency can be observed in most animal species (6). Known examples of this are

Table 1 New proposed maximum limits of copper in complete animal feed[b]

Target species, animal category	R[a]	1.5 × R	Background	NPMC[b]	CAMC[b]
Chickens for fattening, reared for laying	8	12	10	25	25
Laying hens, breeder hens	8	12	10	25	25
Turkeys for fattening, 0–8 weeks of age	10	15	10	25	25
Turkeys for fattening, from 8 weeks of age onward	6	9	10	25	25
Other poultry	8	12	10	25	25
Piglets, weaned	8	12	10	25	170
Pigs for fattening	6	9	10	25	25
Sows	10	15	10	25	25
Calves, milk replacer	10	15	5	15[c]	15
Cattle for fattening	8.8[b]	13.2	10	30[d]	35
Dairy cows	8.8–13.2[b]	13.2–19.8	10	30	35
Sheep	7[b]	10.6	10	15[e]	15
Goats	7–22[b]	10.6–33	10	35	25
Horses	8.8[b]	13.2	10	25	25
Rabbits	5	7.5	10	25	25
Salmonids	5	7.5	10	25	25
Other fish	8	12	10	25	25
Crustaceans				50	50
Dogs	12	15.6[f]	10	25	25
Cats	10	13[f]	10	25	25

[a]R, requirement.
[b]NPMC, newly proposed total maximum contents of copper in complete feed (4); CAMC, currently authorized maximum content of copper in complete feed (3).
[c]Because copper in milk-based diets shows a high bioavailability and does not contain substantial amounts of copper antagonists, the background level (5 mg/kg) is not added to the allowance (15 mg/kg).
[d]Considering cattle feeding on pasture, a potentially high amount of copper antagonists in forage is taken into account.
[e]NPMC is limited by the Mineral Tolerance of Animals (MTL); dietary concentrations above 15 mg/kg could provoke chronic copper poisoning (CCP).
[f]No requirement data available; the allowance (12 and 10 mg/kg for dogs and cats, respectively) is therefore only multiplied by 1.3 to consider different bioavailability of copper supplements.
[g]Adjusted from dry matter to complete feed with 88% dry matter.
[b]Source: reference 4.

paraqueratosis in swine (7) and growth deficiencies in feathering and skeletal development in poultry (8). Zinc is an essential trace element, and zinc deficiency might be related to malabsorption of this metal compound. Similarly, Friesian cows and bull terrier dogs have been shown to have genetic syndromes related to zinc malabsorption (9, 10).

Most of the absorption of zinc occurs in the small intestine, and feed components such as phytates may hamper the absorption in monogastric species, while low molecular weight binding ligands such as citrate, picolinate, EDTA, and amino acids such as histidine and glutamate were shown to increase the absorption of zinc (11).

Zinc is mainly metabolized in the liver, and the main zinc deposit is in bone. Measurement of zinc in bone may be used to determine zinc status or utilization, while measurement of zinc in hair may be used for diagnostic purposes. Zinc concentrations in plasma are not reliable because zinc binds extensively to proteins.

Since zinc is mainly excreted in feces, it is the variable zinc excretion that together with absorption maintains zinc homeostasis in the body. These processes also influence the seepage of zinc from manure into the environment. Zinc absorption and bioavailability are influenced by the feed composition; not only the plant component but also high concentrations of other metals such as copper, nickel, and iron may lead to zinc deficiency. Therefore, formulations of feed need to take into account other feed components that might interfere with zinc absorption and bioavailability.

Toxicity to zinc is low in general, and tolerance to high levels of zinc has been observed. However, ruminants, especially young and pregnant animals, are more susceptible to the effects of excess zinc compared to pigs or poultry. Zinc toxicity has been observed in steers and heifers, but tolerance seems to be higher in dairy cows. Sheep may develop symptoms of excess zinc in their diet, manifesting as symptoms ranging from weakness and jaundice to abortions and stillbirth. Horses, especially young and pregnant animals, are among the most sensitive to excess zinc in the diet and react with lameness and osteochondrosis. Pigs are among the most zinc-tolerant animal species, and it has been shown that even though they can exhibit symptoms of toxicity, it depends on the exposure time to excess zinc diet and the relation of other components of the diet such as calcium. Therefore, in some countries, high zinc concentrations are allowed for therapeutic purposes (12).

Zinc is naturally occurring in agricultural produce, but the levels vary greatly. The content of zinc in natural products depends on the zinc concentration in the soil and the conditions that might influence zinc uptake by plants. Some zinc may also be added due to deposition on plants, soil contamination, and processing. Similar to copper, the available concentrations in raw materials vary and are relatively low in relation to the animal requirements. Therefore, zinc supplementation to animal feed is common (12). However, supplementation has been at relatively high levels, and several organizations have indicated that these levels could be lowered to reduce the impact on environment (12, 13).

For requirements in different animal species and age groups as well as current and proposed supplementation levels, please consult the data in Table 2 (12).

Zinc additives

For supplementation of feed, a number of additives are utilized, including zinc oxide, zinc chloride monohydrate, zinc sulfate monohydrate, zinc sulfate heptahydrate, zinc chelate of amino acids hydrate, zinc acetate dihydrate, and zinc lactate trihydrate, which fall under EEC number E6 (3). In regard to therapeutic use, the products used are similar but require a prescription if regulation permits. In the European Union, this usage has been allowed in some countries but it will be discontinued because the Committee for Veterinary Medicine Products at the European Medicines Agency has recommended that market authorizations be withdrawn for existing products, and new products will be refused largely due to environmental risks and acknowledgement of the risk for of coselection (14).

Therapeutic use of zinc

Zinc may be used in some countries under prescription for treatment and metaphylaxis of diarrheal disease in young animals such as postweaning piglets. Zinc supplements are normally given in the form of premixes used in feed or drinking water. The most relevant zinc forms for this practice are zinc oxide, zinc chloride, and zinc sulfate. For example, in Denmark and Belgium, veterinarians have until recently prescribed zinc oxide supplementation of up to 2,500 ppm for weaning pigs for up to 14 days after weaning, which is much more than the maximum concentration allowed in pig feed—250 ppm in the European Union, with the usual concentrations ranging between 50 and 125 ppm (15–17). Similarly, in other countries around the world, the therapeutic use of zinc is relatively widespread (18), and doses for therapeutic use are between 1,000 and 3,000 ppm for up to 2 to 3 weeks (19). This is contradictory to the fact that these high doses given over a long period may cause toxicity. The use of therapeutic concentrations of zinc has been considered beneficial for the

Table 2 New proposed maximum limits of zinc in complete feed[f]

Target species, animal category	R[a]	1.5 × R	Background	NPMC[b]	CAMC[c]
Chickens for fattening, reared for laying	40–50	60–75	30	100	150
Laying hens, breeder hens	45	67.5	30	100	150
Turkeys for fattening, 0–8 weeks of age	70	105	30	120	150
Turkeys for fattening, from 8 weeks of age onward	50	75	30	120	150
Other poultry	40, 60, 60	80	30	100	150
Piglet below 11 kg weight	100	150	30	150	150
Piglet, weaned above 11 kg weight	80	120	30	150	150
Pigs for fattening	60	90	30	100	150
Sows	50–100	75–150	30	150	150
Calves, milk replacer	40	60	30	100	200
Cattle for fattening	35[d]	53	30	100	150
Dairy cows, dairy heifer	44[d]	66	30	100	150
Sheep	40[d]	60	30	100	150
Goats	31[d]	47	30	100	150
Horses	44[d]	66	30	100	150
Rabbits	70	105	50	150	150
Salmonids	50	75	60	150	200
Other fish	20	30	60	100	200
Dogs		100[e]	70	150	250
Cats		75[e]	70	150	250

[a]R, requirement.
[b]NPMC, newly proposed total maximum contents of zinc in complete feed (13).
[c]CAMC, currently authorized maximum content of zinc in complete feed (3).
[d]Adjusted from dry matter to complete feed with 88% dry matter.
[e]Allowance, taken as 1.5 times the requirement.
[f]Source: reference 13.

reduction and prevention of postweaning diarrhea in weaners and postweaning scouring (20). However, the growth promotion effects are not well understood (12).

According to the risk assessments released at the end of 2016, the benefits of the therapeutic use of zinc compounds in animal production do not outweigh the environmental risks, and additionally, there is an acknowledged risk for coselection of antibiotic resistance; therefore the Committee for Veterinary Medicine Products has recommended the withdrawal of existing market authorizations for veterinary products containing zinc and refusal of approval for new formulations. This recommendation has been backed by the EU Commission, and phase-out is expected in the coming years. Therefore, such products will not be available for therapeutic purposes in the European Union member states in the future (14).

Other Metallic Compounds for Therapeutic Purposes

Arsenic is a metalloid compound that is naturally present in rocks but is present in low amounts in soil and water. The presence of arsenic in the environment may also occur due to human industrial activity (mining, burning nonferrous metals, burning fossil fuel, or use in fertilizers, pesticides, insecticides, etc.). Unlike copper and zinc, arsenic is not thought to be an essential trace element, and therefore supplementation in feed is not considered for nutritional purposes. Arsenic and inorganic arsenic compounds are considered toxic and carcinogenic, while other arsenic-derived compounds are considered either "possibly carcinogenic to humans" or "not classifiable as to their carcinogenicity to humans" (21). However, there have been reports of beneficial effects in cancer therapy, and therefore arsenic might have some unexpected beneficial effects (22). Additionally, exposure to inorganic arsenic in drinking water has been linked to a reduction in breast cancer (23).

Organic arsenical compounds are active against coccidia and other parasites, so they have been used in poultry production to reduce coccidial infection and promote growth. However, even though roxarsone, arsanilic acid, and nitarsone are organic compounds and are thought to be less toxic, it was noticed that their usage led to the increased occurrence of inorganic arsenic residues in liver detected by improved analytical methods, and they have therefore been under scrutiny. These compounds were widely used in the United States and have only recently been banned, starting with a ban on roxarsone, carbasone, and arsanilic acid in 2013, which was followed by a ban on the use of nitarsone for histomoniasis in turkeys in 2015. However, the widespread use and subsequent exposure to arsenic in humans was determined through a significant association between arsenic content in urine and poultry intake in a study performed in the United States between 2003 and 2010 (24). Because these compounds are now banned in the United States and the European Union, it is important to focus on other places in the world where this type of supplementation is still ongoing (25, 26), both to avoid consumption of arsenic by humans and to avoid pollution of the environment around farms (27).

Effect of Supplementation on Microflora and Organs

Copper

It has been generally assumed that copper does not affect the normal bacterial flora, but an extensive literature study found that in piglets and growing pigs, low copper concentrations (<50 mg/kg feed) affected the microbiota in the gastrointestinal tract. Similarly, 100 to 250 mg/kg copper sulfate was found to significantly change the microbial community structure. In poultry (broilers), supplementation with copper, even at low concentrations (<50 mg/kg feed), appeared to affect the microbiota in the gastrointestinal tract. In particular, the *Clostridia* population seemed to be affected even at low concentrations. At higher concentrations (>200 mg/kg feed), inorganic or organic bound copper also appeared to affect the population of lactobacilli and coliforms in broilers (28). Furthermore, the reduction of the pH of the gizzard content may cause severe gizzard erosion (4).

The risk assessments made for copper salt supplements (including copper carbonate) in relation to human consumption have concluded that a maximum residue level is not needed because it seems unlikely that copper salts, when used according to the specifications in veterinary medicine settings, are likely to cause harm in humans through consumption of residues contained in food of animal origin (29).

Zinc

The main consensus regarding zinc supplementation is that it does not appear to have major consequences on the microflora and organs. However, recent studies demonstrated that the effect observed might be due to the regulation of factors related to the immune response leading to a reduction of stem cell factor expression in the small intestine and causing a reduction in the number of mast cells and histamine release.

These findings may have important implications for the prevention of weaning-associated diarrhea in piglets (30). However, a number of studies suggest that changes in the stress response may also indicate a more profound effect of therapeutic zinc supplementation that might affect the immune response (31).

The risk assessments made for zinc supplements in relation to human consumption have concluded that a maximum residue level is not needed because it seems unlikely that zinc salts, when used according to the specifications in veterinary medicine settings, are likely to cause harm in humans through consumption of residues contained in food of animal origin (32).

Usage Data and Distribution

High amounts of zinc additives are used for medical purposes in piglet production in Europe. As an example: European pig production was 248 million heads in 2008 (EURO-25 in 2008); 30% of these were produced in Denmark and Belgium. A percentage piglets were most likely given feed containing 2.5 g Zn/kg in the first 14 days after weaning. If daily feed consumption is 0.4 kg in the first week and 0.5 kg in the second week, the zinc consumed amounts to approximately 1,312 tons per year (13).

A similar scenario can be found in the United States. Here, as in Europe, zinc is fed to newly weaned pigs at high dietary levels of 2.0 to 3.0 g/kg feed (19). Assuming a mean of 2.5 g/kg and the same feed intake during the first 14 days after weaning as stated above for Europe, the 113.8 million pigs raised for slaughter in 2016 (33) would have consumed approximately 1,800 tons of zinc.

Taking Denmark as an example of a major pig-producing country using zinc by prescription, it was observed that the consumption of zinc oxide prescribed by Danish veterinarians has increased over the past 10 years, from ~150 tons in 2005 to ~500 tons in 2014. In this time period, the total consumption of zinc oxide tripled, while pig production increased by only 14% (15, 20). Another example of a European country using zinc oxide for therapeutic purposes is Belgium, where the use of zinc oxide in therapeutic doses in piglets administered for 2 weeks after weaning has been allowed only since September 2013. In Belgium, zinc oxide has become an alternative for colistin, which was previously used in weaned piglets. The data for 2014 and 2015 show a substantial increase in the use of this metal compound, with 81,964 kg and 87,199 kg of zinc oxide, respectively, consumed in Belgium. Simultaneously, the Belgian authorities noticed a decrease in the use of polymyxins (colistin) from 5.8 mg/PCU (population correction unit, which is defined as a measure of biomass, where 1 PCU is equivalent to 1 kg of biomass of livestock or slaughtered animals) in 2012, when zinc oxide was not available, to 3.3 mg/PCU in 2014, and a further 51% decrease was noticed in 2015 (16, 34). As mentioned above, the market authorizations for zinc products will be withdrawn for use for therapeutic purposes following the decision taken by European Medicines Agency, and therefore we expect a sharp drop in the consumption of this compound in the European Union. Because the use of zinc compounds is not exclusive to Europe and is quite widespread in North America (18) and other regions, some therapeutic use might remain, depending on local regulations. Reducing the amount of zinc to a dietary requirement of 100 mg/kg for newly weaned pigs would reduce the yearly zinc consumption in pig farming by over 90% (35).

It has been shown that high zinc supplementation after weaning until pigs reached 12 kg, followed by high copper supplementation until they reached about 25 kg in body weight was both cost-effective and promoted the best growth. Suggested therapeutic copper levels of 100 to 250 mg/kg are 95 to 98% above the dietary requirement for this age group (19, 35).

Environmental Concerns from Use of Metals in Agriculture: Metal Ecotoxicity

The extensive supplementation of feed with these compounds and the additional practices of therapeutic and/or growth promoter usage are not innocuous. Most of these compounds are excreted by the animals and end up in the environment, where their accumulation can have major consequences (36) because these are not degradable and will increase the concentration in the environment, especially in soils amended with slurry/manure from animal production (37). For example, Denmark, which is one of the largest pig-producing countries in the world and uses metals in animal production, has maintained a national monitoring program of heavy metals in the environment for the last 28 years to better understand the effects of these practices on the environment. The values and analyses published in 2016 indicate that the use of pig slurry has led to a significant increase in the concentrations of copper and zinc in soil (38).

Furthermore, the data show that 45% of the analyzed soils have reached zinc levels above the predicted no-effect concentrations (PNEC), while for copper, only one soil sample was above the PNEC. Continued agricultural use of zinc is expected to increase the levels, and larger areas will have soil exceeding the PNEC. Furthermore, the authors noted that the current situa-

tion raises concerns regarding the aquatic environment because the current use of zinc and copper in agriculture might lead to leaching of these metals into water and negatively affect aquatic species (37, 38).

In addition, at the European level, zinc is one of the compounds studied as part of risk assessments regarding the environmental pollution of heavy metals. These reports focus on aspects related to manufacturing of zinc products. A number of studies looking at the accumulation of zinc in soils due to agricultural use are also mentioned, and although these studies are relatively different in scope and methodology, they all agree that zinc will accumulate in soils in a significant manner, and increasing areas will exceed the critical concentrations. However, the time this will take varies and therefore needs to be assessed at the regional level (39). Taking into account these aspects and also acknowledging the risk for coselection, the European authorities have been alerted and are conducting ongoing collection of information for environmental risk assessment of heavy metals as part of veterinary medicinal products. The Committee for Veterinary Medicine Products has therefore concluded that the benefits do not outweigh the risks, and the risk for the environment justifies withdrawing the market authorizations for the therapeutic usage of zinc compounds (34).

Alternatives

As mentioned above, zinc and copper cannot be replaced since they are essential trace elements, but the concentrations can be reduced and adjusted to the essential requirements to avoid overuse. Similarly, in the future, the use of those metals at high concentrations for therapeutic purposes will be discontinued at least in the European Union, not only because of the added pressure leading to selection of bacterial resistance to copper and zinc and subsequently coselection of antibiotic-resistance genes, but mainly because of environmental concerns. Antimicrobials are alternatives for this therapeutic use but are not viable options since there are a number of ongoing efforts to reduce antimicrobial consumption in animals. Replacement should go hand in hand with improvement of management practices to reduce the need for the use of metals or other compounds during the weaning period.

DETECTION OF HEAVY METAL RESISTANCE

In recent years, the identification and/or characterization of strains of bacteria of animal origin that have reduced susceptibility or increased tolerance to heavy

Table 4   C(

Heavy meta

Copper

Zinc

ity, indicatir
negative bac
been identifi
for both cop

Chromoso
defense sy!
Due to the
Earth's histo
iron-sulfur c
oxygen spec
deal with th(
targets of co
cytoplasm i

metals has gained a lot of attention, and therefore, an increasing number of studies include heavy metal susceptibility or tolerance testing. The Web of Science database was searched systematically for articles between January 2005 and December 2016 using the search terms "heavy+ metal+ resistance+ animal" and "heavy+ metal+ resistance+ bacteria+ MIC". This resulted in the retrieval of 278 articles, of which only 23 reported MIC data on bacterial isolates of animal origin, including fish. These studies were reviewed and revealed a number of weaknesses, which can impact the quality of the results or the conclusions made. Here, we will highlight the major pitfalls that make comparisons of studies challenging.

Several methods, such as disc diffusion, agar dilution, and microbroth dilution, have been used in metal tolerance assays. Disc diffusion, the use of paper discs impregnated with a specific heavy metal salt concentration placed on agar plates spread with bacteria, was rarely used (only two studies [40, 41]). Agar and microbroth dilution were the most common methods to determine an isolate's MIC to a particular heavy metal. Both methods are based on a dilution series of the heavy metal that is incorporated into either molten agar or liquid broth. The methodology is similar to that used for antibiotic susceptibility testing, where the dilution series is typically 2-fold dilutions rather an exponential serial dilution. While most studies use the lowest concentration at which there is inhibition of visible growth, a few studies use optical density measurements to determine the presence of bacterial growth (42, 43).

As previously described by Hasman et al. (44), the choice of media and the pH of that media are crucial factors that can influence the detection of metal resistance levels. For example, certain components in complex media can sequester free metal ions, reducing the concentration available for the bacteria. Therefore, it is advisable to use standardized media such as Mueller Hinton, which has been extensively validated for use in antibiotic susceptibility testing. Of the 23 studies included in this analysis and described using agar dilution (*n* = 18), up to six different media were used. While Mueller Hinton agar was the most common, brain heart infusion agar (45), Luria Bertani agar (46), nutrient agar (47, 48), and tryptic soy agar (49, 50) were also used. As previously mentioned, the pH of the medium can influence the detection of metal resistance. For example, pH values above 5.5 can cause zinc sulfate in complex media to precipitate, thereby reducing the concentration of the metal that the bacteria have to encounter. Furthermore, addition of metals into the medium can change the final pH, which can affect bacterial growth. Therefore, it is strongly recommended that after supplementation of the metal, the media is adjusted accordingly to ensure optimal bacterial growth and avoid misleading results. Only seven articles noted that pH adjustments were performed. However, even in studies where adjustments were reported, the pH value was not always consistent; e.g., for $CuSO_4$ in Mueller-Hinton agar, a range of pH values were used by the different studies (pH 7, 7.2, and 7.4) (51–55). It is recommended that when using Mueller Hinton agar or broth, the adjusted pH should be as follows: zinc chloride, pH = 5.5; copper sulfate, pH = 7.2; sodium arsenate, cadmium acetate, and silver nitrate, pH = 7.4 (51, 56).

Studies wanting to categorize bacterial isolates as susceptible or resistant to a particular heavy metal on the basis of their MICs or inhibition zone diameters require approved interpretive criteria. There are no clinical breakpoints for heavy metals. Therefore, epidemiological cutoff values are based on previous studies reporting the MIC distributions for a particular bacterial species. Five studies used a control strain, e.g., the laboratory strain *Escherichia coli* K12 or C600, and strains were considered resistant if the MIC values exceeded that of the control strain (57–61). While this could be a reasonable approach to characterize reduced heavy metal susceptibility among bacterial isolates, the control strain should belong to the same bacterial species as the test isolates. Akinbowale et al. (59) used *E. coli* K12 to describe resistance in *Aeromonas* spp. and *Pseudomonas* spp. While all isolates are Gram negative, there are intrinsic differences between the species that can affect the interpretation of the results.

Increased metal tolerance to zinc and copper has been described in many bacterial species. Initially, these resistant bacterial species were detected among environmental bacteria isolated from areas with high concentrations of heavy metals. Due to the use of heavy metals in food-producing animals and the association of heavy metal resistance with antimicrobial resistance as a result of co-selection, many studies have investigated the levels of reduced susceptibility (Table 3) and the associated genes in a number of bacterial species isolated from food-producing animals (Table 4).

MECHANISMS OF METAL HOMEOSTASIS AND RESISTANCE

Metal homeostasis is a delicate balance of ensuring that a cell's requirement for essential metals is met to ensure proper cell function while at the same time limiting the amount of metal in the cell to avoid toxicity. The

Table 3   B

Metal

Copper

Zinc

ability to b
homeostas:
of metal tr:
ganism's li
to metals.

Copper

As in othe
changed wi
ment durir
came availa
sulfides an
With life
and the lir
karyotes ut
enzymes. C
protect cell
its cytotoxi
the generati
conditions (

Copper u|

In contrast
ber of cop|
exception c
oxidase, loc
brane. Ther

one, CopB, belonging to the "classical" P_{1B-1}-ATPases removing excess Cu(I) from the cytoplasm, while CopA belongs to the FixI/CopA2-like ATPases that are important for proper assembly of membrane-bound Cu-containing enzymes (85, 87, 96). P_{1B}-ATPases have been identified to be involved in copper resistance in several Gram-positive bacteria (97, 98).

Similarly, in Gram-negative bacteria, P_{1B-1}-ATPases have been shown to be involved in expelling excess copper from the cytoplasm. The best characterized are the chromosomally encoded copper homeostasis systems from *E. coli*, including *copA* encoding the P_{1B}-ATPase CopA (99–101). In *E. coli*, *copA* is part of the CueR-regulon. The repressor CueR binds Cu(I) at zeptomolar concentrations and regulates the expression of *copA* and *cueO* (100, 102–105). While CopA in *E. coli* expels Cu(I) from the cytoplasm (106, 107), Cu(I) would now still be in the periplasm to cause damage to the cell. This necessitates CueO, which is a periplasmic multicopper oxidase that has been shown to oxidize Cu(I) into the less toxic Cu(II). CueO also oxidized enterobactin, enabling further sequestration of copper (108–116). The presence of genes encoding homologs of CopA and CueO is widespread among members of the *Enterobacteriaceae*, and this two-pronged approach appears to be a common strategy for copper detoxification (under "normal" aerobic circumstances) (49, 117–121). However, for CueO to be active, the organism requires the presence of oxygen. In the digestive tract of humans and/or animals, limited or no oxygen is available [and Cu(I) is also more stable than in an oxygenated environment]. Therefore, other strategies to keep the periplasm safe from copper toxicity need to be in place (99, 122). In *E. coli*, the CBA transport complex CusCBA is involved in Cu detoxification of the periplasm in the absence of CueO (99, 100, 123). Expression of *cusCFBA* is regulated by the two-component regulatory system CusRS, with CusS being a membrane-bound sensor kinase that detects periplasmic copper and relays the information to the cytoplasmic response regulator CusR, regulating *cusCFBA* expression (124, 125). It was found that in an anaerobic environment, expression was induced at much lower copper concentrations than in the presence of oxygen (100). The CusCBA complex is composed of the resistance nodulation cell division (RND)-protein CusA in the cytoplasmic membrane, the outer membrane factor (OMF) CusC in the outer membrane, and the membrane fusion protein CusB stabilizing the complex. Three molecules of CusA form a complex creating a "vestibule," which forms a funnel to the channel formed by the CusC trimer. Cu(I) enters the funnel in the periplasm and via CusC is expelled into the surrounding medium. Cu(I) transport is energized via the proton gradient across the cytoplasmic membrane (101, 126–131). While CBA transport systems have been described for different types of heavy metals and organic compounds (including antibiotics), the presence of the periplasmic protein CusF is unique to transport systems involved in copper and silver transport (123). CusF could either act as a periplasmic chaperon delivering the metal ion to the CBA transport complex or function as a regulator of the transport (132–139). An alternative system for protection of the periplasm against copper-mediated toxicity under anaerobic conditions can be found in *Salmonella*. Here, the copper tolerance is linked to the presence of the periplasmic protein CueP. Expression of *cueP* in a *cus*-deletion strain of *E. coli* can partially restore its copper resistance under anaerobic conditions (120, 140–143). CueP seems to be confined to members of the genera *Citrobacter* and *Salmonella*.

Copper resistance systems encoded on mobile elements

Genomic islands involved in copper resistance of *Enterobacteria*

A plasmid-bound copper resistance determinant in *Enterobacteria* was first described on plasmid pRJ1004 from *E. coli* (144, 145). Copper resistance encoded on this plasmid is linked to the presence of the *pco* system, which encodes a two-component regulatory system, PcoRS, as well as to the structural proteins involved in copper resistance: PcoA, a periplasmic multicopper oxidase, the outer membrane protein PcoB, the inner membrane protein PcoD, and two periplasmic proteins, PcoC and PcoE (146–149). Expression of *pcoE* is regulated via a chromosomally encoded system, CusRS (124, 149), while expression of *pcoABCD* is regulated by PcoRS (147). Periplasmic PcoE is able to sequester excess copper, giving the cell temporary protection from the toxic effects of copper (149). Periplasmic PcoC also binds copper but is able to transfer it to membrane-bound PcoD to catalyze Cu(I) uptake into the cell. Once in the cytoplasm, Cu(I) is incorporated into the multicopper oxidase PcoA, which is then exported into the periplasm via the twin-arginine translocation pathway. Once in the periplasm, PcoA detoxifies Cu(I) by either oxidation of catechol siderophores and subsequent sequestration of Cu(I) or oxidation of Cu(I) to Cu(II). Cu(II) might be removed from the periplasm via PcoB (Fig. 1) (101, 146, 148, 150, 151). Located adjacent to *pco* on pRJ1004 is a *sil* determinant (150, 151). The *sil* determinant was first identified on plasmid pMG101

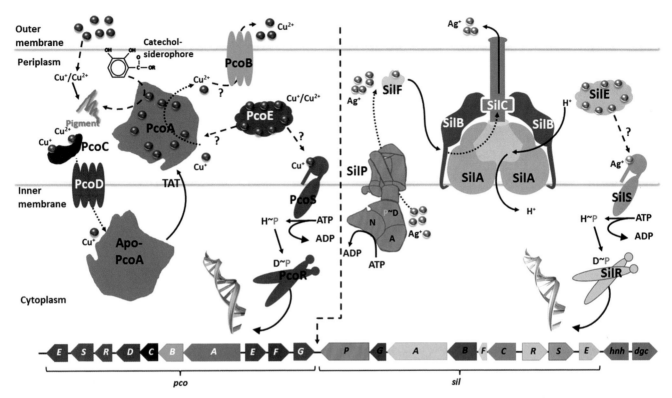

Figure 1 Copper fitness (or pathogenicity) island in *Enterobacteriaceae*. Genes and protein products of the enterobacterial copper fitness island composed of the *pco-* and *sil*-determinants. The genes, including their transcriptional/translational direction, are indicated below the illustration of the proposed or experimentally determined function of the proteins encoded by the *pco/sil* system. Refer to text for details. (Reprinted with permission [171].)

from *Salmonella enterica* serovar Typhimurium and was shown to confer silver resistance (152, 153). Expression of the structural genes of the *sil* determinant is regulated by the two-component regulatory system SilRS. In the presence of silver, *silCFBA* is expressed forming the SilCBA efflux complex (similar to CusCBA), allowing for the export of Ag(I) and Cu(I) from the periplasm. SilF is a periplasmic protein (like CusF) that is able to bind Ag(I) and either shuttles Ag(I) to the transport complex as substrate for export or could act as a regulatory protein of the function of SilCBA. In addition to the RND-dependent transporter SilCBA, the P_{1B-1}-ATPases SilP, the periplasmic protein SilE, and a periplasmic protein, SilG, of unknown function are encoded as part of the *sil* determinant. Like PcoE, SilE is able to bind metal ions [Ag(I) and Cu(I)] and protect the periplasm from short-term metal stress. The P_{1B-1}-ATPase SilP transports silver ions from the cytoplasm into the periplasm, from where they can be removed via SilCBA (150, 151, 153, 154). In contrast to copper, silver ions cannot undergo redox reactions, and therefore oxidation of Ag(I) as a detoxification mechanism is not an

option for the cell. However, the entire *sil* resistance determinant also confers resistance to Cu(I). The overall 20-gene cluster *pco/sil* has been referred to as a copper-pathogenicity island (150) or a copper homeostasis and silver resistance island (151) (Fig. 1). The entire gene cluster has been identified in isolates of *E. coli* and *S.* Typhimurium, including *E. coli* O104:H4 from pigs fed a high-copper diet (155, 156).

Analysis of the available completed genome and plasmid sequences of *Enterobacteria* (Table 5) revealed that the *pco/sil* gene cluster is frequently flanked by *Tn7*-like elements, allowing for transfer of the gene cluster (154, 157). Recent sequencing of *E. coli* J53 (pMG101) (NCTC 50110) showed that the *pco/sil* cluster has integrated from pMG101 (152, 153) into the bacterium's genome (154). Interestingly, in some genera (*Citrobacter, Kosakonia,* and *Raoultella*), all of the identified *pco/sil* sequences are chromosomally encoded, while in others (*Klyvera* and *Serratia*), the sequences are carried only on plasmids. In most of the genera containing the *pco/sil* determinant, it can be carried on plasmids as well as on the bacterial chromo-

Table 5 Distribution of *pco/sil* and yersiniabactin biosynthesis genes among *Enterobacteriaceae*

Genus[a]	Number of sequences analyzed[b]	Occurrence of copper/silver tolerance determinants				
		pco[c]	*sil*[d]	*pco/sil*[e]	Yersiniabactin synthesis[f]	*pco/silP* and yersiniabactin synthesis[g]
Citrobacter	60 genomes	10	10	10	3	0
	50 plasmids	0	0	0	0	
Cronobacter	29 genomes	1	1	1	0	0
	22 plasmids	6	6	6	0	
Enterobacter	167 genomes	22	28	21	0	0
	121 plasmids	6	7	6	0	
Escherichia	946 genomes	33	31	30	121	18
	901 plasmids	7	11	7	0	
Klebsiella	674 genomes	2	3	2	82	30
	628 plasmids	92	92	91	2	
Kluyvera	6 genomes	0	0	0	0	0
	4 plasmids	1	1	1	0	
Kosakonia	10 genomes	1	1	1	0	0
	4 plasmids	0	0	0	0	
Pantoea	66 genomes	0	0	0	0	0
	61 plasmids	0	1	0	0	
Raoultella	9 genomes	1	1	1	4	1
	8 plasmids	0	0	0	0	
Salmonella	602 genomes	14	13	13	5	0
	369 plasmids	4	6	4	7	
Serratia	64 genomes	0	0	0	0	0
	27 plasmids	2	2	2	0	
Yersinia	192 genomes	0	0	0	33	0
	153 plasmids	0	0	0	0	

[a]Genera of *Enterobacteriaceae* harboring *pco*, *sil*, and/or *ybt*.
[b]Number of completed genomic and plasmid sequences of respective genera available for Microbial Genome BLAST (http://blast.ncbi.nlm.nih.gov; accessed 13 September 2017).
[c]Analysis (blastn) using *pco* from pRJ1004 (GenBank accession number X83541.1 [146]) as query.
[d]Analysis (blastn) using *sil* from pMG101 (GenBank accession number NG_035131.1 -[153]) as query.
[e]Analysis (blastn) using *pco* (GenBank accession number X83541.1; [146]) and *sil* (accession number KC146966.1 [151]) from pRJ1004 as query.
[f]Analysis (tblastn) using Ybt peptide/polyketide synthetase HMWP1 (GenBank accession number AAC69588.1 [246]) as query.
[g]Number of strains harboring *pco/sil* and *ybt* with determinant being located on chromosome and/or plasmid, respectively.

some, including strains that harbor a copy on each location. While in most cases the entire 20-gene cluster *pco/sil* is present, some strains of *Enterobacter*, *Escherichia*, *Klebsiella*, *Pantoea*, and *Salmonella* contain only one of the two resistance determinants, *pco* or *sil* (Table 5).

Another strategy of *Enterobacteriaceae* to protect against the toxic effects of copper is the use of siderophores, especially yersiniabactin (158). The presence of the genes encoding the yersiniabactin synthesis pathway has previously been described as a virulence factor, but its presence in copper-resistant isolates indicates its importance in protection from copper toxicity. Yersiniabactin biosynthesis has been found in strains of *E. coli*, *Salmonella*, *Yersinia pestis*, and *Klebsiella pneumoniae*, including *E. coli* isolates from livestock fed high-copper diets (155, 159–163). Analysis of available completed

genome and plasmid sequences of *Enterobacteriaceae* revealed the presence of the yersiniabactin biosynthesis pathways in the genera *Citrobacter* and *Raoultella*, in addition to the previously known genera. While commonly encoded on the bacterial chromosome, in some genera the yersiniabactin biosynthesis genes are located on plasmids as well (Table 5). Some strains of *E. coli* (including strains of enterohemorrhagic *E. coli* O104: H4), *K. pneumoniae*, and *Raoultella* have both the *pco/sil* gene cluster and the yersiniabactin biosynthesis determinant (Table 5).

Genomic islands involved in copper resistance of *Enterococcus*

In addition to Gram-negative bacteria, Gram-positive bacteria of the genus *Enterococcus* have frequently been isolated from livestock and shown to have high copper resistance (52, 121, 164, 165). Copper resistance in *Enterococcus* has been shown to be plasmid encoded and can be transferred via conjugation (121, 166–169). The first gene that could be linked to the plasmid-encoded copper resistance determinant in *Enterococcus* was *tcrB*. TcrB is a member of the P_{1B}-ATPases of copper transporters, but due to the presence of a histidine-rich cytoplasmic N-terminus, a CPH-motif in transmembrane helix VI, and an MSXST-motif, it would be predicted to belong to the P_{1B-3}-ATPase subfamily utilizing Cu(II) as substrate. TcrB is encoded as part of the *tcrYAZB* operon, which encodes TcrA, an additional P_{1B}-ATPase of the P_{1B-1}-ATPase subfamily with Cu(I) as the transported substrate, a cytoplasmic copper chaperon TcrZ, and TcrY, a copper-dependent regulator (150, 166, 170). Approximately 62% of *Enterococcus* strains that harbor transferrable copper resistance contained not only *tcrYAZB* but also *cueO*. This is in contrast to the strains analyzed in another study, where 22% only had *tcrB* and 16% encoded for CueO (121).

Sequence analysis of copper-resistant *Enterococcus faecalis* showed the presence of *tcrZAYB* and *cueO* as part of a larger gene cluster that also encoded a two-component regulatory system, CusRS, and an additional transcriptional regulator, CopY. Directly adjacent to *copY*, an additional P_{1B-1}-ATPase named CopA is encoded, leading to the prediction of *copA* expression being regulated by CopY. Genes encoding several putative metal-binding proteins possibly serving as metal chaperones in the copper detoxification process are also in close proximity. The genes *cusRS* are directly downstream of *cueO*, suggesting regulation by this two-component regulatory system. Since the P_{1B}-ATPases TcrA, TcrB, and CopA export copper ions from the cytoplasm, regulation of the respective genes by cytoplasmic copper-dependent regulators, CopY and TcrY, seems logical. In contrast, CueO, located just outside the cytoplasmic membrane, oxidizing Cu(I) to the less toxic Cu(II), appears to be regulated by CusRS sensing environmental copper concentrations (Fig. 2) (42, 150, 171). Other strains of *E. faecalis* and *Enterococcus faecium* contain related copper-resistance islands that vary slightly in the presence and arrangement of some of the genes in the copper-resistance island. These changes are probably at least in part due to the large number of putative transposons encoded in this region. BLAST analysis of the *E. faecium* HF50105 genome revealed a similar gene region in 5 of the 149 completed plasmid sequences of members of the genus *Enterococcus*, two belonging to *Enterococcus durans*, two to *E. faecium*, and one to *Enterococcus gallinarum*. No chromosomally encoded copper-resistance island could be identified. Further sequence analysis showed that this gene cluster is only present in the genus *Enterococcus* but not in other *Firmicutes*.

Zinc

Zinc bioavailability has changed drastically in course of Earth's history. The greater bioavailability of zinc after the Great Oxidation Event is reflected in the increased use of zinc in eukaryotes (62, 63, 172). Zinc serves as a structural or catalytic component in hundreds of proteins and is one of the most abundant transition metals in a cell. The total amount of zinc in an *E. coli* cell was determined to be in a range similar to the cellular concentrations of calcium and iron (173). However, free Zn(II) in the cytoplasm is essentially nonexistent, since the Zn(II) regulators ZntR (efflux) and Zur (uptake) respond to free Zn(II) concentrations of 10^{-16} M in *E. coli* (173). This shows that bacteria very tightly control the uptake and efflux of Zn(II) to ensure proper cellular function while avoiding metal toxicity.

Zinc uptake

At least three systems (ABC-transporter, ZIP transporter, and phosphate-bound uptake) have been described to be involved in bacterial zinc uptake. Best understood are the systems involved in zinc uptake of *E. coli*. Under zinc-limiting conditions, *E. coli* utilizes the ABC (ATP-binding cassette) transporter ZnuABC. ZnuA is a zinc-binding protein located in the periplasm. ZnuB spans the cytoplasmic membrane and forms the channel to transport Zn(II) into the cytoplasm. ZnuC is bound to the cytoplasmic site on ZnuB, providing the energy for Zn(II)-transport via ATP hydrolysis (174, 175). Expression of the *znu* operon is regulated by Zur, which binds cytoplasmic Zn(II) and acts as repressor of *znu* by blocking the RNA polymerase from binding to the −10 region of the *znuC* promoter. Half-maximal repression by Zur *in vitro* has been shown to occur at a concentration of $2.0 (\pm 0.1) \times 10^{-16}$ M free Zn(II), indicating that the presence of any free Zn(II) in the cell effectively turns off Zn(II) uptake by ZnuABC (173, 176–178). While genes encoding ZnuABC homologs have been identified in the genomes of many bacteria, it is absent in the genome of *Cupriavidus metallidurans* CH34, a bacterium originally isolated from a zinc decantation tank (179–181).

Under nonlimiting zinc conditions, *E. coli* utilizes a different uptake system, ZupT, the first identified bacterial member of the ZIP (ZRT-, IRT-like protein [ZRT, zinc-regulated transporter; IRT, iron-regulated transporter]) family of transport proteins (75, 182). Genes encoding ZupT have been identified in members of

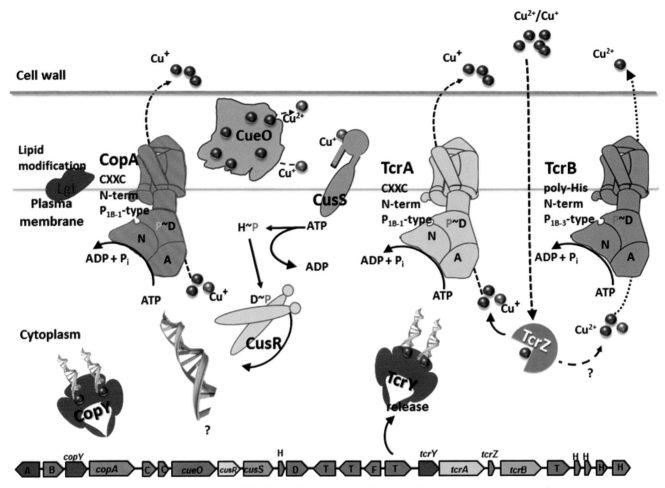

Figure 2 Copper fitness island in *Enterococcus*. Genes and proposed protein products of the copper island in *Enterococcus faecium* HF50105 (GenBank accession number AITS01000024). The genes, including their transcriptional/translational direction, are indicated below the illustration of the proposed function of the proteins. (Refer to text for details.) Adjacent to and separating the genes involved in copper resistance are genes encoding prolipoprotein diacylglyceryl transferase (A), integral membrane protein (B), predicted metal-binding protein/chaperone (C), hypothetical protein (H), transposase (T), and disrupted P-type ATPase (F) that have been identified. (Reprinted with permission [171].)

many bacterial phyla. In *E. coli*, *zupT* is expressed constitutively at a low level, and expression is therefore independent of external zinc availability. In contrast, in *C. metallidurans*, *zupT* expression is regulated by FurC, decreasing the amount of transporter under high zinc conditions and thereby limiting Zn(II) uptake (74, 181). It is not known if or how *zupT* expression is regulated in other microorganisms. While initially described as a zinc uptake system in *E. coli*, ZupT has broad substrate specificity and is also able to take up other metals, including Fe(II), Co(II), and Mn(II). Cadmium and copper also cross the cytoplasmic membrane via ZupT-mediated unspecific uptake (74). Several amino acids have been identified to contribute to ZupT's substrate

specificity (73). In uropathogenic *E. coli* as well as *S. enterica*, ZupT plays an important role in bacterial virulence, especially in the absence of *znu* (175, 183).

Under nonlimiting conditions, zinc can also enter *E. coli* as a metal-phosphate complex via PitA (inorganic phosphate uptake system) (184, 185). Magnesium uptake systems have been shown to have a broad substrate spectrum and are able to transport Zn(II) in addition to Mg(II) (180, 186–188). The presence of both zinc uptake systems is very common among bacteria.

Zinc efflux

Zinc resistance in bacteria is facilitated via efflux (189, 190). At least four systems (P_{1B}-type ATPases, CDF transporters, 2-TM-GxN transporters, and CBA efflux systems) involved in transporting Zn(II) out of the cell have been identified. These systems can be encoded chromosomally or on plasmids.

The most effective transporters that export Zn(II) out of the cell are soft-metal P_{1B}-type ATPases. Members of this family of membrane proteins contain six to eight transmembrane helices and cytoplasmic domains involved in ATP binding and hydrolysis as well as metal-binding domains. Based on structural features and the resulting substrate spectra, several subfamilies can be differentiated. Zn(II) is exported by members of the P_{1B-2}-ATPase subgroup (83, 86). The best-characterized member of this group is ZntA from *E. coli* (191, 192). Members of this subgroup possess eight transmembrane helices, with a conserved CPC motif and Asp as transmembrane metal-binding sites. ZntA has a broad substrate specificity and can also transport Pb(II) and Cd(II), as can other members of this P_{1B-2}-ATPase subgroup. Additionally, other metals such as Co(II), Ni(II), and Cu(II) bind to the transmembrane metal-binding domain, However, when these metals are bound, no ATP hydrolysis or transport takes place (193). Zn(II)-transporting ATPases can be chromosomally encoded, such as ZntA from *E. coli*, or encoded on plasmids, such as CadA from *Staphylococcus aureus* (191, 194, 195). Expression of *zntA* of *E. coli* is regulated by the MerR-like regulator ZntR. In the absence of Zn(II), apo-ZntR binds to the *zntA* promoter, repressing transcription. In the presence of Zn(II) in the cytoplasm, Zn-ZntR acts as a transcriptional activator and allows for transcription of *zntA*. *In vitro* analysis of ZntR affinity to Zn(II) revealed that concentration in the femtomolar range is required for ZntR to bind. However, *in vivo* studies identified ZntR responding to cytoplasmic free Zn(II) concentrations in the nanomolar range (173, 196). On the *E. coli* chromosome, *zntR* and *zntA* are not located in the same gene cluster (197). In contrast, on plasmid pI258 of *S. aureus*, the genes encoding the P_{1B-2}-ATPase and its regulator are organized in an operon, *cadCA*. CadC is a member of the ArsR/SmtB-family and represses transcription in the absence of Zn(II), Cd(II), or Pb(II) (198). P_{1B-2}-ATPases are highly efficient at removing Zn(II) from the cytoplasm, and deletion of the respective genes usually results in Zn(II) sensitivity of the organism (189, 191). Another P_{1B-2}-ATPase of *Staphylococcus* is CzrC, which can be found in some methicillin-resistant strains encoded as part of SCC*mec* (staphylococcal cassette chromosome *mec*) (51, 199, 200). While often associated with SCC*mec*, *czrC* has also been identified in *mecA*-negative strains and on plasmids of *S. aureus*

(201). Initially identified in *S. aureus*, *czrC* has also been found in isolates of other *Staphylococcus* species: *S. haemolyticus*, *S. epidermitis*, *S. lentus*, *S. hominis*, and *S. hyicus* (51, 199, 201–204). Out of the 489 completed *Staphylococcus* genomes in the NCBI database (as of 1 November 2017), 15 carry *czrC* (9 *S. aureus*, 1 *S. condimenti*, 3 *S. epidermis*, and 2 *S. simulans*), while the gene is not found on any of the 483 *Staphylococcus* plasmid sequences. While to date, the regulation of *czrC* expression has not yet been studied, it is likely regulated by an ArsR-like regulator encoded directly upstream of *czrC*.

A second family of membrane transporters linked to bacterial zinc export are cation diffusion facilitator (CDF) proteins, which contain six transmembrane helices with a C- and N-terminus located in the cytoplasm. *E. coli* contains two genes encoding CDF proteins. Both transporters, ZitB and FieF, have been shown to be involved in Zn(II) transport (205, 206). While deletion of *zitB* alone does not impact *E. coli*'s ability to handle elevated concentrations of Zn(II), a double mutant defective in both ZitB and the P_{1B-2}-ATPase ZntA exhibits higher zinc sensitivity than a mutant strain defective only in ZntA (205). While no increase in zinc sensitivity was observed after deletion of *fieF*, everted membrane vesicles of *E. coli* GR362 (deficient in ZnuABC, ZupT, ZntA, ZntB, and ZitB) expressing *fieF* accumulated ^{65}Zn(II). This transport was energized via the proton gradient, as has been shown for other CDF proteins (206). Using reporter gene fusion, expression of both genes, *zitB* and *fieF*, was found to be induced by Zn(II) and to a lesser extent by Cd(II). However, later analysis showed that mRNA levels of *zitB* remain constant after addition of Zn(II) and are elevated, but still independent of Zn(II) concentration, in a *zntA* deletion strain (196, 205, 206). It has been suggested that ZitB is involved in maintaining zinc homeostasis under "normal" conditions, while ZntA confers zinc resistance. CDF proteins involved in Zn(II) transport have been identified in many bacterial species. In *S. aureus*, the chromosomally encoded CDF transporter has been named ZntA and is encoded in an operon encoding ZntR in addition to ZntA. ZntA-null mutants were zinc sensitive, and expression of the operon was Zn(II) dependent and regulated by ZntR (207, 208).

First identified in *S.* Typhimurium, ZntB is a member of the 2-TM-GxN family of membrane transporters. This transporter family is widely found in bacteria, and ZntB-like proteins have been identified in many *Proteobacteria*. Deletion of *zntB* rendered *S.* Typhimurium more sensitive to Zn(II) and Cd(II). ZntB has two transmembrane helixes with the ~270-amino acid

N-terminus and the small C-terminus located in the cytoplasm. ZntB forms a pentamer, forming a cytoplasmic funnel. Each soluble domain monomer of ZntB binds three Zn^{2+}, one in the funnel, while full-length ZntB binds four Zn^{2+} (209–213). In *Agrobacterium tumefaciens*, *zntB* is constitutively expressed but does not seem to contribute to the bacterium's metal tolerance (214).

In contrast to the zinc efflux systems described so far, CBA efflux systems are protein complexes composed of a central transporter of the RND family, a membrane fusion protein, and an OMF. CBA efflux systems are involved in the transport of mono- and divalent heavy metals as well as organic compounds. The RND protein has 12 transmembrane helixes and two large periplasmic domains, which interact with the OMF. Both the RND and the OMF function as homotrimers, forming a channel starting in the periplasmic vestibule of the RND and reaching across the outer membrane via the OMF. The membrane fusion protein (hexamer) interacts with the RND protein and the OMF (190, 215, 216).

Of interest here are members of the heavy metal efflux (HME) family. Members of the HME-RND family are involved in the export of heavy metals, and several subfamilies can be differentiated based on sequence motifs and resulting metal substrates. Zn(II) transport has been credited to the HME1 subfamily (217). The best-characterized member of this family is CzcA from *C. metallidurans* CH34. The *czc* gene cluster is encoded on plasmid pMOL30 of *C. metallidurans* CH34 and allows growth in the presence of Co(II), Zn(II), and Cd(II), increasing the MIC by factors of 10, 25, and 100, respectively, compared to the plasmid-free strain AE104 (218). While export of the metal ions from the cytoplasm was assumed and data indicate transport by CzcA across the cytoplasmic membrane, the fact that a CDF protein as well as a P_{1B-4}-ATPase are encoded as part of the *czc* gene cluster in addition to the two-component regulatory system CzcRS, which monitors the metal content within the periplasm, points toward export of the majority of metal ions from the periplasm into the surrounding environment by CzcCBA. As indicated, the CzcCBA system from *C. metallidurans* CH34 is the best-characterized zinc transporting CBA system to date. The structure of CzcCBA has not yet been solved (189, 215, 216, 219–224). The first structure of an RND protein was solved for AcrB, a multidrug transporter from *E. coli* (225, 226). To date, additional structures of RND transporters have been solved, including ZneA from *C. metallidurans* CH34. ZneA was shown to actively transport Zn(II) across the membrane

via conformational changes within the three ZneA protomers. ZneA interacts with ZneB (membrane fusion protein) and ZneC (OMF) to form the membrane-spanning transport complex. The structure of ZneB was also shown to undergo conformational changes during export of the metal ions, reminiscent of CusB. However, the involvement of ZneCAB in zinc homeostasis of *C. metallidurans* CH34 is not understood (227, 228). Compared to CDF and P_{1B}-type ATPases, CBA efflux systems are not as frequently present on bacterial genomes in bacterial handling of excess zinc.

Copper and Zinc Resistance Determinants: Link to Bacterial Virulence

In addition to these specific metal resistance determinants, there are numerous other genes that improve survival under elevated copper or zinc concentrations. This overview does not go into detail regarding these rather unspecific genes, but we refer the reader to a recent excellent study as an example (229).

The involvement of zinc and copper in bacterial killing is a recent important finding that is of relevance to understanding potential public health challenges arising from feeding livestock copper and zinc supplements. Professional phagocytes such as macrophages engulf pathogens and destroy them through elevation of Zn^{2+} and Cu^+ concentrations in the phagosome, along with other mechanisms (oxidative burst, induction of Fe^{2+}, and Mn^{2+} efflux) (230).

However, it is probable that the mechanisms macrophages use to kill infectious agents evolved in protozoa long before multicellular life arose and the need for macrophages appeared (231). This hypothesis was strengthened showing that copper (and probably zinc) poisoning is used in the model amoeba *Dictyostelium discoideum* to kill bacterial prey (232). Bacteria, in turn, were not just inert prey, and some succeeded in bypassing and resisting phagocytic cells by developing a number of strategies to avoid the protozoan killing mechanisms such as counteracting resistance systems specific for Zn and Cu and possibly other antimicrobial metals. This main concept of ongoing evolution driven by protozoan predation could explain the ongoing evolution of pathogens such as methicillin-resistant *S. aureus*, vancomycin-resistant *Enterococcus*, and extended spectrum beta-lactamase-producing *E. coli*, all of which pose a very important public health problem (233). Farmed animals such as pigs and poultry receive additional Zn and Cu in their diets due to supplementing elements in compound feed as well as medical remedies. Enteral bacteria in farmed animals have been shown to develop resistance to trace elements such as

Zn and Cu. Resistance to Zn is often linked with resistance to methicillin in staphylococci, and Zn supplementation to animal feed may increase the proportion of multiresistant *E. coli* in the gut. Resistance to Cu in bacteria, enterococci in particular, is often associated with resistance to antimicrobial drugs such as macrolides and glycopeptides (e.g., vancomycin). Since Cu and Zn have an important role in protozoan predation, these metal resistances could make survival of these bacteria much more likely. These strains could then become pathogens after transfer to humans (234, 235).

CONCLUSIONS

Copper and zinc have been widely used in livestock feed both as growth promoters and as necessary supplements. In many countries the use of these metals appears to have increased due to a ban on the use of antibiotics. They are effective growth promoters, but it is not entirely clear how this is achieved. The potential negative impacts include zinc and copper contamination in the environment but more importantly the potential of coselecting antibiotic-resistance genes and possibly generating more pathogenic strains of medically relevant bacteria.

Citation. Rensing C, Moodley A, Cavaco LM, McDevitt SF. 2018. Resistance to metals used in agricultural production. Microbiol Spectrum 6(2):ARBA-0025-2017.

References

1. **Suttle NF.** 2010. *Mineral Nutrition of Livestock*, 4th ed. CABI Publishing, Wallingford, United Kingdom. p 283–342.

2. **European Commission Scientific Committee for Animal Nutrition (SCAN).** 2003. Opinion of the Scientific Committee for Animal Nutrition on the use of copper in feedingstuffs.

3. **European Commission.** 2003. Commission Regulation (EC) no 1334/2003 of 25 July 2003. Amending the conditions for authorisation of a number of additives in feedingstuffs belonging to the group of trace elements.

4. **EFSA Panel on Additives and Products or Substances used in Animal Feed (FEEDAP).** 2016. Revision of the currently authorised maximum copper content in complete feed. *EFSA J* 14:e04563.

5. **European Medicines Agency (EMA), Committee for Veterinary Medicinal Products (CVMP).** 1998. Copper chloride, copper gluconate, copper heptanoate, copper oxide, copper methionate, copper sulfate and dicopper oxide: Summary Report. EMEA/MRL/431/98-FINAL.

6. **Todd WR, Elvehjem CA, Hart EB.** 1980. Nutrition classics. The American Journal of Physiology. Volume 107, 1934, pages 146–156. "Zinc in the nutrition of the rat" by W.R. Todd, C.A. Elvehjem and E.B. Hart. *Nutr Rev* 38:151–154.

7. **Tucker HF, Salmon WD.** 1955. Parakeratosis or zinc deficiency disease in the pig. *Proc Soc Exp Biol Med* 88: 613–616.

8. **O'Dell BL, Newberne PM, Savage JE.** 1958. Significance of dietary zinc for the growing chicken. *J Nutr* 65: 503–518.

9. **Chesters JK.** 1983. Zinc metabolism in animals: pathology, immunology and genetics. *J Inherit Metab Dis* 6 (Suppl 1):34–38.

10. **Jezyk PF, Haskins ME, MacKay-Smith WE, Patterson DF.** 1986. Lethal acrodermatitis in bull terriers. *J Am Vet Med Assoc* 188:833–839.

11. **Hambidge KM, Casey CE, Krebs NF.** 1986. Zinc, p 1–137. *In* Mertz W (ed), *Trace Elements in Human and Animal Nutrition*, vol 2. Academic Press, San Diego, CA.

12. **European Commission's Scientific Committee for Animal Nutrition (SCAN).** 2003. Opinion of the Scientific Committee for Animal Nutrition on the use of zinc in feedingstuffs.

13. **EFSA Panel on Additives and Products or Substances Used in Animal Feed (FEEDAP).** 2014. Scientific Opinion on the potential reduction of the currently authorised maximum zinc content in complete feed. *EFSA J* 12:3668.

14. **European Medicines Agency (EMA).** 2016. Committee for Medicinal Products for Veterinary Use (CVMP) meeting 6–8 December 2016. http://www.ema.europa.eu/ema/index.jsp?curl=pages/news_and_events/events/2015/09/event_detail_001206.jsp&mid=WC0b01ac058004d5c3

15. **DANMAP.** 2014. *Use of Antimicrobial Agents and Occurrence of Antimicrobial Resistance in Bacteria from Food Animals, Food and Humans in Denmark.* DANMAP, Copenhagen, Denmark.

16. **BelVetSAC.** 2015. Belgian Veterinary Surveillance of Antibacterial Consumption National consumption report.

17. **BelVetSAC.** 2014. Belgian Veterinary Surveillance of Antibacterial Consumption National consumption report.

18. **Slifierz M.** 2016. The effects of zinc therapy on the coselection of methicillin-resistance in livestock-associated *Staphylococcus aureus* and the bacterial ecology of the porcine microbiota. PhD thesis. University of Guelph, Guelph, Canada.

19. **Jacela JY, DeRouchey JM, Tokach MD, Goodband RD, Nelssen JL, Renter DG, Dritz SS.** 2010. Feed additives for swine: fact sheets–high dietary levels of copper and zinc for young pigs, and phytase. *J Swine Health Prod* 18:87–91.

20. **Poulsen HD.** 1995. Zinc oxide for weanling piglets. *Acta Agriculturae Scandinavica* 45:159–167.

21. **European Food Safety Authority.** 2014. Dietary exposure to inorganic arsenic. *EFSA J* 12:3597.

22. **Antman KH.** 2001. Introduction: the history of arsenic trioxide in cancer therapy. *Oncologist* 6(Suppl 2):1–2.

23. **Smith AH, Marshall G, Yuan Y, Steinmaus C, Liaw J, Smith MT, Wood L, Heirich M, Fritzemeier RM, Pegram MD, Ferreccio C.** 2014. Rapid reduction in

breast cancer mortality with inorganic arsenic in drinking water. *EBioMedicine* 1:58–63.

24. Nigra AE, Nachman KE, Love DC, Grau-Perez M, Navas-Acien A. 2017. Poultry consumption and arsenic exposure in the U.S. population. *Environ Health Perspect* 125:370–377.

25. Caldas D, Pestana IA, Almeida MG, Henry FC, Salomão MSMB, de Souza CMM. 2016. Risk of ingesting As, Cd, and Pb in animal products in north Rio de Janeiro state, Brazil. *Chemosphere* 164:508–515.

26. Zhang XY, Zhou MY, Li LL, Jiang YJ, Zou XT. 2017. Effects of arsenic supplementation in feed on laying performance, arsenic retention of eggs and organs, biochemical indices and endocrine hormones. *Br Poult Sci* 58:63–68.

27. Xi GF, Zhou SB, Ding HC, Yao CX, Kong JJ. 2014. Characteristics of arsenic content in the livestock farms' surrounding environment in Shanghai suburbs. *Huan Jing Ke Xue* 35:1928–1932. (In Chinese.)

28. Jensen BB. 2016. Extensive literature search on the 'effects of copper intake levels in the gut microbiota profile of target animals, in particular piglets'. *EFSA Supporting Publications* 13:1024E-n/a.

29. European Medicines Agency (EMA), Committee for Veterinary Medicinal Products (CVMP). 2016. European public MRL assessment report (EPMAR): copper carbonate (all food producing species). EMA/CVMP/758734/2015.

30. Ou D, Li D, Cao Y, Li X, Yin J, Qiao S, Wu G. 2007. Dietary supplementation with zinc oxide decreases expression of the stem cell factor in the small intestine of weanling pigs. *J Nutr Biochem* 18:820–826.

31. Schulte JN, Brockmann GA, Kreuzer-Redmer S. 2016. Feeding a high dosage of zinc oxide affects suppressor of cytokine gene expression in *Salmonella* Typhimurium infected piglets. *Vet Immunol Immunopathol* 178:10–13.

32. European Medicines Agency (EMA), Committee for Veterinary Medicinal Products (CVMP). 1996. Zinc salts. EMEA/MRL/113/96-FINAL:

33. United States Department of Agriculture (USDA). 2017. Livestock slaughter 2016 summary. USDA National Agricultural Statistics Service, Washington, DC.

34. European Medicines Agency (EMA), European Surveillance of Veterinary Antimicrobial Consumption (ESVAC). 2016. Sales of veterinary antimicrobial agents in 29 European countries in 2014. EMA/61769/2016.

35. National Research Council, Committee on Nutrient Requirements of Swine. 2012. *Nutrient Requirements of Swine*. National Academies Press, Washington, DC.

36. Stolte J, Tesfai M, Øygarden L, Kværnø S, Keizer J, Verheijen F, Panagos P, Ballabio C, Hessel R (ed). 2016. *Soil Threats in Europe*. EUR 27607 EN doi: 10.2788/488054. (print); doi:10.2788/828742 (online).

37. Jensen J, Larsen MM, Bak J. 2016. National monitoring study in Denmark finds increased and critical levels of copper and zinc in arable soils fertilized with pig slurry. *Environ Pollut* 214:334–340.

38. Bak JL, Jensen J, Larsen MM. 2015. Belysning af kobber- og zinkindholdet i jord. Indhold og udvikling i kvadratnettet og måling på udvalgte brugstyper. Aarhus Universitet, DCE – Nationalt Center for Miljø og Energi, 72 s. - Videnskabelig rapport fra DCE - Nationalt Center for Miljø og Energi nr. 159.

39. Joint Research Center (JRC) European Union. 2010. Risk assessment report. CAS: 7440-66-6; EINECS No: 231-175-3 ZINC METAL.

40. Johnson TJ, Siek KE, Johnson SJ, Nolan LK. 2005. DNA sequence and comparative genomics of pAPEC-O2-R, an avian pathogenic *Escherichia coli* transmissible R plasmid. *Antimicrob Agents Chemother* 49: 4681–4688.

41. Salem AZM, Ammar H, Lopez S, Gohar YM, González JS. 2011. Sensitivity of ruminal bacteria isolates of sheep, cattle and buffalo to some heavy metals. *Anim Feed Sci Technol* 163:143–149.

42. Chen S, Li X, Sun G, Zhang Y, Su J, Ye J. 2015. Heavy metal induced antibiotic resistance in bacterium LSJC7. *Int J Mol Sci* 16:23390–23404.

43. Henriques I, Tacão M, Leite L, Fidalgo C, Araújo S, Oliveira C, Alves A. 2016. Co-selection of antibiotic and metal(loid) resistance in Gram-negative epiphytic bacteria from contaminated salt marshes. *Mar Pollut Bull* 109:427–434.

44. Hasman H, Franke S, Rensing C. 2005. Resistance to metals used in agricultural production, p 99–114. *In* Aarestrup FM, Wegener HC (ed), *Antimicrobial Resistance in Bacteria of Animal Origin*. ASM Press, Washington, DC.

45. Jacob ME, Fox JT, Nagaraja TG, Drouillard JS, Amachawadi RG, Narayanan SK. 2010. Effects of feeding elevated concentrations of copper and zinc on the antimicrobial susceptibilities of fecal bacteria in feedlot cattle. *Foodborne Pathog Dis* 7:643–648.

46. Bednorz C, Oelgeschläger K, Kinnemann B, Hartmann S, Neumann K, Pieper R, Bethe A, Semmler T, Tedin K, Schierack P, Wieler LH, Guenther S. 2013. The broader context of antibiotic resistance: zinc feed supplementation of piglets increases the proportion of multi-resistant *Escherichia coli* in vivo. *Int J Med Microbiol* 303:396–403.

47. Toroglu S, Dincer S. 2009. Heavy metal resistances of *Enterobacteriaceae* from Aksu River (Turkey) polluted with different sources. *Asian J Chem* 21:411–420.

48. Kumar PA, Joseph B, Patterson J. 2011. Antibiotic and heavy metal resistance profile of pathogens isolated from infected fish in Tuticorin, south-east coast of India. *Indian J Fish* 58:121–125.

49. Deredjian A, Colinon C, Brothier E, Favre-Bonté S, Cournoyer B, Nazaret S. 2011. Antibiotic and metal resistance among hospital and outdoor strains of *Pseudomonas aeruginosa*. *Res Microbiol* 162:689–700.

50. Wei LS, Musa N, Wee W. 2010. Bacterial flora from a healthy freshwater Asian sea bass (*Lates calcarifer*) fingerling hatchery with emphasis on their antimicrobial and heavy metal resistance pattern. *Vet Arh* 80:411–420.

51. Cavaco LM, Hasman H, Stegger M, Andersen PS, Skov R, Fluit AC, Ito T, Aarestrup FM. 2010. Cloning and occurrence of *czrC*, a gene conferring cadmium and zinc resistance in methicillin-resistant *Staphylococcus aureus* CC398 isolates. *Antimicrob Agents Chemother* 54: 3605–3608.

52. Fard RM, Heuzenroeder MW, Barton MD. 2011. Antimicrobial and heavy metal resistance in commensal enterococci isolated from pigs. *Vet Microbiol* 148:276–282.

53. Medardus JJ, Molla BZ, Nicol M, Morrow WM, Rajala-Schultz PJ, Kazwala R, Gebreyes WA. 2014. In-feed use of heavy metal micronutrients in U.S. swine production systems and its role in persistence of multidrug-resistant salmonellae. *Appl Environ Microbiol* 80:2317–2325.

54. Mourão J, Marçal S, Ramos P, Campos J, Machado J, Peixe L, Novais C, Antunes P. 2016. Tolerance to multiple metal stressors in emerging non-typhoidal MDR *Salmonella* serotypes: a relevant role for copper in anaerobic conditions. *J Antimicrob Chemother* 71:2147–2157.

55. Amachawadi RG, Scott HM, Vinasco J, Tokach MD, Dritz SS, Nelssen JL, Nagaraja TG. 2015. Effects of in-feed copper, chlortetracycline, and tylosin on the prevalence of transferable copper resistance gene, *tcrB*, among fecal enterococci of weaned piglets. *Foodborne Pathog Dis* 12:670–678.

56. Aarestrup FM, Hasman H. 2004. Susceptibility of different bacterial species isolated from food animals to copper sulphate, zinc chloride and antimicrobial substances used for disinfection. *Vet Microbiol* 100:83–89.

57. Hacioglu N, Tosunoglu M. 2014. Determination of antimicrobial and heavy metal resistance profiles of some bacteria isolated from aquatic amphibian and reptile species. *Environ Monit Assess* 186:407–413.

58. Fang L, Li X, Li L, Li S, Liao X, Sun J, Liu Y. 2016. Co-spread of metal and antibiotic resistance within ST3-IncHI2 plasmids from *E. coli* isolates of food-producing animals. *Sci Rep* 6:25312.

59. Akinbowale OL, Peng H, Grant P, Barton MD. 2007. Antibiotic and heavy metal resistance in motile aeromonads and pseudomonads from rainbow trout (*Oncorhynchus mykiss*) farms in Australia. *Int J Antimicrob Agents* 30:177–182.

60. He Y, Jin L, Sun F, Hu Q, Chen L. 2016. Antibiotic and heavy-metal resistance of *Vibrio parahaemolyticus* isolated from fresh shrimps in Shanghai fish markets, China. *Environ Sci Pollut Res Int* 23:15033–15040.

61. Hu Q, Chen L. 2016. Virulence and antibiotic and heavy metal resistance of *Vibrio parahaemolyticus* isolated from crustaceans and shellfish in Shanghai, China. *J Food Prot* 79:1371–1377.

62. Williams RJ, Fraústo Da Silva JJ. 2003. Evolution was chemically constrained. *J Theor Biol* 220:323–343.

63. Hong Enriquez RP, Do TN. 2012. Bioavailability of metal ions and evolutionary adaptation. *Life (Basel)* 2: 274–285.

64. Macomber L, Imlay JA. 2009. The iron-sulfur clusters of dehydratases are primary intracellular targets of copper toxicity. *Proc Natl Acad Sci USA* 106:8344–8349.

65. Dupont CL, Grass G, Rensing C. 2011. Copper toxicity and the origin of bacterial resistance: new insights and applications. *Metallomics* 3:1109–1118.

66. Chillappagari S, Seubert A, Trip H, Kuipers OP, Marahiel MA, Miethke M. 2010. Copper stress affects iron homeostasis by destabilizing iron-sulfur cluster formation in *Bacillus subtilis*. *J Bacteriol* 192:2512–2524.

67. Chillappagari S, Miethke M, Trip H, Kuipers OP, Marahiel MA. 2009. Copper acquisition is mediated by YcnJ and regulated by YcnK and CsoR in *Bacillus subtilis*. *J Bacteriol* 191:2362–2370.

68. Hirooka K, Edahiro T, Kimura K, Fujita Y. 2012. Direct and indirect regulation of the *ycnKJI* operon involved in copper uptake through two transcriptional repressors, YcnK and CsoR, in *Bacillus subtilis*. *J Bacteriol* 194:5675–5687.

69. Yamada-Ankei T, Iwasaki H, Mori T. 1977. Production of copper coproporphyrin III by *Bacillus cereus*. I. Purification and identification of copper coproporphyrin III. *J Biochem* 81:835–842.

70. Balasubramanian R, Kenney GE, Rosenzweig AC. 2011. Dual pathways for copper uptake by methanotrophic bacteria. *J Biol Chem* 286:37313–37319.

71. Teitzel GM, Geddie A, De Long SK, Kirisits MJ, Whiteley M, Parsek MR. 2006. Survival and growth in the presence of elevated copper: transcriptional profiling of copper-stressed *Pseudomonas aeruginosa*. *J Bacteriol* 188:7242–7256.

72. Whiting GC, Rowbury RJ. 1995. Increased resistance of *Escherichia coli* to acrylic acid and to copper ions after cold-shock. *Lett Appl Microbiol* 20:240–242.

73. Taudte N, Grass G. 2010. Point mutations change specificity and kinetics of metal uptake by ZupT from *Escherichia coli*. *Biometals* 23:643–656.

74. Grass G, Franke S, Taudte N, Nies DH, Kucharski LM, Maguire ME, Rensing C. 2005. The metal permease ZupT from *Escherichia coli* is a transporter with a broad substrate spectrum. *J Bacteriol* 187:1604–1611.

75. Guerinot ML. 2000. The ZIP family of metal transporters. *Biochim Biophys Acta* 1465:190–198.

76. Cha JS, Cooksey DA. 1993. Copper hypersensitivity and uptake in *Pseudomonas syringae* containing cloned components of the copper resistance operon. *Appl Environ Microbiol* 59:1671–1674.

77. Fitch MW, Graham DW, Arnold RG, Agarwal SK, Phelps P, Speitel GE Jr, Georgiou G. 1993. Phenotypic characterization of copper-resistant mutants of *Methylosinus trichosporium* OB3b. *Appl Environ Microbiol* 59: 2771–2776.

78. Anttila J, Heinonen P, Nenonen T, Pino A, Iwaï H, Kauppi E, Soliymani R, Baumann M, Saksi J, Suni N, Haltia T. 2011. Is coproporphyrin III a copper-acquisition compound in *Paracoccus denitrificans*? *Biochim Biophys Acta* 1807:311–318.

79. DiSpirito AA, Zahn JA, Graham DW, Kim HJ, Larive CK, Derrick TS, Cox CD, Taylor A. 1998. Copper-binding compounds from *Methylosinus trichosporium* OB3b. *J Bacteriol* 180:3606–3613.

80. Kim HJ, Graham DW, DiSpirito AA, Alterman MA, Galeva N, Larive CK, Asunskis D, Sherwood PM. 2004. Methanobactin, a copper-acquisition compound from methane-oxidizing bacteria. *Science* 305:1612–1615.

81. Zahn JA, DiSpirito AA. 1996. Membrane-associated methane monooxygenase from *Methylococcus capsulatus* (Bath). *J Bacteriol* 178:1018–1029.

82. Nicolaisen K, Hahn A, Valdebenito M, Moslavac S, Samborski A, Maldener I, Wilken C, Valladares A, Flores E, Hantke K, Schleiff E. 2010. The interplay between siderophore secretion and coupled iron and copper transport in the heterocyst-forming cyanobacterium *Anabaena* sp. PCC 7120. *Biochim Biophys Acta* 1798: 2131–2140.

83. Argüello JM. 2003. Identification of ion-selectivity determinants in heavy-metal transport P_{1B}-type ATPases. *J Membr Biol* 195:93–108.

84. Argüello JM, González-Guerrero M. 2008. Cu^+-ATPases brake system. *Structure* 16:833–834.

85. Argüello JM, González-Guerrero M, Raimunda D. 2011. Bacterial transition metal $P_{(1B)}$-ATPases: transport mechanism and roles in virulence. *Biochemistry* 50: 9940–9949.

86. Argüello JM, Eren E, González-Guerrero M. 2007. The structure and function of heavy metal transport P_{1B}-ATPases. *Biometals* 20:233–248.

87. Raimunda D, González-Guerrero M, Leeber BW III, Argüello JM. 2011. The transport mechanism of bacterial Cu^+-ATPases: distinct efflux rates adapted to different function. *Biometals* 24:467–475.

88. Rosenzweig AC, Argüello JM. 2012. Toward a molecular understanding of metal transport by P(1B)-type ATPases. *Curr Top Membr* 69:113–136.

89. Solioz M, Odermatt A, Krapf R. 1994. Copper pumping ATPases: common concepts in bacteria and man. *FEBS Lett* 346:44–47.

90. Solioz M, Vulpe C. 1996. CPx-type ATPases: a class of P-type ATPases that pump heavy metals. *Trends Biochem Sci* 21:237–241.

91. Odermatt A, Suter H, Krapf R, Solioz M. 1992. An ATPase operon involved in copper resistance by *Enterococcus hirae*. *Ann N Y Acad Sci* 671(1 Ion-Motive AT): 484–486.

92. Solioz M, Odermatt A. 1995. Copper and silver transport by CopB-ATPase in membrane vesicles of *Enterococcus hirae*. *J Biol Chem* 270:9217–9221.

93. Solioz M, Stoyanov JV. 2003. Copper homeostasis in *Enterococcus hirae*. *FEMS Microbiol Rev* 27:183–195.

94. Odermatt A, Krapf R, Solioz M. 1994. Induction of the putative copper ATPases, CopA and CopB, of *Enterococcus hirae* by Ag^+ and Cu^{2+}, and Ag^+ extrusion by CopB. *Biochem Biophys Res Commun* 202:44–48.

95. Odermatt A, Solioz M. 1995. Two trans-acting metalloregulatory proteins controlling expression of the copper-ATPases of *Enterococcus hirae*. *J Biol Chem* 270:4349–4354.

96. González-Guerrero M, Raimunda D, Cheng X, Argüello JM. 2010. Distinct functional roles of homologous Cu^+

97. Gaballa A, Cao M, Helmann JD. 2003. Two MerR homologues that affect copper induction of the *Bacillus subtilis copZA* operon. *Microbiology* 149:3413–3421.

98. Reyes A, Leiva A, Cambiazo V, Méndez MA, González M. 2006. Cop-like operon: structure and organization in species of the *Lactobacillale* order. *Biol Res* 39:87–93.

99. Grass G, Rensing C. 2001. Genes involved in copper homeostasis in *Escherichia coli*. *J Bacteriol* 183:2145–2147.

100. Outten FW, Huffman DL, Hale JA, O'Halloran TV. 2001. The independent cue and cus systems confer copper tolerance during aerobic and anaerobic growth in *Escherichia coli*. *J Biol Chem* 276:30670–30677.

101. Rensing C, Grass G. 2003. *Escherichia coli* mechanisms of copper homeostasis in a changing environment. *FEMS Microbiol Rev* 27:197–213.

102. Outten FW, Outten CE, Hale J, O'Halloran TV. 2000. Transcriptional activation of an *Escherichia coli* copper efflux regulon by the chromosomal MerR homologue, cueR. *J Biol Chem* 275:31024–31029.

103. Petersen C, Møller LB. 2000. Control of copper homeostasis in *Escherichia coli* by a P-type ATPase, CopA, and a MerR-like transcriptional activator, CopR. *Gene* 261: 289–298.

104. Stoyanov JV, Hobman JL, Brown NL. 2001. CueR (YbbI) of *Escherichia coli* is a MerR family regulator controlling expression of the copper exporter CopA. *Mol Microbiol* 39:502–511.

105. Changela A, Chen K, Xue Y, Holschen J, Outten CE, O'Halloran TV, Mondragón A. 2003. Molecular basis of metal-ion selectivity and zeptomolar sensitivity by CueR. *Science* 301:1383–1387.

106. Rensing C, Fan B, Sharma R, Mitra B, Rosen BP. 2000. CopA: An *Escherichia coli* Cu(I)-translocating P-type ATPase. *Proc Natl Acad Sci USA* 97:652–656.

107. Fan B, Rosen BP. 2002. Biochemical characterization of CopA, the *Escherichia coli* Cu(I)-translocating P-type ATPase. *J Biol Chem* 277:46987–46992.

108. Grass G, Rensing C. 2001. CueO is a multi-copper oxidase that confers copper tolerance in *Escherichia coli*. *Biochem Biophys Res Commun* 286:902–908.

109. Kim C, Lorenz WW, Hoopes JT, Dean JF. 2001. Oxidation of phenolate siderophores by the multi-copper oxidase encoded by the *Escherichia coli yacK* gene. *J Bacteriol* 183:4866–4875.

110. Roberts SA, Weichsel A, Grass G, Thakali K, Hazzard JT, Tollin G, Rensing C, Montfort WR. 2002. Crystal structure and electron transfer kinetics of CueO, a multicopper oxidase required for copper homeostasis in *Escherichia coli*. *Proc Natl Acad Sci USA* 99:2766–2771.

111. Roberts SA, Wildner GF, Grass G, Weichsel A, Ambrus A, Rensing C, Montfort WR. 2003. A labile regulatory copper ion lies near the T1 copper site in the multicopper oxidase CueO. *J Biol Chem* 278:31958–31963.

efflux ATPases in *Pseudomonas aeruginosa*. *Mol Microbiol* 78:1246–1258.

112. Grass G, Thakali K, Klebba PE, Thieme D, Müller A, Wildner GF, Rensing C. 2004. Linkage between catecholate siderophores and the multicopper oxidase CueO in *Escherichia coli*. *J Bacteriol* **186**:5826–5833.

113. Singh SK, Grass G, Rensing C, Montfort WR. 2004. Cuprous oxidase activity of CueO from *Escherichia coli*. *J Bacteriol* **186**:7815–7817.

114. Sakurai T, Kataoka K. 2007. Basic and applied features of multicopper oxidases, CueO, bilirubin oxidase, and laccase. *Chem Rec* **7**:220–229.

115. Djoko KY, Chong LX, Wedd AG, Xiao Z. 2010. Reaction mechanisms of the multicopper oxidase CueO from *Escherichia coli* support its functional role as a cuprous oxidase. *J Am Chem Soc* **132**:2005–2015.

116. Singh SK, Roberts SA, McDevitt SF, Weichsel A, Wildner GF, Grass GB, Rensing C, Montfort WR. 2011. Crystal structures of multicopper oxidase CueO bound to copper(I) and silver(I): functional role of a methionine-rich sequence. *J Biol Chem* **286**:37849–37857.

117. Lim SY, Joe MH, Song SS, Lee MH, Foster JW, Park YK, Choi SY, Lee IS. 2002. CuiD is a crucial gene for survival at high copper environment in *Salmonella enterica* serovar Typhimurium. *Mol Cells* **14**:177–184.

118. Kosman DJ. 2010. Multicopper oxidases: a workshop on copper coordination chemistry, electron transfer, and metallophysiology. *J Biol Inorg Chem* **15**:15–28.

119. Rademacher C, Moser R, Lackmann JW, Klinkert B, Narberhaus F, Masepohl B. 2012. Transcriptional and posttranscriptional events control copper-responsive expression of a *Rhodobacter capsulatus* multicopper oxidase. *J Bacteriol* **194**:1849–1859.

120. Nies DH, Herzberg M. 2013. A fresh view of the cell biology of copper in enterobacteria. *Mol Microbiol* **87**:447–454.

121. Silveira E, Freitas AR, Antunes P, Barros M, Campos J, Coque TM, Peixe L, Novais C. 2014. Co-transfer of resistance to high concentrations of copper and first-line antibiotics among *Enterococcus* from different origins (humans, animals, the environment and foods) and clonal lineages. *J Antimicrob Chemother* **69**:899–906.

122. Padilla-Benavides T, George Thompson AM, McEvoy MM, Argüello JM. 2014. Mechanism of ATPase-mediated Cu⁺ export and delivery to periplasmic chaperones: the interaction of *Escherichia coli* CopA and CusF. *J Biol Chem* **289**:20492–20501.

123. Franke S, Grass G, Rensing C, Nies DH. 2003. Molecular analysis of the copper-transporting efflux system CusCFBA of *Escherichia coli*. *J Bacteriol* **185**:3804–3812.

124. Munson GP, Lam DL, Outten FW, O'Halloran TV. 2000. Identification of a copper-responsive two-component system on the chromosome of *Escherichia coli* K-12. *J Bacteriol* **182**:5864–5871.

125. Franke S, Grass G, Nies DH. 2001. The product of the *ybdE* gene of the *Escherichia coli* chromosome is involved in detoxification of silver ions. *Microbiology* **147**:965–972.

126. Bagai I, Liu W, Rensing C, Blackburn NJ, McEvoy MM. 2007. Substrate-linked conformational change in the periplasmic component of a Cu(I)/Ag(I) efflux system. *J Biol Chem* **282**:35695–35702.

127. Su CC, Yang F, Long F, Reyon D, Routh MD, Kuo DW, Mokhtari AK, Van Ornam JD, Rabe KL, Hoy JA, Lee YJ, Rajashankar KR, Yu EW. 2009. Crystal structure of the membrane fusion protein CusB from *Escherichia coli*. *J Mol Biol* **393**:342–355.

128. Long F, Su CC, Zimmermann MT, Boyken SE, Rajashankar KR, Jernigan RL, Yu EW. 2010. Crystal structures of the CusA efflux pump suggest methionine-mediated metal transport. *Nature* **467**:484–488.

129. Kulathila R, Kulathila R, Indic M, van den Berg B. 2011. Crystal structure of *Escherichia coli* CusC, the outer membrane component of a heavy metal efflux pump. *PLoS One* **6**:e15610.

130. Su CC, Long F, Zimmermann MT, Rajashankar KR, Jernigan RL, Yu EW. 2011. Crystal structure of the CusBA heavy-metal efflux complex of *Escherichia coli*. *Nature* **470**:558–562.

131. Kim EH, Nies DH, McEvoy MM, Rensing C. 2011. Switch or funnel: how RND-type transport systems control periplasmic metal homeostasis. *J Bacteriol* **193**:2381–2387.

132. Loftin IR, Franke S, Roberts SA, Weichsel A, Héroux A, Montfort WR, Rensing C, McEvoy MM. 2005. A novel copper-binding fold for the periplasmic copper resistance protein CusF. *Biochemistry* **44**:10533–10540.

133. Kittleson JT, Loftin IR, Hausrath AC, Engelhardt KP, Rensing C, McEvoy MM. 2006. Periplasmic metal-resistance protein CusF exhibits high affinity and specificity for both CuI and AgI. *Biochemistry* **45**:11096–11102.

134. Xue Y, Davis AV, Balakrishnan G, Stasser JP, Staehlin BM, Focia P, Spiro TG, Penner-Hahn JE, O'Halloran TV. 2008. Cu(I) recognition via cation-pi and methionine interactions in CusF. *Nat Chem Biol* **4**:107–109.

135. Bagai I, Rensing C, Blackburn NJ, McEvoy MM. 2008. Direct metal transfer between periplasmic proteins identifies a bacterial copper chaperone. *Biochemistry* **47**:11408–11414.

136. Bersch B, Derfoufi KM, De Angelis F, Auquier V, Ekendé EN, Mergeay M, Ruysschaert JM, Vandenbussche G. 2011. Structural and metal binding characterization of the C-terminal metallochaperone domain of membrane fusion protein SilB from *Cupriavidus metallidurans* CH34. *Biochemistry* **50**:2194–2204.

137. Mealman TD, Bagai I, Singh P, Goodlett DR, Rensing C, Zhou H, Wysocki VH, McEvoy MM. 2011. Interactions between CusF and CusB identified by NMR spectroscopy and chemical cross-linking coupled to mass spectrometry. *Biochemistry* **50**:2559–2566.

138. Chacón KN, Mealman TD, McEvoy MM, Blackburn NJ. 2014. Tracking metal ions through a Cu/Ag efflux pump assigns the functional roles of the periplasmic proteins. *Proc Natl Acad Sci USA* **111**:15373–15378.

139. Meir A, Natan A, Moskovitz Y, Ruthstein S. 2015. EPR spectroscopy identifies Met and Lys residues that are essential for the interaction between the CusB N-terminal domain and metallochaperone CusF. *Metallomics* 7:1163–1172.

140. Pontel LB, Soncini FC. 2009. Alternative periplasmic copper-resistance mechanisms in Gram negative bacteria. *Mol Microbiol* 73:212–225.

141. Osman D, Waldron KJ, Denton H, Taylor CM, Grant AJ, Mastroeni P, Robinson NJ, Cavet JS. 2010. Copper homeostasis in *Salmonella* is atypical and copper-CueP is a major periplasmic metal complex. *J Biol Chem* 285: 25259–25268.

142. Yun BY, Piao S, Kim YG, Moon HR, Choi EJ, Kim YO, Nam BH, Lee SJ, Ha NC. 2011. Crystallization and preliminary X-ray crystallographic analysis of *Salmonella* Typhimurium CueP. *Acta Crystallogr Sect F Struct Biol Cryst Commun* 67:675–677.

143. Yoon BY, Yeom JH, Kim JS, Um SH, Jo I, Lee K, Kim YH, Ha NC. 2014. Direct ROS scavenging activity of CueP from *Salmonella enterica* serovar Typhimurium. *Mol Cells* 37:100–108.

144. Williams JR, Morgan AG, Rouch DA, Brown NL, Lee BT. 1993. Copper-resistant enteric bacteria from United Kingdom and Australian piggeries. *Appl Environ Microbiol* 59:2531–2537.

145. Tetaz TJ, Luke RK. 1983. Plasmid-controlled resistance to copper in *Escherichia coli*. *J Bacteriol* 154:1263–1268.

146. Brown NL, Barrett SR, Camakaris J, Lee BT, Rouch DA. 1995. Molecular genetics and transport analysis of the copper-resistance determinant (*pco*) from *Escherichia coli* plasmid pRJ1004. *Mol Microbiol* 17:1153–1166.

147. Rouch DA, Brown NL. 1997. Copper-inducible transcriptional regulation at two promoters in the *Escherichia coli* copper resistance determinant *pco*. *Microbiology* 143:1191–1202.

148. Lee SM, Grass G, Rensing C, Barrett SR, Yates CJ, Stoyanov JV, Brown NL. 2002. The Pco proteins are involved in periplasmic copper handling in *Escherichia coli*. *Biochem Biophys Res Commun* 295:616–620.

149. Zimmermann M, Udagedara SR, Sze CM, Ryan TM, Howlett GJ, Xiao Z, Wedd AG. 2012. PcoE: a metal sponge expressed to the periplasm of copper resistance *Escherichia coli*. Implication of its function role in copper resistance. *J Inorg Biochem* 115:186–197.

150. Hao X, Lüthje FL, Qin Y, McDevitt SF, Lutay N, Hobman JL, Asiani K, Soncini FC, German N, Zhang S, Zhu YG, Rensing C. 2015. Survival in amoeba: a major selection pressure on the presence of bacterial copper and zinc resistance determinants? Identification of a "copper pathogenicity island". *Appl Microbiol Biotechnol* 99:5817–5824.

151. Staehlin BM, Gibbons JG, Rokas A, O'Halloran TV, Slot JC. 2016. Evolution of a heavy metal homeostasis/resistance island reflects increasing copper stress in Enterobacteria. *Genome Biol Evol* 8:811–826.

152. McHugh GL, Moellering RC, Hopkins CC, Swartz MN. 1975. *Salmonella typhimurium* resistant to silver nitrate, chloramphenicol, and ampicillin. *Lancet* 1:235–240.

153. Gupta A, Matsui K, Lo JF, Silver S. 1999. Molecular basis for resistance to silver cations in *Salmonella*. *Nat Med* 5:183–188.

154. Randall CP, Gupta A, Jackson N, Busse D, O'Neill AJ. 2015. Silver resistance in Gram-negative bacteria: a dissection of endogenous and exogenous mechanisms. *J Antimicrob Chemother* 70:1037–1046.

155. Lüthje FL, Hasman H, Aarestrup FM, Alwathnani HA, Rensing C. 2014. Genome sequences of two copper-resistant *Escherichia coli* strains isolated from copper-fed pigs. *Genome Announc* 2:e01341.

156. Qin Y, Hasman H, Aarestrup FM, Alwathnani HA, Rensing C. 2014. Genome sequences of three highly copper-resistant *Salmonella enterica* subsp. I serovar Typhimurium strains isolated from pigs in Denmark. *Genome Announc* 2:e01334-14.

157. Peters JE, Fricker AD, Kapili BJ, Petassi MT. 2014. Heteromeric transposase elements: generators of genomic islands across diverse bacteria. *Mol Microbiol* 93:1084–1092.

158. Chaturvedi KS, Henderson JP. 2014. Pathogenic adaptations to host-derived antibacterial copper. *Front Cell Infect Microbiol* 4:3.

159. Schubert S, Dufke S, Sorsa J, Heesemann J. 2004. A novel integrative and conjugative element (ICE) of *Escherichia coli*: the putative progenitor of the *Yersinia* high-pathogenicity island. *Mol Microbiol* 51:837–848.

160. Rakin A, Schneider L, Podladchikova O. 2012. Hunger for iron: the alternative siderophore iron scavenging systems in highly virulent *Yersinia*. *Front Cell Infect Microbiol* 2:151/1.

161. Aviv G, Tsyba K, Steck N, Salmon-Divon M, Cornelius A, Rahav G, Grassl GA, Gal-Mor O. 2014. A unique megaplasmid contributes to stress tolerance and pathogenicity of an emergent *Salmonella enterica* serovar Infantis strain. *Environ Microbiol* 16:977–994.

162. Chaturvedi KS, Hung CS, Giblin DE, Urushidani S, Austin AM, Dinauer MC, Henderson JP. 2014. Cupric yersiniabactin is a virulence-associated superoxide dismutase mimic. *ACS Chem Biol* 9:551–561.

163. Fodah RA, Scott JB, Tam HH, Yan P, Pfeffer TL, Bundschuh R, Warawa JM. 2014. Correlation of *Klebsiella pneumoniae* comparative genetic analyses with virulence profiles in a murine respiratory disease model. *PLoS One* 9:e107394.

164. Freitas AR, Coque TM, Novais C, Hammerum AM, Lester CH, Zervos MJ, Donabedian S, Jensen LB, Francia MV, Baquero F, Peixe L. 2011. Human and swine hosts share vancomycin-resistant *Enterococcus faecium* CC17 and CC5 and *Enterococcus faecalis* CC2 clonal clusters harboring Tn1546 on indistinguishable plasmids. *J Clin Microbiol* 49:925–931.

165. Zhang S, Wang D, Wang Y, Hasman H, Aarestrup FM, Alwathnani HA, Zhu YG, Rensing C. 2015. Genome sequences of copper resistant and sensitive *Enterococcus faecalis* strains isolated from copper-fed pigs in Denmark. *Stand Genomic Sci* 10:35-015-0021-1.

166. Hasman H, Aarestrup FM. 2002. *tcrB*, a gene conferring transferable copper resistance in *Enterococcus faecium*: occurrence, transferability, and linkage to macrolide and glycopeptide resistance. *Antimicrob Agents Chemother* **46**:1410–1416.

167. Amachawadi RG, Shelton NW, Jacob ME, Shi X, Narayanan SK, Zurek L, Dritz SS, Nelssen JL, Tokach MD, Nagaraja TG. 2010. Occurrence of *tcrB*, a transferable copper resistance gene, in fecal enterococci of swine. *Foodborne Pathog Dis* **7**:1089–1097.

168. Amachawadi RG, Scott HM, Alvarado CA, Mainini TR, Vinasco J, Drouillard JS, Nagaraja TG. 2013. Occurrence of the transferable copper resistance gene *tcrB* among fecal enterococci of U.S. feedlot cattle fed copper-supplemented diets. *Appl Environ Microbiol* **79**: 4369–4375.

169. Pasquaroli S, Di Cesare A, Vignaroli C, Conti G, Citterio B, Biavasco F. 2014. Erythromycin- and copper-resistant *Enterococcus hirae* from marine sediment and co-transfer of *erm(B)* and *tcrB* to human *Enterococcus faecalis*. *Diagn Microbiol Infect Dis* **80**:26–28.

170. Hasman H. 2005. The *tcrB* gene is part of the *tcrYAZB* operon conferring copper resistance in *Enterococcus faecium* and *Enterococcus faecalis*. *Microbiology* **151**: 3019–3025.

171. Rensing C, Alwathnani HA, McDevitt SF. 2016. The copper metallome in prokaryotic cells, p 161–173. *In* de Bruijn FJ (ed), *Stress and Environmental Regulation of Gene Expression and Adaptation in Bacteria*. John Wiley & Sons, Inc., Hoboken, NJ.

172. Hedges SB, Chen H, Kumar S, Wang DY, Thompson AS, Watanabe H. 2001. A genomic timescale for the origin of eukaryotes. *BMC Evol Biol* **1**:4.

173. Outten CE, O'Halloran TV. 2001. Femtomolar sensitivity of metalloregulatory proteins controlling zinc homeostasis. *Science* **292**:2488–2492.

174. Patzer SI, Hantke K. 1998. The ZnuABC high-affinity zinc uptake system and its regulator Zur in *Escherichia coli*. *Mol Microbiol* **28**:1199–1210.

175. Sabri M, Houle S, Dozois CM. 2009. Roles of the extraintestinal pathogenic *Escherichia coli* ZnuACB and ZupT zinc transporters during urinary tract infection. *Infect Immun* **77**:1155–1164.

176. Patzer SI, Hantke K. 2000. The zinc-responsive regulator Zur and its control of the *znu* gene cluster encoding the ZnuABC zinc uptake system in *Escherichia coli*. *J Biol Chem* **275**:24321–24332.

177. Sigdel TK, Easton JA, Crowder MW. 2006. Transcriptional response of *Escherichia coli* to TPEN. **188**: 6709–6713.

178. Gilston BA, Wang S, Marcus MD, Canalizo-Hernández MA, Swindell EP, Xue Y, Mondragón A, O'Halloran TV. 2014. Structural and mechanistic basis of zinc regulation across the *E. coli* Zur regulon. *PLoS Biol* **12**: e1001987.

179. Mergeay M, Nies D, Schlegel HG, Gerits J, Charles P, Van Gijsegem F. 1985. *Alcaligenes eutrophus* CH34 is a facultative chemolithotroph with plasmid-bound resistance to heavy metals. *J Bacteriol* **162**:328–334.

180. Kirsten A, Herzberg M, Voigt A, Seravalli J, Grass G, Scherer J, Nies DH. 2011. Contributions of five secondary metal uptake systems to metal homeostasis of *Cupriavidus metallidurans* CH34. *J Bacteriol* **193**: 4652–4663.

181. Herzberg M, Bauer L, Nies DH. 2014. Deletion of the *zupT* gene for a zinc importer influences zinc pools in *Cupriavidus metallidurans* CH34. *Metallomics* **6**:421–436.

182. Grass G, Wong MD, Rosen BP, Smith RL, Rensing C. 2002. ZupT is a Zn(II) uptake system in *Escherichia coli*. *J Bacteriol* **184**:864–866.

183. Cerasi M, Liu JZ, Ammendola S, Poe AJ, Petrarca P, Pesciaroli M, Pasquali P, Raffatellu M, Battistoni A. 2014. The ZupT transporter plays an important role in zinc homeostasis and contributes to *Salmonella enterica* virulence. *Metallomics* **6**:845–853.

184. Jackson RJ, Binet MR, Lee LJ, Ma R, Graham AI, McLeod CW, Poole RK. 2008. Expression of the PitA phosphate/metal transporter of *Escherichia coli* is responsive to zinc and inorganic phosphate levels. *FEMS Microbiol Lett* **289**:219–224.

185. Beard SJ, Hashim R, Wu G, Binet MR, Hughes MN, Poole RK. 2000. Evidence for the transport of zinc (II) ions via the pit inorganic phosphate transport system in *Escherichia coli*. *FEMS Microbiol Lett* **184**: 231–235.

186. Webb M. 1970. Interrelationships between the utilization of magnesium and the uptake of other bivalent cations by bacteria. *Biochim Biophys Acta* **222**:428–439.

187. Krom BP, Huttinga H, Warner JB, Lolkema JS. 2002. Impact of the Mg(2+)-citrate transporter CitM on heavy metal toxicity in *Bacillus subtilis*. *Arch Microbiol* **178**: 370–375.

188. Knoop V, Groth-Malonek M, Gebert M, Eifler K, Weyand K. 2005. Transport of magnesium and other divalent cations: evolution of the 2-TM-GxN proteins in the MIT superfamily. *Mol Genet Genomics* **274**:205–216.

189. Legatzki A, Grass G, Anton A, Rensing C, Nies DH. 2003. Interplay of the Czc system and two P-type ATPases in conferring metal resistance to *Ralstonia metallidurans*. *J Bacteriol* **185**:4354–4361.

190. Nies DH. 2007. How cells control zinc homeostasis. *Science* **317**:1695–1696.

191. Rensing C, Mitra B, Rosen BP. 1998. A Zn(II)-translocating P-type ATPase from *Proteus mirabilis*. *Biochem Cell Biol* **76**:787–790.

192. Rensing C, Ghosh M, Rosen BP. 1999. Families of soft-metal-ion-transporting ATPases. *J Bacteriol* **181**:5891–5897.

193. Sharma R, Rensing C, Rosen BP, Mitra B. 2000. The ATP hydrolytic activity of purified ZntA, a Pb(II)/Cd (II)/Zn(II)-translocating ATPase from *Escherichia coli*. *J Biol Chem* **275**:3873–3878.

194. Smith K, Novick RP. 1972. Genetic studies on plasmid-linked cadmium resistance in *Staphylococcus aureus*. *J Bacteriol* **112**:761–772.

195. Nucifora G, Chu L, Misra TK, Silver S. 1989. Cadmium resistance from *Staphylococcus aureus* plasmid pI258 *cadA* gene results from a cadmium-efflux ATPase. *Proc Natl Acad Sci USA* 86:3544–3548.

196. Wang D, Hosteen O, Fierke CA. 2012. ZntR-mediated transcription of *zntA* responds to nanomolar intracellular free zinc. *J Inorg Biochem* 111:173–181.

197. Blattner FR, Plunkett G III, Bloch CA, Perna NT, Burland V, Riley M, Collado-Vides J, Glasner JD, Rode CK, Mayhew GF, Gregor J, Davis NW, Kirkpatrick HA, Goeden MA, Rose DJ, Mau B, Shao Y. 1997. The complete genome sequence of *Escherichia coli* K-12. *Science* 277:1453–1462.

198. Yoon KP, Silver S. 1991. A second gene in the *Staphylococcus aureus cadA* cadmium resistance determinant of plasmid pI258. *J Bacteriol* 173:7636–7642.

199. Argudín MA, Butaye P. 2016. Dissemination of metal resistance genes among animal methicillin-resistant coagulase-negative staphylococci. *Res Vet Sci* 105:192–194.

200. Slifierz MJ, Park J, Friendship RM, Weese JS. 2014. Zinc-resistance gene CzrC identified in methicillin-resistant *Staphylococcus hyicus* isolated from pigs with exudative epidermitis. *Can Vet J* 55:489–490.

201. Vandendriessche S, Vanderhaeghen W, Larsen J, de Mendonça R, Hallin M, Butaye P, Hermans K, Haesebrouck F, Denis O. 2014. High genetic diversity of methicillin-susceptible *Staphylococcus aureus* (MSSA) from humans and animals on livestock farms and presence of SCCmec remnant DNA in MSSA CC398. *J Antimicrob Chemother* 69:355–362.

202. Vandendriessche S, Vanderhaeghen W, Soares FV, Hallin M, Catry B, Hermans K, Butaye P, Haesebrouck F, Struelens MJ, Denis O. 2013. Prevalence, risk factors and genetic diversity of methicillin-resistant *Staphylococcus aureus* carried by humans and animals across livestock production sectors. *J Antimicrob Chemother* 68:1510–1516.

203. Agersø Y, Hasman H, Cavaco LM, Pedersen K, Aarestrup FM. 2012. Study of methicillin resistant *Staphylococcus aureus* (MRSA) in Danish pigs at slaughter and in imported retail meat reveals a novel MRSA type in slaughter pigs. *Vet Microbiol* 157:246–250.

204. Nair R, Thapaliya D, Su Y, Smith TC. 2014. Resistance to zinc and cadmium in *Staphylococcus aureus* of human and animal origin. *Infect Control Hosp Epidemiol* 35(Suppl 3):S32–S39.

205. Grass G, Fan B, Rosen BP, Franke S, Nies DH, Rensing C. 2001. ZitB (YbgR), a member of the cation diffusion facilitator family, is an additional zinc transporter in *Escherichia coli*. *J Bacteriol* 183:4664–4667.

206. Grass G, Otto M, Fricke B, Haney CJ, Rensing C, Nies DH, Munkelt D. 2005. FieF (YiiP) from *Escherichia coli* mediates decreased cellular accumulation of iron and relieves iron stress. *Arch Microbiol* 183:9–18.

207. Xiong A, Jayaswal RK. 1998. Molecular characterization of a chromosomal determinant conferring resistance to zinc and cobalt ions in *Staphylococcus aureus*. *J Bacteriol* 180:4024–4029.

208. Singh VK, Xiong A, Usgaard TR, Chakrabarti S, Deora R, Misra TK, Jayaswal RK. 1999. ZntR is an autoregulatory protein and negatively regulates the chromosomal zinc resistance operon *znt* of *Staphylococcus aureus*. *Mol Microbiol* 33:200–207.

209. Van Pham ST, Engman H, Dahlgren LG, Cornvik T, Eshaghi S. 2010. A systematic approach to isolate mono-disperse membrane proteins: purification of zinc transporter ZntB. *Protein Expr Purif* 72:48–54.

210. Papp-Wallace KM, Maguire ME. 2007. Bacterial homologs of eukaryotic membrane proteins: the 2-TM-GxN family of Mg(2+) transporters. *Mol Membr Biol* 24: 351–356.

211. Caldwell AM, Smith RL. 2003. Membrane topology of the ZntB efflux system of *Salmonella enterica* serovar Typhimurium. *J Bacteriol* 185:374–376.

212. Wan Q, Ahmad MF, Fairman J, Gorzelle B, de la Fuente M, Dealwis C, Maguire ME. 2011. X-ray crystallography and isothermal titration calorimetry studies of the *Salmonella* zinc transporter ZntB. *Structure* 19: 700–710.

213. Worlock AJ, Smith RL. 2002. ZntB is a novel Zn^{2+} transporter in *Salmonella enterica* serovar Typhimurium. *J Bacteriol* 184:4369–4373.

214. Chaoprasid P, Nookabkaew S, Sukchawalit R, Mongkolsuk S. 2015. Roles of *Agrobacterium tumefaciens* C58 ZntA and ZntB and the transcriptional regulator ZntR in controlling $Cd^{2+}/Zn^{2+}/Co^{2+}$ resistance and the peroxide stress response. *Microbiology* 161: 1730–1740.

215. Nies DH, Silver S. 1995. Ion efflux systems involved in bacterial metal resistances. *J Ind Microbiol* 14:186–199.

216. Legatzki A, Franke S, Lucke S, Hoffmann T, Anton A, Neumann D, Nies DH. 2003. First step towards a quantitative model describing Czc-mediated heavy metal resistance in *Ralstonia metallidurans*. *Biodegradation* 14:153–168.

217. Nies DH. 2003. Efflux-mediated heavy metal resistance in prokaryotes. *FEMS Microbiol Rev* 27:313–339.

218. Nies D, Mergeay M, Friedrich B, Schlegel HG. 1987. Cloning of plasmid genes encoding resistance to cadmium, zinc, and cobalt in *Alcaligenes eutrophus* CH34. *J Bacteriol* 169:4865–4868.

219. Saier MH Jr, Tam R, Reizer A, Reizer J. 1994. Two novel families of bacterial membrane proteins concerned with nodulation, cell division and transport. *Mol Microbiol* 11:841–847.

220. Diels L, Dong Q, van der Lelie D, Baeyens W, Mergeay M. 1995. The *czc* operon of *Alcaligenes eutrophus* CH34: from resistance mechanism to the removal of heavy metals. *J Ind Microbiol* 14:142–153.

221. Grosse C, Anton A, Hoffmann T, Franke S, Schleuder G, Nies DH. 2004. Identification of a regulatory pathway that controls the heavy-metal resistance system Czc via promoter *czcNp* in *Ralstonia metallidurans*. *Arch Microbiol* 182:109–118.

222. Zoropogui A, Gambarelli S, Covès J. 2008. CzcE from *Cupriavidus metallidurans* CH34 is a copper-binding protein. *Biochem Biophys Res Commun* 365:735–739.

223. Scherer J, Nies DH. 2009. CzcP is a novel efflux system contributing to transition metal resistance in *Cupriavidus metallidurans* CH34. *Mol Microbiol* 73:601–621.

224. von Rozycki T, Nies DH. 2009. *Cupriavidus metallidurans*: evolution of a metal-resistant bacterium. *Antonie van Leeuwenhoek* 96:115–139.

225. Symmons MF, Bokma E, Koronakis E, Hughes C, Koronakis V. 2009. The assembled structure of a complete tripartite bacterial multidrug efflux pump. *Proc Natl Acad Sci USA* 106:7173–7178.

226. Murakami S, Nakashima R, Yamashita E, Matsumoto T, Yamaguchi A. 2006. Crystal structures of a multidrug transporter reveal a functionally rotating mechanism. *Nature* 443:173–179.

227. De Angelis F, Lee JK, O'Connell JD III, Miercke LJ, Verschueren KH, Srinivasan V, Bauvois C, Govaerts C, Robbins RA, Ruysschaert JM, Stroud RM, Vandenbussche G. 2010. Metal-induced conformational changes in ZneB suggest an active role of membrane fusion proteins in efflux resistance systems. *Proc Natl Acad Sci USA* 107:11038–11043.

228. Pak JE, Ekendé EN, Kifle EG, O'Connell JD III, De Angelis F, Tessema MB, Derfoufi KM, Robles-Colmenares Y, Robbins RA, Goormaghtigh E, Vandenbussche G, Stroud RM. 2013. Structures of intermediate transport states of ZneA, a Zn(II)/proton antiporter. *Proc Natl Acad Sci USA* 110:18484–18489.

229. Vaccaro BJ, Lancaster WA, Thorgersen MP, Zane GM, Younkin AD, Kazakov AE, Wetmore KM, Deutschbauer A, Arkin AP, Novichkov PS, Wall JD, Adams MW. 2016. Novel metal cation resistance systems from mutant fitness analysis of denitrifying *Pseudomonas stutzeri*. *Appl Environ Microbiol* 82:6046–6056.

230. Djoko KY, Ong CL, Walker MJ, McEwan AG. 2015. The role of copper and zinc toxicity in innate immune defense against bacterial pathogens. *J Biol Chem* 290:18954–18961.

231. German N, Doyscher D, Rensing C. 2013. Bacterial killing in macrophages and amoeba: do they all use a brass dagger? *Future Microbiol* 8:1257–1264.

232. Hao X, Lüthje F, Rønn R, German NA, Li X, Huang F, Kisaka J, Huffman D, Alwathnani HA, Zhu YG, Rensing C. 2016. A role for copper in protozoan grazing: two billion years selecting for bacterial copper resistance. *Mol Microbiol* 102:628–641.

233. Poole K. 2017. At the nexus of antibiotics and metals: the impact of Cu and Zn on antibiotic activity and resistance. *Trends Microbiol* 25:820–832.

234. Molmeret M, Horn M, Wagner M, Santic M, Abu Kwaik Y. 2005. Amoebae as training grounds for intracellular bacterial pathogens. *Appl Environ Microbiol* 71:20–28.

235. Chandrangsu P, Rensing C, Helmann JD. 2017. Metal homeostasis and resistance in bacteria. *Nat Rev Microbiol* 15:338–350.

236. Tan H, Deng Z, Cao L. 2009. Isolation and characterization of actinomycetes from healthy goat faeces. *Lett Appl Microbiol* 49:248–253.

237. Choudhury P, Kumar R. 1998. Multidrug- and metal-resistant strains of *Klebsiella pneumoniae* isolated from *Penaeus monodon* of the coastal waters of deltaic Sundarban. *Can J Microbiol* 44:186–189.

238. Dutta GN, Devriese LA. 1981. Sensitivity and resistance to growth promoting agents in animal lactobacilli. *J Appl Bacteriol* 51:283–288.

239. Siddaramappa S, Challacombe JF, Duncan AJ, Gillaspy AF, Carson M, Gipson J, Orvis J, Zaitshik J, Barnes G, Bruce D, Chertkov O, Detter JC, Han CS, Tapia R, Thompson LS, Dyer DW, Inzana TJ. 2011. Horizontal gene transfer in *Histophilus somni* and its role in the evolution of pathogenic strain 2336, as determined by comparative genomic analyses. *BMC Genomics* 12:570.

240. Deus D, Krischek C, Pfeifer Y, Sharifi AR, Fiegen U, Reich F, Klein G, Kehrenberg C. 2017. Comparative analysis of the susceptibility to biocides and heavy metals of extended-spectrum β-lactamase-producing *Escherichia coli* isolates of human and avian origin, Germany. *Diagn Microbiol Infect Dis* 88:88–92.

241. Agga GE, Scott HM, Amachawadi RG, Nagaraja TG, Vinasco J, Bai J, Norby B, Renter DG, Dritz SS, Nelssen JL, Tokach MD. 2014. Effects of chlortetracycline and copper supplementation on antimicrobial resistance of fecal *Escherichia coli* from weaned pigs. *Prev Vet Med* 114:231–246.

242. Campos J, Cristino L, Peixe L, Antunes P. 2016. MCR-1 in multidrug-resistant and copper-tolerant clinically relevant *Salmonella* 1,4,[5],12:i:- and S. Rissen clones in Portugal, 2011 to 2015. *Euro Surveill* 21:30270.

243. Gómez-Sanz E, Kadlec K, Feßler AT, Zarazaga M, Torres C, Schwarz S. 2013. Novel erm(T)-carrying multiresistance plasmids from porcine and human isolates of methicillin-resistant *Staphylococcus aureus* ST398 that also harbor cadmium and copper resistance determinants. *Antimicrob Agents Chemother* 57:3275–3282.

244. Argudín MA, Lauzat B, Kraushaar B, Alba P, Agerso Y, Cavaco L, Butaye P, Porrero MC, Battisti A, Tenhagen BA, Fetsch A, Guerra B. 2016. Heavy metal and disinfectant resistance genes among livestock-associated methicillin-resistant *Staphylococcus aureus* isolates. *Vet Microbiol* 191:88–95.

245. Cavaco LM, Hasman H, Aarestrup FM, Wagenaar JA, Graveland H, Veldman K, Mevius D, Fetsch A, Tenhagen B-A, Concepcion Porrero M, Dominguez L, Granier SA, Jouy E, Butaye P, Kaszanyitzky E, Dán A, Zmudzki J, Battisti A, Franco A, Schwarz S, Gutierrez M, Weese JS, Cui S, Pomba C, Members of MRSA-CG. 2011. Zinc resistance of *Staphylococcus aureus* of animal origin is strongly associated with methicillin resistance. *Vet Microbiol* 150:344–348.

246. Gehring AM, DeMoll E, Fetherston JD, Mori I, Mayhew GF, Blattner FR, Walsh CT, Perry RD. 1998. Iron acquisition in plague: modular logic in enzymatic biogenesis of yersiniabactin by *Yersinia pestis*. *Chem Biol* 5:573–586.

Antimicrobial Resistance in Bacteria from Livestock and Companion Animals
Edited by Frank Møller Aarestrup, Stefan Schwarz, Jianzhong Shen, and Lina Cavaco
© 2018 American Society for Microbiology, Washington, DC
doi:10.1128/microbiolspec.ARBA-0006-2017

Resistance of Bacteria to Biocides

6

Jean-Yves Maillard[1]

BIOCIDE USAGE

Chemical biocides have been used for centuries for making water and foodstuff safe to consume, for treating wounds, and for preserving materials since well before the discovery of microorganisms. Today chemical biocides are heavily used in a wide range of applications and environments including the consumer product, water, wastewater, and food industries; goods manufacturing; the pharmaceutical industry; the health care and veterinary sectors; and the oil and gas industries (1). This wide range of applications reflects the versatility of biocide products for environmental disinfection, product preservation, and antisepsis (2). In Europe it is difficult to estimate the quantity of chemical biocides that are used in products or imported (1), although in 2006 the market for biocides was estimated to be €10 billion to €11 billion (1). It is, however, clear that the usage of chemical biocides is continuing to increase, particularly in consumer products. This increased usage may be partly due to consumers' increased awareness of microbial contamination and infection. The rise in antibiotic resistance in bacteria might also have impacted on the usage of biocides, at least in the health care and veterinary settings (3). Widespread media coverage of issues of hospital cleanliness and "superbugs" have also contributed to better-informed customers, providing better marketing arguments for manufacturers and distributors of biocidal products (3). Alongside a better-informed public, the global increase in antimicrobial resistance in bacteria is forcing decision makers to tackle this growing issue. One of the recommended interventions is better hygiene and control of bacteria on surfaces in health care settings but also in animal husbandry (4).

In health care settings biocides are heavily used for the disinfection of environmental surfaces and medical devices and for antisepsis. The growing number of studies highlighting the presence, and at times persistence, of bacterial pathogens, including multidrug-resistant ones, on surfaces despite the use of decontamination (5–14) acknowledges that microorganisms can survive on surfaces and be transmitted to patients, staff, and inanimate objects (15), thus finally emphasizing the importance of controlling the microbial burden on surfaces. This newly found appreciation for controlling microbial pathogens on surfaces has led to an explosion of surface disinfection products and their marketing (16–18), contributing to a higher concentration of biocides eventually released in the environment.

The ability of biocides or biocidal products to decrease the microbial bioburden on surfaces is also highly relevant in animal husbandry, farm buildings, barns, equipment, and vehicles, where their use should contribute to reducing the spread of pathogens. This also includes their use to prevent infectious outbreaks from spreading from farms; for example, large quantities of biocides are being sprayed in the environment and on vehicles in an attempt to decrease the spread of animal viral diseases (19). The heavy use of biocidal products where heavy soiling is present, in particular, their use on vehicle wheels and undercarriages, deserves better scrutiny of its efficacy in preventing potential outbreaks.

The use of biocidal products also includes the disinfection of various environmental surfaces, antibiofouling, the preservation of building materials, and water and wastewater treatment. Biocides play an important role as food preservatives and for controlling microbial contaminants that may enter the food chain during food production. As mentioned previously, one growing area for biocide manufacturers is consumer products, including the preservation of cosmetics, but more recently, personal care products, household products, and textiles.

In Europe, the incorporation of biocides in products and the use of chemical biocides in general is heavily regulated (20), with the consequence that fewer bio-

[1]Cardiff School of Pharmacy and Pharmaceutical Sciences, Cardiff University, Cardiff CF10 3NB United Kingdom.

cides are available for manufacturers to use. This restriction on the number and type of chemical biocides available for manufacturers has, however, not reduced the number of biocidal products and biocide applications. On the contrary, awareness of the role of microorganisms in contamination, infection, or the production of odors, together with the growing threat of bacterial resistance to chemotherapeutic antibiotics, has resulted in the biocidal product market expanding. In Europe, the amounts of chemical biocides used per application is difficult to measure (1). Chemical biocides used in diverse applications eventually find their way to the environment (1). For example, high concentrations of triclosan have been found in river and wastewater effluents (1.4 to 40,000 ng/liter in surface water, up to 85,000 ng/liter in wastewater, and up to 133,000 µg/kg in biosolids from wastewater treatment plants) (20–23). There should be little doubt that chemical biocides even at a low concentration (i.e., sub-MIC level) will exert a selective pressure on microorganisms (18, 24–26), which should be monitored where biocidal products are heavily used (18, 27). The increase in the use of biocides and biocidal products might aggravate the possible link between biocide usage and emergence of antimicrobial resistance in bacteria (1, 3, 18, 28), although there is no doubt that overall biocide usage has brought immense benefit to human and animal health (1–3, 29).

This article explores reports of bacterial resistance to biocides and our current knowledge of the mechanisms of bacterial resistance. It also reflects on the effect of biocides' interactions with bacteria that may lead to a change in susceptibility to antimicrobials. This article does not cover bacterial biofilms.

BIOCIDE RESISTANCE: A QUESTION OF DEFINITIONS

One of the main issues when dealing with bacterial resistance is the definition of "resistance." This definition is linked with the test protocols to measure resistance, and these protocols are described later. There are many definitions of resistance to biocides, some of which describe only a small decrease in susceptibility (18, 28, 31–34). This contrasts with the definition of bacterial resistance to chemotherapeutic antibiotics, which reflects clinical resistance. With biocides the terms "resistance," "tolerance," "decreased susceptibility," "reduced susceptibility," "insusceptibility," and "acquired reduced susceptibility" are used. Such diversity in terms reflects a lack of consensus within the scientific community and is contributing to a degree of confusion in our understanding of bacterial resistance to biocides.

From a practical point of view, a bacterium surviving in a biocidal product is resistant to that product, whatever the concentration of biocide is in the product.

Many papers have used the term "reduced susceptibility," which is based on the measurement of the MIC or the minimum bactericidal concentration. A biocide or biocide product at its in-use concentration may, however, still be effective (18, 35). One of the main difficulties is to determine what fold-difference in MIC or minimum bactericidal concentration reflects a change that will be significant in practice, i.e., a decrease in biocide effectiveness. This is likely to be biocide/biocidal product dependent.

From an academic perspective, other definitions of bacterial resistance have been used: (i) a bacterial strain that is not killed by a biocide concentration to which the majority of the bacterial species are susceptible and (ii) bacterial cells in a culture that survive biocide exposure that kills the majority of the bacterial population in that culture. This latest definition has been used mainly to identify specific mechanisms of biocide resistance in bacteria following stepwise exposure to a specific biocide.

Empirically, bacterial resistance to biocides has been labeled as intrinsic, a natural property of the bacterium, or acquired, following the acquisition of resistance genes or following mutations (36). These definitions still hold true, although the concept of transient resistance, following the expression of a mechanism(s) in response to a direct selective pressure, recognizes that the effect of a biocide on a bacterium may be more complex and short-lived as long as the biocide, exerting a selective pressure, is present (24, 25).

What appears to be more of a concern is the ability of a bacterium to become clinically resistant to an antibiotic(s) following exposure to a biocide/biocidal product. Such cross-resistance has been raised by the European Commission following reports from the Scientific Committee on Emerging and Newly Identified Health Risks (1, 37) and the Scientific Committee on Consumer Safety (38). The Biocidal Product Regulation (20), which regulates the commercialization of biocidal products on the European market, now mentions the potential issue of bacterial resistance and cross-resistance following biocide application. In the United States, the Federal Drug Administration (FDA) recently proposed several rules based on the concern about bacterial resistance linked to the use of certain chemical biocides (39). Demonstrating that a chemical biocide or a biocidal product will not give rise to resistance in bacteria is a question not only of definition but also of methodology.

OCCURRENCE OF BACTERIAL RESISTANCE TO BIOCIDES

Bacterial resistance to biocides and biocidal products has now been well documented in the literature, although examples are often anecdotal where a specific product was investigated. Biocides are a very diverse group of chemicals (1). Surprisingly, bacterial resistance has been studied with only a few biocides. For biocidal products, the formulation will help and hopefully optimize the delivery of the biocide(s) and/or negate some undesirable effects such as corrosiveness of surfaces, pungent smell, poor stability, or toxicity. Components of the formulations may also have a profound effect on biocide efficacy, either increasing or, on occasion, decreasing efficacy. In the peer-reviewed literature, formulations have rarely been studied in the past, although recently, several studies concerned the effect of formulated biocides on bactericidal efficacy (3, 18, 40, 41). Bacterial resistance has been investigated *in vitro* against several chemical classes, including phenolics (e.g., triclosan) (42–49), cationic biocides (e.g., chlorhexidine, quaternary ammonium compounds, particularly cetylpyridinium chloride, and benzalkonium chloride) (50–56), isothiazolinones (57), and more reactive biocides such as iodophors (58), alkylating agents (e.g., glutaraldehyde) (59–64), and several oxidizing compounds (65–68). Studies often differed in their methodology, rendering the comparison of results difficult (1, 18). Using realistic *in vitro* protocols to generate bacteria resistant to a specific biocide is not straightforward either (69). Investigations can generally be divided into four categories:

1. *In vitro* testing of bacterial resistance to a specific biocide, often involving training the bacteria to survive increasing concentrations of a biocide (46–48, 57, 69–73)
2. Studies reporting the isolation of environmental isolates resistant to specific biocides. These investigations principally concern environmental bacterial isolates from, for example, health care settings, manufacturing, and slaughterhouses and include biocides such as glutaraldehyde (59–62, 74), chlorine dioxide (65), chlorhexidine (75–79), triclosan (48, 80), quaternary ammonium compounds (79, 81–83), alcohol, and iodine (75)
3. Studies reporting the contamination of biocidal products principally used in health care settings and possible associations with infection outbreaks and pseudo-outbreaks (74, 84–89)
4. *In situ* studies reporting the impact on bacterial resistance of using specific biocidal products (90–93)

One criticism of *in vitro* studies is that they might not reflect the way bacteria encounter a biocide/biocidal product in practice (3, 69). For example, the use of stepwise training, i.e., the passaging of bacteria in increasing concentrations of a biocide, does not reflect conditions *in situ*. These studies have, however, yielded many insights on bacterial resistance mechanisms (46–48, 57, 69–71, 94). Another issue is that the development and nature of resistance to a biocide depend on the bacterial isolates investigated. Ciusa and colleagues (95) reported that bacterial strains from standard culture collection were not necessarily appropriate to study mechanisms of resistance to triclosan because they did not reflect the level and type of mutations observed with clinical isolates when exposed to bisphenol. This study also highlighted that valuable information is being learned through the study of large numbers of isolates (in this study 1,388 *Staphylococcus aureus* isolates were used) and questioned studies reporting the use of a single isolate (95).

The study of environmental isolates rather than standard culture collection strains yields important and probably more relevant information in terms of expressed mechanisms of resistance. Such investigations reiterate that bacteria can express multiple mechanisms at the same time and that some mechanisms responsible for a stable biocide-resistant phenotype are still unknown. Martin et al. (96) described a vegetative *Bacillus subtilis* endoscope washer isolate with stable resistance to the in-use concentration of chlorine dioxide and hydrogen peroxide, but also to peracetic acid (96, 97). Although this isolate is a good biofilm producer, the mechanisms responsible for the observed level of resistance to these oxidizing agents have not all been identified (96). Other studies that have isolated bacteria from environments where antimicrobials are heavily used identified a decrease in biocide susceptibility (81, 82, 95, 98) in some but not all isolates when compared to counterpart bacteria from standard culture collection (95, 98).

Studies reporting bacterial growth in biocidal products and subsequent infections or pseudo-infections have been very helpful in identifying the risks associated with some products and practices (89). Reported incidents often result from the inappropriate application of a product or the inappropriate preparation of a product, including the use of contaminated tap water, topping up of stock solutions, use of diluted products or inappropriate dilution, and inappropriate storage conditions. Some microorganisms, notably *Pseudomonas* spp., *Burkholderia* spp., and atypical mycobacteria can, however, contaminate the stock solution of a product because of their intrinsic resistance to the product (89). The preconceived idea that bacterial resistance occurs more readily in less reactive biocides such as phenolics (e.g., triclosan) and cationic biocides (e.g., chlorhexidine) rather than reactive ones such as alkylating and oxidizing agents does not hold true. For example, there have been many studies on atypical mycobacterial (*Mycobacterium chelonae*) resistance to 2% glutaraldehyde, which is used for the high-level disinfection of medical devices (59–64). It was speculated that these bacteria arose from a decrease in the effective concentration of glutaraldehyde (i.e., <2%) (60). Fisher et al. (99) reported the presence of glutaraldehyde-resistant atypical mycobacteria associated with endoscope reprocessing systems. Outbreaks of *M. chelonae* linked to endoscope reprocessing using glutaraldehyde have been described since 1991 (100). The more recent nosocomial outbreaks of *Mycobacterium abscessus* subsp. *massiliense* in Brazil, however, identified an isolate that was resistant to both 2% glutaraldehyde and first-line antimycobacterial antibiotics, highlighting the existence of cross-resistance mechanisms that remain to be identified (74).

Studies of the effect of biocidal product applications on emerging bacterial resistance in the community or health care settings remain scarce. These studies usually highlight the difficulty in data interpretation, notably in relation to the definition of "bacterial resistance." The few *in situ* studies nevertheless provide interesting insight on the long-term usage of selected biocidal products. Two studies from Cole and colleagues failed to show any cross-resistance between antibiotics and antibacterial wash products (91, 92). Likewise, Aiello et al. (90) failed to show any statistically significant correlation between the use of triclosan-containing product and reduced susceptibility to antibiotics. A study of benzalkonium chloride-containing product usage in

households, however, found a correlation between elevated QAC MIC and bacterial resistance to antibiotics (93).

There should be no doubt that bacteria have a great ability to survive biocide exposure and that the inappropriate use or preparation of biocidal products can result in bacterial resistance. The reporting of cross-resistance between biocides and unrelated chemicals such as chemotherapeutic antibiotics is increasing as scientists focus more on this possibility.

MECHANISMS OF BACTERIAL RESISTANCE

Biocides and biocidal products induce stress on the bacterial cell. In response, a bacterium expresses several mechanisms to prevent the detrimental effect caused by a biocide. These mechanisms aim to decrease the biocide concentration sufficiently that it is no longer damaging to the bacterial cells and include the ability of the bacterium to repair damages. If damage cannot be repaired efficiently or worsens, for example, because of high metabolic activity, the bacterial cell will be committed to a lethal pathway (Table 1). By some accounts that the maintenance of the cytoplasmic pH is key in that pathway (101, 102). Overall, our understanding of the bacterial mechanisms in place to decrease the susceptibility of a bacterium to biocides has improved, but they remain poorly studied. There is no doubt that bacteria have a plethora of mechanisms at their disposal and that often several mechanisms contribute together to the observed resistance phenotype. Our understanding of the effect of biocide interaction with bacteria and especially the stress response effect on gene expression remains poor. Examples given in the literature are often anecdotal. Understanding and measuring the expression of mechanisms following a biocide or biocidal product interaction with a bacterium has become

Table 1 Levels of biocide interactions with a bacterial cell

Exposure	Interactions	Types of damage	Events
Short exposure	Disruption of the transmembrane PMF leading to an uncoupling of oxidative phosphorylation and inhibition of active transport across the membrane		Reversible
	Inhibition of respiration or catabolic/anabolic reactions		
Prolonged exposure	Disruption of metabolic processes		Reversible
	Disruption of replication		
	Loss of membrane integrity resulting in leakage of essential intracellular constituents (K^+, inorganic phosphate, pentoses, nucleotides and nucleosides, proteins)	Imbalance of pHi	Irreversible
	Coagulation of intracellular materials	Commitment to cell death (autocidal pathway)	
	Lysis	Cell death	

important because it underlies the principle of the observed transient phenotypic changes in bacteria and the cross-resistance mechanisms between antimicrobials.

Mechanisms that Decrease the Concentration of Antimicrobials in Bacteria

Bacteria can use several mechanisms to decrease the lethal or inhibitory concentration of a biocide. Biocides have multiple target sites against the bacterial structure and as such they are often regarded as nonspecific. The sum of the damage caused to multiple target sites and the importance of the target sites defines whether the interaction will lead to a lethal or inhibitory effect (Table 1) (3, 101–105). Decreasing a damaging concentration of a biocide/biocidal product will enable the target bacteria to survive. It should be recognized that a low concentration (sub-MIC) of a biocide will affect the bacteria and, notably, trigger mechanisms to further decrease the biocide concentration. It is now well established in *in vitro* laboratory experiments but also in practice that a low concentration of a biocide will give rise to bacteria that are less susceptible to the biocide, enabling at times the survival of the bacteria in products (60, 89, 96).

Furthermore, biocides are used in complex formulations (i.e., the biocidal product) in practice, yet the effect of a biocidal product on bacterial resistance is not often tested (3, 18, 41, 76, 81). Excipients such as surfactants, chelators, and wetting agents may have a direct effect on the bacterial cell structure and increase the efficacy of a biocide. Arguably, there is sometimes incompatibility between a biocide and an excipient, effectively reducing the bactericidal activity of the product.

Reducing biocide penetration

The effect of bacterial cell structure to prevent or reduce the penetration of antimicrobials has been well established, notably with bacterial endospores (106), Gram-negative bacteria, and mycobacteria (103, 104). The presence of the lipopolysaccharide layer in Gram-negative bacteria has been well documented for its role in decreasing the activity of several membrane active agents such as quaternary ammonium compounds and biguanides. Evidence of the role of lipopolysaccharide in decreasing the activity of a membrane active agent has often been indirect with the use of permeabilizing agents such as chelators and the use of bacterial protoplasts (103, 105, 107, 108). Genetic alterations of the bacterial membrane with, for example, transposon mutagenesis have also provided some important information on biocide/bacterial cell interactions (109). In mycobacteria, in the presence of mycolic acid associated

with the arabinogalactan/arabinomannan cell wall, the lipid-rich outer cell wall is responsible for the lack of penetration of many antimicrobials (61, 104, 110–113). Likewise, porins have been shown to play an important role in the activity of glutaraldehyde and *ortho*-phthalaldehyde in mycobacteria (114). Reducing the expression of porins has been associated with reduced biocide and antibiotic efficacy (115, 116). Changes in bacterial cell membrane and cell wall composition following biocide exposure have been associated with a reduction in biocide activity (94, 115–120). Membrane alterations include membrane protein composition (57, 115, 121, 122), fatty acids (115, 123–127), and phospholipid content (128). A change in membrane potential has also been associated with a decrease in biocide susceptibility in *Pseudomonas aeruginosa* (129).

Efflux pumps

Efflux pumps, which are widespread in bacteria, contribute to decreasing the concentration of antimicrobials that penetrate the bacterial cells. The effect of active efflux on antimicrobial activity has been particularly well documented in *S. aureus* (130–139), *P. aeruginosa* (140–145), *Escherichia coli* (46, 82, 94, 146–149), *Salmonella enterica* serovar Typhimurium (150, 151), and *Acinetobacter baumannii* (116, 152). Five main classes of efflux pumps have been reported (Fig. 1) (153; 160): the drug/metabolite transporter superfamily, the major facilitator superfamily, the ATP-binding cassette family, the resistance-nodulation-division family, and the multidrug and toxic compound extrusion family.

The ability of efflux pumps alone to confer resistance to biocides/biocidal products is questionable, and it is likely that efflux pumps are part of several mechanisms used by a bacterium to survive biocide/biocidal product exposure (3, 83, 155). Some studies investigating triclosan claimed, however, that efflux was responsible for high-level resistance to the bisphenol (142, 144). Studies of bacterial isolates from environments where antimicrobials are heavily used, notably biguanides and QAC, have identified a high prevalence of efflux genes (e.g., *qacA/B*, *norA*, *nor B*, *smr*) in isolates that showed a decreased susceptibility to biocides (77–79, 82, 135).

Efflux can be induced by some antimicrobials (153, 156, 161). The expression of an efflux pump can increase following antimicrobial exposure, not necessarily by inducing the efflux pumps but by affecting global gene regulators, notably *marA* and *soxS* (46, 162). The effect of triclosan on bacteria has been particularly well studied with regard to efflux (46, 49, 140–142, 163, 164). In *S. enterica* serovar Typhimurium, overexpression of efflux results in decreased anti-

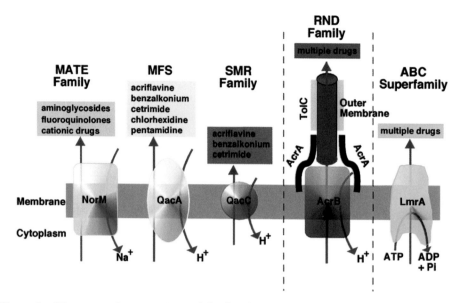

Figure 1 Diagrammatic comparison of the five families of efflux pumps (reproduced from reference 153). MATE, multidrug and toxic compound extrusion; MFS, major facilitator superfamily; SMR, •••; RND, resistance-nodulation-division; ABC, ATP-binding cassette.

microbial susceptibility (162–165). Overexpression of efflux pumps resulting in decreased biocide efficacy has also been described in *Stenotrophomonas maltophilia* with the overexpression of SmedEF (166); in *E. coli* with the overexpression of *acrAB*, *marA*, or *soxS* (46, 49, 162); and in *Campylobacter jejuni* overexpressing CmeB (167). The extent of efflux pumps and their role in bacteria are continuously evolving in the literature. Triggering overexpression of efflux in bacteria following biocide exposure is a concern that is debated later in this article.

Enzymatic degradation

Some bacteria can produce enzymes that degrade biocides. The presence of catalase and superoxide dismutase, for example, has been shown to decrease bacterial susceptibility to oxidizing agents (66, 168). The production of enzymes alone conferring resistance to a biocide is, however, doubtful. This would suggest that enzymatic activity is high and that enzymes are not themselves affected by the biocide. It is more likely that the production of detoxifying enzymes contributes to the battery of mechanisms available to the bacteria to survive biocide injuries (96).

Other examples of enzymatic activity conferring decreased susceptibility to a biocide include the parabens (169, 170), aldehydes (171), and metallic ions. In the latter case the ions are reduced to the inactive metal (34).

Physiological and Metabolic Changes

Bacterial metabolism can be associated with antimicrobial efficacy in that bacteria with a high metabolism are more susceptible to antimicrobials than those with no metabolic activity (172). Exposure of a bacteria to a physical or chemical process, such as a biocide/biocidal product, results in a mixed population of dead, injured, and uninjured bacteria. In the food industry, the recovery of injured bacteria is considered essential (173). This is not so when the efficacy of a biocide treatment is measured. Standard efficacy tests do not consider the effect of the recovery media and incubation conditions post-biocide treatment. The impact of resuscitated injured bacteria following treatment has been exemplified by the dual use of traditional plate counting on a rich nonselective recovery media such as tryptone soy agar and the use of the Bioscreen microbial growth analyzer, which measures bacterial growth in liquid (174). The ability of a bacterium to repair injuries is likely to play an important role when resistance is considered. As shown in Table 1, initial damage caused by a biocide is reversible. In practice, where incubation conditions posttreatment favor recovery from injury, repairs can be visualized with an extended lag phase (173). Biocide exposure has, however, been linked to a decreased growth rate and extended lag phase in bacteria (172, 175–177) because of a direct action of the biocide on the bacterial cells, although in many studies the ability of bacteria to repair injuries was not considered. Change in metabolic pathways has been particularly well exemplified with *S. enterica* exposure to triclosan. The bisphenol at a low concentration has been shown to target specifically the enoyl acyl carrier reductase in bacteria, which affects fatty acid lipid synthesis in the target bacteria (47, 177–179). Webber et al. (180) showed that *S. enterica* could alter its metabolic pathway to produce pyruvate and fatty acids following triclosan exposure. This change was part of a "triclosan resistance network" involving the expression of distinct mechanisms (180). Curiao and colleagues reported similar findings, evoking multiple pathways in the adaptation of *S. enterica* to triclosan and other biocides such as chlorhexidine and benzalkonium chloride (181).

Codling and colleagues (109) showed that in *Serratia marcescens*, the disruption of biosynthetic and metabolic pathways of the bacterium increased bacterial susceptibility to a QAC. A change in metabolic processes following exposure to biocides has also been observed in other bacteria, including *S. aureus* (182) and *P. aeruginosa* (183). The full impact of a change in metabolic pathways on decreasing biocide/biocidal product efficacy has not been assessed, nor has the reproducibility of such a change when exposed to specific antimicrobials. At present, such observations have been bacteria/biocide specific.

Mutations

Mutations in bacteria are by nature random but can be driven by the continuous presence of a selective pressure, notably the presence of antimicrobials. Although

it is widely recognized that the presence of chemotherapeutic antibiotics will drive target site mutations, there are far fewer examples with biocides. Mutations resulting from a biocide exposure have been mainly described with triclosan in several bacteria (43, 178, 180, 184–190). Mutations are linked to the use of triclosan at a low concentration and concern the enoyl-acyl reductase carrier protein (47, 179, 186, 191–193). In Salmonella biocide exposure resulted in mutations included de-repression of multidrug efflux pump AcrAB-TolC, and *rpoA*, which controls the RNA polymerase α-subunit (190). Interestingly, the investigation of 1,388 *S. aureus* clinical isolates' response to triclosan exposure identified several mutations that were similar among the isolates (Fig. 2) but not comparable to those observed with the standard culture collection strain (95). Recent observations questioned the choice of a culture collection strain to study biocide resistance. Standard strains have been widely used in biocide resistance studies with the comparability of results between studies in mind. From Ciusa et al. (95), it appears that standard strains and clinical isolates do not behave the same way. Stepwise training protocols that rely on passaging bacteria in increasing concentrations of biocides have yielded bacteria with decreased susceptibility or resistance to a given biocide but may be criticized for not reflecting real-world conditions (3). Many *in vitro* studies have investigated genetic changes in standard culture collection strains following biocide exposure. The work of Ciusa et al. (95) addresses the appropriateness of this approach and would favor the use of en-

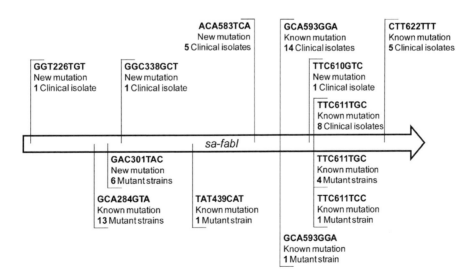

Figure 2 Schematic map of mutations in the *Staphylococcus aureus fabI* (*sa-fabI*) and *Staphylococcus haemolyticus fabI* (*sh-fabI*) genes. Mutations in *sa-fabI* are reported on a schematic map. Mutations detected in clinical isolates are mapped above the sequence, while mutations selected *in vitro* are shown below the sequence. (Reproduced from reference 95.)

vironmental isolates that have been exposed to a biocide/biocidal product.

INDUCTION OF GENE EXPRESSION CONFERRING BACTERIAL RESISTANCE

Biocide exposure even at a low concentration produces a stress on the target bacteria, even if the bacteria are intrinsically resistant to the biocide. The bacterial response to the stress will lead to a change in gene expression (24, 109, 116, 155, 162–167, 181, 194–196), particularly that of regulatory genes (46, 49, 68, 149, 162, 180, 197). The concentration of a biocide that is available to interact with the target bacteria is thus paramount (2, 3, 105, 198, 199), since a low, nonlethal concentration will not kill the bacterium but will undoubtedly produce a stress response. An indication of stress response is given by investigating the bacterial growth curve in the presence of a biocide at different concentrations. Increased lag phase or decreases in bacterial doubling time are indicators of a bacteria/biocide interaction and may reflect the induction/expression of mechanisms enabling the bacteria to decrease the toxicity of the biocide (28, 72, 172) and, as mentioned, allow earlier repair of injuries. Some bacterial mechanisms that play a role in decreasing the susceptibility to biocides are controlled by global regulators such as soxS and marA (46, 49, 146, 162). Antibiotic resistance mechanisms are also controlled by the same regulators (168, 200), which leads to the concern that biocide exposure can trigger antibiotic resistance. The induction of gene expression of global regulators leading to the expression of several mechanisms in bacterial resistance might not, however, be particularly problematic for the use of biocidal products since such expression might be transient. Some studies have shown that a decrease in bacterial susceptibility to biocides and sometimes to antibiotics was transient and only observed in the presence of the biocide (24, 25, 155).

As mentioned earlier, the efficient repair of sublethal injuries may play an important role in bacterial survival of biocide exposure. However, bacteria's ability to repair damage following biocide exposure has received little attention (195, 201, 202). In E. coli polyhexamethylene biguanide alters the expression of several genes, notably rhs, involved in repairing nucleic acid (202). The involvement of effective DNA repair mechanisms has been proposed to explain the high-level resistance of an environmental isolate of B. subtilis to several oxidizing agents (96). Efficient DNA repair mechanisms enable Deinococcus radiodurans to survive ionizing and UV radiation and exposure to chemicals that damage nucleic acid (203). In Lactobacillus pentosus, strains that have adapted to sublethal concentrations of antimicrobials overexpressed ribosomal proteins and glutamyl tRNA synthetase, which was interpreted as a response to damaged proteins directly caused by the antimicrobial exposure (195).

CROSS-RESISTANCE

Exposure to a biocide/biocidal product can lead to a stress response involving the expression of global gene regulators and ultimately the expression of nonspecific mechanisms enabling bacterial survival (116, 155, 156, 162, 181, 190, 200, 204–211). The link between biocide usage and antibiotic resistance has led to many discussions with conflicting evidence; some studies support a link, while others fail to identify any cross-resistance (1, 24, 25, 48, 73, 78, 79, 81, 82, 90–93, 98, 196, 212–220). Where cross-resistance between biocide exposure and antibiotic resistance was identified, suggested common resistance mechanisms included overexpression of efflux (18, 82, 153, 156, 161), changes in bacterial cell wall permeability (115, 117), and changes in bacterial metabolism (180). Differences in protocols to (i) grow test bacteria, (ii) expose test bacteria to the biocide/biocidal product, and (iii) measure resistance to biocides and antibiotics contribute to differences in reported observations of the biocide's effect on antibiotic resistance (18). Although the evidence is mainly in vitro based, the few in situ studies conducted also reported conflicting information about the association between the usage of biocidal products at home and an increase in antibiotic resistance among environmental isolates (89–93). It is worth noting, however, the study from Duarte and colleagues (74) reporting a post-surgical outbreak of a M. abscessus subsp. massiliense-resistant clone resistant to 2% glutaraldehyde and resistant to frontline antimycobacterial antibiotics.

There should be no doubt that bacteria have the capacity to express mechanisms that will lead to decreased susceptibility to both biocides/biocidal products and chemotherapeutic antibiotics. The question remains as to how commonly cross- resistance occurs in practice and what triggers emerging resistance in the first place. For example, efflux can easily be triggered in bacteria, not only by biocides but by a wide range of stimuli, such as spices and essential oil. (221).

MEASURING BACTERIAL RESISTANCE

One of the most important aspects of biocide/biocidal product resistance is how to measure bacterial resistance and cross-resistance. This has become even more pressing with the publication in Europe of the Biocidal Product Regulation (20), which asks manufacturers to demonstrate that their biocidal product will not cause emerging bacterial resistance. Likewise, in North America the FDA (39) issued a final rule on the safety and effectiveness of antibacterial soaps, effectively banning the use of certain biocides for that application. Rules concerning benzalkonium chloride, benzethonium chloride, and chloroxylenol, biocides that are commonly used in several products, deferred. One major issue for manufacturers is that neither the Biocidal Product Regulation nor the FDA indicate what appropriate tests should be conducted to demonstrate the safety of biocidal products where bacterial resistance is concerned.

MIC determination has often been used as a marker for resistance (18, 28, 69–71, 183, 219), although the validity of MIC to measure bacterial resistance has been questioned (1, 3, 18) mainly since in practice, biocides are often used at concentrations exceeding the MIC (120) and biocides are used as part of a formulation whose ingredients will impact on product efficacy (3, 18, 76). MIC could, however, be used as a trend indicator (3, 18, 25, 28, 76, 198, 199, 222, 223). It is thus unfortunate that some studies measure an increase in bacterial resistance in terms of MIC (28, 224). Other studies have used a prevalue biocide concentration above which the environmental isolates were considered to be resistant. For example, Lavilla Lerma and colleagues used a threshold biocide concentration of 0.025 µg/ml at which any bacterial growth was considered bacterial resistance to the biocide (81). Furthermore, resistance has sometimes been defined as a small increase (e.g., 2-fold) in MIC. This definition remains questionable, especially when using a standard protocol such as a broth microdilution method (225) because a 2-fold change might only reflect a 1-dilution difference. The determination of changes in minimum biocidal concentration might be more appropriate, because this indicates a change in the lethal effect of the biocide (18, 223). Some studies have looked at a change in inactivation kinetics. Such protocols, although very useful because they determine the ability of a biocide/biocidal product to kill target bacteria over time, are very cumbersome and time-consuming and would not be able to be used routinely (3, 18).

The determination of a change in the susceptibility profile to chemotherapeutic antibiosis is somewhat easier to perform because the protocols used can follow well-established standards that provide clear guidance but also breakpoints for selected bacteria/antibiotics (226, 227). It is, however, clear that the clinical signifi-

cance should be reported rather than reporting a mere change in the antibiotic zone of inhibition.

Measuring a change in the susceptibility profile to determine a prediction of the risk associated with biocidal product usage is acceptable if the exposure of the target bacterium to the biocidal product is realistic, i.e., if it reflects *in situ* exposure of bacteria with the biocidal products, encompassing dilution of the product upon usage if necessary, extended contact time for residual activity, etc. (18, 25). The test bacterial inoculum preparation needs to be strictly controlled to ensure reproducibility of the assay. When a significant change (here significant means a ≥10-fold change) in susceptibility profile is recorded (25, 222), the nature of this change, whether transient or permanent, needs to be established (18, 25, 223).

A protocol to predict the change in susceptibility profile of target bacteria following exposure to a biocide/biocidal product has been proposed (18). The use of such a protocol established the effect of various biocidal products on *S. enterica* (223), *E. coli*, and *S. aureus* (25). In these studies, triclosan was used as a positive control (25, 223). Triclosan is the most studied biocide in terms of interaction with bacteria. Studies have repeatedly show amended bacterial susceptibility profile to triclosan and antibiotics following exposure to the bisphenol. (23, 25, 228).

CONCLUSIONS

Biocidal products are useful compounds to control microbial contamination and kill pathogens. A biocidal concentration that will not kill the target bacteria will, regardless of the method of application, cause a stress response, which will lead to the expression of mechanisms that enable bacterial survival (3, 18, 28, 173). The concentration of biocide available to interact with the target bacteria is thus paramount. In the veterinary field, the presence of organic matter at the point of the biocidal product application, contributes to reduce the efficacy of the product, and therefore, cleaning the animate or inanimate surface prior to use of the biocidal product should be indicated but might not be practical.

Biocidal products are heavily used for veterinary applications, notably in animal husbandry, disinfection of udders in dairy animals, and in fish farming (1). Despite an increasing use of biocidal products, information related to the occurrence of bacterial resistance in these environments remains scarce (55, 73, 150, 229, 230). Nevertheless, with the growing knowledge and evidence of bacterial resistance in environments where biocides/biocidal products are heavily used, environmental surveillance has been timidly proposed to study the potential spread and occurrence of resistant bacteria (27, 73, 77).

With an increase in biocidal product usage, emerging bacterial resistance is possible, but to date, the risk associated with biocidal product usage has not been measured, mainly because of the lack of standard protocols. The only protocol to date has not yet been widely used against a small number of bacteria (18, 25, 223). The reproducibility of the data obtained may also depend on the bacterial species investigated (24). Such a predictive protocol also relies on using appropriate test parameters that reflect the biocidal product usage in practice (25, 223). Overall, investigating the biocidal effect on bacterial resistance should be welcome because it provides a better understanding of the biocide-bacteria interactions and should contribute to the development of more performant and safer biocidal products. This is particularly pertinent with the increased usage of biocidal products and the usage conditions in animal husbandry.

Citation. Maillard J-Y. 2018. Resistance of bacteria to biocides. Microbiol Spectrum 6(2):ARBA-0006-2017.

References

1. Scientific Committee on Emerging and Newly Identified Health Risks (SCENIHR). 2009. The antibiotic resistance effect of biocides. http://ec.europa.eu/health/ph_risk/committees/04_scenihr/docs/scenihr_o_021.pdf. Accessed January 2017.

2. Maillard J-Y. 2005. Usage of antimicrobial biocides and products in the healthcare environment: efficacy, policies, management and perceived problems. *Ther Clin Risk Manag* 1:340–370.

3. Maillard J-Y, Denyer SP. 2009. Emerging bacterial resistance following biocide exposure: should we be concerned? *Chim Oggi* 27:26–28.

4. O'Neill J. 2016. *Tackling Drug-Resistant Infections Globally: Final Report and Recommendations. The Review on Antimicrobial Resistance.* HM Government, London, United Kingdom.

5. Otter JA, Yezli S, French GL. 2011. The role played by contaminated surfaces in the transmission of nosocomial pathogens. *Infect Control Hosp Epidemiol* 32:687–699.

6. Lawley TD, Clare S, Deakin LJ, Goulding D, Yen JL, Raisen C, Brandt C, Lovell J, Cooke F, Clark TG, Dougan G. 2010. Use of purified *Clostridium difficile* spores to facilitate evaluation of health care disinfection regimens. *Appl Environ Microbiol* 76:6895–6900.

7. Teunis PF, Moe CL, Liu P, Miller SE, Lindesmith L, Baric RS, Le Pendu J, Calderon RL. 2008. Norwalk virus: how infectious is it? *J Med Virol* 80:1468–1476.

8. Boyce JM, Potter-Bynoe G, Chenevert C, King T. 1997. Environmental contamination due to methicillin-resistant *Staphylococcus aureus*: possible infection control implications. *Infect Control Hosp Epidemiol* 18:622–627.

9. Bhalla A, Pultz NJ, Gries DM, Ray AJ, Eckstein EC, Aron DC, Donskey CJ. 2004. Acquisition of nosocomial pathogens on hands after contact with environmental surfaces near hospitalized patients. *Infect Control Hosp Epidemiol* 25:164–167.

10. Vonberg RP, Kuijper EJ, Wilcox MH, Barbut F, Tüll P, Gastmeier P, van den Broek PJ, Colville A, Coignard B, Daha T, Debast S, Duerden BI, van den Hof S, van der Kooi T, Maarleveld HJ, Nagy E, Notermans DW, O'Driscoll J, Patel B, Stone S, Wiuff C, European C difficile-Infection Control Group, European Centre for Disease Prevention and Control (ECDC). 2008. Infection control measures to limit the spread of *Clostridium difficile*. *Clin Microbiol Infect* 14(Suppl 5):2–20.

11. Kramer A, Schwebke I, Kampf G. 2006. How long do nosocomial pathogens persist on inanimate surfaces? A systematic review. *BMC Infect Dis* 6:130–138.

12. Fawley WN, Wilcox MH. 2001. Molecular epidemiology of endemic *Clostridium difficile* infection. *Epidemiol Infect* 126:343–350.

13. Talon D. 1999. The role of the hospital environment in the epidemiology of multi-resistant bacteria. *J Hosp Infect* 43:13–17.

14. Hota B. 2004. Contamination, disinfection, and cross-colonization: are hospital surfaces reservoirs for nosocomial infection? *Clin Infect Dis* 39:1182–1189.

15. Cheeseman KE, Denyer SP, Hosein IK, Williams GJ, Maillard J-Y. 2009. Evaluation of the bactericidal efficacy of three different alcohol hand rubs against 57 clinical isolates of *S. aureus*. *J Hosp Infect* 72:319–325.

16. Williams GJ, Denyer SP, Hosein IK, Hill DW, Maillard J-Y. 2009. Limitations of the efficacy of surface disinfection in the healthcare setting. *Infect Control Hosp Epidemiol* 30:570–573.

17. Siani H, Cooper C, Maillard J-Y. 2011. Efficacy of "sporicidal" wipes against *Clostridium difficile*. *Am J Infect Control* 39:212–218.

18. Maillard J-Y, Bloomfield S, Coelho JR, Collier P, Cookson B, Fanning S, Hill A, Hartemann P, McBain AJ, Oggioni M, Sattar S, Schweizer HP, Threlfall J. 2013. Does microbicide use in consumer products promote antimicrobial resistance? A critical review and recommendations for a cohesive approach to risk assessment. *Microb Drug Resist* 19:344–354.

19. Department for Environment, Food & Rural Affairs. 2012. Controlling disease in farm animals. https://www.gov.uk/guidance/controlling-disease-in-farm-animals. Accessed January 2017.

20. Pedrouzo M, Borrull F, Marcé RM, Pocurull E. 2009. Ultra-high-performance liquid chromatography-tandem mass spectrometry for determining the presence of eleven personal care products in surface and wastewaters. *J Chromatogr A* 1216:6994–7000.

21. Kumar KS, Priya SM, Peck AM, Sajwan KS. 2010. Mass loadings of triclosan and triclocarbon from four wastewater treatment plants to three rivers and landfill

in Savannah, Georgia, USA. *Arch Environ Contam Toxicol* 58:275–285.

22. Wilson B, Chen RF, Cantwell M, Gontz A, Zhu J, Olsen CR. 2009. The partitioning of triclosan between aqueous and particulate bound phases in the Hudson River Estuary. *Mar Pollut Bull* 59:207–212.

23. Scientific Committee on Consumer Safety. 2010. Opinion on triclosan antimicrobial resistance. http://ec.europa.eu/health//sites/health/files/scientific_committees/consumer_safety/docs/sccs_o_054.pdf. Accessed January 2017.

24. Knapp L, Rushton L, Stapleton H, Sass A, Stewart S, Amezquita A, McClure P, Mahenthiralingam E, Maillard J-Y. 2013. The effect of cationic microbicide exposure against *Burkholderia cepacia* complex (Bcc); the use of *Burkholderia lata* strain 383 as a model bacterium. *J Appl Microbiol* 115:1117–1126.

25. Wesgate R, Grasha P, Maillard J-Y. 2016. Use of a predictive protocol to measure the antimicrobial resistance risks associated with biocidal product usage. *Am J Infect Control* 44:458–464.

26. Oggioni MR, Furi L, Coelho JR, Maillard JY, Martínez JL. 2013. Recent advances in the potential interconnection between antimicrobial resistance to biocides and antibiotics. *Expert Rev Anti Infect Ther* 11:363–366.

27. Cookson B. 2005. Clinical significance of emergence of bacterial antimicrobial resistance in the hospital environment. *J Appl Microbiol* 99:989–996.

28. Maillard J-Y. 2007. Bacterial resistance to biocides in the healthcare environment: should it be of genuine concern? *J Hosp Infect* 65(Suppl 2):60–72.

29. Siani H, Maillard J-Y. 2015. Best practice in healthcare environment decontamination. *Eur J Clin Microbiol Infect Dis* 34:1–11.

30. Chapman JS. 1998. Characterizing bacterial resistance to preservatives and disinfectants. *Int Biodeter Biodeg* 41:241–245.

31. Chapman JS, Diehl MA, Fearnside KB. 1998. Preservative tolerance and resistance. *Int J Cosmet Sci* 20:31–39.

32. Hammond SA, Morgan JR, Russell AD. 1987. Comparative susceptibility of hospital isolates of Gram-negative bacteria to antiseptics and disinfectants. *J Hosp Infect* 9:255–264.

33. Russell AD. 2003. Biocide use and antibiotic resistance: the relevance of laboratory findings to clinical and environmental situations. *Lancet Infect Dis* 3:794–803.

34. Cloete TE. 2003. Resistance mechanisms of bacteria to antimicrobial compounds. *Int Biodeter Biodegrad* 51:277–282.

35. Dettenkofer M, Wenzler S, Amthor S, Antes G, Motschall E, Daschner FD. 2004. Does disinfection of environmental surfaces influence nosocomial infection rates? A systematic review. *Am J Infect Control* 32:84–89.

36. Poole K. 2002. Mechanisms of bacterial biocide and antibiotic resistance. *J Appl Microbiol* 92(Suppl):55S–64S.

37. Scientific Committee on Emerging and Newly Identified Health Risks (SCENIHR). 2010. Research strategy to address the knowledge gaps on the antimicrobial resistance effects of biocides. http://ec.europa.eu/health/scientific_committees/emerging/docs/scenihr_o_028.pdf. Accessed January 2017.

38. Scientific Committee on Consumer Safety (SCCS). 2010. Opinion on triclosan antimicrobial resistance. http://ec.europa.eu/health//sites/health/files/scientific_committees/consumer_safety/docs/sccs_o_054.pdf. Accessed January 2017.

39. U.S. Food and Drug Administration. 2016. Safety and effectiveness of consumer antiseptics; topical antimicrobial drug products for over-the-counter human use. http://www.fda.gov/NewsEvents/Newsroom/PressAnnouncements/ucm517478.htm. Accessed January 2017.

40. Lavilla Lerma L, Benomar N, Casado Muñoz MC, Gálvez A, Abriouel H. 2015. Correlation between antibiotic and biocide resistance in mesophilic and psychrotrophic *Pseudomonas* spp. isolated from slaughterhouse surfaces throughout meat chain production. *Food Microbiol* 51:33–44.

41. Cowley NL, Forbes S, Amézquita A, McClure P, Humphreys GJ, McBain AJ. 2015. Effects of formulation on microbicide potency and mitigation of the development of bacterial insusceptibility. *Appl Environ Microbiol* 81:7330–7338.

42. Sasatsu M, Shimizu K, Noguchi N, Kono M. 1993. Triclosan-resistant *Staphylococcus aureus*. *Lancet* 341:756.

43. Heath RJ, Yu YT, Shapiro MA, Olson E, Rock CO. 1998. Broad spectrum antimicrobial biocides target the FabI component of fatty acid synthesis. *J Biol Chem* 273:30316–30320.

44. Bamber AI, Neal TJ. 1999. An assessment of triclosan susceptibility in methicillin-resistant and methicillin-sensitive *Staphylococcus aureus*. *J Hosp Infect* 41:107–109.

45. Randall LP, Cooles SW, Piddock LJ, Woodward MJ. 2004. Effect of triclosan or a phenolic farm disinfectant on the selection of antibiotic-resistant *Salmonella enterica*. *J Antimicrob Chemother* 54:621–627.

46. McMurry LM, Oethinger M, Levy SB. 1998. Overexpression of *marA*, *soxS*, or *acrAB* produces resistance to triclosan in laboratory and clinical strains of *Escherichia coli*. *FEMS Microbiol Lett* 166:305–309.

47. McMurry LM, McDermott PF, Levy SB. 1999. Genetic evidence that InhA of *Mycobacterium smegmatis* is a target for triclosan. *Antimicrob Agents Chemother* 43:711–713.

48. Cottell A, Denyer SP, Hanlon GW, Ochs D, Maillard JY. 2009. Triclosan-tolerant bacteria: changes in susceptibility to antibiotics. *J Hosp Infect* 72:71–76.

49. Curiao T, Marchi E, Viti C, Oggioni MR, Baquero F, Martinez JL, Coque TM. 2015. Polymorphic variation in susceptibility and metabolism of triclosan-resistant mutants of *Escherichia coli* and *Klebsiella pneumoniae* clinical strains obtained after exposure to biocides and antibiotics. *Antimicrob Agents Chemother* 59:3413–3423.

50. Adair FW, Geftic SG, Gelzer J. 1971. Resistance of *Pseudomonas* to quaternary ammonium compounds. II. Cross-resistance characteristics of a mutant of *Pseudomonas aeruginosa*. *Appl Microbiol* 21:1058–1063.

51. **Russell AD.** 2002. Introduction of biocides into clinical practice and the impact on antibiotic-resistant bacteria. *J Appl Microbiol* **92**(Suppl):121S–135S.

52. **Chapman JS.** 2003. Disinfectant resistance mechanisms, cross-resistance, and co-resistance. *Int Biodeter Biodegrad* **51**:271–276.

53. **Stickler DJ.** 1974. Chlorhexidine resistance in *Proteus mirabilis*. *J Clin Pathol* **27**:284–287.

54. **Gillespie MT, May JW, Skurray RA.** 1986. Plasmid-encoded resistance to acriflavine and quaternary ammonium compounds in methicillin-resistant *Staphylococcus aureus*. *FEMS Microbiol Lett* **34**:47–51.

55. **Randall LP, Cooles SW, Sayers AR, Woodward MJ.** 2001. Association between cyclohexane resistance in *Salmonella* of different serovars and increased resistance to multiple antibiotics, disinfectants and dyes. *J Med Microbiol* **50**:919–924.

56. **Romão CMCPA, Faria YN, Pereira LR, Asensi MD.** 2005. Susceptibility of clinical isolates of multiresistant *Pseudomonas aeruginosa* to a hospital disinfectant and molecular typing. *Mem Inst Oswaldo Cruz* **100**:541–548.

57. **Winder CL, Al-Adham IS, Abdel Malek SM, Buultjens TE, Horrocks AJ, Collier PJ.** 2000. Outer membrane protein shifts in biocide-resistant *Pseudomonas aeruginosa* PAO1. *J Appl Microbiol* **89**:289–295.

58. **O'Rourke E, Runyan D, O'Leary J, Stern J.** 2003. Contaminated iodophor in the operating room. *Am J Infect Control* **31**:255–256.

59. **Griffiths PA, Babb JR, Bradley CR, Fraise AP.** 1997. Glutaraldehyde-resistant *Mycobacterium chelonae* from endoscope washer disinfectors. *J Appl Microbiol* **82**:519–526.

60. **van Klingeren B, Pullen W.** 1993. Glutaraldehyde resistant mycobacteria from endoscope washers. *J Hosp Infect* **25**:147–149.

61. **Manzoor SE, Lambert PA, Griffiths PA, Gill MJ, Fraise AP.** 1999. Reduced glutaraldehyde susceptibility in *Mycobacterium chelonae* associated with altered cell wall polysaccharides. *J Antimicrob Chemother* **43**:759–765.

62. **Fraud S, Maillard J-Y, Russell AD.** 2001. Comparison of the mycobactericidal activity of *ortho*- phthalaldehyde, glutaraldehyde and other dialdehydes by a quantitative suspension test. *J Hosp Infect* **48**:214–221.

63. **Walsh SE, Maillard J-Y, Russell AD, Hann AC.** 2001. Possible mechanisms for the relative efficacies of *ortho*-phthalaldehyde and glutaraldehyde against glutaraldehyde-resistant *Mycobacterium chelonae*. *J Appl Microbiol* **91**:80–92.

64. **Nomura K, Ogawa M, Miyamoto H, Muratani T, Taniguchi H.** 2004. Antibiotic susceptibility of glutaraldehyde-tolerant *Mycobacterium chelonae* from bronchoscope washing machines. *Am J Infect Control* **32**:185–188.

65. **Martin DJH, Denyer SP, McDonnell G, Maillard J-Y.** 2008. Resistance and cross-resistance to oxidising agents of bacterial isolates from endoscope washer disinfectors. *J Hosp Infect* **69**:377–383.

66. **Greenberg JT, Demple B.** 1989. A global response induced in *Escherichia coli* by redox-cycling agents overlaps with that induced by peroxide stress. *J Bacteriol* **171**:3933–3939.

67. **Greenberg JT, Monach P, Chou JH, Josephy PD, Demple B.** 1990. Positive control of a global antioxidant defense regulon activated by superoxide-generating agents in *Escherichia coli*. *Proc Natl Acad Sci USA* **87**: 6181–6185.

68. **Dukan S, Touati D.** 1996. Hypochlorous acid stress in *Escherichia coli*: resistance, DNA damage, and comparison with hydrogen peroxide stress. *J Bacteriol* **178**: 6145–6150.

69. **Walsh SE, Maillard J-Y, Russell AD, Catrenich CE, Charbonneau DL, Bartolo RG.** 2003. Development of bacterial resistance to several biocides and effects on antibiotic susceptibility. *J Hosp Infect* **55**:98–107.

70. **Tattawasart U, Maillard J-Y, Furr JR, Russell AD.** 1999. Development of resistance to chlorhexidine diacetate and cetylpyridinium chloride in *Pseudomonas stutzeri* and changes in antibiotic susceptibility. *J Hosp Infect* **42**:219–229.

71. **Thomas L, Maillard J-Y, Lambert RJW, Russell AD.** 2000. Development of resistance to chlorhexidine diacetate in *Pseudomonas aeruginosa* and the effect of a "residual" concentration. *J Hosp Infect* **46**:297–303.

72. **Thomas L, Russell AD, Maillard J-Y.** 2005. Antimicrobial activity of chlorhexidine diacetate and benzalkonium chloride against *Pseudomonas aeruginosa* and its response to biocide residues. *J Appl Microbiol* **98**:533–543.

73. **Molina-González D, Alonso-Calleja C, Alonso-Hernando A, Capita R.** 2014. Effect of sub-lethal concentrations of biocides on the susceptibility to antibiotics of multidrug resistant *Salmonella enterica* strains. *Food Control* **40**:329–334.

74. **Duarte RS, Lourenço MCS, Fonseca LS, Leão SC, Amorim EL, Rocha IL, Coelho FS, Viana-Niero C, Gomes KM, da Silva MG, Lorena NS, Pitombo MB, Ferreira RM, Garcia MH, de Oliveira GP, Lupi O, Vilaça BR, Serradas LR, Chebabo A, Marques EA, Teixeira LM, Dalcolmo M, Senna SG, Sampaio JL.** 2009. Epidemic of postsurgical infections caused by *Mycobacterium massiliense*. *J Clin Microbiol* **47**:2149–2155.

75. **Wisplinghoff H, Schmitt R, Wöhrmann A, Stefanik D, Seifert H.** 2007. Resistance to disinfectants in epidemiologically defined clinical isolates of *Acinetobacter baumannii*. *J Hosp Infect* **66**:174–181.

76. **Bock LJ, Wand ME, Sutton JM.** 2016. Varying activity of chlorhexidine-based disinfectants against *Klebsiella pneumoniae* clinical isolates and adapted strains. *J Hosp Infect* **93**:42–48.

77. **Liu Q, Zhao H, Han L, Shu W, Wu Q, Ni Y.** 2015. Frequency of biocide-resistant genes and susceptibility to chlorhexidine in high-level mupirocin-resistant, methicillin-resistant *Staphylococcus aureus* (MuH MRSA). *Diagn Microbiol Infect Dis* **82**:278–283.

78. **Hijazi K, Mukhopadhya I, Abbott F, Milne K, Al-Jabri ZJ, Oggioni MR, Gould IM.** 2016. Susceptibility to

chlorhexidine amongst multidrug-resistant clinical isolates of *Staphylococcus epidermidis* from bloodstream infections. *Int J Antimicrob Agents* **48:**86–90.

79. Conceição T, Coelho C, de Lencastre H, Aires-de-Sousa M. 2015. High prevalence of biocide resistance determinants in *Staphylococcus aureus* isolates from three African countries. *Antimicrob Agents Chemother* **60:**678–681.

80. Lear JC, Maillard J-Y, Dettmar PW, Goddard PA, Russell AD. 2002. Chloroxylenol- and triclosan-tolerant bacteria from industrial sources. *J Ind Microbiol Biotechnol* **29:**238–242.

81. Lavilla Lerma L, Benomar N, Gálvez A, Abriouel H. 2013. Prevalence of bacteria resistant to antibiotics and/or biocides on meat processing plant surfaces throughout meat chain production. *Int J Food Microbiol* **161:**97–106.

82. Grande Burgos MJ, Fernández Márquez ML, Pérez Pulido R, Gálvez A, Lucas López R. 2016. Virulence factors and antimicrobial resistance in *Escherichia coli* strains isolated from hen egg shells. *Int J Food Microbiol* **238:**89–95.

83. Martínez-Suárez JV, Ortiz S, López-Alonso V. 2016. Potential impact of the resistance to quaternary ammonium disinfectants on the persistence of *Listeria monocytogenes* in food processing environments. *Front Microbiol* **7:**638.

84. Sanford JP. 1970. Disinfectants that don't. *Ann Intern Med* **72:**282–283.

85. Prince J, Ayliffe GAJ. 1972. In-use testing of disinfectants in hospitals. *J Clin Pathol* **25:**586–589.

86. Bridges K, Lowbury EJL. 1977. Drug resistance in relation to use of silver sulphadiazine cream in a burns unit. *J Clin Pathol* **30:**160–164.

87. Klasen HJ. 2000. A historical review of the use of silver in the treatment of burns. II. Renewed interest for silver. *Burns* **26:**131–138.

88. Reiss I, Borkhardt A, Füssle R, Sziegoleit A, Gortner L. 2000. Disinfectant contaminated with *Klebsiella oxytoca* as a source of sepsis in babies. *Lancet* **356:**310.

89. Weber DJ, Rutala WA, Sickbert-Bennett EE. 2007. Outbreaks associated with contaminated antiseptics and disinfectants. *Antimicrob Agents Chemother* **51:**4217–4224.

90. Aiello AE, Marshall B, Levy SB, Della-Latta P, Larson E. 2004. Relationship between triclosan and susceptibilities of bacteria isolated from hands in the community. *Antimicrob Agents Chemother* **48:**2973–2979.

91. Cole EC, Addison RM, Rubino JR, Leese KE, Dulaney PD, Newell MS, Wilkins J, Gaber DJ, Wineinger T, Criger DA. 2003. Investigation of antibiotic and antibacterial agent cross-resistance in target bacteria from homes of antibacterial product users and nonusers. *J Appl Microbiol* **95:**664–676.

92. Cole EC, Addison RM, Dulaney PD, Leese KE, Madanat HM, Guffey AM. 2011. Investigation of antibiotic and antibacterial susceptibility and resistance in *Staphylococcus* form the skin of users and non-users of antibacterial wash products in home environments. *Int J Microbiol Res* **3:**90–96.

93. Carson RT, Larson E, Levy SB, Marshall BM, Aiello AE. 2008. Use of antibacterial consumer products containing quaternary ammonium compounds and drug resistance in the community. *J Antimicrob Chemother* **62:**1160–1162.

94. Alonso-Calleja C, Guerrero-Ramos E, Alonso-Hernando A, Capita R. 2015. Adaptation and cross-adaptation of *Escherichia coli* ATCC 12806 to several food-grade biocides. *Food Control* **56:**86–94.

95. Ciusa ML, Furi L, Knight D, Decorosi F, Fondi M, Raggi C, Coelho JR, Aragones L, Moce L, Visa P, Freitas AT, Baldassarri L, Fani R, Viti C, Orefici G, Martinez JL, Morrissey I, Oggioni MR, BIOHYPO Consortium. 2012. A novel resistance mechanism to triclosan that suggests horizontal gene transfer and demonstrates a potential selective pressure for reduced biocide susceptibility in clinical strains of *Staphylococcus aureus*. *Int J Antimicrob Agents* **40:**210–220.

96. Martin DJH, Wesgate RL, Denyer SP, McDonnell G, Maillard J-Y. 2015. *Bacillus subtilis* vegetative isolate surviving chlorine dioxide exposure: an elusive mechanism of resistance. *J Appl Microbiol* **119:**1541–1551.

97. Bridier A, Le Coq D, del Pilar Sanchez-Vizuete M, Aymerich S, Meylheuc T, Maillard J-Y, Thomas V, Dubois-Brissonnet F, Briandet R. 2012. Biofilms of a *Bacillus subtilis* endoscope WD isolate that protect *Staphylococcus aureus* from peracetic acid. *PLoS One* **7:**e44506.

98. Lear JC, Maillard J-Y, Dettmar PW, Goddard PA, Russell AD. 2006. Chloroxylenol- and triclosan-tolerant bacteria from industrial sources: susceptibility to antibiotics and other biocides. *Int Biodeter Biodegrad* **57:**51–56.

99. Fisher CW, Fiorello A, Shaffer D, Jackson M, McDonnell GE. 2012. Aldehyde-resistant mycobacteria bacteria associated with the use of endoscope reprocessing systems. *Am J Infect Control* **40:**880–882.

100. Alvarado CJ, Stolz SM, Maki DG, Centers for Disease Control (CDC). 1991. Nosocomial infection and pseudoinfection from contaminated endoscopes and bronchoscopes—Wisconsin and Missouri. *MMWR Morb Mortal Wkly Rep* **40:**675–678.

101. Denyer SP, Stewart GSAB. 1998. Mechanisms of action of disinfectants. *Int Biodeter Biodegrad* **41:**261–268.

102. Maillard J-Y. 2002. Bacterial target sites for biocide action. *J Appl Microbiol* **92(Suppl):**16S–27S.

103. Denyer SP, Maillard J-Y. 2002. Cellular impermeability and uptake of biocides and antibiotics in Gram-negative bacteria. *J Appl Microbiol* **92(Suppl):**35S–45S.

104. Lambert PA. 2002. Cellular impermeability and uptake of biocides and antibiotics in Gram-positive bacteria and mycobacteria. *J Appl Microbiol* **92(Suppl):**46S–54S.

105. McDonnell G, Russell AD. 1999. Antiseptics and disinfectants: activity, action, and resistance. *Clin Microbiol Rev* **12:**147–179.

106. Leggett MJ, Schwarz JS, Burke PA, Mcdonnell G, Denyer SP, Maillard J-Y. 2015. Resistance to and killing by the sporicidal microbicide peracetic acid. *J Antimicrob Chemother* **70:**773–779.

107. Munton TJ, Russell AD. 1970. Effect of glutaraldehyde on protoplasts of *Bacillus megaterium*. *J Gen Microbiol* **63**:367–370.

108. Ayres HM, Payne DN, Furr JR, Russell AD. 1998. Effect of permeabilizing agents on antibacterial activity against a simple *Pseudomonas aeruginosa* biofilm. *Lett Appl Microbiol* **27**:79–82.

109. Codling CE, Jones BV, Mahenthiralingam E, Russell AD, Maillard J-Y. 2004. Identification of genes involved in the susceptibility of *Serratia marcescens* to polyquaternium-1. *J Antimicrob Chemother* **54**:370–375.

110. Walsh SE, Maillard J-Y, Russell AD, Hann AC. 2001. Possible mechanisms for the relative efficacies of *ortho*-phthalaldehyde and glutaraldehyde against glutaraldehyde-resistant *Mycobacterium chelonae*. *J Appl Microbiol* **91**:80–92.

111. McNeil MR, Brennan PJ. 1991. Structure, function and biogenesis of the cell envelope of mycobacteria in relation to bacterial physiology, pathogenesis and drug resistance; some thoughts and possibilities arising from recent structural information. *Res Microbiol* **142**:451–463.

112. Broadley SJ, Jenkins PA, Furr JR, Russell AD. 1995. Potentiation of the effects of chlorhexidine diacetate and cetylpyridinium chloride on mycobacteria by ethambutol. *J Med Microbiol* **43**:458–460.

113. Fraud S, Hann AC, Maillard J-Y, Russell AD. 2003. Effects of ortho-phthalaldehyde, glutaraldehyde and chlorhexidine diacetate on *Mycobacterium chelonae* and *Mycobacterium abscessus* strains with modified permeability. *J Antimicrob Chemother* **51**:575–584.

114. Svetlíková Z, Skovierová H, Niederweis M, Gaillard J-L, McDonnell G, Jackson M. 2009. Role of porins in the susceptibility of *Mycobacterium smegmatis* and *Mycobacterium chelonae* to aldehyde-based disinfectants and drugs. *Antimicrob Agents Chemother* **53**:4015–4018.

115. Tattawasart U, Maillard JY, Furr JR, Russell AD, Russell AD. 2000. Outer membrane changes in *Pseudomonas stutzeri* resistant to chlorhexidine diacetate and cetylpyridinium chloride. *Int J Antimicrob Agents* **16**:233–238.

116. Fernández-Cuenca F, Tomás M, Caballero-Moyano FJ, Bou G, Martínez-Martínez L, Vila J, Pachón J, Cisneros JM, Rodríguez-Baño J, Pascual Á, Spanish Group of Nosocomial Infections (GEIH) from the Spanish Society of Clinical Microbiology and Infectious Diseases (SEIMC) and the Spanish Network for Research in Infectious Diseases (REIPI), Spanish Group of Nosocomial Infections GEIH from the Spanish Society of Clinical Microbiology and Infectious Diseases SEIMC and the Spanish Network for Research in Infectious Diseases REIPI. 2015. Reduced susceptibility to biocides in *Acinetobacter baumannii*: association with resistance to antimicrobials, epidemiological behaviour, biological cost and effect on the expression of genes encoding porins and efflux pumps. *J Antimicrob Chemother* **70**:3222–3229.

117. Tattawasart U, Hann AC, Maillard J-Y, Furr JR, Russell AD. 2000. Cytological changes in chlorhexidine-resistant isolates of *Pseudomonas stutzeri*. *J Antimicrob Chemother* **45**:145–152.

118. Braoudaki M, Hilton AC. 2005. Mechanisms of resistance in *Salmonella enterica* adapted to erythromycin, benzalkonium chloride and triclosan. *Int J Antimicrob Agents* **25**:31–37.

119. Pagès JM, James CE, Winterhalter M. 2008. The porin and the permeating antibiotic: a selective diffusion barrier in Gram-negative bacteria. *Nat Rev Microbiol* **6**:893–903.

120. Nikaido H. 2003. Molecular basis of bacterial outer membrane permeability revisited. *Microbiol Mol Biol Rev* **67**:593–656.

121. Gandhi PA, Sawant AD, Wilson LA, Ahearn DG. 1993. Adaptation and growth of *Serratia marcescens* in contact lens disinfectant solutions containing chlorhexidine gluconate. *Appl Environ Microbiol* **59**:183–188.

122. Brözel VS, Cloete TE. 1994. Resistance of *Pseudomonas aeruginosa* to isothiazolone. *J Appl Bacteriol* **76**:576–582.

123. Jones MV, Herd TM, Christie HJ. 1989. Resistance of *Pseudomonas aeruginosa* to amphoteric and quaternary ammonium biocides. *Microbios* **58**:49–61.

124. Méchin L, Dubois-Brissonnet F, Heyd B, Leveau JY. 1999. Adaptation of *Pseudomonas aeruginosa* ATCC 15442 to didecyldimethylammonium bromide induces changes in membrane fatty acid composition and in resistance of cells. *J Appl Microbiol* **86**:859–866.

125. Guérin-Méchin L, Dubois-Brissonnet F, Heyd B, Leveau JY. 1999. Specific variations of fatty acid composition of *Pseudomonas aeruginosa* ATCC 15442 induced by quaternary ammonium compounds and relation with resistance to bactericidal activity. *J Appl Microbiol* **87**:735–742.

126. Guérin-Méchin L, Dubois-Brissonnet F, Heyd B, Leveau JY. 2000. Quaternary ammonium compound stresses induce specific variations in fatty acid composition of *Pseudomonas aeruginosa*. *Int J Food Microbiol* **55**:157–159.

127. Tkachenko O, Shepard J, Aris VM, Joy A, Bello A, Londono I, Marku J, Soteropoulos P, Peteroy-Kelly MA. 2007. A triclosan-ciprofloxacin cross-resistant mutant strain of *Staphylococcus aureus* displays an alteration in the expression of several cell membrane structural and functional genes. *Res Microbiol* **158**:651–658.

128. Boeris PS, Domenech CE, Lucchesi GI. 2007. Modification of phospholipid composition in *Pseudomonas putida* A ATCC 12633 induced by contact with tetradecyltrimethylammonium. *J Appl Microbiol* **103**:1048–1054.

129. Bruinsma GM, Rustema-Abbing M, van der Mei HC, Lakkis C, Busscher HJ. 2006. Resistance to a polyquaternium-1 lens care solution and isoelectric points of *Pseudomonas aeruginosa* strains. *J Antimicrob Chemother* **57**:764–766.

130. Lyon BR, Skurray R. 1987. Antimicrobial resistance of *Staphylococcus aureus*: genetic basis. *Microbiol Rev* **51**:88–134.

131. Tennent JM, Lyon BR, Midgley M, Jones IG, Purewal AS, Skurray RA. 1989. Physical and biochemical characterization of the *qacA* gene encoding antiseptic and disinfectant resistance in *Staphylococcus aureus*. *J Gen Microbiol* **135**:1–10.

132. Littlejohn TG, Paulsen IT, Gillespie MT, Tennent JM, Midgley M, Jones IG, Purewal AS, Skurray RA. 1992. Substrate specificity and energetics of antiseptic and disinfectant resistance in *Staphylococcus aureus*. *FEMS Microbiol Lett* **74**:259–265.

133. Leelaporn A, Paulsen IT, Tennent JM, Littlejohn TG, Skurray RA. 1994. Multidrug resistance to antiseptics and disinfectants in coagulase-negative staphylococci. *J Med Microbiol* **40**:214–220.

134. Heir E, Sundheim G, Holck AL. 1998. The *Staphylococcus qacH* gene product: a new member of the SMR family encoding multidrug resistance. *FEMS Microbiol Lett* **163**:49–56.

135. Heir E, Sundheim G, Holck AL. 1999. The *qacG* gene on plasmid pST94 confers resistance to quaternary ammonium compounds in staphylococci isolated from the food industry. *J Appl Microbiol* **86**:378–388.

136. Rouch DA, Cram DS, DiBerardino D, Littlejohn TG, Skurray RA. 1990. Efflux-mediated antiseptic resistance gene *qacA* from *Staphylococcus aureus*: common ancestry with tetracycline- and sugar-transport proteins. *Mol Microbiol* **4**:2051–2062.

137. Huet AA, Raygada JL, Mendiratta K, Seo SM, Kaatz GW. 2008. Multidrug efflux pump overexpression in *Staphylococcus aureus* after single and multiple *in vitro* exposures to biocides and dyes. *Microbiology* **154**:3144–3153.

138. Schindler BD, Kaatz GW. 2016. Multidrug efflux pumps of Gram-positive bacteria. *Drug Resist Updat* **27**:1–13.

139. Santos Costa S, Viveiros M, Rosato AE, Melo-Cristino J, Couto I. 2015. Impact of efflux in the development of multidrug resistance phenotypes in *Staphylococcus aureus*. *BMC Microbiol* **15**:232.

140. Chuanchuen R, Beinlich K, Hoang TT, Becher A, Karkhoff-Schweizer RR, Schweizer HP. 2001. Cross-resistance between triclosan and antibiotics in *Pseudomonas aeruginosa* is mediated by multidrug efflux pumps: exposure of a susceptible mutant strain to triclosan selects nfxB mutants overexpressing MexCD-OprJ. *Antimicrob Agents Chemother* **45**:428–432.

141. Chuanchuen R, Narasaki CT, Schweizer HP. 2002. The MexJK efflux pump of *Pseudomonas aeruginosa* requires OprM for antibiotic efflux but not for efflux of triclosan. *J Bacteriol* **184**:5036–5044.

142. Mima T, Joshi S, Gomez-Escalada M, Schweizer HP. 2007. Identification and characterization of TriABC-OpmH, a triclosan efflux pump of *Pseudomonas aeruginosa* requiring two membrane fusion proteins. *J Bacteriol* **189**:7600–7609.

143. Schweizer HP. 1998. Intrinsic resistance to inhibitors of fatty acid biosynthesis in *Pseudomonas aeruginosa* is due to efflux: application of a novel technique for generation of unmarked chromosomal mutations for the study of efflux systems. *Antimicrob Agents Chemother* **42**:394–398.

144. Chuanchuen R, Karkhoff-Schweizer RR, Schweizer HP. 2003. High-level triclosan resistance in *Pseudomonas aeruginosa* is solely a result of efflux. *Am J Infect Control* **31**:124–127.

145. Morita Y, Murata T, Mima T, Shiota S, Kuroda T, Mizushima T, Gotoh N, Nishino T, Tsuchiya T. 2003. Induction of mexCD-oprJ operon for a multidrug efflux pump by disinfectants in wild-type *Pseudomonas aeruginosa* PAO1. *J Antimicrob Chemother* **51**:991–994.

146. Moken MC, McMurry LM, Levy SB. 1997. Selection of multiple-antibiotic-resistant (mar) mutants of *Escherichia coli* by using the disinfectant pine oil: roles of the *mar* and *acrAB* loci. *Antimicrob Agents Chemother* **41**:2770–2772.

147. Nishino K, Yamaguchi A. 2001. Analysis of a complete library of putative drug transporter genes in *Escherichia coli*. *J Bacteriol* **183**:5803–5812.

148. Lomovskaya O, Lewis K. 1992. *Emr*, an *Escherichia coli* locus for multidrug resistance. *Proc Natl Acad Sci USA* **89**:8938–8942.

149. Davin-Regli A, Bolla JM, James CE, Lavigne JP, Chevalier J, Garnotel E, Molitor A, Pagès JM. 2008. Membrane permeability and regulation of drug "influx and efflux" in enterobacterial pathogens. *Curr Drug Targets* **9**:750–759.

150. Randall LP, Cooles SW, Coldham NG, Penuela EG, Mott AC, Woodward MJ, Piddock LJ, Webber MA. 2007. Commonly used farm disinfectants can select for mutant *Salmonella enterica* serovar Typhimurium with decreased susceptibility to biocides and antibiotics without compromising virulence. *J Antimicrob Chemother* **60**:1273–1280.

151. Webber MA, Randall LP, Cooles S, Woodward MJ, Piddock LJ. 2008. Triclosan resistance in *Salmonella enterica* serovar Typhimurium. *J Antimicrob Chemother* **62**:83–91.

152. Rajamohan G, Srinivasan VB, Gebreyes WA. 2010. Novel role of *Acinetobacter baumannii* RND efflux transporters in mediating decreased susceptibility to biocides. *J Antimicrob Chemother* **65**:228–232.

153. Piddock LJ. 2006. Clinically relevant chromosomally encoded multidrug resistance efflux pumps in bacteria. *Clin Microbiol Rev* **19**:382–402.

154. Noguchi N, Suwa J, Narui K, Sasatsu M, Ito T, Hiramatsu K, Song JH. 2005. Susceptibilities to antiseptic agents and distribution of antiseptic-resistance genes *qacA/B* and *smr* of methicillin-resistant *Staphylococcus aureus* isolated in Asia during 1998 and 1999. *J Med Microbiol* **54**:557–565.

155. Sánchez MB, Decorosi F, Viti C, Oggioni MR, Martínez JL, Hernández A. 2015. Predictive studies suggest that the risk for the selection of antibiotic resistance by biocides is likely low in *Stenotrophomonas maltophilia*. *PLoS One* **10**:e0132816.

156. Poole K. 2007. Efflux pumps as antimicrobial resistance mechanisms. *Ann Med* **39**:162–176.

157. Brown MH, Paulsen IT, Skurray RA. 1999. The multi-drug efflux protein NorM is a prototype of a new family of transporters. *Mol Microbiol* **31:**394–395.

158. Borges-Walmsley MI, Walmsley AR. 2001. The structure and function of drug pumps. *Trends Microbiol* **9:**71–79.

159. Poole K. 2001. Multidrug resistance in Gram-negative bacteria. *Curr Opin Microbiol* **4:**500–508.

160. Poole K. 2002. Outer membranes and efflux: the path to multidrug resistance in Gram-negative bacteria. *Curr Pharm Biotechnol* **3:**77–98.

161. Buffet-Bataillon S, Tattevin P, Maillard J-Y, Bonnaure-Mallet M, Jolivet-Gougeon A. 2016. Efflux pump induction by quaternary ammonium compounds and fluoroquinolone resistance in bacteria. *Future Microbiol* **11:**81–92.

162. Bailey AM, Constantinidou C, Ivens A, Garvey MI, Webber MA, Coldham N, Hobman JL, Wain J, Woodward MJ, Piddock LJ. 2009. Exposure of *Escherichia coli* and *Salmonella enterica* serovar Typhimurium to triclosan induces a species-specific response, including drug detoxification. *J Antimicrob Chemother* **64:**973–985.

163. Randall LP, Cooles SW, Coldham NG, Penuela EG, Mott AC, Woodward MJ, Piddock LJ, Webber MA. 2007. Commonly used farm disinfectants can select for mutant *Salmonella enterica* serovar Typhimurium with decreased susceptibility to biocides and antibiotics without compromising virulence. *J Antimicrob Chemother* **60:**1273–1280.

164. Webber MA, Randall LP, Cooles S, Woodward MJ, Piddock LJ. 2008. Triclosan resistance in *Salmonella enterica* serovar Typhimurium. *J Antimicrob Chemother* **62:**83–91.

165. Buckley AM, Webber MA, Cooles S, Randall LP, La Ragione RM, Woodward MJ, Piddock LJ. 2006. The AcrAB-TolC efflux system of *Salmonella enterica* serovar Typhimurium plays a role in pathogenesis. *Cell Microbiol* **8:**847–856.

166. Sánchez P, Moreno E, Martinez JL. 2005. The biocide triclosan selects *Stenotrophomonas maltophilia* mutants that overproduce the SmeDEF multidrug efflux pump. *Antimicrob Agents Chemother* **49:**781–782.

167. Pumbwe L, Randall LP, Woodward MJ, Piddock LJV. 2004. Expression of the efflux pump genes *cmeB*, *cmeF* and the porin gene *porA* in multiple-antibiotic-resistant *Campylobacter jejuni*. *J Antimicrob Chemother* **54:**341–347.

168. Demple B. 1996. Redox signaling and gene control in the *Escherichia coli* soxRS oxidative stress regulon: a review. *Gene* **179:**53–57.

169. Hutchinson J, Runge W, Mulvey M, Norris G, Yetman M, Valkova N, Villemur R, Lepine F. 2004. *Burkholderia cepacia* infections associated with intrinsically contaminated ultrasound gel: the role of microbial degradation of parabens. *Infect Control Hosp Epidemiol* **25:**291–296.

170. Valkova N, Lépine F, Valeanu L, Dupont M, Labrie L, Bisaillon JG, Beaudet R, Shareck F, Villemur R. 2001. Hydrolysis of 4-hydroxybenzoic acid esters (parabens) and their aerobic transformation into phenol by the resistant *Enterobacter cloacae* strain EM. *Appl Environ Microbiol* **67:**2404–2409.

171. Kümmerle N, Feucht HH, Kaulfers PM. 1996. Plasmid-mediated formaldehyde resistance in *Escherichia coli*: characterization of resistance gene. *Antimicrob Agents Chemother* **40:**2276–2279.

172. Gomez Escalada M, Russell AD, Maillard J-Y, Ochs D. 2005. Triclosan- bacteria interactions: single or multiple target sites? *Lett Appl Microbiol* **41:**476–481.

173. Wu VCH. 2008. A review of microbial injury and recovery methods in food. *Food Microbiol* **25:**735–744.

174. Lambert RJW, van der Ouderaa M-LH. 1999. An investigation into the differences between the Bioscreen and the traditional plate count disinfectant test methods. *J Appl Microbiol* **86:**689–694.

175. Brown MRW, Williams P. 1985. Influence of substrate limitation and growth phase on sensitivity to antimicrobial agents. *J Antimicrob Chemother* **15**(Suppl A):7–14.

176. Wright NE, Gilbert P. 1987. Influence of specific growth rate and nutrient limitation upon the sensitivity of *Escherichia coli* towards chlorhexidine diacetate. *J Appl Bacteriol* **62:**309–314.

177. Gomez Escalada M, Harwood JL, Maillard J-Y, Ochs D. 2005. Triclosan inhibition of fatty acid synthesis and its effect on growth of *E. coli* and *Ps. aeruginosa*. *J Antimicrob Chemother* **55:**879–882.

178. McMurry LM, Oethinger M, Levy SB. 1998. Triclosan targets lipid synthesis. *Nature* **394:**531–532.

179. Levy CW, Roujeinikova A, Sedelnikova S, Baker PJ, Stuitje AR, Slabas AR, Rice DW, Rafferty JB. 1999. Molecular basis of triclosan activity. *Nature* **398:**383–384.

180. Webber MA, Coldham NG, Woodward MJ, Piddock LJV. 2008. Proteomic analysis of triclosan resistance in *Salmonella enterica* serovar Typhimurium. *J Antimicrob Chemother* **62:**92–97.

181. Curiao T, Marchi E, Grandgirard D, León-Sampedro R, Viti C, Leib SL, Baquero F, Oggioni MR, Martinez JL, Coque TM. 2016. Multiple adaptive routes of *Salmonella enterica* Typhimurium to biocide and antibiotic exposure. *BMC Genomics* **17:**491.

182. Seaman PF, Ochs D, Day MJ. 2007. Small-colony variants: a novel mechanism for triclosan resistance in methicillin-resistant *Staphylococcus aureus*. *J Antimicrob Chemother* **59:**43–50.

183. Abdel-Malek SM, Al-Adham IS, Winder CL, Buultjens TE, Gartland KM, Collier PJ. 2002. Antimicrobial susceptibility changes and T-OMP shifts in pyrithione-passaged planktonic cultures of *Pseudomonas aeruginosa* PAO1. *J Appl Microbiol* **92:**729–736.

184. Parikh SL, Xiao G, Tonge PJ. 2000. Inhibition of InhA, the enoyl reductase from *Mycobacterium tuberculosis*, by triclosan and isoniazid. *Biochemistry* **39:**7645–7650.

185. Chen Y, Pi B, Zhou H, Yu Y, Li L. 2009. Triclosan resistance in clinical isolates of *Acinetobacter baumannii*. *J Med Microbiol* **58:**1086–1091.

186. Zhu L, Lin J, Ma J, Cronan JE, Wang H. 2010. Triclosan resistance of Pseudomonas aeruginosa PAO1 is due to FabV, a triclosan-resistant enoyl-acyl carrier protein reductase. *Antimicrob Agents Chemother* **54:** 689–698.

187. Heath RJ, Li J, Roland GE, Rock CO. 2000. Inhibition of the *Staphylococcus aureus* NADPH-dependent enoyl-acyl carrier protein reductase by triclosan and hexachlorophene. *J Biol Chem* **275:**4654–4659.

188. Slater-Radosti C, Van Aller G, Greenwood R, Nicholas R, Keller PM, DeWolf WE Jr, Fan F, Payne DJ, Jaworski DD. 2001. Biochemical and genetic characterization of the action of triclosan on *Staphylococcus aureus*. *J Antimicrob Chemother* **48:**1–6.

189. Massengo-Tiassé RP, Cronan JE. 2008. *Vibrio cholerae* FabV defines a new class of enoyl-acyl carrier protein reductase. *J Biol Chem* **283:**1308–1316.

190. Webber MA, Whitehead RN, Mount M, Loman NJ, Pallen MJ, Piddock LJV. 2015. Parallel evolutionary pathways to antibiotic resistance selected by biocide exposure. *J Antimicrob Chemother* **70:**2241–2248.

191. Roujeinikova A, Levy CW, Rowsell S, Sedelnikova S, Baker PJ, Minshull CA, Mistry A, Colls JG, Camble R, Stuitje AR, Slabas AR, Rafferty JB, Pauptit RA, Viner R, Rice DW. 1999. Crystallographic analysis of triclosan bound to enoyl reductase. *J Mol Biol* **294:**527–535.

192. Stewart MJ, Parikh S, Xiao G, Tonge PJ, Kisker C. 1999. Structural basis and mechanism of enoyl reductase inhibition by triclosan. *J Mol Biol* **290:**859–865.

193. Heath RJ, Rubin JR, Holland DR, Zhang E, Snow ME, Rock CO. 1999. Mechanism of triclosan inhibition of bacterial fatty acid synthesis. *J Biol Chem* **274:**11110–11114.

194. McCay PH, Ocampo-Sosa AA, Fleming GTA. 2010. Effect of subinhibitory concentrations of benzalkonium chloride on the competitiveness of *Pseudomonas aeruginosa* grown in continuous culture. *Microbiology* **156:** 30–38.

195. Casado Muñoz MC, Benomar N, Ennahar S, Horvatovich P, Lavilla Lerma L, Knapp CW, Gálvez A, Abriouel H. 2016. Comparative proteomic analysis of a potentially probiotic *Lactobacillus pentosus* MP-10 for the identification of key proteins involved in antibiotic resistance and biocide tolerance. *Int J Food Microbiol* **222:**8–15.

196. Casado Muñoz MC, Benomar N, Lavilla Lerma L, Knapp CW, Gálvez A, Abriouel H. 2016. Biocide tolerance, phenotypic and molecular response of lactic acid bacteria isolated from naturally-fermented Aloreña table to different physico-chemical stresses. *Food Microbiol* **60:**1–12.

197. Jang H-J, Chang MW, Toghrol F, Bentley WE. 2008. Microarray analysis of toxicogenomic effects of triclosan on *Staphylococcus aureus*. *Appl Microbiol Biotechnol* **78:**695–707.

198. Cerf O, Carpentier B, Sanders P. 2010. Tests for determining in-use concentrations of antibiotics and disinfectants are based on entirely different concepts: "resistance" has different meanings. *Int J Food Microbiol* **136:**247–254.

199. Russell AD, McDonnell G. 2000. Concentration: a major factor in studying biocidal action. *J Hosp Infect* **44:**1–3.

200. Koutsolioutsou A, Peña-Llopis S, Demple B. 2005. Constitutive *soxR* mutations contribute to multiple-antibiotic resistance in clinical *Escherichia coli* isolates. *Antimicrob Agents Chemother* **49:**2746–2752.

201. Mokgatla RM, Gouws PA, Brözel VS. 2002. Mechanisms contributing to hypochlorous acid resistance of a *Salmonella* isolate from a poultry-processing plant. *J Appl Microbiol* **92:**566–573.

202. Allen MJ, White GF, Morby AP. 2006. The response of *Escherichia coli* to exposure to the biocide polyhexamethylene biguanide. *Microbiology* **152:**989–1000.

203. Slade D, Radman M. 2011. Oxidative stress resistance in *Deinococcus radiodurans*. *Microbiol Mol Biol Rev* **75:**133–191.

204. Daniels C, Ramos JL. 2009. Adaptive drug resistance mediated by root-nodulation-cell division efflux pumps. *Clin Microbiol Infect* **15**(Suppl 1):32–36.

205. Maseda H, Hashida Y, Konaka R, Shirai A, Kourai H. 2009. Mutational upregulation of a resistance-nodulation-cell division-type multidrug efflux pump, SdeAB, upon exposure to a biocide, cetylpyridinium chloride, and antibiotic resistance in *Serratia marcescens*. *Antimicrob Agents Chemother* **53:**5230–5235.

206. Walsh C, Fanning S. 2008. Antimicrobial resistance in foodborne pathogens: a cause for concern? *Curr Drug Targets* **9:**808–815.

207. Li XZ, Nikaido H. 2009. Efflux-mediated drug resistance in bacteria: an update. *Drugs* **69:**1555–1623.

208. Oethinger M, Kern WV, Goldman JD, Levy SB. 1998. Association of organic solvent tolerance and fluoroquinolone resistance in clinical isolates of *Escherichia coli*. *J Antimicrob Chemother* **41:**111–114.

209. Pomposiello PJ, Bennik MH, Demple B. 2001. Genome-wide transcriptional profiling of the *Escherichia coli* responses to superoxide stress and sodium salicylate. *J Bacteriol* **183:**3890–3902.

210. Fraise AP. 2002. Biocide abuse and antimicrobial resistance: a cause for concern? *J Antimicrob Chemother* **49:** 11–12.

211. Langsrud S, Sidhu MS, Heir E, Holck AL. 2003. Bacterial disinfectant resistance: a challenge for the food industry. *Int Biodeter Biodegrad* **51:**283–290.

212. Braoudaki M, Hilton AC. 2004. Adaptive resistance to biocides in *Salmonella enterica* and *Escherichia coli* O157 and cross-resistance to antimicrobial agents. *J Clin Microbiol* **42:**73–78.

213. Braoudaki M, Hilton AC. 2004. Low level of cross-resistance between triclosan and antibiotics in *Escherichia coli* K-12 and *E. coli* O55 compared to *E. coli* O157. *FEMS Microbiol Lett* **235:**305–309.

214. Gilbert P, McBain AJ. 2003. Potential impact of increased use of biocides in consumer products on prevalence of antibiotic resistance. *Clin Microbiol Rev* **16:**189–208.

215. Russell AD. 2004. Bacterial adaptation and resistance to antiseptics, disinfectants and preservatives is not a new phenomenon. *J Hosp Infect* **57:**97–104.

216. **Alonso-Hernando A, Capita R, Prieto M, Alonso-Calleja C.** 2009. Comparison of antibiotic resistance patterns in *Listeria monocytogenes* and *Salmonella enterica* strains pre-exposed and exposed to poultry decontaminants. *Food Control* 20:1108–1111.

217. **Weber DJ, Rutala WA.** 2006. Use of germicides in the home and the healthcare setting: is there a relationship between germicide use and antibiotic resistance? *Infect Control Hosp Epidemiol* 27:1107–1119.

218. **Pumbwe L, Skilbeck CA, Wexler HM.** 2007. Induction of multiple antibiotic resistance in *Bacteroides fragilis* by benzene and benzene-derived active compounds of commonly used analgesics, antiseptics and cleaning agents. *J Antimicrob Chemother* 60:1288–1297.

219. **Lara HH, Ayala-Nunez NV, Turrent LDCI, Padilla CR.** 2010. Bactericidal effect of silver nanoparticles against multidrug-resistant bacteria. *World J Microbiol Biotechnol* 26:615–621.

220. **Peyrat MB, Soumet C, Maris P, Sanders P.** 2008. Phenotypes and genotypes of *Campylobacter* strains isolated after cleaning and disinfection in poultry slaughterhouses. *Vet Microbiol* 128:313–326.

221. **Gilbert P, McBain AJ, Bloomfield SF.** 2002. Biocide abuse and antimicrobial resistance: being clear about the issues. *J Antimicrob Chemother* 50:137–139, author reply 139–140.

222. **Lear JC, Maillard J-Y, Dettmar PW, Goddard PA, Russell AD.** 2006. Chloroxylenol- and triclosan-tolerant bacteria from industrial sources: susceptibility to antibiotics and other biocides. *Int Biodeter Biodegrad* 57:51–56.

223. **Knapp L, Amézquita A, McClure P, Stewart S, Maillard J-Y.** 2015. Development of a protocol for predicting bacterial resistance to microbicides. *Appl Environ Microbiol* 81:2652–2659.

224. **Sundheim G, Langsrud S, Heir E, Holck AL.** 1998. Bacterial resistance to disinfectants containing quaternary ammonium compounds. *Int Biodeter Biodegrad* 41:235–239.

225. **International Organization for Standardization.** 2006. ISO: 20776-1. Clinical laboratory testing and *in vitro* diagnostic test systems: susceptibility testing of infectious agents and evaluation of performance of antimicrobial susceptibility test devices. Part 1. Reference method for testing the *in vitro* activity of antimicrobial agents against rapidly growing aerobic bacteria involved in infectious diseases. British Standard Institute, London, United Kingdom.

226. **European Committee on Antimicrobial Susceptibility Testing (EUCAST).** 2014. Breakpoint tables for interpretation of MICs and zone diameters. Version 4.0. 2014. http://www.eucast.org/fileadmin/src/media/PDFs/EUCAST_files/Breakpoint_tables/v_6.0_Breakpoint_table.pdf. Accessed January 2017.

227. **Andrews JM, BSAC Working Party on Susceptibility Testing.** 2009. BSAC standardized disc susceptibility testing method (version 8). *J Antimicrob Chemother* 64:454–489.

228. **Saleh S, Haddadin RNS, Baillie S, Collier PJ.** 2011. Triclosan: an update. *Lett Appl Microbiol* 52:87–95.

229. **Gradel KO, Randall L, Sayers AR, Davies RH.** 2005. Possible associations between *Salmonella* persistence in poultry houses and resistance to commonly used disinfectants and a putative role of *mar*. *Vet Microbiol* 107:127–138.

230. **Chuanchuen R, Pathanasophon P, Khemtong S, Wannaprasat W, Padungtod P.** 2008. Susceptibilities to antimicrobials and disinfectants in *Salmonella* isolates obtained from poultry and swine in Thailand. *J Vet Med Sci* 70:595–601.

Antimicrobial Resistance in Bacteria from Livestock and Companion Animals
Edited by Frank Møller Aarestrup, Stefan Schwarz, Jianzhong Shen, and Lina Cavaco
© 2018 American Society for Microbiology, Washington, DC
doi:10.1128/microbiolspec.ARBA-0010-2017

Antimicrobial Resistance among Staphylococci of Animal Origin

7

Stefan Schwarz,[1] Andrea T. Feßler,[1] Igor Loncaric,[2] Congming Wu,[3]
Kristina Kadlec,[4] Yang Wang,[3] and Jianzhong Shen[3]

INTRODUCTION

During the past decades, several review articles and book chapters focused on the genetic basis of antimicrobial resistance in staphylococci. Some articles included staphylococci of human and animal origin (1–4), while others focused on either staphylococci of animal origin in general (5, 6) or on specific animal-associated staphylococci such as *Staphylococcus pseudintermedius* (7), bovine *Staphylococcus aureus*, porcine *Staphylococcus hyicus*, and canine *S. pseudintermedius* (8) or livestock-associated methicillin-resistant *S. aureus* (LA-MRSA) (9). As inhabitants of the skin or the mucosal surfaces, staphylococci of animal origin do not live in genetic isolation but are in close contact with a wide variety of other bacteria in the same animal host. Under such conditions and given a high bacterial density in the different compartments, genetic material can be exchanged not only between staphylococci in intraspecies and interspecies exchange events, but also between staphylococci and other Gram-positive bacteria in so-called intergenus exchange processes. Previous studies have shown that staphylococci can act either as donors or as recipients of resistance genes in these events (9). In addition, staphylococci may also be transferred to other animals or humans either by direct contact or by contact with excretions of the animals, e.g., by sneezing, coughing, or licking. Moreover, indirect transmission, e.g., via dust, aerosols, or a contaminated environment, may also play a role in the dissemination of staphylococci. A comparison of the resistance genes detected in human staphylococci and in animal staphylococci (6) revealed that both groups of staphylococci share a large number of resistance genes, whereas only comparatively small numbers of resistance genes have been found exclusively in either human or animal staphylococci (Fig. 1).

This article summarizes the latest information on resistance genes and resistance-mediating mutations detected in staphylococci of animal origin. It represents a completely revised and updated version of a review that we published in 2013 (6). Since different detection methods may give different results, preference is given to those genes for which nucleotide sequence data have been deposited in databases, i.e., the National Center for Biotechnology Information (NCBI) (https://www.ncbi.nlm.nih.gov/nuccore/) or the European Bioinformatics Institute (EMBL-EBI) (https://www.ebi.ac.uk/) (6, 10, 11). The data presented in this article focus on resistance genes and resistance-mediating mutations detected in staphylococci from healthy and diseased animals, whereas those found in staphylococci—in particular, methicillin-resistant *S. aureus* (MRSA)—from food of animal origin have been excluded because this was the topic of a recent review (12).

RESISTANCE TO β-LACTAM ANTIBIOTICS

Two resistance mechanisms mainly account for β-lactam resistance in staphylococci: (i) enzymatic inactivation by the *blaZ*- or *bla*$_{ARL}$-encoded β-lactamases and (ii) target site replacement by the gene products of the *mecA*, *mecB* (formerly *mecA*$_m$), or *mecC* (formerly *mecA*$_{LGA251}$) genes (Table 1).

The *blaZ-blaI-blaR1* operon was identified on transposon Tn*552* (13), which has been detected on plas-

[1]Institute of Microbiology and Epizootics, Centre of Infection Medicine, Department of Veterinary Medicine, Freie Universität Berlin, 14163 Berlin, Germany; [2]Institute of Microbiology, University of Veterinary Medicine, A-1210 Vienna, Austria; [3]Beijing Advanced Innovation Center for Food Nutrition and Human Health, College of Veterinary Medicine, China Agricultural University, Beijing, 100193, China; [4]Institute of Farm Animal Genetics, Friedrich-Loeffler-Institut, 31535 Neustadt-Mariensee, Germany.

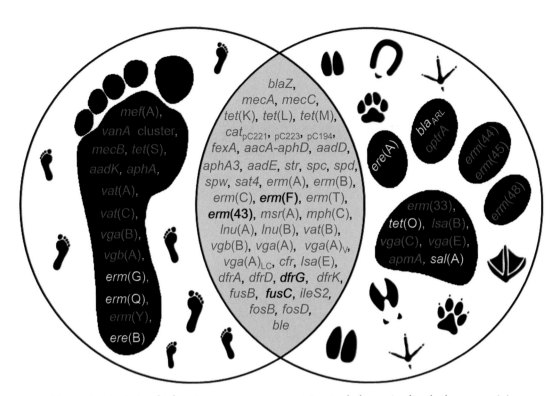

Figure 1 Antimicrobial resistance genes present in staphylococci of only human origin (left), only animal origin (right), and both origins (gray-shaded area in the middle). The genes depicted in red are associated with mobile genetic elements. Please see the text for the function of the different resistance genes. It should be noted that the tetracycline resistance genes *tet*(S) and *tet*(W), both coding for ribosome protective proteins, have recently been identified in staphylococci isolated from retail ground meat (284), and another *tet* gene, *tet*(38), coding for an efflux pump of the major facilitator superfamily, was identified in a *Staphylococcus* isolate of not further specified origin (285). For antimicrobial resistance genes present only in staphylococci of human origin, please see references 1–6.

mids as well as in the chromosomal DNA (1). The *blaZ*-encoded β-lactamase confers resistance to penicillins except isoxazolyl-penicillins. The *blaZ* gene has been detected in *S. aureus*, coagulase-negative staphylococci (CoNS), and *S. hyicus* from cases of bovine mastitis (14–18). The *blaZ* gene has also been described in *S. hyicus* isolates from pigs with exudative epidermitis (19). This gene was also present in *S. aureus* from zoo animals and wildlife (20). Moreover, the *blaZ* gene was also present in most MRSA and methicillin-susceptible (but penicillin/ampicillin-resistant) *S. aureus* from food-producing animals (21–30) and from various European wildlife species (31). Furthermore, the *blaZ* gene was present in staphylococci of canine and feline origin (32), including both methicillin-resistant and methicillin-susceptible *S. pseudintermedius* (33–36) (Table 2).

Whole-genome sequencing of the penicillin-resistant *Staphylococcus arlettae* strain SAN1670 from bovine mastitis milk led to the identification of a novel β-lactamase operon consisting of the β-lactamase-encoding

gene bla_{ARL}, the antirepressor-encoding gene $blaR1_{ARL}$, and the repressor-encoding gene $blaI_{ARL}$ (37). The functionality of bla_{ARL} was demonstrated by gene expression in *S. aureus*. The bla_{ARL} operon was located in the chromosomal DNA. It was detected in 10 additional unrelated strains, suggesting that it may be responsible for intrinsic penicillin resistance in *S. arlettae*. A GenBank search revealed more unique potential β-lactamases in *Staphylococcus* species (37).

The *mec* genes code for alternative penicillin-binding proteins with a strongly reduced affinity to virtually all β-lactam antibiotics, except some anti-MRSA cephalosporins, such as ceftobiprole and ceftaroline, which are approved only for use in human medicine. Staphylococci of animal origin expressing the *mecA* gene should be considered resistant to all β-lactam antibiotics approved for veterinary applications. Whether the same is true for isolates carrying *mecC* needs to be confirmed (6). The *mecA* and *mecC* genes are part of a mobile genetic island called the "staphylococcal cassette chromosome *mec*" (SCC*mec*). Currently, at least 13 major types of SCC*mec* elements plus various subtypes have been described in staphylococci (38–41).

Numerous studies have identified *mecA* genes as part of various SCC*mec* elements in staphylococci of animal origin, and several highly informative reviews have been published (42–50). Moreover, other studies focused on MRSA from pigs (21–23, 51–54), cattle (24, 55–62), sheep (27, 62), goats (62, 63), llamas and alpacas (62), poultry (28–30, 64, 65), horses (25, 66–68), and dogs and cats (69–73) but also from pet animals, including guinea pigs and rabbits and exotic animals such as turtles, parrots, and bats (70). Moreover, *mecA*-mediated methicillin resistance has become rather common in canine and feline *S. pseudintermedius* (34–36, 74–79). Hassler et al. (80) reported the presence of the *mecA* gene in an *S. hyicus* isolate. The *mecA* gene has also been detected in a number of methicillin-resistant CoNS from various animal species, e.g., cattle (81–83), pigs (81, 84, 85), chickens (81, 85, 86), turkeys (81), ducks (81, 85), a goose (81), horses (87–91), dogs and cats (89, 91, 92), as well as sheep and goats (81). In a convenience sample of *S. aureus* (*n* = 124) from European wildlife, six *mecA*-carrying isolates were recovered, one from a European brown hare and the remaining five from rooks (31) (Table 2). It should be noted that *Staphylococcus sciuri* and *Staphylococcus vitulinus* may carry *mecA* alleles that do not confer β-lactam resistance (93). Thus, the detection of *mecA* in isolates of these species should always be accompanied by phenotypic confirmation of oxacillin resistance.

The *mecC* gene was initially identified in *S. aureus* from humans and cattle (94, 95). Further screening for this gene identified it in *S. aureus* from cattle in France (96), goats in Austria (62), and a cat in Norway (97). A study from the United Kingdom identified it in *S. aureus* isolates from a dog, brown rats, a rabbit, a common seal, sheep, and a chaffinch (98, 99). In Germany, Walther et al. (100) identified it in *S. aureus* from cats, dogs, and a guinea pig. Screening of wildlife identified the *mecC* gene not only in MRSA from a European otter and a European brown hare, but also in a *Staphylococcus stepanovicii* from a Eurasian lynx (101). In another study of European wildlife (31), eight *mecC*-positive MRSA isolates were identified: two from European brown hares, four from hedgehogs, one from a red fox, and one from a fallow deer. In addition, *mecC*-carrying *S. aureus* isolates were also found in wood mice (102), red deer (103), white stork nestlings (104), and an Indian flying fox (20) (Table 2). Although identified in 2011, screening of strain collections revealed that the oldest *mecC*-carrying *S. aureus*

isolate dates back to 1975 (105). In recent years, two new *mecC* allotypes have been identified: *mecC1* in *Staphylococcus xylosus* from bovine mastitis (106) and *mecC2* in *Staphylococcus saprophyticus* from a common shrew (107).

Most recently, the *mecB* gene, originally designated *mecA*$_m$, which is part of a methicillin resistance gene complex often associated with transposon Tn*6045* in *Macrococcus caseolyticus*, has been detected on a multi-resistance plasmid in a human cefoxitin-resistant *S. aureus* isolate (108).

Moreover, reduced susceptibility to oxacillin was also observed in *mecA*- and *mecC*-negative *S. aureus* isolates from horses, but the resistance mechanism was not determined (68). Reasons for reduced susceptibility to oxacillin might be the overproduction of a β-lactamase, mutations in penicillin-binding proteins as described for *S. aureus* from human clinical cases (109), or decreased expression of *femA* and *femB* genes (110).

RESISTANCE TO TETRACYCLINES

In animal staphylococci, resistance to tetracyclines is often mediated by the genes *tet*(K) and *tet*(L), which code for membrane-associated efflux proteins of the major facilitator superfamily. In addition, the gene *tet*(M), which codes for a ribosome-protective protein, is also found frequently (Table 1) (111).

The Tet(K) and Tet(L) proteins exhibit 14 transmembrane domains and are composed of 459 and 458 amino acids (aa), respectively (111). The analysis of 228 tetracycline-resistant staphylococcal isolates from pigs, cattle, horses, dogs, cats, rabbits, guinea pigs, mink, turkeys, ducks, and pigeons identified the *tet*(K) gene in 110 isolates including 23 *S. hyicus*, 17 *S. xylosus*, 12 *Staphylococcus epidermidis*, 11 *Staphylococcus haemolyticus*, 11 *Staphylococcus lentus*, seven *Staphylococcus warneri*, six *S. sciuri*, six *S. aureus*, five *S. intermedius* group isolates, four *Staphylococcus simulans*, three *Staphylococcus hominis*, two *S. arlettae*, and single isolates of *Staphylococcus capitis*, *Staphylococcus chromogenes*, and *S. saprophyticus* (112). In addition, the *tet*(K) gene was found in combination with the gene *tet*(M) in eight *S. intermedius* group isolates and two *S. lentus* isolates. In contrast, the gene *tet*(L) was detected as the only *tet* gene in 14 isolates which comprised eight *S. sciuri*, two *S. aureus*, two *S. xylosus*, and single *S. lentus* and *S. hyicus* isolates. Furthermore, *tet*(L) was identified together with *tet*(M) in a single *S. aureus* and two *S. intermedius* group isolates but also together with *tet*(O) in a single *S. xylosus* isolate

Table 1 Resistance genes detected in staphylococci of animal origin[a]

Resistance to ...	Mechanism	Gene	Localization[b]	Mobile genetic element	Accession no. (or reference if there is no accession no.)
β-Lactams	Enzymatic inactivation (β-lactamase)	*blaZ*	Tn, P, C	Tn*552*	X52734
		bla$_{ARL}$	C	Unknown	KY363215
	Target site replacement (alternative penicillin binding proteins)	*mecA*	C	SCC*mec*	AB033763
		mecC (*mecA*$_{LGA251}$)	C	SCC*mec*	FR823292 FR821779
Tetracyclines (except minocycline and glycylcyclines)	Active efflux (major facilitator superfamily)	*tet*(K)	P	pT181	J01764.1 S67449
		tet(L)	P	pKKS25	FN390947
Tetracyclines (including minocycline but excluding glycylcyclines)	Target site protection (ribosome protective protein)	*tet*(M)	Tn, C	Tn*916*	M21136.1
		tet(O)	Unknown	Unknown	112
Nonfluorinated phenicols	Enzymatic inactivation (acetyltransferase)	*cat*$_{pC221}$	P	pC221	NC_006977
		cat$_{pC223}$	P	pC223	NC_005243
		cat$_{pC194}$	P	pC194	NC_002013
	Active efflux (major facilitator superfamily)	*fexA*$_V$	Tn, C	Tn*558*	HF679552
All phenicols	Active efflux (major facilitator superfamily)	*fexA*	Tn, P, C	Tn*558*	AM086211.1
Aminoglycosides (gentamicin, kanamycin, tobramycin, amikacin)	Enzymatic inactivation (acetyltransferase and phospotransferase)	*aacA-aphD*	Tn, P, C	Tn*4001*	GU565967
Aminoglycosides (kanamycin, neomycin, tobramycin)	Enzymatic inactivation (adenyltransferase)	*aadD*	P, C	pUB110 pKKS825	M37273.1 NC_013034.2
Aminoglycosides (kanamycin, neomycin, amikacin)	Enzymatic inactivation (phospotransferase)	*aphA3*	Tn, P, C	Tn*5405*	AB699882.1
Aminoglycosides (streptomycin)	Enzymatic inactivation (adenyltransferase)	*aadE*	Tn, P, C	Tn*5405*	AB699882.1
		str	P	pS194	NC_005564
Aminocyclitols (spectinomycin)	Enzymatic inactivation (adenyltransferase)	*spc*	Tn, P, C	Tn*554*	X03216.1
		spw	P, C	pV7037	JX560992.1
		spd	P	pDJ91S	KC895984
Aminocyclitols/aminoglycosides (apramycin, decreased susceptibility to gentamicin)	Enzymatic inactivation (acetyltransferase)	*apmA*	P	pAFS11 pKKS49	FN806789.3 HE611647.1
Streptothricins	Enzymatic inactivation (acetyltransferase)	*sat4*	Tn, P	Tn*5405*	AB699882.1
Macrolides. lincosamides, streptogramin B	Target site modification (rRNA methylase)	*erm*(A)	Tn, P, C	Tn*554*	X03216.1
		erm(B)	Tn, P	Tn*917*	FN806789.3
		erm(C)	P	pE194 pNE131	V01278.1 M12730.1
		erm(F)	Unknown	Unknown	164, 205
		erm(T)	P	pKKS25	FN390947.1
		erm(33)	P	pSCFS1	AJ313523
		erm(43)	C	Unknown	HE650138
		erm(44)	C	Prophage ΦJW4341	HG796218.2
		erm(44)$_v$	C	Unknown	KJ728533.1
		erm(45)	GI	Genomic island	LN680996.1
		erm(48)	P	pJW2311	LT223129

(Continued)

Table 1   *(Continued)*

Resistance to ...	Mechanism	Gene	Localization[b]	Mobile genetic element	Accession no. (or reference if there is no accession no.)
Macrolides, streptogramin B	Target site protection (ribosome protective ABC-F protein)	*msr*(A)	C, P	pMS97	NG_048001.1 AB013298.1
Macrolides	Enzymatic inactivation (phospotransferase)	*mph*(C)	C, P	pMS97	AB013298.1
	Enzymatic inactivation (esterase)	*ere*(A)	Unknown	Unknown	194
Lincosamides	Enzymatic inactivation (nucleotidyltransferase)	*lnu*(A)	P	pBMSa1	AY541446 JQ861958.1
		lnu(B)	P, C	pV7037	JX560992.1 JQ861959.1
	Target site protection (ribosome protective ABC-F protein)	*lsa*(B)	P	pSCFS1	KU510528.1
Streptogramin A	Enzymatic inactivation (acetyltransferase)	*vat*(B)	P	pIP1156	U19459.1
Streptogramin B	Enzymatic inactivation (hydrolase)	*vgb*(B)	P	pIP1714	AF015628.1
Lincosamides, pleuromutilines, streptogramin A	Target site protection (ribosome protective ABC-F protein)	*vga*(A)	Tn, P	Tn*5406*	M90056.1 FN806791.1
		vga(A)$_{LC}$	P	p131A	KX712120
		vga(A)$_V$	C	Unknown	AF186237
		vga(C)	P	pKKS825	NC_013034.2
		vga(E)	Tn	Tn*6133*	FR772051.1
		vga(E)$_v$	P	pSA-7	KF540226.1
		lsa(E)	P, C	pV7037	JX560992.1
		sal(A)	C	Unknown	KC693025.1
All phenicols, lincosamides, oxazolidinones, pleuromutilins, streptogramin A	Target site modification (rRNA methylase)	*cfr*	P, C	pSCFS1	AJ879565.1
Oxazolidinones, all phenicols	Target site protection (ribosome protective ABC-F protein)	*optrA*	P, C	pWo28-3	KT601170.1 KX447572.1
Trimethoprim	Target replacement (trimethoprim-resistant dihydrofolate reductase)	*dfrA* (*dfrS1*)	Tn, P, C	Tn*4003*	GU565967.1
		dfrD	C	Unknown	KX149097.1
		dfrG	C	Unknown	NG_047756.1
		dfrK	Tn, P, C	Tn*559*, pKKS2187	FN390947
Fusidic acid	Target site protection (ribosome protective protein)	*fusB*	P	p11819-97 pUB101	NC_017350.1 NC_005127.1
		fusC	P, C	SCC*mec*	HE980450.1
Mupirocin	Target replacement (mupirocin-insensitive isoleucyl-tRNA synthase)	*ileS2* (*mupA, ileS*)	P	pPR5	HQ625438.1
Bleomycin	Bleomycin binding protein	*ble*	P, C	pUB110	NC_001384.1
Fosfomycin	Fosfomycin thiol transferase	*fosB*	Unknown	Unknown	164
		fosD	P	pJP2	KC989517

[a]Modified from references 6 and 114.
[b]Tn (transposon), P (plasmid), C (chromosome).

Table 2 Examples of the distribution of resistance genes in staphylococci from different animals

Resistance genes	Bacterial species[a]	Animal host species (reference)
blaZ	*S. aureus*	Pig (21–23, 158, 177), cattle (14–17, 24, 55), sheep (27), horse (25, 68, 88), donkey (26), dog (32, 73), cat (32, 73), chicken (28–30), turkey (28, 226), European wildlife species (rook, red fox, marmot, mouflon, harbor porpoise, moose, badger, red deer, roe deer, wild boar, brown hare, vole) (31), naked mole rat (20), red squirrel (20), Eurasian lynx (20)
	SIG	Cat (32, 35, 79), dog (32–34, 36, 38, 79, 160)
	CoNS	Pig (147, 177), cattle (15, 17, 18), horse (88), dog (32), cat (147)
	S. hyicus	Pig (19, 147), cattle (18)
*bla*ₐᵣₗ	CoNS	Cattle (37)
mecA	*S. aureus*	Pig (21–23, 51–54, 150, 207, 218), cattle (24, 55–62, 163), sheep (27, 62), goat (62, 63), horse (25, 66–68, 74, 90), llama (62), alpaca (62), dog (70–74, 91, 196), cat (69, 70, 73, 74, 196), chicken (28–30, 64, 65), turkey (28, 227), guinea pig (70), rabbit (70), turtle (70), parrot (70), bat (70), European brown hare (31), rook (31), Eurasian lynx (20)
	SIG	Horse (74, 75), donkey (75), dog (34, 36, 74, 75, 78, 79, 92), cat (35, 38, 74–77, 79), parrot (75)
	CoNS	Pig (81, 84, 85, 218), cattle (81–83, 91, 211), sheep (81), goat (81), horse (87–91), dog (89, 91, 92), cat (91), chicken (81, 85, 86, 207), turkey (81), duck (81, 85), goose (81)
	S. hyicus	Pig (80)
mecC (*mecA*ₗ𝒈ₐ₂₅₁)	*S. aureus*	Cattle (94, 96), sheep (98), cat (97, 100), goat (62), dog (98, 100), brown rat (98), rabbit (98), common seal (98), chaffinch (98, 99), guinea pig (100), European otter (101), European brown hare (31, 101), hedgehog (31), red fox (31), fallow deer (31), wood mouse (102), red deer (103), white stork nestling (104), Indian flying fox (20)
	CoNS	Cattle (106), Eurasian lynx (101), common shrew (107)
tet(K)	*S. aureus*	Pig (21, 23, 160, 177), cattle (24, 112), sheep (27), horse (112), dog (73), cat (73, 112), chicken (28, 29), poultry (186), rabbit (112, 198), rook (31), harbor porpoise (31), wild boar (31), brown hare (31), naked mole rat (20)
	SIG	Dog (34, 36, 38, 78, 79, 117, 160), cat (35, 79)
	CoNS	Pig (118, 120, 147, 177), cattle (164, 211), horse (88, 112), dog (120), cat (112), turkey (112), poultry (186), duck (112), pigeon (112), bank vole (119), common shrew (119, 122), rabbit (112), guinea pig (112)
	S. hyicus	Pig (19, 112, 118, 147), poultry (186)
tet(L)	*S. aureus*	Pig (21, 123–126, 160, 161, 177, 207, 218), cattle (24), chicken (28, 29), turkey (28), white-face whistling duck (20)
	CoNS	Pig (118, 120, 128, 177, 218), cattle (164), dog (120), turkey (112), duck (112), guinea pig (112), rabbit (112), pigeon (112)
	S. hyicus	Pig (19, 23, 118, 147)
tet(M)	*S. aureus*	Pig (21, 22, 160, 177), cattle (24, 55), horse (25), donkey (26), dog (72, 73) chicken (28–30), turkey (28, 227), poultry (186)
	SIG	Dog (33, 34, 36, 38, 78, 79, 112), cat (35, 79, 112, 129), pigeon (112), mink (112)
	CoNS	Pig (118, 120, 177), cattle (164), horse (88), dog (120), cat (130), pigeon (112)
	S. hyicus	Pig (147)
tet(O)	SIG	Dog (112)
	CoNS	Mink (112)
*cat*ₚ𝒸₂₂₁	*S. aureus*	Cattle (135, 136), rook (31), red squirrel (20)
	SIG	dog (34, 36, 38, 79, 117, 138, 139), cat (35, 79)
	CoNS	cattle (144), horse (88, 142), dog (116, 143), mink (145)
	S. hyicus	Pig (140, 141)
*cat*ₚ𝒸₂₂₃	*S. aureus*	Cattle (136)
	CoNS	Horse (88), dog (146), mink (145)
*cat*ₚ𝒸₁₉₄	CoNS	Pig (147), dog (143)
*fexA*ᵥ	SIG	Dog (154)
fexA	*S. aureus*	Pig (21, 22, 150, 152, 207), cattle (24, 60), horse (152), marmot (31)
	SIG	Pig (151)

(Continued)

Table 2 *(Continued)*

Resistance genes	Bacterial species[a]	Animal host species (reference)
	CoNS	Pig (151, 153, 167), cattle (148, 152, 164); duck (167), chicken (167)
	S. hyicus	Pig (153)
aacA-aphD	*S. aureus*	Pig (21, 22, 160–162), cattle (24, 163), goat (62), alpaca (62), horse (25, 68, 88, 165), chicken (28, 29, 30), turkey (28), rook (31)
	SIG	Dog (34, 36, 78, 79, 160), cat (35, 79, 160)
	CoNS	Pig (86, 151, 167), cattle (164), horse (88), cat (166), chicken (85, 159, 167), duck (85, 167)
aadD	*S. aureus*	Pig (21, 22, 124), cattle (24, 55, 126), horse (25), dog (73), cat (73), turkey (28), chicken (29, 30) rook (31)
	CoNS	Pig (128), cattle (164), horse (88), duck (167) chicken (167), bird (169)
aphA3	*S. aureus*	Pig (22) cattle (24, 163), horse (25, 68), sheep (27), rook (31)
	SIG	Dog (34, 36, 38, 171), cat (35)
	CoNS	Cattle (164), horse (88)
aadE	*S. aureus*	Pig (161, 162, 207), sheep (27)
	SIG	Dog (34, 36, 38, 171), cat (35, 171)
	CoNS	Pig (169), cattle (164), horse (88)
	S. hyicus	Pig (19, 147)
str	*S. aureus*	Pig (23, 177)
	CoNS	Pig (169, 177), cattle (144), horse (88), dog (169, 208)
	S. hyicus	Pig (141, 176)
spc	*S. aureus*	Pig (21, 23, 207), cattle (24), chicken (28), turkey (28, 227)
	CoNS	Pig (147), cattle (164, 180), cat (147)
	S. hyicus	Pig (147)
spw	*S. aureus*	Pig (161, 181)
	S. hyicus	Pig (147)
spd	*S. aureus*	Pig (182, 183), cattle (182), horse (182), chicken (182, 183), rat (182)
	CoNS	Pig (147)
	S. hyicus	Pig (147)
apmA	*S. aureus*	Pig (184, 185), cattle (126, 164, 184), chicken (30)
	CoNS	Cattle (164)
sat4	*S. aureus*	Horse (25), rook (31)
	CoNS	Cattle (164), horse (88)
	SIG	Dog (34, 36, 38, 171), cat (171)
erm(A)	*S. aureus*	Pig (21–23, 160, 187), cattle (24, 55, 60), horse (25), donkey (26), dog (73), cat (73), dog/cat (187), chicken (28), turkey (28, 29, 227), poultry (186, 190), red fox (31)
	SIG	Dog (187, 188), cat (187), pigeon (189)
	CoNS	Cattle (164, 191), cat (147), poultry (186, 190)
	S. hyicus	Pig (19, 147, 187)
erm(B)	*S. aureus*	Pig (21, 161, 162, 187), cattle (24, 126, 194), dog (187, 188), cat (187), chicken (29), turkey (28, 227), poultry (190), brown hare (31)
	SIG	Dog (33, 34, 36, 38, 74, 79, 171, 172, 188), cat (35, 80, 171), dog/cat (187)
	CoNS	Pig (85, 167), cattle (164, 193, 194), horses (88), chicken (85, 167), poultry (190), turkey (191), duck (85, 167), poultry (190), mink (192)
	S. hyicus	Pig (19, 147, 187, 188)
erm(C)	*S. aureus*	Pig (21–23, 89, 187), cattle (24, 55, 194, 195) horse (25, 68), donkey (26) dog (72, 196), cat (196), dog/cat (187), sheep (27), goat (62), chicken (28–30, 197), turkey (28), poultry (186, 190), rabbits (195, 198), wild boar (31)
	SIG	Dog (78, 117, 188), carrier pigeon (195)
	CoNS	Pig (147, 191, 195), cattle (164, 193, 194), sheep (195), horse (88, 195), dogs (195, 203), cat (195), chicken (85, 167, 195), turkey (191), poultry (190), carrier pigeon (195, 204), bank vole (201), rodents/insectivores (202), parrot (195), guinea pig (195)
	S. hyicus	Pig (19, 147, 187, 195, 199, 200)

(Continued)

Table 2 *(Continued)*

Resistance genes	Bacterial species[a]	Animal host species (reference)
erm(F)	SIG	Dog (205)
	CoNS	Cattle (164), not further specified animal (205)
erm(T)	*S. aureus*	Pig (126), cattle (24), chicken (28–30), turkey (28)
	CoNS	Cattle (164)
erm(33)	*S. aureus*	Pig (207)
	CoNS	Cattle (180, 206)
erm(43)	CoNS	Dog (208), chicken (208)
erm(44)	CoNS	Cattle (209)
erm(45)	CoNS	Cattle (211)
erm(48)	CoNS	Cattle (212)
msr(A)	*S. aureus*	Cattle (194), horse (68), dog/cat (187), poultry (190)
	SIG	Dog/cat (187)
	CoNS	Pig (191), cattle (164, 191, 193, 194), turkey (191), rodents/insectivores (202)
	S. hyicus	Cattle (194)
mph(C)	*S. aureus*	Cattle (194), horse (68), dog/cat (187)
	CoNS	Pig (191), cattle (164, 191, 193, 194, 209), sheep (208), horse (88), turkey (191), chicken (208), rodents/insectivores (202)
ere(A)	*S. aureus*	Cattle (194)
	CoNS	Cattle (194)
lnu(A)	*S. aureus*	Pig (22, 218, 219), cattle (55, 193, 195, 217), turkey (28)
	SIG	Dog (34)
	CoNS	Pig (218), cattle (164, 194, 220)
	S. hyicus	Pig (187), cattle (194)
lnu(B)	*S. aureus*	Pig (161, 162, 207)
	S. hyicus	Pig (147)
lsa(B)	CoNS	Pig (153), cattle (180)
vat(B)	CoNS	Poultry (186)
vgb(B)	CoNS	Poultry (186)
vga(A) + variants	*S. aureus*	Pig (21, 23, 207, 219, 228), cattle (24, 194), dog (73), cat (219, 232), chicken (29), turkey (28)
[*vga*(A)$_V$, *vga*	CoNS	Cattle (164, 194, 230)
(A)$_{LC}$]	*S. hyicus*	Pig (147)
vga(C)	*S. aureus*	Pig (124, 228), cattle (24)
	S. hyicus	Pig (147)
vga(E)	*S. aureus*	Pig (226), cattle (227), turkey (28, 227)
vga(E)$_v$	CoNS	Pig (231)
lsa(E)	*S. aureus*	Pig (161, 162, 207), cattle (230),
	CoNS	cattle (230), dog (232)
	S. hyicus	Pig (147)
sal(A)	CoNS	Cattle (230), cat (232), dog (232)
cfr	*S. aureus*	Pig (22, 150–152, 207, 241), cattle (60), horse (152), marmot (31)
	CoNS	Pig (85, 151, 153, 167), cattle (83, 152, 164, 180, 234), chicken (85, 167), duck (85, 167)
	S. hyicus	Pig (153)
optrA	CoNS	Pig (241–244)
dfrA (*dfrS1*)	*S. aureus*	Pig (22) horse (25, 68, 88), dog (73), rook (31)
	CoNS	Cattle (163), horse (88)
dfrD	*S. aureus*	Pig (22)
	CoNS	Cattle (163), horse (88)
dfrG	*S. aureus*	Pig (21–23, 177), horse (68)
	SIG	Dog (34, 36, 38, 79), cat (35, 79)
	CoNS	Pig (177), cattle (164)

(Continued)

Table 2   *(Continued)*

Resistance genes	Bacterial species[a]	Animal host species (reference)
dfrK	S. aureus	Pig (21, 22, 123–126, 218, 245), cattle (24), horse (68), chicken (28–30), turkey (28)
	CoNS	Cattle (164)
	S. hyicus	Pig (185)
fusB	S. aureus	Sheep (27)
	CoNS	Cattle (164, 248)
fusC	S. aureus	Donkey (26)
	SIG	Dog (33)
ileS2 (mupA, ileS)	SIG	Dog (254, 255)
fosB	S. aureus	Horse (25), dog (73), cat (73), European wildlife species (brown hare, gray partridge, red fox, marmot, mouflon, wild boar, harbor porpoise, rook, moose, badger, red deer, roe deer, chamois, mute swan, red kite, green woodpecker, common magpie, great tit, whitetailed eagle, tawny owl, golden eagle, bank vole, wild cat) (31)
	CoNS	Cattle (164)
fosD	CoNS	Duck (167)

[a]SIG, *Staphylococcus intermedius* group; CoNS, coagulase-negative staphylococci.

(112). In addition, the *tet*(K) gene has also been identified in methicillin-susceptible *S. aureus* (MSSA) from chickens (28), turkeys (28), and a naked mole rat (20) (Table 2).

The genes *tet*(K) and *tet*(L) are often located on plasmids. The *tet*(K)-carrying plasmids usually display a structure similar to the 4.4-kb plasmid pT181 (113, 114) and rarely carry additional resistance genes. Such plasmids have been identified in staphylococci of animal origin including coagulase-positive (*S. aureus, S. intermedius/pseudintermedius*), coagulase-variable (*S. hyicus*), and various CoNS (e.g., *Staphylococcus cohnii, S. epidermidis, Staphylococcus equorum, S. haemolyticus, S. saprophyticus, S. sciuri, S. warneri,* and *S. xylosus*) (112, 115–120). The small *tet*(K)-carrying plasmid pT181 can be integrated via IS*431* into the J1 region of SCC*mec* elements commonly found in LA-MRSA (40, 121) or via IS*257* into larger plasmids (114). The 6,913-bp plasmid pSTE2 from *S. lentus* obtained from a common shrew harbors *tet*(K) and the macrolide-lincosamide-streptogramin B (MLS$_B$) resistance gene *erm*(C) (122). Detailed structural analysis suggested that plasmid pSTE2 developed from pT181- and pPV141-like ancestor plasmids by cointegrate formation at the staphylococcal recombination site RS$_A$ (122). Plasmids that carry the *tet*(L) gene have been found among *S. aureus* (in particular, among LA-MRSA ST398) (21, 24, 123–126), *S. hyicus,* and CoNS, such as *S. epidermidis, S. lentus, S. sciuri,* and *S. xylosus,* of animal origin (112, 118) (Table 3). In contrast to *tet*(K)-carrying plasmids, those carrying *tet*(L) range in size between 5.5 and >40 kb and often harbor one or more additional resistance genes (114, 118, 124–128).

In addition, tetracycline resistance via *tet*(M) is also commonly observed in staphylococci of animal origin, whereas *tet*(O) genes have been detected very rarely in staphylococci (112). The *tet*(M) genes are commonly located on conjugative transposons of enterococcal origin, such as Tn*916* or Tn*1545* (111). The *tet*(M) and *tet*(O) gene products represent ribosome protective proteins which mediate resistance to all tetracyclines, including minocycline (Table 1). The analysis of the aforementioned 228 tetracycline-resistant staphylococci obtained from diverse animal sources identified *tet*(M) genes as the sole *tet* genes in 89 *S. intermedius* group isolates (112). Further studies confirmed that tetracycline resistance in *S. intermedius/S. pseudintermedius* was almost exclusively based on the presence of a *tet*(M) gene (7, 34, 35, 79, 112, 129). The *tet*(M) gene was also present in MSSA from chickens and turkeys (28–30). The *tet*(O) gene has so far only been detected in a single *S. pseudintermedius* isolate and in combination with a *tet*(L) gene in a single *S. xylosus* isolate (112). Studies of LA-MRSA from pigs, cattle, and chickens and ducks showed that such strains—regardless of their origin—often carried the genes *tet*(M), *tet*(K), and *tet*(L) in various combinations with two or all three *tet* genes being present in the same isolate (21, 22, 24, 28–30) (Table 2). While *tet*(M) genes are commonly found in the chromosomal DNA of staphylococci, a plasmid-borne *tet*(M) gene as part of a largely truncated Tn*916* was identified on the 28,743-bp multiresistance plasmid pSWS47 from a feline *S. epidermidis* ST5 isolate (130) (Table 3)

In a recent study (108), a *tet*(S) gene, also coding for a ribosome-protective protein, was identified on a multiresistance plasmid in a human clinical *mecB*-carrying *S. aureus* isolate.

RESISTANCE TO PHENICOLS

Resistance to nonfluorinated (e.g., chloramphenicol) or fluorinated (e.g., florfenicol) phenicols among animal staphylococci is mediated by (i) enzymatic inactivation via chloramphenicol acetyltransferases, (ii) active efflux via exporters of the major facilitator superfamily, (iii) target site modification via the rRNA methylase Cfr (131), or (iv) ribosome protection by the ABC-F protein OptrA.

So far, three types of chloramphenicol acetyltransferases have been identified among staphylococci (Table 1) (3, 114, 131). The corresponding *cat* genes have been named according to the plasmids on which they were first identified: *cat*$_{pC221}$, *cat*$_{pC223}$, and *cat*$_{pC194}$ (132–135). These *cat* genes code for Cat monomers of 215, 215, and 216 aa, respectively, which form the trimeric mature Cat enzyme (131). In staphylococci of animal origin, the *cat*$_{pC221}$ gene has been detected on a wide variety of plasmids in bovine *S. aureus* (136, 137), canine *S. pseudintermedius* (34, 36, 38, 79, 117, 138, 139), porcine *S. hyicus* (140, 141), canine *S. epidermidis* (116), equine (88, 142), canine (143), and bovine *S. sciuri* (144), and mink *S. lentus* (145). Plasmids that carry a *cat*$_{pC223}$ gene have been detected only in bovine *S. aureus* (136), canine *S. haemolyticus* (146), equine *S. xylosus* (88), and mink *S. lentus* (145). In staphylo-

cocci from animals, a *cat*$_{pC194}$-like gene has so far been identified on plasmid pSCS34 from a canine *S. sciuri* isolate (143) and in a porcine *S. equorum* isolate (147) (Table 2). It should be noted that all three chloramphenicol acetyltransferases confer resistance to only nonfluorinated phenicols.

In contrast, the 475-aa FexA protein of the major facilitator superfamily, which consists of 14 transmembrane domains, exports not only nonfluorinated phenicols, but also fluorinated phenicols such as florfenicol (Table 1) (148). The *fexA* gene is located on transposon Tn558 and was first identified in a bovine *S. lentus* isolate (149). This transposon can be located on plasmids (including multiresistance plasmids) (Table 3) and in the chromosomal DNA. The *fexA* gene has also been detected in MRSA from pigs (21, 22, 150–152), cattle (24, 60), and a horse (152) and in *S. aureus* from a marmot (31). This gene has also been identified in various CoNS species including bovine *S. chromogenes*, *S. simulans*, and *S. sciuri* (152) and porcine *S. arlettae*, *S. cohnii*, *S. epidermidis*, *S. equorum*, *S. haemolyticus*, *S. hominis*, *S. hyicus* *S. lentus*, *S. pseudintermedius*, *S. saprophyticus*, *S. sciuri*, *S. simulans*, *S. warneri*, and *S. xylosus* (151–153) (Table 2). A *fexA* variant, *fexA*$_V$, which conferred only chloramphenicol, but not florfenicol, resistance was detected in a canine *S. pseudintermedius* isolate from Spain. The FexA$_V$ protein exhibited two amino acid substitutions, Gly33Ala and Ala37Val, both of which seem to be important for substrate recognition. Site-directed mutagenesis that

Table 3 Examples for multiresistance plasmids among staphylococci from animals

Plasmid	Bacterial species	Host species	Size (kb)	Antimicrobial resistance genes	Other resistance genes	Accession no	Reference
pWo28-3	S. sciuri	Pig	60.563	*optrA*, *cfr*, *fexA*, *ble*, *aacA-aphD*, *aadD*		KT601170.1	241
pJP2	S. rostri	Duck	~50	*erm*(B), *aacA-aphD*, *fosD*, *ble*, *aadD*, *fexA*, *cfr*		KC989517.1	167
pAFS11	S. aureus	Cattle	49.192	*aadD*, *erm*(B), *tet*(L), *dfrK*, *apmA*	*cadD*, *cadX*, *mco*, *copA*	FN806789.3	126
pSCFS6	S. warneri	Pig	~43	*lsa*(B), *cfr*, *fexA*		AM408573.1	153
pV7037	S. aureus	Pig	40.971	*aacA-aphD*, *erm*(B), *tet*(L), *aadE*, *spw*, *lsa*(E), *lnu*(B), Δ*blaZ*	*cadD*, *cadX*	JX560992.1, HF586889.1	161, 162
pSS-01	S. cohnii	Pig	~40	*aacA-aphD*, *fexA*, *cfr*		JF834909.1	151
pJP1-like	S. lentus	Chicken	~40	*aacA-aphD*, *ble*, *aadD*, *fexA*, *cfr*		KF129408	167
pSWS47	S. epidermidis	Cat	28.743	*vga*(A), *aadD*, *tet*(L), *dfrK*, *tet*(M), *blaZ*		HG380319.1	130
pUR1902	S. aureus	Pig	~22	*erm*(T), *tet*(L), *aadD*	*cadD*, *cadX*, *mco*, *copA*	HF583291.1	271
pSCFS1	S. sciuri	Cattle	17.108	*cfr*, *lsa*(B), *erm*(33), *spc*		NC_005076.1	180
pKKS825	S. aureus	Pig	14.365	*aadD*, *tet*(L), *dfrK*, *vga*(C)		FN377602.2	124
pMSA16	S. aureus	Cattle	7.054	*cfr*, *erm*(A)		JQ246438.1	60
pSTS7	S. epidermidis	Pig	~5.5	*tet*(L), *aadD*, *ble*		U35229.1	128

reverted the mutated base pairs to those present in the original *fexA* gene restored the chloramphenicol/florfenicol resistance phenotype (154).

Phenicol resistance may also be based on target site modification via the methylase Cfr or on ribosomal protection via the ABC-F protein OptrA. For more on this, please see the section on resistance to oxazolidinones.

RESISTANCE TO AMINOGLYCOSIDES

Resistance to aminoglycosides is based on a number of inactivating enzymes which differ in their specific substrate spectra (Table 1) (155). In staphylococci of animal origin, the following genes for aminoglycoside-modifying enzymes have been detected so far.

The gene *aacA-aphD* [also known as *aac(6′)-Ie–aph(2″)-Ia*] codes for a bifunctional enzyme of 479 aa that shows acetyltransferase and phosphotransferase activity and confers resistance to gentamicin, kanamycin, tobramycin and—when overexpressed—amikacin (156, 157). This gene is located on transposon Tn*4001*, which consists of a central resistance gene region that is bracketed by two IS*256* elements located in opposite orientations (158). Detailed analysis of *aacA-aphD*-carrying plasmids in avian CoNS isolates, including *S. warneri* and *S. sciuri*, identified truncated Tn*4001* elements in which the terminal IS*256* sequences were in part deleted by the insertion of complete or incomplete copies of IS*257* (159). The *aacA-aphD* gene is widespread in staphylococci of animal origin, including canine and feline *S. pseudintermedius* (34–36, 78, 79, 160), *S. aureus* (mostly MRSA) from pigs (21–23, 160–162), cattle (24, 163, 164), a goat and an alpaca (62), horses (25, 68, 88, 165), chickens and turkeys (28–30), and rooks (31) but also CoNS from dogs (166), pigs (85, 151, 167), poultry (85, 159, 167), and horses (88) (Table 2).

The gene *aadD* [also known as *ant(4′)-Ia*] codes for the 256-aa adenyltransferase, which confers resistance to kanamycin, neomycin, and tobramycin. This gene was initially identified on plasmid pUB110 (168), which is also often integrated in type II SCC*mec* elements. In animal staphylococci, it has been detected—often on plasmids—in LA-MRSA/MSSA from pigs (21, 22, 124), cattle (24, 55), turkeys (28), chickens (29, 30), horses (25), and rooks (31). It has also been identified among CoNS from animals, e.g., in an avian *S. sciuri* isolate (169) and a porcine *S. epidermidis* isolate (128) (Table 2).

The gene *aphA3* [also known as *aph(3′)-IIIa*] codes for a phosphotransferase of 264 aa, which mediates resistance to kanamycin, neomycin, and amikacin (170, 171). In animal staphylococci, this gene was found mainly in canine and feline *S. pseudintermedius* (34–36, 171, 172)

but also in MRSA from pigs (22), cattle (24, 163), sheep (27), horses (25, 68), and rooks (31) (Table 2).

The gene *aadE* [also known as *ant(6)-Ia*] encodes a 302-aa adenyltransferase, which confers streptomycin resistance. Both genes, *aadE* and *aphA3*, together with the streptothricin resistance gene *sat4* are part of transposon Tn*5405* (170). The *aadE* gene seems to be the predominant streptomycin resistance gene in canine and feline *S. pseudintermedius* (34–36, 171). It was also detected in porcine *S. hyicus* (19) and *S. sciuri* (169). The *aadE* gene is also part of multiresistance gene clusters of enterococcal origin found in porcine MRSA ST9 and CC398 (147, 161, 162, 173, 174) and porcine *S. hyicus* (147) (Table 2).

The gene *str* [also known as *aad(6)*] encodes a 282-aa adenyltransferase (175), which mediates streptomycin resistance. Among staphylococci of animal origin, this gene has been identified in porcine MRSA (23), canine and porcine *S. sciuri* (169), in porcine *S. hyicus* (141, 176), in porcine *S. aureus* and *S. rostri* (177), and in bovine *S. sciuri* (144) (Table 2).

RESISTANCE TO AMINOCYCLITOLS

Two aminocyclitol antibiotics, spectinomycin and apramycin, are used in veterinary medicine. Spectinomycin resistance in staphylococci is based on adenyltransferases encoded by the genes *spc*, *spw*, and *spd*, whereas a single gene, *apmA*, has been described so far to code for apramycin resistance in staphylococci.

The gene *spc* [also known as *aad(9)-Ia*] encodes a 260-aa adenyltransferase (Table 1) (178). The gene *spc* is part of the transposon Tn*554* and as such is often found in combination with the also Tn*554*-associated MLS$_B$ resistance gene *erm*(A). A PCR assay for the detection of the physical linkage between these two genes has been developed and applied (24, 179). The gene *spc* has been detected in MRSA from pigs (21, 23), cattle (24), and chickens and turkeys (28). Among CoNS, it was identified on a multiresistance plasmid from bovine *S. sciuri* (180) and in feline *S. simulans* (147). Moreover, it was also detected in a single porcine *S. hyicus* isolate (147).

The gene *spw* codes for an adenyltransferase of 269 aa. It was found as part of a multiresistance gene cluster in MRSA ST398 and ST9 isolates from pigs and chickens (161, 162, 174, 181). The Spw protein had only 64.7% identity to the Tn*554*-associated Spc protein (181). In 2014, a third spectinomycin resistance gene, designated *spd*, was detected (182). The Spd protein codes for an adenyltransferase of 259 aa that shared only 45% sequence identity with the Spw protein. The *spd* gene was initially detected in MRSA ST398 from humans and various animal species (182) and soon thereafter, also in porcine MSSA ST433 (183). Further studies of *S. hyicus* and CoNS from animals identified a variant of the gene *spd* on small plasmids in porcine *S. hyicus*, *S. chromogenes*, and *S. equorum* (147). This gene variant had a 12-bp deletion in the terminal part of the *spd* gene, which, however, had no impact on the high spectinomycin MIC conferred by the gene (147) (Table 2).

The gene *apmA* is the first and so far only apramycin resistance gene in staphylococci (Table 1). It codes for a 274-aa acetyltransferase which confers resistance to apramycin and decreased susceptibility to gentamicin (184). It was detected on large multiresistance plasmids in bovine, porcine, and avian LA-MRSA of CC398 (30, 184) or, in a single case, on a small plasmid that conferred only apramycin resistance in a porcine LA-MRSA of CC398 (185). Argudín and coworkers also found the *apmA* gene in a *S. lentus* isolate from a veal calf (164). Recently, the complete sequence of the *apmA*-carrying plasmid pAFS11 was published and showed that this plasmid carried several antimicrobial resistance genes in combination with cadmium and copper resistance genes and a novel *ica*-like gene cluster (126) (Table 3).

RESISTANCE TO STREPTOTHRICINS

Resistance against streptothricins is mediated by the gene *sat4*, which codes for a 176-aa acetyltransferase protein (Table 1) (170). The *sat4* gene is also part of Tn*5405* and, as such, is commonly detected in staphylococci that also harbor *aphA3* and *aadE*. In staphylococci of animal origin, this gene has been detected in canine and feline *S. pseudintermedius* (34–36, 38, 171, 172), in MRSA CC8 (ST254) from horses in Germany (25), and in MRSA CC1 from rooks in Austria (31). Moreover, it has also been detected in CoNS of bovine (164) and equine origin (88) (Table 2).

RESISTANCE TO MACROLIDES, LINCOSAMIDES, AND STREPTOGRAMINS

Resistance to macrolides, lincosamides, and streptogramins is based on a variety of genes that code for different resistance mechanisms with diverse substrate spectra (Table 1).

Combined Resistance to MLS$_B$

According to the nomenclature center for macrolide, lincosamide, and streptogramin resistance genes (http://

faculty.washington.edu/marilynr/ermweb4.pdf), MLS$_B$ resistance in staphylococci of animal origin is based on the presence of one or more *erm* genes of the classes A, B, C, F, T, 33, 43, 44, 45 and 48 (Table 1). These genes code for methylases that modify the target site A2058 in 23S rRNA and thereby inhibit the binding of MLS$_B$ compounds to the bacterial ribosome.

Of the *erm* genes that have been detected in staphylococci of animal origin, *erm*(A) and *erm*(B) are associated with transposons Tn*554* and Tn*917*/Tn*551*, respectively. Tn*554* has also been frequently found to be integrated into SCC*mec* type II elements. The *erm*(A) gene was found in *S. aureus* (mostly MRSA) from various animal species (21, 22–25, 28, 29, 31, 159, 186, 187) but also in *S. pseudintermedius* from dogs (187, 188) and a pigeon (189). In addition, the *erm*(A) gene was also found in porcine *S. hyicus* (19, 145), feline *S. simulans* (147), bovine *S. equorum*, *S. lentus*, and *S. sciuri* (164), and novobiocin-resistant CoNS from poultry (186). Nawaz and coworkers detected the *erm*(A) gene in all 24 poultry-associated *Staphylococcus* isolates investigated (190). Jaglic et al. identified the gene *erm*(A) in a not further specified CoNS isolate from cattle (191) (Table 2).

The *erm*(B) gene is the most predominant *erm* gene in canine and feline *S. pseudintermedius* (33–36, 38, 78, 171, 172, 187, 188). In addition, the *erm*(B) gene was present in canine *S. aureus* as well as porcine *S. aureus* and *S. hyicus* (19, 21, 147, 161, 162, 187, 188). Moreover, the *erm*(B) gene has also been detected in LA-MRSA from pigs (21), cattle (24), chickens and turkeys (28, 29), and a brown hare (31). It was also found on small plasmids in an *S. lentus* isolate from a mink (192) and in various CoNS from pigs (151). *erm*(B) was also present in *Staphylococcus* spp. from poultry (190). Jaglic et al. detected the gene *erm*(B) in not further specified CoNS isolates from turkeys (191). The *erm*(B) gene was also found in CoNS from pigs (85, 167), cattle (164, 193, 194), horses (88), and chickens and ducks (85, 167) (Table 2).

The gene *erm*(C) is commonly located on small plasmids ranging in size from 2.3 to 4.4 kb that do not carry additional resistance genes. Such plasmids have been identified in *S. aureus* (including MRSA) from pigs (21–23, 89, 187), cattle (24, 55, 194, 195), horses (25), dogs and cats (72, 187, 196), sheep (27), goats (62), poultry (28–30, 186, 190, 197), rabbits (195, 198), and a wild boar (31). The *erm*(C) gene has rarely been detected in canine *S. pseudintermedius* (78, 117, 188) and in avian *S. intermedius* (195), whereas it has been detected in *S. hyicus* (199, 200) and in a wide variety of CoNS, including *S. saprophyticus* and *S. lentus* from rodents and insectivores (201, 202), canine *S. epidermidis* (195, 203), equine *S. xylosus*, porcine *S. haemolyticus* and *S. equorum*, feline *S. warneri*, ovine *S. sciuri*, *Staphylococcus gallinarum* from a chicken, *S. hominis* from a parrot, *S. capitis* from a guinea pig, and *S. lentus* from carrier pigeons (195, 204). Jaglic and coworkers found the gene *erm*(C) in not further specified CoNS isolates from turkeys and pigs (191) (Table 2).

During a study of the host range of the gene *erm*(F) in bacteria of human and animal origin, this methylase gene was detected in isolates of the *S. intermedius* group but also in CoNS of animal origin, such as *S. haemolyticus*, *S. lentus*, and *S. sciuri* (205). The *erm*(F) gene has also been identified in *S. sciuri* isolates from veal calves (164).

The gene *erm*(T) is often found on large multiresistance plasmids and was first identified in staphylococci in 2010 in a porcine MRSA CC398 isolate (125). Since then, it has been identified in MRSA from cattle (24) and chickens and turkeys (28–30). In most cases, the *erm*(T) gene was plasmid-borne and the corresponding plasmids harbored additional resistance genes (Table 3). The *erm*(T) gene has also been detected in bovine CoNS (164) (Table 2).

The gene *erm*(33) is an *in vivo* recombination product between *erm*(A) and *erm*(C) and has been detected on a the multiresistance plasmid pSCFS1 from bovine *S. sciuri* (180, 206). The *erm*(33) gene has also been detected in porcine MRSA ST9 and ST63 isolates from China (207). The gene *erm*(43) has been detected in the chromosomal DNA of *S. lentus* isolates of human, dog, and chicken origin (208). The gene *erm*(44) was found to be associated with a prophage. It was detected in the chromosomal DNA of an *S. xylosus* isolate from bovine mastitis (209). The *erm*(44) gene and a novel *erm*(44) variant, which showed only 84% aa identity, were found in *S. xylosus* and *S. saprophyticus*, respectively, from aquatic environments (210). The gene *erm*(45) was detected in a genomic island in a *Staphylococcus fleurettii* isolate from bovine milk (211) (Table 2). The gene *erm*(48) was identified by whole-genome sequencing of a *S. xylosus* isolate from bovine mastitis milk. It was located on the nonconjugative 49,273-bp plasmid pJW2311, which also carried the macrolide resistance genes *mph*(C) and *msr*(A) (212).

Combined Resistance to Macrolides and Streptogramin B

The *msr*(A) gene codes for a 488-aa ABC-F protein which confers resistance to macrolides and streptogramin B antibiotics (Table 1) (213). ABC-F proteins

are neither fused to transmembrane domains nor are they genetically linked to genes that code for transmembrane proteins in operon structures. Experimental evidence has been published that ABC-F proteins involved in antimicrobial resistance act by protecting the ribosomes from the inhibitory effects of the antimicrobial agents rather than by exporting the respective antimicrobial agents from the bacterial cell (214). The *msr*(A) gene has been detected in *S. aureus* isolates of poultry (190), cattle (194), horse (68), and dog/cat origin (187), in canine *S. pseudintermedius* (187), and in various species of CoNS from pigs (191), cattle (164, 191, 194), turkeys (191), and rodents and insectivores (202). This gene was also found in bovine *S. hyicus* (194) (Table 2).

Resistance to Macrolides Only

The gene *mph*(C) codes for a macrolide phosphotransferase of 299 aa which confers only resistance to macrolides (Table 1) (88, 202, 215). However, it should be noted that *mph*(C) is often linked to *msr*(A) and that the Mph(C) phosphotransferase alone confers only low-level resistance to macrolides (193). The *mph*(C) gene has been detected in a canine *S. aureus* isolate (187). Moreover, *mph*(C) was also detected in CoNS from pigs (191), horses (88), cattle (164, 191, 193, 194, 209), sheep (208), chickens (208), turkeys (191), and rodents and insectivores (202). It should be noted that *mph*(C) gene variants, whose gene products do not confer macrolide resistance, have been identified in *S. lentus*, *S. sciuri*, and *S. cohnii* from animal sources (202) (Table 2).

The gene *ere*(A) codes for a macrolide esterase that confers resistance to macrolides. This gene was identified in *S. aureus* and in CoNS, including *S. chromogenes*, *S. haemolyticus*, *S. epidermidis*, and *S. hyicus*, all from cases of bovine mastitis (194).

Resistance to Lincosamides Only

The gene *lnu*(A) encodes a lincosamide nucleotidyltransferase of 161 aa (Table 1) (216). This gene is often located on small plasmids. The *lnu*(A) gene was identified in *S. aureus*, including MRSA from dairy cattle (217), pigs (22, 218, 219), and a turkey (28) and a methicillin-resistant canine *S. pseudintermedius* isolate (34) but also from various CoNS species, including *S. epidermidis*, *S. chromogenes*, *S. simulans*, *S. haemolyticus*, *S. warneri*, *S. sciuri*, and *S. equorum* of bovine origin (164, 193, 195, 220) and a methicillin-resistant *S. sciuri* isolate of porcine origin (218). Moreover, the *lnu*(A) gene was also detected in porcine and bovine *S. hyicus* isolates (187, 194) (Table 2).

The gene *lnu*(B) codes for a lincosamide nucleotidyl-transferase of 267 aa (Table 1) and usually occurs in the genera *Streptococcus* and *Enterococcus* (187). Recently, it has been detected as part of multiresistance gene clusters on a plasmid as well as in the chromosomal DNA of porcine and avian MRSA ST9 isolates from China (161, 162, 173, 174) and porcine *S. hyicus* (147) (Table 2).

The gene *lnu*(E) was originally found in porcine *Streptococcus suis* but was shown to be functionally active after cloning and expression in *S. aureus*. This gene confers only low-level resistance to lincomycin (221).

The plasmid-borne *lsa*(B) gene encodes a 492-aa ABC-F protein which has been reported to confer decreased susceptibility to lincosamides (180, 214) (Table 1). This gene has also been detected in a bovine *S. sciuri* isolate and porcine *S. simulans* and *S. warneri* isolates (153, 180).

Resistance to Streptogramin A Only

Inactivation of streptogramin A antibiotics in staphylococci is mediated by *vat*(A), *vat*(B), or *vat*(C) genes, which code for acetyltransferases of 219, 212, or 212 aa, respectively (3). Among them, only the *vat*(B) gene has been identified in two *S. xylosus* isolates of poultry origin (Table 1) (186). It should be noted that resistance to streptogramin A can also be mediated by *vga*, *lsa* and *sal* genes; for more on this, please see the section on pleuromutilin resistance (Table 2).

Resistance to Streptogramin B Only

The genes *vgb*(A) and *vgb*(B) code for streptogramin B lyases, also known as streptogramin B lactonases or steptogramin B lactone hydrolases, of 299 and 295 aa, respectively (3, 222). The two *vat*(B)-positive *S. xylosus* isolates from poultry also carried a *vgb*(B) gene (186) (Tables 1 and 2).

RESISTANCE TO PLEUROMUTILINS

The ABC-F proteins specified by the genes *vga*(A), *vga*(A)$_{LC}$, *vga*(B), *vga*(C), and *vga*(E) exhibit sizes of 522, 522, 552, 522, and 524 aa, respectively (124, 223–229). All of them mediate resistance to streptogramin A antibiotics, whereas the Vga(C) and Vga(E) proteins as well as certain Vga(A) proteins also confer resistance to lincosamides and pleuromutilins (Table 1) (124, 219, 224–229) by protecting the ribosomes from the inhibitory effects of the corresponding antimicrobial agents (214). In staphylococci of animal origin, *vga*(A) gene variants have been identified not only in *S. aureus* (mostly MRSA) from pigs (21, 23, 228), cat-

tle (24), and chickens and turkeys (28, 29), but also in CoNS from cattle (164, 194, 230) and *S. hyicus* from pigs (147). Moreover, the gene *vga*(C) was detected in MRSA from pigs (125, 228) and cattle (24) as well as in porcine *S. hyicus* (147), whereas the gene *vga*(E) was identified in MRSA from pigs (226), cattle (227), and chickens and turkeys (28, 227). A novel variant of the *vga*(E) gene, which codes for an ABC-F protein of 524 aa, was found on the same 5,585-bp plasmid in independent porcine *S. cohnii* and *S. simulans* isolates (231). The variant gene shared 85.7% nucleotide sequence identity with the original *vga*(E) gene, and the variant protein shared 85.3% amino acid sequence identity with the original Vga(E) protein (Table 2).

The *lsa*(E) gene, which also mediates combined resistance to pleuromutilins, lincosamides, and streptogramin A, has been detected in MRSA from pigs and poultry (161, 162, 173, 207), MRSA from cattle (230), CoNS from cattle (230) and dogs (232), and *S. hyicus* from pigs (147). This gene codes for an ABC-F protein of 494 aa. The *lsa*(E) gene, together with the genes *lnu*(B), *aadE*, and *spw*, forms the core component of a multiresistance gene cluster which most likely originates from *Enterococcus faecalis* (173) (Table 2).

The gene *sal*(A), originally described as a lincosamide-streptogramin A resistance gene (233), has also been shown to confer pleuromutilin resistance (230). This gene codes for an ABC-F protein of 541 aa which is only distantly related to the Vga and Lsa proteins.

A survey of pleuromutilin resistance genes among bovine MRSA and CoNS identified two *S. haemolyticus* and single *S. xylosus*, *S. lentus*, and *S. hominis* isolates as *vga*(A)-positive. Twelve *S. aureus*, two *S. warneri*, and single *S. lentus* and *S. xylosus* isolates carried the *lsa*(E) gene. Moreover, single *S. aureus*, *S. haemolyticus*, *S. xylosus*, and *S. epidermidis* isolates were positive for both genes, *vga*(A) and *lsa*(E). The *sal*(A) gene was found in one *S. sciuri* isolate (230). Although the *sal*(A) gene was believed to be restricted to *S. sciuri*, a recent study of pleuromutilin resistance genes among staphylococci from pets identified the *sal*(A) gene not only in the chromosomal DNA of feline and canine *S. sciuri*, but also in a feline *S. haemolyticus* and in canine *S. epidermidis* and *S. xylosus* isolates (232). Moreover, that study identified the *lsa*(E) gene in a novel variant of the aforementioned multiresistance gene cluster in a canine *S. epidermidis* isolate and a *vga*(A)$_{LC}$ gene on a plasmid in a feline *S. haemolyticus* isolate (232).

Pleuromutilin resistance can also be conferred by the methyltransferase Cfr; for more on this, see the following section on resistance to oxazolidinones.

RESISTANCE TO OXAZOLIDINONES

Oxazolidinones are not approved for veterinary use but may be used in non-food-producing animals via the Animal Medicinal Drug Use Clarification Act of 1994 in the United States or similar regulations in other countries. Only two transferable oxazolidinone resistance genes, *cfr* and *optrA*, are currently known to occur in staphylococci of animal origin.

The gene *cfr* was initially identified on a multiresistance plasmid in a bovine *S. sciuri* isolate (234). It codes for an rRNA methylase of 349 aa, which methylates the adenine at position 2503 in the 23S rRNA (235). Because this adenine residue is located in the overlapping binding region of phenicols, lincosamides, oxazolidinones, pleuromutilins, and streptogramin A antibiotics, methylation of A2503 interferes with the binding and correct positioning of these antimicrobial agents. Thus, Cfr confers a penta-resistance phenotype which includes the aforementioned classes of antimicrobial agents (Table 1) (236). Because oxazolidinones are last-resort antimicrobial agents in human medicine and the gene *cfr* confers transferable oxazolidinone resistance, there is growing interest in the dissemination of this gene (237–239).

In staphylococci of animal origin, the *cfr* gene has been detected in *S. aureus* (including MRSA) from pigs (22, 150–152, 207), cattle (60), a horse (152), and a marmot (31) and in porcine *S. hyicus* (153). The CoNS species in which *cfr* was detected include bovine *S. lentus, S. simulans,* and *S. sciuri* (83, 152, 234), porcine *S. arlettae, S. cohnii, S. haemolyticus, S. hyicus, S. lentus, S. saprophyticus, S. sciuri, S. simulans,* and *S. warneri* (85, 150–153), chicken *S. cohnii, S. lentus,* and *S. sciuri*; and duck *S. arlettae, S. rostri,* and *S. sciuri* (85, 167) (Table 2). Although the *cfr* gene is most often located on plasmids in staphylococci (239) (Table 3), it has also been detected to be integrated via insertion sequences into a SCC*mec* cassette in a porcine ST9 MRSA isolate (207).

The *optrA* gene codes for an ABC-F protein of 655 aa, which mediates resistance not only to the oxazolidinones linezolid and tedizolid, but also to fluorinated and nonfluorinated phenicols (240). This gene was recently identified in enterococci from humans and animals (240). Soon thereafter, the *optrA* gene was detected on plasmids and in the chromosomal DNA of porcine, canine, and feline *S. sciuri* isolates (241–244). These plasmids harbored additional resistance genes which may favor coselection and persistence of *optrA* (241–244). Most recently, the *optrA* gene was detected in *S. simulans* from household pigs in rural China (244) (Table 2).

RESISTANCE TO TRIMETHOPRIM

Resistance to trimethoprim is based on any of the four genes *dfrA* (also known as *dfrS1*), *dfrD, dfrG,* and *dfrK* (9), which code for trimethoprim-resistant dihydrofolate reductases of 161, 166, 165, and 163 aa, respectively (Table 1).

The Tn*4003*-associated gene *dfrA* is most widespread among staphylococci from humans (1). In staphylococci of animal origin, it has rarely been found. There are few reports about its occurrence in *S. aureus* (mostly MRSA) from pigs (22), horses (25, 68, 88), dogs (73), and rooks (31). The gene *dfrD* has been detected even more rarely in animal staphylococci. There is only a single report, which describes its occurrence together with *dfrA* in a single porcine MRSA isolate (22). The genes *dfrA* and *dfrD* have also been found in CoNS from cattle (164) and horses (88). In contrast, the gene *dfrG* seems to be the predominant *dfr* gene in canine and feline *S. pseudintermedius* (34–36, 79). It has also been detected in MRSA (21–23), MSSA (177), and the coagulase-negative *S. rostri* (177), all from pigs, but also in bovine CoNS (164). The gene *dfrK* was initially found on multiresistance plasmids from porcine MRSA ST398, where it was linked to the tetracycline resistance gene *tet*(L) (124–126) (Table 3). Later, the *dfrK* gene was also identified as part of the transposon Tn*559* in a porcine MSSA CC398 isolate (245). PCR assays have been developed and applied to differentiate between its linkage with *tet*(L) and its location within Tn*559* (24, 179). The *dfrK* gene has been found not only in MRSA from pigs (21–23), cattle (24), horses (68), and chickens and turkeys (28–30), but also in a porcine *S. hyicus* isolate (185) and in CoNS from cattle (164) (Table 2).

RESISTANCE TO FUSIDIC ACID

Resistance to fusidic acid is based on the expression of the genes *fusB* (*far1*) and *fusC,* which code for cytoplasmatic proteins of 213 and 212 aa (246) or on single point mutations in the *fusA* gene (Table 1). It has been shown that the FusB protein binds to the staphylococcal elongation factor G (EF-G) and thereby protects the translation system from inhibition by fusidic acid (247). Fusidic acid resistance in animal staphylococci has rarely been detected. The *fusB* gene has been found in MRSA isolates from sheep (27) and in single isolates of *S. epidermidis, S. haemolyticus,* and *S. hominis* from cattle (164, 248). Few reports describe the presence of *fusC* in *S. aureus* from donkeys (26) and in canine *S. pseudintermedius* (33) (Table 2). Loeffler et al. identified six MRSA isolates from cats and dogs with high MICs of fusidic acid (≥ 512 mg/liter), but no information is available about the corresponding resistance genes (249).

RESISTANCE TO MUPIROCIN

Resistance to mupirocin in staphylococci is commonly due to a mupirocin-insensitive isoleucyl-tRNA synthase of 1,024 aa, encoded by the gene *ileS2*, also known as *ileS* or *mupA* (Table 1) (250, 251). Although a small number of mupirocin-resistant MRSA/MSSA isolates from dogs have been reported (252, 253), no information about the corresponding resistance genes is available. In 2013, the *ileS2* gene was identified in a canine *S. pseudintermedius* isolate (254), where it was located together with the aminoglycoside resistance gene *aacA-aphD* on a conjugative plasmid. In another study, only 1 of 581 *S. pseudintermedius* isolates was resistant to mupirocin and also carried the high-level mupirocin resistance gene *ileS2* on a plasmid (255) (Table 2).

FLUOROQUINOLONE RESISTANCE

Fluoroquinolone resistance in staphylococci is mainly based on mutations that resulted in amino acid substitutions in the quinolone-resistance-determining regions of the topoisomerase genes *gyrA*, *gyrB*, *grlA*, and *grlB*. Such mutations have been described in *S. pseudintermedius* (7, 38). A few studies reported such mutations in naturally occurring *S. aureus* from animals and food of animal origin (256–258). A detailed description of the known mutations in *S. aureus* from animals is given in reference 4. So far, no plasmid-mediated quinolone resistance genes have been detected in staphylococci.

RIFAMPICIN RESISTANCE

Rifampicin interacts with the β subunit of the bacterial RNA polymerase encoded by the *rpoB* gene. While numerous mutations in the *rpoB* gene have been detected in clinical *S. aureus* isolates from humans and laboratory strains, little information is currently available about rifampicin-resistance-mediating mutations in staphylococci from animals (258). Within the *rpoB* gene of porcine MRSA ST9, mutations were found at the following positions: Asp471Tyr, Ala473Glu, His481Asn, and Ser529Leu (258). It became apparent that not all mutations had the same effect on the rifampicin MICs and that occasionally isolates with two or three *rpoB* mutations exhibited higher MICs than isolates with a single *rpoB* mutation (258). A detailed description of the known rifampicin-resistance-mediating mutations

in *S. aureus* from animals is given in reference 4. Another study identified *rpoB* mutations in multidrug-resistant *S. pseudintermedius* isolates from dogs (259). In that study, single mutations were detected at positions Gln513Leu, Ala522Asp, His526Arg, His5256Pro, His526Tyr, and Ser531Leu, whereas double mutations included the positions Ser508Asn + Ser509Pro and Ser509Pro + Asp516Asn (259).

MISCELLANEOUS RESISTANCE PROPERTIES

Resistance to bleomycin encoded by the gene *ble* is commonly associated with the aminoglycoside resistance gene *aadD* (168). Both *aadD* and *ble* are located on small plasmids of the type pUB110, which are also integrated into certain types of SCC*mec* cassettes (39) and into larger plasmids (3, 114).

In contrast to the situation in humans, fully vancomycin-resistant staphylococci have so far not been isolated from animals. However, porcine MRSA ST9 isolates from China which displayed reduced vancomycin susceptibility (260) and porcine vancomycin-intermediate MRSA ST398/t9538 isolates from Brazil (261) have been described.

Sulfonamide resistance is known to occur in staphylococci (1, 4). However, in contrast to *Enterobacteriaceae*, no specific sulfonamide resistance genes have been identified in staphylococci so far. In contrast, sulphonamide resistance is believed to result from (i) mutations in the dihydropteroate synthase genes, which change the affinity of the corresponding enzymes to sulfonamides, (ii) overexpression of sulfonamide-susceptible dihydropteroate synthase genes, or (iii) increased production of *p*-aminobenzoic acid (1).

Fosfomycin resistance in staphylococci was found to be encoded by the gene *fosD*, which codes for a 139-aa fosfomycin thiol transferase. This gene was detected on a ca. 50-kb multiresistance plasmid of a *S. rostri* isolate of duck origin. This plasmid also harbored the resistance genes *erm*(B), *aacA-aphD*, *cfr*, *ble*, *aadD*, and *fexA* (169). The fosfomycin resistance gene *fosB* was detected in an *S. epidermidis* isolate from a veal calf (163) and in *S. aureus* from horses (25), dogs (73), cats (73), and European wildlife species (31) (Table 2).

Resistance to heavy metals in staphylococci has been known of for more than 30 years (1). A review on metal resistance (262) provides additional information. Witte et al. (263) investigated *S. aureus* of human and animal origin for its resistance to mercury and cadmium. Mercury resistance was detected in human isolates, but the isolates from cattle, pigs, chicken, and sheep were classified as susceptible. In comparison, cadmium resistance was detected among isolates from humans and cattle. An analysis of 32 porcine and 20 bovine *S. hyicus* isolates revealed that cadmium resistance was present in 28 and 16 isolates, respectively (264). However, there was no information on the genetic basis of the cadmium resistance. In 2010, Aarestrup et al. (265) found a correlation between methicillin resistance and decreased susceptibility to zinc in porcine LA-MRSA CC398, and subsequently Cavaco et al. (266) identified the cadmium and zinc resistance gene *czrC* within the type V SCC*mec* element. When the *czrC* gene was cloned and transferred in *S. aureus* RN4220, it conferred a 4-fold increase of the zinc chloride MIC and an 8-fold increase of the cadmium MIC (267). The strong correlation of the presence of the *czrC* gene with MRSA CC398 was confirmed when testing porcine and bovine MRSA and MSSA isolates from 10 European countries, Canada, and China (267). In 2011, novel SCC*mec* elements were described to occur in MRSA CC398, which carried numerous metal resistance genes, including *cadDX* (cadmium resistance), *arsRBC* and *arsDARBC* (arsenic resistance), *copB* (copper resistance), and *czrC* (cadmium/zinc resistance) (268). Moreover, resistance to heavy metals was seen among LA-MRSA, and the resistance genes *arsA*, *cadD*, *copB*, and *czrC* were identified (269). In another study, 130 methicillin-resistant CoNS from pigs and veal calves were investigated for the presence of metal resistance genes, and almost half of the isolates carried metal resistance genes (*czrC* 5.4%, *copB* 38.5%, *cadD* 7.7%, *arsA* 26.2%), regardless of their SCC*mec* type (270). Cadmium and copper resistance genes were also detected on multiresistance plasmids from Spanish porcine MRSA isolates. They harbored the functional *cadD*/*cadX* cadmium resistance operon and/or the multicopper oxidase gene *mco* and the ATPase copper transport gene *copA* on plasmids that also carried the antimicrobial resistance genes *aadD* and/or *erm*(T) and *tet*(L) (271). A novel multiresistance plasmid from bovine MRSA ST398 that harbored the antimicrobial resistance genes *aadD*, *tet*(L), *dfrK*, *erm*(B), and *apmA* together with a novel biofilm gene cluster and the metal resistance operons *cadD*/*cadX* and *copA*/*mco* was recently sequenced (126). These examples show that metal resistance and antimicrobial resistance can easily be coselected. In this regard, it is important to know that the increased use of metals in livestock animals, especially zinc in pigs, may coselect for methicillin resistance in staphylococci.

Resistance to biocides is also detected frequently among staphylococci. The reader is referred elsewhere for a review (272) that provides detailed information

on the mechanisms of biocide resistance and the genes involved. In staphylococci of animal origin, *qac* genes that confer resistance to quaternary ammonium compounds were identified in staphylococci from cattle (*qacA/B*, *smr*, *qacG*, and *qacJ*) and goats (*qacA/B* and *smr*). In many cases, these genes were located on plasmids (273). Another study identified the genes *qacC/D* among 3/86 non-CC398 MRSA isolates originating from pigs (269). The resistance genes *qacG* and *qacC* were identified in 3/79 and 1/79 porcine CC30 *S. aureus* isolates, respectively (274). A study from Portugal identified the biocide resistance genes *qacG* and *qacJ* in 13/74 and 1/74 MRSA CC398 isolates from pigs, respectively, while 4/74 MRSA isolates (3 CC5 from dogs and humans and 1 CC22 from a dog) had insertions in the −10 motif of the *norA* promoter (275). Slifierz et al. found that MRSA from pigs with benzalkonium MICs of ≥2 mg/liter carried at least one of the biocide resistance genes *qacG*, *qacH*, *qacA/B*, and *smr*, with about one-third of the isolates harboring the combination *qacG*-*qacH*-*smr* (276). A study of methicillin-resistant staphylococci from horses identified *S. haemolyticus* and *S. cohnii* subsp. *cohnii* isolates that carried plasmid-borne *qacA* and *sh-fabI* or *qacB* and *qacH*-like genes, respectively (277).

Resistance to antimicrobial peptides has rarely been investigated in staphylococci of animal origin. A study of the *in vitro* activity of human and animal cathelicidins against LA-MRSA revealed that none of the 14 most common antimicrobial resistance genes affected the antimicrobial activity of the cathelicidins (278). In a follow-up study, MICs of *S. aureus* field isolates for the cathelicidins LL-37, mCRAMP, CAP18, BMAP-27, and BMAP-28 in the presence and absence of different efflux pump inhibitors were determined (279). After blocking resistance-nodulation-cell division-type efflux pumps with 1-(1-naphthylmethyl)-piperazine, the MICs for CAP18, but not those for the other cathelicidins tested, were significantly decreased. In good correlation with these data, significantly decreased MICs for CAP18 and BMAP-27 were observed for SecDF knockout mutants. In addition, the MIC values increased again after reintroducing a cloned *secDF* via plasmid complementation. These results indicated involvement of SecDF in reduced efficacy of species-specific cathelicidins against *S. aureus* (279).

RESISTANCE DATA OF ANIMAL STAPHYLOCOCCI

Percentages of resistant staphylococci are presented in numerous publications. However, as described elsewhere (280), the results are only comparable when the same antimicrobial susceptibility testing methodology and the same interpretive criteria are used. Moreover, the most reliable results are obtained if the tested isolates were obtained following a defined sampling plan that secures sufficient numbers of isolates and avoids the inclusion of multiple members of the same bacterial clone. As such, the most reliable results are obtained from national monitoring programs. A survey of national monitoring programs in the veterinary sector, however, revealed that staphylococci of animal origin are only rarely part of national monitoring programs (281). Table 4 presents data obtained from the Swedish SVARM (282) and the German Germ-Vet (283) programs. Both programs followed the standards for broth microdilution of the Clinical and Laboratory Standards Institute (CLSI) and CLSI-approved clinical breakpoints for the evaluation of the results. As can be seen from this example, striking differences were seen for the different staphylococcal species from infections of the different animal species. This observation emphasizes the need for detailed analyses that include the staphylococcal species, the animal host, and the site of infection.

CONCLUSIONS AND PERSPECTIVES

The data presented in this chapter show that staphylococci from animals harbor a wide range of resistance genes and resistance-mediating mutations. For most resistance properties, several resistance genes, which account for the same resistance trait, such as the various *erm*, *tet*, or *cat* genes, have been detected in staphylococci. Moreover, staphylococci of animal origin have been shown to simultaneously carry two or three resistance genes that specify the same resistance phenotype. Examples are the carriage of the *tet*(M), *tet*(K), and *tet*(L) genes or the *erm*(A), *erm*(B), *erm*(C), or *erm*(T) genes in various combinations in LA-MRSA from pigs, cattle, and poultry (21, 24, 28–30). Since one of these genes is sufficient to confer tetracycline or MLS$_B$ resistance, respectively, the simultaneous presence of two or three of these *tet* or *erm* genes may be explained by their acquisition at different times and their location on plasmids that carry other resistance genes.

The analysis of the resistance genes present in animal staphylococci has also identified genes that confer resistance to antimicrobial agents, such as florfenicol or apramycin, that are approved for the treatment of infections in livestock other than those caused by staphylococci. However, it needs to be understood that the applied antimicrobial agents not only target the causa-

tive agents of an infection, but also put the physiological microbiota in the respective body compartments under selective pressure. As a consequence, staphylococci which live as commensals on the skin or the mucosal surfaces may also acquire resistance genes that allow their survival in the presence of antimicrobial agents such as florfenicol and apramycin. The observation that florfenicol resistance genes such as *fexA* and *cfr* have been detected as the only phenicol resistance genes among MRSA from cattle and pigs might reflect the use of florfenicol for the control of respiratory tract infections in these animal species.

This observation also showed that the use of antimicrobial agents adds to the presence of antimicrobial resistance genes in animal staphylococci. However, there is no linear correlation between antimicrobial use and the presence of resistance properties or resistance genes. In this regard, coselection and persistence of resistance genes in the absence of a direct selective pressure need to be taken into account, especially since many mobile genetic elements carry more than a single antimicrobial resistance gene (1–6) (Table 3). In this regard, genes that confer resistance to heavy metals or disinfectants and that are located on the same multiresistance plasmid or SCC*mec* cassette, may also contribute to the coselection process. Thus, measures such as the ban or the limitation of use of certain antimicrobial agents do not necessarily result in a decrease or loss of resistance properties/genes. To make an educated guess about what to expect from such measures, it is indispensable to know which resistance genes are physically linked to other resistance genes or are part of resistance gene clusters that are commonly cotransferred (Table 3). Hence, detailed analyses of multiresistance plasmids or multiresistance gene clusters in staphylococci further our understanding of processes such as coselection and persistence of resistance.

Finally, the data presented in this article has shown that staphylococci of animal origin do not exist in genetic isolation. Instead, they share resistance genes with staphylococci of human origin but also with other bacteria, such as *Bacillus* spp., *Enterococcus* spp., *Streptococcus* spp., *Lactococcus* spp., and *Lactobacillus* spp. Database searches revealed that some of the resistance genes found in staphylococci of animal origin, such as *aacA-aphD*, *erm*(B), and *tet*(M) are widespread among Gram-positive bacteria, while others, such as *apmA*, *erm*(33), *erm*(43), *lsa*(B), *vga*(C), *vga*(E), and *vgb*(B) have not yet been detected in bacteria other than staphylococci.

In summary, coagulase-positive, -variable, and -negative staphylococci of animal origin harbor a wide

Table 4 Resistance rates to selected antimicrobial agents among staphylococci of animal origin

Antimicrobial agent	Staphylococcal species	Origin	Year	Isolates tested	Resistant isolates (%)	Country	Reference
Penicillin	*S. aureus*	Horses – skin infection	2016	75	15 (20.0)	Sweden	282
	S. schleiferi	Dogs – various infections	2016	163	3 (1.8)	Sweden	282
	S. felis	Cats – various infections	2016	277	39 (14.1)	Sweden	282
	S. aureus	Poultry – various infections	2014	35	23 (65.7)	Germany	283
	SIG[c]	Dogs – skin/soft tissue infections	2014	59	47 (79.7)	Germany	283
	S. aureus	Cattle – mastitis	2015	363	94 (25.9)	Germany	283
	S. hyicus	Pigs – various infections	2015	39	30 (76.9)	Germany	283
Oxacillin	*S. aureus*	Horses – skin infection	2016	75	0 (0.0)	Sweden	282
	S. schleiferi	Dogs – various infections	2016	163	0 (0.0)	Sweden	282
	S. felis	Cats – various infections	2016	277	0 (0.0)	Sweden	282
	S. aureus	Poultry – various infections	2014	35	3 (8.6)	Germany	283
	SIG	Dogs – skin/soft tissue infections	2014	57	11 (19.3)	Germany	283
	S. aureus	Cattle – mastitis	2015	363	15 (4.1)	Germany	283
	S. hyicus	Pigs – various infections	2015	39	0 (0.0)	Germany	283
Tetracycline	*S. aureus*	Horses – skin infection	2016	75	1 (1.3)	Sweden	282
	S. schleiferi	Dogs – various infections	2016	163	6 (3.7)	Sweden	282
	S. felis	Cats – various infections	2016	277	2 (0.7)	Sweden	282
	S. aureus	Poultry – various infections	2014	59	23 (65.7)	Germany	283
	SIG	Dogs – skin/soft tissue infections	2014	59	23 (39.0)	Germany	283
	S. aureus	Cattle – mastitis	2015	363	53 (14.6)	Germany	283
	S. hyicus	Pigs – various infections	2015	39	15 (38.5)	Germany	283
Erythromycin	*S. aureus*	Horses – skin infection	2016	75	0 (0.0)	Sweden	282
	S. schleiferi	Dogs – various infections	2016	163	9 (5.5)	Sweden	282
	S. felis	Cats – various infections	2016	277	46 (16.6)	Sweden	282
	S. aureus	Poultry – various infections	2014	35	17 (48.6)	Germany	283
	SIG	Dogs – skin/soft tissue infections	2014	59	26 (44.1)	Germany	283
	S. aureus	Cattle – mastitis	2015	363	29 (8.0)	Germany	283
	S. hyicus	Pigs – various infections	2015	39	8 (20.5)	Germany	283
Clindamycin	*S. aureus*	Horses – skin infection	2016	75	2 (2.7)	Sweden	282
	S. schleiferi	Dogs – various infections	2016	163	12 (7.4)	Sweden	282
	S. felis	Cats – various infections	2016	277	19 (6.9)	Sweden	282
	S. aureus	Poultry – various infections	2014	35	17 (48.6)[a]	Germany	283
	SIG	Dogs – skin/soft tissue infections	2014	59	23 (39.0)	Germany	283
	S. aureus	Cattle – mastitis	2015	363	32 (8.8)[a]	Germany	283
	S. hyicus	Pigs – various infections	2015	39	13 (33.3)[a]	Germany	283
Gentamicin	*S. aureus*	Horses – skin infection	2016	75	3 (4.0)	Sweden	282
	S. schleiferi	Dogs – various infections	2016	163	1 (0.6)	Sweden	282
	S. felis	Cats – various infections	2016	277	2 (0.7)	Sweden	282
	S. aureus	Poultry – various infections	2014	35	1 (2.9)	Germany	283
	SIG	Dogs – skin/soft tissue infections	2014	59	5 (8.5)	Germany	283
	S. aureus	Cattle – mastitis	2015	363	3 (0.8)	Germany	283
	S. hyicus	Pigs – various infections	2015	39	2 (5.1)	Germany	283
Enrofloxacin	*S. aureus*	Horses – skin infection	2016	35	1 (2.9)	Sweden	282
	S. schleiferi	Dogs – various infections	2016	55	11 (20.0)	Sweden	282
	S. felis	Cats – various infections	2016	97	0 (0.0)	Sweden	282
	S. aureus	Poultry – various infections	2014	35	26 (74.3)[b]	Germany	283
	SIG	Dogs – skin/soft tissue infections	2014	59	9 (15.3)[b]	Germany	283
	S. aureus	Cattle – mastitis	2015	363	28 (7.7)[b]	Germany	283
	S. hyicus	Pigs – various infections	2015	39	7 (17.9)[b]	Germany	283

[a]Isolates showing an MIC of ≥4 mg/liter.
[b]Isolates showing an MIC of ≥1 mg/liter.
[c]SIG, *S. intermedius* group (*S. intermedius*, *S. pseudintermedius*, and *S. delphini*).

range of resistance genes. The analysis of these resistance genes and their genetic environment, including the mobile genetic elements on which resistance genes are located, clearly point toward gene exchange events within the Gram-positive resistance gene pool. Growing interest in staphylococci of animal origin accompanied by a growing number of available whole-genome sequences will surely identify additional resistance genes and resistance-mediating mutations in the future and thereby broaden our knowledge in this field.

Acknowledgments. We apologize in advance to all the investigators whose research could not be appropriately cited owing to space limitations. The work of ATF, KK, and SS on staphylococci from 2011 to 2016 was financially supported by the German Federal Ministry of Education and Research (BMBF) through the German Aerospace Center (DLR), grant numbers 01KI1014D (MedVet-Staph I) and 01KI1014E (MedVet-Staph II). Since 2017, staphylococcal research by ATF and SS has been funded by the Federal Ministry of Education and Research (BMBF) under project number 01KI1727D as part of the Research Network Zoonotic Infectious Diseases. Since 2018, research on LA-MRSA by ATF, SS, YW, and CW has been supported by the German Research Foundation (DFG) and the National Natural Science Foundation of China (NSFC) under grant numbers SCHW 382/11-1 and 31761133022, respectively.

Citation. Schwarz S, Feßler AT, Loncaric I, Wu C, Kadlec K, Wang Y, Shen J. 2018. Antimicrobial resistance among staphylococci of animal origin. Microbiol Spectrum 6(4):ARBA-0010-2017.

References

1. Lyon BR, Skurray R. 1987. Antimicrobial resistance of *Staphylococcus aureus*: genetic basis. *Microbiol Rev* **51:** 88–134.

2. Jensen SO, Lyon BR. 2009. Genetics of antimicrobial resistance in *Staphylococcus aureus*. *Future Microbiol* **4:** 565–582.

3. Schwarz S, Feßler AT, Hauschild T, Kehrenberg C, Kadlec K. 2011. Plasmid-mediated resistance to protein biosynthesis inhibitors in staphylococci. *Ann N Y Acad Sci* **1241:**82–103.

4. Feßler AT, Li J, Kadlec K, Wang Y, Schwarz S. 2018. Antimicrobial resistance properties of *Staphylococcus aureus*, p 57–86. *In* Fetsch A (ed), *Staphylococcus aureus – a Foodborne Pathogen: Epidemiology, Detection, Characterization, Prevention and Control.* Academic Press, London, United Kingdom.

5. Aarestrup FM, Schwarz S. 2006. Antimicrobial resistance in staphylococci and streptococci of animal origin, p 187–212. *In* Aarestrup FM (ed), *Antimicrobial Resistance in Bacteria of Animal Origin.* ASM Press, Washington, DC.

6. Wendlandt S, Feßler AT, Monecke S, Ehricht R, Schwarz S, Kadlec K. 2013. The diversity of antimicrobial resistance genes among staphylococci of animal origin. *Int J Med Microbiol* **303:**338–349.

7. Kadlec K, Schwarz S. 2012. Antimicrobial resistance of *Staphylococcus pseudintermedius*. *Vet Dermatol* **23:** 276–282, e55.

8. Werckenthin C, Cardoso M, Martel J-L, Schwarz S. 2001. Antimicrobial resistance in staphylococci from animals with particular reference to bovine *Staphylococcus aureus*, porcine *Staphylococcus hyicus*, and canine *Staphylococcus intermedius*. *Vet Res* **32:**341–362.

9. Kadlec K, Feßler AT, Hauschild T, Schwarz S. 2012. Novel and uncommon antimicrobial resistance genes in livestock-associated methicillin-resistant *Staphylococcus aureus*. *Clin Microbiol Infect* **18:**745–755.

10. van Hoek AH, Mevius D, Guerra B, Mullany P, Roberts AP, Aarts HJ. 2011. Acquired antibiotic resistance genes: an overview. *Front Microbiol* **2:**203.

11. Roberts MC, Schwarz S, Aarts HJ. 2012. Erratum: acquired antibiotic resistance genes: an overview. *Front Microbiol* **3:**384.

12. Wendlandt S, Schwarz S, Silley P. 2013. MRSA: a foodborne pathogen? *Annu Rev Food Sci Technol* **4:** 117–139.

13. Rowland SJ, Dyke KG. 1989. Characterization of the staphylococcal β-lactamase transposon Tn552. *EMBO J* **8:**2761–2773.

14. Vesterholm-Nielsen M, Olhom Larsen M, Olsen JE, Aarestrup FM. 1999. Occurrence of the *blaZ* gene in penicillin resistant *Staphylococcus aureus* isolated from bovine mastitis in Denmark. *Acta Vet Scand* **40:**279–286.

15. Yazdankhah SP, Sørum H, Oppegaard H. 2000. Comparison of genes involved in penicillin resistance in staphylococci of bovine origin. *Microb Drug Resist* **6:** 29–36.

16. Haveri M, Suominen S, Rantala L, Honkanen-Buzalski T, Pyörälä S. 2005. Comparison of phenotypic and genotypic detection of penicillin G resistance of *Staphylococcus aureus* isolated from bovine intramammary infection. *Vet Microbiol* **106:**97–102.

17. Olsen JE, Christensen H, Aarestrup FM. 2006. Diversity and evolution of *blaZ* from *Staphylococcus aureus* and coagulase-negative staphylococci. *J Antimicrob Chemother* **57:**450–460.

18. Sawant AA, Gillespie BE, Oliver SP. 2009. Antimicrobial susceptibility of coagulase-negative *Staphylococcus* species isolated from bovine milk. *Vet Microbiol* **134:** 73–81.

19. Aarestrup FM, Jensen LB. 2002. Trends in antimicrobial susceptibility in relation to antimicrobial usage and presence of resistance genes in *Staphylococcus hyicus* isolated from exudative epidermitis in pigs. *Vet Microbiol* **89:**83–94.

20. Feßler AT, Thomas P, Mühldorfer K, Grobbel M, Brombach J, Eichhorn I, Monecke S, Ehricht S, Schwarz S. Phenotypic and genotypic characteristics of *Staphylococcus aureus* isolates from zoo and wild animals. *Vet Microbiol* **218:**98–103.

21. Kadlec K, Ehricht R, Monecke S, Steinacker U, Kaspar H, Mankertz J, Schwarz S. 2009. Diversity of antimicrobial resistance pheno- and genotypes of methicillin-

resistant *Staphylococcus aureus* ST398 from diseased swine. *J Antimicrob Chemother* 64:1156–1164.

22. Argudín MA, Tenhagen BA, Fetsch A, Sachsenröder J, Käsbohrer A, Schroeter A, Hammerl JA, Hertwig S, Helmuth R, Bräunig J, Mendoza MC, Appel B, Rodicio MR, Guerra B. 2011. Virulence and resistance determinants of German *Staphylococcus aureus* ST398 isolates from nonhuman sources. *Appl Environ Microbiol* 77:3052–3060.

23. Overesch G, Büttner S, Rossano A, Perreten V. 2011. The increase of methicillin-resistant *Staphylococcus aureus* (MRSA) and the presence of an unusual sequence type ST49 in slaughter pigs in Switzerland. *BMC Vet Res* 7:30.

24. Feßler A, Scott C, Kadlec K, Ehricht R, Monecke S, Schwarz S. 2010. Characterization of methicillin-resistant *Staphylococcus aureus* ST398 from cases of bovine mastitis. *J Antimicrob Chemother* 65:619–625.

25. Walther B, Monecke S, Ruscher C, Friedrich AW, Ehricht R, Slickers P, Soba A, Wleklinski CG, Wieler LH, Lübke-Becker A. 2009. Comparative molecular analysis substantiates zoonotic potential of equine methicillin-resistant *Staphylococcus aureus*. *J Clin Microbiol* 47:704–710.

26. Gharsa H, Ben Sallem R, Ben Slama K, Gómez-Sanz E, Lozano C, Jouini A, Klibi N, Zarazaga M, Boudabous A, Torres C. 2012. High diversity of genetic lineages and virulence genes in nasal *Staphylococcus aureus* isolates from donkeys destined to food consumption in Tunisia with predominance of the ruminant associated CC133 lineage. *BMC Vet Res* 8:203.

27. Gharsa H, Ben Slama K, Lozano C, Gómez-Sanz E, Klibi N, Ben Sallem R, Gómez P, Zarazaga M, Boudabous A, Torres C. 2012. Prevalence, antibiotic resistance, virulence traits and genetic lineages of *Staphylococcus aureus* in healthy sheep in Tunisia. *Vet Microbiol* 156:367–373.

28. Monecke S, Ruppelt A, Wendlandt S, Schwarz S, Slickers P, Ehricht R, Jäckel SC. 2013. Genotyping of *Staphylococcus aureus* isolates from diseased poultry. *Vet Microbiol* 162:806–812.

29. Wendlandt S, Kadlec K, Feßler AT, Monecke S, Ehricht R, van de Giessen AW, Hengeveld PD, Huijsdens X, Schwarz S, van Duijkeren E. 2013. Resistance phenotypes and genotypes of methicillin-resistant *Staphylococcus aureus* isolates from broiler chickens at slaughter and abattoir workers. *J Antimicrob Chemother* 68:2458–2463.

30. Wendlandt S, Kadlec K, Feßler AT, Mevius D, van Essen-Zandbergen A, Hengeveld PD, Bosch T, Schouls L, Schwarz S, van Duijkeren E. 2013. Transmission of methicillin-resistant *Staphylococcus aureus* isolates on broiler farms. *Vet Microbiol* 167:632–637.

31. Monecke S, Gavier-Widén D, Hotzel H, Peters M, Guenther S, Lazaris A, Loncaric I, Müller E, Reissig A, Ruppelt-Lorz A, Shore AC, Walter B, Coleman DC, Ehricht R. 2016. Diversity of *Staphylococcus aureus* isolates in European wildlife. *PLoS One* 11:e0168433.

32. Malik S, Christensen H, Peng H, Barton MD. 2007. Presence and diversity of the β-lactamase gene in cat and dog staphylococci. *Vet Microbiol* 123:162–168.

33. Norström M, Sunde M, Tharaldsen H, Mørk T, Bergsjø B, Kruse H. 2009. Antimicrobial resistance in *Staphylococcus pseudintermedius* in the Norwegian dog population. *Microb Drug Resist* 15:55–59.

34. Perreten V, Kadlec K, Schwarz S, Grönlund Andersson U, Finn M, Greko C, Moodley A, Kania SA, Frank LA, Bemis DA, Franco A, Iurescia M, Battisti A, Duim B, Wagenaar JA, van Duijkeren E, Weese JS, Fitzgerald JR, Rossano A, Guardabassi L. 2010. Clonal spread of methicillin-resistant *Staphylococcus pseudintermedius* in Europe and North America: an international multi-centre study. *J Antimicrob Chemother* 65:1145–1154.

35. Kadlec K, Schwarz S, Perreten V, Andersson UG, Finn M, Greko C, Moodley A, Kania SA, Frank LA, Bemis DA, Franco A, Iurescia M, Battisti A, Duim B, Wagenaar JA, van Duijkeren E, Weese JS, Fitzgerald JR, Rossano A, Guardabassi L. 2010. Molecular analysis of methicillin-resistant *Staphylococcus pseudintermedius* of feline origin from different European countries and North America. *J Antimicrob Chemother* 65:1826–1828.

36. Gómez-Sanz E, Torres C, Lozano C, Sáenz Y, Zarazaga M. 2011. Detection and characterization of methicillin-resistant *Staphylococcus pseudintermedius* in healthy dogs in La Rioja, Spain. *Comp Immunol Microbiol Infect Dis* 34:447–453.

37. Andreis SN, Perreten V, Schwendener S. 2017. Novel β-Lactamase *bla*ARL in *Staphylococcus arlettae*. *MSphere* 2:e00117-17.

38. Descloux S, Rossano A, Perreten V. 2008. Characterization of new staphylococcal cassette chromosome *mec* (SCC*mec*) and topoisomerase genes in fluoroquinolone- and methicillin-resistant *Staphylococcus pseudintermedius*. *J Clin Microbiol* 46:1818–1823.

39. Black CC, Solyman SM, Eberlein LC, Bemis DA, Woron AM, Kania SA. 2009. Identification of a predominant multilocus sequence type, pulsed-field gel electrophoresis cluster, and novel staphylococcal chromosomal cassette in clinical isolates of *mecA*-containing, methicillin-resistant *Staphylococcus pseudintermedius*. *Vet Microbiol* 139:333–338.

40. International Working Group on the Classification of Staphylococcal Cassette Chromosome Elements (IWG-SCC). 2009. Classification of staphylococcal cassette chromosome *mec* (SCC*mec*): guidelines for reporting novel SCC*mec* elements. *Antimicrob Agents Chemother* 53:4961–4967.

41. Wu Z, Li F, Liu D, Xue H, Zhao X. 2015. Novel type XII staphylococcal cassette chromosome *mec* harboring a new cassette chromosome recombinase, CcrC2. *Antimicrob Agents Chemother* 59:7597–7601.

42. Cuny C, Friedrich A, Kozytska S, Layer F, Nübel U, Ohlsen K, Strommenger B, Walther B, Wieler L, Witte W. 2010. Emergence of methicillin-resistant *Staphylococcus aureus* (MRSA) in different animal species. *Int J Med Microbiol* 300:109–117.

43. Loeffler A, Lloyd DH. 2010. Companion animals: a reservoir for methicillin-resistant *Staphylococcus aureus* in the community? *Epidemiol Infect* 138:595–605.

44. Vanderhaeghen W, Hermans K, Haesebrouck F, Butaye P. 2010. Methicillin-resistant *Staphylococcus aureus*

(MRSA) in food production animals. *Epidemiol Infect* **138:**606–625.

45. Weese JS. 2010. Methicillin-resistant *Staphylococcus aureus* in animals. *ILAR J* **51:**233–244.

46. Weese JS, van Duijkeren E. 2010. Methicillin-resistant *Staphylococcus aureus* and *Staphylococcus pseudintermedius* in veterinary medicine. *Vet Microbiol* **140:**418–429.

47. Graveland H, Duim B, van Duijkeren E, Heederik D, Wagenaar JA. 2011. Livestock-associated methicillin-resistant *Staphylococcus aureus* in animals and humans. *Int J Med Microbiol* **301:**630–634.

48. Fitzgerald JR. 2012. Livestock-associated *Staphylococcus aureus*: origin, evolution and public health threat. *Trends Microbiol* **20:**192–198.

49. Fluit AC. 2012. Livestock-associated *Staphylococcus aureus*. *Clin Microbiol Infect* **18:**735–744.

50. Pantosti A. 2012. Methicillin-resistant *Staphylococcus aureus* associated with animals and its relevance to human health. *Front Microbiol* **3:**127.

51. Voss A, Loeffen F, Bakker J, Klaassen C, Wulf M. 2005. Methicillin-resistant *Staphylococcus aureus* in pig farming. *Emerg Infect Dis* **11:**1965–1966.

52. de Neeling AJ, van den Broek MJ, Spalburg EC, van Santen-Verheuvel MG, Dam-Deisz WD, Boshuizen HC, van de Giessen AW, van Duijkeren E, Huijsdens XW. 2007. High prevalence of methicillin resistant *Staphylococcus aureus* in pigs. *Vet Microbiol* **122:**366–372.

53. van Duijkeren E, Jansen MD, Flemming SC, de Neeling H, Wagenaar JA, Schoormans AH, van Nes A, Fluit AC. 2007. Methicillin-resistant *Staphylococcus aureus* in pigs with exudative epidermitis. *Emerg Infect Dis* **13:** 1408–1410.

54. Wagenaar JA, Yue H, Pritchard J, Broekhuizen-Stins M, Huijsdens X, Mevius DJ, Bosch T, Van Duijkeren E. 2009. Unexpected sequence types in livestock associated methicillin-resistant *Staphylococcus aureus* (MRSA): MRSA ST9 and a single locus variant of ST9 in pig farming in China. *Vet Microbiol* **139:**405–409.

55. Monecke S, Kuhnert P, Hotzel H, Slickers P, Ehricht R. 2007. Microarray based study on virulence-associated genes and resistance determinants of *Staphylococcus aureus* isolates from cattle. *Vet Microbiol* **125:**128–140.

56. Vanderhaeghen W, Cerpentier T, Adriaensen C, Vicca J, Hermans K, Butaye P. 2010. Methicillin-resistant *Staphylococcus aureus* (MRSA) ST398 associated with clinical and subclinical mastitis in Belgian cows. *Vet Microbiol* **144:**166–171.

57. Holmes MA, Zadoks RN. 2011. Methicillin resistant *S. aureus* in human and bovine mastitis. *J Mammary Gland Biol Neoplasia* **16:**373–382.

58. Spohr M, Rau J, Friedrich A, Klittich G, Fetsch A, Guerra B, Hammerl JA, Tenhagen BA. 2011. Methicillin-resistant *Staphylococcus aureus* (MRSA) in three dairy herds in southwest Germany. *Zoonoses Public Health* **58:**252–261.

59. Feßler AT, Olde Riekerink RG, Rothkamp A, Kadlec K, Sampimon OC, Lam TJ, Schwarz S. 2012. Characterization of methicillin-resistant *Staphylococcus aureus* CC398 obtained from humans and animals on dairy farms. *Vet Microbiol* **160:**77–84.

60. Wang XM, Zhang WJ, Schwarz S, Yu SY, Liu H, Si W, Zhang RM, Liu S. 2012. Methicillin-resistant *Staphylococcus aureus* ST9 from a case of bovine mastitis carries the genes *cfr* and *erm*(A) on a small plasmid. *J Antimicrob Chemother* **67:**1287–1289.

61. Juhász-Kaszanyitzky E, Jánosi S, Somogyi P, Dán A, van der Graaf-van Bloois L, van Duijkeren E, Wagenaar JA. 2007. MRSA transmission between cows and humans. *Emerg Infect Dis* **13:**630–632.

62. Schauer B, Krametter-Frötscher R, Knauer F, Ehricht R, Monecke S, Feßler AT, Schwarz S, Grunert T, Spergser J, Loncaric I. 2018. Diversity of methicillin-resistant *Staphylococcus aureus* (MRSA) isolated from Austrian ruminants and New World camelids. *Vet Microbiol* **215:** 77–82.

63. Chu C, Yu C, Lee Y, Su Y. 2012. Genetically divergent methicillin-resistant *Staphylococcus aureus* and *sec*-dependent mastitis of dairy goats in Taiwan. *BMC Vet Res* **8:**39.

64. Nemati M, Hermans K, Lipinska U, Denis O, Deplano A, Struelens M, Devriese LA, Pasmans F, Haesebrouck F. 2008. Antimicrobial resistance of old and recent *Staphylococcus aureus* isolates from poultry: first detection of livestock-associated methicillin-resistant strain ST398. *Antimicrob Agents Chemother* **52:**3817–3819.

65. Persoons D, Van Hoorebeke S, Hermans K, Butaye P, de Kruif A, Haesebrouck F, Dewulf J. 2009. Methicillin-resistant *Staphylococcus aureus* in poultry. *Emerg Infect Dis* **15:**452–453.

66. Cuny C, Strommenger B, Witte W, Stanek C. 2008. Clusters of infections in horses with MRSA ST1, ST254, and ST398 in a veterinary hospital. *Microb Drug Resist* **14:**307–310.

67. van Duijkeren E, Moleman M, Sloet van Oldruitenborgh-Oosterbaan MM, Multem J, Troelstra A, Fluit AC, van Wamel WJ, Houwers DJ, de Neeling AJ, Wagenaar JA. 2010. Methicillin-resistant *Staphylococcus aureus* in horses and horse personnel: an investigation of several outbreaks. *Vet Microbiol* **141:**96–102.

68. Sieber S, Gerber V, Jandova V, Rossano A, Evison JM, Perreten V. 2011. Evolution of multidrug-resistant *Staphylococcus aureus* infections in horses and colonized personnel in an equine clinic between 2005 and 2010. *Microb Drug Resist* **17:**471–478.

69. Sing A, Tuschak C, Hörmansdorfer S. 2008. Methicillin-resistant *Staphylococcus aureus* in a family and its pet cat. *N Engl J Med* **358:**1200–1201.

70. Walther B, Wieler LH, Friedrich AW, Hanssen AM, Kohn B, Brunnberg L, Lübke-Becker A. 2008. Methicillin-resistant *Staphylococcus aureus* (MRSA) isolated from small and exotic animals at a university hospital during routine microbiological examinations. *Vet Microbiol* **127:**171–178.

71. Nienhoff U, Kadlec K, Chaberny IF, Verspohl J, Gerlach GF, Schwarz S, Simon D, Nolte I. 2009. Transmission of methicillin-resistant *Staphylococcus aureus* strains

between humans and dogs: two case reports. *J Antimicrob Chemother* 64:660–662.

72. Coelho C, Torres C, Radhouani H, Pinto L, Lozano C, Gómez-Sanz E, Zaragaza M, Igrejas G, Poeta P. 2011. Molecular detection and characterization of methicillin-resistant *Staphylococcus aureus* (MRSA) isolates from dogs in Portugal. *Microb Drug Resist* 17:333–337.

73. Haenni M, Saras E, Châtre P, Médaille C, Bes M, Madec JY, Laurent F. 2012. A USA300 variant and other human-related methicillin-resistant *Staphylococcus aureus* strains infecting cats and dogs in France. *J Antimicrob Chemother* 67:326–329.

74. Ruscher C, Lübke-Becker A, Wleklinski CG, Soba A, Wieler LH, Walther B. 2009. Prevalence of methicillin-resistant *Staphylococcus pseudintermedius* isolated from clinical samples of companion animals and equidaes. *Vet Microbiol* 136:197–201.

75. Ruscher C, Lübke-Becker A, Semmler T, Wleklinski CG, Paasch A, Soba A, Stamm I, Kopp P, Wieler LH, Walther B. 2010. Widespread rapid emergence of a distinct methicillin- and multidrug-resistant *Staphylococcus pseudintermedius* (MRSP) genetic lineage in Europe. *Vet Microbiol* 144:340–346.

76. Nienhoff U, Kadlec K, Chaberny IF, Verspohl J, Gerlach GF, Kreienbrock L, Schwarz S, Simon D, Nolte I. 2011. Methicillin-resistant *Staphylococcus pseudintermedius* among dogs admitted to a small animal hospital. *Vet Microbiol* 150:191–197.

77. Nienhoff U, Kadlec K, Chaberny IF, Verspohl J, Gerlach GF, Schwarz S, Kreienbrock L, Nolte I, Simon D. 2011. Methicillin-resistant *Staphylococcus pseudintermedius* among cats admitted to a veterinary teaching hospital. *Vet Microbiol* 153:414–416.

78. Wang Y, Yang J, Logue CM, Liu K, Cao X, Zhang W, Shen J, Wu C. 2012. Methicillin-resistant *Staphylococcus pseudintermedius* isolated from canine pyoderma in North China. *J Appl Microbiol* 112:623–630.

79. Kadlec K, Weiß S, Wendlandt S, Schwarz S, Tonpitak W. 2016. Characterization of canine and feline methicillin-resistant *Staphylococcus pseudintermedius* (MRSP) from Thailand. *Vet Microbiol* 194:93–97.

80. Hassler C, Nitzsche S, Iversen C, Zweifel C, Stephan R. 2008. Characteristics of *Staphylococcus hyicus* strains isolated from pig carcasses in two different slaughterhouses. *Meat Sci* 80:505–510.

81. Zhang Y, Agidi S, LeJeune JT. 2009. Diversity of staphylococcal cassette chromosome in coagulase-negative staphylococci from animal sources. *J Appl Microbiol* 107:1375–1383.

82. Feßler AT, Billerbeck C, Kadlec K, Schwarz S. 2010. Identification and characterization of methicillin-resistant coagulase-negative staphylococci from bovine mastitis. *J Antimicrob Chemother* 65:1576–1582.

83. Vanderhaeghen W, Vandendriessche S, Crombé F, Nemeghaire S, Dispas M, Denis O, Hermans K, Haesebrouck F, Butaye P. 2013. Characterization of methicillin-resistant non-*Staphylococcus aureus* staphylococci carriage isolates from different bovine populations. *J Antimicrob Chemother* 68:300–307.

84. Tulinski P, Fluit AC, Wagenaar JA, Mevius D, van de Vijver L, Duim B. 2012. Methicillin-resistant coagulase-negative staphylococci on pig farms as a reservoir of heterogeneous staphylococcal cassette chromosome *mec* elements. *Appl Environ Microbiol* 78:299–304.

85. Wang Y, He T, Schwarz S, Zhao Q, Shen Z, Wu C, Shen J. 2013. Multidrug resistance gene *cfr* in methicillin-resistant coagulase-negative staphylococci from chickens, ducks, and pigs in China. *Int J Med Microbiol* 303: 84–87.

86. Kawano J, Shimizu A, Saitoh Y, Yagi M, Saito T, Okamoto R. 1996. Isolation of methicillin-resistant coagulase-negative staphylococci from chickens. *J Clin Microbiol* 34:2072–2077.

87. Yasuda R, Kawano J, Matsuo E, Masuda T, Shimizu A, Anzai T, Hashikura S. 2002. Distribution of *mecA*-harboring staphylococci in healthy mares. *J Vet Med Sci* 64:821–827.

88. Schnellmann C, Gerber V, Rossano A, Jaquier V, Panchaud Y, Doherr MG, Thomann A, Straub R, Perreten V. 2006. Presence of new *mecA* and *mph*(C) variants conferring antibiotic resistance in *Staphylococcus* spp. isolated from the skin of horses before and after clinic admission. *J Clin Microbiol* 44:4444–4454.

89. Bagcigil FA, Moodley A, Baptiste KE, Jensen VF, Guardabassi L. 2007. Occurrence, species distribution, antimicrobial resistance and clonality of methicillin- and erythromycin-resistant staphylococci in the nasal cavity of domestic animals. *Vet Microbiol* 121:307–315.

90. De Martino L, Lucido M, Mallardo K, Facello B, Mallardo M, Iovane G, Pagnini U, Tufano MA, Catalanotti P. 2010. Methicillin-resistant staphylococci isolated from healthy horses and horse personnel in Italy. *J Vet Diagn Invest* 22:77–82.

91. van Duijkeren E, Box AT, Heck ME, Wannet WJ, Fluit AC. 2004. Methicillin-resistant staphylococci isolated from animals. *Vet Microbiol* 103:91–97.

92. Kania SA, Williamson NL, Frank LA, Wilkes RP, Jones RD, Bemis DA. 2004. Methicillin resistance of staphylococci isolated from the skin of dogs with pyoderma. *Am J Vet Res* 65:1265–1268.

93. Monecke S, Müller E, Schwarz S, Hotzel H, Ehricht R. 2012. Rapid microarray-based identification of different *mecA* alleles in staphylococci. *Antimicrob Agents Chemother* 56:5547–5554.

94. García-Álvarez L, Holden MT, Lindsay H, Webb CR, Brown DF, Curran MD, Walpole E, Brooks K, Pickard DJ, Teale C, Parkhill J, Bentley SD, Edwards GF, Girvan EK, Kearns AM, Pichon B, Hill RL, Larsen AR, Skov RL, Peacock SJ, Maskell DJ, Holmes MA. 2011. Meticillin-resistant *Staphylococcus aureus* with a novel *mecA* homologue in human and bovine populations in the UK and Denmark: a descriptive study. *Lancet Infect Dis* 11:595–603.

95. Shore AC, Deasy EC, Slickers P, Brennan G, O'Connell B, Monecke S, Ehricht R, Coleman DC. 2011. Detection of staphylococcal cassette chromosome *mec* type XI carrying highly divergent *mecA*, *mecI*, *mecR1*, *blaZ*, and *ccr* genes in human clinical isolates of clonal com-

plex 130 methicillin-resistant *Staphylococcus aureus*. *Antimicrob Agents Chemother* 55:3765–3773.

96. Laurent F, Chardon H, Haenni M, Bes M, Reverdy ME, Madec JY, Lagier E, Vandenesch F, Tristan A. 2012. MRSA harboring *mecA* variant gene *mecC*, France. *Emerg Infect Dis* 18:1465–1467.

97. Medhus A, Slettemeås J, Marstein L, Larssen K, Sunde M. 2013. MRSA with the novel *mecC* gene variant isolated from a cat suffering from chronic conjunctivitis. *J Antimicrob Chemother* 68:968–969.

98. Paterson GK, Larsen AR, Robb A, Edwards GE, Pennycott TW, Foster G, Mot D, Hermans K, Baert K, Peacock SJ, Parkhill J, Zadoks RN, Holmes MA. 2012. The newly described *mecA* homologue, *mecA*$_{LGA251}$, is present in methicillin-resistant *Staphylococcus aureus* isolates from a diverse range of host species. *J Antimicrob Chemother* 67:2809–2813.

99. Robb A, Pennycott T, Duncan G, Foster G. 2013. *Staphylococcus aureus* carrying divergent *mecA* homologue (*mecA*$_{LGA251}$) isolated from a free-ranging wild bird. *Vet Microbiol* 162:300–301.

100. Walther B, Wieler LH, Vincze S, Antão E-M, Brandenburg A, Stamm I, Kopp PA, Kohn B, Semmler T, Lübke-Becker A. 2012. MRSA variant in companion animals. *Emerg Infect Dis* 18:2017–2020.

101. Loncaric I, Kübber-Heiss A, Posautz A, Stalder GL, Hoffmann D, Rosengarten R, Walzer C. 2013. Characterization of methicillin-resistant *Staphylococcus* spp. carrying the *mecC* gene, isolated from wildlife. *J Antimicrob Chemother* 68:2222–2225.

102. Gómez P, González-Barrio D, Benito D, García JT, Viñuela J, Zarazaga M, Ruiz-Fons F, Torres C. 2014. Detection of methicillin-resistant *Staphylococcus aureus* (MRSA) carrying the *mecC* gene in wild small mammals in Spain. *J Antimicrob Chemother* 69:2061–2064.

103. Gómez P, Lozano C, González-Barrio D, Zarazaga M, Ruiz-Fons F, Torres C. 2015. High prevalence of methicillin-resistant *Staphylococcus aureus* (MRSA) carrying the *mecC* gene in a semi-extensive red deer (*Cervus elaphus hispanicus*) farm in Southern Spain. *Vet Microbiol* 177:326–331.

104. Gómez P, Lozano C, Camacho MC, Lima-Barbero JF, Hernández JM, Zarazaga M, Höfle Ú, Torres C. 2016. Detection of MRSA ST3061-t843-*mecC* and ST398-t011-*mecA* in white stork nestlings exposed to human residues. *J Antimicrob Chemother* 71:53–57.

105. Paterson GK, Harrison EM, Holmes MA. 2014. The emergence of *mecC* methicillin-resistant *Staphylococcus aureus*. *Trends Microbiol* 22:42–47.

106. Harrison EM, Paterson GK, Holden MT, Morgan FJ, Larsen AR, Petersen A, Leroy S, De Vliegher S, Perreten V, Fox LK, Lam TJ, Sampimon OC, Zadoks RN, Peacock SJ, Parkhill J, Holmes MA. 2013. A *Staphylococcus xylosus* isolate with a new *mecC* allotype. *Antimicrob Agents Chemother* 57:1524–1528.

107. Małyszko I, Schwarz S, Hauschild T. 2014. Detection of a new *mecC* allotype, *mecC2*, in methicillin-resistant *Staphylococcus saprophyticus*. *J Antimicrob Chemother* 69:2003–2005.

108. Becker K, van Alen S, Idelevich EA, Schleimer N, Seggewiß J, Mellmann A, Kaspar U, Peters G. 2018. Plasmid-encoded transferable *mecB*-mediated methicillin resistance in *Staphylococcus aureus*. *Emerg Infect Dis* 24:242–248.

109. Ba X, Harrison EM, Edwards GF, Holden MT, Larsen AR, Petersen A, Skov RL, Peacock SJ, Parkhill J, Paterson GK, Holmes MA. 2014. Novel mutations in penicillin-binding protein genes in clinical *Staphylococcus aureus* isolates that are methicillin resistant on susceptibility testing, but lack the *mec* gene. *J Antimicrob Chemother* 69:594–597.

110. Berger-Bächi B, Tschierske M. 1998. Role of *fem* factors in methicillin resistance. *Drug Resist Updat* 1:325–335.

111. Roberts MC. 1996. Tetracycline resistance determinants: mechanisms of action, regulation of expression, genetic mobility, and distribution. *FEMS Microbiol Rev* 19:1–24.

112. Schwarz S, Roberts MC, Werckenthin C, Pang Y, Lange C. 1998. Tetracycline resistance in *Staphylococcus* spp. from domestic animals. *Vet Microbiol* 63:217–227.

113. Khan SA, Novick RP. 1983. Complete nucleotide sequence of pT181, a tetracycline-resistance plasmid from *Staphylococcus aureus*. *Plasmid* 10:251–259.

114. Schwarz S, Shen J, Wendlandt S, Feßler AT, Wang Y, Kadlec K, Wu CM. 2014. Plasmid-mediated antimicrobial resistance in staphylococci and other firmicutes. *Microbiol Spectr* 2: 10.1128/microbiolspec.PLAS-0020-2014.

115. Schwarz S, Blobel H. 1990. Isolation and restriction endonuclease analysis of a tetracycline resistance plasmid from *Staphylococcus hyicus*. *Vet Microbiol* 24:113–122.

116. Schwarz S, Cardoso M, Grölz-Krug S, Blobel H. 1990. Common antibiotic resistance plasmids in *Staphylococcus aureus* and *Staphylococcus epidermidis* from human and canine infections. *Zentralbl Bakteriol* 273:369–377.

117. Greene RT, Schwarz S. 1992. Small antibiotic resistance plasmids in *Staphylococcus intermedius*. *Zentralbl Bakteriol* 276:380–389.

118. Schwarz S, Noble WC. 1994. Tetracycline resistance genes in staphylococci from the skin of pigs. *J Appl Bacteriol* 76:320–326.

119. Hauschild T, Kehrenberg C, Schwarz S. 2003. Tetracycline resistance in staphylococci from free-living rodents and insectivores. *J Vet Med B Infect Dis Vet Public Health* 50:443–446.

120. Hauschild T, Stepanović S, Dakić I, Djukić S, Ranin L, Jezek P, Schwarz S. 2007. Tetracycline resistance and distribution of *tet* genes in members of the *Staphylococcus sciuri* group isolated from humans, animals and different environmental sources. *Int J Antimicrob Agents* 29:356–358.

121. Larsen J, Clasen J, Hansen JE, Paulander W, Petersen A, Larsen AR, Frees D. 2016. Copresence of *tet*(K) and *tet*(M) in livestock-associated methicillin-resistant *Staphylococcus aureus* clonal complex 398 is associated with increased fitness during exposure to sublethal con-

centrations of tetracycline. *Antimicrob Agents Chemother* 60:4401–4403.

122. Hauschild T, Lüthje P, Schwarz S. 2005. Staphylococcal tetracycline-MLS$_B$ resistance plasmid pSTE2 is the product of an RS$_A$-mediated *in vivo* recombination. *J Antimicrob Chemother* 56:399–402.

123. Kadlec K, Schwarz S. 2009. Identification of a novel trimethoprim resistance gene, *dfrK*, in a methicillin-resistant *Staphylococcus aureus* ST398 strain and its physical linkage to the tetracycline resistance gene *tet*(L). *Antimicrob Agents Chemother* 53:776–778.

124. Kadlec K, Schwarz S. 2009. Novel ABC transporter gene, *vga*(C), located on a multiresistance plasmid from a porcine methicillin-resistant *Staphylococcus aureus* ST398 strain. *Antimicrob Agents Chemother* 53:3589–3591.

125. Kadlec K, Schwarz S. 2010. Identification of a plasmid-borne resistance gene cluster comprising the resistance genes *erm*(T), *dfrK*, and *tet*(L) in a porcine methicillin-resistant *Staphylococcus aureus* ST398 strain. *Antimicrob Agents Chemother* 54:915–918.

126. Feßler AT, Zhao Q, Schoenfelder S, Kadlec K, Brenner Michael G, Wang Y, Ziebuhr W, Shen J, Schwarz S. 2017. Complete sequence of a plasmid from a bovine methicillin-resistant *Staphylococcus aureus* harbouring a novel *ica*-like gene cluster in addition to antimicrobial and heavy metal resistance genes. *Vet Microbiol* 200:95–100.

127. Schwarz S, Cardoso M, Wegener HC. 1992. Nucleotide sequence and phylogeny of the *tet*(L) tetracycline resistance determinant encoded by plasmid pSTE1 from *Staphylococcus hyicus*. *Antimicrob Agents Chemother* 36:580–588.

128. Schwarz S, Gregory PD, Werckenthin C, Curnock S, Dyke KG. 1996. A novel plasmid from *Staphylococcus epidermidis* specifying resistance to kanamycin, neomycin and tetracycline. *J Med Microbiol* 45:57–63.

129. Schwarz S, Wang Z. 1993. Tetracycline resistance in *Staphylococcus intermedius*. *Lett Appl Microbiol* 17:88–91.

130. Weiß S, Kadlec K, Feßler AT, Schwarz S. 2014. Complete sequence of a multiresistance plasmid from a methicillin-resistant *Staphylococcus epidermidis* ST5 isolated in a small animal clinic. *J Antimicrob Chemother* 69:847–859.

131. Schwarz S, Kehrenberg C, Doublet B, Cloeckaert A. 2004. Molecular basis of bacterial resistance to chloramphenicol and florfenicol. *FEMS Microbiol Rev* 28:519–542.

132. Horinouchi S, Weisblum B. 1982. Nucleotide sequence and functional map of pC194, a plasmid that specifies inducible chloramphenicol resistance. *J Bacteriol* 150:815–825.

133. Brenner DG, Shaw WV. 1985. The use of synthetic oligonucleotides with universal templates for rapid DNA sequencing: results with staphylococcal replicon pC221. *EMBO J* 4:561–568.

134. Projan SJ, Kornblum J, Moghazeh SL, Edelman I, Gennaro ML, Novick RP. 1985. Comparative sequence and functional analysis of pT181 and pC221, cognate plasmid replicons from *Staphylococcus aureus*. *Mol Gen Genet* 199:452–464.

135. Smith MC, Thomas CD. 2004. An accessory protein is required for relaxosome formation by small staphylococcal plasmids. *J Bacteriol* 186:3363–3373.

136. Cardoso M, Schwarz S. 1992. Chloramphenicol resistance plasmids in *Staphylococcus aureus* isolated from bovine subclinical mastitis. *Vet Microbiol* 30:223–232.

137. Cardoso M, Schwarz S. 1992. Nucleotide sequence and structural relationships of a chloramphenicol acetyltransferase encoded by the plasmid pSCS6 from *Staphylococcus aureus*. *J Appl Bacteriol* 72:289–293.

138. Schwarz S, Spies U, Cardoso M. 1991. Cloning and sequence analysis of a plasmid-encoded chloramphenicol acetyltransferase gene from *Staphylococcus intermedius*. *J Gen Microbiol* 137:977–981.

139. Schwarz S, Werckenthin C, Pinter L, Kent LE, Noble WC. 1995. Chloramphenicol resistance in *Staphylococcus intermedius* from a single veterinary centre: evidence for plasmid and chromosomal location of the resistance genes. *Vet Microbiol* 43:151–159.

140. Schwarz S, Cardoso M, Blobel H. 1989. Plasmid-mediated chloramphenicol resistance in *Staphylococcus hyicus*. *J Gen Microbiol* 135:3329–3336.

141. Schwarz S, Noble WC. 1994. Structure and putative origin of a plasmid from *Staphylococcus hyicus* that mediates chloramphenicol and streptomycin resistance. *Lett Appl Microbiol* 18:281–284.

142. Schwarz S, Cardoso M, Blobel H. 1990. Detection of a novel chloramphenicol resistance plasmid from "equine" *Staphylococcus sciuri*. *Zentralbl Veterinarmed B* 37:674–679.

143. Hauschild T, Stepanović S, Vuković D, Dakić I, Schwarz S. 2009. Occurrence of chloramphenicol resistance and corresponding resistance genes in members of the *Staphylococcus sciuri* group. *Int J Antimicrob Agents* 33:383–384.

144. Schwarz S, Grölz-Krug S. 1991. A chloramphenicol-streptomycin-resistance plasmid from a clinical strain of *Staphylococcus sciuri* and its structural relationships to other staphylococcal resistance plasmids. *FEMS Microbiol Lett* 66:319–322.

145. Schwarz S. 1994. Emerging chloramphenicol resistance in *Staphylococcus lentus* from mink following chloramphenicol treatment: characterisation of the resistance genes. *Vet Microbiol* 41:51–61.

146. Schwarz S, Cardoso M. 1991. Molecular cloning, purification, and properties of a plasmid-encoded chloramphenicol acetyltransferase from *Staphylococcus haemolyticus*. *Antimicrob Agents Chemother* 35:1277–1283.

147. Wendlandt S, Kadlec K, Schwarz S. 2015. Four novel plasmids from *Staphylococcus hyicus* and CoNS that carry a variant of the spectinomycin resistance gene *spd*. *J Antimicrob Chemother* 70:948–949.

148. Kehrenberg C, Schwarz S. 2004. *fexA*, a novel *Staphylococcus lentus* gene encoding resistance to florfenicol and chloramphenicol. *Antimicrob Agents Chemother* 48:615–618.

149. Kehrenberg C, Schwarz S. 2005. Florfenicol-chloramphenicol exporter gene *fexA* is part of the novel transposon Tn*558*. *Antimicrob Agents Chemother* **49:** 813–815.

150. Kehrenberg C, Cuny C, Strommenger B, Schwarz S, Witte W. 2009. Methicillin-resistant and -susceptible *Staphylococcus aureus* strains of clonal lineages ST398 and ST9 from swine carry the multidrug resistance gene *cfr*. *Antimicrob Agents Chemother* **53:**779–781.

151. Wang Y, Zhang W, Wang J, Wu C, Shen Z, Fu X, Yan Y, Zhang Q, Schwarz S, Shen J. 2012. Distribution of the multidrug resistance gene *cfr* in *Staphylococcus* species isolates from swine farms in China. *Antimicrob Agents Chemother* **56:**1485–1490.

152. Kehrenberg C, Schwarz S. 2006. Distribution of florfenicol resistance genes *fexA* and *cfr* among chloramphenicol-resistant *Staphylococcus* isolates. *Antimicrob Agents Chemother* **50:**1156–1163.

153. Kehrenberg C, Aarestrup FM, Schwarz S. 2007. IS*21-558* insertion sequences are involved in the mobility of the multiresistance gene *cfr*. *Antimicrob Agents Chemother* **51:**483–487.

154. Gómez-Sanz E, Kadlec K, Feßler AT, Zarazaga M, Torres C, Schwarz S. 2013. A novel *fexA* variant from a canine *Staphylococcus pseudintermedius* isolate that does not confer florfenicol resistance. *Antimicrob Agents Chemother* **57:**5763–5766.

155. Ramirez MS, Tolmasky ME. 2010. Aminoglycoside modifying enzymes. *Drug Resist Updat* **13:**151–171.

156. Ferretti JJ, Gilmore KS, Courvalin P. 1986. Nucleotide sequence analysis of the gene specifying the bifunctional 6′-aminoglycoside acetyltransferase 2″-aminoglycoside phosphotransferase enzyme in *Streptococcus faecalis* and identification and cloning of gene regions specifying the two activities. *J Bacteriol* **167:**631–638.

157. Rouch DA, Byrne ME, Kong YC, Skurray RA. 1987. The *aacA-aphD* gentamicin and kanamycin resistance determinant of Tn*4001* from *Staphylococcus aureus*: expression and nucleotide sequence analysis. *J Gen Microbiol* **133:**3039–3052.

158. Byrne ME, Rouch DA, Skurray RA. 1989. Nucleotide sequence analysis of IS*256* from the *Staphylococcus aureus* gentamicin-tobramycin-kanamycin-resistance transposon Tn*4001*. *Gene* **81:**361–367.

159. Lange CC, Werckenthin C, Schwarz S. 2003. Molecular analysis of the plasmid-borne *aacA/aphD* resistance gene region of coagulase-negative staphylococci from chickens. *J Antimicrob Chemother* **51:**1397–1401.

160. Schwarz S, Kadlec K, Strommenger B. 2008. Methicillin-resistant *Staphylococcus aureus* and *Staphylococcus pseudintermedius* detected in the BfT-GermVet monitoring programme 2004–2006 in Germany. *J Antimicrob Chemother* **61:**282–285.

161. Wendlandt S, Li B, Ma Z, Schwarz S. 2013. Complete sequence of the multi-resistance plasmid pV7037 from a porcine methicillin-resistant *Staphylococcus aureus*. *Vet Microbiol* **166:**650–654.

162. Li B, Wendlandt S, Yao J, Liu Y, Zhang Q, Shi Z, Wei J, Shao D, Schwarz S, Wang S, Ma Z. 2013. Detection

and new genetic environment of the pleuromutilin-lincosamide-streptogramin A resistance gene *lsa*(E) in methicillin-resistant *Staphylococcus aureus* of swine origin. *J Antimicrob Chemother* **68:**1251–1255.

163. Turutoglu H, Hasoksuz M, Ozturk D, Yildirim M, Sagnak S. 2009. Methicillin and aminoglycoside resistance in *Staphylococcus aureus* isolates from bovine mastitis and sequence analysis of their *mecA* genes. *Vet Res Commun* **33:**945–956.

164. Argudín MA, Vanderhaeghen W, Butaye P. 2015. Diversity of antimicrobial resistance and virulence genes in methicillin-resistant non-*Staphylococcus aureus* staphylococci from veal calves. *Res Vet Sci* **99:**10–16.

165. Cuny C, Kuemmerle J, Stanek C, Willey B, Strommenger B, Witte W. 2006. Emergence of MRSA infections in horses in a veterinary hospital: strain characterisation and comparison with MRSA from humans. *Euro Surveill* **11:**44–47.

166. Sidhu MS, Oppegaard H, Devor TP, Sørum H. 2007. Persistence of multidrug-resistant *Staphylococcus haemolyticus* in an animal veterinary teaching hospital clinic. *Microb Drug Resist* **13:**271–280.

167. He T, Wang Y, Schwarz S, Zhao Q, Shen J, Wu C. 2014. Genetic environment of the multi-resistance gene *cfr* in methicillin-resistant coagulase-negative staphylococci from chickens, ducks, and pigs in China. *Int J Med Microbiol* **304:**257–261.

168. McKenzie T, Hoshino T, Tanaka T, Sueoka N. 1987. Correction. A revision of the nucleotide sequence and functional map of pUB110. *Plasmid* **17:**83–85.

169. Hauschild T, Vuković D, Dakić I, Jezek P, Djukić S, Dimitrijević V, Stepanović S, Schwarz S. 2007. Aminoglycoside resistance in members of the *Staphylococcus sciuri* group. *Microb Drug Resist* **13:**77–84.

170. Derbise A, Dyke KG, el Solh N. 1996. Characterization of a *Staphylococcus aureus* transposon, Tn*5405*, located within Tn*5404* and carrying the aminoglycoside resistance genes, *aphA-3* and *aadE*. *Plasmid* **35:**174–188.

171. Boerlin P, Burnens AP, Frey J, Kuhnert P, Nicolet J. 2001. Molecular epidemiology and genetic linkage of macrolide and aminoglycoside resistance in *Staphylococcus intermedius* of canine origin. *Vet Microbiol* **79:**155–169.

172. Ben Zakour NL, Bannoehr J, van den Broek AH, Thoday KL, Fitzgerald JR. 2011. Complete genome sequence of the canine pathogen *Staphylococcus pseudintermedius*. *J Bacteriol* **193:**2363–2364.

173. Wendlandt S, Lozano C, Kadlec K, Gómez-Sanz E, Zarazaga M, Torres C, Schwarz S. 2013. The enterococcal ABC transporter gene *lsa*(E) confers combined resistance to lincosamides, pleuromutilins and streptogramin A antibiotics in methicillin-susceptible and methicillin-resistant *Staphylococcus aureus*. *J Antimicrob Chemother* **68:**473–475.

174. Wendlandt S, Li J, Ho J, Porta MA, Feßler AT, Wang Y, Kadlec K, Monecke S, Ehricht R, Boost M, Schwarz S. 2014. Enterococcal multiresistance gene cluster in methicillin-resistant *Staphylococcus aureus* from vari-

ous origins and geographical locations. *J Antimicrob Chemother* 69:2573–2575.

175. Projan SJ, Moghazeh S, Novick RP. 1988. Nucleotide sequence of pS194, a streptomycin-resistance plasmid from *Staphylococcus aureus*. *Nucleic Acids Res* 16: 2179–2187.

176. Schwarz S, Blobel H. 1990. A new streptomycin-resistance plasmid from *Staphylococcus hyicus* and its structural relationship to other staphylococcal resistance plasmids. *J Med Microbiol* 32:201–205.

177. Stegmann R, Perreten V. 2010. Antibiotic resistance profile of *Staphylococcus rostri*, a new species isolated from healthy pigs. *Vet Microbiol* 145:165–171.

178. Murphy E. 1985. Nucleotide sequence of a spectinomycin adenyltransferase AAD(9) determinant from *Staphylococcus aureus* and its relationship to AAD(3′′) (9). *Mol Gen Genet* 200:33–39.

179. Feßler AT, Kadlec K, Hassel M, Hauschild T, Eidam C, Ehricht R, Monecke S, Schwarz S. 2011. Characterization of methicillin-resistant *Staphylococcus aureus* isolates from food and food products of poultry origin in Germany. *Appl Environ Microbiol* 77:7151–7157.

180. Kehrenberg C, Ojo KK, Schwarz S. 2004. Nucleotide sequence and organization of the multiresistance plasmid pSCFS1 from *Staphylococcus sciuri*. *J Antimicrob Chemother* 54:936–939.

181. Wendlandt S, Li B, Lozano C, Ma Z, Torres C, Schwarz S. 2013. Identification of the novel spectinomycin resistance gene *spw* in methicillin-resistant and methicillin-susceptible *Staphylococcus aureus* of human and animal origin. *J Antimicrob Chemother* 68:1679–1680.

182. Jamrozy DM, Coldham NG, Butaye P, Fielder MD. 2014. Identification of a novel plasmid-associated spectinomycin adenyltransferase gene *spd* in methicillin-resistant *Staphylococcus aureus* ST398 isolated from animal and human sources. *J Antimicrob Chemother* 69:1193–1196.

183. Wendlandt S, Feßler AT, Kadlec K, van Duijkeren E, Schwarz S. 2014. Identification of the novel spectinomycin resistance gene *spd* in a different plasmid background among methicillin-resistant *Staphylococcus aureus* CC398 and methicillin-susceptible *S. aureus* ST433. *J Antimicrob Chemother* 69:2000–2003.

184. Feßler AT, Kadlec K, Schwarz S. 2011. Novel apramycin resistance gene *apmA* in bovine and porcine methicillin-resistant *Staphylococcus aureus* ST398 isolates. *Antimicrob Agents Chemother* 55:373–375.

185. Kadlec K, Feßler AT, Couto N, Pomba CF, Schwarz S. 2012. Unusual small plasmids carrying the novel resistance genes *dfrK* or *apmA* isolated from methicillin-resistant or -susceptible staphylococci. *J Antimicrob Chemother* 67:2342–2345.

186. Aarestrup FM, Agersø Y, Ahrens P, Jørgensen JC, Madsen M, Jensen LB. 2000. Antimicrobial susceptibility and presence of resistance genes in staphylococci from poultry. *Vet Microbiol* 74:353–364.

187. Lüthje P, Schwarz S. 2007. Molecular basis of resistance to macrolides and lincosamides among staphylococci and streptococci from various animal sources

collected in the resistance monitoring program BfT-GermVet. *Int J Antimicrob Agents* 29:528–535.

188. Eady EA, Ross JI, Tipper JL, Walters CE, Cove JH, Noble WC. 1993. Distribution of genes encoding erythromycin ribosomal methylases and an erythromycin efflux pump in epidemiologically distinct groups of staphylococci. *J Antimicrob Chemother* 31:211–217.

189. Werckenthin C, Schwarz S. 2000. Molecular analysis of the translational attenuator of a constitutively expressed *erm*(A) gene from *Staphylococcus intermedius*. *J Antimicrob Chemother* 46:785–788.

190. Nawaz MS, Khan SA, Khan AA, Khambaty FM, Cerniglia CE. 2000. Comparative molecular analysis of erythromycin-resistance determinants in staphylococcal isolates of poultry and human origin. *Mol Cell Probes* 14:311–319.

191. Jaglic Z, Vlkova H, Bardon J, Michu E, Cervinkova D, Babak V. 2012. Distribution, characterization and genetic bases of erythromycin resistance in staphylococci and enterococci originating from livestock. *Zoonoses Public Health* 59:202–211.

192. Werckenthin C, Schwarz S, Dyke K. 1996. Macrolide-lincosamide-streptogramin B resistance in *Staphylococcus lentus* results from the integration of part of a transposon into a small plasmid. *Antimicrob Agents Chemother* 40:2224–2225.

193. Lüthje P, Schwarz S. 2006. Antimicrobial resistance of coagulase-negative staphylococci from bovine subclinical mastitis with particular reference to macrolide-lincosamide resistance phenotypes and genotypes. *J Antimicrob Chemother* 57:966–969.

194. Li L, Feng W, Zhang Z, Xue H, Zhao X. 2015. Macrolide-lincosamide-streptogramin resistance phenotypes and genotypes of coagulase-positive *Staphylococcus aureus* and coagulase-negative staphylococcal isolates from bovine mastitis. *BMC Vet Res* 11:168.

195. Lodder G, Werckenthin C, Schwarz S, Dyke K. 1997. Molecular analysis of naturally occuring *erm*C-encoding plasmids in staphylococci isolated from animals with and without previous contact with macrolide/lincosamide antibiotics. *FEMS Immunol Med Microbiol* 18:7–15.

196. Strommenger B, Kehrenberg C, Kettlitz C, Cuny C, Verspohl J, Witte W, Schwarz S. 2006. Molecular characterization of methicillin-resistant *Staphylococcus aureus* strains from pet animals and their relationship to human isolates. *J Antimicrob Chemother* 57:461–465.

197. Wendlandt S, Kadlec K, Feßler AT, van Duijkeren E, Schwarz S. 2014. Two different *erm*(C)-carrying plasmids in the same methicillin-resistant *Staphylococcus aureus* CC398 isolate from a broiler farm. *Vet Microbiol* 171:382–387.

198. Vancraeynest D, Hermans K, Martel A, Vaneechoutte M, Devriese LA, Haesebrouck F. 2004. Antimicrobial resistance and resistance genes in *Staphylococcus aureus* strains from rabbits. *Vet Microbiol* 101:245–251.

199. Schwarz S, Wegener H, Blobel H. 1990. Plasmid-encoded resistance to macrolides and lincosamides in *Staphylococcus hyicus*. *J Appl Bacteriol* 69:845–849.

200. Schwarz S, Lange C, Werckenthin C. 1998. Molecular analysis of the macrolide-lincosamide resistance gene region of a novel plasmid from *Staphylococcus hyicus*. *J Med Microbiol* **47**:63–70.

201. Hauschild T, Lüthje P, Schwarz S. 2006. Characterization of a novel type of MLS$_B$ resistance plasmid from *Staphylococcus saprophyticus* carrying a constitutively expressed *erm*(C) gene. *Vet Microbiol* **115**:258–263.

202. Hauschild T, Schwarz S. 2010. Macrolide resistance in *Staphylococcus* spp. from free-living small mammals. *Vet Microbiol* **144**:530–531.

203. Schwarz S, Blobel H. 1990. Isolation of a plasmid from "canine" *Staphylococcus epidermidis* mediating constitutive resistance to macrolides and lincosamides. *Comp Immunol Microbiol Infect Dis* **13**:209–216.

204. Lodder G, Schwarz S, Gregory P, Dyke K. 1996. Tandem duplication in *ermC* translational attenuator of the macrolide-lincosamide-streptogramin B resistance plasmid pSES6 from *Staphylococcus equorum*. *Antimicrob Agents Chemother* **40**:215–217.

205. Chung WO, Werckenthin C, Schwarz S, Roberts MC. 1999. Host range of the *ermF* rRNA methylase gene in bacteria of human and animal origin. *J Antimicrob Chemother* **43**:5–14.

206. Schwarz S, Kehrenberg C, Ojo KK. 2002. *Staphylococcus sciuri* gene *erm*(33), encoding inducible resistance to macrolides, lincosamides, and streptogramin B antibiotics, is a product of recombination between *erm*(C) and *erm*(A). *Antimicrob Agents Chemother* **46**:3621–3623.

207. Li D, Wu C, Wang Y, Fan R, Schwarz S, Zhang S. 2015. Identification of multiresistance gene *cfr* in methicillin-resistant *Staphylococcus aureus* from pigs: plasmid location and integration into a staphylococcal cassette chromosome *mec* complex. *Antimicrob Agents Chemother* **59**:3641–3644.

208. Schwendener S, Perreten V. 2012. New MLS$_B$ resistance gene *erm*(43) in *Staphylococcus lentus*. *Antimicrob Agents Chemother* **56**:4746–4752.

209. Wipf JR, Schwendener S, Perreten V. 2014. The novel macrolide-lincosamide-streptogramin B resistance gene *erm*(44) is associated with a prophage in *Staphylococcus xylosus*. *Antimicrob Agents Chemother* **58**:6133–6138.

210. Wendlandt S, Heß S, Li J, Feßler AT, Wang Y, Kadlec K, Gallert C, Schwarz S. 2015. Detection of the macrolide-lincosamide-streptogramin B resistance gene *erm*(44) and a novel *erm*(44) variant in staphylococci from aquatic environments. *FEMS Microbiol Ecol* **91**:fiv090.

211. Wipf JR, Schwendener S, Nielsen JB, Westh H, Perreten V. 2015. The new macrolide-lincosamide-streptogramin B resistance gene *erm*(45) is located within a genomic island in *Staphylococcus fleurettii*. *Antimicrob Agents Chemother* **59**:3578–3581.

212. Wipf JRK, Riley MC, Kania SA, Bemis DA, Andreis S, Schwendener S, Perreten V. 2017. New macrolide-lincosamide-streptogramin B resistance gene *erm*(48) on the novel plasmid pJW2311 in *Staphylococcus xylosus*. *Antimicrob Agents Chemother* **61**:e00066–e17.

213. Ross JI, Eady EA, Cove JH, Cunliffe WJ, Baumberg S, Wootton JC. 1990. Inducible erythromycin resistance in staphylococci is encoded by a member of the ATP-binding transport super-gene family. *Mol Microbiol* **4**:1207–1214.

214. Sharkey LK, Edwards TA, O'Neill AJ. 2016. ABC-F proteins mediate antibiotic resistance through ribosomal protection. *MBio* **7**:e01975.

215. Matsuoka M, Endou K, Kobayashi H, Inoue M, Nakajima Y. 1998. A plasmid that encodes three genes for resistance to macrolide antibiotics in *Staphylococcus aureus*. *FEMS Microbiol Lett* **167**:221–227.

216. Brisson-Noël A, Courvalin P. 1986. Nucleotide sequence of gene *linA* encoding resistance to lincosamides in *Staphylococcus haemolyticus*. *Gene* **43**:247–253.

217. Loeza-Lara PD, Soto-Huipe M, Baizabal-Aguirre VM, Ochoa-Zarzosa A, Valdez-Alarcón JJ, Cano-Camacho H, López-Meza JE. 2004. pBMSa1, a plasmid from a dairy cow isolate of *Staphylococcus aureus*, encodes a lincomycin resistance determinant and replicates by the rolling-circle mechanism. *Plasmid* **52**:48–56.

218. Lozano C, Aspiroz C, Sáenz Y, Ruiz-García M, Royo-García G, Gómez-Sanz E, Ruiz-Larrea F, Zarazaga M, Torres C. 2012. Genetic environment and location of the *lnu*(A) and *lnu*(B) genes in methicillin-resistant *Staphylococcus aureus* and other staphylococci of animal and human origin. *J Antimicrob Chemother* **67**:2804–2808.

219. Lozano C, Aspiroz C, Rezusta A, Gómez-Sanz E, Simon C, Gómez P, Ortega C, Revillo MJ, Zarazaga M, Torres C. 2012. Identification of novel *vga*(A)-carrying plasmids and a Tn*5406*-like transposon in meticillin-resistant *Staphylococcus aureus* and *Staphylococcus epidermidis* of human and animal origin. *Int J Antimicrob Agents* **40**:306–312.

220. Lüthje P, von Köckritz-Blickwede M, Schwarz S. 2007. Identification and characterization of nine novel types of small staphylococcal plasmids carrying the lincosamide nucleotidyltransferase gene *lnu*(A). *J Antimicrob Chemother* **59**:600–606.

221. Zhao Q, Wendlandt S, Li H, Li J, Wu C, Shen J, Schwarz S, Wang Y. 2014. Identification of the novel lincosamide resistance gene *lnu*(E) truncated by IS*Enfa5-cfr*-IS*Enfa5* insertion in *Streptococcus suis*: de novo synthesis and confirmation of functional activity in *Staphylococcus aureus*. *Antimicrob Agents Chemother* **58**:1785–1788.

222. Roberts MC, Sutcliffe J, Courvalin P, Jensen LB, Rood J, Seppala H. 1999. Nomenclature for macrolide and macrolide-lincosamide-streptogramin B resistance determinants. *Antimicrob Agents Chemother* **43**:2823–2830.

223. Allignet J, El Solh N. 1997. Characterization of a new staphylococcal gene, *vgaB*, encoding a putative ABC transporter conferring resistance to streptogramin A and related compounds. *Gene* **202**:133–138.

224. Haroche J, Allignet J, Buchrieser C, El Solh N. 2000. Characterization of a variant of *vga*(A) conferring resistance to streptogramin A and related compounds. *Antimicrob Agents Chemother* **44**:2271–2275.

225. Gentry DR, McCloskey L, Gwynn MN, Rittenhouse SF, Scangarella N, Shawar R, Holmes DJ. 2008. Genetic characterization of Vga ABC proteins conferring reduced susceptibility of *Staphylococcus aureus* to pleuromutilins. *Antimicrob Agents Chemother* 52:4507–4509.

226. Schwendener S, Perreten V. 2011. New transposon Tn*6133* in methicillin-resistant *Staphylococcus aureus* ST398 contains *vga*(E), a novel streptogramin A, pleuromutilin, and lincosamide resistance gene. *Antimicrob Agents Chemother* 55:4900–4904.

227. Hauschild T, Feßler AT, Kadlec K, Billerbeck C, Schwarz S. 2012. Detection of the novel *vga*(E) gene in methicillin-resistant *Staphylococcus aureus* CC398 isolates from cattle and poultry. *J Antimicrob Chemother* 67:503–504.

228. Kadlec K, Pomba CF, Couto N, Schwarz S. 2010. Small plasmids carrying *vga*(A) or *vga*(C) genes mediate resistance to lincosamides, pleuromutilins and streptogramin A antibiotics in methicillin-resistant *Staphylococcus aureus* ST398 from swine. *J Antimicrob Chemother* 65:2692–2693.

229. Novotna G, Janata J. 2006. A new evolutionary variant of the streptogramin A resistance protein, Vga(A)$_{LC}$, from *Staphylococcus haemolyticus* with shifted substrate specificity towards lincosamides. *Antimicrob Agents Chemother* 50:4070–4076.

230. Wendlandt S, Kadlec K, Feßler AT, Schwarz S. 2015. Identification of ABC transporter genes conferring combined pleuromutilin-lincosamide-streptogramin A resistance in bovine methicillin-resistant *Staphylococcus aureus* and coagulase-negative staphylococci. *Vet Microbiol* 177:353–358.

231. Li J, Li B, Wendlandt S, Schwarz S, Wang Y, Wu C, Ma Z, Shen J. 2014. Identification of a novel *vga*(E) gene variant that confers resistance to pleuromutilins, lincosamides and streptogramin A antibiotics in staphylococci of porcine origin. *J Antimicrob Chemother* 69:919–923.

232. Deng F, Wang H, Liao Y, Li J, Feßler AT, Michael GB, Schwarz S, Wang Y. 2017. Detection and genetic environment of pleuromutilin-lincosamide-streptogramin A resistance genes in staphylococci isolated from pets. *Front Microbiol* 8:234.

233. Hot C, Berthet N, Chesneau O. 2014. Characterization of *sal*(A), a novel gene responsible for lincosamide and streptogramin A resistance in *Staphylococcus sciuri*. *Antimicrob Agents Chemother* 58:3335–3341.

234. Schwarz S, Werckenthin C, Kehrenberg C. 2000. Identification of a plasmid-borne chloramphenicol-florfenicol resistance gene in *Staphylococcus sciuri*. *Antimicrob Agents Chemother* 44:2530–2533.

235. Kehrenberg C, Schwarz S, Jacobsen L, Hansen LH, Vester B. 2005. A new mechanism for chloramphenicol, florfenicol and clindamycin resistance: methylation of 23S ribosomal RNA at A2503. *Mol Microbiol* 57:1064–1073.

236. Long KS, Poehlsgaard J, Kehrenberg C, Schwarz S, Vester B. 2006. The Cfr rRNA methyltransferase confers resistance to phenicols, lincosamides, oxazolidinones, pleuromutilins, and streptogramin A antibiotics. *Antimicrob Agents Chemother* 50:2500–2505.

237. Witte W, Cuny C. 2011. Emergence and spread of *cfr*-mediated multiresistance in staphylococci: an interdisciplinary challenge. *Future Microbiol* 6:925–931.

238. Michael GB, Freitag C, Wendlandt S, Eidam C, Feßler AT, Lopes GV, Kadlec K, Schwarz S. 2015. Emerging issues in antimicrobial resistance of bacteria from food-producing animals. *Future Microbiol* 10:427–443.

239. Shen J, Wang Y, Schwarz S. 2013. Presence and dissemination of the multiresistance gene *cfr* in Gram-positive and Gram-negative bacteria. *J Antimicrob Chemother* 68:1697–1706.

240. Wang Y, Lv Y, Cai J, Schwarz S, Cui L, Hu Z, Zhang R, Li J, Zhao Q, He T, Wang D, Wang Z, Shen Y, Li Y, Feßler AT, Wu C, Yu H, Deng X, Xia X, Shen J. 2015. A novel gene, *optrA*, that confers transferable resistance to oxazolidinones and phenicols and its presence in *Enterococcus faecalis* and *Enterococcus faecium* of human and animal origin. *J Antimicrob Chemother* 70:2182–2190.

241. Li D, Wang Y, Schwarz S, Cai J, Fan R, Li J, Feßler AT, Zhang R, Wu C, Shen J. 2016. Co-location of the oxazolidinone resistance genes *optrA* and *cfr* on a multiresistance plasmid from *Staphylococcus sciuri*. *J Antimicrob Chemother* 71:1474–1478.

242. Fan R, Li D, Wang Y, He T, Feßler AT, Schwarz S, Wu C. 2016. Presence of the *optrA* gene in methicillin-resistant *Staphylococcus sciuri* of porcine origin. *Antimicrob Agents Chemother* 60:7200–7205.

243. Fan R, Li D, Feßler AT, Wu C, Schwarz S, Wang Y. 2017. Distribution of *optrA* and *cfr* in florfenicol-resistant *Staphylococcus sciuri* of pig origin. *Vet Microbiol* 210:43–48.

244. Sun C, Zhang P, Ji X, Fan R, Chen B, Wang Y, Schwarz S, Wu C. Presence and molecular characteristics of oxazolidinone resistance in staphylococci from household animals in rural China. *J Antimicrob Chemother*. (Epub ahead of print.)

245. Kadlec K, Schwarz S. 2010. Identification of the novel *dfrK*-carrying transposon Tn*559* in a porcine methicillin-susceptible *Staphylococcus aureus* ST398 strain. *Antimicrob Agents Chemother* 54:3475–3477.

246. O'Neill AJ, McLaws F, Kahlmeter G, Henriksen AS, Chopra I. 2007. Genetic basis of resistance to fusidic acid in staphylococci. *Antimicrob Agents Chemother* 51:1737–1740.

247. O'Neill AJ, Chopra I. 2006. Molecular basis of *fusB*-mediated resistance to fusidic acid in *Staphylococcus aureus*. *Mol Microbiol* 59:664–676.

248. Yazdankhah SP, Asli AW, Sørum H, Oppegaard H, Sunde M. 2006. Fusidic acid resistance, mediated by *fusB*, in bovine coagulase-negative staphylococci. *J Antimicrob Chemother* 58:1254–1256.

249. Loeffler A, Baines SJ, Toleman MS, Felmingham D, Milsom SK, Edwards EA, Lloyd DH. 2008. *In vitro* activity of fusidic acid and mupirocin against coagulase-positive staphylococci from pets. *J Antimicrob Chemother* 62:1301–1304.

250. Hodgson JE, Curnock SP, Dyke KG, Morris R, Sylvester DR, Gross MS. 1994. Molecular characterization of the gene encoding high-level mupirocin resistance in *Staphylococcus aureus* J2870. *Antimicrob Agents Chemother* 38:1205–1208.

251. Needham C, Rahman M, Dyke KG, Noble WC. 1994. An investigation of plasmids from *Staphylococcus aureus* that mediate resistance to mupirocin and tetracycline. *Microbiology* 140:2577–2583.

252. Fulham KS, Lemarie SL, Hosgood G, Dick HL. 2011. *In vitro* susceptibility testing of meticillin-resistant and meticillin-susceptible staphylococci to mupirocin and novobiocin. *Vet Dermatol* 22:88–94.

253. Manian FA. 2003. Asymptomatic nasal carriage of mupirocin-resistant, methicillin-resistant *Staphylococcus aureus* (MRSA) in a pet dog associated with MRSA infection in household contacts. *Clin Infect Dis* 36: e26–e28.

254. Matanovic K, Pérez-Roth E, Pintarić S, Šeol Martinec B. 2013. Molecular characterization of high-level mupirocin resistance in *Staphylococcus pseudinter-medius*. *J Clin Microbiol* 51:1005–1007.

255. Godbeer SM, Gold RM, Lawhon SD. 2014. Prevalence of mupirocin resistance in *Staphylococcus pseudinter-medius*. *J Clin Microbiol* 52:1250–1252.

256. Wipf JR, Perreten V. 2016. Methicillin-resistant *Staphylococcus aureus* isolated from dogs and cats in Switzerland. *Schweiz Arch Tierheilkd* 158:443–450.

257. Hauschild T, Feßler AT, Billerbeck C, Wendlandt S, Kaspar H, Mankertz J, Schwarz S, Kadlec K. 2012. Target gene mutations among methicillin-resistant *Staphylococcus aureus* and methicillin-susceptible *S. aureus* with elevated MICs of enrofloxacin obtained from diseased food-producing animals or food of animal origin. *J Antimicrob Chemother* 67:1791–1793.

258. Li J, Feßler AT, Jiang N, Fan R, Wang Y, Wu C, Shen J, Schwarz S. 2016. Molecular basis of rifampicin resistance in multiresistant porcine livestock-associated MRSA. *J Antimicrob Chemother* 71:3313–3315.

259. Kadlec K, van Duijkeren E, Wagenaar JA, Schwarz S. 2011. Molecular basis of rifampicin resistance in methicillin-resistant *Staphylococcus pseudintermedius* isolates from dogs. *J Antimicrob Chemother* 66:1236–1242.

260. Kwok GM, O'Donoghue MM, Doddangoudar VC, Ho J, Boost MV. 2013. Reduced vancomycin susceptibility in porcine ST9 MRSA isolates. *Front Microbiol* 4:316.

261. Moreno LZ, Dutra MC, Moreno M, Ferreira TS, Silva GF, Matajira CE, Silva AP, Moreno AM. 2016. Vancomycin-intermediate livestock-associated methicillin-resistant *Staphylococcus aureus* ST398/t9538 from swine in Brazil. *Mem Inst Oswaldo Cruz* 111:659–661.

262. Rensing C, Moodley A, Cavaco LM, McDevitt SF. 2018. Resistance to metals used in agricultural production. *Microbiol Spectr* 6(2).

263. Witte W, Van Dip N, Hummel R. 1980. Resistance against mercury and cadmium by *Staphylococcus aureus* of diverse ecological origin. *Z Allg Mikrobiol* 20:517–521. (In German.)

264. Schwarz S, Blobel H. 1989. Plasmids and resistance to antimicrobial agents and heavy metals in *Staphylococcus hyicus* from pigs and cattle. *Zentralbl Veterinarmed B* 36:669–673.

265. Aarestrup FM, Cavaco L, Hasman H. 2010. Decreased susceptibility to zinc chloride is associated with methicillin resistant *Staphylococcus aureus* CC398 in Danish swine. *Vet Microbiol* 142:455–457.

266. Cavaco LM, Hasman H, Stegger M, Andersen PS, Skov R, Fluit AC, Ito T, Aarestrup FM. 2010. Cloning and occurrence of *czrC*, a gene conferring cadmium and zinc resistance in methicillin-resistant *Staphylococcus aureus* CC398 isolates. *Antimicrob Agents Chemother* 54:3605–3608.

267. Cavaco LM, Hasman H, Aarestrup FM, Wagenaar JA, Graveland H, Veldman K, Mevius D, Fetsch A, Tenhagen B-A, Concepcion Porrero M, Dominguez L, Granier SA, Jouy E, Butaye P, Kaszanyitzky E, Dán A, Zmudzki J, Battisti A, Franco A, Schwarz S, Gutierrez M, Weese JS, Cui S, Pomba C, Members of MRSA-CG. 2011. Zinc resistance of *Staphylococcus aureus* of animal origin is strongly associated with methicillin resistance. *Vet Microbiol* 150:344–348.

268. Li S, Skov RL, Han X, Larsen AR, Larsen J, Sørum M, Wulf M, Voss A, Hiramatsu K, Ito T. 2011. Novel types of staphylococcal cassette chromosome *mec* elements identified in clonal complex 398 methicillin-resistant *Staphylococcus aureus* strains. *Antimicrob Agents Chemother* 55:3046–3050.

269. Argudín MA, Lauzat B, Kraushaar B, Alba P, Agerso Y, Cavaco L, Butaye P, Porrero MC, Battisti A, Tenhagen BA, Fetsch A, Guerra B. 2016. Heavy metal and disinfectant resistance genes among livestock-associated methicillin-resistant *Staphylococcus aureus* isolates. *Vet Microbiol* 191:88–95.

270. Argudín MA, Butaye P. 2016. Dissemination of metal resistance genes among animal methicillin-resistant coagulase-negative staphylococci. *Res Vet Sci* 105:192–194.

271. Gómez-Sanz E, Kadlec K, Feßler AT, Zarazaga M, Torres C, Schwarz S. 2013. Novel *erm*(T)-carrying multiresistance plasmids from porcine and human isolates of methicillin-resistant *Staphylococcus aureus* ST398 that also harbor cadmium and copper resistance determinants. *Antimicrob Agents Chemother* 57:3275–3282.

272. Maillard J-Y. 2018. Resistance of bacteria to biocides. *Microbiol Spectr* 6(2).

273. Bjorland J, Steinum T, Kvitle B, Waage S, Sunde M, Heir E. 2005. Widespread distribution of disinfectant resistance genes among staphylococci of bovine and caprine origin in Norway. *J Clin Microbiol* 43:4363–4368.

274. Seier-Petersen MA, Nielsen LN, Ingmer H, Aarestrup FM, Agersø Y. 2015. Biocide susceptibility of *Staphylococcus aureus* CC398 and CC30 isolates from pigs and identification of the biocide resistance genes, *qacG* and *qacC*. *Microb Drug Resist* 21:527–536.

275. Couto N, Belas A, Kadlec K, Schwarz S, Pomba C. 2015. Clonal diversity, virulence patterns and antimicrobial and biocide susceptibility among human, animal and environmental MRSA in Portugal. *J Antimicrob Chemother* 70:2483–2487.

276. Slifierz MJ, Friendship RM, Weese JS. 2015. Methicillin-resistant *Staphylococcus aureus* in commercial swine herds is associated with disinfectant and zinc usage. *Appl Environ Microbiol* 81:2690–2695.

277. Couto N, Belas A, Tilley P, Couto I, Gama LT, Kadlec K, Schwarz S, Pomba C. 2013. Biocide and antimicrobial susceptibility of methicillin-resistant staphylococcal isolates from horses. *Vet Microbiol* 166:299–303.

278. Blodkamp S, Kadlec K, Gutsmann T, Naim HY, von Köckritz-Blickwede M, Schwarz S. 2016. *In vitro* activity of human and animal cathelicidins against livestock-associated methicillin-resistant *Staphylococcus aureus*. *Vet Microbiol* 194:107–111.

279. Blodkamp S, Kadlec K, Gutsmann T, Quiblier C, Naim HY, Schwarz S, von Köckritz-Blickwede M. 2017. Effects of SecDF on the antimicrobial functions of cathelicidins against *Staphylococcus aureus*. *Vet Microbiol* 200:52–58.

280. Watts JL, Sweeney MT, Lubbers BV. 2018. Antimicrobial susceptibility testing of bacteria of veterinary origin. *Microbiol Spectr* 6(2).

281. Silley P, Simjee S, Schwarz S. 2012. Surveillance and monitoring of antimicrobial resistance and antibiotic consumption in humans and animals. *Rev Sci Tech* 31:105–120.

282. Swedres-Svarm. 2016. *Consumption of Antibiotics and Occurrence of Resistance in Sweden*. Public Health Agency of Sweden and National Veterinary Institute, Solna/Uppsala, Sweden.

283. BVL. 2017. *BVL-Report 11.5; Berichte zu den Resistenzmonitoringstudien 2014 und 2015*. https://www.bvl.bund.de/DE/09_Untersuchungen/01_Aufgaben/03_Nationales%20Resistenz-Monitoring/untersuchungen_NatResistenzmonitoring_node.html.

284. Guran HS, Kahya S. 2015. Species diversity and pheno- and genotypic antibiotic resistance patterns of staphylococci isolated from retail ground meats. *J Food Sci* 80:M1291–M1298.

285. Truong-Bolduc QC, Dunman PM, Strahilevitz J, Projan SJ, Hooper DC. 2005. MgrA is a multiple regulator of two new efflux pumps in *Staphylococcus aureus*. *J Bacteriol* 187:2395–2405.

Antimicrobial Resistance in Bacteria from Livestock and Companion Animals
Edited by Frank Møller Aarestrup, Stefan Schwarz, Jianzhong Shen, and Lina Cavaco
© 2018 American Society for Microbiology, Washington, DC
doi:10.1128/microbiolspec.ARBA-0008-2017

Antimicrobial Resistance in *Streptococcus* spp.

8

Marisa Haenni[1], Agnese Lupo[1], and Jean-Yves Madec[1]

TAXONOMIC OVERVIEW OF STREPTOCOCCI

More than 60 *Streptococcus* species have been recognized so far. Some of these, such as *S. pyogenes*, *S. agalactiae*, *S. equi*, *S. canis*, and *S. iniae*, produce hemolytic factors and, when cultivated on solid media containing blood, can be classified as beta-hemolytic. However, nonhemolytic variants can also be observed (1). Isolates belonging to other species, such as *S. dysgalactiae* subsp. *dysgalactiae*, *S. pneumoniae*, *S. mutans*, *S. salivarius*, *S. sanguinis*, *S. gordonii*, *S. mitis*, and *S. oralis*, produce hydrogen peroxide that partially lyses the erythrocytes, with the subsequent oxidation of the heme group resulting in a greenish pigment in the medium that is often interpreted as alpha-hemolysis. This oxidation process is influenced by several cultivation conditions and is variably evident. For this reason, it is preferable to consider those latter-mentioned species as nonhemolytic. The truly nonhemolytic species, mainly encompassing *S. gallolyticus* (formerly *S. bovis*), were also named gamma-hemolytic. A classification of *Streptococcus* species proposed by Rebecca Lancefield in the 1930s was based on the antigenic reaction of the cell wall-associated carbohydrates and remains classically used (2). On the basis of this approach, streptococci are distributed into groups ranging from A to W, depending on the antibodies recognizing the specific carbohydrates of a definite streptococcal species. Nevertheless, the whole picture is sometimes complicated by the fact that several antibodies can react with isolates belonging to the same species. For instance, depending on the isolates, *S. dysgalactiae* subsp. *equisimilis* may be classified as belonging to the C or G group, while it may also be classified, even though less commonly, as group A or L (3); isolates from *S. phocae* may belong to either the C or G group; isolates from

S. infantarius are sporadically considered as group D; isolates from *S. anginosus* are indifferently classified as group A, C, G, F, or N; isolates from *S. constellatus* subsp. *constellatus* belong to either group F or N; sporadic isolates belonging to *S. constellatus* subsp. *pharyngis* can be considered as group C; isolates from the *S. intermedius* species can be considered as group N; and finally, isolates belonging to *S. porcinus* are classified in either group P, U, or V.

In the following sections, the most relevant *Streptococcus* species responsible for diseases in animals and/ or humans will be summarized. The relative resistances to selected antibiotics will be discussed in the sections on macrolides-lincosamides-streptogramins B tetracyclines, beta-lactam resistance, fluoroquinolone resistance, and integrative and conjugative elements (ICEs).

Group A

Streptococci have diverse ecological origins, and certain species are exclusively adapted to a unique host as exemplified by the beta-hemolytic *S. pyogenes*, which is considered as the most pathogenic type of streptococcus for humans, together with *S. pneumoniae*, and is responsible for pharyngitis, erysipelas, and other invasive diseases such as soft tissue infection, rheumatic fever, glomerulonephritis, and streptococcal toxic shock syndrome (STSS) (4, 5). The finding of *S. pyogenes* in animals has been debated. According to Copperman (6), pets could have been the source of contagious pharyngitis (6), but no expansion of these findings has been reported, supporting the hypothesis that humans are the exclusive reservoir of *S. pyogenes*.

Group B

The beta-hemolytic *S. agalactiae*, or group B streptococci, according to the Lancefield's classification, is a

---

[1]Université de Lyon—ANSES, Unité Antibiorésistance et Virulence Bactériennes, Lyon, France.

commensal of the human intestinal and urogenital tract and is infamous as a human pathogen causing severe diseases such as pneumonia, sepsis, and meningitis in newborns and pregnant women; recently, its pathogenic importance in elderly and immunocompromised patients has been re-evaluated (7). *S. agalactiae* is also an animal pathogen and has been reported from a variety of hosts such as fish with meningoencephalitis (8), camels with mastitis and joints infections (9), and horses with unspecified disease or death (10). Classically, *S. agalactiae* has been associated with mastitis in cows (11), and the zoonotic potential of *S. agalactiae* is debated. On one side, genomic comparative approaches highlight a specific host adaptation of *S. agalactiae* isolates causing infections (12); on the other side, infections of humans from consumption of fish infected by *S. agalactiae* has recently been documented (13). Also, experimental infections of fish with *S. agalactiae* isolates of human origin have resulted in fish death (14). Globally, the hygienic control measures implemented for controlling contagious bovine mastitis have contributed to a sharply decreased prevalence of *S. agalactiae* in the veterinary sector (15, 16).

Group D
Group D streptococci were divided into two diverging groups in the early 1980s: *S. feacalis* and *S. faecium*, which were renamed *Enterococcus faecalis* and *Enterococcus faecium* (17). Since then, several new species have been added to the *Enterococcus* genus (18), which will not be discussed in this review.

Formerly, *S. bovis* was included in the viridans group of streptococci, and its taxonomy has been reviewed in several studies. Overall, several previously identified *S. bovis* isolates were classified as group D according to Lancefield's reaction, as shown in Table 1. Molecular evidence has provided the basis for the classification of the former *S. bovis* isolates into five species: *S. gallolyticus* subsp. *gallolyticus*, *S. gallolyticus* subsp. *pasteurianus*, *S. gallolyticus* subsp. *macedonicus*, *S. infantarius* subsp. *infantarius*, and *S. lutetiensis* (19). Isolates belonging to *S. gallolyticus* subsp. *gallolyticus* have been found as commensals of the gastrointestinal tract of humans and animals but also cause invasive diseases such as sepsis, endocarditis, arthritis, and meningitis in both humans and animals (Table 1). The transmission of *S. gallolyticus* subsp. *gallolyticus* between animals and humans has been reported (20), highlighting the zoonotic potential of this species. *S. gallolyticus* subsp. *pasteurianus* is an emergent infective agent in human medicine that is responsible for sepsis, bone and joint infections, and meningitis (21–23). In birds, this

bacterium is responsible for similar diseases (24, 25). *S. lutetiensis* has rarely been associated with infective endocarditis and sepsis (26).

Group E
In Lancefield's group E, *S. porcinus* is typically associated with sepsis, endocarditis, pneumonia, and lymphadenitis in swine (27). Infections sustained by *S. porcinus* have also occurred in humans (28); however, *S. porcinus* isolates infecting humans seem to have a different origin when compared to *S. porcinus* isolates of nonhuman sources (29).

Groups C and G
S. dysgalactiae subsp. *dysgalactiae* belongs to Lancefield's group C and G and plays a major role in mastitis (30). On rare occasions, it has also been found in necrotic tissues of fish and in humans, as responsible for various diseases (Table 1). In the same Lancefield's groups, *S. dysgalactiae* subsp. *equisimilis* is a beta-hemolytic bacterium found associated with strangles-like diseases in horses and with arthritis and endocarditis in swine. Unfortunately, this species is also associated with invasive diseases in humans, such as STSS and sepsis (Table 1). *S. equi* subsp. *zooepidemicus* organisms react with group C and G Lancefield's antigens as well. This organism is commonly found in bovine mastitis (90, 94, 137; also see Table and Table 3) and has sporadically been found associated with mastitis in sheep (31) and is most prevalent in equine infective diseases as the causative agent of joint and respiratory tract infections (32). This species also causes severe infections in humans in association with the consumption of contaminated dairy products (33). Transmission of *S. canis* isolates belonging to Lancefield's group C and G between pets and humans seems conceivable (34). This bacterium is responsible for arthritis in cats and humans (35) and endocarditis and skin, soft tissue, and urinary tract infections in dogs and humans. Skin lesions seem to represent the entry portal for establishing infections in humans (34, 36). In contrast, *S. equi* subsp. *equi*, belonging to Lancefield's groups C and G and responsible for strangles disease in horses, is exclusively animal adapted (32).

Group R
S. suis is a major pathogen for swine and causes meningitis, endocarditis, sepsis, arthritis, and pneumonia. In humans, *S. suis* is mostly responsible for meningitis and STSS. It is a well-recognized zoonotic agent, and indeed, human exposure to swine and swine-derived food products is a risk factor for infection by *S. suis* (37, 38).

Table 1 Overview of streptococci causative of infections in humans and animals[a]

Lancefield group	Hemolysin	Species	Host	Associated disease	References
B	Beta	*S. agalactiae*	Human	Sepsis, meningitis, pneumonia, joint and urinary tract infections	7, 11, 199, 200
			Cows, camels, horses, dolphins, fish	Mastitis, joint infection, meningitis, death	
C	Alpha	*S. dysgalactiae* subsp. *dysgalactiae*	Humans	Endocarditis, joint infection, cellulitis	48, 201, 202
			Fish, cows	Tissue necrosis, mastitis	
	Beta	*S. dysgalactiae* subsp. *equisimilis*	Humans	STSS, sepsis, soft tissue infections, pneumonia, pharyngitis	33, 203–210
			Swine, seals, horses	Arthritis, endocarditis, lymphadenitis, joint infection, strangles-like disease, respiratory tract infection	
	Beta	*S. equi* subsp. *equi*	Horses	Strangles disease	32
	Beta	*S. equi* subsp. *zooepidemicus*	Humans	Nephritis, STSS	33
			Sheep, horses	Mastitis, lymphadenitis, joint and respiratory infections, endometritis	31, 32, 211
	Beta	*S. phocae*	Fish, seals	Respiratory infections, abortions, sepsis	212
D		*S. gallolyticus* spp. *gallolyticus*	Humans	Sepsis, endocarditis, arthritis, meningitis	213–216
			Koalas, birds	Intestinal colonizer, endocarditis, sepsis	
		S. gallolyticus spp. *pasteurianus*	Humans	Sepsis, bone and joint infections, meningitis	21–25
			Birds	Sepsis, meningitis	
E	Beta	*S. porcinus*	Humans	Urinary tract, placenta, and wound infections, sepsis	27, 28, 217, 218
			Swine	Endocarditis, respiratory tract infection, sepsis	
G	Beta	*S. canis*	Humans	Skin, soft-tissue and respiratory infections, sepsis	34, 35, 219, 220
			Dogs, cats	Skin, soft-tissue, and urinary tract infections, otitis, arthritis, STSS	
R	Nonhemolytic/beta	*S. suis*	Humans	Sepsis, meningitis, endocarditis, STSS	37, 221–225
			Swine, boars, rabbits	Sepsis, meningitis, pneumonia, arthritis	
Undefined	Beta	*S. iniae*	Humans	Soft-tissue infection	48, 49
			Dolphins, fish	Abscess, streptococcosis, sepsis	226–231
		S. uberis/ *S. parauberis*	Cows, horses	Mastitis	11, 16, 30, 43

[a]Isolates belonging to *S. dysgalactiae* subsp. *equisimilis* react with antigen G with comparable prevalence of antigen C reaction, whereas reaction with antigens A and L are less common; isolates belonging to *S. phocae* react also with antigen G; isolates belonging to *S. porcinus* react also with antigens P, U, and V. Nonhemolytic variant can be recovered among isolates of *S. agalactiae* and *S. dysgalactiae* subsp. *equisimilis*.

The production of a capsule seems to have a major role in pathogenesis, and capsular types 2 and 14 are the most prevalent among *S. suis* isolates that cause disease in humans (39).

Non-Lancefield Streptococci
All other streptococci lacking the Lancefield antigens are thus considered non-Lancefield (or nontypable) streptococci. Several are frequently encountered in animals and are detailed below.

S. uberis
If hygienic measures have been effective to control the dissemination of *S. agalactiae*, the same cannot be said for *S. uberis*, which remains a major animal pathogen and a leading cause of mastitis in cattle (15, 16). This

nonserotypable organism has an environmental origin, possesses a flexible metabolism, and is almost exclusively adapted to cattle (40). Infections can occur by a variety of strains, which in some cases are able to persist and propagate among different cows within a herd (41, 42). Rarely, it has been responsible for mastitis in heifers, and even more rarely it has been isolated from shrimps (43–45). The control of *S. uberis* propagation is more challenging than that of other *Streptococcus* spp. probably because of its ability, among others, to survive on bedding material (46, 47).

S. iniae

Another nonserotypable species is *S. iniae*, which was primarily isolated from diseased dolphins and was subsequently confirmed as a major fish pathogen and as responsible for soft tissue infections in humans with zoonotic features (Table 1) (48–52).

S. pneumoniae

S. pneumoniae is a major streptococcal pathogen of humans and is responsible for serious infections such as pneumonia and meningitis; reports of infections in animals are extremely rare and concern horses with respiratory tract infections (53). A recent publication also reported *S. pneumoniae*, probably of human origin, in wild and captive chimpanzees (54). The spread of this pathogen due to the migration of infected animals to other communities or the reintroduction into wild populations of formerly captive animals might be a real danger.

Viridans streptococci

These organisms were defined as viridans because of the hemolytic features described above that produce a greenish pigmentation on blood agar, their absence of Lancefield antigens, and their resistance to the chemical compound optochin. Generally, viridans streptococci are implicated in the establishment of dental caries, arthritis, and infective endocarditis in humans (50–52).

Certain *Streptococcus* species, including *S. sobrinus* and *S. mutans*, the first representative of the mutans group; *S. salivarius*, *S. vestibularis*, and *S. infantarius* from the salivarius group; the anginosus group, including *S. anginosus*, *S. constellatus*, and *S. intermedius*; the sanguinus group, including *S. sanguinis*, *S. parasanguinis*, and *S. gordonii*; and most species of the mitis group, including *S. mitis*, *S. oralis*, *S. cristatus*, *S. infantis*, and *S. peroris*, have exclusive human adaptation; others have been found only in animal hosts, such as *S. macacae* from monkeys, *S. ferus* from wild rodents, *S. orisratti* from rats, and *S. hyointestinalis* and *S. hyovaginalis* from swine, with no associated

diseases (55–59). Three species of the viridans group, namely *S. sobrinus*, *S. criceti*, and *S. ratti*, have been reported from humans and experimental rats, whereas *S. alactolyticus* has been found in swine, dogs, and humans (56, 60, 61); *S. downei* was isolated first from a monkey and more recently from human dental plaque (62, 63). Another species of the viridans group, *S. pluranimalium*, has been reported rarely. It was first reported in 1999 from bovine mastitis, and few clinical human cases have been reported since then (64, 65).

This brief introduction does not pretend to be exhaustive. The reviews by Póntigo et al. and Facklam provide a comprehensive nomenclature and classification of streptococci based on molecular and phenotypic features, respectively (1, 66).

EVOLUTION OF ANTIMICROBIAL RESISTANCE IN VETERINARY STREPTOCOCCI

Monitoring Programs

Prevalence data on antimicrobial resistance were principally obtained through dedicated studies performed at the scale of a region, a country, or a consortium of countries. However, only monitoring programs can give an evolutionary picture of antimicrobial resistance rates over time. Consequently, surveillance systems are highly valuable to follow trends and detect emergent resistant phenotypes.

Several national surveillance and monitoring programs in veterinary medicine exist in Europe (67), including the Monitoring of Antimicrobial Resistance and Antibiotic Usage in Animals in the Netherlands program, the Swedish Veterinary Antimicrobial Resistance Monitoring program (SVARM), the Danish Integrated Antimicrobial Resistance Monitoring and Research Program, the German Resistance Monitoring in Veterinary Medicine program, and the French surveillance network for antimicrobial resistance in pathogenic bacteria of animal origin (RESAPATH). Two similar programs cover the North American continent, the National Antimicrobial Resistance Monitoring System for Enteric Bacteria in the United States and the Canadian Integrated Program for Antimicrobial Resistance Surveillance, and one reports Japanese data (the Japanese Veterinary Antimicrobial Resistance Monitoring program). An additional industry-based pan-European monitoring program commissioned by the Executive Animal Health Study Center investigates pathogens from farm (VetPath) and companion animals (ComPath). In addition to the recurrently criticized lack of harmonization (67, 68), a major feature of most programs is their main focus on bacteria of animal origin but of relevance for human health, such as zoonotics and commensal indicators. Accordingly, streptococci of animal origin were poorly included, and data on their resistance to antimicrobials remain limited at a global scale. Indeed, only two monitoring programs reported data on a long-term basis: the Monitoring of Antimicrobial Resistance and Antibiotic Usage in Animals in the Netherlands program from 2002 to 2008 and RESAPATH from 2006 until today. Other programs such as the Swedish Veterinary Antimicrobial Resistance Monitoring program (in 2002), the German Resistance Monitoring in Veterinary Medicine program, and ComPath/VetPath have also documented antimicrobial resistance in streptococci, but on a sporadic basis.

Different Methodologies to Determine Antibiotic Resistance

Standard surveillance programs rely on phenotypic methods that are used in routine diagnostic laboratories. The most frequently used methods are antibiograms performed by disc diffusion and MIC performed by broth microdilution. These techniques generate qualitative or quantitative results, respectively, that are then interpreted according to official guidelines (EUCAST, CLSI, Antibiogram Committee of the French Microbiology Society (CA-SFM), etc.) so that the studied isolates can be classified as susceptible, intermediate, or resistant to the tested antibiotics. In the surveillance systems, the genotypic techniques are only optionally implemented as a second-line characterization.

This traditional approach may be disrupted by the democratization of next-generation sequencing methodologies. Recently, several publications proved the usefulness of large-scale genomic analyses for the efficient detection of resistance mechanisms and capsular types (69), for the sequence-based prediction of beta-lactam resistance using the penicillin-binding protein (PBP) transpeptidase signatures (70), and for the prediction of the antimicrobial profile and its potential evolution toward resistance over time (71). This is, of course, not an exhaustive list of publications using next-generation sequencing, especially in a field that is progressing very rapidly. There are still a couple of drawbacks to the direct implementation of next-generation sequencing in diagnostic laboratories, including the time needed to generate results (which exceeds the 48 hours traditionally needed for phenotypic testing) and the price. However, this methodology is so powerful that it will undoubtedly be used in monitoring programs, at least for long-term surveillance purposes.

Evolution of Resistance in *Streptococcus* spp.

The main *Streptococcus* species studied through monitoring programs were *S. uberis* and *S. dysgalactiae* isolated from bovine mastitis. *S. agalactiae* is also still considered a major streptococcal pathogen associated with bovine subclinical and mild to moderate clinical mastitis, but its incidence has drastically fallen in the past 20 years due to hygiene measures and guidelines for good practices. Consequently, *S. agalactiae* is now only rarely isolated from cattle mastitis, and the numbers are too small to be reliably reported. The evolution of antimicrobial resistance thus focuses on *S. uberis* and *S. dysgalactiae*. Here, we review data on resistance to the main antibiotics used in the treatment of animal infections due to *S. uberis* and *S. dysgalactiae*, i.e., penicillin G, tetracyclines, erythromycin, lincomycin, enrofloxacin, and streptomycin.

Evolution of Antimicrobial Resistance in the Netherlands

The Monitoring of Antimicrobial Resistance and Antibiotic Usage in Animals in the Netherlands program reported antimicrobial resistance data on streptococci isolates collected from milk in the context of intramammary infections, but the monitoring of these pathogens stopped in 2008. From 2002 to 2008, the overall prevalence of resistance was quite stable for most antibiotics, with a seemingly upward trend for a few (72). Resistance to beta-lactams (represented by penicillin G and cefalotin) was only detected in rare cases of *S. uberis* and was absent in *S. dysgalactiae*. The highest rates of resistance were for tetracyclines (around 40% for *S. uberis* and 70% for *S. dysgalactiae*) and lincomycin (also around 40% for *S. uberis* and 25% for *S. dysgalactiae*). The discrepancy between the prevalence of tetracycline resistance in *S. dysgalactiae* compared to *S. uberis* is in accordance with what has been reported in other monitoring programs (see below) and numerous studies (see "Prevalence of Resistance to Macrolides among Streptococci of Bovine Origin" below). Resistance to erythromycin (around 20% for *S. uberis* and 10% for *S. dysgalactiae*) was systematically lower than for lincomycin, suggesting a significant prevalence of non-*erm*-mediated mechanisms of resistance.

RESAPATH, the Ongoing French Monitoring Program

RESAPATH is the only ongoing and long-term monitoring program for, among other topics, resistance to antimicrobials in streptococci in Europe. For *S. uberis*, from 2006 to 2015, antimicrobial resistance was tested on 600 to 1,500 isolates, depending on the nature of the antibiotics, and the global trend was quite stable for all antibiotics (Fig. 1). The highest prevalence of resistance was observed for enrofloxacin, which may be explained by the intrinsic low-level resistance of streptococci to fluoroquinolones. Indeed, in the RESAPATH network, resistance is defined as the addition of both resistant and intermediate phenotypes, which may lead to the over-estimation of the prevalence of resistance in the case of fluoroquinolones. For erythromycin and lincomycin, the resistance rates decreased from 24% to 17% between 2006 and 2007, were stable during next 6 years until 2013, and increased again in 2014 to 2015 up to around 22% of resistant isolates. Both curves matched perfectly, indicating a cross-resistance to macrolides-lincosamides involving *erm* genes (see "Resistance to Macrolides, Lincosamides, and Streptogramin B" below). Tetracycline resistance is following a very slow upward trend (from 14% in 2006 to 21% in 2015), to be confirmed in the coming years. Finally, streptomycin is the antibiotic presenting the lowest prevalence of resistance (from 11 to 16% over the 10-year period of 2006 to 2015), albeit the highest among resistance to aminoglycosides. Indeed, rates of resistance to kanamycin and gentamicin only reached 5% and 3%, respectively, in 2015. However, these resistances are of major importance since they may result in the loss of synergy between aminoglycosides and beta-lactams, which is a frequently used combination in veterinary practice. Taken together, these data show globally high basal levels of resistance of streptococci to antimicrobials in 2006 and a slight but increasing prevalence, which will have to be monitored in the near future.

The number of *S. dysgalactiae* isolates that can be considered for global trends in prevalence is around 10 times lower than for *S. uberis* (25 compared to 235 isolates), so that the prevalence rates are subject to wider variations. However, the rates observed are different though more stable than for *S. uberis*. The antibiotic with the highest prevalence of resistance by far was tetracyclines. Up to 85% of the *S. dysgalactiae* isolates were resistant to this drug, which is in accordance with what has been reported in other studies (see "Prevalence of Resistance to Macrolides among Streptococci of Bovine Origin" below). Enrofloxacin presents fluctuating resistance rates of around 50%. Finally, erythromycin, lincomycin, and streptomycin present a stable prevalence of around 22%, 12%, and 6%, respectively. The 10% discrepancy between erythromycin and lincomycin resistance rates deserves special attention since it may signal a divergence in the resistance mechanisms involved compared to *S. uberis*.

Though originating from two countries only, these evolution rates constitute a starting point to address the issue of resistance in *Streptococcus* spp. in veterinary medicine. In line with these trends, the next sections will detail the epidemiology and mechanisms of resistance of the antibiotics mentioned above.

RESISTANCE TO MACROLIDES, LINCOSAMIDES, AND STREPTOGRAMIN B

Erythromycin was the first macrolide discovered in 1952 by McGuire as a natural product originating from *Streptomyces erythreus*. The other macrolides were derived from erythromycin by semi-synthesis, and their core unit consists of a lactone ring that can be constituted by 14, 15, and 16 carbon atoms. These molecules are bacteriostatic in staphylococci and bactericidal in streptococci, inhibiting the protein translocation by binding to the 23S or 50S ribosomal subunit at peculiar residues (i.e., the guanine 2505, the uridine 2609, and the adenines 2058, 2059, and 2062) (73). Macrolides have a broad spectrum of action, being effective against Gram-positive and Gram-negative bacteria and intracellular pathogens, and are reputed as valuable agents for their good pharmacodynamics properties, their relatively few side effects, and their good penetration in tissues. Lincosamides, including lincomycin and clindamycin, together with streptogramin B, including pristinamycin and quinupristin, are structurally unrelated to macrolides, but they have a common mechanism of action and, as a consequence, resistance to all these classes of antibiotics is crossed. In addition to the treatment of infections caused by intracellular pathogens, the usage of macrolides and lincosamides in human clinics is principally dedicated to the treatment of uncomplicated infections in patients who are allergic to beta-lactams. In veterinary medicine, macrolides and lincosamides are available as in-feed and injectable formulations and are used for the treatment of a variety of diseases ranging from respiratory tract infections to infective mastitis in food-producing animals, especially swine and cattle (74, 75). Frequently, macrolides and lincosamides are used in combination with other drugs such as aminoglycosides, ampicillin, colistin, tetracyclines, sulfonamides, and trimethoprim (76). Certain macrolides were also used as growth promoters (council regulation EC2821/98, 17 December 1998). Unfortunately, shortly after the introduction of macrolides in human therapy, resistant isolates were recovered; the emergence of resistant isolates has also occurred in animals. In the following subsections we will describe the most common mechanisms of resistance to

A.

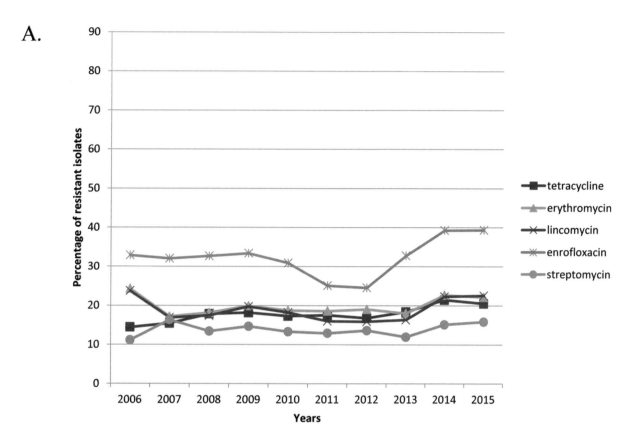

B.

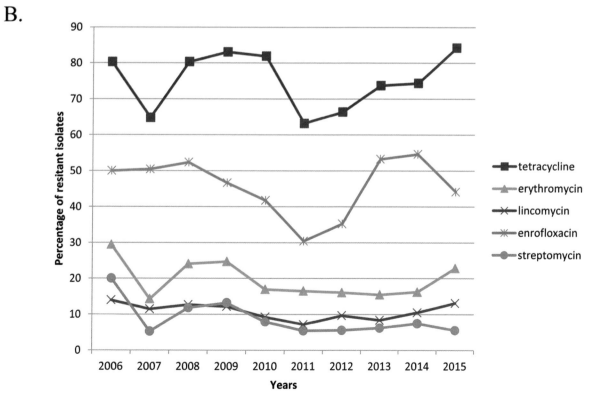

Figure 1   Ten-year evolution of resistance in France in (A) *S. uberis* and (B) *S. dysgalactiae*.

macrolides, lincosamides, and streptogramins B found in streptococci of animal origin.

Macrolides, Lincosamides, and Streptogramins B Resistance Determinants

Target modification
Ribosomal mutation in the residues crucial to the binding of macrolides results in cross-resistance to all macrolides, lincosamides, and streptogramins B conferring the so-called MLSb phenotype. Human clinical isolates with such mutations have been sporadically observed, probably because this mechanism requires mutations in all the operon copies encoding the ribosomal subunits.

Target protection
The methylation of the adenine at position 2058 is enough to confer an MLSb resistance phenotype. This reaction is mediated by the methylases encoded by the *erm* (erythromycin ribosome methylation) gene family, originated by the natural producers of macrolides. In the presence of an Erm methylase, resistance to lincosamides and streptogramin B can be either constitutive or induced by the presence of erythromycin (73). Overall, this mechanism is the most prevalent method conferring resistance to macrolides in human and veterinary clinical isolates. Currently, about 40 variants of the *erm* gene have been reported, with *erm*(B) gene being the most prevalent (77). It is often located on mobile genetic elements (MGEs) and associated with genes conferring resistance to tetracyclines (see below). These two factors have consistently contributed to the dissemination of resistance to macrolides (78).

Efflux
The second most common mechanism of resistance to macrolides in streptococci is represented by the efflux mediated by the Mef efflux pumps. The *mefA* gene was described for the first time in *S. pyogenes*, and other variants have been reported since then that are principally represented by *mefE* and *mefI* (79). These efflux systems confer resistance to 14- and 15-carbon atom macrolides only, determining an M phenotype. Transcription of *mef* genes is coupled with the expression of *msr* genes encoding for an ATP-dependent efflux system. The presence of *mef* genes seems to be necessary to confer macrolide resistance (80). Genes of the *mef* family are often located on genetic units that can transfer by transformation, such as the MEGA (macrolide efflux genetic assembly) element harboring the *mefE* gene and conjugative transposons such as the Tn*1207.3* harboring the *mefA* variant and the 5216IQ composite

element harboring the *mefI* gene (81–83). With a lower prevalence, the *mreA* efflux pump has been reported as well (84). Finally, genes of the *lsa* family have been described, conferring cross-resistance to lincosamides, streptogramin A and pleuromutilins. These genes, encoding ATP-binding proteins, most likely promote the efflux of the antibiotics (192).

Drug modification
Lincosamides can be inactivated by adenylation in position 3 by a 3-lincosamide-O-nucleotidyltransferase encoded by the *linB* gene conferring an L phenotype (85). The *linB* gene was first found in a clinical isolate of *E. faecium*. Its origin remains unknown because no similar sequence has been found in natural lincosamide producers. The *linB* gene was reported sporadically; however, its transfer to *S. agalactiae* has occurred and has been reported from a human clinical isolate in Canada (86). After the first description, the *linB* gene was renamed *lnuB*. Later, Achard et al. unveiled the mechanism behind the lincomycin resistance in an *S. agalactiae* isolate that was surprisingly susceptible to clindamycin. It consisted of a novel nucleotidyltransferase encoded by the *lnuC* gene (87). The LnuD-adenylating clindamycin was later discovered in *S. uberis* (88).

Inactivation of macrolides can also be caused by phosphotransferases encoded by the *mph* gene families with differential affinity for the different macrolide types and lincosamides according to the variant of the *mph* gene expressed (89).

Prevalence of Resistance to Macrolides among Streptococci of Bovine Origin
Studies of the resistance to macrolides in streptococci of bovine origin have focused on isolates responsible for clinical and subclinical mastitis. During an investigation of different streptococcal species from bovine mastitis during 2002 to 2003 in Portugal, Rato et al. found a constitutive MLSb phenotype in 11/60 *S. agalactiae* isolates; among those, 10 isolates were positive for the presence of an *erm*(B) gene and one harbored an *erm*(A) gene (90). Among *S. dysgalactiae* subsp. *dysgalactiae* isolates, 4/18 demonstrated a constitutive MLSb phenotype, with the presence of *erm*(A) and *erm*(B) in 1 and 3 isolates, respectively, whereas all the MLSb-resistant *S. uberis* isolates (8/30) harbored an *erm*(B) gene. An L phenotype was demonstrated in 11 isolates, 3 belonging to *S. dysgalactiae* subsp. *dysgalactiae* and 8 to *S. uberis* species, all of them harboring an *lnuB* gene. In 2005, Duarte et al. found that 8.5% (9/38) of *S. agalactiae* isolates from Brazil were resistant

to erythromycin with a constitutive MLSb phenotype. All of the isolates harbored an *erm*(B) and an *mreA* gene; six of these coharbored *erm*(A) and were co-resistant to tetracyclines (29). Contemporaneously, Dogan et al. reported a 3.6% prevalence of erythromycin-resistant isolates among 83 *S. agalactiae* from bovines in New York. The resistance was mediated by Erm(B) in all isolates, and coresistance to tetracyclines was observed as well (91). A study from China was published in 2012 on 55 *S. agalactiae* isolates recovered from bovine mastitis during an undetermined period and reported a 23.5% rate of resistance to erythromycin. All isolates harbored the *erm*(B) gene (92). Pinto et al. analyzed 29 *S. agalactiae* isolates collected between 1980 and 2006 in Brazil. They found that 27% of the isolates were resistant to erythromycin, with *erm*(B) as the most prevalent gene, followed by the *erm*(A) variant. In this study, the presence of a *mef* allele was reported as well (93).

More recently, our investigation of 76 *S. agalactiae* isolates demonstrated an MLSb phenotype in eight isolates, including four isolates with a constitutive phenotype and four with an inducible phenotype. Six isolates harbored an *erm*(B) gene, and the two remaining ones harbored the *erm*(A) variant. In the same study, 4/32 isolates of *S. dysgalactiae* demonstrated the presence of an *erm*(B) gene; in this case also, the constitutive or inducible phenotypes were equally distributed (94). The *erm*(B) gene has also been confirmed as the most common gene conferring resistance to macrolides among *S. dysgalactiae* isolates; for instance, it was present in 4/4 isolates detected in dairy herds in the southwestern United States (95). We conducted a study to characterize the erythromycin resistance of 125 isolates of *S. uberis* collected from bovine mastitis during 2007 to 2008 in France. Overall, 111/125 isolates demonstrated an MLSb phenotype, constitutive in 42.3% of the isolates and inducible in the remaining ones. An *erm*(B) gene was present in all isolates. In this collection, 14 isolates demonstrated an L phenotype and harbored an *lnuB* gene. In one isolate, the less common *lnuD* gene was found as well (96). Contemporaneously, another study, conducted on dairy cows in Mayenne, France, confirmed MLSb resistance in 12 (12/55, 22%) *S. uberis* isolates, which all were positive for the *erm*(B) gene. An *lnuB* gene was present in four isolates with the L phenotype (97). In *S. uberis*, emergence of the *mphB* gene was documented in 2008 (98), but propagation of this mechanism has not occurred in a large scale.

Among others, the German Resistance Monitoring in Veterinary Medicine program has provided extensive data from Germany from 2007 to 2010 (Table 2). Sev-

eral other studies from different parts of the world and based on the phenotypic characterization of mastitis isolates provided a comprehensive picture of the problematic link to the rise of resistance to macrolides in streptococci causing mastitis. An overview is provided in Table 2, and for exhaustive reports on temporal and geographical evolution of macrolide and lincosamide resistance in streptococci, we suggest the reports from Hendriksen et al. in 2008 and Thomas et al. in 2015 (99, 100). Overall, the lowest prevalence of macrolide and lincosamide resistance was observed in Sweden (101), and large differences in prevalence were observed among countries. However, no major variation was observed from one year to another in a single country.

Prevalence of Resistance to Macrolides among Streptococci of Porcine Origin

Macrolides, lincosamides, and streptogramins B are widely used for the treatment of infections in swine. Unfortunately, it appears that the usage of these drugs has influenced the emergence of resistance in *S. suis* (102). High rates of resistance to these drugs were observed over time, ranging from 52% (11/21 isolates) in the first observation in Norway in 1986 (103) to 94% (216/226 isolates) in Korea during 2010 to 2013 (104). The most prevalent genetic determinant is the *erm*(B) gene, whereas *mef*A/E were sporadically detected in human isolates (105). Often, such resistances occur together with tetracycline resistance (see below). *S. suis* may also act as a reservoir of lincosamide resistance genes, as exemplified by the emergence of the *lnuE* gene, previously identified in *S. suis*, in staphylococcal isolates (106). The report from Hendriksen et al. shows a certain variability of erythromycin resistance in *S. suis* among European countries during 2002 to 2004 (107). In addition, other streptococcal species were rarely found to cause diseases in swine. Within the framework of the BfT-GermVET program, Lüthje and Schwarz reported the presence of *S. dysgalactiae* subsp. *equisimilis* in diseased swine, with 21 isolates demonstrating resistance to macrolides. Among those, 13 harbored an *erm*(B) gene, one an *erm*(B) gene together with *mefA* and *msrD*, and one a *lnuB* gene (108).

In all, such an alarming prevalence of macrolide resistance in a relevant zoonotic pathogen such as *S. suis* highlights the need to prevent infections through appropriate hygienic measures.

Prevalence of Resistance to Macrolides among Streptococci from Non-Food-Producing Animals

In Brazil, six isolates of *S. dysgalactiae* subsp. *equisimilis* from horses were included in a study of antimicrobial

Table 2 Erythromycin and lincosamide resistance in streptococci in animal hosts[a]

Animal host	Country	Year	Bacterial species	No. of isolates	Genetic determinants									Percentage of resistance (%) to		Reference
					mefA	mefE	msr	ermA	ermB	lnuB	lnuD	mph	mreA	M	L	
Cattle	USA	ND	S. dysgalactiae	152										10	25.6	136
			S. uberis	133										9	42.9	
Cattle	France		S. uberis	55	0				12					22		97
Cattle	USA	ND	S. dysgalactiae	4	0	0		0	4	4				100		95
			S. uberis	20	0	0		0	12					60		
Cattle	China	ND	S. agalactiae	55	0			0	13					23.5		92
Cattle	Brazil	1980–2006	S. agalactiae	29	5			4	7	0				31	20.7	93
Cattle	France	1984–2008	S. agalactiae	76	0			2	6					10.1		94
			S. dysgalactiae	32	0			0	4					ND		
			S. uberis	101	0			0	75	5	1			ND		
Cattle	Brazil	1995–2000	S. agalactiae	38	0			6	9	0			9	8.5	8.5	29
Cattle	France	1995–2000	S. agalactiae	8										0	0	134
			S. dysgalactiae	41										16.7	11.9	
			S. uberis	50										28	36	
Cattle	Argentina	1999–2003	S. agalactiae	36										16.7	19.4	232
			S. dysgalactiae	8										12.5	12.5	
Cattle	USA	2000–2002	S. agalactiae	83	0			0	3					3.6		91
Cattle	Portugal	2002–2003	S. agalactiae	60	0			1	10	0				18.3	18.3	90
			S. dysgalactiae	18	0			1	3	3				22.2	38.9	
			S. uberis	30	0			0	8	8				26.7	26.7	
Cattle	Sweden	2002–2003	S. agalactiae	6										16.7	16.7	133
			S. dysgalactiae	152										0	0.7	
			S. uberis	113										0	0	

Source	Country	Years of isolation	Species	No. of isolates	No. tested	No. R (M)	No. R (L)	% M	% L	Reference
Cattle	Korea	2004–2008	*S. agalactiae*	5				0	60	233
			S. bovis group	24				12.5	33.3	
			S. uberis	99				34.3	41.4	
			S. oralis	30				36.7	36.7	
			S. salivarius	13				0	69.2	
			S. intermedius	7				42.8	71.4	
Cattle	Turkey	ND	*S. agalactiae*	5				0	40	169
			S. uberis	18				11	17	
Cattle	France	2007–2008	*S. uberis*	125			0	ND	ND	96
Cattle	Estonia	2007–2009	*S. agalactiae*		111		0	1.3	6.2	168
			S. dysgalactiae				3	6.7	7.8	
			S. uberis				0	8.2	6.6	
Cattle	Germany	2007–2010	*S. agalactiae*	101	15	13	2	16.8	ND	234
			S. dysgalactiae	100	10	1	2	11	ND	
			S. uberis	102	5	2	2	17.6	ND	
Cattle	Switzerland	2010–2012	*S. dysgalactiae*	46				2.2	2.2	238
			S. uberis	208				10.6	10.6	
Cattle	Switzerland	2011–2013	*S. dysgalactiae*	213				ND	37.4	167
			S. uberis	1,228				ND	49.7	
Swine	EU	1987–1997	*S. suis*	404				55.3		139
Swine	Denmark	1989–2002	*S. suis*	103	39			40.8		237
Swine	France	1996–2000	*S. suis*	110				78.2	78.2	235
Swine	Belgium	1999–2000	*S. suis*	87	62		0	71	71	236
Swine	Spain	1999–2001	*S. suis*	151				90.7	87.4	143
Swine	Italy	2003–2007	*S. suis*	57	44		0	81	81	140
Swine	China	2005–2007	*S. suis*	421		18		67.2	68.4	142
Swine	China	2005–2012	*S. suis*	96	35	51		38.5	38.5	170
Swine	China	2008–2010	*S. suis*	106	70	51	0	67.9	67.9	146
Swine	Brazil	2009–2010	*S. suis*	260				46.5	84.6	144
Swine	Korea	2010–2013	*S. suis*	227	218		39	94	95.6	104

aND, not determined; M, macrolides; L, lincosamides.

resistance in humans, and prevalence data on resistance to macrolides were similar in isolates from the two sectors (109). In Germany, an *S. equi* subsp. *zooepidemicus* isolate with an M phenotype was recovered from a horse and harbored a *mefA* and an *msrD* gene. *S. canis* resistant to macrolides, mostly with an MLSb phenotype, has been reported from diseased dogs in Denmark and Germany (110). From dogs and cats, six *S. dysgalactiae* subsp. *equisimilis* macrolide-resistant isolates were found in Germany with five isolates harboring an *erm*(B) gene and one harboring a *mefA* and a *msrD* gene (108).

TETRACYCLINES

Tetracyclines, which were discovered in the late 1940s, are bacteriostatic antibiotics that block bacterial protein synthesis by preventing the attachment of aminoacyl-tRNA to the ribosomal acceptor A site (111). Because of their broad-spectrum activity against both Gram-positive and Gram-negative bacteria, they rapidly became one of the most widely used antibiotics (112), and consequently, the first resistant isolate was reported in 1953 in *Shigella dysenteriae* (113). Tetracycline resistance rapidly and broadly disseminated in bacteria of human, animal, and environmental origin and is now considered one of the most frequently seen resistances to antimicrobials (114). In humans, tetracyclines have largely been supplanted by beta-lactams, while they remain one of the main classes of antibiotics used in veterinary medicine (115–117). In animals, tetracyclines are also considered as growth-promoting factors when mixed with food at subtherapeutic levels, in order for food-producing animals to gain weight more quickly (111). This practice was banned in Europe at the latest on 1 January 2006 since it can promote resistance selection, as exemplified by the increase of vancomycin-resistant enterococci in animals through the use of the glycopeptide avoparcin (118). However, growth promoters are still authorized in many countries worldwide, such as in the United States, and tetracycline is again the most frequently used antibiotic class (117). The past and present excessive use of tetracyclines first of all hampers the efficacy of these molecules, but may also have unexpected side effects such as the selection of hypervirulent *S. agalactiae* clones worldwide and increasing numbers of neonate infections (119).

Tetracycline Resistance Determinants

A total of 46 *tet* or *otr* genes have been identified as tetracycline resistance determinants in 126 genera (120, 121). They are commonly divided into two main groups characterized by their mode of action: the genes coding for efflux proteins and those coding for ribosomal protection enzymes (120). In *Streptococcus* spp., *tet*(K), *tet*(L), *tet*(M), *tet*(O), *tet*(Q), and *tet*(T) are the most frequently reported genes (111, 113, 121). Tet(K) and Tet(L) code for membrane-associated efflux systems that share nearly 60% amino acid identity (111) and confer resistance to tetracycline but not to minocycline. The *tet*(K) gene was discovered on a pT181 plasmid in *Staphylococcus aureus* (122), whereas *tet*(L) was found associated with small non-conjugative plasmids in streptococci (123). In contrast, Tet(M), Tet(O), Tet(S), Tet(Q), Tet(T), and the more recently identified Tet(W) are enzymes that protect the ribosome from the action of tetracycline, a mechanism conferring resistance to all available antibiotics of the tetracycline family. The *tet*(M) gene was concomitantly identified with *tet*(L) on streptococcal plasmids (123). It has now been extensively detected and studied in both Gram-negative and Gram-positive species and is often found on ICEs of the Tn*916*-Tn*1545* family (124–127). Since the Tn*916*-Tn*1545* elements also encode, among others, resistance to erythromycin and kanamycin, these mobile determinants promote the emergence of multiresistant isolates, as exemplified by their frequent association with the *tet*(M) and *erm*(B) resistance genes in streptococci isolates (120). The dissemination of the remaining protecting enzymes—Tet(O) (which was first discovered in *Campylobacter coli* [128]), Tet(S) (discovered in *Listeria monocytogenes* [129]), Tet(Q) (first described in *Bacteroides* species [130]), and the closely related Tet(T) (first detected in *S. pyogenes* [131])—was less efficient than the diffusion of Tet(M), probably because of the localization of the corresponding genes, which have never been reported on conjugative transposons such as Tn*916* and Tn*1545*, mentioned above. Of note, Tet(M), Tet(O), Tet(S), and Tet(Q) are closely related since they share around 78% sequence identity (113), even though they can easily be differentiated using specific primers. Tet(W) is the latest protection enzyme detected in streptococci and was first identified in *Butyrivibrio fibrisolvens* (132).

Prevalence of Tetracycline Resistance among Streptococci of Bovine or Ovine Origin

Most studies reporting tetracycline resistance in isolates of bovine or ovine origin were performed on *S. uberis*, *S. dysgalactiae*, and *S. agalactiae* in the context of clinical or subclinical mastitis. Tetracycline is often the antibiotic presenting the highest prevalence of resistance. When considering the CLSI breakpoints which categorize as tetracycline resistant all isolates presenting an

MIC of >4 mg/liter, resistance rates in *S. uberis* ranged from 1.8 to 4% in Sweden between 2002 and 2009 up to 60% in Portugal in 2003 (90, 101, 133), with intermediate prevalence of 12.9 to 22% in France, 15% in England, 27.1% in the United States (1997 to 1999), and 44% in Italy (99, 134–136). In *S. dysgalactiae* prevalence is overall higher, ranging from 6% in Sweden to 76.6% in the Netherlands and 100% in Portugal and France (90, 94). Prevalence rate figures are less frequently available for *S. agalactiae* but also suggest a very high frequency of tetracycline resistance, with 33.4% in Sweden in 2002 and 37.5% in France in 2000 (133, 134).

Only a few studies have reported the molecular characterization of *tet* resistance genes (Table 3) in streptococci of bovine origin. When reported, the *tet* genes did not have a bacterial specificity and were often described in combination, such as *tet*(M)/*tet*(O), *tet*(M)/*tet*(K), or *tet*(O)/*tet*(K) (90, 94, 137, 138).

Most studies detailed here were performed in Europe in the 2000s. Having a better and updated view of the evolution of resistance in veterinary streptococci would require monitoring of tetracycline resistance in bacteria from animal origins at a larger scale.

Prevalence of Tetracycline Resistance among Streptococci of Porcine Origin

In line with *S. suis* being the major *Streptococcus* spp. in swine, numerous publications have reported antimicrobial resistance in this pathogen, mostly in diseased animals. Tetracycline, as already noted for streptococci of bovine or ovine origin, is often the antibiotic presenting the highest prevalence of resistance. The lowest rates were reported in the oldest European isolates studied (no resistance in Danish isolates collected in 1967 to 1981 and 7.7% in Swedish isolates collected in 1992 to 1997) and in the context of the ARBAO-II study performed in 2002 to 2004 (48% resistance in the Netherlands and 52.2% in Denmark in 2003) (102, 107). Higher rates were then reported in the United States (66.7% in 1986), Spain (68.0% in 2004), Poland (64.0% in 2004), Japan (86.9%), Italy (89.5%), and a pan-European study (75.1%) (107, 139–141). Several studies showed resistance rates greater than 90%, with 91.7%, 95.4% and 97.9% in China, Spain, and Brazil, respectively (142–144).

A few molecular studies detailed the *tet* genes responsible for the phenotypic resistance detected. Tet(O) is by far the most commonly detected enzyme in *S. suis*, while Tet(M) has also been reported (Table 3), either alone or in association with other Tet determinants, in particluar Tet(O). The distribution of these *tet* genes

may also vary depending on the serotype, but further work on larger cohorts is needed to have statistically relevant data. The *tet*(W) gene was repeatedly reported in *S. suis*, initially in a human patient in Italy, but then also in pig isolates (140, 145, 146). Of note, the only occurrence of *tet*(B) in streptococci was reported in 17 *S. suis* isolates (17/111, 15%) in the United States (147).

Tetracycline Resistance among Other Streptococci

Tetracycline resistance in *S. canis* was reported from diseased cats and dogs, with a prevalence of 32.1% in France, 23.5% in Japan, and 27% in Portugal (including a few isolates from horses and humans) (34, 148, 149). In these studies, tetracycline resistance was due principally to the presence of the *tet*(M) and *tet*(O) genes, alone or in combination. A study performed in Belgium on healthy individually owned cats and groups of cats noted a higher prevalence of tetracycline resistance in a cattery (52%) compared to individual animals (22.2%), most likely due to the clonal transmission of resistant strains in the cattery (150).

BETA-LACTAM RESISTANCE

Beta-lactams are the largest family of antibiotics available in both human and veterinary medicine. All members of this family act on the bacterial cell wall by covalently blocking the PBPs and thus impairing the continuous building of this protecting structure. Currently, bacterial resistance to the last generations of beta-lactams is one of the most challenging issues in both human and animal medicine. The key threats are the worldwide emergence and dissemination of inactivating enzymes such as extended-spectrum beta-lactamases, cephalosporinases (AmpCs), and carbapenemases in Gram-negative bacteria. All these resistance determinants are carried by plasmids and thus display a high capacity to efficiently disseminate in an intra- or interspecies manner. In Gram-positive bacteria, methicillin-resistant *S. aureus*—which possesses an additional PBP2A presenting a decreased affinity to beta-lactams—remains an issue in human medicine, despite the fact that its prevalence in hospitals has been considerably reduced in the past decades with improvements of hygiene measures. In veterinary medicine, methicillin-resistant *Staphylococcus pseudintermedius* is known to cause serious treatment challenges because of its associated multiresistance. However, the success of both methicillin-resistant *S. aureus* and methicillin-resistant *S. pseudintermedius* is more due to epidemic bursts of

Table 3 Distribution of the tetracycline resistance genes in streptococci in animal hosts

Animal host	Country	Year	Bacterial species	No. of isolates	Efflux		Ribosomal protection			No. of TetR isolates[b]	Percentage of resistance (%)	Reference
					tet(K)	tet(L)	tet(M)	tet(O)	tet(S)			
Cattle	USA	1990	*S. agalactiae*	39	0	0	NT[a]	7	NT	10	25.6	137
			S. dysgalactiae	21	1	1	NT	1	NT	9	42.9	
			S. uberis	11	1		NT	1	NT	2	18.2	
Cattle	France	1984–2008	*S. agalactiae*	76	NT	NT	16	13	1	30	39.5	94
			S. dysgalactiae	32	NT	NT	5	4	4	32	100.0	
			S. uberis	101	NT	NT	23	36	3	62	61.4	
Cattle	Portugal	2002–2003	*S. agalactiae*	60	34	NT	13	20	0	34	56.7	90
			S. dysgalactiae	18	0	NT	6	6	0	18	100.0	
			S. uberis	30	0	NT	2	9	8	18	60.0	
Ovine	Italy	2004–2014	*S. uberis*	51	9	NT	12	12	NT	18	35.3	138
Pig	USA	1986	*S. suis*	21	0	0	5	NT	NT	14	66.7	103
Pig	Denmark	1989–2002	*S. suis*	103	NT	0	11	6	0	25	24.3	237
Pig	Italy	2003–2007	*S. suis*	57	0	0	2	38	0	51	89.5	140
Pig	China	2005–2012	*S. suis*	62	NT	NT	53	42	NT	57	91.9	170
			S. suis	34	NT	NT	24	9	NT	28	82.4	
Pig	China	2008–2010	*S. suis*	106	NT	2	16	86	1	105	99.1	146
Dog/cat	France	2010	*S. canis*	112	NT	1	31	16	5	36	32.1	148
Dog/cat	Japan	2015	*S. canis*	68	0	0	13	10	NT	16	23.5	149
Dog/cat/horse/human[c]	Portugal	2000–2010	*S. canis*	85	NT	1	11	8	1	23	27.0	34

[a]NT, not tested.
[b]Discrepancies between the number of tetracycline-resistant isolates and the genes identified may be due to either unidentified genes or to isolates presenting an association of two or three *tet* genes.
[c]Human isolates could not be individualized.

successful clones than to the mobilization of the *mecA*-carrying cassette.

Streptococci are unique among the major pathogens in the sense that they are incapable of acquiring any exogenous beta-lactam resistance genes. However, they can progressively mutate their own PBPs. Indeed, no isolate carrying a beta-lactamase (such as Gram-negative bacteria) or a new PBP (such as staphylococci) has been described yet, and a few species, including *S. pyogenes*, are even unable to develop decreased susceptibility to beta-lactams *in vitro* (151).

Beta-Lactam Resistance in Streptococci

To achieve beta-lactam resistance, streptococci sequentially modify their PBPs, specifically the class B PBP2B and PBP2X (and the class A PBP1A in the more resistant isolates). This was particularly exemplified in *S. pneumoniae*, the only *Streptococcus* spp. for which penicillin-resistance was successfully achieved and widely disseminated, where both mutated and mosaic PBPs were reported. Other less-documented genes were sporadically reported as PBP-independent penicillin-resistance mechanisms. These include the *MurMN* operon encoding enzymes that are responsible for the biosynthesis of branched muropeptide components (152), the *ciaRH* operon, a two-component signal-transducing system (153), the *adr* gene coding for a peptidoglycan O-acetyltransferase (154), the *stkP* gene encoding a serine/threonine kinase (155), the *pstS* gene encoding a subunit of a phosphate ABC transporter (156), and the *spr1178* gene encoding for a putative iron permease (157). Penicillin-resistant *S. pneumoniae* has widely disseminated through the success of a limited number of serotypes, selected mainly by the excessive use of antibiotics (158), but the prevalence of this resistance has considerably decreased since the early 2000s by both the reduced consumption of antibiotics and the marketing of efficient vaccines (159, 160). The presence and characterization of mutated PBPs in isolates presenting decreased susceptibilities to beta-lactam were also reported in *S. agalactiae* of human origin (69, 161, 162). Recently, a classification of *S. agalactiae* was proposed which takes into account the different mutations in the PBPs (163).

In veterinary medicine, *Streptococcus* isolates presenting full penicillin resistance have only rarely been reported, and only a few molecular studies were conducted either on laboratory strains or on field isolates presenting reduced susceptibility to beta-lactams. The presence of three groups of PBPs (PBP 1, PBP 2, and PBP 3) was demonstrated in *S. suis*, and PBP modifications were strongly suggested to be responsible for pen-

icillin G-resistant phenotypes in both *in vitro* mutants and field isolates (164). In *S. uberis*, Haenni et al. (165) showed that both a quality control strain and field strains were capable of developing a 60-fold MIC increase after 30 cycles of exposure to penicillin G. This increase was due to the accumulation of mutations in the class B (PBP 2B and PBP 2X) and A (PBP 1A) enzymes, including the systematic presence of the two specific $E_{381}K$ and $Q_{554}E$ mutations in the PBP 2X. Interestingly, PBP analysis of seven field strains collected in Switzerland, France, and Holland and presenting MICs of 0.25 to 0.5 mg/liter also revealed the systematic presence of these two key mutations (165). However, none of the tested strains (selected either *in vitro* or by treatment on farms) could achieve full resistance, since their MICs only reached 0.25 to 2 mg/liter, which is still considered intermediately resistant.

Phenotypic Reports on Beta-Lactam Activity in Bovine Mastitis

In veterinary medicine, beta-lactam resistance has mostly been documented in bovine streptococci, namely *S. uberis*, *S. dysgalactiae*, and *S. agalactiae*. Data were gathered in cases of clinical and subclinical mastitis, a pathology for which the first-line treatment is beta-lactams. Comparison between studies can be difficult because of the heterogeneity of the methods (disc diffusion, agar diffusion, broth microdilution) and the guidelines used. If no interpretation was inferred, an isolate was considered resistant when the MIC was ≥4 mg/liter according to the CLSI breakpoints.

Most studies based on the determination of MICs report the absence of penicillin G resistance in *S. uberis* and *S. dysgalactiae*, even though isolates presenting decreased susceptibilities (0.25 to 0.5 mg/liter) were regularly reported. In France, such nonsusceptible isolates were reported in 2002, with 14.0% of the *S. uberis* showing an MIC of 0.25 mg/liter (134), and a shift toward decreased susceptibilities was suggested in 2010 based on the comparison of disk diffusion and MIC results (166). In Sweden, two studies performed successively in 2003 (133) and 2008 to 2009 (101) showed a slight shift over the years toward decreased susceptibility, with 6.0% of the *S. uberis* isolates displaying an MIC of 0.25 mg/liter and 10.0% of the *S. dysgalactiae* isolates displaying an MIC of 0.12 mg/liter in 2009, whereas only 0.9% of the *S. uberis* isolates had an MIC of 0.25 mg/liter, and all the *S. dysgalactiae* isolates were fully susceptible (MIC, <0.06 mg/liter) in 2003. In the United States, one true resistant *S. dysgalactiae* isolate (MIC, 4 mg/liter) was detected over 152 strains tested, whereas 6.8% of the *S. uberis* isolates presented

MICs of 0.5 mg/liter to penicillin, and one strain displayed an MIC of 1 mg/liter (136). The VetPath data (multicenter European data) collected between 2002 and 2006 showed no true resistance, but 29.8% of isolates presented decreased susceptibility (MICs ranging from 0.25 mg/liter to 1 mg/liter) (100). Though without any MIC values, other studies also reported data on beta-lactam resistance in veterinary streptococci, often with a very low prevalence of resistance. One pan-European study performed in 2002 to 2004 showed very low levels (0 to 3.9%) of penicillin resistance (99). A Swiss study detected susceptibilities to ampicillin of 92.3% for *S. uberis* and 94.8% for *S. dysgalactiae* from cows sampled in 2011 to 2013 (167). Kalmus et al. showed 0 to 0.4% resistance to penicillin G, ampicillin, and cefalotin in Estonia between 2007 and 2009 (168). In France, 12.9% of the *S. uberis* and 1.4% of the *S. dysgalactiae* presented resistance patterns to oxacillin, but these were not confirmed by MIC determination (135). In Turkey, 94% of the *S. uberis* isolates showed susceptibility to penicillin G (169).

These different data confirm beta-lactams as efficient antibiotics against streptococci isolated from bovine mastitis. However, this slow but clear shift of strains from full toward decreased susceptibility will have to be surveyed in the future. Beta-lactam resistance development in streptococci surely does not present the same dynamic as in Gram-negative bacteria, where plasmids play a major role. However, this should not hide rampant and silent acquisition of beta-lactam resistance in streptococci of animal origin, which may one day limit the therapeutic arsenal available for veterinarians.

Beta-Lactam Resistance Outside the Context of Cattle Mastitis

Antibiotic resistance was also monitored in *S. suis* isolated from pigs, and several studies reported the absence of resistance to any beta-lactams. Nevertheless, isolates presenting particularly high MICs to penicillin G were also recurrently reported, with unfortunately, no concomitant molecular work on the underlying mechanisms of resistance. Indeed, 4% of the Spanish isolates displayed MICs ranging from 4 to 16 mg/liter, whereas two Chinese studies reported 2.1% and 9.5% of isolates with an MIC of ≥4 mg/liter (142, 143, 170). In the Netherlands, 0.5% and 0.3% of over 1,163 isolates of *S. suis* tested were considered resistant to penicillin G and ampicillin between 2013 and 2015 (171). In Japan, Poland, and Portugal, resistance was reported in 0.9%, 8.1%, and 13.0% of the isolates, re-

spectively (107, 141). However, despite these cases, beta-lactams can still be recommended as first-line antibiotics for the treatment of *S. suis*.

Aside from *S. suis* and streptococci isolated from bovine mastitis, reports of veterinary streptococci are quite rare. Beta-lactam resistance was described once in *S. dysgalactiae* subspecies *equisimilis* isolated from swine in Brazil and in four studies of *S. canis* isolated from pets and horses in France, Japan, Belgium, and Portugal (34, 148–150, 172), and these five studies found full susceptibility of all isolates to penicillin G.

FLUOROQUINOLONE RESISTANCE

Quinolones are not active against streptococci, because of their intrinsic resistance. However, fluoroquinolones may be an alternative to beta-lactam antibiotics to treat streptococcal infections. The main agents used in veterinary medicine are enrofloxacin, marbofloxacin, danofloxacin, and the more recent pradofloxacin.

Resistance to fluoroquinolones is generally mediated by point mutations in the quinolone resistance-determinants regions of the *gyrA* and *parC* genes (173). Furthermore, plasmidic *qnr* genes participate in the dissemination of low-level resistance, but they have never been reported in streptococci. Efflux pumps also play a role in fluoroquinolone resistance, as has been proved for the SatAB, an ABC transporter, in *S. suis* (174).

Fluoroquinolone-Resistance Phenotypes

Resistance to fluoroquinolones has rarely been reported in veterinary streptococci. Moreover, in the fluoroquinolone family, there is a wide variability of the agents tested (enrofloxacin and ciprofloxacin are the most frequently used), thus making comparisons among studies difficult.

A 1.5% prevalence of resistance to enrofloxacin in *S. uberis* and 5.5% in *S. dysgalactiae* was reported in France in 2010 (135). In the same bacterial species, MICs ranging from 0.5 to 2 mg/liter were observed in Sweden (101). These apparently elevated MICs are constitutive of streptococci, which have a basal MIC higher than that of *Enterobacteriaceae* or staphylococci. In a study performed between 1994 and 2001, the same range of MICs was reported, and no increase in the resistance rate was observed over the years (175). Except for three resistant strains (MIC, 4 mg/liter), all *S. uberis* and *S. dysgalactiae* isolates collected in a multicenter European study presented MICs to marbofloxacin ranging from 0.25 to 2 mg/liter (176). In *S. suis*, the resistance rates to enrofloxacin determined in a pan-European study performed in 2009 to 2012 and to ciprofloxacin determined in Japan in 1987 to 1996 were very similar: 0.7% and 0.3%, respectively (177). Enrofloxacin resistance was also observed in *S. canis* in France, where MICs ranged from 0.25 to 2 mg/liter (148). *Streptococcus* spp. isolated from cats and dogs were studied through the ComPath European network: no resistance was reported in dermatological samples, whereas 1.8% of the cats and 4.0% of the dogs presenting with a respiratory tract infection carried enrofloxacin-resistant streptococci (178, 179).

ROLE OF THE ICES IN THE EVOLUTION OF RESISTANCE

MGEs play a major role in the dissemination of antibiotic resistance genes. MGEs mostly comprise conjugative plasmids, transposons, phages, and ICEs (initially named conjugative transposons). ICEs are chromosomal, self-transmissible MGEs that are capable of promoting their excision, conjugation, and site-specific integration in a recipient cell (180, 181). One of the most emblematic members of the ICEs is the Tn*916*-Tn*1545* family, which carries *tet*(M) and other antibiotic resistance genes (126, 127, 182, 183).

ICEs have been widely reported in streptococci, and they were recently detected in all *Streptococcus* spp. for which at least one complete genome was available, with *S. suis* being the most "colonized" species (184, 185). In human clinical streptococcal isolates, *erm* and *tet* resistance genes were recurrently reported on ICEs, such as *erm*(B) on ICE*Sp1116* and *erm*(TR)-*tet*(O) on ICE*Sp2905* in *S. pyogenes* (186, 187), *erm*(TR) on ICE*Sag*TR7 in *S. agalactiae* (188), and *erm*(B) and *tet*(O) on ICE*SsD9* in *S. suis* (189). Interestingly, resistance genes can also be mobilized by coresident ICEs, as demonstrated by the mobilization of an *erm*(T)-carrying plasmid in *S. dysgalactiae* subsp. *equisimilis* (190). Other antibiotic resistance determinants can also be found on ICEs, as exemplified by the presence of *tet*(M) and a chloramphenicol acetyl-transferase on ICE*Sp23FST81* from *S. agalactiae* (191), lincosamide resistance (*lsa* genes) on different ICEs in *S. agalactiae* (192), and a multidrug resistance cluster on ICE*Ssu*NC28 carried by *S. suis* (193). Moreover, ICEs originating from different streptococcal species may form hybrids that can further transfer *in vitro* to a third streptococcal species (194). This illustrates the wide distribution and the plasticity of these MGEs and thus their role in the dissemination of resistance genes. Finally, resistance determinants may be adjacent to—and not inside—an ICE. This is exemplified by the first vancomycin-resistance determinants in streptococci, the *vanG*

operons, which were identified in one *S. agalactiae* and two *S. anginosus* isolates (195). These *vanG* operons were immediately followed by a large chromosomal element named ICE-r (ICE-like sequences). A plausible hypothesis is that the integration of ICE-r in the streptococcal chromosome may have favored the subsequent integration of the *vanG* element.

Except for elements from the Tn*916*-Tn*1545* family which were broadly reported in different streptococcal species originating from diverse animal hosts (9, 94, 170, 196), ICEs carrying resistance genes have rarely been reported in streptococci from animal origin. Indeed, only the mosaic *tet*(O/W/32/O) carried on ICE*Ssu32457* in *S. suis*, which could then be transferred to *S. pneumoniae*, *S. pyogenes*, and *S. agalactiae* (197), as well as the lincomycin-resistance gene *lsa* (192) were described on such MGEs. This will likely change in the near future, since new research perspectives are emerging with the democratized access to high-throughput sequencing technologies and the subsequent databases (185, 198).

CONCLUSION

In veterinary medicine streptococci are frequent pathogens not only in food-producing but also in companion animals. However, as far as public health is concerned, there are few situations in which streptococci of animal origin may cause risk for humans, and vice-versa. Among those, *S. suis* and, to a lesser extent, *S. agalactiae* are likely the most relevant examples, and are both considered zoonotic pathogens. Studies of resistance to antimicrobials in streptococci of animal origin have largely focused on tetracyclines and macrolides/lincosamides, which are widely used in the animal sector globally. Accordingly, high resistance rates to these molecules have frequently been observed, which is also in line with specific niches covering major animal diseases, such as cattle mastitis of streptococcal origin. Molecular investigations highlighted the diversity of the resistance genes of the *tet* and *erm* families, together with the pivotal role of the ICEs. Nonetheless, most data originate from Europe, and there is a need for larger prevalence and molecular studies on a global scale. Of note, despite the wide use of penicillins to treat streptococcal infections, resistance to beta-lactams does not appear to be a crucial issue in veterinary streptococci, in contrast to what has been observed with the human-specific *S. pneumoniae*. In all, as in humans, antimicrobial resistance in *Streptococcus* of animal origin may largely differ depending on the *Streptococcus* sp. and therefore should not be considered as a whole.

Citation. Haenni M, Lupo A, Madec J-Y. 2018. Antimicrobial resistance in *Streptococcus* spp. Microbiol Spectrum 6(2): ARBA-0008-2017.

References

1. **Póntigo F, Moraga M, Flores SV.** 2015. Molecular phylogeny and a taxonomic proposal for the genus *Streptococcus*. *Genet Mol Res* **14**:10905–10918.

2. **Lancefield RC, Freimer EH.** 1966. Type-specific polysaccharide antigens of group B streptococci. *J Hyg (Lond)* **64**:191–203.

3. **Tanaka D, Isobe J, Watahiki M, Nagai Y, Katsukawa C, Kawahara R, Endoh M, Okuno R, Kumagai N, Matsumoto M, Morikawa Y, Ikebe T, Watanabe H, Working Group for Group A Streptococci in Japan.** 2008. Genetic features of clinical isolates of *Streptococcus dysgalactiae* subsp. *equisimilis* possessing Lancefield's group A antigen. *J Clin Microbiol* **46**:1526–1529.

4. **Brouwer S, Barnett TC, Rivera-Hernandez T, Rohde M, Walker MJ.** 2016. *Streptococcus pyogenes* adhesion and colonization. *FEBS Lett* **590**:3739–3757.

5. **Carapetis JR, Steer AC, Mulholland EK, Weber M.** 2005. The global burden of group A streptococcal diseases. *Lancet Infect Dis* **5**:685–694.

6. **Copperman SM.** 1982. Cherchez le chien: household pets as reservoirs of persistent or recurrent streptococcal sore throats in children. *N Y State J Med* **82**:1685–1687.

7. **Farley MM.** 2001. Group B streptococcal disease in nonpregnant adults. *Clin Infect Dis* **33**:556–561.

8. **Olivares-Fuster O, Klesius PH, Evans J, Arias CR.** 2008. Molecular typing of *Streptococcus agalactiae* isolates from fish. *J Fish Dis* **31**:277–283.

9. **Fischer A, Liljander A, Kaspar H, Muriuki C, Fuxelius HH, Bongcam-Rudloff E, de Villiers EP, Huber CA, Frey J, Daubenberger C, Bishop R, Younan M, Jores J.** 2013. Camel *Streptococcus agalactiae* populations are associated with specific disease complexes and acquired the tetracycline resistance gene *tetM* via a Tn*916*-like element. *Vet Res (Faisalabad)* **44**:86.

10. **Yildirim AO, Lämmler C, Weiss R.** 2002. Identification and characterization of *Streptococcus agalactiae* isolated from horses. *Vet Microbiol* **85**:31–35.

11. **McDonald TJ, McDonald JS.** 1976. Streptococci isolated from bovine intramammary infections. *Am J Vet Res* **37**:377–381.

12. **Brochet M, Couvé E, Zouine M, Vallaeys T, Rusniok C, Lamy MC, Buchrieser C, Trieu-Cuot P, Kunst F, Poyart C, Glaser P.** 2006. Genomic diversity and evolution within the species *Streptococcus agalactiae*. *Microbes Infect* **8**:1227–1243.

13. **Rajendram P, Mar Kyaw W, Leo YS, Ho H, Chen WK, Lin R, Pratim P, Badaruddin H, Ang B, Barkham T, Chow A.** 2016. Group B streptococcus sequence type 283 disease linked to consumption of raw fish, Singapore. *Emerg Infect Dis* **22**:1974–1977.

14. **Evans JJ, Klesius PH, Pasnik DJ, Bohnsack JF.** 2009. Human *Streptococcus agalactiae* isolate in Nile tilapia (*Oreochromis niloticus*). *Emerg Infect Dis* **15**:774–776.

15. **Bradley A.** 2002. Bovine mastitis: an evolving disease. *Vet J* **164**:116–128.

16. **Leigh JA.** 1999. *Streptococcus uberis*: a permanent barrier to the control of bovine mastitis? *Vet J* **157**:225–238.

17. **Schleifer KH, Kilpper-Bälz R.** 1984. Transfer of *Streptococcus faecalis* and *Streptococcus faecium* to the genus *Enterococcus* nom. rev. as *Enterococcus faecalis* comb. nov. and *Enterococcus faecium* comb. nov. *Int J Syst Evol Microbiol* **34**:31–34.

18. **Köhler W.** 2007. The present state of species within the genera *Streptococcus* and *Enterococcus*. *Int J Med Microbiol* **297**:133–150.

19. **Ben-Chetrit E, Wiener-Well Y, Kashat L, Yinnon AM, Assous MV.** 2016. *Streptococcus bovis* new taxonomy: does subspecies distinction matter? *Eur J Clin Microbiol Infect Dis* **36(2)**:387.

20. **Dumke J, Hinse D, Vollmer T, Schulz J, Knabbe C, Dreier J.** 2015. Potential transmission pathways of *Streptococcus gallolyticus* subsp. *gallolyticus*. *PLoS One* **10**: e0126507.

21. **Gherardi G, Palmieri C, Marini E, Pompilio A, Crocetta V, Di Bonaventura G, Creti R, Facinelli B.** 2016. Identification, antimicrobial resistance and molecular characterization of the human emerging pathogen *Streptococcus gallolyticus* subsp. *pasteurianus*. *Diagn Microbiol Infect Dis* **86**:329–335.

22. **Sheng WH, Chuang YC, Teng LJ, Hsueh PR.** 2014. Bacteraemia due to *Streptococcus gallolyticus* subspecies *pasteurianus* is associated with digestive tract malignancies and resistance to macrolides and clindamycin. *J Infect* **69**:145–153.

23. **Sturt AS, Yang L, Sandhu K, Pei Z, Cassai N, Blaser MJ.** 2010. *Streptococcus gallolyticus* subspecies *pasteurianus* (biotype II/2), a newly reported cause of adult meningitis. *J Clin Microbiol* **48**:2247–2249.

24. **Barnett J, Ainsworth H, Boon JD, Twomey DF.** 2008. *Streptococcus gallolyticus* subsp. *pasteurianus* septicaemia in goslings. *Vet J* **176**:251–253.

25. **Li M, Gu C, Zhang W, Li S, Liu J, Qin C, Su J, Cheng G, Hu X.** 2013. Isolation and characterization of *Streptococcus gallolyticus* subsp. *pasteurianus* causing meningitis in ducklings. *Vet Microbiol* **162**:930–936.

26. **Marmolin ES, Hartmeyer GN, Christensen JJ, Nielsen XC, Dargis R, Skov MN, Knudsen E, Kemp M, Justesen US.** 2016. Bacteremia with the bovis group streptococci: species identification and association with infective endocarditis and with gastrointestinal disease. *Diagn Microbiol Infect Dis* **85**:239–242.

27. **Wessman GE.** 1986. Biology of the group E streptococci: a review. *Vet Microbiol* **12**:297–328.

28. **Facklam R, Elliott J, Pigott N, Franklin AR.** 1995. Identification of *Streptococcus porcinus* from human sources. *J Clin Microbiol* **33**:385–388.

29. **Duarte RS, Barros RR, Facklam RR, Teixeira LM.** 2005. Phenotypic and genotypic characteristics of *Streptococcus porcinus* isolated from human sources. *J Clin Microbiol* **43**:4592–4601.

30. Jonsson P, Olsson SO, Olofson AS, Fälth C, Holmberg O, Funke H. 1991. Bacteriological investigations of clinical mastitis in heifers in Sweden. *J Dairy Res* 58: 179–185.

31. Cuccuru C, Meloni M, Sala E, Scaccabarozzi L, Locatelli C, Moroni P, Bronzo V. 2011. Effects of intramammary infections on somatic cell score and milk yield in Sarda sheep. *N Z Vet J* 59:128–131.

32. Timoney JF. 2004. The pathogenic equine streptococci. *Vet Res* 35:397–409.

33. Hashikawa S, Iinuma Y, Furushita M, Ohkura T, Nada T, Torii K, Hasegawa T, Ohta M. 2004. Characterization of group C and G streptococcal strains that cause streptococcal toxic shock syndrome. *J Clin Microbiol* 42:186–192.

34. Pinho MD, Matos SC, Pomba C, Lübke-Becker A, Wieler LH, Preziuso S, Melo-Cristino J, Ramirez M. 2013. Multilocus sequence analysis of *Streptococcus canis* confirms the zoonotic origin of human infections and reveals genetic exchange with *Streptococcus dysgalactiae* subsp. *equisimilis*. *J Clin Microbiol* 51:1099–1109.

35. Iglauer F, Kunstýr I, Mörstedt R, Farouq H, Wullenweber M, Damsch S. 1991. *Streptococcus canis* arthritis in a cat breeding colony. *J Exp Anim Sci* 34:59–65.

36. Lacave G, Coutard A, Troché G, Augusto S, Pons S, Zuber B, Laurent V, Amara M, Couzon B, Bédos JP, Pangon B, Grimaldi D. 2016. Endocarditis caused by *Streptococcus canis*: an emerging zoonosis? *Infection* 44:111–114.

37. Goyette-Desjardins G, Auger JP, Xu J, Segura M, Gottschalk M. 2014. *Streptococcus suis*, an important pig pathogen and emerging zoonotic agent: an update on the worldwide distribution based on serotyping and sequence typing. *Emerg Microbes Infect* 3:e45.

38. Segura M, Calzas C, Grenier D, Gottschalk M. 2016. Initial steps of the pathogenesis of the infection caused by *Streptococcus suis*: fighting against nonspecific defenses. *FEBS Lett* 590:3772–3799.

39. Taniyama D, Sakurai M, Sakai T, Kikuchi T, Takahashi T. 2016. Human case of bacteremia due to *Streptococcus suis* serotype 5 in Japan: the first report and literature review. *IDCases* 6:36–38.

40. Ward PN, Holden MT, Leigh JA, Lennard N, Bignell A, Barron A, Clark L, Quail MA, Woodward J, Barrell BG, Egan SA, Field TR, Maskell D, Kehoe M, Dowson CG, Chanter N, Whatmore AM, Bentley SD, Parkhill J. 2009. Evidence for niche adaptation in the genome of the bovine pathogen *Streptococcus uberis*. *BMC Genomics* 10:54–71.

41. Phuektes P, Mansell PD, Dyson RS, Hooper ND, Dick JS, Browning GF. 2001. Molecular epidemiology of *Streptococcus uberis* isolates from dairy cows with mastitis. *J Clin Microbiol* 39:1460–1466.

42. Wilesmith JW, Francis PG, Wilson CD. 1986. Incidence of clinical mastitis in a cohort of British dairy herds. *Vet Rec* 118:199–204.

43. Compton CW, Heuer C, Parker K, McDougall S. 2007. Epidemiology of mastitis in pasture-grazed peripartum dairy heifers and its effects on productivity. *J Dairy Sci* 90:4157–4170.

44. Hasson KW, Wyld EM, Fan Y, Lingsweiller SW, Weaver SJ, Cheng J, Varner PW. 2009. Streptococcosis in farmed *Litopenaeus vannamei*: a new emerging bacterial disease of penaeid shrimp. *Dis Aquat Organ* 86:93–106.

45. Parker KI, Compton C, Anniss FM, Weir A, Heuer C, McDougall S. 2007. Subclinical and clinical mastitis in heifers following the use of a teat sealant precalving. *J Dairy Sci* 90:207–218.

46. Dodd FH. 1983. Mastitis: progress on control. *J Dairy Sci* 66:1773–1780.

47. Zehner MM, Farnsworth RJ, Appleman RD, Larntz K, Springer JA. 1986. Growth of environmental mastitis pathogens in various bedding materials. *J Dairy Sci* 69: 1932–1941.

48. Koh TH, Sng LH, Yuen SM, Thomas CK, Tan PL, Tan SH, Wong NS. 2009. Streptococcal cellulitis following preparation of fresh raw seafood. *Zoonoses Public Health* 56:206–208.

49. Weinstein MR, Litt M, Kertesz DA, Wyper P, Rose D, Coulter M, McGeer A, Facklam R, Ostach C, Willey BM, Borczyk A, Low DE. 1997. Invasive infections due to a fish pathogen, *Streptococcus iniae*. S. *iniae* Study Group. *N Engl J Med* 337:589–594.

50. Nilson B, Olaison L, Rasmussen M. 2016. Clinical presentation of infective endocarditis caused by different groups of non-beta haemolytic streptococci. *Eur J Clin Microbiol Infect Dis* 35:215–218.

51. Simón-Soro A, Mira A. 2015. Solving the etiology of dental caries. *Trends Microbiol* 23:76–82.

52. Yombi J, Belkhir L, Jonckheere S, Wilmes D, Cornu O, Vandercam B, Rodriguez-Villalobos H. 2012. *Streptococcus gordonii* septic arthritis: two cases and review of literature. *BMC Infect Dis* 12:215–220.

53. Burrell MH, Mackintosh ME, Taylor CE. 1986. Isolation of *Streptococcus pneumoniae* from the respiratory tract of horses. *Equine Vet J* 18:183–186.

54. Köndgen S, Calvignac-Spencer S, Grützmacher K, Keil V, Mätz-Rensing K, Nowak K, Metzger S, Kiyang J, Becker AL, Deschner T, Wittig RM, Lankester F, Leendertz FH. 2017. Evidence for human *Streptococcus pneumoniae* in wild and captive chimpanzees: a potential threat to wild populations. *Sci Rep* 7:14581.

55. Beighton D, Hayday H. 1982. The streptococcal flora of the tongue of the monkey *Macaca fascicularis*. *Arch Oral Biol* 27:331–335.

56. Devriese LA, Hommez J, Pot B, Haesebrouck F. 1994. Identification and composition of the streptococcal and enterococcal flora of tonsils, intestines and faeces of pigs. *J Appl Bacteriol* 77:31–36.

57. Devriese LA, Pot B, Vandamme P, Kersters K, Collins MD, Alvarez N, Haesebrouck F, Hommez J. 1997. *Streptococcus hyovaginalis* sp. nov. and *Streptococcus thoraltensis* sp. nov., from the genital tract of sows. *Int J Syst Bacteriol* 47:1073–1077.

58. Freedman ML, Coykendall AL, O'Neill EM. 1982. Physiology of "mutans-like" *Streptococcus ferus* from wild rats. *Infect Immun* 35:476–482.

59. Zhu H, Willcox MD, Knox KW. 2000. A new species of oral *Streptococcus* isolated from Sprague-Dawley rats,

Streptococcus orisratti sp. nov. *Int J Syst Evol Microbiol* **50:**55–61.

60. Rinkinen ML, Koort JM, Ouwehand AC, Westermarck E, Björkroth KJ. 2004. *Streptococcus alactolyticus* is the dominating culturable lactic acid bacterium species in canine jejunum and feces of four fistulated dogs. *FEMS Microbiol Lett* **230:**35–39.

61. Toepfner N, Shetty S, Kunze M, Orlowska-Volk M, Krüger M, Berner R, Hentschel R. 2014. Fulminant neonatal sepsis due to *Streptococcus alactolyticus*: a case report and review. *APMIS* **122:**654–656.

62. Beighton D, Russell RR, Hayday H. 1981. The isolation of characterization of *Streptococcus mutans* serotype h from dental plaque of monkeys (*Macaca fascicularis*). *J Gen Microbiol* **124:**271–279.

63. Yoo SY, Kim KJ, Lim SH, Kim KW, Hwang HK, Min BM, Choe SJ, Kook JK. 2005. First isolation of *Streptococcus downei* from human dental plaques. *FEMS Microbiol Lett* **249:**323–326.

64. Aryasinghe L, Sabbar S, Kazim Y, Awan LM, Khan HK. 2014. *Streptococcus pluranimalium*: a novel human pathogen? *Int J Surg Case Rep* **5:**1242–1246.

65. Devriese LA, Vandamme P, Collins MD, Alvarez N, Pot B, Hommez J, Butaye P, Haesebrouck F. 1999. *Streptococcus pluranimalium* sp. nov., from cattle and other animals. *Int J Syst Bacteriol* **49:**1221–1226.

66. Facklam R. 2002. What happened to the streptococci: overview of taxonomic and nomenclature changes. *Clin Microbiol Rev* **15:**613–630.

67. Silley P, Simjee S, Schwarz S. 2012. Surveillance and monitoring ofantimicrobial resistance and antibiotic consumption in humans and animals. *Rev Sci Tech* **31:**105–120.

68. de Jong A, Thomas V, Klein U, Marion H, Moyaert H, Simjee S, Vallé M. 2013. Pan-European resistance monitoring programmes encompassing food-borne bacteria and target pathogens of food-producing and companion animals. *Int J Antimicrob Agents* **41:**403–409.

69. Metcalf BJ, Chochua S, Gertz RE Jr, Hawkins PA, Ricaldi J, Li Z, Walker H, Tran T, Rivers J, Mathis S, Jackson D, Glennen A, Lynfield R, McGee L, Beall B, Active Bacterial Core surveillance team. 2017. Short-read whole genome sequencing for determination of antimicrobial resistance mechanisms and capsular serotypes of current invasive *Streptococcus agalactiae* recovered in the USA. *Clin Microbiol Infect* **23:**574e577–574e514.

70. Li Y, Metcalf BJ, Chochua S, Li Z, Gertz RE Jr, Walker H, Hawkins PA, Tran T, Whitney CG, McGee L, Beall BW. 2016. Penicillin-binding protein transpeptidase signatures for tracking and predicting beta-lactam resistance levels in *Streptococcus pneumoniae*. *MBio* **7:**pii e00756-16.

71. Mobegi FM, Cremers AJ, de Jonge MI, Bentley SD, van Hijum SA, Zomer A. 2017. Deciphering the distance to antibiotic resistance for the pneumococcus using genome sequencing data. *Sci Rep* **7:**42808.

72. MARAN. 2009. Monitoring of Antimicrobial Resistance and Antibiotic Usage in Animals in The Netherlands in 2008. CIDC-Lelystad, Lelystad, The Netherlands.

73. Leclercq R. 2002. Mechanisms of resistance to macrolides and lincosamides: nature of the resistance elements and their clinical implications. *Clin Infect Dis* **34:**482–492.

74. Collignon P, Powers JH, Chiller TM, Aidara-Kane A, Aarestrup FM. 2009. World Health Organization ranking of antimicrobials according to their importance in human medicine: a critical step for developing risk management strategies for the use of antimicrobials in food production animals. *Clin Infect Dis* **49:**132–141.

75. Edmondson PW. 1989. An economic justification of "blitz" therapy to eradicate *Streptococcus agalactiae* from a dairy herd. *Vet Rec* **125:**591–593.

76. Pyörälä S, Baptiste KE, Catry B, van Duijkeren E, Greko C, Moreno MA, Pomba MC, Rantala M, Ružauskas M, Sanders P, Threlfall EJ, Torren-Edo J, Törneke K. 2014. Macrolides and lincosamides in cattle and pigs: use and development of antimicrobial resistance. *Vet J* **200:**230–239.

77. De Mouy D, Cavallo JD, Leclercq R, Fabre R, AFICORPI-BIO Network. Association de Formation Continue en Pathologie Infectieuse des Biologistes. 2001. Antibiotic susceptibility and mechanisms of erythromycin resistance in clinical isolates of *Streptococcus agalactiae*: French multicenter study. *Antimicrob Agents Chemother* **45:**2400–2402.

78. Puopolo KM, Klinzing DC, Lin MP, Yesucevitz DL, Cieslewicz MJ. 2007. A composite transposon associated with erythromycin and clindamycin resistance in group B *Streptococcus*. *J Med Microbiol* **56:**947–955.

79. Cai Y, Kong F, Gilbert GL. 2007. Three new macrolide efflux (*mef*) gene variants in *Streptococcus agalactiae*. *J Clin Microbiol* **45:**2754–2755.

80. Ambrose KD, Nisbet R, Stephens DS. 2005. Macrolide efflux in *Streptococcus pneumoniae* is mediated by a dual efflux pump (*mel* and *mef*) and is erythromycin inducible. *Antimicrob Agents Chemother* **49:**4203–4209.

81. Gay K, Stephens DS. 2001. Structure and dissemination of a chromosomal insertion element encoding macrolide efflux in *Streptococcus pneumoniae*. *J Infect Dis* **184:**56–65.

82. Mingoia M, Vecchi M, Cochetti I, Tili E, Vitali LA, Manzin A, Varaldo PE, Montanari MP. 2007. Composite structure of *Streptococcus pneumoniae* containing the erythromycin efflux resistance gene *mefI* and the chloramphenicol resistance gene *catQ*. *Antimicrob Agents Chemother* **51:**3983–3987.

83. Santagati M, Iannelli F, Cascone C, Campanile F, Oggioni MR, Stefani S, Pozzi G. 2003. The novel conjugative transposon *tn1207.3* carries the macrolide efflux gene *mef*(A) in *Streptococcus pyogenes*. *Microb Drug Resist* **9:**243–247.

84. Clancy J, Dib-Hajj F, Petitpas JW, Yuan W. 1997. Cloning and characterization of a novel macrolide efflux gene, *mreA*, from *Streptococcus agalactiae*. *Antimicrob Agents Chemother* **41:**2719–2723.

85. Bozdogan B, Berrezouga L, Kuo MS, Yurek DA, Farley KA, Stockman BJ, Leclercq R. 1999. A new resistance gene, *linB*, conferring resistance to lincosamides

by nucleotidylation in *Enterococcus faecium* HM1025. *Antimicrob Agents Chemother* 43:925–929.

86. de Azavedo JC, McGavin M, Duncan C, Low DE, McGeer A. 2001. Prevalence and mechanisms of macrolide resistance in invasive and noninvasive group B streptococcus isolates from Ontario, Canada. *Antimicrob Agents Chemother* 45:3504–3508.

87. Achard A, Villers C, Pichereau V, Leclercq R. 2005. New *lnu*(C) gene conferring resistance to lincomycin by nucleotidylation in *Streptococcus agalactiae* UCN36. *Antimicrob Agents Chemother* 49:2716–2719.

88. Petinaki E, Guérin-Faublée V, Pichereau V, Villers C, Achard A, Malbruny B, Leclercq R. 2008. Lincomycin resistance gene *lnu*(D) in *Streptococcus uberis*. *Antimicrob Agents Chemother* 52:626–630.

89. Chesneau O, Tsvetkova K, Courvalin P. 2007. Resistance phenotypes conferred by macrolide phosphotransferases. *FEMS Microbiol Lett* 269:317–322.

90. Rato MG, Bexiga R, Florindo C, Cavaco LM, Vilela CL, Santos-Sanches I. 2013. Antimicrobial resistance and molecular epidemiology of streptococci from bovine mastitis. *Vet Microbiol* 161:286–294.

91. Dogan B, Schukken YH, Santisteban C, Boor KJ. 2005. Distribution of serotypes and antimicrobial resistance genes among *Streptococcus agalactiae* isolates from bovine and human hosts. *J Clin Microbiol* 43:5899–5906.

92. Gao J, Yu FQ, Luo LP, He JZ, Hou RG, Zhang HQ, Li SM, Su JL, Han B. 2012. Antibiotic resistance of *Streptococcus agalactiae* from cows with mastitis. *Vet J* 194:423–424.

93. Pinto TC, Costa NS, Vianna Souza AR, Silva LG, Corrêa AB, Fernandes FG, Oliveira IC, Mattos MC, Rosado AS, Benchetrit LC. 2013. Distribution of serotypes and evaluation of antimicrobial susceptibility among human and bovine *Streptococcus agalactiae* strains isolated in Brazil between 1980 and 2006. *Braz J Infect Dis* 17:131–136.

94. Haenni M, Saras E, Bertin S, Leblond P, Madec JY, Payot S. 2010. Diversity and mobility of integrative and conjugative elements in bovine isolates of *Streptococcus agalactiae*, *S. dysgalactiae* subsp. *dysgalactiae*, and *S. uberis*. *Appl Environ Microbiol* 76:7957–7965.

95. Loch IM, Glenn K, Zadoks RN. 2005. Macrolide and lincosamide resistance genes of environmental streptococci from bovine milk. *Vet Microbiol* 111:133–138.

96. Haenni M, Saras E, Chaussière S, Treilles M, Madec JY. 2011. *ermB*-mediated erythromycin resistance in *Streptococcus uberis* from bovine mastitis. *Vet J* 189:356–358.

97. Schmitt-Van de Leemput E, Zadoks RN. 2007. Genotypic and phenotypic detection of macrolide and lincosamide resistance in *Streptococcus uberis*. *J Dairy Sci* 90:5089–5096.

98. Achard A, Guérin-Faublée V, Pichereau V, Villers C, Leclercq R. 2008. Emergence of macrolide resistance gene *mph*(B) in *Streptococcus uberis* and cooperative effects with *rdmC*-like gene. *Antimicrob Agents Chemother* 52:2767–2770.

99. Hendriksen RS, Mevius DJ, Schroeter A, Teale C, Meunier D, Butaye P, Franco A, Utinane A, Amado A, Moreno M, Greko C, Stärk K, Berghold C, Myllyniemi AL, Wasyl D, Sunde M, Aarestrup FM. 2008. Prevalence of antimicrobial resistance among bacterial pathogens isolated from cattle in different European countries: 2002–2004. *Acta Vet Scand* 50:28–38.

100. Thomas V, de Jong A, Moyaert H, Simjee S, El Garch F, Morrissey I, Marion H, Vallé M. 2015. Antimicrobial susceptibility monitoring of mastitis pathogens isolated from acute cases of clinical mastitis in dairy cows across Europe: VetPath results. *Int J Antimicrob Agents* 46:13–20.

101. Persson Y, Nyman AK, Grönlund-Andersson U. 2011. Etiology and antimicrobial susceptibility of udder pathogens from cases of subclinical mastitis in dairy cows in Sweden. *Acta Vet Scand* 53:36.

102. Aarestrup FM, Rasmussen SR, Artursson K, Jensen NE. 1998. Trends in the resistance to antimicrobial agents of *Streptococcus suis* isolates from Denmark and Sweden. *Vet Microbiol* 63:71–80.

103. Wasteson Y, Høie S, Roberts MC. 1994. Characterization of antibiotic resistance in *Streptococcus suis*. *Vet Microbiol* 41:41–49.

104. Gurung M, Tamang MD, Moon DC, Kim SR, Jeong JH, Jang GC, Jung SC, Park YH, Lim SK. 2015. Molecular basis of resistance to selected antimicrobial agents in the emerging zoonotic pathogen *Streptococcus suis*. *J Clin Microbiol* 53:2332–2336.

105. Palmieri C, Varaldo PE, Facinelli B. 2011. *Streptococcus suis*, an emerging drug-resistant animal and human pathogen. *Front Microbiol* 2:235–241.

106. Zhao Q, Wendlandt S, Li H, Li J, Wu C, Shen J, Schwarz S, Wang Y. 2014. Identification of the novel lincosamide resistance gene *lnu*(E) truncated by IS*Enfa5*-*cfr*-IS*Enfa5* insertion in *Streptococcus suis*: de novo synthesis and confirmation of functional activity in *Staphylococcus aureus*. *Antimicrob Agents Chemother* 58:1785–1788.

107. Hendriksen RS, Mevius DJ, Schroeter A, Teale C, Jouy E, Butaye P, Franco A, Utinane A, Amado A, Moreno M, Greko C, Stärk KD, Berghold C, Myllyniemi AL, Hoszowski A, Sunde M, Aarestrup FM. 2008. Occurrence of antimicrobial resistance among bacterial pathogens and indicator bacteria in pigs in different European countries from year 2002–2004: the ARBAO-II study. *Acta Vet Scand* 50:19–29.

108. Lüthje P, Schwarz S. 2007. Molecular basis of resistance to macrolides and lincosamides among staphylococci and streptococci from various animal sources collected in the resistance monitoring program BfT-GermVet. *Int J Antimicrob Agents* 29:528–535.

109. Silva LG, Genteluci GL, Corrêa de Mattos M, Glatthardt T, Sá Figueiredo AM, Ferreira-Carvalho BT. 2015. Group C *Streptococcus dysgalactiae* subsp. *equisimilis* in south-east Brazil: genetic diversity, resistance profile and the first report of human and equine isolates belonging to the same multilocus sequence typing lineage. *J Med Microbiol* 64:551–558.

110. Pedersen K, Pedersen K, Jensen H, Finster K, Jensen VF, Heuer OE. 2007. Occurrence of antimicrobial resistance in bacteria from diagnostic samples from dogs. *J Antimicrob Chemother* **60:**775–781.

111. Chopra I, Roberts M. 2001. Tetracycline antibiotics: mode of action, applications, molecular biology, and epidemiology of bacterial resistance. *Microbiol Mol Biol Rev* **65:**232–260.

112. Speer BS, Shoemaker NB, Salyers AA. 1992. Bacterial resistance to tetracycline: mechanisms, transfer, and clinical significance. *Clin Microbiol Rev* **5:**387–399.

113. Roberts MC. 1996. Tetracycline resistance determinants: mechanisms of action, regulation of expression, genetic mobility, and distribution. *FEMS Microbiol Rev* **19:**1–24.

114. Kazimierczak KA, Rincon MT, Patterson AJ, Martin JC, Young P, Flint HJ, Scott KP. 2008. A new tetracycline efflux gene, *tet*(40), is located in tandem with *tet*(O/32/O) in a human gut firmicute bacterium and in metagenomic library clones. *Antimicrob Agents Chemother* **52:**4001–4009.

115. Moulin G, Cavalié P, Pellanne I, Chevance A, Laval A, Millemann Y, Colin P, Chauvin C, Antimicrobial Resistance ad hoc Group of the French Food Safety Agency. 2008. A comparison of antimicrobial usage in human and veterinary medicine in France from 1999 to 2005. *J Antimicrob Chemother* **62:**617–625.

116. Report UOH. 2015. Joint report on human and animal antibiotic use, sales and resistance, 2013. https://www.gov.uk/government/collections/antimicrobial-resistance-amr-information-and-resources.

117. FDA. 2014. 2012 Summary report on antimicrobials sold or distributed for use in food-producing animals. FDA, Washington, DC. http://www.fda.gov/downloads/ForIndustry/UserFees/AnimalDrugUserFeeActADUFA/-UCM416983.pdf.

118. van den Bogaard AE, Bruinsma N, Stobberingh EE. 2000. The effect of banning avoparcin on VRE carriage in The Netherlands. *J Antimicrob Chemother* **46:**146–148.

119. Da Cunha V, Davies MR, Douarre PE, Rosinski-Chupin I, Margarit I, Spinali S, Perkins T, Lechat P, Dmytruk N, Sauvage E, Ma L, Romi B, Tichit M, Lopez-Sanchez MJ, Descorps-Declere S, Souche E, Buchrieser C, Trieu-Cuot P, Moszer I, Clermont D, Maione D, Bouchier C, McMillan DJ, Parkhill J, Telford JL, Dougan G, Walker MJ, Holden MTG, Poyart C, Glaser P, Glaser P, DEVANI Consortium. 2014. *Streptococcus agalactiae* clones infecting humans were selected and fixed through the extensive use of tetracycline. *Nat Commun* **5:**4544.

120. Roberts MC. 2005. Update on acquired tetracycline resistance genes. *FEMS Microbiol Lett* **245:**195–203.

121. Roberts MC, Schwarz S. 2016. Tetracycline and phenicol resistance genes and mechanisms: importance for agriculture, the environment, and humans. *J Environ Qual* **45:**576–592.

122. Khan SA, Novick RP. 1983. Complete nucleotide sequence of pT181, a tetracycline-resistance plasmid from *Staphylococcus aureus*. *Plasmid* **10:**251–259.

123. Burdett V, Inamine J, Rajagopalan S. 1982. Heterogeneity of tetracycline resistance determinants in *Streptococcus*. *J Bacteriol* **149:**995–1004.

124. Hartley DL, Jones KR, Tobian JA, LeBlanc DJ, Macrina FL. 1984. Disseminated tetracycline resistance in oral streptococci: implication of a conjugative transposon. *Infect Immun* **45:**13–17.

125. Courvalin P, Carlier C. 1987. Tn*1545*: a conjugative shuttle transposon. *Mol Gen Genet* **206:**259–264.

126. Clewell DB, Flannagan SE, Jaworski DD, Clewell DB. 1995. Unconstrained bacterial promiscuity: the Tn*916*-Tn*1545* family of conjugative transposons. *Trends Microbiol* **3:**229–236.

127. Rice LB. 1998. Tn*916* family conjugative transposons and dissemination of antimicrobial resistance determinants. *Antimicrob Agents Chemother* **42:**1871–1877.

128. Sougakoff W, Papadopoulou B, Nordmann P, Courvalin P. 1987. Nucleotide sequence and distribution of gene *tetO* encoding tetracycline resistance in *Campylobacter coli*. *FEMS Microbiol Lett* **44:**153–159.

129. Charpentier E, Gerbaud G, Courvalin P. 1993. Characterization of a new class of tetracycline-resistance gene *tet*(S) in *Listeria monocytogenes* BM4210. *Gene* **131:**27–34.

130. Fletcher HM, Macrina FL. 1991. Molecular survey of clindamycin and tetracycline resistance determinants in *Bacteroides* species. *Antimicrob Agents Chemother* **35:**2415–2418.

131. Clermont D, Chesneau O, De Cespédès G, Horaud T. 1997. New tetracycline resistance determinants coding for ribosomal protection in streptococci and nucleotide sequence of *tet*(T) isolated from *Streptococcus pyogenes* A498. *Antimicrob Agents Chemother* **41:**112–116.

132. Barbosa TM, Scott KP, Flint HJ. 1999. Evidence for recent intergeneric transfer of a new tetracycline resistance gene, *tet*(W), isolated from *Butyrivibrio fibrisolvens*, and the occurrence of *tet*(O) in ruminal bacteria. *Environ Microbiol* **1:**53–64.

133. Bengtsson B, Unnerstad HE, Ekman T, Artursson K, Nilsson-Ost M, Waller KP. 2009. Antimicrobial susceptibility of udder pathogens from cases of acute clinical mastitis in dairy cows. *Vet Microbiol* **136:**142–149.

134. Guérin-Faublée V, Tardy F, Bouveron C, Carret G. 2002. Antimicrobial susceptibility of *Streptococcus* species isolated from clinical mastitis in dairy cows. *Int J Antimicrob Agents* **19:**219–226.

135. Botrel MA, Haenni M, Morignat E, Sulpice P, Madec JY, Calavas D. 2010. Distribution and antimicrobial resistance of clinical and subclinical mastitis pathogens in dairy cows in Rhône-Alpes, France. *Foodborne Pathog Dis* **7:**479–487.

136. Rossitto PV, Ruiz L, Kikuchi Y, Glenn K, Luiz K, Watts JL, Cullor JS. 2002. Antibiotic susceptibility patterns for environmental streptococci isolated from bovine mastitis in central California dairies. *J Dairy Sci* **85:**132–138.

137. Brown MB, Roberts MC. 1991. Tetracycline resistance determinants in streptococcal species isolated from the bovine mammary gland. *Vet Microbiol* **29:**173–180.

138. Lollai SA, Ziccheddu M, Duprè I, Piras D. 2016. Characterization of resistance to tetracyclines and aminoglycosides of sheep mastitis pathogens: study of the effect of gene content on resistance. *J Appl Microbiol* 121:941–951.

139. Wisselink HJ, Veldman KT, Van den Eede C, Salmon SA, Mevius DJ. 2006. Quantitative susceptibility of *Streptococcus suis* strains isolated from diseased pigs in seven European countries to antimicrobial agents licensed in veterinary medicine. *Vet Microbiol* 113:73–82.

140. Princivalli MS, Palmieri C, Magi G, Vignaroli C, Manzin A, Camporese A, Barocci S, Magistrali C, Facinelli B. 2009. Genetic diversity of *Streptococcus suis* clinical isolates from pigs and humans in Italy (2003–2007). *Euro Surveill* 14:pii=19310. http://www.eurosurveillance.org/content/10.2807/ese.14.33.19310-en.

141. Kataoka Y, Yoshida T, Sawada T. 2000. A 10-year survey of antimicrobial susceptibility of *Streptococcus suis* isolates from swine in Japan. *J Vet Med Sci* 62:1053–1057.

142. Zhang C, Ning Y, Zhang Z, Song L, Qiu H, Gao H. 2008. *In vitro* antimicrobial susceptibility of *Streptococcus suis* strains isolated from clinically healthy sows in China. *Vet Microbiol* 131:386–392.

143. Vela AI, Moreno MA, Cebolla JA, González S, Latre MV, Domínguez L, Fernández-Garayzábal JF. 2005. Antimicrobial susceptibility of clinical strains of *Streptococcus suis* isolated from pigs in Spain. *Vet Microbiol* 105:143–147.

144. Soares TC, Paes AC, Megid J, Ribolla PE, Paduan KS, Gottschalk M. 2014. Antimicrobial susceptibility of *Streptococcus suis* isolated from clinically healthy swine in Brazil. *Can J Vet Res* 78:145–149.

145. Manzin A, Palmieri C, Serra C, Saddi B, Princivalli MS, Loi G, Angioni G, Tiddia F, Varaldo PE, Facinelli B. 2008. *Streptococcus suis* meningitis without history of animal contact, Italy. *Emerg Infect Dis* 14:1946–1948.

146. Chen L, Song Y, Wei Z, He H, Zhang A, Jin M. 2013. Antimicrobial susceptibility, tetracycline and erythromycin resistance genes, and multilocus sequence typing of *Streptococcus suis* isolates from diseased pigs in China. *J Vet Med Sci* 75:583–587.

147. Chander Y, Oliveira SR, Goyal SM. 2011. Identification of the *tet*(B) resistance gene in *Streptococcus suis*. *Vet J* 189:359–360.

148. Haenni M, Hourquet C, Saras E, Madec JY. 2015. Genetic determinants of antimicrobial resistance in *Streptococcus canis* in France. *J Glob Antimicrob Resist* 3:142–143.

149. Tsuyuki Y, Kurita G, Murata Y, Goto M, Takahashi T. 2017. Identification of group G streptococci isolates from companion animals in Japan and their antimicrobial resistance. *Jpn J Infect Dis* 70:394–398.

150. Moyaert H, De Graef EM, Haesebrouck F, Decostere A. 2006. Acquired antimicrobial resistance in the intestinal microbiota of diverse cat populations. *Res Vet Sci* 81:1–7.

151. Pérez-Trallero E, Fernández-Mazarrasa C, García-Rey C, Bouza E, Aguilar L, García-de-Lomas J, Baquero F, Spanish Surveillance Group for Respiratory Pathogens. 2001. Antimicrobial susceptibilities of 1,684 *Streptococcus pneumoniae* and 2,039 *Streptococcus pyogenes* isolates and their ecological relationships: results of a 1-year (1998–1999) multicenter surveillance study in Spain. *Antimicrob Agents Chemother* 45:3334–3340.

152. Filipe SR, Tomasz A. 2000. Inhibition of the expression of penicillin resistance in *Streptococcus pneumoniae* by inactivation of cell wall muropeptide branching genes. *Proc Natl Acad Sci USA* 97:4891–4896.

153. Guenzi E, Gasc AM, Sicard MA, Hakenbeck R. 1994. A two-component signal-transducing system is involved in competence and penicillin susceptibility in laboratory mutants of *Streptococcus pneumoniae*. *Mol Microbiol* 12:505–515.

154. Crisóstomo MI, Vollmer W, Kharat AS, Inhülsen S, Gehre F, Buckenmaier S, Tomasz A. 2006. Attenuation of penicillin resistance in a peptidoglycan O-acetyl transferase mutant of *Streptococcus pneumoniae*. *Mol Microbiol* 61:1497–1509.

155. Dias R, Félix D, Caniça M, Trombe MC. 2009. The highly conserved serine threonine kinase StkP of *Streptococcus pneumoniae* contributes to penicillin susceptibility independently from genes encoding penicillin-binding proteins. *BMC Microbiol* 9:121.

156. Soualhine H, Brochu V, Ménard F, Papadopoulou B, Weiss K, Bergeron MG, Légaré D, Drummelsmith J, Ouellette M. 2005. A proteomic analysis of penicillin resistance in *Streptococcus pneumoniae* reveals a novel role for PstS, a subunit of the phosphate ABC transporter. *Mol Microbiol* 58:1430–1440.

157. Fani F, Leprohon P, Légaré D, Ouellette M. 2011. Whole genome sequencing of penicillin-resistant *Streptococcus pneumoniae* reveals mutations in penicillin-binding proteins and in a putative iron permease. *Genome Biol* 12: R115.

158. Goldstein FW. 1999. Penicillin-resistant *Streptococcus pneumoniae*: selection by both beta-lactam and non-beta-lactam antibiotics. *J Antimicrob Chemother* 44: 141–144.

159. Anonymous. 2008. Recent trends in antimicrobial resistance among *Streptococcus pneumoniae* and *Staphylococcus aureus* isolates: the French experience. *Euro Surveill* 13:pii=19035. http://eurosurveillance.org/content/10.2807/ese.13.46.19035-en.

160. Dagan R, Klugman KP. 2008. Impact of conjugate pneumococcal vaccines on antibiotic resistance. *Lancet Infect Dis* 8:785–795.

161. Kimura K, Suzuki S, Wachino J, Kurokawa H, Yamane K, Shibata N, Nagano N, Kato H, Shibayama K, Arakawa Y. 2008. First molecular characterization of group B streptococci with reduced penicillin susceptibility. *Antimicrob Agents Chemother* 52:2890–2897.

162. Nagano N, Nagano Y, Kimura K, Tamai K, Yanagisawa H, Arakawa Y. 2008. Genetic heterogeneity in *pbp* genes among clinically isolated group B streptococci with reduced penicillin susceptibility. *Antimicrob Agents Chemother* 52:4258–4267.

163. Kimura K, Nagano N, Arakawa Y. 2015. Classification of group B streptococci with reduced β-lactam susceptibility (GBS-RBS) based on the amino acid substitutions in PBPs. *J Antimicrob Chemother* **70**:1601–1603.

164. Cain D, Malouin F, Dargis M, Harel J, Gottschalk M. 1995. Alterations in penicillin-binding proteins in strains of *Streptococcus suis* possessing moderate and high levels of resistance to penicillin. *FEMS Microbiol Lett* **130**:121–127.

165. Haenni M, Galofaro L, Ythier M, Giddey M, Majcherczyk P, Moreillon P, Madec JY. 2010. Penicillin-binding protein gene alterations in *Streptococcus uberis* isolates presenting decreased susceptibility to penicillin. *Antimicrob Agents Chemother* **54**:1140–1145.

166. Haenni M, Saras E, Madec JY. 2010. Demonstration of a shift towards penicillin resistance in the *Streptococcus uberis* population. *J Med Microbiol* **59**:993–995.

167. Rüegsegger F, Ruf J, Tschuor A, Sigrist Y, Rosskopf M, Hässig M. 2014. Antimicrobial susceptibility of mastitis pathogens of dairy cows in Switzerland. *Schweiz Arch Tierheilkd* **156**:483–488.

168. Kalmus P, Aasmäe B, Kärssin A, Orro T, Kask K. 2011. Udder pathogens and their resistance to antimicrobial agents in dairy cows in Estonia. *Acta Vet Scand* **53**:4.

169. Bal EB, Bayar S, Bal MA. 2010. Antimicrobial susceptibilities of coagulase-negative staphylococci (CNS) and streptococci from bovine subclinical mastitis cases. *J Microbiol* **48**:267–274.

170. Zhang C, Zhang Z, Song L, Fan X, Wen F, Xu S, Ning Y. 2015. Antimicrobial resistance profile and genotypic characteristics of *Streptococcus suis* capsular type 2 isolated from clinical carrier sows and diseased pigs in China. *BioMed Res Int* **2015**:284303.

171. van Hout J, Heuvelink A, Gonggrijp M. 2016. Monitoring of antimicrobial susceptibility of *Streptococcus suis* in the Netherlands, 2013–2015. *Vet Microbiol* **194**:5–10.

172. Moreno LZ, da Costa BL, Matajira CE, Gomes VT, Mesquita RE, Silva AP, Moreno AM. 2016. Molecular and antimicrobial susceptibility profiling of *Streptococcus dysgalactiae* isolated from swine. *Diagn Microbiol Infect Dis* **86**:178–180.

173. Drlica K, Zhao X. 1997. DNA gyrase, topoisomerase IV, and the 4-quinolones. *Microbiol Mol Biol Rev* **61**:377–392.

174. Escudero JA, San Millan A, Gutierrez B, Hidalgo L, La Ragione RM, AbuOun M, Galimand M, Ferrándiz MJ, Domínguez L, de la Campa AG, Gonzalez-Zorn B. 2011. Fluoroquinolone efflux in *Streptococcus suis* is mediated by SatAB and not by SmrA. *Antimicrob Agents Chemother* **55**:5850–5860.

175. Meunier D, Acar JF, Martel JL, Krocmer S, Vallé M. 2004. Seven years survey of susceptibility to marbofloxacin of bovine pathogenic strains from eight European countries. *Int J Antimicrob Agents* **24**:268–278.

176. Kroemer S, Galland D, Guérin-Faublée V, Giboin H, Woehrlé-Fontaine F. 2012. Survey of marbofloxacin susceptibility of bacteria isolated from cattle with respiratory disease and mastitis in Europe. *Vet Rec* **170**:53.

177. El Garch F, de Jong A, Simjee S, Moyaert H, Klein U, Ludwig C, Marion H, Haag-Diergarten S, Richard-Mazet A, Thomas V, Siegwart E. 2016. Monitoring of antimicrobial susceptibility of respiratory tract pathogens isolated from diseased cattle and pigs across Europe, 2009–2012: VetPath results. *Vet Microbiol* **194**:11–22.

178. Morrissey I, Moyaert H, de Jong A, El Garch F, Klein U, Ludwig C, Thiry J, Youala M. 2016. Antimicrobial susceptibility monitoring of bacterial pathogens isolated from respiratory tract infections in dogs and cats across Europe: ComPath results. *Vet Microbiol* **191**:44–51.

179. Ludwig C, de Jong A, Moyaert H, El Garch F, Janes R, Klein U, Morrissey I, Thiry J, Youala M. 2016. Antimicrobial susceptibility monitoring of dermatological bacterial pathogens isolated from diseased dogs and cats across Europe (ComPath results). *J Appl Microbiol* **121**:1254–1267.

180. Burrus V, Pavlovic G, Decaris B, Guédon G. 2002. Conjugative transposons: the tip of the iceberg. *Mol Microbiol* **46**:601–610.

181. Wozniak RA, Waldor MK. 2010. Integrative and conjugative elements: mosaic mobile genetic elements enabling dynamic lateral gene flow. *Nat Rev Microbiol* **8**:552–563.

182. Santoro F, Vianna ME, Roberts AP. 2014. Variation on a theme; an overview of the Tn*916*/Tn*1545* family of mobile genetic elements in the oral and nasopharyngeal streptococci. *Front Microbiol* **5**:535–545.

183. Roberts AP, Mullany P. 2011. Tn*916*-like genetic elements: a diverse group of modular mobile elements conferring antibiotic resistance. *FEMS Microbiol Rev* **35**:856–871.

184. Ambroset C, Coluzzi C, Guédon G, Devignes MD, Loux V, Lacroix T, Payot S, Leblond-Bourget N. 2016. New insights into the classification and integration specificity of *Streptococcus* integrative conjugative elements through extensive genome exploration. *Front Microbiol* **6**:1483–1504.

185. Huang J, Ma J, Shang K, Hu X, Liang Y, Li D, Wu Z, Dai L, Chen L, Wang L. 2016. Evolution and diversity of the antimicrobial resistance associated mobilome in *Streptococcus suis*: a probable mobile genetic elements reservoir for other streptococci. *Front Cell Infect Microbiol* **6**:118.

186. Brenciani A, Tiberi E, Morici E, Oryasin E, Giovanetti E, Varaldo PE. 2012. ICE*Sp1116*, the genetic element responsible for *erm*(B)-mediated, inducible resistance to erythromycin in *Streptococcus pyogenes*. *Antimicrob Agents Chemother* **56**:6425–6429.

187. Giovanetti E, Brenciani A, Tiberi E, Bacciaglia A, Varaldo PE. 2012. ICE*Sp2905*, the *erm*(TR)-*tet*(O) element of *Streptococcus pyogenes*, is formed by two independent integrative and conjugative elements. *Antimicrob Agents Chemother* **56**:591–594.

188. Mingoia M, Morici E, Marini E, Brenciani A, Giovanetti E, Varaldo PE. 2016. Macrolide resistance gene *erm*(TR) and *erm*(TR)-carrying genetic elements in *Streptococcus agalactiae*: characterization of ICE*Sag*TR7, a new composite element containing IME*Sp2907*. *J Antimicrob Chemother* **71**:593–600.

189. Huang K, Song Y, Zhang Q, Zhang A, Jin M. 2016. Characterisation of a novel integrative and conjugative element ICESsD9 carrying *erm*(B) and *tet*(O) resistance determinants in *Streptococcus suis*, and the distribution of ICESsD9-like elements in clinical isolates. *J Glob Antimicrob Resist* 7:13–18.

190. Palmieri C, Magi G, Creti R, Baldassarri L, Imperi M, Gherardi G, Facinelli B. 2013. Interspecies mobilization of an *erm*T-carrying plasmid of *Streptococcus dysgalactiae* subsp. *equisimilis* by a coresident ICE of the ICE*Sa*2603 family. *J Antimicrob Chemother* 68:23–26.

191. Croucher NJ, Walker D, Romero P, Lennard N, Paterson GK, Bason NC, Mitchell AM, Quail MA, Andrew PW, Parkhill J, Bentley SD, Mitchell TJ. 2009. Role of conjugative elements in the evolution of the multidrug-resistant pandemic clone *Streptococcus pneumoniae*[Spain23F] ST81. *J Bacteriol* 191:1480–1489.

192. Douarre PE, Sauvage E, Poyart C, Glaser P. 2015. Host specificity in the diversity and transfer of *lsa* resistance genes in group B *Streptococcus*. *J Antimicrob Chemother* 70:3205–3213.

193. Huang K, Zhang Q, Song Y, Zhang Z, Zhang A, Xiao J, Jin M. 2016. Characterization of spectinomycin resistance in *Streptococcus suis* leads to two novel insights into drug resistance formation and dissemination mechanism. *Antimicrob Agents Chemother* 60:6390–6392.

194. Marini E, Palmieri C, Magi G, Facinelli B. 2015. Recombination between *Streptococcus suis* ICESsu32457 and *Streptococcus agalactiae* ICESa2603 yields a hybrid ICE transferable to *Streptococcus pyogenes*. *Vet Microbiol* 178:99–104.

195. Srinivasan V, Metcalf BJ, Knipe KM, Ouattara M, McGee L, Shewmaker PL, Glennen A, Nichols M, Harris C, Brimmage M, Ostrowsky B, Park CJ, Schrag SJ, Frace MA, Sammons SA, Beall B. 2014. *vanG* element insertions within a conserved chromosomal site conferring vancomycin resistance to *Streptococcus agalactiae* and *Streptococcus anginosus*. *MBio* 5:e01386-14.

196. Meng F, Kanai K, Yoshikoshi K. 2009. Structural characterization of Tn916-like element in *Streptococcus parauberis* serotype II strains isolated from diseased Japanese flounder. *Lett Appl Microbiol* 48:770–776.

197. Palmieri C, Magi G, Mingoia M, Bagnarelli P, Ripa S, Varaldo PE, Facinelli B. 2012. Characterization of a *Streptococcus suis tet*(O/W/32/O)-carrying element transferable to major streptococcal pathogens. *Antimicrob Agents Chemother* 56:4697–4702.

198. Richards VP, Zadoks RN, Pavinski Bitar PD, Lefébure T, Lang P, Werner B, Tikofsky L, Moroni P, Stanhope MJ. 2012. Genome characterization and population genetic structure of the zoonotic pathogen, *Streptococcus canis*. *BMC Microbiol* 12:293–309.

199. Bekele T, Molla B. 2001. Mastitis in lactating camels (*Camelus dromedarius*) in Afar Region, north-eastern Ethiopia. *Berl Munch Tierarztl Wochenschr* 114:169–172.

200. Evans JJ, Pasnik DJ, Klesius PH, Al-Ablani S. 2006. First report of *Streptococcus agalactiae* and *Lactococcus garvieae* from a wild bottlenose dolphin (*Tursiops truncatus*). *J Wildl Dis* 42:561–569.

201. Jordal S, Glambek M, Oppegaard O, Kittang BR. 2015. New tricks from an old cow: infective endocarditis caused by *Streptococcus dysgalactiae* subsp. *dysgalactiae*. *J Clin Microbiol* 53:731–734.

202. Nomoto R, Munasinghe LI, Jin DH, Shimahara Y, Yasuda H, Nakamura A, Misawa N, Itami T, Yoshida T. 2004. Lancefield group C *Streptococcus dysgalactiae* infection responsible for fish mortalities in Japan. *J Fish Dis* 27:679–686.

203. Hilmarsdóttir I, Valsdóttir F. 2007. Molecular typing of beta-hemolytic streptococci from two patients with lower-limb cellulitis: identical isolates from toe web and blood specimens. *J Clin Microbiol* 45:3131–3132.

204. Kawata K, Minakami T, Mori Y, Katsumi M, Kataoka Y, Ezawa A, Kikuchi N, Takahashi T. 2003. rDNA sequence analyses of *Streptococcus dysgalactiae* subsp. *equisimilis* isolates from pigs. *Int J Syst Evol Microbiol* 53:1941–1946.

205. Lopardo HA, Vidal P, Sparo M, Jeric P, Centron D, Facklam RR, Paganini H, Pagniez NG, Lovgren M, Beall B. 2005. Six-month multicenter study on invasive infections due to *Streptococcus pyogenes* and *Streptococcus dysgalactiae* subsp. *equisimilis* in Argentina. *J Clin Microbiol* 43:802–807.

206. Nei T, Akutsu K, Shima A, Tsuboi I, Suzuki H, Yamamoto T, Tanaka K, Shinoyama A, Kojima Y, Washio Y, Okawa S, Sonobe K, Norose Y, Saito R. 2012. A case of streptococcal toxic shock syndrome due to group G streptococci identified as *Streptococcus dysgalactiae* subsp. *equisimilis*. *J Infect Chemother* 18:919–924.

207. Savini V, Catavitello C, Talia M, Manna A, Pompetti F, Di Bonaventura G, Di Giuseppe N, Febbo F, Balbinot A, Di Zacomo S, Esattore F, D'Antonio D. 2008. Beta-lactam failure in treatment of two group G *Streptococcus dysgalactiae* subsp. *equisimilis* pharyngitis patients. *J Clin Microbiol* 46:814–816.

208. Siljander T, Karppelin M, Vähäkuopus S, Syrjänen J, Toropainen M, Kere J, Vuento R, Jussila T, Vuopio-Varkila J. 2008. Acute bacterial, nonnecrotizing cellulitis in Finland: microbiological findings. *Clin Infect Dis* 46:855–861.

209. Wajima T, Morozumi M, Hanada S, Sunaoshi K, Chiba N, Iwata S, Ubukata K. 2016. Molecular characterization of invasive *Streptococcus dysgalactiae* subsp. *equisimilis*, Japan. *Emerg Infect Dis* 22:247–254.

210. Zoric M, Nilsson E, Lundeheim N, Wallgren P. 2009. Incidence of lameness and abrasions in piglets in identical farrowing pens with four different types of floor. *Acta Vet Scand* 51:23–32.

211. Casagrande Proietti P, Bietta A, Coppola G, Felicetti M, Cook RF, Coletti M, Marenzoni ML, Passamonti F. 2011. Isolation and characterization of β-haemolytic-streptococci from endometritis in mares. *Vet Microbiol* 152:126–130.

212. Imai D, Jang S, Miller M, Conrad PA. 2009. Characterization of beta-hemolytic streptococci isolated from southern sea otters (*Enhydra lutris nereis*) stranded along the California coast. *Vet Microbiol* 136:378–381.

213. García-País MJ, Rabuñal R, Armesto V, López-Reboiro M, García-Garrote F, Coira A, Pita J, Rodríguez-

Macías AI, López-Álvarez MJ, Alonso MP, Corredoira J. 2016. *Streptococcus bovis* septic arthritis and osteomyelitis: a report of 21 cases and a literature review. *Semin Arthritis Rheum* 45:738–746.

214. Osawa R, Sly LI. 1991. Phenotypic characterization of CO2-requiring strains of *Streptococcus bovis* from koalas. *Appl Environ Microbiol* 57:3037–3039.

215. Sekizaki T, Nishiya H, Nakajima S, Nishizono M, Kawano M, Okura M, Takamatsu D, Nishino H, Ishiji T, Osawa R. 2008. Endocarditis in chickens caused by subclinical infection of *Streptococcus gallolyticus* subsp. *gallolyticus*. *Avian Dis* 52:183–186.

216. van Samkar A, Brouwer MC, Pannekoek Y, van der Ende A, van de Beek D. 2015. *Streptococcus gallolyticus* meningitis in adults: report of five cases and review of the literature. *Clin Microbiol Infect* 21:1077–1083.

217. Katsumi M, Kataoka Y, Takahashi T, Kikuchi N, Hiramune T. 1997. Bacterial isolation from slaughtered pigs associated with endocarditis, especially the isolation of *Streptococcus suis*. *J Vet Med Sci* 59:75–78.

218. O'Sullivan T, Friendship R, Blackwell T, Pearl D, McEwen B, Carman S, Slavić D, Dewey C. 2011. Microbiological identification and analysis of swine tonsils collected from carcasses at slaughter. *Can J Vet Res* 75:106–111.

219. Miller CW, Prescott JF, Mathews KA, Betschel SD, Yager JA, Guru V, DeWinter L, Low DE. 1996. Streptococcal toxic shock syndrome in dogs. *J Am Vet Med Assoc* 209:1421–1426.

220. Reissmann S, Friedrichs C, Rajkumari R, Itzek A, Fulde M, Rodloff AC, Brahmadathan KN, Chhatwal GS, Nitsche-Schmitz DP. 2010. Contribution of *Streptococcus anginosus* to infections caused by groups C and G streptococci, southern India. *Emerg Infect Dis* 16:656–663.

221. Hatrongjit R, Kerdsin A, Gottschalk M, Takeuchi D, Hamada S, Oishi K, Akeda Y. 2015. First human case report of sepsis due to infection with *Streptococcus suis* serotype 31 in Thailand. *BMC Infect Dis* 15:392–399.

222. Mancini F, Adamo F, Creti R, Monaco M, Alfarone G, Pantosti A, Ciervo A. 2016. A fatal case of streptococcal toxic shock syndrome caused by *Streptococcus suis* carrying *tet* (40) and *tet* (O/W/32/O), Italy. *J Infect Chemother* 22:774–776.

223. Sánchez del Rey V, Fernández-Garayzábal JF, Briones V, Iriso A, Domínguez L, Gottschalk M, Vela AI. 2013. Genetic analysis of *Streptococcus suis* isolates from wild rabbits. *Vet Microbiol* 165:483–486.

224. Sánchez del Rey V, Fernández-Garayzábal JF, Domínguez L, Gottschalk M, Vela AI. 2016. Screening of virulence-associated genes as a molecular typing method for characterization of *Streptococcus suis* isolates recovered from wild boars and pigs. *Vet J* 209:108–112.

225. Staats JJ, Feder I, Okwumabua O, Chengappa MM. 1997. *Streptococcus suis*: past and present. *Vet Res Commun* 21:381–407.

226. Anshary H, Kurniawan RA, Sriwulan S, Ramli R, Baxa DV. 2014. Isolation and molecular identification of the etiological agents of streptococcosis in Nile tilapia (*Oreochromis niloticus*) cultured in net cages in Lake Sentani, Papua, Indonesia. *Springerplus* 3:627–638.

227. Bonar CJ, Wagner RA. 2003. A third report of "golf ball disease" in an Amazon River dolphin (*Inia geoffrensis*) associated with *Streptococcus iniae*. *J Zoo Wildl Med* 34:296–301.

228. Chou L, Griffin MJ, Fraites T, Ware C, Ferguson H, Keirstead N, Brake J, Wiles J, Hawke JP, Kearney MT, Getchell RG, Gaunt P, Soto E. 2014. Phenotypic and genotypic heterogeneity among *Streptococcus iniae* isolates recovered from cultured and wild fish in North America, Central America and the Caribbean islands. *J Aquat Anim Health* 26:263–271.

229. El Aamri F, Padilla D, Acosta F, Caballero M, Roo J, Bravo J, Vivas J, Real F. 2010. First report of *Streptococcus iniae* in red porgy (*Pagrus pagrus*, L.). *J Fish Dis* 33:901–905.

230. Figueiredo HC, Netto LN, Leal CA, Pereira UP, Mian GF. 2012. *Streptococcus iniae* outbreaks in Brazilian Nile tilapia (*Oreochromis niloticus* L:) farms. *Braz J Microbiol* 43:576–580.

231. Keirstead ND, Brake JW, Griffin MJ, Halliday-Simmonds I, Thrall MA, Soto E. 2014. Fatal septicemia caused by the zoonotic bacterium *Streptococcus iniae* during an outbreak in Caribbean reef fish. *Vet Pathol* 51:1035–1041.

232. Denamiel G, Llorente P, Carabella M, Rebuelto M, Gentilini E. 2005. Anti-microbial susceptibility of *Streptococcus* spp. isolated from bovine mastitis in Argentina. *J Vet Med B Infect Dis Vet Public Health* 52: 125–128.

233. Nam HM, Lim SK, Kang HM, Kim JM, Moon JS, Jang KC, Joo YS, Kang MI, Jung SC. 2009. Antimicrobial resistance of streptococci isolated from mastitic bovine milk samples in Korea. *J Vet Diagn Invest* 21:698–701.

234. Entorf M, Feßler AT, Kaspar H, Kadlec K, Peters T, Schwarz S. 2016. Comparative erythromycin and tylosin susceptibility testing of streptococci from bovine mastitis. *Vet Microbiol* 194:36–42.

235. Marie J, Morvan H, Berthelot-Hérault F, Sanders P, Kempf I, Gautier-Bouchardon AV, Jouy E, Kobisch M. 2002. Antimicrobial susceptibility of *Streptococcus suis* isolated from swine in France and from humans in different countries between 1996 and 2000. *J Antimicrob Chemother* 50:201–209.

236. Martel A, Baele M, Devriese LA, Goossens H, Wisselink HJ, Decostere A, Haesebrouck F. 2001. Prevalence and mechanism of resistance against macrolides and lincosamides in *Streptococcus suis* isolates. *Vet Microbiol* 83: 287–297.

237. Tian Y, Aarestrup FM, Lu CP. 2004. Characterization of *Streptococcus suis* serotype 7 isolates from diseased pigs in Denmark. *Vet Microbiol* 103:55–62.

238. Overesch G, Stephan R, Perreten V. 2013. Antimicrobial susceptibility of gram-positive udder pathogens from bovine mastitis milk in Switzerland. *Schweiz Arch Tierheilkd* 155:339–350.

Antimicrobial Resistance in Bacteria from Livestock and Companion Animals
Edited by Frank Møller Aarestrup, Stefan Schwarz, Jianzhong Shen, and Lina Cavaco
© 2017 American Society for Microbiology, Washington, DC
doi:10.1128/microbiolspec.ARBA-0032-2018

Antimicrobial Resistance in *Enterococcus* spp. of animal origin

9

Carmen Torres,[1] Carla Andrea Alonso,[1] Laura Ruiz-Ripa,[1]
Ricardo León-Sampedro,[2,3] Rosa del Campo,[2,4] and Teresa M. Coque[2,3]

INTRODUCTION

Enterococcus species are natural inhabitants of the intestinal tract in humans and animals, and due to their ubiquity in human and animal feces and their persistence in the environment, enterococci are considered indicators of fecal contamination in water (1). Moreover, enterococci serve as important key indicator bacteria for several human and veterinary resistance surveillance systems.

During the evisceration process at slaughterhouses, fecal enterococci can contaminate food products of animal origin. Some studies reported that over 90% of food samples of animal origin are contaminated with enterococci at the slaughterhouse, mostly with *Enterococcus faecalis*, followed by *Enterococcus faecium* (1, 2). In addition, enterococci are opportunistic pathogens which have become one of the main causes of nosocomial and community-acquired human infections, including septicemia, endocarditis, and urinary tract infections, among others (3).

The genus *Enterococcus* presently contains over 50 species, and *E. faecalis* and *E. faecium* are the predominant isolated species, accounting for more than 80% of isolates. In addition, these two species are considered the third- and fourth-most prevalent nosocomial pathogens worldwide (4). Other *Enterococcus* species, such as *E. hirae*, *E. avium*, *E. durans*, *E. gallinarum*, *E. casseliflavus*, and *E. raffinosus*, are rare causes of human clinical infections and are thought to be more opportunistic in nature than *E. faecium* and *E. faecalis* (5–10). *E. faecalis* and *E. faecium* are also the most representative enterococcal species detected in the human intestine, whereas other species, such as *E. durans* and

E. avium, are occasionally detected (11). The most commonly encountered enterococcal species in the guts of animals are *E. faecalis*, *E. faecium*, *E. hirae*, and *E. durans*; other species are also detected sporadically or in particular age groups (such as *E. cecorum* in older poultry) (11, 12). Several members of the genus *Enterococcus* can cause bovine mastitis, endocarditis, septicemia and amyloid encephalopathy with sudden death in chickens (13), and diarrhea in dogs, cats, pigs, and rats (12). In the past decade, *E. cecorum* has emerged as an important poultry pathogen, associated with arthritis and osteomyelitis (14–15).

The intrinsic resistance of these bacteria to several antimicrobial agents has compromised the choice of therapeutic options to treat enterococcal infections. Those intrinsic resistances confer resistance to semisynthetic penicillins (low-level resistance), aminoglycosides (low-level resistance), vancomycin (*E. gallinarum*, *E. casseliflavus*, and *E. flavescens*), and polymyxins and streptogramins (*E. faecalis*) (11). Moreover, enterococci frequently acquire antimicrobial resistance genes through plasmids and/or transposons. The antibiotic resistances in *Enterococcus* species have been reviewed previously (3, 16–18), with focuses on specific agents (such as vancomycin [19–22] or aminoglycosides [23]) or sources (livestock/food [24–26]). The zoonotic transmission potential of antimicrobial-resistant enterococci has also been reviewed (27). In this review, we update the available knowledge on the prevalence and molecular mechanisms of antimicrobial resistance in enterococcal isolates from a wide range of animals (livestock, pets, and wildlife) and animal-derived food, with

[1]Biochemistry and Molecular Biology Unit, University of La Rioja, 26006 Logroño, Spain; [2]Department of Microbiology, Ramón y Cajal University Hospital, Ramón y Cajal Health Research Institute (IRYCIS), Madrid, Spain; [3]Centro de Investigación Biomédica en Red de Epidemiología y Salud Pública (CIBER-ESP), Madrid, Spain; [4]Red Española de Investigación en Patología Infecciosa (REIPI), Instituto de Salud Carlos III, Madrid, Spain.

particular emphasis on beta-lactams, vancomycin, and linezolid. Furthermore, we outline the major clonal lineages and plasmids responsible for antimicrobial resistance in *Enterococcus* from farm and companion animals.

DIVERSITY OF ENTEROCOCCAL SPECIES IN THE ANIMAL INTESTINAL TRACT

Enterococci are ubiquitous bacteria in the gastrointestinal tract of humans and a wide range of animals (mammals, reptiles, birds, and some invertebrates). In addition, they are commonly found in vegetables, water, soil, and food derived from animals (including fermented and dairy products) (11). Enterococci are classified as lactic acid bacteria and are highly adaptable to different environmental conditions. They survive over a wide range of temperature (10 to 45°C), and pH (4.8 to 9.6) and are able to grow at high salt concentrations (up 6.5% NaCl). Most of them can hydrolyze esculin in the presence of 40% bile salts, a characteristic used for phenotypic identification processes (11). These and other properties explain the utilization of enterococci in diverse roles; for instance, they have been used as probiotics, starter cultures, biopreservatives, and indicators of fecal contamination of water and sanitary quality of food (28–30).

Genomic analysis revealed that members of the genus *Enterococcus* have a low G+C content, ranging from 34.29 to 44.75% (31). For a long time, *Enterococcus* species were considered streptococci of Lancefield group D. In 1984, application of nucleic hybridization and 16S rRNA sequencing led to a reclassification of *Streptococcus faecium* and *Streptococcus faecalis* in the genus *Enterococcus* (32). Currently, this genus includes around 50 species (33). Many of them were discovered in this century, mostly recovered from nonhuman sources, such as plants (*E. plantarum*, *E. ureilyticus*), water (*E. quebecensis*, *E. rivorum*, *E. ureasiticus*), animals (*E. canis*, *E. phoeniculicola*, *E. devriesei*), and food products (*E. thailandicus*, *E. italicus*) (34–42).

A recent genomic study which compared the concatenated nucleotide sequences of the core genes of 37 enterococci belonging to a variety of species divided these strains into 6 branches: (i) the *E. faecium* branch (containing *E. faecium*, *E. mundtii*, *E. durans*, *E. hirae*, *E. ratti*, *E. villorum*, *E. thailandicus*, *E. phoeniculicola*), (ii) the *E. faecalis* branch (*E. faecalis*, *E. termitis*, *E. quebecensis*, *E. moraviensis*, *E. caccae*, *E. haemoperoxidus*, *E. silesiacus*), (iii) the *E. dispar* branch (*E. dispar*, *E. canintestini*, *E. asini*), (iv) the *E. casseliflavus* branch (*E. casseliflavus*, *E. gallinarum*, *E. aquimarinus*,

E. saccharolyticus, *E. italicus*, *E. sulfureus*, *E. cecorum*, *E. columbae*), (v) the *E. pallens* branch (*E. pallens*, *E. hermanniensis*, *E. devriesei*, *E. gilvus*, *E. malodoratus*, *E. avium*, *E. raffinosus*), and (vi) the *E. canis* branch, which contained only one strain (31). Results showed that most strains from human and other mammals were clustered into the *E. faecium*, *E. faecalis*, *E. dispar*, and *E. pallens* branches, whereas the majority of the bird isolates belonged to the *E. casseliflavus* branch.

In 1963, Mundt and colleagues carried out a survey of the occurrence of enterococci among animals living in the wild environment (43). They obtained enterococci from the feces of 71% of the studied mammals, 86% of the reptiles, and 32% of the birds. In addition, patterns of food and animal species dependence were observed. In general, enterococci were only isolated sporadically in samples recovered from herbivorous mammals. However, they were abundant in rodents, bats, and larger animals with omnivorous or carnivorous diets (43), but as demonstrated in several other reports, the differences in the proportions of enterococci in each niche, as well as the species distributions, varied not only according to the diet, but also according to seasonal changes, individual characteristics (gender, age), and geographic location (11, 44).

In general, *E. faecium*, *E. faecalis*, *E. hirae*, and *E. durans* are the most prevalent enterococcal species in the gastrointestinal tract of humans and other mammals (11). *E. cecorum* is also a relevant member of the normal enterococcal microbiota in the gut of farm and pet animals (cattle, pigs, dogs, cats) and birds (poultry and pigeons) (45–47). However, in chickens, a significant age-dependent increase in gut colonization has been reported for this species. *E. cecorum* has been found to be a dominant part of the enterococcal gastrointestinal microbiota in mature chickens (48). Some other species, such as *E. gallinarum* and *E. avium*, which were first described in chickens, have not been frequently detected among enterococcal gut populations in poultry (49, 50).

In cattle and swine, the proportions of the enterococcal species vary across studies. *E. faecium*, *E. durans*, *E. hirae*, and *E. faecalis* were unanimously found in different surveys (46, 50–52). In some works, *E. faecalis* was the predominant enterococcal species in the gut of bovines and swines (46, 53). In others, *E. hirae* and *E. faecium* were described as the more abundant bacteria in both livestock species (44, 51, 52). As observed, variations between geographical regions might explain these differences in the composition of the enterococcal populations (44). *E. casseliflavus*, *E. gallinarum*, *E. avium*, and *E. cecorum* have also been reported as part of the bovine and swine microbiota, but they were present in lower proportions (46, 50, 51). Additionally, some minoritary species, such as *E. villorum* and *E. thailandicus*, have been sporadically detected in feces from cattle and pigs (52, 54, 55).

The enterococcal microbiota of the intestinal tract of dogs and cats showed a predominance of *E. faecalis* and *E. faecium*, followed by *E. hirae* (56–59). *E. avium* has been commonly isolated in canines and also, although in smaller proportions, in feline feces (56, 57). Other species, such as *E. durans*, *E. gallinarum*, *E. casseliflavus*, *E. cecorum*, and *E. raffinosus*, have been occasionally reported (56, 58, 59). In addition, some newly characterized species were isolated from anal swabs and chronic otitis externa (*E. canis*) and fecal samples (*E. canintestini*) of dogs (34, 60).

Enterococci are also normal residents of the gut of a wide range of free-living animals. In pigeons, the predominant species is *E. columbae* and, to a lesser extent, *E. cecorum*. However, *E. faecium* and *E. faecalis* are rare in these birds (61). Another study reported a high prevalence of enterococci among three species of coraciiform birds (74%), with a dominance of *E. faecalis*, followed by *E. casseliflavus* (62). In Portugal, *E. faecium* was the most frequently encountered species in buzzard fecal samples (63), and *E. faecium*, *E. durans*, and *E. gallinarum* were found in the feces of a variety of wild birds (64). The enterococcal gut microbiota has also been analyzed in wild marine species. *E. faecium* was identified as the most abundant species in echinoderms collected from Azorean waters. Minor species, such as *E. hirae*, *E. faecalis*, and *E. gallinarum*, were also detected (65). In a recent study in southern Brazil, different wild marine animals were analyzed using real-time quantitative PCR to identify and quantify enterococci in feces. These bacteria were found in all the studied animal species, with a dominance of *E. faecalis* and *E. mundtii* in most of the marine mammals; *E. faecalis* in green turtles, Magellanic penguins, and albatross; and *E. hirae* and *E. gallinarum* in white-backed stilts (66). Enterococci are also a relevant part of the facultative anaerobic microbiota of the gastrointestinal tract of large wild mammals (wolf, wildboar, deer, etc.) and rodents (67–69).

Administration of antibiotics in both human and animal medicine may shift the gut microbial community, allowing drug-resistant strains (e.g., vancomycin-resistant enterococci) to proliferate dramatically. Because many enterococcal infections are caused by normal inhabitants of the gastrointestinal tract that become opportunistic pathogens, the selection of antibiotic-resistant strains raises the risk of developing difficult-to-treat infections. The following sections give an overview of the mechanisms and prevalence of antimicrobial resistance in enterococci in the animal setting.

ANTIMICROBIAL RESISTANCE IN ENTEROCOCCI OF ANIMALS AND FOODS OF ANIMAL ORIGIN

Beta-Lactam Resistance

Enterococci are intrinsically resistant to cephalosporins and present a natural reduced susceptibility to penicillins, due to the expression of low-affinity penicillin binding proteins (PBPs) that bind weakly to beta-lactam antibiotics. For this reason, the MICs for penicillins are higher in enterococci than in streptococci or other Gram-positive organisms, which do not produce chromosomally encoded low-affinity PBPs (17). *E. faecalis* isolates normally exhibit lower MIC values for penicillins than *E. faecium* (18).

All enterococci have at least five PBPs, and six putative PBP genes have been detected by genomic analysis in *E. faecalis* and *E. faecium* (class A: *ponA*, *pbpF*, *pbpZ*; class B: *pbp5*, *pbpA*, *pbpB*) (18). The expression of the species-specific chromosomally located *pbp5* gene, which encodes PBP5, with low affinity binding for penicillins and cephalosporins, is associated with intrinsic resistance to beta-lactams. In *E. faecium*, the *pbp5* gene is included within an operon, together with two other genes that are also implicated in cell wall synthesis (*psr* and *ftsW*) (18).

Acquired (enhanced) resistance for penicillins (penicillin or ampicillin) has been frequently detected among clinical *E. faecium* isolates, being rare in *E. faecalis*. High-level ampicillin resistance in *E. faecium* (MIC, ≥128 µg/ml) has been associated with increased production of PBP5 (requiring a higher concentration of the agent to saturate the active site) or with specific amino acid changes in its sequence, which make the low-affinity PBP5 even less susceptible to inhibition by penicillins (70, 71). The amino acid substitutions near the Ser-Thr-Phe-Lys, Ser-Asp-Ala, and Lys-Thr-Gly motifs, which are part of the active-site cavity, seem to be the most significant ones (16).

Combinations of specific amino acid changes in the C-terminal transpeptidase domain of PBP5 (especially the substitution Met-485-Ala/Thr, but also the changes Ala-499-Ile/Thr, Glu-629-Val, and Pro-667-Ser), and the insertion of serine or aspartic acid after position 466, have been associated with ampicillin resistance in *E. faecium* isolates (72–76). It has been found that single substitutions at positions 485, 499, 629, and

466-insertion have only slight influence on ampicillin MIC, but when combined, the effect increases. Mutations in genes encoding other species-specific proteins that participate in cell wall synthesis may also slightly increase the MIC value (76).

Two distinct allelic forms have been identified when the whole sequence of the *pbp5* gene is considered, which differ in 5% of the sequence, yielding two types of PBP5 (PBP5-S and PBP5-R) with changes in 21 amino acid residues. PBP5-S is usually detected in community-associated ampicillin-susceptible *E. faecium* isolates (MIC of usually ≤2 µg/ml), and PBP5-R is usually detected in hospital-associated ampicillin-resistant isolates (MIC of usually ≥16 µg/ml) (77, 78). A hybrid-like type of PBP5 (PBP5-S/R), with a sequence between the other two types, has been observed in some isolates, with a MIC for ampicillin of around 4 µg/ml (77, 78).

Considering the population structure of *E. faecium*, two main lineages have been postulated in humans: (i) subclade A1, hospital-associated, enriched in mobile genetic elements, usually implicated in human infections, and in most cases, ampicillin-resistant (MIC, ≥16 µg/ml) with the consensus allele *pbp5*-R, and (ii) clade B: community-associated, detected in isolates from healthy humans (not implicated in infections), generally ampicillin-susceptible (MIC, ≤2 µg/ml), and harboring the consensus allele *pbp5*-S. The subclade A2 includes *E. faecium* isolates mostly from animal settings, exhibits a wide range of ampicillin MIC values (0.5 to 128 µg/ml), and generally carries the hybrid-like *pbp5* allele (*pbp5*-S/R) (72, 78, 79). In addition to amino acid sequence alteration in PBP5, elevated levels of this protein are also observed in highly ampicillin-resistant isolates of clade A (subclade A1 and part of A2), but not in the ampicillin-susceptible isolates of subclade A2 and clade B, suggesting a differential regulation process in each clade. The upstream region of *pbp5* seems to have a role in the level of expression of the gene (72).

In *E. faecalis*, acquired ampicillin resistance is unusual but is generally mediated by mutations in *pbp4* (27, 80). Selected strains of *E. faecalis* produce a plasmid-mediated beta-lactamase that is similar to the enzyme produced by *Staphylococcus aureus* (17, 81), encoded by the *blaZ* gene, although some polymorphisms in this gene have also been detected in some isolates. This beta-lactamase is expressed in a constitutive way in *E. faecalis*, in contrast to the inducible production in *S. aureus*. The enzyme is produced in low amounts in *E. faecalis*, and for this reason, the strain can appear as ampicillin susceptible when the MIC is tested *in vitro*. In any case, this mechanism of resistance is very infrequently seen in *E. faecalis*. Very unusual beta-lactamase-producing *E. faecium* strains have also been reported (82). Chromosomal beta-lactamase-encoding genes conferring ampicillin resistance have also been detected in *E. faecium* isolates (83).

The *in vitro* transferability of *pbp5* in *E. faecium* isolates (84), which suggests a mechanism by which high-level ampicillin resistance conferred by mutated *pbp5* alleles could be disseminated among clinical isolates, has been reported. Moreover, Novais *et al.* (85) demonstrated *in vitro* ampicillin-resistance transference by conjugation in 28% of the *E. faecium* isolates from a pig farm environment, although the genetic basis of this transference was not determined. Codiversification of the *E. faecium* core genome and *pbp5* has been recently analyzed, showing evidence of *pbp5* horizontal transfer (86).

Various studies have evaluated the prevalence of penicillin or ampicillin resistance in enterococci from food-producing animals, pets, or wild animals, as well as in those from food of animal origin. For *E. faecium*, the prevalence of resistance is variable depending on the country and the type of animal. Reflecting this, no resistant *E. faecium* isolates were detected in a surveillance study performed in a cattle population at slaughter in Australia (87), but a rate of 30% resistance was detected in isolates of poultry in Portugal (88). For pets, the following ampicillin resistance rates were reported among *E. faecium* isolates: 63% and 37% in dogs and cats, respectively, in the United States and 3% in pets in Portugal (58, 88). Moreover, ampicillin-resistant *E. faecium* isolates were detected in 23% of the dogs screened in a cross-sectional study in the United Kingdom and in 76% of the dogs analyzed in a longitudinal study in Denmark (89). Most of these resistant isolates belonged to the hospital-adapted clonal complex CC17. Frequencies of ampicillin resistance in the range of 4.5 to 7.7% have been detected in *E. faecium* isolates recovered from wild animals (wild boar, Iberian wolf, and gilt-head seabream) (74, 90, 91), but no resistant isolates were detected in Iberian lynx (92).

A surveillance study was performed analyzing the prevalence of antimicrobial resistance in 21,077 *Enterococcus* isolates obtained from retail meat samples in the United States between 2002 and 2014, through the National Antimicrobial Resistance Monitoring System (NARMS) (2). A low frequency of ampicillin resistance was detected among *E. faecium* isolates from ground beef and pork chops (4% and 2.7%, respectively), but higher percentages were detected in retail chicken (26%), and even higher in ground turkey (62.6%). Bortolaia *et al.* (25) reviewed ampicillin resistance data reported in European countries (Denmark, Sweden, The Netherlands, Slovenia) and the United States for *E. faecium* isolates recovered from poultry meat, comparing them to human isolates in the same countries (93–95). Human isolates showed very high rates of ampicillin resistance in all countries (>80%), but resistance in food isolates was significantly lower than in those of humans. Of note is the detection of 10% ampicillin resistance in *E. faecium* of (imported) broiler meat in Denmark and >50% resistance in isolates of turkey meat in the United States. Almost no ampicillin-resistant *E. faecalis* isolates (with very few exceptions) have been reported in animals or food of animal origin.

Glycopeptide Resistance

Mechanism of resistance

Vancomycin and teicoplanin are important members of the glycopeptide family and are used for the treatment of severe human infections. Avoparcin, another member of this family, has been extensively used in the past as a growth-promoter in food-producing animals in many countries.

The mechanism of action of glycopeptides is the inhibition of the synthesis of the bacterial cell wall, by the link to the D-Ala-D-Ala terminus of the pentapeptide precursor of the peptidoglycan, preventing crosslinking of the peptidoglycan chain and inhibiting cell wall synthesis. The main mechanism of glycopeptide resistance in enterococci implicates the alteration of the peptidoglycan synthesis pathway. In this sense, the terminus D-Ala-D-Ala of the pentapeptide to which vancomycin binds is modified to D-Ala-D-Lac (causing high-level vancomycin resistance; MIC, >64 μg/ml) or to D-Ala-D-Ser (low-level vancomycin resistance; MIC, 4 to 32 μg/ml). These modified cell-wall precursors bind glycopeptides with reduced affinity (about 1,000-fold and 7-fold for D-Lac and D-Ser substitutions, respectively) (18, 22).

The first vancomycin-resistant enterococci (VRE) with an acquired mechanism of resistance were detected three decades ago in clinical *E. faecium* isolates in France and the United Kingdom (96, 97). Since then, VRE have been extensively described in hospitals worldwide; they have been seen especially frequently in the United States since the 1990, mostly in patients in intensive care units, and at lower levels in Europe since the 2000s (21). According to surveillance data from the European Centre for Disease Prevention and Control (EARS-Net), the European Union/European Economic Area population-weighted mean percentage

of vancomycin resistance in *E. faecium* was 11.8% in 2016, and national percentages ranged from 0 to 46.3%; the prevalence of vancomycin resistance for *E. faecalis* was lower (98).

Vancomycin resistance is mediated by *van* operons, which encode the modified peptidoglycan precursors. To date, eight *van* operons have been identified in enterococci mediating acquired vancomycin resistance (*vanA*, *vanB*, *vanD*, *vanE*, *vanG*, *vanL*, *vanM*, and *vanN*), and one additional operon in intrinsic vancomycin resistance (*vanC*) (18, 19, 99–102). Three variants of the gene *vanC* have been described (*vanC1*, *vanC2*, and *vanC3*), intrinsic to *E. gallinarum*, *E. casseliflavus*, and *E. flavescens*, respectively. Moreover, different subtypes have been identified for *vanB* (*vanB1*, *vanB2*, and *vanB3*), *vanD* (*vanD1* to *vanD5*) and *vanG* (*vanG1*, *vanG2*) (100, 103, 104). An additional variant, *vanF*, has also been described, but until now only in the environmental microorganism *Paenibacillus popilliae* (105).

vanA and *vanB* are the most frequent genotypes among VRE with acquired resistance mechanisms of humans and animals, mostly among *E. faecalis* and *E. faecium*. The genotypes *vanD*, *vanE*, *vanG*, *vanL*, *vanM*, and *vanN* are very unusual in VRE isolates, and *E. faecalis* (*vanE/G/L*) and *E. faecium* (*vanD/M/N*) are the most common carriers (22).

The *vanA* operon is associated with the transposon Tn*1546* and includes seven open reading frames transcribed under two different promoters (106). Regulation is mediated by a *vanS-vanR* (sensor-kinase-response regulator) two-component system, transcribed with a common promoter (107). The remaining genes are transcribed from a second promoter (22). The proteins encoded by *vanH* (dehydrogenase that converts pyruvate into lactate) and *vanA* (ligase that forms a D-Ala-D-Lac dipeptide) modify the synthesis of peptidoglycan precursors; moreover, the proteins encoded by both *vanX* (dipeptidase that cleaves D-Ala-D-Ala) and *vanY* (D,D-carboxipeptidase), interrupt the formation of the D-Ala-D-Ala end of the pentapeptide, and the *vanZ* gene is related to teicoplanin resistance (22, 108). Different insertion elements (ISs) can be included in the *vanA* operon, rendering different variants (109).

The *vanB* operon has been associated with different transposons (Tn*1547*, Tn*1549*, and Tn*5382*). Tn*1549* is widely prevalent among *vanB*-type enterococci, usually located in the chromosome and less frequently on plasmids (22). The structure of the *vanB* operon is similar to that of *vanA*, with two promoters and seven open reading frames, but with important differences, mostly in the two-component signaling regulatory system (encoded by *vanR~B~* and *vanS~B~*) and in the absence of a homolog of *vanZ* (substituted by *vanW*, of unknown function); consequently, *vanB* enterococci show vancomycin resistance (high or low level) but teicoplanin susceptibility (22, 108). The structure of the different *van* operons and their mechanisms of action have been extensively reviewed in previous studies (17–19, 21, 22, 108, 110).

Origin of vancomycin resistance
Partially preassembled glycopeptide resistance-associated gene clusters present in environmental organisms are suggested as the source of the vancomycin resistance genes in VRE (105, 111). The environmental organism *P. popilliae*, carrier of a *vanF* variant with high similarity at the amino acid level to *vanA*, has been suggested as the potential origin of vancomycin resistance in enterococci. To a lesser extent, this role could also be attributed to glycopeptide-producing organisms (e.g., the vancomycin-producing organism *Amycolatopsis orientalis*), which require these genes to inhibit the action of produced glycopeptides (111). Nevertheless, the genes in these organisms are probably not the direct source of the enterococcal vancomycin resistance genes since they are similar but not identical; in this sense, transference could have occurred from a common ancestral bacterium or via one or more bacterial intermediaries. In addition, considering the differences in G+C content, as well as the sequence homology among different organisms, it is possible that the genes of the *van* cluster could have more than one origin (111).

Historical aspects related to glycopeptide resistance
During the 1990s, VRE with the *vanA* genotype emerged in food-producing animals, healthy humans, food products, and environmental samples throughout Europe and other countries; this emergence was linked to the use of the glycopeptide avoparcin since the mid-1970s, in subtherapeutic concentrations, as an animal growth promoter (22, 26, 112, 113). This hypothesis was tested in poultry flocks and pig herds receiving or not receiving avoparcin, confirming the significant role of avoparcin in VRE selection in the animals (112, 113). This association was also corroborated in an animal model with young chickens receiving avoparcin supplementation (114). Avoparcin was banned as a growth promoter in the European Union in 1997, and a clear decrease in VRE fecal carriage in food-producing animals and healthy humans was observed (115), as well as in food-derived products. Nevertheless, VRE persisted in the animal setting many years after the

avoparcin ban (116, 117). A similar situation happened in Taiwan after the ban of avoparcin in 2000 that resulted in a clear decrease of VRE prevalence in chickens, although it still persisted in this animal population (118). In dogs, high rates of fecal VRE carriage were reported before the avoparcin ban in the European Union (119), although no VRE was detected in dogs in Spain a decade after the ban (120). The frequency of human infection by VRE in the European Union was low during the period of high prevalence in animals, but an increase in the frequency of VRE-related human infections was evidenced since 1999 (22).

The situation in the United States and Canada was completely different than that in the European Union. Avoparcin use has never been approved in animal production in those countries, and VRE was not reported in animals until the end of the 2000s (20, 76, 121, 122). Nevertheless, in North America, VRE was a frequent cause of human infections, especially in patients in intensive care units, which was attributed to the high use of vancomycin in humans (22, 123). The differences in VRE prevalence in humans and animals in the European Union and the United States before and after the avoparcin ban in the European Union introduce some doubts about the possible routes of transmission of VRE determinants between animals and humans (22, 124).

Different theories have been postulated to explain the persistence of VRE in food-producing animals after the avoparcin ban in the European Union and in other countries, such as coselection by the use of other antimicrobials (e.g., erythromycin and tetracycline). It has been shown that *vanA* and *erm*(B) genes (the latter implicated in erythromycin resistance) are frequently located in the same transferable plasmids (113). Moreover, the gene *tcrB*, implicated in copper resistance, has been detected in pig *E. faecium* isolates in the same plasmid as *vanA* and *erm*(B) (125). However, the presence of plasmid addition systems in the same plasmid that carries the *vanA* gene could force bacteria to retain the resistance (125).

VRE in food-producing animals and food of animal origin
Tables 1 and 2 summarize the papers that have been published related to the prevalence and mechanisms of vancomycin resistance in enterococci isolated from food-producing animals and food of animal origin, respectively, as well as the genetic lineages of the isolates (when available). The data are organized by animal species (poultry, pigs, and cattle, among others) and by the year the isolates were recovered. Many of the studies

were performed in European countries, but studies in the American, African and Asian countries, as well as Australia and New Zealand are also included.

Most of the surveys of food-producing animals reported *E. faecium* as the major species of the genus *Enterococcus* exhibiting acquired resistance to vancomycin, in most cases with the *vanA* genotype. However, *vanA*-containing *E. faecalis* isolates, and to a lesser extent *E. durans* and *E. hirae* isolates, have also been frequently detected in food-producing animals (Table 1) (27, 85, 87, 114, 121, 122, 125–165). Other enterococcal species have occasionally been reported as *vanA* carriers, such as *E. mundtii* in poultry in Hungary (130) and *E. casseliflavus* in cattle in France (158) and in horses and swine in Italy (159). Available data indicate that *vanA* was, by far, the main gene responsible for acquired VRE in food-producing animals worldwide, regardless of the species. Nevertheless, *vanB* (and especially the *vanB2* variant) was occasionally detected. The first detection of *vanB2* in animals was in a vancomycin-resistant *E. hirae* isolate recovered from a pig in Spain in 2008 (145); later, *vanB*-positive *E. faecium* and *E. faecalis* isolates were detected in poultry in Czech Republic (132) and in *Enterococcus* species in pigs in South Africa (147). Moreover, *vanC1* was detected as an acquired gene in isolates of *E. faecium*, *E. faecalis*, and *E. mundtii* in poultry in Australia (140). In most of the studies, VRE were detected when a selective protocol with media supplemented with vancomycin was used (Table 1). Resistance frequencies varied depending on the type of animals tested (poultry, 0 to 77%; pigs, 0 to 25.3%; cattle, 0 to 0.5%), the year the study was performed, the country, and the protocol used for VRE recovery (see Table 1). *vanA*-containing enterococci have also been detected in ostriches and mullet fish in Portugal (prevalence of resistance of 7.4% and 3.9%, respectively) (164). In eight of the reviewed papers in which VRE were detected in food-producing animals, the multilocus sequence typing (MLST) data were provided for *vanA*-positive *E. faecium* (most isolates) or *E. faecalis* isolates. A wide variety of sequence types were identified among the *E. faecium* isolates from poultry and pigs (>30 sequence types) (27, 85, 121, 122, 127, 129, 144, 156). Also, the lineage sequence type 6 (ST6) (CC2) was identified in *E. faecalis* of pig origin (85).

The *E. faecium* species carrier of the *vanA* gene was the most frequent VRE detected in food of animal origin. Nevertheless, *vanA*-containing *E. faecalis*, *E. durans*, and *E. hirae* isolates were also frequently detected in these types of samples (Table 2) (2, 118, 128, 133, 162, 166–194). VRE with the *vanB* gene was

found in *E. faecium* isolates from veal and chicken in Spain (ST17-*vanB2*) (188) and in different types of food in Greece (*vanB2/3*) and Spain (*vanB*) (181, 190). The identification of the unusual *vanN* gene in five *E. faecium* isolates from chicken meat in Japan is interesting, showing a low level of vancomycin resistance (MIC, 12 µg/ml) (177). Also notable is the unusual detection of *vanA*-containing *E. cecorum* isolates in chicken samples in Japan (168), *vanA*-positive *E. gallinarum* in fish in Egypt (193), and *vanC1*-positive *E. faecalis* isolates from sheep milk samples in Spain (192). The frequencies of detection of VRE with acquired resistance in food samples were variable (Table 1). In chicken and pork food samples analyzed from 1996 to 1999, the prevalence was in the range of 4.2 to 34% (Table 2), with a few exceptions (1.3%) (167). Very high frequencies were detected in different types of food in Korea (44%) (133), but no VRE were found in the studies performed in the United States (2, 171, 185). In some cases, isolates showing a phenotype usually associated with the *vanB* genotype (high-level resistance to vancomycin, susceptibility to teicoplanin) were detected in *Enterococcus* strains harboring the *vanA* gene (118, 168, 173).

VRE in companion animals
Table 3 shows the detection of VRE with acquired mechanisms of resistance in companion animals. *vanA*-containing *E. faecium* is a unique type of VRE with acquired resistance reported in dogs and cats (136, 145, 195–202). These isolates, recovered from fecal samples from 1996 to 2003, were found in the United States, Spain, and Portugal, with variable frequencies of detection (ranging from 2.8 to 22.7%) (136, 145, 195, 196). No VRE were detected in studies performed in the following years (Table 3), not even in sick dogs (197, 200). Vancomycin-resistant *E. faecium* and *E. durans* isolates were detected in fecal samples of equids obtained in 2007 to 2008 (prevalence 4.4%) in a study performed in Portugal (202).

VRE in free-living animals
Table 3 also shows the detection of VRE with acquired mechanisms of resistance in free-living animals, including different species of mammals and birds (136, 165, 203–226). Many studies have been performed with this type of animal, including in various countries in Europe, the Americas (United States, Canada, and Brazil), and Africa (Tunisia and Tanzania). The most frequently detected mechanism of resistance was *vanA*, mainly among *E. faecium* isolates, followed by *E. faecalis* (*E. durans* and *E. hirae* were infrequently detected).

Table 1 Summary of reports about detection of VRE with acquired mechanisms of resistance in healthy food-producing animals

Animal species	Year of recovery of tested isolates	Country	% Prevalence[a]	Species ST (CC)[b] (genotype)	Vancomycin selection method	Reference
Poultry	1996	Spain	11/15	*E. hirae/E. faecium* (*vanA*)	+	114
Poultry	1997	Netherlands	29 (poultry and farmers)	*E. faecium/E. durans/E. hirae* (*vanA*) *E. faecalis* (*vanA*)	+	126
Poultry	1997	Norway	0.8–4.6	*E. faecium* ST26/ST146/ST195/ST242/ ST248/ST9/ST241/ST244/ ST245 (*vanA*)	+	127
Poultry	1997–1998	Spain	16	*E. durans* (*vanA*)	+	128
Poultry	1998–1999	Norway	34	*E. faecium* (*vanA*)	+	125
Poultry	2000–2007	Sweden	<1 (2000), 40 (2005), 30 (2006–2007)	*E. faecium* ST13/ST370/ST310 (*vanA*)	+	129
Poultry	2001–2004	Hungary	8.6 (2001), 23 (2002), 0 (2003–2007)	*E. faecium/E. durans/ E. mundtii* (*vanA*)	+	130
Poultry	2002–2003	New Zealand	5.8	*E. faecium/E. faecalis/E. durans* (*vanA*)	+	131
Poultry	2002–2004	Czech Republic	2.1	*E. faecium* (*vanA*), *E. faecium/ E. faecalis* (*vanB*)	–	132
Poultry	2003	Korea	1.4	*E. faecium* (*vanA*)	+	133
Poultry	2003–2004	Canada	0		–	134
Poultry	2003–2004	Canada	0		–	135
Poultry	2004	Portugal	9.2	*E. faecium/E. durans/E. hirae* (*vanA*)	+	136
Poultry	2005	Hungary	1.1	*E. faecium/E. faecalis* (*vanA*)	+	137
Poultry	2005–2008	Greece	14.4	*E. faecium* (*vanA*)	+	138
Poultry	2009	Germany	17.6	*Enterococcus* spp. (*vanA*)	+	139
Poultry	2000	Australia	8.6	*E. faecium/E. mundtii/ E. faecalis* (*vanC1*)	+	140
	2008–2009		0	-	+	
Poultry	2010	Denmark	47	*E. faecium* ST10/ST12/ST22/ST26/ ST38/ST157/ST417/ST520/ST587/ ST784/ST785/ST839/ST840/ST841/ ST842 (*vanA*)	+	27
Poultry	2010–2011	Germany	0		–	141
Poultry	2013–2014	Poland	0.11	NS[c]	–	142
Poultry	NS	Italy	8.7	NS	–	143
Poultry	NS	Sweden	55–70 (few samples)	*E. faecium*- ST310- (*vanA*)	+	144
Pigs	1998	Spain	6.1	*E. faecium* (*vanA*), *E. hirae* (*vanB2*)	+	145
Pigs	1998–1999	Spain	8.0	*E. faecium* (NS), *E. hirae* (NS), *E. durans* (NS)	+	146
Pigs and farm facilities	2006–2007	Portugal	5	*E. faecium* ST132/ST185 (CC5) (*vanA*), *E. faecium* ST443 (*vanA*), *E. faecalis* ST6 (CC2) (*vanA*)	+	85
Pigs	2009	USA	10.9	*E. faecium* ST5/ST6/ST185 (CC5) (*vanA*)	+	121
Pigs	2009–2010	USA	8.2	*E. faecium* ST5/ST6/ST185 (CC5) (*vanA*)	+	122
Pigs	2014	South Africa	NS	*Enterococcus* spp. (*vanB*)	–	147
Pigs	NS	Australia	0		NS	148
Poultry and pigs	1998–1999	Costa Rica	14.8 (poultry), 10.9 (pigs)	*E. faecium/E. faecalis/E. durans/ E. hirae* (*vanA*)	+	149

(Continued)

Table 1 *(Continued)*

Animal species	Year of recovery of tested isolates	Country	% Prevalence[a]	Species ST (CC)[b] (genotype)	Vancomycin selection method	Reference
Poultry and pigs	1998–2000	European countries	8.2	*E. faecium/E. faecalis/E. hirae* (*vanA*)	+	150
Poultry and pigs	2002	UK and Wales	24 (poultry), 5 (pigs)	*E. faecium* (*vanA*)	+	151
Poultry and pigs	2005	France	1.6 (poultry), 6.2 (pigs)	*E. faecium/E. faecalis/Enterococcus* spp. (*vanA*)	+	152
Poultry and pigs	2009	China	0		–	153
Poultry and cattle	2014	Nigeria	0		–	154
Poultry and cattle	NS	Ethiopia	30–54	NS	–	155
Poultry, pigs, cattle	2008–2013	China	0.2 (pigs), 0 (poultry), 0 (cattle)	*E. faecium* ST6 (CC5) (*vanA*)	+	156
Poultry, pigs, cattle	NS[a]	Austria	47.8 (poultry), 0.5 (cattle), 0 (pigs)	*E. faecium/E. durans* (*vanA*)	+	157
Cattle	2003–2004 (healthy cattle)–2006 (sick cattle)	France	0.1 (healthy cattle), 0.4 (sick cattle)	*E. faecium/E. faecalis/E. casseliflavus* (*vanA*)	+	158
Cattle	NS[a]	Australia	0		–	87
Equines and swine	2005	Italy	6.7 (equine), 16.1 (swine)	*E. faecium/E. faecalis/E. casseliflavus* (*vanA*)	+	159
Sheep, pigs, cattle	2008–2009	Portugal	25.3 (pigs), 2.7 (sheep), 0 (cattle)	*E. faecium/E. hirae* (*vanA*)	+	160
Farm animals	1998–2003	USA	0		+	161
Farm animals	2000–2001	Korea	0.67	*E. faecium* (*vanA*)	+	162
Farm animals	2001	Korea	16.7 (chicken), 1.9 (pigs), 0 (cattle)	*E. faecium* (*vanA*)	+	163
Ostriches	2009–2010	Portugal	7.4	*E. durans* (*vanA*)	+	164
Mullet fish	2006–2007	Portugal	3.9	*E. faecium* (*vanA*)	+	165

[a]Some characteristics (year of isolation, or type of samples) are included in parenthesis.
[b]ST (CC), sequence type (clonal complex), if data are available.
[c]NS, not specified.

Occasionally, enterococci were found to be *vanB* carriers: two small mammals (*Rattus rattus*) harbored *vanB2*-containing *E. faecalis* ST6 isolates in Spain (204), and *E. faecium vanB* was detected in wild game meat, also in Spain (226). The frequencies of detection of *vanA*-containing enterococci in wild animals ranged from 0 to 13.5%, with the highest values detected in red foxes, seagulls, and buzzards in Portugal (9 to 13.5%) (216, 220, 222). Interestingly, *vanA*-containing *E. faecium* isolates detected were ascribed to different sequence types included in the high-risk clonal complex CC17 (ST18, ST262, ST273, ST280, ST313, ST362, ST412, ST448, and ST555). These isolates were

detected in corvids in the United States and in mullet fish, gilt-head seabream, seagulls, buzzards, partridges, red foxes, and Iberian wolves in Portugal (Table 3).

Resistance to Linezolid

The widespread occurrence of VRE in many countries makes it necessary to look for other therapeutic options, and linezolid is an important one. This oxazolidinone, introduced in 2000 in the United States and in 2001 in the United Kingdom, is an important agent for the treatment not only of VRE, but also of other Gram-positive bacteria, such as methicillin-resistant *S. aureus*.

Table 2 Summary of reports about detection of VRE with acquired mechanisms of resistance in food samples of animal origin

Origin of the food sample	Year of recovery of tested isolates	Country	% Prevalence[a]	Species-ST (CC)[b] (genotype)	Vancomycin selection method	Reference
Chicken	1995–1996	Japan	3.0	*E. faecium/E. faecalis* (*vanA*)	–	166
Chicken	1997–1998	Spain	27.2	*E. faecium/E. faecalis/E. durans/ E. hirae* (*vanA*)	+	128
Chicken	1997–1998	Belgium	1.3	*E. faecium* (NS[c])	–	167
Chicken	2000–2001	Korea	60 (15 samples)	*E. faecium* (*vanA*)	+	162
Chicken	2000–2003	Taiwan	13.7 (2000), 3.7 (2003) (*E. faecalis*), 3.4 (2000)– 0 (2003) (*E. faecium*)	*E. faecium/E. faecalis* (*vanA*)	+	118
Chicken	2009	Japan	4.5 (22 samples)	*E. cecorum* (*vanA*)	+	168
Chicken	2009	Colombia	3.7	NS[c]	–	169
Chicken	2009–2010	Turkey	0	–	–	170
Chicken	NS	USA	0	–	–	171
Chicken	NS	UK	18.5	NS	+	172
Food and poultry	1999–2001	Portugal	34.0	*E. faecium/E. faecalis/ Enterococcus* spp. (*vanA*)	+	173
Chicken and pork	1996–1997	Germany	12.3	*E. faecium/E. durans/E. faecalis/ E. hirae* (*vanA*)	+	174
Chicken and pork	1997–1998	Italy	15.9 (1997), 8.1 (1998) (poultry product) 4.2 (1997), 6.9 (1998) (pork products)	*E. faecium/E. faecalis/E. durans/ E. hirae* (*vanA*)	+	175
Chicken and pork	1999	France	10.2	*E. faecium/E. durans* (*vanA*)	+	176
Chicken and pork	2011	Japan	0.6 (chicken meat)	*E. faecium* (*vanN*)	+	177
Various types of food	2000–2002	Germany	0		–	178
Various types of food	2010	Argentina	7.5	*E. faecium* (*vanA*)	–	179
Various types of food	2010	Iran	NS	*E. faecium* ST669 (*vanA*)	+	180
Various types of food	2010–2012	Greece	21.9	*E. faecium* (*vanA*), *E. faecium* (*vanA* + *van*B2/3), *E. faecium* (*van*B2/3)	+	181
Various types of food	2012	Italy	3.53	NS	–	182
Various types of food	NS	Spain	5.4	NS	–	183
Various meats	1997–1998	Italy	14.6 (1997), 8.0 (1998)	*E. faecium/E. faecalis/E. durans/ E. hirae* (*vanA*)	+	184
Various meats	2001–2002	USA	0		–	185
Various meats	2003	Korea	44	*E. faecium* (*vanA*)	+	133
Various meats and feces	2004–2006	Japan	0		+	186
Various meats	2007–2008	Canada	0		–	187
Various meats	2007–2009	Spain	3.9	*E. faecium* ST78 (CC17)/ST425 (*vanA*), *E. durans/E. hirae* (*vanA*), *E. faecium* ST17 (CC17) (*van*B2)	+	188
Various meats	NS	Canada	0		–	189
Various meats	NS	Spain	19.4	*E. faecium/E. durans/E. hirae* (*vanA*), *E. faecium* (*vanB*)	+	190
Retail meats	2002–2014	USA	0		–	2
Cheese	2005	France	0		+	191
Milk (sheep)	NS	Spain	1.7	*E. faecalis* ST168 (*vanC1*)	–	192
Shellfish	NS	UK	2.7	NS	–	172
Fish (Tilapia)	NS	Egypt	37.5 (8 samples)	*E. faecalis/E. gallinarum* (*vanA*)	–	193
Frozen food	NS	Thailand	9.7	NS	–	194

[a]Some characteristics (year of isolation or type of samples) are included in parenthesis.
[b]ST (CC), Sequence type (clonal complex), if data are available.
[c]NS, not specified.

Linezolid resistance is still unusual among enterococci but has emerged in recent years in human and animal isolates (227). Mutations in the central loop of domain V of the 23S rDNA is the most common mechanism of resistance in enterococci, the amino acid change G2576T being the predominant one, although other changes have also been described (G2505A, U2500A, G2447U, C2534U, and G2603U) (18). *E. faecalis* and *E. faecium* possess four and six 23S rDNA alleles per genome, respectively, and depending on the number of mutated versus wild-type alleles per genome, these correlate with the level of resistance of the isolates (227). In some cases, this mechanism appears during the course of treatment with oxazolidinones, and nosocomial transmission of linezolid-resistant enterococci has been reported (228). Linezolid-resistant *E. faecalis* and *E. gallinarum* isolates of swine origin were detected in China (MIC, 8 to 16 μg/ml), and the nucleic acid change G2576T was identified in the 23S rDNA of these isolates (229). Mutations in the ribosomal proteins L3, L4, and L22 can confer decreased susceptibility to linezolid in enterococci and staphylococci (230).

In recent years, there has been concern about the emergence of transferable resistance to linezolid, associated with the acquisition of the *cfr* gene or with the recently described *optr*A gene. The *cfr* gene has been detected in enterococci of both human and animal origin (231) and encodes an rRNA methyltransferase that modifies the adenine residue at position 2503 in domain V of the 23S rRNA; it confers resistance to oxazolidinones, phenicols, lincosamides, pleuromutilins, and streptogramin A (the phenotype named PhLOPS$_A$) (18). Among oxazolidinones, linezolid is mostly affected by *cfr*; tedizolid, a new compound of this family, showed increased activity in *cfr*-positive enterococci, so these isolates are susceptible to this agent. Table 4 summarizes the data published until now in relation to linezolid resistance mechanisms in enterococci of animal and food origin, as well as in enterococci of environmental origin (229, 232–241).

The *cfr* gene was identified for the first time in enterococci in 2011, specifically in an *E. faecalis* isolate recovered on a dairy farm in China (232). Since then, *cfr* has been detected in human clinical *E. faecalis* isolates (242), as well as in swine *E. casseliflavus*, *E. gallinarum*, and *E. faecalis* isolates in China and Brazil (233–235) and in a cattle *E. faecalis* isolate in China (234). A second variant of the *cfr* gene, named *cfr*(B), has been described in *E. faecium* isolates of human origin. This new plasmid-located variant is more similar to a *cfr*-like gene of *Clostridium difficile* than to the *cfr*

genes of staphylococci or other enterococcal species (243, 244), and it has so far not been detected in enterococci of animal origin.

The novel *optr*A gene confers transferable resistance to oxazolidinones (both linezolid and telizolid) and phenicoles (chloramphenicol and florfenicol) and has been detected in *E. faecalis* and *E. faecium* isolates of both human and animal origin (236). This gene encodes an ABC transporter and has been detected more frequently in *E. faecalis* than in *E. faecium* isolates and more frequently in isolates from food-producing animals (pigs and chickens) than in those of human origin (236). The *optr*A gene has been detected both in chromosomal and in plasmidic locations in animal and human *E. faecalis* and *E. faecium* isolates. As shown in Table 4, *optr*A-positive enterococci have been detected in food-producing animals (poultry, pigs, and occasionally, cattle) in Asiatic countries, mostly in *E. faecalis* and *E. faecium* belonging to many different sequence types, and sporadically in *E. gallinarum*. The prevalence of *optr*A-positive enterococci represents 10% and 5.7% of total *E. faecalis* and *E. faecium* isolates, respectively, obtained from fecal samples of poultry and pigs in a study performed in China (236). In a recent study carried out in Korea, 11,659 *E. faecalis* and *E. faecium* isolates obtained from fecal and carcass samples of healthy cattle, pigs, and chickens from farms and slaughter houses from 2003 to 2014 were tested for linezolid resistance, detecting a rate of resistance of 0.33%, mainly attributed to *optr*A carriage (238). The *optr*A gene has also been detected in sporadic isolates of *E. faecalis* and *E. faecium* (*n* = 3) obtained in meat samples in Denmark (imported poultry and veal), which represented <0.1% of total enterococci recovered from these samples (239). In Colombia, *optr*A has been detected in three *E. faecalis* isolates from poultry meat, coharboring the *fexA*, *tet*(L), and *lsa*(A) resistance genes (240). Both *cfr* and *optr*A have been detected in VRE isolates of human origin (245), but not in animal isolates so far.

The *optr*A gene has also been detected in two *E. faecalis* isolates of the lineage ST86 recovered from urban wastewater in Tunisia, accounting for 1% of all chloramphenicol-resistant enterococci tested (241); *optr*A was located within a transferable mosaic plasmid, which also contained the *fexA* and *erm*(A) genes.

At least 12 and 5 polymorphic variants of the *optr*A gene have been detected among human and animal enterococci, respectively (237, 246–248). The wild OptrA type (OptrA$_{E349}$) and the variants Tyr176Asp + Lys3Glu-Gly393Asp or Thr481Pro or Thr112Lys or Gly393Asp have been found in animal isolates (237,

Table 3 Summary of reports about detection of VRE with acquired mechanisms of resistance in companion and free-living animals

Animal species	Isolation year	Country	% Prevalence[a]	Species-ST (CC)[b] (genotype)	Vancomycin selection method	Reference
Companion animals						
Dogs (sick)	1996–1998	USA	2.8	*E. faecium* (*vanA*)	–	195
Dogs/cats	1998	Spain	22.7 (22 samples)	*E. faecium* (*vanA*)	+	145
Dogs	1998–2003	Spain	12.6	*E. faecium* (*vanA*)	+	196
Dogs/cats	2003	Portugal	2.6 (dogs) 0 (cats)	*E. faecium* (*vanA*)	+	136
Dogs (sick)	2008–2009	USA	0		–	197
Dogs	2009	Spain	0		+	120
Dogs/cats (antibiotic-treated)	2011–2012	Japan	0		–	198
Dogs/cats	2014	Egypt	0		–	199
Dogs (sick)	NS[c]	Portugal	0		–	200
Dogs/cats	NS	Turkey	3.8 (dogs) 0 (cats)	NS[c]	–	201
Equids	2007–2008	Portugal	4.4	*E. faecium*/*E. durans* (*vanA*)	+	202
Free-living animals						
Wild mammals	1997–2000	England	1.2 (badgers) 4.6 (woodmice)	*E. faecium* (*vanA*)	–	203
Wild animals	2004	Portugal	0		+	136
Wild animals	2008–2013	Spain	2.0	*E. faecium*-ST915 (*vanA*), *E. faecalis* ST6 (CC2) (*vanB2*)	+	204
Wild animals	2012	Poland	14.9	NS	–	205
Wild animals	2014–2015	Spain	0.3	*E. faecium* ST993 (*vanA*)	+	206
Wild birds	2006–2010	Portugal	2.7	*E. faecium*/*E. durans* (*vanA*)	+	207
Wild birds	2009–2010	Portugal	1.3	*E. faecium*/*E. durans*/*E. hirae* (*vanA*)	+	208
Wild birds	2010	Portugal	0.7	*E. faecalis* (*vanA*)		209
Wild birds	2012	Tunisia	3.6	*E. faecium* (*vanA*)	+	210
Corvids (American crows)	2012	USA	2.5	*E. faecium* ST18 (CC17)/ST555 (CC17)/ST749/ST750/ST751/ST752–(*vanA*), *E. faecalis* ST179 (CC16)/ST16 (CC16)/ST6 (CC2) (*vanA*)	+	211
Corvids (American crows)	2012–2015	USA	2.7	*E. faecium*-ST362/ST412 (CC17)-(*vanA*)	+	212
Corvids	2012–2013	Canada	0.7	*E. faecium* ST448 (*vanA*)	+	213
Corvids	2013	Slovakia	1.3	*E. faecium* ST917/ST6 (CC5) (*vanA*)	+	214
Wild boars	2005–2006	Portugal	3	*E. faecium* (*vanA*)	+	215
Mullets fish	2006–2007	Portugal	3.8	*E. faecium* ST273 (CC17)/ST280 (CC17) (*vanA*)	+	165
Seagulls	2007	Portugal	10.5	*E. faecium*-ST5 (CC17)-(*vanA*), *E. durans*-(*vanA*)	+	216
Gilt-head seabream	2007	Portugal	5.9	*E. faecium* ST273 (CC17)/ST313 (CC17)/ST76 (*vanA*), *E. faecalis* ST6 (CC2) (*vanA*), *E. durans* (*vanA*)	+	217
Wild rabbits	2007–2008	Portugal	3.9	*E. faecium*-(*vanA*)	+	218
Pigeons	2007–2008	Brazil	0		–	219
Buzzards	2007–2009	Portugal	9	*E. faecium* ST273 (CC17)/ST5 (*vanA*), *E. durans* (*vanA*)	+	220
Partridges	2015–2016	Portugal	2	*E. faecium*-ST18(CC17)/ST448(CC17)/ST139(CC5)-(*vanA*)	+	221

(Continued)

Table 3 *(Continued)*

Animal species	Isolation year	Country	% Prevalence[a]	Species-ST (CC)[b] (genotype)	Vancomycin selection method	Reference
Red foxes	2008–2009	Portugal	13.5	*E. faecium* ST262 (CC17)/ST273 (CC17) (*vanA*), *E. durans* (*vanA*)	+	222
Iberian wolf, Iberian lynx	2008–2010	Portugal	0.5 (Iberian wolf) 0 (Iberian lynx)	*E. faecium* ST18 (CC17)/ST573 (*vanA*)	+	223
Buffalo, wildebeest, zebra	2010–2011	Tanzania	2.8 (buffalo) 20 (zebra) 2.5 (wildebeest)	NS	+	224
Camels	NS	Spain	0		–	225
Wild game meat	NS	Spain	30.9	*E. faecium/E. faecalis/E. durans* (*vanA*), *E. faecium* (*vanB*)	–	226

[a]Some characteristics (year of isolation, type of samples) are included in parenthesis.
[b]ST (CC), sequence type (clonal complex), if data are available.
[c]NS, not specified.

246). Functional *cfr* and *optrA* genes have been identified in both enterococci and *S. aureus*. In most of the animal isolates, *optrA* is located close to other genes, as is the case of *fexA* (implicated in phenicol resistance) and a novel *erm*(A)-like gene. This *erm*(A)-like gene encodes an rRNA methylase, which shows 85.2% amino acid identity to the Erm(A) protein of transposon Tn554 of *S. aureus* (237).

Most of the *cfr*-positive enterococci of food-producing animals (>90%) showed a MIC for linezolid of ≥8 μg/ml, but two *E. faecalis* isolates presented a MIC of 4 μg/ml. *optrA*-positive isolates of food-producing animal and food origin showed a linezolid MIC in the range of 2 to >8 μg/ml, presenting 19% of the isolates' MICs in the range of 2 to 4 μg/ml (categorized as susceptible according to EUCAST breakpoints and susceptible-intermediate according to CLSI) (Table 4). It is interesting to note that *cfr*- and *optrA*-positive enterococci could appear as linezolid-susceptible, probably leading to an underestimation of their actual incidence.

Oxazolidinones are not used in food-producing animals. Nevertheless, the emergent detection in these animals of linezolid-resistant enterococci carrying the *optrA* gene in transferable plasmids, linked to resistance genes for antibiotics commonly used in animals (phenicols, tetracyclines, lincosamides, and aminoglycosides), suggests its role in the coselection of multi-resistant bacteria, which poses a risk for public health.

To summarize, transferable linezolid resistance genes, mostly *optrA*, have been detected in enterococci of food-producing animals and food of animal origin in various European, South American, and Asian countries, but so far not in Africa. These mechanisms of resistance have not been detected so far, to our knowledge, in pets or in wild animals.

Resistance to Aminoglycosides

Enterococci are intrinsically resistant to clinically achievable concentrations of aminoglycosides due to their low cell wall permeability. In addition, some species, such as *E. faecium* [*aac(6′)-Ii*], *E. durans* [*aac(6′)-Id*], and *E. hirae* [*aac(6′)-Ih*], intrinsically express a chromosomal-encoded acetyltransferase that confers resistance to tobramycin, kanamycin, and amikacin (249). The chromosomally encoded methyltransferase EfmM has been exceptionally described in an *E. faecium* isolate (250) codifying resistance to kanamycin and tobramycin. Acquired resistances to aminoglycosides are detected in strains from both animals and humans and usually confer a high level of resistance to gentamicin, kanamycin, and streptomycin.

High-level resistance to gentamicin in enterococcal isolates of animal origin was first described in 1998 in Denmark (251) and in 2001 in the United States (252). The acquired genetic mechanisms identified in animal isolates are identical to those described in human isolates. The most frequent ones are the bifunctional enzyme encoded by *aac(6′)-Ie-aph(2″)-Ia* (conferring resistance to gentamicin, kanamycin, amikacin, netilmicin, and tobramycin) and *aph(3)-IIIa* (conferring resistance to kanamycin and amikacin) (23, 253). High-level gentamicin resistance can also be due to the expression of the unusual *aph(2″)-Ic*, *aph(2″)-Id*, *aph (2″)-Ie*, and *aph(2″)-Ib* genes (17, 23); *aph(2‴)-Ic* seems to be more frequent in enterococci of animal origin, and some farm animals could be a reservoir of this gene (252). High-level resistance to streptomycin is

Table 4 Mechanisms implicated in linezolid resistance in enterococci of animals, food of animal origin, and the environment

Origin	Species	Sample	Year of isolation	Country	Number of linezolid resistant isolates (%)	Linezolid MIC (μg/ml)	Mechanism of linezolid resistance (genetic location, number of isolates)[a]	ST (number of isolates)[b]	Characteristics (number of isolates)	Reference
Food-producing animals										
Cattle	E. faecalis	Feces	2009	China	1	4	cfr (P)		fexB-linked	232
Pigs	E. faecalis	Feces	2009	China	1 (0.3% of E. faecalis)	4	cfr (P)	ST21	fexA (in a different plasmid)	233
Pigs	E. faecalis	Rectal swabs	2013	Brazil	5 (2% of E. faecalis)	8->8	cfr (5)	ST591 (2); ST29, ST590, ST592 (1 each)		234
Pigs	E. gallinarum (n = 1), E. casseliflavus (n = 24)	Rectal swabs	2012	China	25 (31.5% of florfenicol-resistant enterococci)	8–16	Mutation in ribosomal L3 protein (V149I) (1) cfr (25) (C,1; P, 8)		fexA-linked (5), fexA-fexB-linked (1)	235
Poultry and pigs	E. faecalis	Feces	2012–2013	China	20 (10% of E. faecalis of animal origin)	2[c]–8	optrA (C, 8; P, 9; P/C, 3)	ST21 (2); ST27, ST59, ST74, ST93, ST116, ST256, ST330, ST403, ST475, ST476, ST480, ST593, ST618, ST619, ST620, ST621, ST622, ST623 (1 each)	fexA-linked (14), fexB-linked (2), fexA-fexB-linked (1) optrA amino acid changes: Y176D, T481P (2); K3E, Y176D, G393D (1); T112K, Y176D (2); Y176D, G393D (1)	236, 237
Poultry and pigs	E. faecium	Feces	2005, 2009, 2012, 2014	China	5 (5.7% of E. faecium of animal origin)	4[d]–8	optrA (C, 1; P/C, 4)	ST957 (2); ST32, ST184, ST29 (1 each)	fexB-linked (4)	236, 237

	Species	Sample	Year	Country	No. (%)	MIC	Mechanism	ST	*fexA*/other	Reference
Poultry and pigs	*E. faecalis*	Feces and carcass	2008, 2012, 2014	Korea	12 (0.2% of *E. faecalis*)	8→16	*optrA* (12)	ST21 (4); ST49 (2); ST16, ST32, ST256, ST403, ST728, ST729 (1 each)	*fexA*-linked (11)	238
Poultry and cattle	*E. faecium*	Feces and carcass	2008, 2010, 2012–2014	Korea	27 (0.7% of *E. faecium*)	8→16	*optrA* (23) Mutation in ribosomal L4 protein (N130K) (7)	ST195 (6); ST32 (2); ST157 (2); ST1171 (2); ST1168 (2); ND (4); ST8, ST120, ST121, ST236, ST241, ST1166, ST1167, ST1169, ST1170 (1 each)	*fexA*-linked (19)	238
Pigs	*E. faecalis* (n = 5), *E. gallinarum* (n = 1)			China	6 (17.14% of enterococci)	8–16	23S rRNA mutation: G2576T	ST29, ST146, ST220, ST283, ST535		229
Meat										
Cattle	*E. faecalis*	Danish veal	2015	Denmark	1 (<0.1% of *E. faecalis*)	8	*optrA* (P)	ST22	*fexA*-linked	239
Poultry	*E. faecium*	Imported turkey and broiler meat	2012, 2013	Denmark	2 (<0.1% of *E. faecium*)	8	*optrA* (P, 1)	ST22, ST873	*fexA*-linked	239
Poultry	*E. faecalis*	Meat	2010–2011	Colombia	3 (0.5% of enterococci)	8	*optrA* (P, 3)	ST59 (2), ST489	*fexA*-linked	240
Environment										
Wastewater	*E. faecalis*	Urban wastewater treatment plant	2014	Tunisia	2 (1% of chloramphenicol-resistant enterococci)	4	*optrA* (P)	ST86 (2)	*fexA*-linked (2), *optrA* amino acid changes: M1L (2), K3E (1) and I622M (1)	241

[a]P, plasmid; C, chromosome.
[b]ND, not determined.
[c]Five *optrA*-positive *E. faecalis* isolates showed a linezolid MIC of 2 µg/ml, and five isolates showed an MIC of 4 µg/ml.
[d]Two *optrA*-positive *E. faecium* isolates showed a linezolid MIC of 4 mcg/ml.

commonly caused by punctual ribosomal mutations, although acquisition of some modifying enzymes has been also described [*ant(3″)-Ia* and *ant(6′)-Ia*]. Table 5 summarizes papers (from 2013 to 2017) that analyzed the rates of antimicrobial resistance (high level to gentamicin and others such as tetracycline, erythromycin, and ciprofloxacin) in enterococcal isolates from animals (65, 15, 87, 90, 92, 135, 141, 143, 147, 153, 154, 198, 205, 209, 254–276).

Resistance to Tetracycline

This family of antimicrobials integrates several antibacterial active compounds (277), although tetracycline, chlortetracycline, oxytetracycline, and doxycycline are the most used in veterinary. Despite Roberts' extensive 1996 review about tetracycline resistance mechanisms (278), a more recent update was published in 2005 (279). Almost 60 tetracycline resistance genes have been described, although the most frequent ones in *Enterococcus* are those implicated in ribosomal protection [*tet*(M), *tet*(O), *tet*(S)], efflux, or enzymatic inactivation [*tet*(K), *tet*(L)]. In *Enterococcus*, as occurs in other Gram-positive microorganisms, the ribosomal protection protein mechanism encoded by the *tet*(M) gene is the most frequent, independent of the origin of the strains. The transferability of the tetracycline resistance determinants in the absence of plasmids has been described (280); the Tn*916*/Tn*1545* conjugative transposon family carrying the *tet*(M) gene is responsible, usually in combination with *erm*(B).

Resistance to Macrolides/ Lincosamines/Streptogramins

Numerous chemically diverse compounds are integrated into the macrolide family, with erythromycin being the most representative. Resistance to this antibiotic was immediately reported after its introduction in human clinical use in 1952; moreover, enterococci are intrinsically resistant to clindamycin and lincomycin. Tylosin, spiramycin, and virginiamycin were widely used in pigs and other animals before the European Union limited their use. After the ban, erythromycin resistance in *Enterococcus* strains from animals decreased spectacularly (281), demonstrating the link between consumption of the antibiotic and the increase in resistance rates, even in different environments.

Chromosomal intrinsic resistance to macrolides by *msr*(A) and to lincosamides by *linB* in *E. faecium* has been described (282, 283). Acquired resistance to macrolides can be codified by various genetic determinants (up to 92 have been described) (284), although the most common worldwide is *erm*(B), usually carried by

Tn*917*, which is widespread in human and animal isolates. Other relevant genes in the genus *Enterococcus* are the efflux genes *mef*(A), conferring resistance to macrolides, *vgb*(A), conferring resistance to virginiamycin, *lnu*(B), conferring resistance to lincosamide, and *vat*(D) and *vat*(E), conferring resistance to streptogramins.

Resistance to Quinolones

Fluoroquinolones have reduced antimicrobial activity against enterococci, with levofloxacin and moxifloxacin being the most active compounds. Acquired resistance is the consequence of mutations in the *gyrA* and *parC* genes (285, 286, 287) or the acquisition of the *qnr* genes (287). Efflux pumps such as EmeA for *E. faecalis* (288) and NorA-like for *E. faecium* (289) have also been described, although their frequency is low. Resistance to ciprofloxacin is a conserved feature among the high-risk *E. faecium* CC17 clone linked to nosocomial outbreaks (290) and among almost all isolates with resistance to glycopeptides. Fluoroquinolones have never been used as growth promoters, although their use for veterinary therapy is common.

MOLECULAR EPIDEMIOLOGY AND POPULATION STRUCTURE OF ENTEROCOCCI IN FARM AND COMPANION ANIMALS

Epidemiological studies of farm and companion animals were originally driven by the interest in establishing a relationship between antibiotic-resistant isolates from human and nonhuman hosts. At present, the resistance phenotypes of clinical relevance that may be linked to animals mainly comprise resistance to ampicillin, gentamicin, quinupristin-dalfopristin, vancomycin, and linezolid.

Molecular typing of enterococci strains has been performed by different methods, including pulsed field gel electrophoresis (PFGE), amplified fragment length polymorphism (AFLP), MLST, cgMLST, Bayesian analysis of population structure (BAPS) and whole-genome sequencing (WGS) (revised in 291).

The emergence of VRE in European food-producing animals and food of animal origin in the early 1990s (128, 291, 292–296), as well as in the feces of healthy volunteers and food handlers (297–299), led to surveillance studies in the community setting that suggested a relationship between the extensive use of animal growth promoters in veterinary medicine (e.g., avoparcin and tylosin), the colonization pressure in animals, and the subsequent transmission to human hosts throughout the food chain (300, 301).

The first report of VRE in nonhuman hosts occurred in 1993 in the United Kingdom and documented the similarity between isolates of different origins (300). This study was followed by others, which confirmed the similarity of VRE strains from humans and farm animals exposed to avoparcin in different European countries (26, 292, 302–305). The potential selection of antibiotic-resistant enterococci by antibiotics led to the ban of avoparcin as an animal growth promoter in Sweden in 1986, Denmark and Switzerland in 1995, and in the rest of the European countries 2 years later (Commission Directive 97/6/EC). By 1999, other antibiotics (such as bacitracin, virginiamycin, and tylosin) were also banned as growth promoters for healthy animals in Europe, and this was followed in 2006 by a ban on all antibiotics as growth promoters. In this way, Europe led the first intervention against VRE at a global level. In contrast to western countries, the use of antimicrobials in livestock and poultry, as well as the standard policies on antimicrobial use, varies significantly among Asian countries (reviewed in 306). In Korea, avoparcin was used in the management of poultry and swine from 1983 to 1997 but was banned thereafter to reduce exposure of humans to VRE (133). After several years of avoparcin discontinuance in Korea, the prevalence of VRE in Korean livestock was investigated, and some studies reported that the VRE incidence rate in chicken samples was higher than that in pig samples (163, 307).

The ban led to a significant reduction of VRE colonization in animals, foods, and fecal samples of community-based people in different countries. However, VRE was recovered in feces of animals and humans years later, reflecting the important effects of previous livestock practices in the population structure of enterococci in animals.

Most information came from the species *E. faecium* and *E. faecalis*, the predominant species in the gastrointestinal tract of mammals, along with *E. hirae*, *E. durans*, and *E. cecorum* (11, 45, 46).

E. faecium
PFGE remained the "gold standard" for molecular typing of *E. faecium* until the recent introduction of WGS-based epidemiology (291, 308). By using PFGE, clonal dissemination of *E. faecium* strains with clinically relevant phenotypes (ampicillin, gentamicin, quinupristin-dalfopristin, and vancomycin) has been extensively documented between animals from the same or different farms and has also been suggested between animals and humans (309, 310). The data vary greatly among geographic areas and are normally associated with the use of antibiotics.

Ecological differentiation of *E. faecium* has been documented in epidemiological studies using AFLP, MLST, and/or BAPS (311–314). AFLP analysis originally revealed different subpopulations (or ecotypes) corresponding to hospitalized patients, community-based people, and farm animals, including veal calves, poultry, and swine (311, 315). Later, MLST results using eBURST confirmed the split of *E. faecium* into host-specific subgroups, one from hospitalized patients (originally termed clonal complex 17 [CC17]) and others from domesticated animals (291, 316). More recently, BAPS analysis allowed the partitioning of 519 sequence types of 1,720 *E. faecium* isolates into 13 nonoverlapping groups. Again, BAPS groups were significantly associated with isolates from hospitalized patients (BAPS 3-3) and farm animals (BAPS 2-1 and 2-4) (313). More recently, single-nucleotide polymorphism-based phylogenetic analysis of WGS data split *E. faecium* into isolates causing infections (clade A1), isolates from healthy humans (clade B), and isolates from healthy humans and animals (clade A2) (79). Clade A1 mostly comprises isolates from hospitalized humans associated with lineages 17 (including ST16 and ST17), 18 (ST18), and 78 (ST78 and ST192), although isolates from animals have been extensively reported (89, 304, 313). The ST78 isolates show putative evolutionary hallmarks with respect to pets (dogs and cats) and poultry isolates and diversified mainly through recombination and acquisition or loss of mobile genetic elements, which eventually led to adaptation to different ecological niches. Thus, ecological distinction is not absolute, and the main zoonotic risk linked to *E. faecium* isolates is represented by transfer of mobile genetic elements harboring antimicrobial resistance genes.

Poultry
E. faecium isolates resistant to macrolides, quinupristin-dalfoprisitin, or other streptogramins were extensively reported in poultry farms, revealing high heterogeneity of PFGE types and sequence types, although some similar patterns were eventually detected on farms in Europe, the United States, and Asia (317–319). Clonal dissemination of VRE of the *E. faecium* species (VREfm) in poultry farms exposed to antibiotics before and after the avoparcin ban (109, 302) were documented in European and Asian countries, with sequence types belonging to CC9 or CC96 being predominant in Europe and Malaysia, respectively (320). A dramatic increase of VREfm in Sweden from 2000 to 2009 was due to the clonal expansion of the clone ST310, despite the absence of selection by antibiotics in this country, where the use of antibiotics as animal growth promoters has

Table 5 Summary of articles on the antimicrobial resistance in *Enterococcus* isolated from animals from 2013 to 2017

Animal	Country	Enterococcal specie	Percentage of resistance to[a]				Reference
			TET	ERY	HLR-GEN	CIP	
Food-producing and farm animals							
Camels	Tunisia	*Enterococcus* spp.	4	11	0	ND	254
Chickens and pigs	China	*Enterococcus* spp.	92.5	72.8	30	ND	153
Aquaculture	Spain	*E. faecalis*	0	5	ND	62	255
		E. faecium	5	37	ND	26	
Rainbow trout	Spain	*Enterococcus* spp.	27.1	41	7	0	256
Marine aquaculture	Italy	*Enterococcus* spp.	66	25	0	ND	257
Tibetan pigs	Tibet	*E. faecalis*	93.5	93.5	0	0	258
		E. faecium	44.4	20	0	0	
Farm animals	Argentina	*E. faecalis*	100	50	0	ND	259
Chickens	Southeast Asian countries	*E. faecalis*	69.2	70.9	11.1	17.9	260
		E. faecium	92.2	79.4	13.9	82.8	
Poultry	Italy	*Enterococcus* spp.	65.2	87.8	60	70.4	143
Beef and sheep	Tunisia	*E. faecalis*	15	30	2.5	22.5	261
Pigs	South Africa	*E. faecalis*	ND	100	ND	45	147
		E. faecium	ND	98.3	ND	94.1	
Poultry	Germany	*E. faecalis*	82	70	98	14	141
		E. faecium	67	89	89	72	
Poultry	Nigeria	*Enterococcus* spp.	81.6	100	20	ND	262
Chicken and turkey	Canada	*Enterococcus* spp.	94	64–74	8–15	2–8	135
Fish and seafood	Switzerland	*E. faecalis*	16	ND	4	0	263
Infection in poultry	Poland	*E. cecorum*	29	51	1	ND	15
Poultry and cattle	Nigeria	*Enterococcus* spp.	61	61	32.7	9.7	154
Mastitis in cows	China	*Enterococcus* spp.	6.7	ND	50	25	264
Cattle	Australia	*E. faecalis*	7.3	10.4	0	ND	87
		E. faecium	11.7	8.3	0	ND	
Pigs	Nigeria	*E. faecalis*	60	68.7	85	0.5	265
		E. faecium	20	31.5	40	7.4	
Donkey	Spain	*E. faecium*	68	44	0	60	266
Pets and companion animals							
Healthy dogs and cats	Japan	*Enterococcus* spp.	ND	40	44	25	267
Hospitalized dogs	Korea	*E. faecalis*	64.3	50	7.1	0	268
		E. faecium	66.7	44.4	33.3	55.6	
Antibiotic-treated dogs and cats	Japan	*E. faecalis*	58	52	38	30	198
		E. faecium	15	28	21	8	
Various animals	Poland	*E. faecalis*	36	48	ND	38	205
		E. faecium	7	60	ND	46	
Healthy cats and dogs	Italy	*Enterococcus* spp.	97.4	81.7	40.8	7.8	269
Wild animals							
Iberian lynx	Spain	*Enterococcus* spp.	33	30	4	7	92
Iberian wolf	Portugal	*Enterococcus* spp.	55	22	1	15	90
Echinoderms	Portugal	*E. faecium*	31.7	33	0.8	30.8	65
Red foxes	Portugal	*E. faecalis*	81	36	18	ND	270
		E. faecium	96	56	12	ND	
Wild birds	Portugal	*E. faecalis*	32.3	15.3	0	15.3	209
		E. faecium	45	15	0	32.5	
Eurasian otter	Portugal	*E. faecalis*	32	ND	52	ND	271
		E. faecium	78	ND	11	ND	
House flies	USA	*E. faecalis*	60	18	5	0	272

(Continued)

Table 5   *(Continued)*

Animal	Country	Enterococcal specie	Percentage of resistance to[a]				Reference
			TET	ERY	HLR-GEN	CIP	
Wild birds	Tunisia	*E. faecalis*	33	33	50	66	261
		E. faecium	16	53	11	38	
Wild fur seals	Brazil	*E. faecalis*	0	25	0	10	273
Wild marine animals	Brazil	*Enterococcus* spp.	14.5	32.2	0	20.9	274
Seafood	Tunisia	*E. faecalis*	42.9	38.1	14.3	52.4	275
		E. faecium	18.2	27.3	0	63.6	
House flies	Thailand	*Enterococcus* spp.	75	42.5	ND	ND	276

[a]TET, tetracycline; ERY, erythromycin; HLR-GEN, high-level resistance to gentamicin; CIP, ciprofloxacin.

been forbidden since 1986 (129). A Danish study showed a high rate of VREfm in Danish farms after the 15-year ban of avoparcin, with different sequence types and the presence of an ST842 clone in 36 flocks analyzed corresponding to eight farms broadly distributed across the country (85). Recently, clonally unrelated *E. faecium* isolates resistant to linezolid emerged on farms in China (236, 237). Common PFGE profiles or sequence types between humans and broilers have also been documented (321–323), but the human health risk associated with the presence of *E. faecium* in poultry meat is under debate (25).

Swine

VREfm has been extensively reported in pig farms in European countries before and after the avoparcin ban (113, 324, 325). Clonal spread of VREfm was documented in Denmark, Norway, Finland (113), Switzerland (326), Portugal (304), and Spain (327), with predominance of sequence types belonging to the CC5 lineage (ST5, ST6, ST185). The persistence of VREfm in pig farms after the avoparcin ban was associated later with the use of tylosin, which facilitated the coselection of strains resistant to both glycopeptides and macrolides due to the presence of both *vanA* and *erm*(B) genes in the same plasmid (113). VREfm was also detected in county fairs in Michigan from 2008 to 2010, which represents the first and only report of VREfm in livestock in the United States to date (121, 122). In Asia, the occurrence varies among countries and is sporadic in China (156). In all these studies, CC5 strains were predominantly identified. A particular ST6 (CC5) clone was identified on farms in different European Union countries and the United States, as well as in healthy volunteers and hospitalized patients, all carrying a Tn*1546* in *orf1* and a G-T point mutation in position 8234 at *vanX* (304, 328). In addition to tylosin, copper is frequently added to pig and cattle feeds, so coloca-

tion of heavy metal resistance determinants has also been demonstrated in Europe and the United States (329, 330). Copper resistance is often associated with resistance to macrolides [*erm*(B)], tetracyclines [*tet*(M)], and glycopeptides (*vanA*). Although clonal dissemination has been reported (330), a great diversity has been observed on farms (331). Major human clones CC9 and CC22 (previously classified as CC17) have also been documented in some studies (85, 332, 333).

Companion animals

A few studies have analyzed the fecal carriage of ampicillin-resistant *E. faecium* (AREfm) and VREfm in companion animals. High rates of AREfm were observed among fecal samples of dogs collected in the United Kingdom and Denmark in 2006 and 2008 (23% and 76%, respectively) (89, 334). Most of these isolates belonged to the major human clonal lineage originally called CC17, which suggested a possible transmission between hosts. Later, de Regt *et al.* demonstrated some unique metabolic features in these CC17 canine isolates that could have facilitated niche adaptation (335). A recent large Dutch country-wide population-based study reported a higher prevalence of fecal carriers of AREfm in dogs and cats than in a healthy human population (25.6%, 5.1%, and 1.5%, respectively). This study concluded that isolates from pets were genetically distinct from those of humans based on the lack of co-occurrence and the cgMLST results (336). Prior antibiotic use and eating raw meat were considered a risk factor for acquiring AREfm in all the available studies (197, 336). Clinical isolates from dogs and cats treated with amoxicillin belong to high clonal complex risks and were similar to those from humans (197, 337).

E. faecalis

A plethora of molecular methods have been used to type this species, including PFGE, AFLP, and MLST. In contrast to *E. faecium*, *E. faecalis* isolated from different sources/hosts cannot be grouped using MLST or AFLP. Studies using MLST data revealed the presence of many sequence types in different hosts, including farm animals, companion animals, and hospitalized patients (338, 339). Moreover, some sequence types are associated with a higher prevalence of antibiotic resistance, represented by ST2, ST8, ST9, ST16, ST40, and ST87 (303, 339, 340), all of them being overrepresented in humans. To date, ST16 has been recovered from humans and farm animals and is considered a zoonotic lineage (25), involved in the spread of resistance to all antibiotics used in animals, including bacitracin, phenicols, oxazolidinones (341). Clonal outbreaks of *E. faecalis* ST82, a common cause of amyloid arthropathy in poultry, have been reported on farms in Denmark, the United States, France, and Germany (342).

Although the detection of more-prevalent *E. faecalis* sequence types in distant geographical locations and different hosts suggests frequent horizontal gene transfer between different host populations (69, 211, 241, 339, 340, 343), some studies using comparative genomics discarded the idea of global transmission (344).

The incongruence in the topologies of the seven MLST gene trees revealed that this species is highly recombinogenic (291, 343). Subsequent analysis of the *E. faecalis* population structure based on MLST data using BAPS also yielded incongruent results and confirmed the lack of host-specific groups or ecotypes (313, 314). This issue was also demonstrated by studies that characterized the phylogenetic diversity of *E. faecalis* using whole genomes (phylogenomics and cgMLST) of clinical, human commensal, and animal isolates and that observed a lack of distinct clustering of isolates according to the source (291, 345).

Additional WGS studies are necessary to characterize and describe the role of animals in the evolution, genetic diversity, and population structure of *E. faecalis*.

PLASMIDS IN ENTEROCOCCI FROM FOODBORNE AND COMPANION ANIMALS

Horizontal gene transfer plays a relevant role in the dissemination of antibiotic resistance in nonhuman hosts, and plasmids play a central role in this dissemination. Classically, plasmid categorization is based on the presence and diversity of their replication machinery (346), which were established by replication-initiator protein (*rep*) schemes (347, 348) identified in Grampositive species to date. In Fig. 1 we show the plasmid content (percentage and diversity of *rep* sequences) of the 67 *E. faecium* and 47 *E. faecalis* genomes of animal

origin obtained from the WGS database of the NCBI. The enterococcal genomes from public databases were classified according to their origin (Table 6), information obtained from the Pathosystems Resource Integration Center (PATRIC) database (349). The *rep* genes obtained by the PlasmidFinder bioinformatics tool (350) belong to plasmid families with theta (RepaA_N, Inc18, Rep3_small tetha) or rolling-circle replication mechanisms (Fig. 1).

Plasmids conferring resistance in enterococci to vancomycin, macrolides, tetracycline, aminoglycosides, and heavy metals (copper, cadmium, bacitracin zinc) have been detected on farms that were exposed to antimicrobials used as growth promoters (avoparcin, virginiamycin, tylosin, or bacitracin zinc), therapeutically (tetracyclines, gentamicin, penicillins), or as dietary supplements (e.g., copper). Antibiotic-resistant plasmids have also been recovered from areas where selection was not apparent. Some emblematic examples are transferable *vanA* in commercial animal husbandry on farms in Michigan, where avoparcin has never been licensed for use in growth promotion (121, 122), and persistent *vanA*-Inc18 plasmids in Norwegian broiler flocks after the ban of some antibiotics. These studies suggest alternative routes of selection, introduction, and spread of *vanA*-type vancomycin resistance, plasmid fitness, and other phenomena (351).

Plasmids Conferring Resistance to Glycopeptides

Tn*1546* (*vanA*), the predominant mechanism of glycopeptide resistance in enterococci, has been successfully disseminated among poultry and swine through plasmids of the Inc18 and RepA_N families, respectively (352, 353). In poultry, an 18- to 25-kb fragment that includes the 10.85 kb of Tn*1546* (*vanA*), is conserved in Inc18 plasmids detected in Norwegian broiler flocks for more than 1 decade (from 1999 to years after the avoparcin ban) and in pIP186, the first Inc18 (*vanA*) plasmid described, in 1986, in an *E. faecium* clinical isolate (354, 355). The persistence of *vanA* plasmids on Norwegian poultry farms is attributed to the toxin-antitoxin system ω-ε-ζ originally described in pRE25, a plasmid of *E. faecalis* that carries resistance to different antibiotic families and is prevalent in animals and foods (127, 354). Analyses of the Tn*1546* insertion sites and plasmid backbones suggest spread of the *vanA* transposon across clonal lines in the broiler industry (125, 354–356). Bortolaia and Guardabassi recently associated the persistence of glycopeptide resistance in Danish poultry flocks after 15 years of the avoparcin ban with a nontransferable 54-kb plasmid in isolates

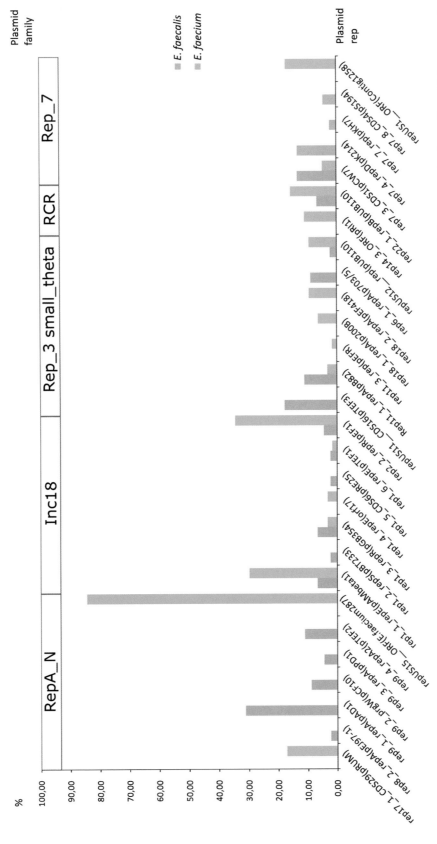

Figure 1 Plasmid gene content of 67 *E. faecium* and 47 *E. faecalis* genomes of animal origin from the NCBI whole-genome database. Plasmid data were obtained by the PlasmidFinder bioinformatics tool. The genomes from the database were classified by source, extracting the isolate information from the Pathosystems Resource Integration Center (PATRIC) database (344). Reps, replicases.

Table 6 *Enterococcus* isolates with animal source from the Genbank database included in the plasmid *rep* genes *in silico* screening

Species	Isolate	MLST	Plasmid rep	Isolation source	Year	Isolation country	Assembly accession
Enterococcus faecalis	PF3		0	Adélie penguin (*Pygoscelis adeliae*)	2010	Antarctica	GCA_000505585.1
	DBH18		1	Mallard duck (*Anas platyrhynchos*)	2005	Spain	GCF_001563075.1
	ATCC 27959	40	0	Cattle	1975	United States	GCA_000395265.1
	ATCC 35038	59	2	Chicken (*Gallus gallus*)	1980		GCA_000392955.1
	ATCC 29212		0	Chicken (*Gallus gallus*)			GCA_900117325.1
	ATCC 29212		2	Chicken (*Gallus gallus*)			GCA_900117335.1
	F1	72	2	Cow	1900		GCA_000393095.1
	ATCC 6055	113	2	Cow	1937		GCA_000393375.1
	ARO1/DG	108	3	Dog (*Canis lupus familiaris*)			GCA_000157275.1
	UCD-PD3		1	*Felis catus*	2015	United States	GCF_001692955.1
	Fly1	101	0	Fruit fly (*Drosophila*)		United States	GCA_000157415.1
	Fly 2	102	1	Fruit fly (*Drosophila*)	2005		GCA_000393215.1
	P9-1		2	Magellanic penguin (*Spheniscus magellanicus*)	2013	Brazil	GCF_001400065.1
	P8-1		3	Magellanic penguin, (*Spheniscus magellanicus*)	2013	Brazil	GCF_001400055.1
	KB1		1	*Mus musculus*	2011	Germany	GCA_002221625.2
	KB1		0	*Mus musculus*	2015	Switzerland	GCF_001689055.1
	7330257-1	16	1	Pig (*Sus scrofa*)	2001	Denmark	GCA_000390805.1
	7330259-5	16	1	Pig (*Sus scrofa*)	2001	Denmark	GCA_000390825.1
	7330948-5	16	1	Pig (*Sus scrofa*)	2001	Denmark	GCA_000390845.1
	7330112-3	16	6	Pig (*Sus scrofa*)	2001	Denmark	GCA_000390765.1
	7430416-3	16	0	Pig (*Sus scrofa*)	2002	Denmark	GCA_000390905.1
	19116	16	1	Pig (*Sus scrofa*)	2002	Denmark	GCA_000390685.1
	7430275-3	16	1	Pig (*Sus scrofa*)	2002	Denmark	GCA_000390865.1
	7430821-4	16	1	Pig (*Sus scrofa*)	2002	Denmark	GCA_000390925.1
	D6	16	0	Pig (*Sus scrofa*)		Denmark	GCA_000157455.1
	7430315-3	35	3	Pig (*Sus scrofa*)	2002	Denmark	GCA_000390885.1
	D1	40	0	Pig (*Sus scrofa*)			GCA_000393575.1
	7330082-2	40	0	Pig (*Sus scrofa*)	2001	Denmark	GCA_000390745.1
	D32	40	1	Pig (*Sus scrofa*)	2001	Denmark	GCA_000281195.1
	D3	47	2	Pig (*Sus scrofa*)			GCA_000392915.1
	7330245-2	47	2	Pig (*Sus scrofa*)	2001	Denmark	GCA_000390785.1
	L9		0	Pig (*Sus scrofa*)	2013	Brazil	GCF_001878735.1
	L12		0	Pig (*Sus scrofa*)	2013	Brazil	GCF_001886675.1
	IBUN9046YE		5	Pig (*Sus scrofa*)	2014	Colombia	GCA_002250145.1
	19		1	Pig (*Sus scrofa*)	2011	Denmark	GCA_000788165.1
	17		1	Pig (*Sus scrofa*)	2011	Denmark	GCA_000788185.1
	1		2	Pig (*Sus scrofa*)	2011	Denmark	GCA_000788175.1
	32		2	Pig (*Sus scrofa*)	2011	Denmark	GCA_000788255.1
	12		3	Pig (*Sus scrofa*)	2011	Denmark	GCA_000788155.1
	18		3	Pig (*Sus scrofa*)	2011	Denmark	GCA_000788235.1
	Enfs51		2	Pig (*Sus scrofa*)	2012	Malaysia	GCF_001806515.1
	P.En250		3	Pig (*Sus scrofa*)	2012	Malaysia	GCF_002009545.1
	P. En090		3	Pig (*Sus scrofa*)	2012	Malaysia	GCF_002009565.1
	Enfs85		5	Pig (*Sus scrofa*)	2012	Malaysia	GCF_002009465.1
	XJ05		1	Sheep (*Ovis aries*)	2002	China	GCF_001263775.1
	OG1X	92	1	Tunicate (*Lissoclinum patella*)	2006	Solomon Islands	GCA_000320305.1
	2924	116	1	Turkey meat	2005	Denmark	GCA_000390725.1

(Continued)

Table 6   *(Continued)*

Species	Isolate	MLST	Plasmid rep	Isolation source	Year	Isolation country	Assembly accession
Enterococcus	E1573	21	1	Bison (*Bison* sp.)	1994	Belgium	GCA_000321765.1
faecium	825		4	Cattle	2004	United States	GCA_002360185.1
	E0045	9	3	Chicken (*Gallus gallus*)	1992	United Kingdom	GCA_000321465.1
	E2134	12	6	Chicken (*Gallus gallus*)	2004	Netherlands	GCA_000322185.1
	VAN 342	22	6	Chicken (*Gallus gallus*)	2010	Denmark	GCA_000395785.1
	VAN 332	38	4	Chicken (*Gallus gallus*)	2010	Denmark	GCA_000395745.1
	VAN 345	38	5	Chicken (*Gallus gallus*)	2010	Denmark	GCA_000395805.1
	E1575	158	4	Chicken (*Gallus gallus*)	1995	Belgium	GCA_000321805.1
	F9730129-1	245	4	Chicken (*Gallus gallus*)	1997	Denmark	GCA_000395965.1
	VAN 335	417	4	Chicken (*Gallus gallus*)	2010	Denmark	GCA_000395765.1
	VAN 219	784	3	Chicken (*Gallus gallus*)	2010	Denmark	GCA_000395705.1
	VAN 222	784	3	Chicken (*Gallus gallus*)	2010	Denmark	GCA_000395725.1
	7527		3	Chicken (*Gallus gallus*)	2003	United States	GCA_002360135.1
	6605		4	Chicken (*Gallus gallus*)	2003	United States	GCA_002360225.1
	5209		6	Chicken (*Gallus gallus*)	2003	United States	GCA_002360255.1
	E1574	27	3	Dog (*Canis lupus familiaris*)	1995	Belgium	GCA_000321785.1
	E4389	78	5	Dog (*Canis lupus familiaris*)		Denmark	GCA_000322425.1
	E4453	192	5	Dog (*Canis lupus familiaris*)			GCA_000239095.2
	E4452	266	5	Dog (*Canis lupus familiaris*)	2008	Netherlands	GCA_000239115.2
	GL3		0	Dromedary	2013	Algeria	GCF_001277795.1
	ICIS 96		5	*Equus caballus*	2014	Russia	GCA_002265255.1
	LS170308		2	*Moschus berezovskii*	2017	China	GCA_002831505.1
	E1622	104	0	Mouse	1959	Netherlands	GCA_000321945.1
	E1576	159	3	Ostrich (*Struthio camelus*)	2001	South Africa	GCA_000321825.1
	E0688	5	4	Pig (*Sus scrofa*)		Spain	GCA_000321605.1
	HF50104	5	2	Pig (*Sus scrofa*)	2008	United States	GCA_000396685.1
	HF50215	5	4	Pig (*Sus scrofa*)	2008	United States	GCA_000396785.1
	A17 Sv1	6	1	Pig (*Sus scrofa*)	1995	Denmark	GCA_000392125.1
	E8sv3	6	1	Pig (*Sus scrofa*)	1995	Denmark	GCA_000392145.1
	9730219-1	6	1	Pig (*Sus scrofa*)	1997	Denmark	GCA_000391945.1
	9730357-1	6	1	Pig (*Sus scrofa*)	1997	Denmark	GCA_000391965.1
	9731352-4	6	2	Pig (*Sus scrofa*)	1997	Denmark	GCA_000392005.1
	9830091-5	6	1	Pig (*Sus scrofa*)	1998	Denmark	GCA_000392025.1
	9830512-2	6	1	Pig (*Sus scrofa*)	1998	Denmark	GCA_000392045.1
	9931110-4	6	3	Pig (*Sus scrofa*)	1999	Denmark	GCA_000392105.1
	7330446-2	6	1	Pig (*Sus scrofa*)	2001	Denmark	GCA_000391825.1
	7330519-3	6	1	Pig (*Sus scrofa*)	2001	Denmark	GCA_000391845.1
	7330884-2	6	1	Pig (*Sus scrofa*)	2001	Denmark	GCA_000391885.1
	7430166-3	6	1	Pig (*Sus scrofa*)	2002	Denmark	GCA_000391905.1
	S658-3	6	1	Pig (*Sus scrofa*)	2002	Denmark	GCA_000395425.1
	HF50204	6	1	Pig (*Sus scrofa*)	2008	United States	GCA_000396765.1
	HF50105	6	3	Pig (*Sus scrofa*)	2008	United States	GCA_000396705.1
	HF50106	6	3	Pig (*Sus scrofa*)	2008	United States	GCA_000396725.1
	9731349-1	82	4	Pig (*Sus scrofa*)	1997	Denmark	GCA_000391985.1
	9930238-2	133	1	Pig (*Sus scrofa*)	1999	Denmark	GCA_000392085.1
	7330381-1	133	1	Pig (*Sus scrofa*)	2001	Denmark	GCA_000391805.1
	E0679	150	2	Pig (*Sus scrofa*)		Belgium	GCA_000321565.1
	E0680	151	3	Pig (*Sus scrofa*)		Germany	GCA_000321585.1
	E1578	160	1	Pig (*Sus scrofa*)	2001	Germany	GCA_000321845.1
	9830565-4	185	1	Pig (*Sus scrofa*)	1998	Denmark	GCA_000392065.1

(Continued)

Table 6 *(Continued)*

Species	Isolate	MLST	Plasmid rep	Isolation source	Year	Isolation country	Assembly accession
	7330614-1	185	1	Pig (*Sus scrofa*)	2001	Denmark	GCA_000391865.1
	HF50203	185	1	Pig (*Sus scrofa*)	2008	United States	GCA_000396745.1
	CICYT-205	437	3	Pig (*Sus scrofa*)		Spain	GCF_001622975.1
	7230532-1		1	Pig (*Sus scrofa*)	2000	Denmark	GCA_000391785.1
	2006-70-121		0	Pig (*Sus scrofa*)	2006	Denmark	GCA_000391765.1
	1970-07-08		0	Pig (*Sus scrofa*)	2011	Denmark	GCA_000767345.1
	70-40-11		1	Pig (*Sus scrofa*)	2011	Denmark	GCA_000804405.1
	70-61-3		1	Pig (*Sus scrofa*)	2011	Denmark	GCA_000767355.1
	1970-08-02		2	Pig (*Sus scrofa*)	2011	Denmark	GCA_000804415.1
	70-36-8		2	Pig (*Sus scrofa*)	2011	Denmark	GCA_000767365.1
	70-61-7		2	Pig (*Sus scrofa*)	2011	Denmark	GCA_000804385.1
	E2071	27	1	Poultry	2001	Denmark	GCA_000322165.1
	FDAARGOS_397		2	Tonsil crypt			GCA_002554355.1
	E0269	9	3	Turkey (*Meleagris gallopavo*)	1996	Netherlands	GCA_000321525.1
	E0164	26	3	Turkey (*Meleagris gallopavo*)	1996	Netherlands	GCA_000321505.1
	M3K31		3	Vulture	2010	Spain	GCF_001039515.1
	58M		1	Wooly mammoth (*Mammuthus primigenius*)	2014	Russia	GCF_001280775.1

that only confer resistance to glycopeptides (27). It is notable that broiler flocks raised in Denmark come from parent birds imported from Sweden, and the high occurrence of VREfm was also observed in Swedish broiler flocks until 2011 (129).

In swine, large plasmids belonging to the RepA_N family (150 to 190 kb, rep$_{pLG1}$), which carry a truncated variant of Tn*1546* and *tcrB* (coding for resistance to copper), have been detected in a pandemic CC5 *E. faecium* clone that has been circulating in swine farms in Spain, Portugal, Denmark, Switzerland, and the United States for decades and in other *E. faecium* lineages of pigs and humans, which suggests transmission (304). These plasmids used to carry the *erm*(B) gene (macrolide resistance) and, eventually, *trcB* (copper resistance) (see below).

Also, sporadic reports have documented the occurrence of strains carrying other *vanB* or *vanN* operons on plasmids in poultry meat (178, 188), farmed game meat and wild game meat (226). Finally, vancomycin-susceptible *E. faecalis* strains carrying *vanC1* on transferable elements (plasmids, transposons, and integrons) have also been reported in cloacal swabs of broilers (357) and feces of diseased pigs from different farms (358). Transmission of species-specific *vanC1* and *vanC2/C3* genes could be currently underestimated given the high prevalence of *E. gallinarum* and *E. casseliflavus*, respectively, in food-producing animals (159, 359–360) and the scarcity of studies that screen *vanC* genes in other species.

Plasmids Conferring Resistance to Macrolides, Streptogramins, and Lincosamides

These plasmids have been extensively recovered in enterococci from poultry and pig farms where macrolides (spiramycin and tylosin) and streptogramins (virginiamycin) were used as growth promoters and pleuromutilins (tiamulin and valnemulin) were used to treat infections. Lincomycin, alone or in combination with spectinomycin, has been widely used to control respiratory and gastrointestinal bacterial pathogens in cattle, swine, poultry, dogs, and cats, and pirlimycin has been only used to treat bovine mastitis cases. Clindamycin is a common therapeutic option for topical infections in dogs and cats.

Macrolides

The most widespread gene that confers resistance to macrolides in enterococci is *erm*(B), which is located in different transposons and plasmids in species of the *Enterococcus*, *Streptococcus*, *Staphylococcus*, and *Clostridium* genera (346, 361). pRE25, a multidrug-resistant plasmid originally recovered from an *E. faecalis* isolate from a sausage sample, is the paradigm of the Inc18 family and has greatly contributed to the spread of *erm*(B) among animals and humans (346, 353, 362). This plasmid encodes resistance to 12 antimicrobials from 5 structural classes (macrolides, lincosamides, streptothricin, chloramphenicol, aminoglycosides) due to the presence of *erm*(B) (macrolide-lincosamide-streptogramin B), cat_{pIP501} (chloramphenicol), and Tn*5405*, which comprises the genes *aadE-sat4-aphA3* (aminoglycoside-streptothricin) (363, 364). The genes carried by pRE25 are present in several animal pathogens, namely, *Streptococcus pyogenes*, *Streptococcus agalactiae*, *S. aureus*, *Bacillus subtilis*, *Campylobacter coli*, *Clostridium perfringens*, and *C. difficile*. The *erm*(B) gene has also been found in small plasmids in poultry samples (365) and in large plasmids in food samples in addition to other genes such as *msr*(C) and *lnu*(B), *tet*(L), and *tet*(W) (366). Its presence in chromosomes is also frequent.

The gene *erm*(A), associated with Tn*554* and commonly found in staphylococci from swine, has also been found in streptococci and sporadic isolates of *E. faecalis* and *E. faecium* from pigs, suggesting transfer events (282, 367). More recently, a novel *erm*(A)-like gene that confers high-level resistance to erythromycin (MIC, >128 µg/ml) has been detected in Inc18 plasmids with genes encoding resistance to phenicols and oxazolidinones (see below). This gene differs from the widespread *erm*(A) gene on Tn*554* and the *erm*(A) gene formerly called *ermTR*, predominant in staphylococci and streptococci, respectively (82 to 85% homology at the amino acid level). This *erm*(A) enterococcal variant has a 116-bp deletion in the translational attenuator (237).

Streptogramins

Genes conferring resistance to streptogramins (acetyltransferases encoded by *satG/vatE* and *satA/vatA* genes and ABC transporters encoded by *vgb/vgbB*) and macrolides [23S rRNA methylases encoded by *erm*(B), *erm*(A), *erm*(C) genes] are observed in a diversity of plasmids and clonal backgrounds. In addition, *vat* genes are often cotranscribed and cotransferred along with *vga*, *vgaB*, *vgb*, *vgbB*, or *erm*(B) genes through transposable elements, some of them previously observed in staphylococci (364, 368–373). Transferability of *vat* genes and streptogramin resistance in *E. faecium* strains through contaminated pork and chicken meat, raw manure, and surface/ground water has been extensively documented (374, 375).

Lincosamides

Resistance to this antibiotic family can be due to the presence of genes coding for ABC transporters or modifying enzymes, most of them located on plasmids and/or transposable elements. These elements have been extensively documented in staphylococci and to a lesser extent in streptococci, *Clostridium*, and other species of Gram-positive bacteria in animals.

ABC transporters that confer resistance to pleuromutilins, lincosamides, and streptogramin A antibiotics (PLS$_A$) include the genes *vga* and *vga*(A)v, *vga*(C), *vga*(E), *vga*(E)v, *eat*(A)v, *sal*(A), *lsa*(A), *lsa*(C), and *lsa*(E). They frequently appear within clusters in plasmids or transferable chromosomal regions previously reported in *S. aureus* (230). A 8,705-bp region flanked by IS*Efa8* and IS*1216*, and comprising genes coding for one or more antibiotics, namely *lnu*(B) (lincosamide), *lsa*(E) (PLS$_A$), *spw* (spectinomycin), *aadE* (streptomycin), and *erm*(B) (macrolide-lincosamide-streptogramin B), is common for plasmids of *S. aureus* (pV7037) and *E. faecium* (pY13, pXD4, pXD5) strains recovered from pigs (230, 376, 377). The pY13 plasmid also contains a copy of the genes *lnu*(B) (lincosamide) and *aphA3* (kanamycin/neomycin) and a second copy of *erm*(B), highlighting the redundancy of determinants in settings under high selective pressure.

Two genes coding for nucleotidyl transferases (*lnu*), which only confer resistance to lincosamides, have been described in *Enterococcus* from swine recovered on Chinese farms (229, 378). *lnu*(G) is part of a 4,738-bp functionally active transposon designated Tn*6260*, which was first detected in an *E. faecalis* isolate of swine origin; this element is similar to others of the Tn*554* family, which includes different antibiotic resistance genes (378). *lnu*(B) has been detected in porcine *E. faecium* isolates, and it has been found in a nonconjugative plasmid linked to the *erm*(B), *lsa*(E), *spw*, *aadE*, and *aphA3* genes, which account for resistance to macrolides, lincosamides, streptogramins, pleuromutilins, streptomycin, spectinomycin, and kanamycin/neomycin (229).

Plasmids Conferring Resistance to Phenicols and Oxazolidinones

Genes coding for resistance to nonfluorinated phenicols (*cat*), nonfluorinated and fluorinated phenicols (*fexA*, *fexB*), and to both phenicols and oxazolidinones (*cfr*, *optrA*) have been detected in enterococcal species from animals, foods, and humans.

The production of chloramphenicol acetyltransferase (CAT) enzymes seems to be the main mechanism of resistance to chloramphenicol, although the number of studies addressing the diversity and the genetic context of *cat* genes in *Enterococcus* is still scarce. The predominant *cat* variants are *cat*(A-7), associated with pRE25-like plasmids of the Inc18 family, which are widely disseminated in food and farm animals, predominantly poultry (241), and *cat*(A-8), also known as *cat*$_{pC223}$, associated with pC223 plasmids originally detected in *S. aureus* that are now predominant in *E. faecalis* from swine. This gene eventually appears in tandem with *tet*(M) and *tet*(L) genes within the transposon Tn*6245*, and relics of this transposon have been observed in plasmids that also carry *fexA* and *optrA* (237). Although isolates positive for the *cat*(A-9) gene have been recently identified in *E. faecalis* from swine, their genetic context has not been characterized (A. Freitas, personal communication).

The florfenicol exporter gene *fexB* was initially detected in nonconjugative plasmids of *E. faecium*, *E. faecalis*, and *E. hirae* isolates collected on Chinese swine farms heavily exposed to florfenicol (379). These plasmids share common regions with the backbone of Inc18 plasmid derivatives (e.g., pVEF4), widely disseminated in Norwegian poultry farms (355). The *fexB* gene is bracketed by IS*1216* and would have been acquired by widespread pRE25-like plasmids, as occurred for other antimicrobial resistance genes flanked by this IS. The *fexB* gene has also been identified in enterococci from other farm animals (bovine) and aquaculture, although the plasmids have not been characterized (241, 380). A different epidemiological landscape occurs for the *fexA* gene, which is located on plasmids (241) and chromosomes (236) of enterococcal animal isolates, often in tandem with the *optrA* gene (237, 241) or the *cfr* gene (235). The *fexA* gene is inserted in the emblematic Tn*554* of staphylococci, although in enterococci traces of this transposon might be absent as a consequence of different events of horizontal gene transfer (237).

Enterococcal plasmids carrying *optrA* have been detected in poultry, swine, and humans. Despite differences in size (30 to 80 kb) and the backbone, all share similar regions upstream and downstream of the *optrA* gene (236, 237, 241). The presence of a novel *erm*(A)-like gene that confers a high level of resistance to erythromycin is notable (237). The genetic context of *optrA* is flanked by copies of IS*1216* in the same or opposite direction, which determine the mobility.

Conjugative and nonconjugative plasmids carrying the *cfr* gene flanked by different ISs (IS*1216*, IS*Enfa4*, IS*Enfa5*, IS*256*) have been described in animal isolates of various Gram-positive species, including enterococci. The nonconjugative pEF-01 (32.2 kb) plasmid represents the first description of a *cfr*-plasmid in this bacterial genus and was identified in a fecal *E. faecalis* isolate of bovine origin collected in 2009 on a Chinese farm (232). This plasmid has three Rep proteins of the Inc18 and Rep3 plasmid families and 9-kb and 6-kb regions which exhibit high similarity with the backbone of *vanA* Inc18 plasmids (pVEF1-2-3), which have been widely isolated on poultry farms (232). Moreover, the *cfr* gene was flanked by IS*1216*, which would facilitate

recombination processes, and the plasmid also contains the *fexA* gene, which provides resistance to phenicols. Conjugative plasmids carrying the *cfr* gene bracketed by IS*Enfa4* copies were isolated from *E. thailandicus* and *E. faecalis* from Chinese swine farms. These are closely related to another emblematic Inc18 plasmid, pAMb1, and contained *erm*(B) and *erm*(A) genes, conferring the MLS$_B$ phenotype and the ω-ε-ζ toxin-antitoxin module, which may promote the persistence of plasmids by encoding a system that kills or prevents the growth of plasmid-free cells (55). This genetic context has also been detected in streptococci and staphylococci and points to independent acquisition events for the *cfr* gene. The *cfr* gene bracketed by two copies of IS*Enfa5* has been documented in *E. gallinarum* and *E. casseliflavus* of swine origin (235).

Plasmids Conferring Resistance to Bacitracin

Bacitracin has been used as an animal growth promoter in China, and recent reports documented *E. faecalis* isolates with high-level resistance to this antibiotic (MIC, ≥256 μg/ml), due to the presence of the *bcrABDR* cluster, which is composed by the *bcrABD* operon and its regulatory gene, *bcrR*. The cluster bracketed by either two, one, or no IS*Enfa1* copies is located on transferable plasmids (341) or chromosomes. The structure IS*Enfa1*-*bcrABDR*-IS*Enfa1* may be circulating and may have been transferred to other species by IS-mediated recombination. A multiresistant 79-kb pheromone-responsive plasmid carrying this IS*Enfa1*-*bcrABDR*-IS*Enfa1* platform as well as *optrA*, *fexA*, Tn*6425* (*cat*$_{pC223}$-*tetM*-*tetL*), Tn*5405* (*aph-sat-str*), and genes for resistance to copper and cadmium seems to be disseminated in Chinese farms (341), frequently associated with *E. faecalis* ST16. This *bcrABDR* cluster is also common in *E. cecorum*, a chicken commensal species (341).

Plasmids Conferring Resistance to Copper

Transferable resistance to copper (*tcrB*) in enterococci has been detected in piglets, calves, poultry, and humans in Europe, Asia, Australia, and North America (148, 331, 368, 381–383). Plasmids carrying *tcrB* are identified in intensively copper-supplemented livestock species, but plasmids with additional linkage with erythromycin [*erm*(B)] and/or vancomycin resistance (*vanA*) genes have only been observed in heavily copper-exposed swine (often with different copper compounds) in European countries where avoparcin was used as growth enhancer in the 1990s (148, 329, 381, 383, 384). The plasmids were detected in several enterococcal species (*E. faecium*, *E. faecalis*, *E. gallinarum*,

E. casseliflavus, E. mundtii, E. hirae), and conjugation has been experimentally demonstrated from *E. faecalis* to *E. faecium* (381). Copper fed to feedlot cattle at a growth-promotion concentration (10 × basal requirement) was associated with increased frequencies of *tcrB*-positive, macrolide-resistant *erm*(B) and, eventually, tetracycline-resistant *tet*(M) enterococci; however, copper susceptibilities were not increased in piglets in which the effect of in-feed tylosin or chlortetracycline was evaluated (382, 385). Cotransmission of *tcrB* and *erm*(B) genes between *E. hirae* from a sediment-derived livestock isolate and *E. faecalis* has been experimentally demonstrated (386). A recent analysis of WGS of *E. faecalis* from copper-supplemented Danish pigs also documented the presence of a chromosomal cluster of genes involved in susceptibility to copper, including the *tcrYAZB* operon, in three of six isolates analyzed, all containing plasmids (387). A detailed characterization of this chromosomal region was not provided, although other authors, who also identified redundancy of copper genes in chromosomes, demonstrated its cotransferability with ampicillin resistance (331).

CONCLUDING REMARKS

This review summarizes the current knowledge concerning the epidemiology and population structure of antibiotic-resistant *Enterococcus* species from food-producing, wild, and companion animals. Members of this genus are normal components of the intestinal microbiota of animals, and some species may also be etiological agents of a wide variety of infections with *E. faecalis* ST16 (considered a zoonotic pathogen) or ST82 (an etiological agent of the amyloid encephalopathy in chickens).

Enterococcus species are frequent contaminants on foods (especially poultry meat), although the risk of transmission from animals to humans through the food chain is based on indirect evidence, and thus, the bacterial load necessary to colonize the human gut remains greatly unknown. The food and animal industries seem to have contributed to the spread of certain pathogenic lineages (*E. faecalis* ST82 and ST16 lineages) and multidrug-resistant strains. Other species adapted to animals seem to act as important reservoirs of adaptive traits (*E. cecorum*). However, transmission of antimicrobial resistance by horizontal gene transfer events represents the main risk of foods contaminated by enterococci. Genes encoding resistance to vancomycin, macrolides, phenicols, and linezolid have been extensively documented in animals, frequently in response to heavy selection by antimicrobials (antibiotics and

heavy metals) used in prophylaxis or as growth promoters. Although the same genes and plasmids may be present in humans and animals, particular plasmid variants are often documented on farms, suggesting certain host specificity and transmission at a local level. Deep analysis of antimicrobial-resistant genes reveals a wide diversity of alleles [e.g., *erm*(A), *optrA, cfr*] and also the frequent presence of ISs (e.g., IS*1216*) that highlight the risk of frequent and independent acquisition and selection events of antimicrobial resistance on farms. More studies are necessary to establish the risks of the emergence and transmission of antibiotic-resistant enterococci from animals to humans.

Acknowledgments. Work in University of La Rioja is financed by project SAF2016-76571-R of the Agencia Estatal de Investigación (AEI) of Spain and the Fondo Europeo de Desarrollo Regional (FEDER). Work in TMC lab is supported by grants funded by the Joint Programming Initiative in Antimicrobial Resistance (JPIAMR Third call, STARCS, JPIAMR2016 AC16/00039 and the European Development Regional Fund "A way to achieve Europe" (ERDF) that cofunds the Spanish R&D National Plan 2012-2019 (PI15-01307), CIBER (CIBER in Epidemiology and Public Health, CIBERESP; CB06/02/0053), and the Regional Government of Madrid (InGeMICS- B2017/BMD-3691). L. Ruiz-Ripa has a predoctoral FPI fellowship of the University of La Rioja, Spain.

Citation. Torres C, Alonso CA, Ruiz-Ripa L, León-Sampedro R, del Campo R, Coque TM. 2018. Antimicrobial resistance in *Enterococcus* spp. Microbiol Spectrum 6(2):ARBA-0032-2018.

References

1. **Boehm AB, Sassoubre LM.** 2014. Enterococci as indicators of environmental fecal contamination. *In* Gilmore MS, Clewell DB, Ike Y, Shankar N (ed), *Enterococci: from Commensals to Leading Causes of Drug Resistant Infection.* Eye and Ear Infirmary, Boston, MA.

2. **Tyson GH, Nyirabahizi E, Crarey E, Kabera C, Lam C, Rice-Trujillo C, McDermott PF, Tate H.** 2017. Prevalence and antimicrobial resistance of enterococci isolated from retail meats in the United States, 2002–2014. *Appl Environ Microbiol* 84:e01902–e01917.

3. **Arias CA, Murray BE.** 2012. The rise of the *Enterococcus:* beyond vancomycin resistance. *Nat Rev Microbiol* 10:266–278.

4. **European Centre for Disease Prevention and Control (ECDC).** 2011. Annual epidemiological report on communicable diseases in Europe. *Euro Surveill* 16:20012.

5. **Iaria C, Stassi G, Costa GB, Di Leo R, Toscano A, Cascio A.** 2005. Enterococcal meningitis caused by *Enterococcus casseliflavus.* First case report. *BMC Infect Dis* 5:3.

6. **Canalejo E, Ballesteros R, Cabezudo J, García-Arata MI, Moreno J.** 2008. Bacteraemic spondylodiscitis caused by *Enterococcus hirae. Eur J Clin Microbiol Infect Dis* 27:613–615.

7. Mastroianni A. 2009. *Enterococcus raffinosus* endocarditis. First case and literature review. *Infez Med* **17**: 14–20.

8. Antonello VS, Zenkner FM, França J, Santos BR. 2010. *Enterococcus gallinarum* meningitis in an immunocompetent host: a case report. *Rev Inst Med Trop São Paulo* **52**:111–112.

9. Escribano JA, Solivera J, Vidal E, Rivin E, Lozano J. 2013. Otogenic cerebellar abscess by *Enterococcus avium*, a very rare infectious agent. *J Neurol Surg A Cent Eur Neurosurg* **74**(Suppl 1):e155–e158.

10. Kenzaka T, Takamura N, Kumabe A, Takeda K. 2013. A case of subacute infective endocarditis and blood access infection caused by *Enterococcus durans*. *BMC Infect Dis* **13**:594.

11. Lebreton F, Willems RJL, Gilmore MS. 2014. *Enterococcus* diversity, origins in nature, and gut colonization. *In* Gilmore MS, Clewell DB, Ike Y, Shankar N (ed), *Enterococci: from Commensals to Leading Causes of Drug Resistant Infection*. Eye and Ear Infirmary, Boston, MA.

12. Aarestrup FM, Butaye P, Witte W. 2002. Nonhuman reservoirs of enterococci, p 1281–1289. *In* Gilmore MS, Clewell DB, Courvalin P, Dunny GM, Murray BE, Rice LB (ed), *The Enterococci: Pathogenesis, Molecular Biology, and Antibiotic Resistance*. ASM Press, Washington, DC.

13. Aarestrup FM (ed). 2006. *Antimicrobial Resistance in Bacteria of Animal Origin*. ASM Press, Washington, DC.

14. Stalker MJ, Brash ML, Weisz A, Ouckama RM, Slavic D. 2010. Arthritis and osteomyelitis associated with *Enterococcus cecorum* infection in broiler and broiler breeder chickens in Ontario, Canada. *J Vet Diagn Invest* **22**:643–645.

15. Dolka B, Chrobak-Chmiel D, Makrai L, Szeleszczuk P. 2016. Phenotypic and genotypic characterization of *Enterococcus cecorum* strains associated with infections in poultry. *BMC Vet Res* **12**:129.

16. Kak V, Chow JM. 2002. Acquired antibiotic resistances in enterococci, p 355–383. *In* Gilmore MS, Clewell B, Courvalin P, Dunny GM, Murray BM, Rice LB (ed), *The Enterococci: Pathogenesis, Molecular Biology, and Antibiotic Resistance*. ASM Press, Washington, DC.

17. Hollenbeck BL, Rice LB. 2012. Intrinsic and acquired resistance mechanisms in *enterococcus*. *Virulence* **3**: 421–433.

18. Miller WR, Munita JM, Arias CA. 2014. Mechanisms of antibiotic resistance in enterococci. *Expert Rev Anti Infect Ther* **12**:1221–1236.

19. Courvalin P. 2006. Vancomycin resistance in Gram-positive cocci. *Clin Infect Dis* **42**(Suppl 1):S25–S34.

20. Nilsson O. 2012. Vancomycin resistant enterococci in farm animals: occurrence and importance. *Infect Ecol Epidemiol* **2**:16959.

21. Cattoir V, Leclercq R. 2013. Twenty-five years of shared life with vancomycin-resistant enterococci: is it time to divorce? *J Antimicrob Chemother* **68**:731–742.

22. Ahmed MO, Baptiste KE. 2017. Vancomycin-resistant enterococci: a review of antimicrobial resistant mechanisms and perspectives of human and animal health. *Microb Drug Resist*. Epub ahead of print.

23. Chow JW. 2000. Aminoglycoside resistance in enterococci. *Clin Infect Dis* **31**:586–589.

24. Hammerum AM, Lester CH, Heuer OE. 2010. Antimicrobial-resistant enterococci in animals and meat: a human health hazard? *Foodborne Pathog Dis* **7**: 1137–1146.

25. Bortolaia V, Espinosa-Gongora C, Guardabassi L. 2016. Human health risks associated with antimicrobial-resistant enterococci and *Staphylococcus aureus* on poultry meat. *Clin Microbiol Infect* **22**:130–140.

26. Hammerum AM. 2012. Enterococci of animal origin and their significance for public health. *Clin Microbiol Infect* **18**:619–625.

27. Bortolaia V, Guardabassi L. 2015. Zoonotic transmission of antimicrobial resistant enterococci: a threat to public health or an overemphasized risk? p 407–431. *In* Sing A (ed), *Zoonoses: Infections Affecting Humans and Animals*. Focus on Public Health Aspects. Springer, New York, NY.

28. Stiles ME, Holzapfel WH. 1997. Lactic acid bacteria of foods and their current taxonomy. *Int J Food Microbiol* **36**:1–29.

29. Lund B, Adamsson I, Edlund C. 2002. Gastrointestinal transit survival of an *Enterococcus faecium* probiotic strain administered with or without vancomycin. *Int J Food Microbiol* **77**:109–115.

30. Foulquié Moreno MR, Sarantinopoulos P, Tsakalidou E, De Vuyst L. 2006. The role and application of enterococci in food and health. *Int J Food Microbiol* **106**:1–24.

31. Zhong Z, Zhang W, Song Y, Liu W, Xu H, Xi X, Menghe B, Zhang H, Sun Z. 2017. Comparative genomic analysis of the genus *Enterococcus*. *Microbiol Res* **196**:95–105.

32. Schleifer KH, Kilpper-Balz R. 1984. Transfer of *Streptococcus faecalis* and *Streptococcus faecium* to the genus *Enterococcus* nom. rev. as *Enterococcus faecalis* comb. nov. and *Enterococcus faecium* comb. nov. *Int J Syst Bacteriol* **34**:31–34.

33. Parte AC. 2014. LPSN: list of prokaryotic names with standing in nomenclature. *Nucleic Acids Res* **42**(D1): D613–D616.

34. De Graef EM, Devriese LA, Vancanneyt M, Baele M, Collins MD, Lefebvre K, Swings J, Haesebrouck F. 2003. Description of *Enterococcus canis* sp. nov. from dogs and reclassification of *Enterococcus porcinus* Teixeira *et al.* 2001 as a junior synonym of *Enterococcus villorum* Vancanneyt *et al.* 2001. *Int J Syst Evol Microbiol* **53**:1069–1074.

35. Law-Brown J, Meyers PR. 2003. *Enterococcus phoeniculicola* sp. nov., a novel member of the enterococci isolated from the uropygial gland of the red-billed woodhoopoe, *Phoeniculus purpureus*. *Int J Syst Evol Microbiol* **53**:683–685.

36. Fortina MG, Ricci G, Mora D, Manachini PL. 2004. Molecular analysis of artisanal Italian cheeses reveals *Enterococcus italicus* sp. nov. *Int J Syst Evol Microbiol* **54**:1717–1721.

37. Švec P, Vancanneyt M, Koort J, Naser SM, Hoste B, Vihavainen E, Vandamme P, Swings J, Björkroth J.

2005. *Enterococcus devriesei* sp. nov., associated with animal sources. *Int J Syst Evol Microbiol* 55:2479–2484.

38. Tanasupawat S, Sukontasing S, Lee JS. 2008. *Enterococcus thailandicus* sp. nov., isolated from fermented sausage ('mum') in Thailand. *Int J Syst Evol Microbiol* 58:1630–1634.

39. Švec P, Vandamme P, Bryndová H, Holochová P, Kosina M, Maslanová I, Sedláček I. 2012. *Enterococcus plantarum* sp. nov., isolated from plants. *Int J Syst Evol Microbiol* 62:1499–1505.

40. Niemi RM, Ollinkangas T, Paulin L, Švec P, Vandamme P, Karkman A, Kosina M, Lindström K. 2012. *Enterococcus rivorum* sp. nov., from water of pristine brooks. *Int J Syst Evol Microbiol* 62:2169–2173.

41. Sistek V, Maheux AF, Boissinot M, Bernard KA, Cantin P, Cleenwerck I, De Vos P, Bergeron MG. 2012. *Enterococcus ureasiticus* sp. nov. and *Enterococcus quebecensis* sp. nov., isolated from water. *Int J Syst Evol Microbiol* 62:1314–1320.

42. Sedláček I, Holochová P, Mašlaňová I, Kosina M, Spröer C, Bryndová H, Vandamme P, Rudolf I, Hubálek Z, Švec P. 2013. *Enterococcus ureilyticus* sp. nov. and *Enterococcus rotai* sp. nov., two urease-producing enterococci from the environment. *Int J Syst Evol Microbiol* 63:502–510.

43. Mundt JO. 1963. Occurrence of enterococci in animals in a wild environment. *Appl Microbiol* 11:136–140.

44. Kühn I, Iversen A, Burman LG, Olsson-Liljequist B, Franklin A, Finn M, Aarestrup F, Seyfarth AM, Blanch AR, Vilanova X, Taylor H, Caplin J, Moreno MA, Dominguez L, Herrero IA, Möllby R. 2003. Comparison of enterococcal populations in animals, humans, and the environment: a European study. *Int J Food Microbiol* 88:133–145.

45. Devriese LA, Ceyssens K, Haesebrouck F. 1991a. Characteristics of *Enterococcus cecorum* strains from the intestines of different animal species. *Lett Appl Microbiol* 12:137–139.

46. Devriese LA, Laurier L, De Herdt P, Haesebrouck F. 1992. Enterococcal and streptococcal species isolated from faeces of calves, young cattle and dairy cows. *J Appl Bacteriol* 72:29–31.

47. Scupham AJ, Patton TG, Bent E, Bayles DO. 2008. Comparison of the cecal microbiota of domestic and wild turkeys. *Microb Ecol* 56:322–331.

48. Gong J, Forster RJ, Yu H, Chambers JR, Wheatcroft R, Sabour PM, Chen S. 2002. Molecular analysis of bacterial populations in the ileum of broiler chickens and comparison with bacteria in the cecum. *FEMS Microbiol Ecol* 41:171–179.

49. Devriese LA, Hommez J, Wijfels R, Haesebrouck F. 1991. Composition of the enterococcal and streptococcal intestinal flora of poultry. *J Appl Bacteriol* 71:46–50.

50. Kojima A, Morioka A, Kijima M, Ishihara K, Asai T, Fujisawa T, Tamura Y, Takahashi T. 2010. Classification and antimicrobial susceptibilities of *Enterococcus* species isolated from apparently healthy food-producing animals in Japan. *Zoonoses Public Health* 57:137–141.

51. Iweriebor BC, Obi LC, Okoh AI. 2016. Macrolide, glycopeptide resistance and virulence genes in *Enterococcus* species isolates from dairy cattle. *J Med Microbiol* 65:641–648.

52. Beukers AG, Zaheer R, Cook SR, Stanford K, Chaves AV, Ward MP, McAllister TA. 2015. Effect of in-feed administration and withdrawal of tylosin phosphate on antibiotic resistance in enterococci isolated from feedlot steers. *Front Microbiol* 6:483.

53. Hwang IY, Ku HO, Lim SK, Park CK, Jung GS, Jung SC, Nam HM. 2009. Species distribution and resistance patterns to growth-promoting antimicrobials of enterococci isolated from pigs and chickens in Korea. *J Vet Diagn Invest* 21:858–862.

54. Vancanneyt M, Snauwaert C, Cleenwerck I, Baele M, Descheemaeker P, Goossens H, Pot B, Vandamme P, Swings J, Haesebrouck F, Devriese LA. 2001. *Enterococcus villorum* sp. nov., an enteroadherent bacterium associated with diarrhoea in piglets. *Int J Syst Evol Microbiol* 51:393–400.

55. Liu Y, Wang Y, Schwarz S, Li Y, Shen Z, Zhang Q, Wu C, Shen J. 2013. Transferable multiresistance plasmids carrying *cfr* in *Enterococcus* spp. from swine and farm environment. *Antimicrob Agents Chemother* 57:42–48.

56. Devriese LA, Cruz Colque JI, De Herdt P, Haesebrouck F. 1992. Identification and composition of the tonsillar and anal enterococcal and streptococcal flora of dogs and cats. *J Appl Bacteriol* 73:421–425.

57. Rodrigues J, Poeta P, Martins A, Costa D. 2002. The importance of pets as reservoirs of resistant *Enterococcus* strains, with special reference to vancomycin. *J Vet Med B Infect Dis Vet Public Health* 49:278–280.

58. Jackson CR, Fedorka-Cray PJ, Davis JA, Barrett JB, Frye JG. 2009. Prevalence, species distribution and antimicrobial resistance of enterococci isolated from dogs and cats in the United States. *J Appl Microbiol* 107:1269–1278.

59. Ben Said L, Dziri R, Sassi N, Lozano C, Ben Slama K, Ouzari I, Torres C, Klibi N. 2017. Species distribution, antibiotic resistance and virulence traits in canine and feline enterococci in Tunisia. *Acta Vet Hung* 65:173–184.

60. Naser SM, Vancanneyt M, De Graef E, Devriese LA, Snauwaert C, Lefebvre K, Hoste B, Svec P, Decostere A, Haesebrouck F, Swings J. 2005. *Enterococcus canintestini* sp. nov., from faecal samples of healthy dogs. *Int J Syst Evol Microbiol* 55:2177–2182.

61. Baele M, Devriese LA, Butaye P, Haesebrouck F. 2002. Composition of enterococcal and streptococcal flora from pigeon intestines. *J Appl Microbiol* 92:348–351.

62. Splichalova P, Svec P, Ghosh A, Zurek L, Oravcova V, Radimersky T, Bohus M, Literak I. 2015. Prevalence, diversity and characterization of enterococci from three coraciiform birds. *Antonie van Leeuwenhoek* 107:1281–1289.

63. Radhouani H, Poeta P, Gonçalves A, Pacheco R, Sargo R, Igrejas G. 2012. Wild birds as biological indicators of environmental pollution: antimicrobial resistance patterns of *Escherichia coli* and enterococci isolated

from common buzzards (*Buteo buteo*). *J Med Microbiol* **61:**837–843.

64. Silva N, Igrejas G, Rodrigues P, Rodrigues T, Gonçalves A, Felgar AC, Pacheco R, Gonçalves D, Cunha R, Poeta P. 2011. Molecular characterization of vancomycin-resistant enterococci and extended-spectrum β-lactamase-containing *Escherichia coli* isolates in wild birds from the Azores Archipelago. *Avian Pathol* **40:**473–479.

65. Marinho C, Silva N, Pombo S, Santos T, Monteiro R, Gonçalves A, Micael J, Rodrigues P, Costa AC, Igrejas G, Poeta P. 2013. Echinoderms from Azores islands: an unexpected source of antibiotic resistant *Enterococcus* spp. and *Escherichia coli* isolates. *Mar Pollut Bull* **69:** 122–127.

66. Medeiros AW, Blaese Amorim D, Tavares M, de Moura TM, Franco AC, d'Azevedo PA, Frazzon J, Frazzon AP. 2017. *Enterococcus* species diversity in fecal samples of wild marine species as determined by real-time PCR. *Can J Microbiol* **63:**129–136.

67. Farnleitner AH, Ryzinska-Paier G, Reischer GH, Burtscher MM, Knetsch S, Kirschner AK, Dirnböck T, Kuschnig G, Mach RL, Sommer R. 2010. *Escherichia coli* and enterococci are sensitive and reliable indicators for human, livestock and wildlife faecal pollution in alpine mountainous water resources. *J Appl Microbiol* **109:**1599–1608.

68. Radhouani H, Igrejas G, Carvalho C, Pinto L, Gonçalves A, Lopez M, Sargo R, Cardoso L, Martinho A, Rego V, Rodrigues R, Torres C, Poeta P. 2011. Clonal lineages, antibiotic resistance and virulence factors in vancomycin-resistant enterococci isolated from fecal samples of red foxes (*Vulpes vulpes*). *J Wildl Dis* **47:** 769–773.

69. Lozano C, González-Barrio D, García JT, Ceballos S, Olea PP, Ruiz-Fons F, Torres C. 2015. Detection of vancomycin-resistant *Enterococcus faecalis* ST6-*vanB2* and *E. faecium* ST915-*vanA* in faecal samples of wild *Rattus rattus* in Spain. *Vet Microbiol* **177:**168–174.

70. Fontana R, Aldegheri M, Ligozzi M, Lopez H, Sucari A, Satta G. 1994. Overproduction of a low-affinity penicillin-binding protein and high-level ampicillin resistance in *Enterococcus faecium*. *Antimicrob Agents Chemother* **38:** 1980–1983.

71. Ligozzi M, Pittaluga F, Fontana R. 1996. Modification of penicillin-binding protein 5 associated with high-level ampicillin resistance in *Enterococcus faecium*. *Antimicrob Agents Chemother* **40:**354–357.

72. Montealegre MC, Roh JH, Rae M, Davlieva MG, Singh KV, Shamoo Y, Murray BE. 2016. Differential penicillin-binding protein 5 (PBP5) levels in the *Enterococcus faecium* clades with different levels of ampicillin resistance. *Antimicrob Agents Chemother* **61:**e02034-16.

73. Jureen R, Top J, Mohn SC, Harthug S, Langeland N, Willems RJ. 2003. Molecular characterization of ampicillin-resistant *Enterococcus faecium* isolates from hospitalized patients in Norway. *J Clin Microbiol* **41:** 2330–2336.

74. Poeta P, Costa D, Igrejas G, Sáenz Y, Zarazaga M, Rodrigues J, Torres C. 2007. Polymorphisms of the *pbp5* gene and correlation with ampicillin resistance in *Enterococcus faecium* isolates of animal origin. *J Med Microbiol* **56:**236–240.

75. Klibi N, Sáenz Y, Zarazaga M, Ben Slama K, Masmoudi A, Ruiz-Larrea F, Boudabous A, Torres C. 2008. Polymorphism in *pbp5* gene detected in clinical *Enterococcus faecium* strains with different ampicillin MICs from a Tunisian hospital. *J Chemother* **20:**436–440.

76. Kristich CJ, Rice LB, Arias CA. 2014. Enterococcal infection treatment and antibiotic resistance. *In* Gilmore MS, Clewell DB, Ike Y, Shankar N (ed), *Enterococci: from Commensals to Leading Causes of Drug Resistant Infection*. Eye and Ear Infirmary, Boston: MA.

77. Galloway-Peña JR, Rice LB, Murray BE. 2011. Analysis of PBP5 of early U.S. isolates of *Enterococcus faecium*: sequence variation alone does not explain increasing ampicillin resistance over time. *Antimicrob Agents Chemother* **55:**3272–3277.

78. Pietta E, Montealegre MC, Roh JH, Cocconcelli PS, Murray BE. 2014. *Enterococcus faecium* PBP5-S/R, the missing link between PBP5-S and PBP5-R. *Antimicrob Agents Chemother* **58:**6978–6981.

79. Lebreton F, van Schaik W, McGuire AM, Godfrey P, Griggs A, Mazumdar V, Corander J, Cheng L, Saif S, Young S, Zeng Q, Wortman J, Birren B, Willems RJ, Earl AM, Gilmore MS. 2013. Emergence of epidemic multidrug-resistant *Enterococcus faecium* from animal and commensal strains. *MBio* **4:**e00534-13.

80. Ono S, Muratani T, Matsumoto T. 2005. Mechanisms of resistance to imipenem and ampicillin in *Enterococcus faecalis*. *Antimicrob Agents Chemother* **49:**2954–2958.

81. Murray BE, Lopardo HA, Rubeglio EA, Frosolono M, Singh KV. 1992. Intrahospital spread of a single gentamicin-resistant, beta-lactamase-producing strain of *Enterococcus faecalis* in Argentina. *Antimicrob Agents Chemother* **36:**230–232.

82. Coudron PE, Markowitz SM, Wong ES. 1992. Isolation of a beta-lactamase-producing, aminoglycoside-resistant strain of *Enterococcus faecium*. *Antimicrob Agents Chemother* **36:**1125–1126.

83. Sarti M, Campanile F, Sabia C, Santagati M, Gargiulo R, Stefani S. 2012. Polyclonal diffusion of beta-lactamase-producing *Enterococcus faecium*. *J Clin Microbiol* **50:**169–172.

84. Rice LB, Carias LL, Rudin S, Lakticová V, Wood A, Hutton-Thomas R. 2005. *Enterococcus faecium* low-affinity *pbp5* is a transferable determinant. *Antimicrob Agents Chemother* **49:**5007–5012.

85. Novais C, Freitas AR, Silveira E, Antunes P, Silva R, Coque TM, Peixe L. 2013. Spread of multidrug-resistant *Enterococcus* to animals and humans: an underestimated role for the pig farm environment. *J Antimicrob Chemother* **68:**2746–2754.

86. Novais C, Tedim AP, Lanza VF, Freitas AR, Silveira E, Escada R, Roberts AP, Al-Haroni M, Baquero F, Peixe L, Coque TM. 2016. Co-diversification of *Enterococcus faecium* core genomes and PBP5: evidences of *pbp5* horizontal transfer. *Front Microbiol* **7:**1581.

87. Barlow RS, McMillan KE, Duffy LL, Fegan N, Jordan D, Mellor GE. 2017. Antimicrobial resistance status

of *Enterococcus* from Australian cattle populations at slaughter. *PLoS One* **12:**e0177728.

88. Poeta P, Costa D, Rodrigues J, Torres C. 2006. Antimicrobial resistance and the mechanisms implicated in faecal enterococci from healthy humans, poultry and pets in Portugal. *Int J Antimicrob Agents* **27:**131–137.

89. Damborg P, Top J, Hendrickx AP, Dawson S, Willems RJ, Guardabassi L. 2009. Dogs are a reservoir of ampicillin-resistant *Enterococcus faecium* lineages associated with human infections. *Appl Environ Microbiol* **75:**2360–2365.

90. Gonçalves A, Igrejas G, Radhouani H, Correia S, Pacheco R, Santos T, Monteiro R, Guerra A, Petrucci-Fonseca F, Brito F, Torres C, Poeta P. 2013. Antimicrobial resistance in faecal enterococci and *Escherichia coli* isolates recovered from Iberian wolf. *Lett Appl Microbiol* **56:**268–274.

91. Barros J, Igrejas G, Andrade M, Radhouani H, López M, Torres C, Poeta P. 2011. Gilthead seabream (*Sparus aurata*) carrying antibiotic resistant enterococci. A potential bioindicator of marine contamination? *Mar Pollut Bull* **62:**1245–1248.

92. Gonçalves A, Igrejas G, Radhouani H, Santos T, Monteiro R, Pacheco R, Alcaide E, Zorrilla I, Serra R, Torres C, Poeta P. 2013. Detection of antibiotic resistant enterococci and *Escherichia coli* in free range Iberian Lynx (*Lynx pardinus*). *Sci Total Environ* **456-457:**115–119.

93. DANMAP. 2014. *Use of antimicrobial agents and occurrence of antimicrobial resistance in bacteria from food animals, food and humans in Denmark.* www.danmap.org.

94. Swedres-Svarm. 2015. *Consumption of antibiotics and occurrence of antibiotic resistance in Sweden.* Solna/Uppsala, Sweden.

95. NethMap-MARAN. 2015. *Monitoring of antimicrobial resistance and antibiotic usage in animals in the Netherlands in 2014.* Nigmegen. SWAB. https://www.swab.nl/nethmap

96. Uttley AH, George RC, Naidoo J, Woodford N, Johnson AP, Collins CH, Morrison D, Gilfillan AJ, Fitch LE, Heptonstall J. 1989. High-level vancomycin-resistant enterococci causing hospital infections. *Epidemiol Infect* **103:**173–181.

97. Leclercq R, Derlot E, Duval J, Courvalin P. 1988. Plasmid-mediated resistance to vancomycin and teicoplanin in *Enterococcus faecium*. *N Engl J Med* **319:**157–161.

98. European Centre for Disease Prevention and Control. 2017. *Antimicrobial resistance surveillance in Europe 2016. Annual report of the European Antimicrobial Resistance Surveillance Network (EARS-Net).* ECDC, Stockholm, Sweden.

99. Lebreton F, Depardieu F, Bourdon N, Fines-Guyon M, Berger P, Camiade S, Leclercq R, Courvalin P, Cattoir V. 2011. D-Ala-D-Ser VanN-type transferable vancomycin resistance in *Enterococcus faecium*. *Antimicrob Agents Chemother* **55:**4606–4612.

100. Boyd DA, Du T, Hizon R, Kaplen B, Murphy T, Tyler S, Brown S, Jamieson F, Weiss K, Mulvey MR.

2006. VanG-type vancomycin-resistant *Enterococcus faecalis* strains isolated in Canada. *Antimicrob Agents Chemother* **50:**2217–2221.

101. Boyd DA, Willey BM, Fawcett D, Gillani N, Mulvey MR. 2008. Molecular characterization of *Enterococcus faecalis* N06-0364 with low-level vancomycin resistance harboring a novel D-Ala-D-Ser gene cluster, vanL. *Antimicrob Agents Chemother* **52:**2667–2672.

102. Xu X, Lin D, Yan G, Ye X, Wu S, Guo Y, Zhu D, Hu F, Zhang Y, Wang F, Jacoby GA, Wang M. 2010. *vanM*, a new glycopeptide resistance gene cluster found in *Enterococcus faecium*. *Antimicrob Agents Chemother* **54:**4643–4647.

103. Depardieu F, Foucault ML, Bell J, Dubouix A, Guibert M, Lavigne JP, Levast M, Courvalin P. 2009. New combinations of mutations in VanD-type vancomycin-resistant *Enterococcus faecium*, *Enterococcus faecalis*, and *Enterococcus avium* strains. *Antimicrob Agents Chemother* **53:**1952–1963.

104. López M, Rezusta A, Seral C, Aspiroz C, Marne C, Aldea MJ, Ferrer I, Revillo MJ, Castillo FJ, Torres C. 2012. Detection and characterization of a ST6 clone of *vanB2-Enterococcus faecalis* from three different hospitals in Spain. *Eur J Clin Microbiol Infect Dis* **31:**257–260.

105. Patel R, Piper K, Cockerill FR III, Steckelberg JM, Yousten AA. 2000. The biopesticide *Paenibacillus popilliae* has a vancomycin resistance gene cluster homologous to the enterococcal VanA vancomycin resistance gene cluster. *Antimicrob Agents Chemother* **44:**705–709.

106. Hegstad K, Mikalsen T, Coque TM, Werner G, Sundsfjord A. 2010. Mobile genetic elements and their contribution to the emergence of antimicrobial resistant *Enterococcus faecalis* and *Enterococcus faecium*. *Clin Microbiol Infect* **16:**541–554.

107. Arthur M, Quintiliani R Jr. 2001. Regulation of VanA- and VanB-type glycopeptide resistance in enterococci. *Antimicrob Agents Chemother* **45:**375–381.

108. Arthur M, Courvalin P. 1993. Genetics and mechanisms of glycopeptide resistance in enterococci. *Antimicrob Agents Chemother* **37:**1563–1571.

109. López M, Sáenz Y, Alvarez-Martínez MJ, Marco F, Robredo B, Rojo-Bezares B, Ruiz-Larrea F, Zarazaga M, Torres C. 2010. Tn1546 structures and multilocus sequence typing of *vanA*-containing enterococci of animal, human and food origin. *J Antimicrob Chemother* **65:**1570–1575.

110. Werner G, Strommenger B, Witte W. 2008. Acquired vancomycin resistance in clinically relevant pathogens. *Future Microbiol* **3:**547–562.

111. Patel R. 2003. Clinical impact of vancomycin-resistant enterococci. *J Antimicrob Chemother* **51**(Suppl 3): iii13–iii21.

112. Bager F, Madsen M, Christensen J, Aarestrup FM. 1997. Avoparcin used as a growth promoter is associated with the occurrence of vancomycin-resistant *Enterococcus faecium* on Danish poultry and pig farms. *Prev Vet Med* **31:**95–112.

113. Aarestrup FM, Kruse H, Tast E, Hammerum AM, Jensen LB. 2000. Associations between the use of antimicrobial agents for growth promotion and the occurrence of resistance among *Enterococcus faecium* from broilers and pigs in Denmark, Finland, and Norway. *Microb Drug Resist* **6:**63–70.

114. Robredo B, Singh KV, Baquero F, Murray BE, Torres C. 1999. From *vanA Enterococcus hirae* to *vanA Enterococcus faecium*: a study of feed supplementation with avoparcin and tylosin in young chickens. *Antimicrob Agents Chemother* **43:**1137–1143.

115. Klare I, Badstübner D, Konstabel C, Böhme G, Claus H, Witte W. 1999. Decreased incidence of VanA-type vancomycin-resistant enterococci isolated from poultry meat and from fecal samples of humans in the community after discontinuation of avoparcin usage in animal husbandry. *Microb Drug Resist* **5:**45–52.

116. Borgen K, Sørum M, Wasteson Y, Kruse H. 2001. VanA-type vancomycin-resistant enterococci (VRE) remain prevalent in poultry carcasses 3 years after avoparcin was banned. *Int J Food Microbiol* **64:**89–94.

117. Bortolaia V, Mander M, Jensen LB, Olsen JE, Guardabassi L. 2015. Persistence of vancomycin resistance in multiple clones of *Enterococcus faecium* isolated from Danish broilers 15 years after the ban of avoparcin. *Antimicrob Agents Chemother* **59:**2926–2929.

118. Lauderdale TL, Shiau YR, Wang HY, Lai JF, Huang IW, Chen PC, Chen HY, Lai SS, Liu YF, Ho M. 2007. Effect of banning vancomycin analogue avoparcin on vancomycin-resistant enterococci in chicken farms in Taiwan. *Environ Microbiol* **9:**819–823.

119. van Belkun A, van den Braak N, Thomassen R, Verbrugh H, Endtz H. 1996. Vancomycin-resistant enterococci in cats and dogs. *Lancet* **348:**1038–1039.

120. López M, Tenorio C, Torres C. 2013. Study of vancomycin resistance in faecal enterococci from healthy humans and dogs in Spain a decade after the avoparcin ban in Europe. *Zoonoses Public Health* **60:**160–167.

121. Donabedian SM, Perri MB, Abdujamilova N, Gordoncillo MJ, Naqvi A, Reyes KC, Zervos MJ, Bartlett P. 2010. Characterization of vancomycin-resistant *Enterococcus faecium* isolated from swine in three Michigan counties. *J Clin Microbiol* **48:**4156–4160.

122. Gordoncillo MJ, Donabedian S, Bartlett PC, Perri M, Zervos M, Kirkwood R, Febvay C. 2013. Isolation and molecular characterization of vancomycin-resistant *Enterococcus faecium* from swine in Michigan, USA. *Zoonoses Public Health* **60:**319–326.

123. Centers for Disease Control and Prevention (CDC). 1993. Nosocomial enterococci resistant to vancomycin: United States, 1989–1993. *MMWR Morb Mortal Wkly Rep* **42:**597–599.

124. Goossens H. 1998. Spread of vancomycin-resistant enterococci: differences between the United States and Europe. *Infect Control Hosp Epidemiol* **19:**546–551.

125. Johnsen PJ, Østerhus JI, Sletvold H, Sørum M, Kruse H, Nielsen K, Simonsen GS, Sundsfjord A. 2005. Persistence of animal and human glycopeptide-resistant enterococci on two Norwegian poultry farms formerly exposed to avoparcin is associated with a widespread plasmid-mediated *vanA* element within a polyclonal *enterococcus faecium* population. *Appl Environ Microbiol* **71:**159–168.

126. van den Bogaard AE, Willems R, London N, Top J, Stobberingh EE. 2002. Antibiotic resistance of faecal enterococci in poultry, poultry farmers and poultry slaughterers. *J Antimicrob Chemother* **49:**497–505.

127. Sørum M, Johnsen PJ, Aasnes B, Rosvoll T, Kruse H, Sundsfjord A, Simonsen GS. 2006. Prevalence, persistence, and molecular characterization of glycopeptide-resistant enterococci in Norwegian poultry and poultry farmers 3 to 8 years after the ban on avoparcin. *Appl Environ Microbiol* **72:**516–521.

128. Robredo B, Singh KV, Baquero F, Murray BE, Torres C. 2000. Vancomycin-resistant enterococci isolated from animals and food. *Int J Food Microbiol* **54:**197–204.

129. Nilsson O, Greko C, Top J, Franklin A, Bengtsson B. 2009. Spread without known selective pressure of a vancomycin-resistant clone of *Enterococcus faecium* among broilers. *J Antimicrob Chemother* **63:**868–872.

130. Ghidán A, Kaszanyitzky EJ, Dobay O, Nagy K, Amyes SG, Rozgonyi F. 2008a. Distribution and genetic relatedness of vancomycin-resistant enterococci (VRE) isolated from healthy slaughtered chickens in Hungary from 2001 to 2004. *Acta Vet Hung* **56:**13–25.

131. Manson JM, Smith JM, Cook GM. 2004. Persistence of vancomycin-resistant enterococci in New Zealand broilers after discontinuation of avoparcin use. *Appl Environ Microbiol* **70:**5764–5768.

132. Kolar M, Pantucek R, Bardon J, Cekanova L, Kesselova M, Sauer P, Vagnerova I, Koukalová D. 2005. Occurrence of vancomycin-resistant enterococci in humans and animals in the Czech Republic between 2002 and 2004. *J Med Microbiol* **54:**965–967.

133. Jung WK, Lim JY, Kwon NH, Kim JM, Hong SK, Koo HC, Kim SH, Park YH. 2007. Vancomycin-resistant enterococci from animal sources in Korea. *Int J Food Microbiol* **113:**102–107.

134. Tremblay CL, Letellier A, Quessy S, Boulianne M, Daignault D, Archambault M. 2011. Multiple-antibiotic resistance of *Enterococcus faecalis* and *Enterococcus faecium* from cecal contents in broiler chicken and turkey flocks slaughtered in Canada and plasmid colocalization of *tetO* and *ermB* genes. *J Food Prot* **74:**1639–1648.

135. Boulianne M, Arsenault J, Daignault D, Archambault M, Letellier A, Dutil L. 2016. Drug use and antimicrobial resistance among *Escherichia coli* and *Enterococcus* spp. isolates from chicken and turkey flocks slaughtered in Quebec, Canada. *Can J Vet Res* **80:**49–59.

136. Poeta P, Costa D, Rodrigues J, Torres C. 2005. Study of faecal colonization by *vanA*-containing *Enterococcus* strains in healthy humans, pets, poultry and wild animals in Portugal. *J Antimicrob Chemother* **55:**278–280.

137. Ghidán A, Dobay O, Kaszanyitzky EJ, Samu P, Amyes SG, Nagy K, Rozgonyi F. 2008. Vancomycin resistant enterococci (VRE) still persist in slaughtered poultry in hungary 8 years after the ban on avoparcin. *Acta Microbiol Immunol Hung* **55:**409–417.

138. Tzavaras I, Siarkou VI, Zdragas A, Kotzamanidis C, Vafeas G, Bourtzi-Hatzopoulou E, Pournaras S, Sofianou D. 2012. Diversity of *vanA*-type vancomycin-resistant *Enterococcus faecium* isolated from broilers, poultry slaughterers and hospitalized humans in Greece. *J Antimicrob Chemother* **67**:1811–1818.

139. Sting R, Richter A, Popp C, Hafez HM. 2013. Occurrence of vancomycin-resistant enterococci in turkey flocks. *Poult Sci* **92**:346–351.

140. Obeng AS, Rickard H, Ndi O, Sexton M, Barton M. 2013. Comparison of antimicrobial resistance patterns in enterococci from intensive and free range chickens in Australia. *Avian Pathol* **42**:45–54.

141. Maasjost J, Mühldorfer K, Hafez HM, Hafez HM, Cortez de Jäckel S. 2015. Antimicrobial susceptibility patterns of *Enterococcus faecalis* an *Enterococcus faecium* isolated from poultry flocks in Germany. *Avian Dis* **59**:143–148.

142. Stępień-Pyśniak D, Marek A, Banach T, Adaszek Ł, Pyzik E, Wilczyński J, Winiarczyk S. 2016. Prevalence and antibiotic resistance of *Enterococcus* strains isolated from poultry. *Acta Vet Hung* **64**:148–163.

143. Bertelloni F, Salvadori C, Moni A, Cerri D, Mani P, Ebani VV. 2015. Antimicrobial resistance in *Enterococcus* spp. isolated from laying hens of backyard poultry floks. *Ann Agric Environ Med* **22**:665–669.

144. Nilsson O, Greko C, Bengtsson B. 2009. Environmental contamination by vancomycin resistant enterococci (VRE) in Swedish broiler production. *Acta Vet Scand* **51**:49.

145. Torres C, Tenorio C, Portillo A, García M, Martínez C, Del Campo R, Ruiz-Larrea F, Zarazaga M. 2003. Intestinal colonization by *vanA*- or *vanB2*-containing enterococcal isolates of healthy animals in Spain. *Microb Drug Resist* **9**(Suppl 1):S47–S52.

146. Herrero IA, Teshager T, Garde J, Moreno MA, Domínguez L. 2000. Prevalence of vancomycin-resistant *Enterococcus faecium* (VREF) in pig faeces from slaughterhouses in Spain. *Prev Vet Med* **47**:255–262.

147. Iweriebor BC, Obi LC, Okoh AI. 2015. Virulence and antimicrobial resistance factors of *Enterococcus* spp. isolated from fecal samples from piggery farms in Eastern Cape, South Africa. *BMC Microbiol* **15**:136.

148. Fard RM, Heuzenroeder MW, Barton MD. 2011. Antimicrobial and heavy metal resistance in commensal enterococci isolated from pigs. *Vet Microbiol* **148**:276–282.

149. Bustamante W, Alpízar A, Hernández S, Pacheco A, Vargas N, Herrera ML, Vargas A, Caballero M, García F. 2003. Predominance of *vanA* genotype among vancomycin-resistant *Enterococcus* isolates from poultry and swine in Costa Rica. *Appl Environ Microbiol* **69**:7414–7419.

150. Kühn I, Iversen A, Finn M, Greko C, Burman LG, Blanch AR, Vilanova X, Manero A, Taylor H, Caplin J, Domínguez L, Herrero IA, Moreno MA, Möllby R. 2005. Occurrence and relatedness of vancomycin-resistant enterococci in animals, humans, and the environment in different European regions. *Appl Environ Microbiol* **71**:5383–5390.

151. García-Migura L, Pleydell E, Barnes S, Davies RH, Liebana E. 2005. Characterization of vancomycin-resistant *Enterococcusfaecium* isolates from broiler poultry and pig farms in England and Wales. *J Clin Microbiol* **43**:3283–3289.

152. Kempf I, Hellard G, Perrin-Guyomard A, Gicquel-Bruneau M, Sanders P, Leclercq R. 2008. Prevalence of high-level vancomycin-resistant enterococci in French broilers and pigs. *Int J Antimicrob Agents* **32**:463–464.

153. Liu Y, Liu K, Lai J, Wu C, Shen J, Wang Y. 2013. Prevalence and antimicrobial resistance of *Enterococcus* species of food animal origin from Beijing and Shandong Province, China. *J Appl Microbiol* **114**:555–563.

154. Ngbede EO, Raji MA, Kwanashie CN, Kwaga JKP. 2017. Antimicrobial resistance and virulence profile of enterococci isolated from poultry and cattle sources in Nigeria. *Trop Anim Health Prod* **49**:451–458.

155. Bekele B, Ashenafi M. 2010. Distribution of drug resistance among enterococci and *Salmonella* from poultry and cattle in Ethiopia. *Trop Anim Health Prod* **42**: 857–864.

156. Ho PL, Lai E, Chan PY, Lo WU, Chow KH. 2013. Rare occurrence of vancomycin-resistant *Enterococcus faecium* among livestock animals in China. *J Antimicrob Chemother* **68**:2948–2949.

157. Eisner A, Feierl G, Gorkiewicz G, Dieber F, Kessler HH, Marth E, Köfer J. 2005. High prevalence of VanA-type vancomycin-resistant enterococci in Austrian poultry. *Appl Environ Microbiol* **71**:6407–6409.

158. Haenni M, Saras E, Châtre P, Meunier D, Martin S, Lepage G, Ménard MF, Lebreton P, Rambaud T, Madec JY. 2009. *vanA* in *Enterococcus faecium*, *Enterococcus faecalis*, and *Enterococcus casseliflavus* detected in French cattle. *Foodborne Pathog Dis* **6**: 1107–1111.

159. de Niederhäusern S, Sabia C, Messi P, Guerrieri E, Manicardi G, Bondi M. 2007. VanA-type vancomycin-resistant enterococci in equine and swine rectal swabs and in human clinical samples. *Curr Microbiol* **55**:240–246.

160. Ramos S, Igrejas G, Rodrigues J, Capelo-Martínez JL, Poeta P. 2012. Genetic characterisation of antibiotic resistance and virulence factors in vanA-containing enterococci from cattle, sheep and pigs subsequent to the discontinuation of the use of avoparcin. *Vet J* **193**: 301–303.

161. Hershberger E, Oprea SF, Donabedian SM, Perri M, Bozigar P, Bartlett P, Zervos MJ. 2005. Epidemiology of antimicrobial resistance in enterococci of animal origin. *J Antimicrob Chemother* **55**:127–130.

162. Song JY, Hwang IS, Eom JS, Cheong HJ, Bae WK, Park YH, Kim WJ. 2005. Prevalence and molecular epidemiology of vancomycin-resistant enterococci (VRE) strains isolated from animals and humans in Korea. *Korean J Intern Med (Korean Assoc Intern Med)* **20**:55–62.

163. Lim SK, Kim TS, Lee HS, Nam HM, Joo YS, Koh HB. 2006. Persistence of *vanA*-type *Enterococcus faecium* in Korean livestock after ban on avoparcin. *Microb Drug Resist* **12**:136–139.

164. Gonçalves A, Poeta P, Silva N, Araújo C, López M, Ruiz E, Uliyakina I, Direitinho J, Igrejas G, Torres C. 2010. Characterization of vancomycin-resistant enterococci isolated from fecal samples of ostriches by molecular methods. *Foodborne Pathog Dis* 7:1133–1136.

165. Araújo C, Torres C, Gonçalves A, Carneiro C, López M, Radhouani H, Pardal M, Igrejas G, Poeta P. 2011. Genetic detection and multilocus sequence typing of vanA-containing *Enterococcus* strains from mullets fish (*Liza ramada*). *Microb Drug Resist* 17:357–361.

166. Yoshimura H, Ishimaru M, Endoh YS, Suginaka M, Yamatani S. 1998. Isolation of glycopeptide-resistant enterococci from chicken in Japan. *Antimicrob Agents Chemother* 42:3333.

167. Butaye P, Van Damme K, Devriese LA, Van Damme L, Bael M, Lauwers S, Haesebrouck F. 2000. *In vitro* susceptibility of *Enterococcus faecium* isolated from food to growth-promoting and therapeutic antibiotics. *Int J Food Microbiol* 54:181–187.

168. Harada T, Kawahara R, Kanki M, Taguchi M, Kumeda Y. 2012. Isolation and characterization of vanA genotype vancomycin-resistant *Enterococcus cecorum* from retail poultry in Japan. *Int J Food Microbiol* 153: 372–377.

169. Donado-Godoy P, Byrne BA, León M, Castellanos R, Vanegas C, Coral A, Arevalo A, Clavijo V, Vargas M, Romero Zuñiga JJ, Tafur M, Pérez-Gutierrez E, Smith WA. 2015. Prevalence, resistance patterns, and risk factors for antimicrobial resistance in bacteria from retail chicken meat in Colombia. *J Food Prot* 78:751–759.

170. Kasimoglu-Dogru A, Gencay YE, Ayaz ND. 2010. Prevalence and antibiotic resistance profiles of *Enterococcus* species in chicken at slaughter level; absence of vanA and vanB genes in *E. faecalis* and *E. faecium*. *Res Vet Sci* 89:153–158.

171. Harwood VJ, Brownell M, Perusek W, Whitlock JE. 2001. Vancomycin-resistant *Enterococcus* spp. isolated from wastewater and chicken feces in the United States. *Appl Environ Microbiol* 67:4930–4933.

172. Wilson IG, McAfee GG. 2002. Vancomycin-resistant enterococci in shellfish, unchlorinated waters, and chicken. *Int J Food Microbiol* 79:143–151.

173. Novais C, Coque TM, Costa MJ, Sousa JC, Baquero F, Peixe LV. 2005. High occurrence and persistence of antibiotic-resistant enterococci in poultry food samples in Portugal. *J Antimicrob Chemother* 56:1139–1143.

174. Lemcke R, Bülte M. 2000. Occurrence of the vancomycin-resistant genes vanA, vanB, vanCl, vanC2 and vanC3 in *Enterococcus* strains isolated from poultry and pork. *Int J Food Microbiol* 60:185–194.

175. Del Grosso M, Caprioli A, Chinzari P, Fontana MC, Pezzotti G, Manfrin A, Giannatale ED, Goffredo E, Pantosti A. 2000. Detection and characterization of vancomycin-resistant enterococci in farm animals and raw meat products in Italy. *Microb Drug Resist* 6: 313–318.

176. Gambarotto K, Ploy MC, Dupron F, Giangiobbe M, Denis F. 2001. Occurrence of vancomycin-resistant enterococci in pork and poultry products from a cattle-rearing area of France. *J Clin Microbiol* 39:2354–2355.

177. Nomura T, Tanimoto K, Shibayama K, Arakawa Y, Fujimoto S, Ike Y, Tomita H. 2012. Identification of VanN-type vancomycin resistance in an *Enterococcus faecium* isolate from chicken meat in Japan. *Antimicrob Agents Chemother* 56:6389–6392.

178. Peters J, Mac K, Wichmann-Schauer H, Klein G, Ellerbroek L. 2003. Species distribution and antibiotic resistance patterns of enterococci isolated from food of animal origin in Germany. *Int J Food Microbiol* 88: 311–314.

179. Delpech G, Pourcel G, Schell C, De Luca M, Basualdo J, Bernstein J, Grenovero S, Sparo M. 2012. Antimicrobial resistance profiles of *Enterococcus faecalis* and *Enterococcus faecium* isolated from artisanal food of animal origin in Argentina. *Foodborne Pathog Dis* 9: 939–944.

180. Talebi M, Sadeghi J, Rahimi F, Pourshafie MR. 2015. Isolation and biochemical fingerprinting of vancomycin-resistant *Enterococcus faecium* from meat, chicken and cheese. *Jundishapur J Microbiol* 8:e15815.

181. Gousia P, Economou V, Bozidis P, Papadopoulou C. 2015. Vancomycin-resistance phenotypes, vancomycin-resistance genes, and resistance to antibiotics of enterococci isolated from food of animal origin. *Foodborne Pathog Dis* 12:214–220.

182. Pesavento G, Calonico C, Ducci B, Magnanini A, Lo Nostro A. 2014. Prevalence and antibiotic resistance of *Enterococcus* spp. isolated from retail cheese, ready-to-eat salads, ham, and raw meat. *Food Microbiol* 41:1–7.

183. Sánchez Valenzuela A, Lavilla Lerma L, Benomar N, Gálvez A, Pérez Pulido R, Abriouel H. 2013. Phenotypic and molecular antibiotic resistance profile of *Enterococcus faecalis* and *Enterococcus faecium* isolated from different traditional fermented foods. *Foodborne Pathog Dis* 10:143–149.

184. Pantosti A, Del Grosso M, Tagliabue S, Macrì A, Caprioli A. 1999. Decrease of vancomycin-resistant enterococci in poultry meat after avoparcin ban. *Lancet* 354:741–742.

185. Hayes JR, English LL, Carter PJ, Proescholdt T, Lee KY, Wagner DD, White DG. 2003. Prevalence and antimicrobial resistance of *Enterococcus* species isolated from retail meats. *Appl Environ Microbiol* 69:7153–7160.

186. Hiroi M, Kawamori F, Harada T, Sano Y, Miwa N, Sugiyama K, Hara-Kudo Y, Masuda T. 2012. Antibiotic resistance in bacterial pathogens from retail raw meats and food-producing animals in Japan. *J Food Prot* 75: 1774–1782.

187. Aslam M, Diarra MS, Checkley S, Bohaychuk V, Masson L. 2012. Characterization of antimicrobial resistance and virulence genes in *Enterococcus* spp. isolated from retail meats in Alberta, Canada. *Int J Food Microbiol* 156:222–230.

188. López M, Sáenz Y, Rojo-Bezares B, Martínez S, del Campo R, Ruiz-Larrea F, Zarazaga M, Torres C. 2009. Detection of vanA and vanB2-containing enterococci

from food samples in Spain, including *Enterococcus faecium* strains of CC17 and the new singleton ST425. *Int J Food Microbiol* **133**:172–178.

189. Jahan M, Krause DO, Holley RA. 2013. Antimicrobial resistance of *Enterococcus* species from meat and fermented meat products isolated by a PCR-based rapid screening method. *Int J Food Microbiol* **163**: 89–95.

190. Guerrero-Ramos E, Molina-González D, Blanco-Morán S, Igrejas G, Poeta P, Alonso-Calleja C, Capita R. 2016a. Prevalence, antimicrobial resistance, and genotypic characterization of vancomycin-resistant enterococci in meat preparations. *J Food Prot* **79**:748–756.

191. Jamet E, Akary E, Poisson MA, Chamba JF, Bertrand X, Serror P. 2012. Prevalence and characterization of antibiotic resistant *Enterococcus faecalis* in French cheeses. *Food Microbiol* **31**:191–198.

192. de Garnica ML, Valdezate S, Gonzalo C, Saez-Nieto JA. 2013. Presence of the *vanC1* gene in a vancomycin-resistant *Enterococcus faecalis* strain isolated from ewe bulk tank milk. *J Med Microbiol* **62**:494–495.

193. Osman KM, Ali MN, Radwan I, ElHofy F, Abed AH, Orabi A, Fawzy NM. 2016. Dispersion of the vancomycin resistance genes *vanA* and *vanC* of *Enterococcus* isolated from Nile Tilapia on retail sale: a public health hazard. *Front Microbiol* **7**:1354.

194. Tansuphasiri U, Khaminthakul D, Pandii W. 2006. Antibiotic resistance of enterococci isolated from frozen foods and environmental water. *Southeast Asian J Trop Med Public Health* **37**:162–170.

195. Simjee S, White DG, McDermott PF, Wagner DD, Zervos MJ, Donabedian SM, English LL, Hayes JR, Walker RD. 2002. Characterization of Tn*1546* in vancomycin-resistant *Enterococcus faecium* isolated from canine urinary tract infections: evidence of gene exchange between human and animal enterococci. *J Clin Microbiol* **40**:4659–4665.

196. Herrero IA, Fernández-Garayzábal JF, Moreno MA, Domínguez L. 2004. Dogs should be included in surveillance programs for vancomycin-resistant enterococci. *J Clin Microbiol* **42**:1384–1385.

197. Ghosh A, Dowd SE, Zurek L. 2011. Dogs leaving the ICU carry a very large multi-drug resistant enterococcal population with capacity for biofilm formation and horizontal gene transfer. *PLoS One* **6**:e22451.

198. Kataoka Y, Umino Y, Ochi H, Harada K, Sawada T. 2014. Antimicrobial susceptibility of enterococcal species isolated from antibiotic-treated dogs and cats. *J Vet Med Sci* **76**:1399–1402.

199. Abdel-Moein KA, El-Hariri MD, Wasfy MO, Samir A. 2017. Occurrence of ampicillin-resistant *Enterococcus faecium* carrying *esp* gene in pet animals: an upcoming threat for pet lovers. *J Glob Antimicrob Resist* **9**:115–117.

200. Oliveira M, Tavares M, Gomes D, Touret T, São Braz B, Tavares L, Semedo-Lemsaddek T. 2016. Virulence traits and antibiotic resistance among enterococci isolated from dogs with periodontal disease. *Comp Immunol Microbiol Infect Dis* **46**:27–31.

201. Gulhan T, Boynukara B, Ciftci A, Sogut MU, Findik A. 2015. Characterization of *Enterococcus faecalis* isolates originating from different sources for their virulence factors and genes, antibiotic resistance patterns, genotypes and biofilm production. *Majallah-i Tahqiqat-i Dampizishki-i Iran* **16**:261–266.

202. Moura I, Radhouani H, Torres C, Poeta P, Igrejas G. 2010. Detection and genetic characterisation of *vanA*-containing *Enterococcus* strains in healthy Lusitano horses. *Equine Vet J* **42**:181–183.

203. Mallon DJ, Corkill JE, Hazel SM, Wilson JS, French NP, Bennett M, Hart CA. 2002. Excretion of vancomycin-resistant enterococci by wild mammals. *Emerg Infect Dis* **8**:636–638.

204. Lozano C, González-Barrio D, García JT, Ceballos S, Olea PP, Ruiz-Fons F, Torres C. 2015. Detection of vancomycin-resistant *Enterococcus faecalis* ST6-vanB2 and *E. faecium* ST915-vanA in faecal samples of wild *Rattus rattus* in Spain. *Vet Microbiol* **177**:168–174.

205. Nowakiewicz A, Ziółkowska G, Zięba P, Kostruba A. 2014. Undomesticated animals as a reservoir of multidrug-resistant *Enterococcus* in eastern Poland. *J Wildl Dis* **50**:645–650.

206. Lozano C, González-Barrio D, Camacho MC, Lima-Barbero JF, de la Puente J, Höfle U, Torres C. 2016. Characterization of fecal vancomycin-resistant enterococci with acquired and intrinsic resistance mechanisms in wild animals, Spain. *Microb Ecol* **72**:813–820.

207. Silva N, Igrejas G, Rodrigues P, Rodrigues T, Gonçalves A, Felgar AC, Pacheco R, Gonçalves D, Cunha R, Poeta P. 2011. Molecular characterization of vancomycin-resistant enterococci and extended-spectrum β-lactamase-containing *Escherichia coli* isolates in wild birds from the Azores Archipelago. *Avian Pathol* **40**:473–479.

208. Silva N, Igrejas G, Felgar A, Gonçalves A, Pacheco R, Poeta P. 2012. Molecular characterization of *vanA*-containing *Enterococcus* from migratory birds: song thrush (*Turdus philomelos*). *Braz J Microbiol* **43**:1026–1029.

209. Santos T, Silva N, Igrejas G, Rodrigues P, Micael J, Rodrigues T, Resendes R, Gonçalves A, Marinho C, Gonçalves D, Cunha R, Poeta P. 2013. Dissemination of antibiotic resistant *Enterococcus* spp. and *Escherichia coli* from wild birds of Azores Archipelago. *Anaerobe* **24**:25–31.

210. Klibi N, Ben Amor I, Rahmouni M, Dziri R, Douja G, Ben Said L, Lozano C, Boudabous A, Ben Slama K, Mansouri R, Torres C. 2015. Diversity of species and antibiotic resistance among fecal enterococci from wild birds in Tunisia. Detection of *vanA*-containing *Enterococcus faecium* isolates. *Eur J Wildl Res* **61**:319–323.

211. Oravcova V, Zurek L, Townsend A, Clark AB, Ellis JC, Cizek A, Literak I. 2014. American crows as carriers of vancomycin-resistant enterococci with *vanA* gene. *Environ Microbiol* **16**:939–949.

212. Roberts MC, No DB, Marzluff JM, Delap JH, Turner R. 2016. Vancomycin resistant *Enterococcus* spp. from crows and their environment in metropolitan Washington State, USA: is there a correlation between

VRE positive crows and the environment? *Vet Microbiol* 194:48–54.

213. Oravcova V, Janecko N, Ansorge A, Masarikova M, Literak I. 2014. First record of vancomycin-resistant *Enterococcus faecium* in Canadian wildlife. *Environ Microbiol Rep* 6:210–211.

214. Oravcova V, Hadelova D, Literak I. 2016. Vancomycin-resistant *Enterococcus faecium* with *vanA* gene isolated for the first time from wildlife in Slovakia. *Vet Microbiol* 194:43–47.

215. Poeta P, Costa D, Igrejas G, Rojo-Bezares B, Sáenz Y, Zarazaga M, Ruiz-Larrea F, Rodrigues J, Torres C. 2007. Characterization of *vanA*-containing *Enterococcus faecium* isolates carrying Tn5397-like and Tn916/Tn1545-like transposons in wild boars (*Sus Scrofa*). *Microb Drug Resist* 13:151–156.

216. Radhouani H, Poeta P, Pinto L, Miranda J, Coelho C, Carvalho C, Rodrigues J, López M, Torres C, Vitorino R, Domingues P, Igrejas G. 2010. Proteomic characterization of *vanA*-containing *Enterococcus* recovered from seagulls at the Berlengas Natural Reserve, W Portugal. *Proteome Sci* 8:48.

217. Barros J, Andrade M, Radhouani H, López M, Igrejas G, Poeta P, Torres C. 2012. Detection of *vanA*-containing *Enterococcus* species in faecal microbiota of gilthead seabream (*Sparus aurata*). *Microbes Environ* 27:509–511.

218. Figueiredo N, Radhouani H, Gonçalves A, Rodrigues J, Carvalho C, Igrejas G, Poeta P. 2009. Genetic characterization of vancomycin-resistant enterococci isolates from wild rabbits. *J Basic Microbiol* 49:491–494.

219. da Silva VL, Caçador NC, da Silva CS, Fontes CO, Garcia GD, Nicoli JR, Diniz CG. 2012. Occurrence of multidrug-resistant and toxic-metal tolerant enterococci in fresh feces from urban pigeons in Brazil. *Microbes Environ* 27:179–185.

220. Radhouani H, Pinto L, Coelho C, Sargo R, Araújo C, López M, Torres C, Igrejas G, Poeta P. 2010. MLST and a genetic study of antibiotic resistance and virulence factors in *vanA*-containing *Enterococcus* from buzzards (*Buteo buteo*). *Lett Appl Microbiol* 50:537–541.

221. Silva V, Igrejas G, Carvalho I, Peixoto F, Cardoso L, Pereira JE, Del Campo R, Poeta P. 2018. Genetic characterization of *vanA*-*Enterococcus faecium* isolates from wild red-legged partridges in Portugal. *Microb Drug Resist* 24:89–94.

222. Radhouani H, Igrejas G, Carvalho C, Pinto L, Gonçalves A, Lopez M, Sargo R, Cardoso L, Martinho A, Rego V, Rodrigues R, Torres C, Poeta P. 2011. Clonal lineages, antibiotic resistance and virulence factors in vancomycin-resistant enterococci isolated from fecal samples of red foxes (*Vulpes vulpes*). *J Wildl Dis* 47:769–773.

223. Gonçalves A, Igrejas G, Radhouani H, López M, Guerra A, Petrucci-Fonseca F, Alcaide E, Zorrilla I, Serra R, Torres C, Poeta P. 2011. Detection of vancomycin-resistant enterococci from faecal samples of Iberian wolf and Iberian lynx, including *Enterococcus faecium* strains of CC17 and the new singleton ST573. *Sci Total Environ* 410-411:266–268.

224. Katakweba AA, Møller KS, Muumba J, Muhairwa AP, Damborg P, Rosenkrantz JT, Minga UM, Mtambo MM, Olsen JE. 2015. Antimicrobial resistance in faecal samples from buffalo, wildebeest and zebra grazing together with and without cattle in Tanzania. *J Appl Microbiol* 118:966–975.

225. Tejedor Junco MT, González-Martin M, Rodríguez González NF, Gutierrez C. 2015. Identification, antimicrobial susceptibility, and virulence factors of *Enterococcus* spp. strains isolated from Camels in Canary Islands, Spain. *Vet Ital* 51:179–183.

226. Guerrero-Ramos E, Cordero J, Molina-González D, Poeta P, Igrejas G, Alonso-Calleja C, Capita R. 2016. Antimicrobial resistance and virulence genes in enterococci from wild game meat in Spain. *Food Microbiol* 53 (Pt B):156–164.

227. Klare I, Fleige C, Geringer U, Thürmer A, Bender J, Mutters NT, Mischnik A, Werner G. 2015. Increased frequency of linezolid resistance among clinical *Enterococcus faecium* isolates from German hospital patients. *J Glob Antimicrob Resist* 3:128–131.

228. Herrero IA, Issa NC, Patel R. 2002. Nosocomial spread of linezolid-resistant, vancomycin-resistant *Enterococcus faecium*. *N Engl J Med* 346:867–869.

229. Si H, Zhang WJ, Chu S, Wang XM, Dai L, Hua X, Dong Z, Schwarz S, Liu S. 2015. Novel plasmid-borne multidrug resistance gene cluster including *lsa*(E) from a linezolid-resistant *Enterococcus faecium* isolate of swine origin. *Antimicrob Agents Chemother* 59:7113–7116.

230. Mendes RE, Deshpande LM, Jones RN. 2014. Linezolid update: stable *in vitro* activity following more than a decade of clinical use and summary of associated resistance mechanisms. *Drug Resist Updat* 17:1–12.

231. Shen J, Wang Y, Schwarz S. 2013. Presence and dissemination of the multiresistance gene *cfr* in Gram-positive and Gram-negative bacteria. *J Antimicrob Chemother* 68:1697–1706.

232. Liu Y, Wang Y, Wu C, Shen Z, Schwarz S, Du XD, Dai L, Zhang W, Zhang Q, Shen J. 2012. First report of the multidrug resistance gene *cfr* in *Enterococcus faecalis* of animal origin. *Antimicrob Agents Chemother* 56:1650–1654.

233. Liu Y, Wang Y, Schwarz S, Wang S, Chen L, Wu C, Shen J. 2014. Investigation of a multiresistance gene *cfr* that fails to mediate resistance to phenicols and oxazolidinones in *Enterococcus faecalis*. *J Antimicrob Chemother* 69:892–898.

234. Filsner PHLN, de Almeida LM, Moreno M, Moreno LZ, Matajira CEC, Silva KC, Pires C, Cerdeira LT, Sacramento AG, Mamizuka EM, Lincopan N, Moreno AM. 2017. Identification of the *cfr* methyltransferase gene in *Enterococcus faecalis* isolated from swine: first report in Brazil. *J Glob Antimicrob Resist* 8:192–193.

235. Liu Y, Wang Y, Dai L, Wu C, Shen J. 2014. First report of multiresistance gene *cfr* in *Enterococcus* species *casseliflavus* and *gallinarum* of swine origin. *Vet Microbiol* 170:352–357.

236. Wang Y, Lv Y, Cai J, Schwarz S, Cui L, Hu Z, Zhang R, Li J, Zhao Q, He T, Wang D, Wang Z, Shen Y, Li Y,

Feßler AT, Wu C, Yu H, Deng X, Xia X, Shen J. 2015. A novel gene, *optrA*, that confers transferable resistance to oxazolidinones and phenicols and its presence in *Enterococcus faecalis* and *Enterococcus faecium* of human and animal origin. *J Antimicrob Chemother* 70:2182–2190.

237. He T, Shen Y, Schwarz S, Cai J, Lv Y, Li J, Feßler AT, Zhang R, Wu C, Shen J, Wang Y. 2016. Genetic environment of the transferable oxazolidinone/phenicol resistance gene *optrA* in *Enterococcus faecalis* isolates of human and animal origin. *J Antimicrob Chemother* 71: 1466–1473.

238. Tamang MD, Moon DC, Kim SR, Kang HY, Lee K, Nam HM, Jang GC, Lee HS, Jung SC, Lim SK. 2017. Detection of novel oxazolidinone and phenicol resistance gene *optrA* in enterococcal isolates from food animals and animal carcasses. *Vet Microbiol* 201:252–256.

239. Cavaco LM, Korsgaard H, Kaas RS, Seyfarth AM, Leekitcharoenphon P, Hendriksen RS. 2017. First detection of linezolid resistance due to the *optrA* gene in enterococci isolated from food products in Denmark. *J Glob Antimicrob Resist* 9:128–129.

240. Cavaco LM, Bernal JF, Zankari E, Léon M, Hendriksen RS, Perez-Gutierrez E, Aarestrup FM, Donado-Godoy P. 2017. Detection of linezolid resistance due to the *optrA* gene in *Enterococcus faecalis* from poultry meat from the American continent (Colombia). *J Antimicrob Chemother* 72:678–683.

241. Freitas AR, Elghaieb H, León-Sampedro R, Abbassi MS, Novais C, Coque TM, Hassen A, Peixe L. 2017. Detection of *optrA* in the African continent (Tunisia) within a mosaic *Enterococcus faecalis* plasmid from urban wastewaters. *J Antimicrob Chemother* 72:3245–3251.

242. Diaz L, Kiratisin P, Mendes RE, Panesso D, Singh KV, Arias CA. 2012. Transferable plasmid-mediated resistance to linezolid due to *cfr* in a human clinical isolate of *Enterococcus faecalis*. *Antimicrob Agents Chemother* 56:3917–3922.

243. Deshpande LM, Ashcraft DS, Kahn HP, Pankey G, Jones RN, Farrell DJ, Mendes RE. 2015. Detection of a new *cfr*-like gene, *cfr*(B), in *Enterococcus faecium* recovered from human specimens in the United States: report from the SENTRY antimicrobial surveillance program. *Antimicrob Agents Chemother* 59:6256–6261.

244. Bender JK, Fleige C, Klare I, Fiedler S, Mischnik A, Mutters NT, Dingle KE, Werner G. 2016. Detection of a *cfr*(B) variant in German *Enterococcus faecium* clinical isolates and the impact on linezolid resistance in *Enterococcus* spp. *PLoS One* 11:e0167042.

245. Lazaris A, Coleman DC, Kearns AM, Pichon B, Kinnevey PM, Earls MR, Boyle B, O'Connell B, Brennan GI, Shore AC. 2017. Novel multiresistance *cfr* plasmids in linezolid-resistant methicillin-resistant *Staphylococcus epidermidis* and vancomycin-resistant *Enterococcus faecium* (VRE) from a hospital outbreak: co-location of *cfr* and *optrA* in VRE. *J Antimicrob Chemother* 72: 3252–3257.

246. Morroni G, Brenciani A, Simoni S, Vignaroli C, Mingoia M, Giovanetti E. 2017. Nationwide surveillance of novel oxazolidinone resistance gene *optrA* in *Enterococcus* isolates in China from 20004 to 2014. *Front Microbiol* 8:1631.

247. Cai J, Wang Y, Schwarz S, Lv H, Li Y, Liao K, Yu S, Zhao K, Gu D, Wang X, Zhang R, Shen J. 2015. Enterococcal isolates carrying the novel oxazolidinone resistance gene *optrA* from hospitals in Zhejiang, Guangdong, and Henan, China, 2010–2014. *Clin Microbiol Infect* 21:1095.e1–1095.e4.

248. Cui L, Wang Y, Lv Y, Wang S, Song Y, Li Y, Liu J, Xue F, Yang W, Zhang J. 2016. Nationwide surveillance of novel oxazolidinone resistance gene *optrA* in *Enterococcus* isolates in China from 2004 to 2014. *Antimicrob Agents Chemother* 60:7490–7493.

249. Del Campo R, Galán JC, Tenorio C, Ruiz-Garbajosa P, Zarazaga M, Torres C, Baquero F. 2005. New aac (6′)-I genes in *Enterococcus hirae* and *Enterococcus durans*: effect on beta-lactam/aminoglycoside synergy. *J Antimicrob Chemother* 55:1053–1055.

250. Galimand M, Schmitt E, Panvert M, Desmolaize B, Douthwaite S, Mechulam Y, Courvalin P. 2011. Intrinsic resistance to aminoglycosides in *Enterococcus faecium* is conferred by the 16S rRNA m5C1404-specific methyltransferase EfmM. *RNA* 17:251–262.

251. Bager F, Emborg HD (ed). 1998. *DANMAP 1997. Consumption of antimicrobial agents and occurrence of antimicrobial resistance in bacteria from food animals, food and humans in Denmark*. National Food Institute, Technical University of Denmark, Søborg, Denmark.

252. Donabedian SM, Thal LA, Hershberger E, Perri MB, Chow JW, Bartlett P, Jones R, Joyce K, Rossiter S, Gay K, Johnson J, Mackinson C, Debess E, Madden J, Angulo F, Zervos MJ. 2003. Molecular characterization of gentamicin-resistant enterococci in the United States: evidence of spread from animals to humans through food. *J Clin Microbiol* 41:1109–1113.

253. Werner G, Coque TM, Franz CM, Grohmann E, Hegstad K, Jensen L, van Schaik W, Weaver K. 2013. Antibiotic resistant enterococci: tales of a drug resistance gene trafficker. *Int J Med Microbiol* 303:360–379.

254. Klibi N, Ben Lagha A, Ben Slama K, Boudabous A, Torres C. 2013. Faecal enterococci from camels in Tunisia: species, antibiotic resistance and virulent genes. *Vet Rec* 172:213.

255. Muñoz-Atienza E, Gómez-Sala B, Araújo C, Campanero C, del Campo R, Hernández PE, Herranz C, Cintas LM. 2013. Antimicrobial activity, antibiotic susceptibility and virulence factors of lactic acid bacteria of aquatic origin intended for use as probiotics in aquaculture. *BMC Microbiol* 13:15.

256. Araújo C, Muñoz-Atienza E, Hernández PE, Herranz C, Cintas LM, Igrejas G, Poeta P. 2015. Evaluation of *Enterococcus* spp. from rainbow trout (*Oncorhynchus mykiss*, Walbaum), feed, and rearing environment against fish pathogens. *Foodborne Pathog Dis* 12:311–322.

257. Di Cesare A, Pasquaroli S, Vignaroli C, Paroncini P, Luna GM, Manso E, Biavasco F. 2014. The marine environment as a reservoir of enterococci carrying resistance and virulence genes strongly associated with clinical strains. *Environ Microbiol Rep* 6:184–190.

258. Li P, Wu D, Liu K, Suolang S, He T, Liu X, Wu C, Wang Y, Lin D. 2014. Investigation of antimicrobial resistance in *Escherichia coli* and enterococci isolated from Tibetan pigs. *PLoS One* 9:e95623.

259. Pantozzi FL, Ibar MP, Nievas VF, Vigo GB, Moredo FA, Giacoboni GI. 2014. Wild-type minimal inhibitory concentration distributions in bacteria of animal origin in Argentina. *Rev Argent Microbiol* 46:34–40.

260. Usui M, Ozawa S, Onozato H, Kuge R, Obata Y, Uemae T, Ngoc PT, Heriyanto A, Chalemchaikit T, Makita K, Muramatsu Y, Tamura Y. 2014. Antimicrobial susceptibility of indicator bacteria isolated from chickens in Southeast Asian countries (Vietnam, Indonesia and Thailand). *J Vet Med Sci* 76:685–692.

261. Klibi N, Aouini R, Borgo F, Ben Said L, Ferrario C, Dziri R, Boudabous A, Torres C, Ben Slama K. 2015. Antibiotic resistance and virulence of faecal enterococci isolated from food-producing animals in Tunisia. *Ann Microbiol* 65:695–702.

262. Ayeni FA, Odumosu BT, Oluseyi AE, Ruppitsch W. 2016. Identification and prevalence of tetracycline resistance in enterococci isolated from poultry in Ilishan, Ogun State, Nigeria. *J Pharm Bioallied Sci* 8:69–73.

263. Boss R, Overesch G, Baumgartner A. 2016. Antimicrobial resistance of *Escherichia coli*, enterococci, *Pseudomonas aeruginosa*, and *Staphylococcus aureus* from raw fish and seafood imported into Switzerland. *J Food Prot* 79:1240–1246.

264. Wu X, Hou S, Zhang Q, Ma Y, Zhang Y, Kan W, Zhao X. 2016. Prevalence of virulence and resistance to antibiotics in pathogenic enterococci isolated from mastitic cows. *J Vet Med Sci* 78:1663–1668.

265. Beshiru A, Igbinosa IH, Omeje FI, Ogofure AG, Eyong MM, Igbinosa EO. 2017. Multi-antibiotic resistant and putative virulence gene signatures in *Enterococcus* species isolated from pig farms environment. *Microb Pathog* 104:90–96.

266. Carvalho I, Campo RD, Sousa M, Silva N, Carrola J, Marinho C, Santos T, Carvalho S, Nóvoa M, Quaresma M, Pereira JE, Cobo M, Igrejas G, Poeta P. 2017. Antimicrobial-resistant *Escherichia coli* and *Enterococcus* spp. isolated from Miranda donkey (*Equus asinus*): an old problem from a new source with a different approach. *J Med Microbiol* 66:191–202.

267. Kataoka Y, Ito C, Kawashima A, Ishii M, Yamashiro S, Harada K, Ochi H, Sawada T. 2013. Identification and antimicrobial susceptibility of enterococci isolated from dogs and cats subjected to differing antibiotic pressures. *J Vet Med Sci* 75:749–753.

268. Chung YS, Kwon KH, Shin S, Kim JH, Park YH, Yoon JW. 2014. Characterization of veterinary hospital-associated isolates of *Enterococcus* species in Korea. *J Microbiol Biotechnol* 24:386–393.

269. Iseppi R, Messi P, Anacarso I, Bondi M, Sabia C, Condò C, de Niederhausern S. 2015. Antimicrobial resistance and virulence traits in *Enterococcus* strains isolated from dogs and cats. *New Microbiol* 38:369–378.

270. Radhouani H, Igrejas G, Gonçalves A, Pacheco R, Monteiro R, Sargo R, Brito F, Torres C, Poeta P. 2013. Antimicrobial resistance and virulence genes in *Escherichia coli* and enterococci from red foxes (*Vulpes vulpes*). *Anaerobe* 23:82–86.

271. Semedo-Lemsaddek T, Nóbrega CS, Ribeiro T, Pedroso NM, Sales-Luís T, Lemsaddek A, Tenreiro R, Tavares L, Vilela CL, Oliveira M. 2013. Virulence traits and antibiotic resistance among enterococci isolated from Eurasian otter (*Lutra lutra*). *Vet Microbiol* 163:378–382.

272. Doud CW, Scott HM, Zurek L. 2014. Role of house flies in the ecology of *Enterococcus faecalis* from wastewater treatment facilities. *Microb Ecol* 67:380–391.

273. Santestevan NA, de Angelis Zvoboda D, Prichula J, Pereira RI, Wachholz GR, Cardoso LA, de Moura TM, Medeiros AW, de Amorin DB, Tavares M, d'Azevedo PA, Franco AC, Frazzon J, Frazzon AP. 2015. Antimicrobial resistance and virulence factor gene profiles of *Enterococcus* spp. isolates from wild *Arctocephalus australis* (South American fur seal) and *Arctocephalus tropicalis* (Subantarctic fur seal). *World J Microbiol Biotechnol* 31:1935–1946.

274. Prichula J, Pereira RI, Wachholz GR, Cardoso LA, Tolfo NC, Santestevan NA, Medeiros AW, Tavares M, Frazzon J, d'Azevedo PA, Frazzon AP. 2016. Resistance to antimicrobial agents among enterococci isolated from fecal samples of wild marine species in the southern coast of Brazil. *Mar Pollut Bull* 105:51–57.

275. Ben Said L, Hamdaoui M, Klibi A, Ben Slama K, Torres C, Klibi N. 2017. Diversity of species and antibiotic resistance in enterococci isolated from seafood in Tunisia. *Ann Microbiol* 67:135–141.

276. Chaiwong T, Srivoramas T, Panya M, Wanram S, Panomket P. 2014. Antibiotic resistance patterns of *Enterococcus* spp. isolated from *Musca domestica* and *Chrysomya megacephala* in ubon Ratchathani. *J Med Assoc Thai* 97(Suppl 4):S1–S6.

277. Chopra I, Roberts M. 2001. Tetracycline antibiotics: mode of action, applications, molecular biology, and epidemiology of bacterial resistance. *Microbiol Mol Biol Rev* 65:232–260.

278. Roberts MC, Sutcliffe J, Courvalin P, Jensen LB, Rood J, Seppala H. 1999. Nomenclature for macrolide and macrolide-lincosamide-streptogramin B resistance determinants. *Antimicrob Agents Chemother* 43:2823–2830.

279. Roberts MC. 2005. Update on acquired tetracycline resistance genes. *FEMS Microbiol Lett* 245:195–203.

280. Franke AE, Clewell DB. 1980. Evidence for conjugal transfer of a *Streptococcus faecalis* tranposon (Tn916) from a chromosomal site in the absence of plasmid DNA. *Cold Spring Harb Symp Quant Biol* 46:7780.

281. Aarestrup FM, Seyfarth AM, Emborg HD, Pedersen K, Hendriksen RS, Bager F. 2001. Effect of abolishment of the use of antimicrobial agents for growth promotion on occurrence of antimicrobial resistance in fecal enterococci from food animals in Denmark. *Antimicrob Agents Chemother* 45:2054–2059.

282. Portillo A, Ruiz-Larrea F, Zarazaga M, Alonso A, Martinez JL, Torres C. 2000. Macrolide resistance genes in *Enterococcus* spp. *Antimicrob Agents Chemother* 44:967–971.

283. Bozdogan B, Berrezouga L, Kuo MS, Yurek DA, Farley KA, Stockman BJ, Leclercq R. 1999. A new resistance gene, *linB*, conferring resistance to lincosamides by nucleotidylation in *Enterococcus faecium* HM1025. *Antimicrob Agents Chemother* 43:925–929.

284. Roberts MC. 1996. Tetracycline resistance determinants: mechanisms of action, regulation of expression, genetic mobility, and distribution. *FEMS Microbiol Rev* 19:1–24.

285. Hooper DC. 2002. Fluoroquinolone resistance among Gram-positive cocci. *Lancet Infect Dis* 2:530–538.

286. López M, Tenorio C, Del Campo R, Zarazaga M, Torres C. 2011. Characterization of the mechanisms of fluoroquinolone resistance in vancomycin-resistant enterococci of different origins. *J Chemother* 23:87–91.

287. Arsène S, Leclercq R. 2007. Role of a *qnr*-like gene in the intrinsic resistance of *Enterococcus faecalis* to fluoroquinolones. *Antimicrob Agents Chemother* 51:3254–3258.

288. Jonas BM, Murray BE, Weinstock GM. 2001. Characterization of *emeA*, a NorA homolog and multidrug resistance efflux pump, in *Enterococcus faecalis*. *Antimicrob Agents Chemother* 45:3574–3579.

289. Oyamada Y, Ito H, Fujimoto K, Asada R, Niga T, Okamoto R, Inoue M, Yamagishi J. 2006. Combination of known and unknown mechanisms confers high-level resistance to fluoroquinolones in *Enterococcus faecium*. *J Med Microbiol* 55:729–736.

290. Werner G, Fleige C, Ewert B, Laverde-Gomez JA, Klare I, Witte W. 2010. High-level ciprofloxacin resistance among hospital-adapted *Enterococcus faecium* (CC17). *Int J Antimicrob Agents* 35:119–125.

291. Guzman Prieto AM, van Schaik W, Rogers MR, Coque TM, Baquero F, Corander J, Willems RJ. 2016. Global emergence and dissemination of enterococci as nosocomial pathogens: attack of the clones? *Front Microbiol* 7:788.

292. van den Bogaard AE, Jensen LB, Stobberingh EE. 1997. Vancomycin-resistant enterococci in turkeys and farmers. *N Engl J Med* 337:1558–1559.

293. Klein G, Pack A, Reuter G. 1998. Antibiotic resistance patterns of enterococci and occurrence of vancomycin-resistant enterococci in raw minced beef and pork in Germany. *Appl Environ Microbiol* 64:1825–1830.

294. Butaye P, Devriese LA, Goossens H, Ieven M, Haesebrouck F. 1999. Enterococci with acquired vancomycin resistance in pigs and chickens of different age groups. *Antimicrob Agents Chemother* 43:365–366.

295. Klare I, Heier H, Claus H, Böhme G, Marin S, Seltmann G, Hakenbeck R, Antanassova V, Witte W. 1995. *Enterococcus faecium* strains with *vanA*-mediated high-level glycopeptide resistance isolated from animal foodstuffs and fecal samples of humans in the community. *Microb Drug Resist* 1:265–272.

296. Wegener HC, Madsen M, Nielsen N, Aarestrup FM. 1997. Isolation of vancomycin resistant *Enterococcus faecium* from food. *Int J Food Microbiol* 35:57–66.

297. Balzereit-Scheuerlein F, Stephan R. 2001. Prevalence of colonisation and resistance patterns of vancomycin-resistant enterococci in healthy, non-hospitalised persons in Switzerland. *Swiss Med Wkly* 131:280–282.

298. Van der Auwera P, Pensart N, Korten V, Murray BE, Leclercq R. 1996. Influence of oral glycopeptides on the fecal flora of human volunteers: selection of highly glycopeptide-resistant enterococci. *J Infect Dis* 173:1129–1136.

299. del Campo R, Ruiz-Garbajosa P, Sánchez-Moreno MP, Baquero F, Torres C, Cantón R, Coque TM. 2003. Antimicrobial resistance in recent fecal enterococci from healthy volunteers and food handlers in Spain: genes and phenotypes. *Microb Drug Resist* 9:47–60.

300. Bates J, Jordens Z, Selkon JB. 1993. Evidence for an animal origin of vancomycin-resistant enterococci. *Lancet* 342:490–491.

301. Nannini E, Murray BE. 2006. Vancomycin resistant enterococci, p 155–188. *In* Fong IW, Drlica K (ed), *Reemergence of Established Pathogens in the 21st Century*. Kluwer Academic, New York, NY.

302. Freitas AR, Novais C, Ruiz-Garbajosa P, Coque TM, Peixe L. 2009. Dispersion of multidrug-resistant *Enterococcus faecium* isolates belonging to major clonal complexes in different Portuguese settings. *Appl Environ Microbiol* 75:4904–4908.

303. Freitas AR, Novais C, Ruiz-Garbajosa P, Coque TM, Peixe L. 2009. Clonal expansion within clonal complex 2 and spread of vancomycin-resistant plasmids among different genetic lineages of *Enterococcus faecalis* from Portugal. *J Antimicrob Chemother* 63:1104–1111.

304. Freitas AR, Coque TM, Novais C, Hammerum AM, Lester CH, Zervos MJ, Donabedian S, Jensen LB, Francia MV, Baquero F, Peixe L. 2011. Human and swine hosts share vancomycin-resistant *Enterococcus faecium* CC17 and CC5 and *Enterococcus faecalis* CC2 clonal clusters harboring Tn*1546* on indistinguishable plasmids. *J Clin Microbiol* 49:925–931.

305. Robredo B, Singh KV, Torres C, Murray BE. 2000. Streptogramin resistance and shared pulsed-field gel electrophoresis patterns in *vanA*-containing *Enterococcus faecium* and *Enterococcus hirae* isolated from humans and animals in Spain. *Microb Drug Resist* 6:305–311.

306. Daniel DS, Lee SM, Dykes GA, Rahman S. 2015. Public health risks of multiple-drug-resistant *Enterococcus* spp. in Southeast Asia. *Appl Environ Microbiol* 81:6090–6097.

307. Seo KS, Lim JY, Yoo HS, Bae WK, Park YH. 2005. Comparison of vancomycin-resistant enterococci isolates from human, poultry and pigs in Korea. *Vet Microbiol* 106:225–233.

308. Howden BP, Holt KE, Lam MM, Seemann T, Ballard S, Coombs GW, Tong SY, Grayson ML, Johnson PD, Stinear TP. 2013. Genomic insights to control the emergence of vancomycin-resistant enterococci. *MBio* 4:e00412-13.

309. Hammerum AM, Lester CH, Neimann J, Porsbo LJ, Olsen KE, Jensen LB, Emborg HD, Wegener HC, Frimodt-Moller N. 2004. A vancomycin-resistant *Enterococcus faecium* isolate from a Danish healthy volunteer, detected 7 years after the ban of avoparcin, is

possibly related to pig isolates. *J Antimicrob Chemother* 53:547–549.

310. van den Bogaard AE, Stobberingh EE. 2000. Epidemiology of resistanceto antibiotics. Links between animals and humans. *Int J Antimicrob Agents* 14:327–335.

311. Willems RJ, Top J, van Den Braak N, van Belkum A, Endtz H, Mevius D, Stobberingh E, van Den Bogaard A, van Embden JD. 2000. Host specificity of vancomycin-resistant *Enterococcus faecium*. *J Infect Dis* 182:816–823.

312. Homan WL, Tribe D, Poznanski S, Li M, Hogg G, Spalburg E, Van Embden JD, Willems RJ. 2002. Multilocus sequence typing scheme for *Enterococcus faecium*. *J Clin Microbiol* 40:1963–1971.

313. Willems RJ, Top J, van Schaik W, Leavis H, Bonten M, Sirén J, Hanage WP, Corander J. 2012. Restricted gene flow among hospital subpopulations of *Enterococcus faecium*. *MBio* 3:e00151-12.

314. Tedim AP, Ruiz-Garbajosa P, Corander J, Rodríguez CM, Cantón R, Willems RJ, Baquero F, Coque TM. 2015. Population biology of intestinal enterococcus isolates from hospitalized and nonhospitalized individuals in different age groups. *Appl Environ Microbiol* 81:1820–1831.

315. Bruinsma N, Willems RJ, van den Bogaard AE, van Santen-Verheuvel M, London N, Driessen C, Stobberingh EE. 2002. Different levels of genetic homogeneity in vancomycin-resistant and -susceptible *Enterococcus faecium* isolates from different human and animal sources analyzed by amplified-fragment length polymorphism. *Antimicrob Agents Chemother* 46:2779–2783.

316. Willems RJ, Top J, van Santen M, Robinson DA, Coque TM, Baquero F, Grundmann H, Bonten MJ. 2005. Global spread of vancomycin-resistant *Enterococcus faecium* from distinct nosocomial genetic complex. *Emerg Infect Dis* 11:821–828.

317. Hwang IY, Ku HO, Lim SK, Lee KJ, Park CK, Jung GS, Jung SC, Park YH, Nam HM. 2010. Distribution of streptogramin resistance genes and genetic relatedness among quinupristin/dalfopristin-resistant *Enterococcus faecium* recovered from pigs and chickens in Korea. *Res Vet Sci* 89:1–4.

318. Donabedian SM, Perri MB, Vager D, Hershberger E, Malani P, Simjee S, Chow J, Vergis EN, Muder RR, Gay K, Angulo FJ, Bartlett P, Zervos MJ. 2006. Quinupristin-dalfopristin resistance in *Enterococcus faecium* isolates from humans, farm animals, and grocery store meat in the United States. *J Clin Microbiol* 44:3361–3365.

319. De Graef EM, Decostere A, De Leener E, Goossens H, Baele M, Haesebrouck F. 2007. Prevalence and mechanism of resistance against macrolides, lincosamides, and streptogramins among *Enterococcus faecium* isolates from food-producing animals and hospital patients in Belgium. *Microb Drug Resist* 13:135–141.

320. Cha JO, Jung YH, Lee HR, Yoo JI, Lee YS. 2012. Comparison of genetic epidemiology of vancomycin-resistant *Enterococcus faecium* isolates from humans and poultry. *J Med Microbiol* 61:1121–1128.

321. Stobberingh E, van den Bogaard A, London N, Driessen C, Top J, Willems R. 1999. Enterococci with glycopep-

tide resistance in turkeys, turkey farmers, turkey slaughterers, and (sub)urban residents in the south of The Netherlands: evidence for transmission of vancomycin resistance from animals to humans? *Antimicrob Agents Chemother* 43:2215–2221.

322. Simonsen GS, Haaheim H, Dahl KH, Kruse H, Løvseth A, Olsvik O, Sundsfjord A. 1998. Transmission of VanA-type vancomycin-resistant enterococci and *vanA* resistance elements between chicken and humans at avoparcin-exposed farms. *Microb Drug Resist* 4:313–318.

323. De Leener E, Martel A, De Graef EM, Top J, Butaye P, Haesebrouck F, Willems R, Decostere A. 2005. Molecular analysis of human, porcine, and poultry *Enterococcus faecium* isolates and their *erm*(B) genes. *Appl Environ Microbiol* 71:2766–2770.

324. Aarestrup FM, Carstensen B. 1998. Effect of tylosin used as a growth promoter on the occurrence of macrolide-resistant enterococci and staphylococci in pigs. *Microb Drug Resist* 4:307–312.

325. Bager F, Madsen M, Christensen J, Aarestrup FM. 1997. Avoparcin used as a growth promoter is associated with the occurrence of vancomycin-resistant *Enterococcus faecium* on Danish poultry and pig farms. *Prev Vet Med* 31:95–112.

326. Boerlin P, Wissing A, Aarestrup FM, Frey J, Nicolet J. 2001. Antimicrobial growth promoter ban and resistance to macrolides and vancomycin in enterococci from pigs. *J Clin Microbiol* 39:4193–4195.

327. Novais C, Coque TM, Boerlin P, Herrero I, Moreno MA, Dominguez L, Peixe L. 2005. Vancomycin-resistant *Enterococcus faecium* clone in swine, Europe. *Emerg Infect Dis* 11:1985–1987.

328. Novais C, Freitas AR, Sousa JC, Baquero F, Coque TM, Peixe LV. 2008. Diversity of Tn*1546* and its role in the dissemination of vancomycin-resistant enterococci in Portugal. *Antimicrob Agents Chemother* 52:1001–1008.

329. Hasman H, Aarestrup FM. 2002. *tcrB*, a gene conferring transferable copper resistance in *Enterococcus faecium*: occurrence, transferability, and linkage to macrolide and glycopeptide resistance. *Antimicrob Agents Chemother* 46:1410–1416.

330. Amachawadi RG, Shelton NW, Shi X, Vinasco J, Dritz SS, Tokach MD, Nelssen JL, Scott HM, Nagaraja TG. 2011. Selection of fecal enterococci exhibiting *tcrB*-mediated copper resistance in pigs fed diets supplemented with copper. *Appl Environ Microbiol* 77:5597–5603.

331. Silveira E, Freitas AR, Antunes P, Barros M, Campos J, Coque TM, Peixe L, Novais C. 2014. Co-transfer of resistance to high concentrations of copper and first-line antibiotics among *Enterococcus* from different origins (humans, animals, the environment and foods) and clonal lineages. *J Antimicrob Chemother* 69:899–906.

332. Freitas AR, Tedim AP, Novais C, Ruiz-Garbajosa P, Werner G, Laverde-Gomez JA, Cantón R, Peixe L, Baquero F, Coque TM. 2010. Global spread of the *hyl* (Efm) colonization-virulence gene in megaplasmids of the *Enterococcus faecium* CC17 polyclonal subcluster. *Antimicrob Agents Chemother* 54:2660–2665.

333. Getachew Y, Hassan L, Zakaria Z, Abdul Aziz S. 2013. Genetic variability of vancomycin-resistant *Enterococcus faecium* and *Enterococcus faecalis* isolates from humans, chickens, and pigs in Malaysia. *Appl Environ Microbiol* 79:4528–4533.

334. Damborg P, Sørensen AH, Guardabassi L. 2008. Monitoring of antimicrobial resistance in healthy dogs: first report of canine ampicillin-resistant *Enterococcus faecium* clonal complex 17. *Vet Microbiol* 132:190–196.

335. de Regt MJ, van Schaik W, van Luit-Asbroek M, Dekker HA, van Duijkeren E, Koning CJ, Bonten MJ, Willems RJ. 2012. Hospital and community ampicillin-resistant *Enterococcus faecium* are evolutionarily closely linked but have diversified through niche adaptation. *PLoS One* 7:e30319.

336. van den Bunt G, Top J, Hordijk J, de Greeff SC, Mughini-Gras L, Corander J, van Pelt W, Bonten MJM, Fluit AC, Willems RJL. Intestinal carriage of ampicillin- and vancomycin-resistant *Enterococcus faecium* in humans, dogs and cats in the Netherlands. *J Antimicrob Chemother*. Epub ahead of print.

337. Marques C, Belas A, Franco A, Aboim C, Gama LT, Pomba C. 2018. Increase in antimicrobial resistance and emergence of major international high-risk clonal lineages in dogs and cats with urinary tract infection: 16 year retrospective study. *J Antimicrob Chemother* 73:377–384.

338. Ruiz-Garbajosa P, Bonten MJM, Robinson DA, Top J, Nallapareddy SR, Torres C, Coque TM, Cantón R, Baquero F, Murray BE, del Campo R, Willems RJL. 2006. Multilocus sequence typing scheme for *Enterococcus faecalis* reveals hospital-adapted genetic complexes in a background of high rates of recombination. *J Clin Microbiol* 44:2220–2228.

339. McBride SM, Fischetti VA, Leblanc DJ, Moellering RC Jr, Gilmore MS. 2007. Genetic diversity among *Enterococcus faecalis*. *PLoS One* 2:e582.

340. Kuch A, Willems RJL, Werner G, Coque TM, Hammerum AM, Sundsfjord A, Klare I, Ruiz-Garbajosa P, Simonsen GS, van Luit-Asbroek M, Hryniewicz W, Sadowy E. 2012. Insight into antimicrobial susceptibility and population structure of contemporary human *Enterococcus faecalis* isolates from Europe. *J Antimicrob Chemother* 67:551–558.

341. Chen MY, Lira F, Liang HQ, Wu RT, Duan JH, Liao XP, Martínez JL, Liu YH, Sun J. 2016. Multilevel selection of *bcr*ABDR-mediated bacitracin resistance in *Enterococcus faecalis* from chicken farms. *Sci Rep* 6:34895.

342. Petersen A, Christensen H, Philipp H-C, Bisgaard M. 2009. Clonality of *Enterococcus faecalis* associated with amyloid arthropathy in chickens evaluated by multilocus sequence typing (MLST). *Vet Microbiol* 134:392–395.

343. Ruiz-Garbajosa P, Cantón R, Pintado V, Coque TM, Willems R, Baquero F, del Campo R. 2006. Genetic and phenotypic differences among *Enterococcus faecalis* clones from intestinal colonisation and invasive disease. *Clin Microbiol Infect* 12:1193–1198.

344. Raven KE, Reuter S, Gouliouris T, Reynolds R, Russell JE, Brown NM, Török ME, Parkhill J, Peacock SJ. 2016. Genome-based characterization of hospital-adapted *Enterococcus faecalis* lineages. *Nat Microbiol* 1:15033.

345. Palmer KL, Godfrey P, Griggs A, Kos VN, Zucker J, Desjardins C, Cerqueira G, Gevers D, Walker S, Wortman J, Feldgarden M, Haas B, Birren B, Gilmore MS. 2012. Comparative genomics of enterococci: variation in *Enterococcus faecalis*, clade structure in *E. faecium*, and defining characteristics of *E. gallinarum* and *E. casseliflavus*. *MBio* 3:e00318-11.

346. Clewell DB, Weaver KE, Dunny GM, Coque TM, Francia MV, Hayes F. 2014. Extrachromosomal and mobile elements in enterococci: transmission, maintenance, and epidemiology. *In* Gilmore MS, Clewell DB, Ike Y, Shankar N (ed), *Enterococci: from Commensals to Leading Causes of Drug Resistant Infection*. Eye and Ear Infirmary, Boston, MA.

347. Jensen LB, Garcia-Migura L, Valenzuela AJS, Løhr M, Hasman H, Aarestrup FM. 2010. A classification system for plasmids from enterococci and other Gram-positive bacteria. *J Microbiol Methods* 80:25–43.

348. Wardal E, Gawryszewska I, Hryniewicz W, Sadowy E. 2013. Abundance and diversity of plasmid-associated genes among clinical isolates of *Enterococcus faecalis*. *Plasmid* 70:329–342.

349. Wattam AR, Abraham D, Dalay O, Disz TL, Driscoll T, Gabbard JL, Gillespie JJ, Gough R, Hix D, Kenyon R, Machi D, Mao C, Nordberg EK, Olson R, Overbeek R, Pusch GD, Shukla M, Schulman J, Stevens RL, Sullivan DE, Vonstein V, Warren A, Will R, Wilson MJC, Yoo HS, Zhang C, Zhang Y, Sobral BW. 2014. PATRIC, the bacterial bioinformatics database and analysis resource. *Nucleic Acids Res* 42(D1):D581–D591.

350. Carattoli A, Zankari E, García-Fernández A, Voldby Larsen M, Lund O, Villa L, Møller Aarestrup F, Hasman H. 2014. *In silico* detection and typing of plasmids using PlasmidFinder and plasmid multilocus sequence typing. *Antimicrob Agents Chemother* 58:3895–3903.

351. Johnsen PJ, Townsend JP, Bøhn T, Simonsen GS, Sundsfjord A, Nielsen KM. 2011. Retrospective evidence for a biological cost of vancomycin resistance determinants in the absence of glycopeptide selective pressures. *J Antimicrob Chemother* 66:608–610.

352. Freitas AR, Tedim AP, Francia MV, Jensen LB, Novais C, Peixe L, Sánchez-Valenzuela A, Sundsfjord A, Hegstad K, Werner G, Sadowy E, Hammerum AM, Garcia-Migura L, Willems RJ, Baquero F, Coque TM. 2016. Multilevel population genetic analysis of *vanA* and *vanB Enterococcus faecium* causing nosocomial outbreaks in 27 countries (1986–2012). *J Antimicrob Chemother* 71:3351–3366.

353. Lanza VF, Tedim AP, Martínez JL, Baquero F, Coque TM. 2015. The plasmidome of *Firmicutes*: impact on the emergence and the spread of resistance to antimicrobials. *Microbiol Spectr* 3:PLAS-0039-2014.

354. Sletvold H, Johnsen PJ, Hamre I, Simonsen GS, Sundsfjord A, Nielsen KM. 2008. Complete sequence of *Enterococcus faecium* pVEF3 and the detection of an

omega-epsilon-zeta toxin-antitoxin module and an ABC transporter. *Plasmid* **60**:75–85.

355. Sletvold H, Johnsen PJ, Wikmark OG, Simonsen GS, Sundsfjord A, Nielsen KM. 2010. Tn*1546* is part of a larger plasmid-encoded genetic unit horizontally disseminated among clonal *Enterococcus faecium* lineages. *J Antimicrob Chemother* **65**:1894–1906.

356. Garcia-Migura L, Hasman H, Svendsen C, Jensen LB. 2008. Relevance of hot spots in the evolution and transmission of Tn*1546* in glycopeptide-resistant *Enterococcus faecium* (GREF) from broiler origin. *J Antimicrob Chemother* **62**:681–687.

357. Moura TM, Cassenego AP, Campos FS, Ribeiro AM, Franco AC, d'Azevedo PA, Frazzon J, Frazzon AP. 2013. Detection of *vanC1* gene transcription in vancomycin-susceptible *Enterococcus faecalis*. *Mem Inst Oswaldo Cruz* **108**:453–456.

358. Schwaiger K, Bauer J, Hörmansdorfer S, Mölle G, Preikschat P, Kämpf P, Bauer-Unkauf I, Bischoff M, Hölzel C. 2012. Presence of the resistance genes *vanC1* and *pbp5* in phenotypically vancomycin and ampicillin susceptible *Enterococcus faecalis*. *Microb Drug Resist* **18**:434–439.

359. Batista Xavier D, Moreno Bernal FE, Titze-de-Almeida R. 2006. Absence of VanA- and VanB-containing enterococci in poultry raised on nonintensive production farms in Brazil. *Appl Environ Microbiol* **72**:3072–3073.

360. Mammina C, Di Noto AM, Costa A, Nastasi A. 2005. VanB-VanC1 *Enterococcus gallinarum*, Italy. *Emerg Infect Dis* **11**:1491–1492.

361. Mikalsen T, Pedersen T, Willems R, Coque TM, Werner G, Sadowy E, van Schaik W, Jensen LB, Sundsfjord A, Hegstad K. 2015. Investigating the mobilome in clinically important lineages of *Enterococcus faecium* and *Enterococcus faecalis*. *BMC Genomics* **16**:282.

362. Teuber M, Schwarz F, Perreten V. 2003. Molecular structure and evolution of the conjugative multiresistance plasmid pRE25 of *Enterococcus faecalis* isolated from a raw-fermented sausage. *Int J Food Microbiol* **88**:325–329.

363. Schwarz FV, Perreten V, Teuber M. 2001. Sequence of the 50-kb conjugative multiresistance plasmid pRE25 from *Enterococcus faecalis* RE25. *Plasmid* **46**:170–187.

364. Werner G, Hildebrandt B, Witte W. 2003. Linkage of *erm*(B) and *aadE-sat4-aphA-3* in multiple-resistant *Enterococcus faecium* isolates of different ecological origins. *Microb Drug Resist* **9**(Suppl 1):S9–S16.

365. Khan AA, Nawaz MS, Khan SA, Steele R. 2002. Detection and characterization of erythromycin-resistant methylase genes in Gram-positive bacteria isolated from poultry litter. *Appl Microbiol Biotechnol* **59**:377–381.

366. Thumu SC, Halami PM. 2014. Phenotypic expression, molecular characterization and transferability of erythromycin resistance genes in *Enterococcus* spp. isolated from naturally fermented food. *J Appl Microbiol* **116**:689–699.

367. Schwaiger K, Bauer J. 2008. Detection of the erythromycin rRNA methylase gene *erm*(A) in *Enterococcus faecalis*. *Antimicrob Agents Chemother* **52**:2994–2995.

368. Werner G, Hildebrandt B, Klare I, Witte W. 2000. Linkage of determinants for streptogramin A, macrolide-lincosamide-streptogramin B, and chloramphenicol resistance on a conjugative plasmid in *Enterococcus faecium* and dissemination of this cluster among streptogramin-resistant enterococci. *Int J Med Microbiol* **290**:543–548.

369. Werner G, Klare I, Heier H, Hinz KH, Böhme G, Wendt M, Witte W. 2000. Quinupristin/dalfopristin-resistant enterococci of the *satA* (*vatD*) and *satG* (*vatE*) genotypes from different ecological origins in Germany. *Microb Drug Resist* **6**:37–47.

370. Hammerum AM, Flannagan SE, Clewell DB, Jensen LB. 2001. Indication of transposition of a mobile DNA element containing the *vat*(D) and *erm*(B) genes in *Enterococcus faecium*. *Antimicrob Agents Chemother* **45**:3223–3225.

371. Jackson CR, Fedorka-Cray PJ, Barrett JB, Hiott LM, Woodley TA. 2007. Prevalence of streptogramin resistance in enterococci from animals: identification of *vatD* from animal sources in the USA. *Int J Antimicrob Agents* **30**:60–66.

372. Jensen LB, Hammerum AM, Aarestrup FM. 2000. Linkage of *vat*(E) and *erm*(B) in streptogamin-resistant *Enterococcus faecium* isolates from Europe. *Antimicrob Agents Chemother* **44**:2231–2232.

373. Jensen LB, Hammerum AM, Bager F, Aarestrup FM. 2002. Streptogramin resistance among *Enterococcus faecium* isolated from production animals in Denmark in 1997. *Microb Drug Resist* **8**:369–374.

374. Sørensen TL, Blom M, Monnet DL, Frimodt-Møller N, Poulsen RL, Espersen F. 2001. Transient intestinal carriage after ingestion of antibiotic-resistant *Enterococcus faecium* from chicken and pork. *N Engl J Med* **345**:1161–1166.

375. Smith DL, Johnson JA, Harris AD, Furuno JP, Perencevich EN, Morris JG Jr. 2003. Assessing risks for a pre-emergent pathogen: virginiamycin use and the emergence of streptogramin resistance in *Enterococcus faecium*. *Lancet Infect Dis* **3**:241–249.

376. Li XS, Dong WC, Wang XM, Hu GZ, Wang YB, Cai BY, Wu CM, Wang Y, Du XD. 2014. Presence and genetic environment of pleuromutilin-lincosamide-streptogramin A resistance gene lsa(E) in enterococci of human and swine origin. *J Antimicrob Chemother* **69**:1424–1426.

377. Wang XM, Li XS, Wang YB, Wei FS, Zhang SM, Shang YH, Du XD. 2015. Characterization of a multidrug resistance plasmid from *Enterococcus faecium* that harbours a mobilized bcrABDR locus. *J Antimicrob Chemother* **70**:609–611.

378. Zhu XQ, Wang XM, Li H, Shang YH, Pan YS, Wu CM, Wang Y, Du XD, Shen JZ. 2017. Novel *lnu*(G) gene conferring resistance to lincomycin by nucleotidylation, located on Tn*6260* from *Enterococcus faecalis* E531. *J Antimicrob Chemother* **72**:993–997.

379. Liu H, Wang Y, Wu C, Schwarz S, Shen Z, Jeon B, Ding S, Zhang Q, Shen J. 2012. A novel phenicol exporter gene, *fexB*, found in enterococci of animal origin. *J Antimicrob Chemother* **67**:322–325.

380. Novais C, Campos J, Freitas AR, Barros M, Silveira E, Coque TM, Antunes P, Peixe L. 2018. Water supply and feed as sources of antimicrobial-resistant *Enterococcus* spp. in aquacultures of rainbow trout (*Oncorhyncus mykiss*), Portugal. *Sci Total Environ* **625:** 1102–1112.

381. Aarestrup FM, Hasman H, Jensen LB, Moreno M, Herrero IA, Domínguez L, Finn M, Franklin A. 2002. Antimicrobial resistance among enterococci from pigs in three European countries. *Appl Environ Microbiol* **68:**4127–4129.

382. Amachawadi RG, Scott HM, Alvarado CA, Mainini TR, Vinasco J, Drouillard JS, Nagaraja TG. 2013. Occurrence of the transferable copper resistance gene *tcrB* among fecal enterococci of U.S. feedlot cattle fed copper-supplemented diets. *Appl Environ Microbiol* **79:** 4369–4375.

383. Kim J, Lee S, Choi S. 2012. Copper resistance and its relationship to erythromycin resistance in *Enterococcus* isolates from bovine milk samples in Korea. *J Microbiol* **50:**540–543.

384. Hasman H, Kempf I, Chidaine B, Cariolet R, Ersbøll AK, Houe H, Bruun Hansen HC, Aarestrup FM. 2006. Copper resistance in *Enterococcus faecium*, mediated by the *tcrB* gene, is selected by supplementation of pig feed with copper sulfate. *Appl Environ Microbiol* **72:**5784–5789.

385. Amachawadi RG, Scott HM, Vinasco J, Tokach MD, Dritz SS, Nelssen JL, Nagaraja TG. 2015. Effects of in-feed copper, chlortetracycline, and tylosin on the prevalence of transferable copper resistance gene, *tcrB*, among fecal enterococci of weaned piglets. *Foodborne Pathog Dis* **12:**670–678.

386. Pasquaroli S, Di Cesare A, Vignaroli C, Conti G, Citterio B, Biavasco F. 2014. Erythromycin- and copper-resistant *Enterococcus hirae* from marine sediment and co-transfer of *erm*(B) and *tcrB* to human *Enterococcus faecalis*. *Diagn Microbiol Infect Dis* **80:**26–28.

387. Zhang S, Wang D, Wang Y, Hasman H, Aarestrup FM, Alwathnani HA, Zhu YG, Rensing C. 2015. Genome sequences of copper resistant and sensitive *Enterococcus faecalis* strains isolated from copper-fed pigs in Denmark. *Stand Genomic Sci* **10:**35.

Antimicrobial Resistance in Bacteria from Livestock and Companion Animals
Edited by Frank Møller Aarestrup, Stefan Schwarz, Jianzhong Shen, and Lina Cavaco
© 2018 American Society for Microbiology, Washington, DC
doi:10.1128/microbiolspec.ARBA-0004-2016

Antimicrobial Resistance in *Rhodococcus equi*

10

Steeve Giguère[1], Londa J. Berghaus[1], and Jennifer M. Willingham-Lane[1]

INTRODUCTION

Rhodococcus equi, a Gram-positive facultative intracellular pathogen, is one of the most important causes of disease in foals between 3 weeks and 5 months of age. *R. equi* has also emerged as a common opportunistic pathogen in immunocompromised people, especially those infected with the human immunodeficiency virus (1–3). Infection in both foals and people is most commonly characterized by life-threatening pyogranulomatous pneumonia, but extrapulmonary infections are also common (3, 4). In foals, extrapulmonary disorders might occur concurrent with or independent of pneumonia, and some foals have multiple extrapulmonary disorders concurrently (5, 6). Because ultrasonographic screening for early detection has become routine practice at many farms endemic for pneumonia caused by *R. equi*, the most frequently recognized form of *R. equi* infection on those farms is a subclinical form in which foals develop sonographic evidence of peripheral pulmonary consolidation or abscessation without manifesting clinical signs (7, 8).

R. equi is commonly cultured from the submaxillary lymph nodes of pigs with granulomatous lymphadenitis. However, the causative role of *R. equi* in these lesions is unclear, because it can be isolated from 3 to 5% of apparently healthy pigs, and experimental infection studies have failed to reproduce granulomatous lymphadenitis (9–11). *R. equi* is also occasionally isolated from abscesses or granulomas in the lymph nodes of cattle (12). It has been cultured from rare cases of pulmonary or extrapulmonary infections in cattle, goats, camelids, dogs, and cats (13–17).

Since the 1980s the standard treatment recommendation for foals infected with *R. equi* has been the combination of a macrolide (erythromycin initially and, more recently, clarithromycin or azithromycin) and

rifampin with, until recently, very few documented instances of resistance to these drugs. This text reviews the available data regarding antimicrobial resistance in *R. equi*, with emphasis on the molecular mechanisms of the recent emergence of resistance to macrolides and rifampin in equine isolates of *R. equi*.

IN VITRO ACTIVITY

In vitro Susceptibility Testing of *R. equi*

Antimicrobial susceptibility testing can be done using a variety of methods, with broth dilution, disk diffusion, and concentration gradient test (Etest) being commonly used by veterinary diagnostic laboratories. The decision regarding which method to use is based on cost, ease of use, and flexibility to meet the needs of the laboratory. The methods all assess inhibition of growth rather than killing of the bacterium as the endpoint. *In vitro* susceptibility tests must be performed using standardized procedures to provide valid and reproducible results. Although numerous studies have investigated the *in vitro* activity of a variety of antimicrobial drugs against *R. equi* over the years, different methods, media, and incubation conditions have been used. A protocol for antimicrobial susceptibility testing of *R. equi* by broth microdilution was recently adopted by the Veterinary Antimicrobial Susceptibility Testing subcommittee of the Clinical and Laboratory Standards Institute (CLSI) and will be included in the upcoming CLSI document (18). The approved protocol recommends a standard inoculum of 1×10^5 CFU/ml, an incubation temperature of $35 \pm 2^{\circ}$C, the use of cation-adjusted Mueller-Hinton broth supplemented with 2% (vol/vol) lysed horse blood, and reading of the results after 24 h (19). This protocol was recently evaluated in 18 laboratories.

[1]Department of Large Animal Medicine, College of Veterinary Medicine, University of Georgia, Athens, GA 30605.

All 18 participating laboratories were able to perform broth microdilution according to guidelines established by the CLSI, with over 98% of all MIC determinations for the *Escherichia coli* quality control strain being within the acceptable range (18). There was more inter-laboratory variability for *R. equi*, with 72 to 100% of all MICs being within the acceptable range (modal MIC ± 1 dilution), with only one laboratory being below 80% (18).

The results generated by *in vitro* susceptibility tests, whether they are determined by disk diffusion, concentration gradient, or dilution methodologies, are usually presented to the clinician by designating the pathogen as susceptible, intermediate, or resistant. Despite adopting a standardized protocol for antimicrobial susceptibility testing, the CLSI has not established interpretive criteria for the classification of isolates of *R. equi* as susceptible, intermediate, or resistant. Therefore, interpretive criteria reported by diagnostic laboratories are extrapolated from criteria established for other bacterial agents and, for most drugs, based on therapeutic concentrations achievable in people or other animal species. The results of broth macrodilution, disk diffusion, and Etest for *in vitro* susceptibility testing of macrolide-susceptible and macrolide-resistant isolates of *R. equi* were compared recently. Categorical agreement between methods ranged between 85.1 and 100% depending on the drug tested (20). Overall, the agreement between Etest and disk diffusion was better than the agreement between broth macrodilution and the agar-based methods (20). Etest tended to overestimate MICs relative to broth macrodilution for clarithromycin and gentamicin and underestimate MICs for erythromycin and doxycycline (20).

MIC and MBC of Drugs Used Against *R. equi*

Drugs with the highest *in vitro* activity against *R. equi* based on MIC are clarithromycin, rifampin, imipenem, telithromycin, erythromycin, gentamicin, apramycin, vancomycin, azithromycin, gamithromycin, doxycycline, enrofloxacin, and linezolid (Table 1). Trimethoprim-sulfonamide combinations are also active *in vitro* against the majority of isolates. Not all macrolides are equally active, with tildipirosin, tilmicosin, tulathromycin, spiramycin, and tylosin being poorly active against *R. equi in vitro*. Most drugs including macrolides and rifampin exert only bacteriostatic activity against *R. equi*, with only amikacin, gentamicin, enrofloxacin, and vancomycin being bactericidal (21). Combinations including a macrolide (erythromycin, clarithromycin, or azithromycin) and either rifampin or doxycycline, and the combination doxycycline-rifampin are highly synergistic against *R. equi in vitro* (21–23). In contrast, combinations containing amikacin and erythromycin, clarithromycin, azithromycin, or rifampin and the combination gentamicin-rifampin are antagonistic *in vitro* (21–23). However, the clinical significance of these *in vitro* findings has not been established.

Mutant Prevention Concentration (MPC)

Given the recent emergence of resistance to macrolides and rifampin among isolates of *R. equi* (see below), the relative propensity of currently available antimicrobial agents to selectively enrich for resistant mutant subpopulations among *R. equi* isolates has been studied. A common way to compare drugs for selective enrichment of resistant mutants is based on measurement of the MPC, which is defined as the drug concentration that prevents selective enrichment of first-step resistant mutants within a large susceptible bacterial population. The range of concentrations between the MIC and the MPC is known as the mutant selection window, which represents the danger zone for emergence of resistant mutants (24). Minimizing the length of time that the drug concentrations remain in the mutant selection window may reduce the likelihood of development of resistance during therapy. Of 10 antimicrobial agents studied (erythromycin, clarithromycin, azithromycin, rifampin, amikacin, gentamicin, enrofloxacin, vancomycin, imipenem, and doxycycline), rifampin had the highest MPC, indicating that rifampin monotherapy is likely to select for resistance (25). However, combining rifampin with erythromycin, clarithromycin, or azithromycin resulted in a profound and significant decrease in MPC (25). The MPC was well above clinically achievable plasma concentrations for most antimicrobial drugs studied (25).

Activity of Drugs Against Intracellular *R. equi*

The ability of *R. equi* to survive and replicate in macrophages is the basis of its pathogenicity, and strains unable to replicate intracellularly are avirulent for foals (26). Many drugs active against *R. equi in vitro* have been hypothesized to be ineffective *in vivo* because of poor cellular uptake and resulting low intracellular concentrations. Studies with facultative intracellular bacterial pathogens have shown that evaluation of the bactericidal activity of antimicrobial agents against intracellular bacteria is more closely associated with *in vivo* efficacy than with traditional *in vitro* susceptibility testing. In one study, clarithromycin was more active than azithromycin, erythromycin, and gamithromycin against intracellular *R. equi* (27). More recently, equine monocyte-derived macrophages were infected

Table 1 MIC data for *R. equi* isolates susceptible to macrolides and rifampin[a]

Antimicrobial classes/agents	n	MIC (g/ml)		
		MIC$_{90}$[b]	MIC$_{50}$[c]	Range
Macrolides/azalides/ketolides				
Azithromycin	264	1	1	0.06–4
Clarithromycin	264	0.06	0.06	0.008–0.5
Erythromycin	263	0.5	0.5	0.06–1
Gamithromycin	30	1	1	0.5–1
Spiramycin	200	32	32	2–64
Telithromycin	25	0.25	0.25	0.25–0.5
Tildipirosin	40	32	16	8–32
Tilmicosin	278	64	32	0.5–>64
Tulathromycin	278	>64	64	8–>64
Tylosin	200	32	32	1–64
Rifamycins				
Rifampin	194	0.12	0.06	0.008–0.25
β-lactams				
Ampicillin	264	8	4	0.06–8
Amoxicillin-clavulanic acid[d]	264	8	4	0.06–16
Penicillin G	200	4	4	0.03–8
Cefazolin	64	16	≤2	≤2–>16
Cefoperazone	200	32	16	2–64
Cefotaxime	200	8	8	0.12–16
Ceftazidime	64	>32	>32	≤0.25–>32
Ceftiofur	278	16	8	0.25–16
Cefquinome	200	4	2	0.12–8
Imipenem	200	0.12	0.12	0.015–0.25
Aminoglycosides				
Amikacin	64	4	≤2	≤2–8
Apramycin	200	0.5	0.25	0.12–8
Gentamicin	264	0.5	0.5	0.12–1
Quinolones				
Enrofloxacin	264	1	1	0.25–4
Nalidixic acid	200	128	128	16–256
Tetracycline				
Tetracycline	264	8	4	0.5–16
Doxycycline	278	1	1	0.25–2
Other classes				
Chloramphenicol	342	16	8	≤4–32
Clindamycin	264	8	2	0.8–8
Florfenicol	200	16	16	4–32
Linezolid	78	1	1	0.5–2
Quinupristin/dalfopristin	200	18	8	0.5–16
Trimethoprim/sulfamethoxazole[e]	342	1	0.5	0.06–>4
Vancomycin	278	0.5	0.5	0.12–1

[a]Adapted from references 27, 43, 49, 57.
[b]MIC that inhibits at least 90% of the isolates tested.
[c]MIC that inhibits at least 50% of the isolates tested.
[d]Expressed as MIC of amoxicillin.
[e]Expressed as MIC of trimethoprim.

with virulent *R. equi* and exposed to erythromycin, clarithromycin, azithromycin, rifampin, ceftiofur, gentamicin, enrofloxacin, vancomycin, imipenem, or doxycycline at concentrations achievable in plasma at clinically recommended dosages in foals. Enrofloxacin, gentamicin, and vancomycin were significantly more active than other drugs against intracellular *R. equi*, whereas doxycycline was the least active drug (21).

EMERGENCE OF RESISTANCE TO MACROLIDES AND RIFAMPIN IN ISOLATES FROM HORSES

The combination of a macrolide such as erythromycin, clarithromycin, or azithromycin with rifampicin has been the mainstay of therapy in foals infected with *R. equi* since the early 1980s (28–30), with only one report of macrolide resistance in foals before 1999 (31). During the same period, reports of rifampin resistance were rare and typically associated with the use of the drug in monotherapy (31–33). Over the past 15 years, however, the incidence of macrolide-resistant *R. equi* from foals has increased considerably, at least in the United States. The overall prevalence of macrolide and rifampin-resistant isolates in Texas and Florida between 1997 and 2008 was 4%, with most resistant isolates being identified after 2001 (34). In the same study, the odds of death were approximately 7 times higher in foals infected with resistant isolates (34). More recently, it has been documented that mass antimicrobial treatment of subclinically affected foals has selected for antimicrobial resistance over time, with isolates of *R. equi* resistant to all macrolides and rifampin now being cultured from the environment and from up to 40% of pneumonic foals at one farm (35). While there was considerable chromosomal heterogeneity among susceptible *R. equi* isolates, macrolide- and rifampin-resistant isolates from the farm were all closely related and formed two distinct genotypic clusters (35). To date, isolates of *R. equi* resistant to macrolides and rifampin have been identified from at least five U.S. states. However, the true prevalence of macrolide- and/or rifampin-resistant *R. equi* in the United States and elsewhere is unknown. Reports of macrolide resistance in veterinary isolates of *R. equi* outside the United States have been extremely rare. There is one report of isolation of a macrolide- and rifampin-resistant strain from a foal in China (36). Resistance to macrolides or rifampin has been reported in 3 to 4% of isolates cultured from people (37).

MOLECULAR BASIS OF DRUG RESISTANCE

Macrolides, Lincosamides, and Streptogramin B

Three main mechanisms account for acquired macrolide resistance in bacteria: rRNA methylation, active efflux, and enzymatic inactivation (38). rRNA methylation and active efflux are the mechanisms responsible for the majority of resistant isolates. Most macrolide-resistance genes are associated with mobile elements and thus have the capacity to spread among strains, species, and bacterial ecosystems. rRNA methylation, encoded by erythromycin-resistant methylase (*erm*) genes, results in cross-resistance to the macrolides, lincosamides, and streptogramin B. Efflux of macrolide antimicrobial agents is mediated by members of the ATP binding cassette family of proteins or by major facilitator superfamily transporters. These proteins pump antimicrobial agents out of the cell or cellular membrane, thereby allowing the bacterial ribosomes to function again. The third and less common mechanism of resistance is due to enzymatic inactivation of macrolides by bacteria (39). A very small proportion of macrolide-resistant bacteria do not carry any of the known acquired macrolide-resistance genes described above. These isolates typically have mutations in the V domain of the 23S rRNA genes and/or the genes coding the ribosomal proteins L4 and L22 (40).

Macrolide resistance in macrolide-resistant isolates of *R. equi* cultured in the United States is caused by *erm*(46), an erythromycin-resistant methylase gene that has been identified only in *R. equi* to date (41). The *erm*(46) gene encodes a predicted methyltransferase that targets the 50S subunit of the bacterial ribosome and is most similar (68 to 69% nucleotide sequence identity) to the mycobacterial rRNA methyltransferases encoded by *erm*(38), *erm*(39), and *erm*(40). The *erm*(46) gene is flanked upstream by an open reading frame encoding a putative AAA-family P-loop ATPase/nucleotide kinase domain, and downstream by an open reading frame encoding a putative integrase/Tra5-like transposase with closely related homologs in other *Actinobacteria*. Erm(46) and its mycobacterial counterparts form a distinct branch within an Erm subclade populated by enzymes from various *Actinobacteria* genera including *Streptomyces*, *Corynebacterium*, and *Micrococcus* (41), suggesting that the *R. equi erm*(46) gene has an actinobacterial origin and was likely horizontally acquired via a transposable mobile element.

There was complete agreement between the macrolide resistance phenotype and detection of the *erm*(46) gene, with 100% of resistant (*n* = 62) and susceptible (*n* = 62) isolates testing positive and negative, respectively (41). Expression of *erm*(46) in the macrolide-susceptible strain 103[+] conferred high-level (>256 g/ml) resistance to all macrolides tested (azithromycin, clarithromycin, erythromycin, gamithromycin, tildipirosin), lincosamides, and streptogramin B (41). Expression of the gene conferred a lower level of resistance (8 to 16 g/ml) to ketolides and to the combination of quinupristin and dalfopristin. Expression of the gene did not confer resistance to aminoglycosides, tetracyclines, glycopeptides, β-lactams, fluoroquinolones, and rifampin. Mating experiments confirmed horizontal transfer of *erm*(46) from resistant to susceptible strains of *R. equi*, with transfer frequencies ranging from 3×10^{-3} to 1×10^{-2} (41). To the authors' knowledge, the presence of *erm* (46) in *R. equi* isolates resistant to macrolides cultured outside the United States has not been examined. Macrolide resistance in an isolate of *R. equi* cultured from a foal in China was associated with an A to G mutation at position 2063 in domain V of the 23S rRNA gene (36). It is unknown if the isolate was also carrying *erm*(46), given that the report was published before the discovery of the gene.

The vast majority of macrolide-resistant *R. equi* isolates identified so far are also resistant to rifampin. There are no known mechanisms of cross-resistance between macrolides and rifampin. Rifampin resistance in *R. equi* has been shown to be the result of mutations in the *rpoB* gene (see below). Selection pressure caused by the combined use of rifampin with a macrolide for the treatment and prevention of *R. equi* infection at endemic horse breeding farms might have coselected for the acquisition of *erm*(46) alongside an *rpoB* mutation in specific strains.

Rifampin

Rifampin resistance in several bacterial genera typically results from the substitution of a limited number of highly conserved amino acids in the RNA polymerase β subunit encoded by the *rpoB* gene. This gene is divided into three regions: clusters I, II, and III. In *Mycobacterium* spp., the vast majority of substitutions conferring rifampin resistance are found in cluster I within an 81-bp resistance-determining region corresponding to codons

507 to 533 (*E. coli* numbering) of the *rpoB* gene. Most substitutions associated with rifampin resistance detected to date in *R. equi* are single substitutions within the same resistance-determining region, with mutations at codons 526 or 531 being the most commonly reported (Table 2) (32, 42, 43). The level of antimicrobial resistance has been reported to be dependent on both the location and the nature of the base substitution. However, different isolates with the same substitution have been found occasionally to have considerably different MICs (43). Rare isolates of *R. equi* resistant to rifampin do not have mutations in the 81-bp resistance-determining region (43). It is possible that such isolates have mutations in other regions of the *rpoB* gene, as reported in a small percentage of rifampin-resistant strains of *Mycobacterium tuberculosis*. Alternatively, resistance in these isolates of *R. equi* might be caused by one or more mechanism(s). Several rifampin-inactivating enzymes have been identified in environmental and pathogenic Gram-positive bacteria such as *Bacillus* spp., *Nocardia* spp., *Mycobacterium smegmatis*, and *Listeria monocytogenes* (44–46). A gene encoding a monooxigenase-like protein was identified in one strain of *R. equi* and shown to confer low-level resistance to rifampin by inactivating the drug (47). The role played by rifampin-inactivating enzymes in rifampin resistance in foals in a clinical setting is unknown.

Fluoroquinolones

Fluoroquinolones are rarely used to treat infections caused by *R. equi* in foals because of the risk of arthropathy (48). *R. equi* is highly resistant to first-generation quinolones such as nalidixic acid. However, resistance to higher-generation fluoroquinolones in clinical use is

Table 2 Mutations in the *rpoB* gene associated with rifampin resistance in *R. equi*[a]

Origin[b]	Country	Rifampin MIC (g/ml)	Substitution	
			Codon[c]	Amino acid exchange
Human	Thailand	8	509	Ser → Pro
Horse	United States	64	513	Gln → Leu
Horse	Germany, France	2–4	516	Asp → Val
Horse	France, United States	128–256	526	His → Asp
Horse	France	8	526	His → Asn
Human, *in vitro*	Thailand, NA[d]	≥256	526	His → Tyr
In vitro	NA	≥256	526	His → Arg
Horse	France, United States	8–128	531	Ser → Leu
Horse	United States	≥256	531	Ser → Phe
Human	Thailand	64	531	Ser → Trp

[a]Adapted from references 32, 42, 43.
[b]Species of origin or *in vitro* mutations generated in the laboratory.
[c]*E. coli* numbering.
[d]NA: not applicable.

rare in equine isolates of *R. equi*, with less than 5% of isolates being classified as resistant to enrofloxacin or ciprofloxacin using CLSI breakpoints for other bacterial agents (MIC ≥ 4 g/ml as resistant), and with most isolates classified as being of intermediate susceptibility (MIC 1 to 2 g/ml) to enrofloxacin and susceptible to ciprofloxacin (43, 49, 50). Resistance to ciprofloxacin appears to be more common in isolates cultured from people, with approximately 85% of isolates classified as susceptible (37, 51). Bacterial resistance to fluoroquinolones can be the result of chromosomal mutations coding for modifications in target subunits of bacterial topoisomerases II and IV, by active efflux, or by alterations in the expression of outer membrane proteins.

The mechanisms of fluoroquinolone resistance have not been studied in clinical isolates of *R. equi*. However, *in vitro* selection for resistance to ciprofloxacin in *R. equi* is typically associated with one of seven identified single amino acid substitutions in the quinolone resistance-determining region of DNA gyrase subunit A (52, 53). Mutants with amino acid substitutions at Ser-83 of GyrA were particularly resistant (MIC > 64 g/ml) (53). In the same study, a single amino acid in the quinolone resistance-determining region of *gyrB* was identified and associated with a lower level of resistance (MIC=4g/ml) (53). Some ciprofloxacin-resistant mutants did not have substitutions in the quinolone resistance-determining region of *gyrA* or *gyrB*, indicating that other fluoroquinolone resistance mechanisms such as efflux pumps or alteration in membrane permeability might also occur. The MPC for enrofloxacin and ciprofloxacin ranged between 32 and 64 g/ml, which is well above concentrations achievable *in vivo*, indicating that monotherapy with fluoroquinolones might result in emergence of resistant mutants (25, 52).

Other Antimicrobial Agents

Resistance to aminoglycosides in clinical use such as gentamicin and amikacin and to glycopeptides such as vancomycin is extremely rare (20, 37, 43, 49). In one study, an inducible glycopeptide-resistance operon (*vanO*) was described in a single isolate of *R. equi* from soil (54). The *vanO* operon had unique gene organization compared to the *vanA* operon in enterococci and displayed structural similarities to putative operon-like clusters detected in actinomycetes (54). The *vanO* operon is located on the chromosome, and attempts at transferring vancomycin resistance by conjugation or transformation were not successful (54). The molecular mechanisms of antimicrobial resistance to other antimicrobial agents in *R. equi* have not been studied. The genome of the *R. equi* reference strain 103S contains an array of putative antimicrobial-resistance determinants, including a variety of antibiotic-inactivation enzymes, β-lactamases, and multidrug efflux systems (55). However, the functionality of these putative determinants has not been confirmed. Isolates of *R. equi* have been reported to be resistant to a variety of antimicrobial agents and drug classes. These findings must be interpreted in the context of the lack of CLSI-approved breakpoints for *R. equi*. Therefore, breakpoints for the classification of isolates of *R. equi* as susceptible, intermediate, or resistant are CLSI breakpoints for other species, and bacterial agents used have not been consistent between studies.

R. equi isolates are typically resistant or of intermediate susceptibility to most β-lactam antimicrobial agents, with the exception of the carbapenems such as imipenem or meropenem (Table 1). Resistance to carbapenems is rare, and low-level imipenem resistance has been associated with an altered penicillin-binding protein pattern (56). Most isolates of *R. equi* are of intermediate susceptibility to tetracyclines and chloramphenicol, and resistance is not uncommon. However, resistance to doxycycline is extremely rare (<1% of isolates) (20, 43, 49). Most isolates of *R. equi* are susceptible to combinations of trimethoprim-sulfonamide, but resistance is not uncommon.

CONCLUSIONS

Our understanding of the molecular mechanisms of macrolide and rifampin resistance in *R. equi* has improved considerably in the past few years. However, further work is needed to assess the overall prevalence of macrolide and rifampin resistance in isolates of *R. equi*. Resistance to other antimicrobial agents such as tetracyclines, chloramphenicol, trimethoprim-sulfa, and fluoroquinolones is not uncommon, and more work is needed to characterize the molecular mechanisms of resistance to these drugs.

Acknowledgments. The authors acknowledge support from the Morris Animal Foundation, the Grayson Jockey Club Research Foundation, and the Hodgson Equine Research Endowment of the University of Georgia.

Citation. Giguère S, Berghaus LJ, Willingham-Lane JM. 2017. Antimicrobial resistance in *Rhodococcus equi*. Microbiol Spectrum 5(5):ARBA-0004-2016.

References

1. **Arlotti M, Zoboli G, Moscatelli GL, Magnani G, Maserati R, Borghi V, Andreoni M, Libanore M, Bonazzi L, Piscina A, Ciammarughi R.** 1996. *Rhodococcus equi* infection in HIV-positive subjects: a retrospective analysis of 24 cases. *Scand J Infect Dis* **28:**463–467.

2. Donisi A, Suardi MG, Casari S, Longo M, Cadeo GP, Carosi G. 1996. *Rhodococcus equi* infection in HIV-infected patients. *AIDS* 10:359–362.

3. Yamshchikov AV, Schuetz A, Lyon GM. 2010. *Rhodococcus equi* infection. *Lancet Infect Dis* 10:350–359.

4. Giguère S, Cohen ND, Chaffin MK, Hines SA, Hondalus MK, Prescott JF, Slovis NM. 2011. *Rhodococcus equi*: clinical manifestations, virulence, and immunity. *J Vet Intern Med* 25:1221–1230.

5. Reuss SM, Chaffin MK, Cohen ND. 2009. Extrapulmonary disorders associated with *Rhodococcus equi* infection in foals: 150 cases (1987–2007). *J Am Vet Med Assoc* 235:855–863.

6. Zink MC, Yager JA, Smart NL. 1986. *Corynebacterium equi* infections in horses, 1958–1984: a review of 131 cases. *Can Vet J* 27:213–217.

7. Slovis NM, McCracken JL, Mundy G. 2005. How to use thoracic ultrasound to screen foals for *Rhodococcus equi* at affected farms. *Proc Am Assoc Equine Pract* 51:274–278.

8. Venner M, Kerth R, Klug E. 2007. Evaluation of tulathromycin in the treatment of pulmonary abscesses in foals. *Vet J* 174:418–421.

9. Komijn RE, Wisselink HJ, Rijsman VM, Stockhofe-Zurwieden N, Bakker D, van Zijderveld FG, Eger T, Wagenaar JA, Putirulan FF, Urlings BA. 2007. Granulomatous lesions in lymph nodes of slaughter pigs bacteriologically negative for *Mycobacterium avium* subsp. *avium* and positive for *Rhodococcus equi*. *Vet Microbiol* 120:352–357.

10. Madarame H, Yaegashi R, Fukunaga N, Matsukuma M, Mutoh K, Morisawa N, Sasaki Y, Tsubaki S, Hasegawa Y, Takai S. 1998. Pathogenicity of *Rhodococcus equi* strains possessing virulence-associated 15- to 17-kDa and 20-kDa antigens: experimental and natural cases in pigs. *J Comp Pathol* 119:397–405.

11. Takai S, Fukunaga N, Ochiai S, Sakai T, Sasaki Y, Tsubaki S. 1996. Isolation of virulent and intermediately virulent *Rhodococcus equi* from soil and sand on parks and yards in Japan. *J Vet Med Sci* 58:669–672.

12. Flynn O, Quigley F, Costello E, O'Grady D, Gogarty A, Mc Guirk J, Takai S. 2001. Virulence-associated protein characterisation of *Rhodococcus equi* isolated from bovine lymph nodes. *Vet Microbiol* 78:221–228.

13. Hong CB, Donahue JM. 1995. *Rhodococcus equi*-associated necrotizing lymphadenitis in a llama. *J Comp Pathol* 113:85–88.

14. Kinne J, Madarame H, Takai S, Jose S, Wernery U. 2011. Disseminated *Rhodococcus equi* infection in dromedary camels (*Camelus dromedarius*). *Vet Microbiol* 149:269–272.

15. Tkachuk-Saad O, Lusis P, Welsh RD, Prescott JF. 1998. *Rhodococcus equi* infections in goats. *Vet Rec* 143:311–312.

16. Bryan LK, Clark SD, Diaz-Delgado J, Lawhon SD, Edwards JF. 2016. *Rhodococcus equi* infections in dogs. *Vet Pathol*.

17. Takai S, Martens RJ, Julian A, Garcia Ribeiro M, Rodrigues de Farias M, Sasaki Y, Inuzuka K, Kakuda T, Tsubaki S, Prescott JF. 2003. Virulence of *Rhodococcus equi* isolated from cats and dogs. *J Clin Microbiol* 41:4468–4470.

18. Riesenberg A, Kaspar H, Feßler AT, Werckenthin C, Schwarz S. 2016. Susceptibility testing of *Rhodococcus equi*: an interlaboratory test. *Vet Microbiol* 194:30–35.

19. Riesenberg A, Feßler AT, Frömke C, Kadlec K, Klarmann D, Kreienbrock L, Werckenthin C, Schwarz S. 2013. Harmonization of antimicrobial susceptibility testing by broth microdilution for *Rhodococcus equi* of animal origin. *J Antimicrob Chemother* 68:2173–2175.

20. Berghaus LJ, Giguère S, Guldbech K, Warner E, Ugorji U, Berghaus RD. 2015. Comparison of Etest, disk diffusion, and broth macrodilution for *in vitro* susceptibility testing of *Rhodococcus equi*. *J Clin Microbiol* 53:314–318.

21. Giguère S, Lee EA, Guldbech KM, Berghaus LJ. 2012. *In vitro* synergy, pharmacodynamics, and postantibiotic effect of 11 antimicrobial agents against *Rhodococcus equi*. *Vet Microbiol* 160:207–213.

22. Nordmann P, Ronco E. 1992. *In-vitro* antimicrobial susceptibility of *Rhodococcus equi*. *J Antimicrob Chemother* 29:383–393.

23. Prescott JF, Nicholson VM. 1984. The effects of combinations of selected antibiotics on the growth of *Corynebacterium equi*. *J Vet Pharmacol Ther* 7:61–64.

24. Blondeau JM. 2009. New concepts in antimicrobial susceptibility testing: the mutant prevention concentration and mutant selection window approach. *Vet Dermatol* 20:383–396.

25. Berghaus LJ, Giguère S, Guldbech K. 2013. Mutant prevention concentration and mutant selection window for 10 antimicrobial agents against *Rhodococcus equi*. *Vet Microbiol* 166:670–675.

26. Giguère S, Hondalus MK, Yager JA, Darrah P, Mosser DM, Prescott JF. 1999. Role of the 85-kilobase plasmid and plasmid-encoded virulence-associated protein A in intracellular survival and virulence of *Rhodococcus equi*. *Infect Immun* 67:3548–3557.

27. Berghaus LJ, Giguère S, Sturgill TL, Bade D, Malinski TJ, Huang R. 2012. Plasma pharmacokinetics, pulmonary distribution, and *in vitro* activity of gamithromycin in foals. *J Vet Pharmacol Ther* 35:59–66.

28. Giguère S, Jacks S, Roberts GD, Hernandez J, Long MT, Ellis C. 2004. Retrospective comparison of azithromycin, clarithromycin, and erythromycin for the treatment of foals with *Rhodococcus equi* pneumonia. *J Vet Intern Med* 18:568–573.

29. Giguère S, Cohen ND, Chaffin MK, Slovis NM, Hondalus MK, Hines SA, Prescott JF. 2011. Diagnosis, treatment, control, and prevention of infections caused by *Rhodococcus equi* in foals. *J Vet Intern Med* 25:1209–1220.

30. Hillidge CJ. 1987. Use of erythromycin-rifampin combination in treatment of *Rhodococcus equi* pneumonia. *Vet Microbiol* 14:337–342.

31. Kenney DG, Robbins SC, Prescott JF, Kaushik A, Baird JD. 1994. Development of reactive arthritis and resistance to erythromycin and rifampin in a foal during

treatment for *Rhodococcus equi* pneumonia. *Equine Vet J* 26:246–248.

32. Fines M, Pronost S, Maillard K, Taouji S, Leclercq R. 2001. Characterization of mutations in the *rpoB* gene associated with rifampin resistance in *Rhodococcus equi* isolated from foals. *J Clin Microbiol* 39:2784–2787.

33. Takai S, Takeda K, Nakano Y, Karasawa T, Furugoori J, Sasaki Y, Tsubaki S, Higuchi T, Anzai T, Wada R, Kamada M. 1997. Emergence of rifampin-resistant *Rhodococcus equi* in an infected foal. *J Clin Microbiol* 35:1904–1908.

34. Giguère S, Lee E, Williams E, Cohen ND, Chaffin MK, Halbert N, Martens RJ, Franklin RP, Clark CC, Slovis NM. 2010. Determination of the prevalence of antimicrobial resistance to macrolide antimicrobials or rifampin in *Rhodococcus equi* isolates and treatment outcome in foals infected with antimicrobial-resistant isolates of *R equi*. *J Am Vet Med Assoc* 237:74–81.

35. Burton AJ, Giguère S, Sturgill TL, Berghaus LJ, Slovis NM, Whitman JL, Levering C, Kuskie KR, Cohen ND. 2013. Macrolide- and rifampin-resistant *Rhodococcus equi* on a horse breeding farm, Kentucky, USA. *Emerg Infect Dis* 19:282–285.

36. Liu H, Wang Y, Yan J, Wang C, He H, Forbes BA. 2014. Appearance of multidrug-resistant virulent *Rhodococcus equi* clinical isolates obtained in China. *J Clin Microbiol* 52:703.

37. McNeil MM, Brown JM. 1992. Distribution and antimicrobial susceptibility of *Rhodococcus equi* from clinical specimens. *Eur J Epidemiol* 8:437–443.

38. Roberts MC. 2004. Resistance to macrolide, lincosamide, streptogramin, ketolide, and oxazolidinone antibiotics. *Mol Biotechnol* 28:47–62.

39. Roberts MC. 2008. Update on macrolide-lincosamide-streptogramin, ketolide, and oxazolidinone resistance genes. *FEMS Microbiol Lett* 282:147–159.

40. Franceschi F, Kanyo Z, Sherer EC, Sutcliffe J. 2004. Macrolide resistance from the ribosome perspective. *Curr Drug Targets Infect Disord* 4:177–191.

41. Anastasi E, Giguère S, Berghaus LJ, Hondalus MK, Willingham-Lane JM, MacArthur I, Cohen ND, Roberts MC, Vazquez-Boland JA. 2015. Novel transferable *erm* (46) determinant responsible for emerging macrolide resistance in *Rhodococcus equi*. *J Antimicrob Chemother* 70:3184–3190.

42. Asoh N, Watanabe H, Fines-Guyon M, Watanabe K, Oishi K, Kositsakulchai W, Sanchai T, Kunsuikmengrai K, Kahintapong S, Khantawa B, Tharavichitkul P, Sirisanthana T, Nagatake T. 2003. Emergence of rifampin-resistant *Rhodococcus equi* with several types of mutations in the rpoB gene among AIDS patients in northern Thailand. *J Clin Microbiol* 41:2337–2340.

43. Riesenberg A, Feßler AT, Erol E, Prenger-Berninghoff E, Stamm I, Böse R, Heusinger A, Klarmann D, Werckenthin C, Schwarz S. 2014. MICs of 32 antimicrobial agents for *Rhodococcus equi* isolates of animal origin. *J Antimicrob Chemother* 69:1045–1049.

44. Quan S, Venter H, Dabbs ER. 1997. Ribosylative inactivation of rifampin by *Mycobacterium smegmatis* is a principal contributor to its low susceptibility to this antibiotic. *Antimicrob Agents Chemother* 41:2456–2460.

45. Spanogiannopoulos P, Waglechner N, Koteva K, Wright GD. 2014. A rifamycin inactivating phosphotransferase family shared by environmental and pathogenic bacteria. *Proc Natl Acad Sci USA* 111:7102–7107.

46. Hoshino Y, Fujii S, Shinonaga H, Arai K, Saito F, Fukai T, Satoh H, Miyazaki Y, Ishikawa J. 2010. Monooxygenation of rifampicin catalyzed by the *rox* gene product of *Nocardia farcinica*: structure elucidation, gene identification and role in drug resistance. *J Antibiot (Tokyo)* 63:23–28.

47. Andersen SJ, Quan S, Gowan B, Dabbs ER. 1997. Monooxygenase-like sequence of a *Rhodococcus equi* gene conferring increased resistance to rifampin by inactivating this antibiotic. *Antimicrob Agents Chemother* 41:218–221.

48. Vivrette S, Bostian A, Bermingham E, Papich MG. 2001. Quinolone induced arthropathy in neonatal foals. *Proc. Am. Assoc. Equine Pract* 47:376–377.

49. Jacks SS, Giguère S, Nguyen A. 2003. *In vitro* susceptibilities of *Rhodococcus equi* and other common equine pathogens to azithromycin, clarithromycin, and 20 other antimicrobials. *Antimicrob Agents Chemother* 47:1742–1745.

50. Giguère S. 2006. Antimicrobial drug use in horses, p 449–462. *In* Giguère S, Prescott JF, Baggot JD, Walker RD, Dowling PM (ed), *Antimicrobial Therapy in Veterinary Medicine*, 4th ed. Blackwell Publishing, Ames IA.

51. Gundelly P, Suzuki Y, Ribes JA, Thornton A. 2016. Differences in *Rhodococcus equi* infections based on immune status and antibiotic susceptibility of clinical isolates in a case series of 12 patients and cases in the literature. *BioMed Res Int* 2016:2737295.

52. Niwa H, Hobo S, Anzai T. 2006. A nucleotide mutation associated with fluoroquinolone resistance observed in *gyrA* of *in vitro* obtained *Rhodococcus equi* mutants. *Vet Microbiol* 115:264–268.

53. Niwa H, Lasker BA. 2010. Mutant selection window and characterization of allelic diversity for ciprofloxacin-resistant mutants of *Rhodococcus equi*. *Antimicrob Agents Chemother* 54:3520–3523.

54. Gudeta DD, Moodley A, Bortolaia V, Guardabassi L. 2014. *vanO*, a new glycopeptide resistance operon in environmental *Rhodococcus equi* isolates. *Antimicrob Agents Chemother* 58:1768–1770.

55. Letek M, González P, Macarthur I, Rodríguez H, Freeman TC, Valero-Rello A, Blanco M, Buckley T, Cherevach I, Fahey R, Hapeshi A, Holdstock J, Leadon D, Navas J, Ocampo A, Quail MA, Sanders M, Scortti MM, Prescott JF, Fogarty U, Meijer WG, Parkhill J, Bentley SD, Vázquez-Boland JA. 2010. The genome of a pathogenic *Rhodococcus*: cooptive virulence underpinned by key gene acquisitions. *PLoS Genet* 6:e1001145.

56. Nordmann P, Nicolas MH, Gutmann L. 1993. Penicillin-binding proteins of *Rhodococcus equi*: potential role in resistance to imipenem. *Antimicrob Agents Chemother* 37:1406–1409.

57. Carlson KL, Kuskie KR, Chaffin KM, Libal MC, Giguère S, Lawhon SD, Cohen ND. 2010. Antimicrobial activity of tulathromycin and 14 other antimicrobials against virulent *Rhodococcus equi in vitro*. *Vet Ther* 11:E1–E9.

Antimicrobial Resistance in Bacteria from Livestock and Companion Animals
Edited by Frank Møller Aarestrup, Stefan Schwarz, Jianzhong Shen, and Lina Cavaco
© 2018 American Society for Microbiology, Washington, DC
doi:10.1128/microbiolspec.ARBA-0031-2017

Antimicrobial Resistance in *Listeria* Species

11

Laura Luque-Sastre,[1] Cristina Arroyo,[2] Edward M. Fox,[3] Barry J. McMahon,[2] Li Bai,[4] Fengqin Li,[4] and Séamus Fanning[1]

Currently, multidrug resistance is not a common feature encountered in *Listeria* species. However, as has been observed with other pathogens of importance to humans, *Listeria* species have the ability to rapidly develop resistance to any antimicrobial agent, a feature that represents an emerging and increasing threat to human and animal health. Isolates of *Listeria* have been reported with varying degrees of resistance to commonly used antibiotics, and the first multidrug-resistant *Listeria* isolate was identified in France in 1988. These isolates developed resistance through a number of well-known mechanisms, including target gene mutations, such as within genes encoding efflux pumps, together with the acquisition of mobile genetic elements. This article will focus, in particular, on describing the mechanisms that confer resistance in *Listeria* species to antibiotics, biocides, and heavy metals.

INTRODUCTION TO THE GENUS *LISTERIA* AND SPECIES

Listeria species are small rod-shaped bacteria, typically 0.5 μm in diameter and 1 to 2 μm in length. They are Gram-positive bacteria, facultative anaerobes, and nonsporulating. They are catalase-positive, oxidase-negative, and motile at low temperatures. They grow at temperatures in the range of 4 to 45°C and pH values of 4.7 to 9.6, and have a low GC content. The genus *Listeria* comprises 17 recognized species: *L. monocytogenes*, *L. ivanovii*, *L. grayi*, *L. innocua*, *L. seeligeri*, *L. welshimeri*, *L. marthii*, *L. fleischmannii*, *L. floridensis*, *L. aquatica*, *L. newyorkensis*, *L. cornellensis*, *L. rocour-*

tiae, *L. weihenstephanensis*, *L. grandensis*, *L. riparia*, and *L. booriae* (Fig. 1) (1). *Listeria* species can be classified into *Listeria sensu stricto* (*L. monocytogenes*, *L. ivanovii*, *L. innocua*, *L. seeligeri*, *L. welshimeri*, and *L. marthii*) and *Listeria sensu lato* (*L. grayi*, *L. fleischmannii*, *L. floridensis*, *L. aquatica*, *L. newyorkensis*, *L. cornellensis*, *L. rocourtiae*, *L. weihenstephanensis*, *L. grandensis*, *L. riparia*, and *L. booriae*) (1).

Phylogenetic studies indicate that the most closely related genus is *Brochothrix*, and there is a relatedness to other Gram-positive bacteria with low GC content, such as *Bacillus*, *Clostridium*, *Enterococcus*, *Staphylococcus*, and *Streptococcus* (2, 3). Orsi and Wiedmann (1) proposed a reclassification of the *Listeria* genus into four genera, *Listeria*, *Mesolisteria*, *Paenilisteria*, and *Murraya* (Fig. 1). The species that belong to the *Mesolisteria* genus are unable to grow at temperatures below 7°C. *Listeria sensu stricto* species and *L. grayi* possess motility genes that enable them to move, in contrast to the rest of the *Listeria* species.

Listeria species can be classified into serotypes based on the serological reactions of listerial somatic antigen (O-antigen) and flagellar antigen (H-antigen) with specific antisera. *L. monocytogenes* can be differentiated into at least 13 serotypes, and these are divided into 4 lineages, I to IV (Table 1) (4). The majority of *L. monocytogenes* isolates cluster into lineages I and II, described by Piffaretti et al. (5). Lineage IV is the most recently identified, and currently few isolates belong to this lineage (6, 7).

L. monocytogenes is an important facultative human foodborne pathogen, and it is the third leading cause

[1]UCD-Centre for Food Safety, UCD School of Public Health, Physiotherapy, and Sports Science, UCD Centre for Molecular Innovation and Drug Discovery, University College Dublin, Belfield, Dublin D04 N2E5, Ireland; [2]UCD School of Agriculture and Food Science, University College Dublin, Belfield, Dublin D04 N2E5, Ireland; [3]CSIRO Agriculture and Food, Werribee, Victoria, Australia; [4]Key Laboratory of Food Safety Risk Assessment of Ministry of Health, China National Center for Food Safety Risk Assessment, Beijing 100021, The Peoples Republic of China.

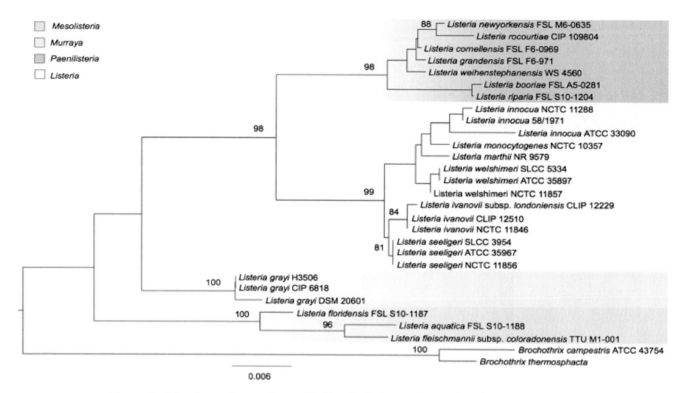

Figure 1 *Listeria* species maximum likelihood phylogenetic tree based on concatenated nucleotide sequences of the 16S rRNA genes from all *Listeria* species. Values on branches represent bootstrap values based on 500 bootstrap replicates; bootstrap values >80% are not displayed. *Listeria* species are color coded according the new genera classification proposed by Orsi et al. (1).

of deaths due to foodborne bacteria the United States (8). *Listeria* outbreaks are distributed globally, causing a significant economic impact on the food industry and public health. This bacterium was first isolated in rabbits and guinea pigs with pronounced monocytosis (9). *Listeria* species are ubiquitous and widespread in the environment. The pathogenicity of *Listeria* species is associated with intercellular replication, and its reservoir extends from the environment to humans and animals, providing an ecological niche (10).

LISTERIA SPECIES IN DOMESTIC ANIMALS AND THE FARM ENVIRONMENT

Listeria species have been isolated from a wide range of domestic and wild animals including mammals, birds, fish, and crustaceans (11, 12). The clinical disease is usually observed in domestic ruminants and humans, though occasionally also in poultry, pigs, rabbits, and other species. Clinical listeriosis in birds is rare, but birds tend to be asymptomatic carriers, because they can ingest this bacterium through contaminated food,

Table 1 *Listeria monocytogenes* lineages and serotype distribution

Lineage	Serotypes	Distribution	Genetic characteristics
I	1/2b, 3b, 4b	Commonly isolated from various sources; overrepresented among human isolates	Lowest diversity among the lineages; lowest levels of recombination among the lineages
II	1/2a, 1/2c, 3a, 3c	Commonly isolated from various sources; overrepresented among food and food-related as well as natural environments	Most diverse, highest recombination levels
III	4a, 4b, 4c	Most isolates obtained from ruminants	Very diverse; recombination levels between those for lineage I and lineage II
IV	4a, 4b, 4c	Most isolates obtained from ruminants	Few isolates analyzed to date

water, bedding, or soil (13). Younger cohorts of bird populations seem to be more susceptible (14). Like rabbits, guinea pigs are also susceptible, and *L. monocytogenes* has also been isolated in canine cutaneous infection (15). There have been reports of symptoms such as miscarriages and septicemia associated with *L. monocytogenes* equine infections (16). The prevalence of *Listeria* in wildlife species ranges from 1 to 60%, although species were mainly captive or domestic (17–19). Less than 1% prevalence was recorded in wild birds and mammals in their natural habitats in Japan (20), while *Listeria* species were recorded in 5% of sampled red fox, beech marten, and raccoon populations in Poland (21). Contact with contaminated silage is believed to be an important transmission vector for livestock infection (22).

Listeria can be classified as a saprophytic bacterium, because its reservoirs are the soil and the intestinal tracts of asymptomatic animals, with soil and fecal contamination resulting in the presence of these bacteria on plants and fodder, particularly silage, along with walls, floors, and drains in the agricultural environment (23, 24).

Evidence indicates that farm systems with cattle species have a higher prevalence of *L. monocytogenes*, including the species that cause human listeriosis, compared to other animals (25). In the addition, it appears that cattle play an important part in the amplification and spread of *L. monocytogenes* in agricultural environments (Fig. 2), while there is evidence of a difference in epidemiology and transmission between ruminant species (25, 26). *L. monocytogenes* can be isolated from cattle farms more frequently during the spring, a feature that may be related to variables including housing with silage feeding during the winter and the application of slurry (27). This would indicate that farmyard environments are reservoirs. The latter feature is not surprising since healthy bovine species with fecal carriage of *L. monocytogenes* as high as 46.3% have been reported (28, 29).

However, the disease ecology caused by *Listeria* species is not fully understood, and fundamental questions regarding the interaction between the hosts, the pathogen, and environment remain to be answered. Specifically, the determinants and mechanisms of transmission from the principal reservoirs, i.e., ruminants, within agricultural ecosystems merit further investigations (30).

OVERVIEW OF THE PATHOGENESIS OF LISTERIOSIS

The genus *Listeria* contains two pathogenic species, *L. monocytogenes* and *L. ivanovii*. However, on rare occasions infections caused by *L. innocua* and *L. seeligeri* have occurred (31, 32). Listeriosis in humans and many vertebrate species, including birds, is caused by *L. monocytogenes*, with *L. ivanovii* infections being specific to ruminants (33). Most infections caused by

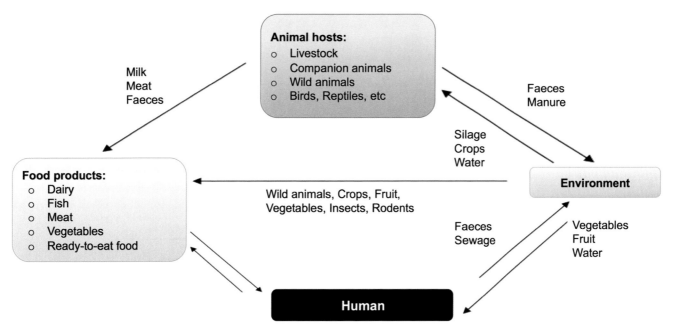

Figure 2 Transmission dynamics of listeriosis involving human and animal hosts. Potential transmission pathways of *Listeria* species are indicated by arrows, and vehicles are represented by colored boxes.

Listeria result from the ingestion of contaminated food such as raw milk, meat, and fish; ready-to-eat meals; unpasteurized dairy products; and uncooked vegetables in humans and from contaminated silage or other sources of feed in animals. The cycle of infection is completed with the liberation of *Listeria* into the environment in the feces. *Listeria* is a saprophyte when it is found in the environment but makes a transition to a physiological state that promotes bacterial survival and replication in host cells (24). *Listeria* has evolved a number of mechanisms to invade and exploit host processes to multiply, spread from cell-to-cell, and evade the immune system without damaging the host cell. The intracellular infectious cycle consists of distinct stages: (i) invasion of the eukaryotic host cell, (ii) escape from the intracellular vacuole, (iii) intercellular proliferation, (iv) actin filament-based intercellular spread, and (v) dissemination to adjacent cells (Fig. 3) (34).

As indicated, *Listeria* is an intracellular pathogen that spreads from cell to cell, and *L. monocytogenes* has evolved mechanisms to evade exposure to the host innate immune defenses. One example of immune eva-sion mechanisms in *L. monocytogenes* is the O-acetyl-transferase (*oatA*), which encodes for O-acetylation of muramic residues contained in the peptidoglycan. OatA increases the bacterial cell wall resistance to antimicrobial compounds such as lysozyme, thereby favoring bacterial persistence in macrophages and virulence *in vivo* (34). However, the host has evolved innate and acquired immunity mechanisms, including the induction of apoptosis and the generation of cytotoxic T-cells that recognize and lyse listeria-infected cells, releasing bacteria into the extracellular space and rendering them susceptible to infiltrating phagocytes (35). (For a more complete description of the bacterial mechanisms underpinning the pathogenesis and virulence of *Listeria*, the following references 33 and 36–39 provide additional information.)

LISTERIOSIS IN FOOD-PRODUCING AND OTHER ANIMALS AND IN HUMANS

Listeria species have been isolated from more than 50 animal species, both domestic and wild (Table 2), with

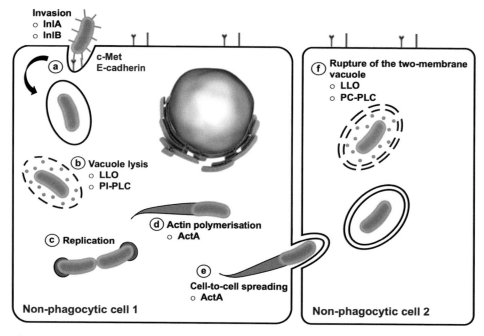

Figure 3 L. monocytogenes *intracellular life cycle.* (a) *Listeria* invades the host cells via a zipper mechanism, by the interaction of surface internalins InlA and InlB with the host cell surface receptors E-cadherin and Met, respectively. (b) *Listeria* escapes from the phagosome before the fusion with the lysosome occurs, by the action of the secreted proteins, the pore-forming toxin LLO, and phosphatidylinositide phospholipase C (PI-PLC). (c) *Listeria* may replicate in the cytosol, and (d) it spreads by actin polymerization, which propels the bacteria unidirectionally, (e) promoting cell-to-cell spreading of *Listeria*. (f) Rupture of the two-membrane vacuole is mainly mediated by the action of LLO and phosphatidylcholine-specific phospholipase C (PC-PLC).

Table 2 Mammals, birds, and other species from which *Listeria* species have been isolated

Mammals	Cats, cattle, chinchillas, deer, dogs, ferrets, foxes, goats, guinea pigs, horses, humans, jackals, lemmings, mice, mink, monkeys, moose, pigs, rabbits, raccoons, rats, sheep, skunks, and voles
Birds	Canaries, chaffinches, chickens, cranes, doves, ducks, eagles, geese, hawks, lorikeets, owls, parrots, partridges, pheasants, pigeons, seagulls, turkeys, white grouse, whitethroat grouse, and wood grouse
Other	Ants, crustaceans, lizards, fish, flies, frogs, snails, ticks and tortoises

presentation of disease varying according to the host (Table 3). Most infections in animals are subclinical, but invasive listeriosis can occur either sporadically or as part of an outbreak (12). Clinical disease is seen most often in domestic ruminants and humans, though occasional cases have been reported in poultry, pigs, rabbits, and other species.

Listeriosis in Food-Producing Domestic Ruminants

In ruminants, infection with *Listeria* and disease are predominantly due to the consumption of spoiled silage contaminated with *L. ivanovii* or *L. monocytogenes*. *Listeria* species can replicate in poorly fermented silage with pH values above 5.5, and these bacteria can reach numbers of up to 10^7 colony-forming units/kg. Other contamination sources apart from silage include barn equipment such as bedding, water, and feeding troughs (40), where bacteria can survive within biofilms. Depending on the number of bacteria ingested, the pathogenic properties of the individual bacterial isolate, and the immune status of the host, listeriosis may present as meningoencephalitis, abortion, or septicemia. It is uncommon for different clinical manifestations to be observed during the same outbreak. The following subsections provide a brief synopsis of the clinical features associated with these presentations.

Meningoencephalitis

Meningoencephalitis (rhombencephalitis) is caused by *L. monocytogenes* and is the most characteristic clinical manifestation of listeriosis in adult ruminants. Indeed, it is among the most common causes of neurological disease in ruminants. A naturally occurring case of ovine meningoencephalitis due to *L. innocua* has also been reported (41). The incubation period is usually 2 to 3 weeks, and the course of the infection is more acute and frequently fatal in sheep and goats (death may occur within 2 to 3 days after the onset of

symptoms) but is subacute to chronic in cattle. Once these bacteria cross the intestinal barrier they can gain access to the central nervous system (CNS) via the blood stream. An alternative route to the CNS is through damaged oral, nasal, or ocular mucosas, where the bacterium can track along the trigeminal nerve terminals with subsequent intraneural direct spread to the brain stem and to further areas of the brain via axonal pathways (42). Clinical presentation depends on the localization and distribution of lesions in the nervous system (30). Early and nonspecific symptoms such as depression and anorexia are followed by neurologic signs, often unilateral, such as facial and tongue paralysis with profuse salivation, nystagmus, absence of palpebral reflex, and dropped ear. The syndrome is known as "circling disease" because it is characterized by a lack of coordination, leaning against objects, head deviation sometimes with head tilt, involuntary torticollis, and walking aimlessly in circles as a result of brainstem lesions. In a further development of the infection, prostration is followed by paddling movements and convulsions before death. The course of the infection is short, extending from 1 to 4 days in sheep and from 1 to 2 weeks in cattle.

Abortion

L. monocytogenes and *L. ivanovii* can gain access to the developing fetus via hematogenous penetration of the placental barrier. Vaginal transmission can also occur. The depression of cell-mediated immunity during advanced pregnancy is thought to play an important role in the development of listeriosis (33). The incubation period can be as short as 1 day, and the outcome of the fetal infection is mainly abortion, though cases of stillbirths have been reported. Abortion occurs in the last trimester of gestation (after 7 months in cattle [approximately 9 months gestation] and 12 weeks in sheep and goats [approximately 20 weeks gestation]),

Table 3 *Listeria* species, hosts, and forms of disease

Species	Host	Forms of disease
L. monocytogenes	Cattle, sheep, goat	Encephalitis, abortion, septicaemia, ocular form
	Cattle	Mastitis (rare)
	Cats, dogs, horses	Abortion, encephalitis (rare)
	Pigs	Encephalitis, abortion, septicaemia
	Birds	Septicaemia
L. ivanovii	Cattle, sheep	Abortion
L. innocua	Sheep	Encephalitis (rare)

and abortion storms are more commonly reported in sheep and goats. In both species, the rates of abortion in a group are low but may reach as high as 15%. Mothers have no other clinical signs, with the exception of fever and anorexia, and it is not known yet why these animals never develop CNS infection or overt septicemic disease (33). If the placenta is retained, metritis may result.

Septicemia

The septicemic form of listeriosis is relatively uncommon in adult ruminants and generally, but not invariably, occurs in the neonate as a consequence of *in utero* infection. It is marked by weakness, depression, inappetence, fever, and death. In this clinical form, multiple *foci* of necrosis in the liver and, less frequently, the spleen may be noted at necropsy.

Other presentations

Mastitis has rarely been associated with *L. monocytogenes* infection and is not as frequent as with *Brucella* species, *Mycobacterium bovis*, *Escherichia coli*, *Staphylococcus* species, or *Streptococcus* species. However, subclinical *L. monocytogenes* mastitis is also reported (43). Gastrointestinal infections can occasionally occur in sheep and goats (44), with dullness, inappetence, pyrexia, diarrhea, and death within 24 hours of clinical signs. Unilateral uveitis and keratoconjunctivitis (ocular listeriosis) are also reported in cattle (45) and are attributed to direct ocular contact with contaminated silage.

In addition to the clinical cases of listeriosis, a significant number of animals within a herd may be subclinically infected and excrete *Listeria* species in their feces, a feature that represents a strong risk factor for contamination of the environment and a means by which the bacterium could gain access to the slaughterhouse (46).

Listeriosis in Other Animals

Birds

Birds are usually subclinical carriers of *L. monocytogenes*. Secretions and excretions from colonized birds are rich sources of these bacteria, and they can play a major role in transmission and spread of *Listeria* species to both humans and animals via the ingestion of contaminated food, feed, water, litter, and soil (13). Outbreaks of listeriosis are occasionally observed in the young animals. Predisposing factors include immunosuppression, wet/damp conditions, moist litters, and cold (47). The most frequent form is septicemia occurring with symptoms including depression, listlessness,

diarrhea, and emaciation. Peracute deaths occur sometimes without other clinical signs (13). The encephalitic form of listeriosis in birds, meningoencephalitis, is a rare occurrence. However, an outbreak of encephalitic listeriosis in red-legged partridges between 8 and 28 days of age has been recently documented (48). Meningoencephalitis in birds is characterized by incoordination, torticollis, stupor, and paresis or paralysis (49). In young geese, both meningoencephalitis and septicaemia can be seen concurrently. Salpingitis is observed in hens during the acute systemic phase (49).

Rabbits

In rabbits, *L. monocytogenes* usually causes abortion during late pregnancy or sudden death. Encephalitis is rare. *L. monocytogenes* was first isolated by Murray et al. as the etiological agent of septicemia in laboratory rabbits and guinea pigs in England in 1926 (9).

Swine

Swine listeriosis is caused by *L. monocytogenes*, but it is uncommon. The primary manifestation is septicemia in young piglets, with death within 3 to 4 days. Encephalitis in adults and abortions are also seen occasionally.

Others

Septicemia and neurologic signs resembling rabies have been reported in dogs, and *L. monocytogenes* has also been isolated in canine cutaneous infection (15). Rare cases of encephalitis or septicemia occur in cats, with typical nonspecific symptoms including depression, inappetence, abdominal pain, vomiting, and diarrhea. In horses, there have been reports of meningoencephalitis, abortions, intrauterine infection, septicemia, and kerato-conjunctivitis associated with *L. monocytogenes* (16). Occasionally, septicemia disease is the usual form of listeriosis in other species, but abortions can also occur.

Listeriosis in Humans

L. monocytogenes is the most commonly reported etiological agent in cases of human listeriosis, though adult meningitis caused by *L. seeligeri* (31), a fatal bacteremia caused by *L. innocua* (32), and various cases of listeriosis caused by *L. ivanovii* (50) have also been reported. The disease mainly affects pregnant women and immunocompromised individuals by either physiological means—due to an immature (in newborns and young children) or suppressed (in the elderly) immune system—by infectious means (arising from immunosuppressive viruses and advanced systemic pathologies), or by iatrogenic means (associated with postchemotherapy or pretransplant immunosuppression). Currently, listeriosis is regarded as a foodborne disease of serious public health concern with a high mortality rate (25 to 30%) and a variable incubation period from 3 to 70 days.

In pregnant women, listeriosis is most commonly noted in the third trimester, but cases have been reported at all stages of pregnancy. The main clinical symptoms documented include mild flu-like symptoms, bloody vaginal discharge, and septicemia, and these may result in premature delivery, abortion, or stillbirth (33). A perinatal listeriosis infection occurs when *L. monocytogenes* crosses the placenta and elicits an infection in the fetus, but cross-infection during delivery is also possible (51). Perinatal infection is classified on the basis of the clinical symptoms observed: an early onset of listeriosis occurs in the fetus or neonate within the first week after delivery and is characterized by a serious septicemia (granulomatosis infantisepticum). Late onset occurs within the 2nd to 4th week of life and is manifested as meningitis with hydrocephalus as sequela (52). In immunocompromised adults, listeriosis can manifest as a rare but severe form of infection including septicemia or encephalitis (meningoencephalitis or rhombencephalitis), with symptoms appearing after 2 to 10 weeks of infection (33, 53).

Healthy individuals (who are immunocompetent) rarely develop clinical signs after infection, though a milder gastroenteritis with fever, abdominal and back pain, headache, and myalgia can occur. The incubation period is reported to extend from 8 to 48 h, and symptoms are typically self-limiting and resolve within 1 to 3 days. Direct transmission of *L. monocytogenes* from animals to humans is reported among farmers, veterinarians, and animal handlers who are in frequent direct contact with colonized animals or healthy carriers. A cutaneous form characterized by a nonpainful, nonpruritic pyogranulomatous rash has been reported in individuals who handle infected newborns, fetuses, or aborted cows or who perform necropsies on septicemic animals (54), while cases of conjunctivitis have been reported in workers in poultry processing plants who handled listeria-positive chickens (13).

CHEMOTHERAPEUTIC OPTIONS FOR THE TREATMENT OF ANIMAL AND HUMAN LISTERIOSIS

Cell-mediated immunity is the main host defense strategy against *Listeria* species and is largely dependent on the action of cytotoxic T-cells—hence the association

between listeriosis and conditions involving impairments of cell-mediated immunity (55). The intracellular lifecycle of this bacterium confounds the efficacy of antimicrobial chemotherapy together with the lack of development of anti-*Listeria* immunity by the host postinfection. However, an anti-listeriolysin O (LLO) neutralizing monoclonal antibody has been reported to increase host resistance to infection in mouse models (56). Anti-LLO antibodies have been shown to help arrest the growth of *Listeria* species within macrophages, and this approach can be used for the serodiagnosis of these infections in humans and animals (57, 58), though it cannot discriminate between a current or previous infection (59), and furthermore, it provides no indication of the duration of this immunity (46).

Antimicrobial chemotherapy is the only viable option for the treatment of listeriosis. For an antibiotic such as a penicillin-based agent to be effective against this bacterium, it must penetrate into the host cell, maintain a high intracellular concentration, and bind to the penicillin-binding protein 3 (PBP3) expressed by *Listeria* species (60). High drug doses and early treatment are essential to treat animals with encephalitis, though if signs of encephalitis are severe, death usually occurs despite the intervention. Treatment in sheep and goats usually has little value soon after the appearance of neurological signs or in chronic cases. According to *The Merck Veterinary Manual* (54), in cattle, chlortetracycline given at a dose of 10 mg/kg body weight per day and administered for 5 days intravenously is effective in the treatment of encephalitis cases. If penicillin G is used, it should be given intramuscularly at 44,000 U/kg body weight per day for 1 to 2 weeks, and the first injection should be accompanied by the same dose given intravenously. Time durations for antimicrobial treatment may vary according to the level of infection. In severe cases, it is often recommended to continue treatment for up to 1 week after the clinical symptoms have disappeared. Supportive care, including the provision of clean housing along with fluids and electrolytes, is an important part of therapy. High-dose dexamethasone (1 mg/kg, given intravenously) at first examination is considered beneficial by some but is controversial and will cause abortion during the last two trimesters in cattle and after day 135 in sheep. Gentamicin has been found to be effective in the treatment of bovine genital listeriosis (61). Other drugs of choice to treat cases of listeriosis in livestock include erythromycin and trimethoprim/sulfamethoxazole. In birds, penicillin, tetracycline, erythromycin, gentamicin, and trimethoprim/sulfamethoxazole may be used successfully to treat the septicemic forms of infection, while treatment of the encephalitic form is usually unsuccessful.

Strategies for vaccine development are currently under study, and these are urgently required to tackle the infection in sheep, though advances in these protocols remain to be validated (12).

In humans, there are specific antimicrobial chemotherapeutic strategies to treat listeriosis depending on the individual and the corresponding diagnosis. Ampicillin or penicillin G combined with an aminoglycoside, classically gentamicin, is the most commonly prescribed treatment for listeriosis (62, 63). However, the combination of trimethoprim/sulfamethoxazole can be used as an alternative treatment. A review by Janakiraman et al. (63) provides information on different treatment options for listeriosis in humans.

RESISTANCE OF *LISTERIA* SPECIES TO DIFFERENT ANTIMICROBIAL AGENTS

Antimicrobial agents have been used in a wide range of settings to eliminate or inhibit bacterial growth. Most of these compounds target unique bacterial cell features including cell wall synthesis, the bacterial membrane, particular stages of protein synthesis, DNA and RNA synthesis, and folic acid metabolism, and depending on the nature of the drug, these can result in bacterial cell death or the inhibition of growth (64).

Bacteria possess two types of resistance: intrinsic, or naturally occurring, resistance and acquired resistance via mutations in chromosomal genes and by horizontal gene transfer (65). Intrinsic resistance usually arises as a result of inherent structural or functional characteristics of the microorganism. An example of intrinsic resistance arises due to the lack of affinity of the antimicrobial compound for its bacterial target in *L. monocytogenes*, and this is found in two cases of β-lactam-based compounds, monobactams and broad-spectrum cephalosporins. In these cases, intrinsic resistance is caused by the low affinity of theses drugs for PBP3, the enzyme that catalyzes the final step during cell wall synthesis. Although a few intrinsic resistance mechanisms in *Listeria* species have been described, most cases of resistance to antimicrobial compounds in this bacterium are due to acquired mechanisms, such as mobile genetic elements including self-transferable plasmids and conjugative transposons (66, 67).

Listeria species are well known for their susceptibility to a wide range of antimicrobial agents. Nonetheless, they possess intrinsic or natural resistance to a select number of antimicrobial compounds. Although natural resistance differs among members of the genus

Listeria, all of the *Listeria* species tested, including *L. monocytogenes*, *L. innocua*, *L. welshimeri*, *L. ivanovii*, *L. grayi*, and *L. seeligeri*, were susceptible or intermediately resistant to aminoglycosides, carbapenems, cefotiam, cefoperazone, first- and second-generation cephalosporins (cefaclor, cefazolin, loracarbef), chloramphenicol, dalfopristin/quinupristin, glycopeptides, lincosamides, macrolides, penicillins (except for oxacillin), and tetracyclines (68). Troxler et al. (68) demonstrated that *L. monocytogenes* and *L. innocua* were naturally resistant to fosfomycin and fusidic acid, whereas other *Listeria* species were found to be naturally resistant only to fusidic acid (Table 4) (68). *Listeria* species differ in their natural susceptibility to co-trimoxazole, fluoroquinolones, fosfomycin, fusidic acid, rifampicin, and trimethoprim (Table 4), while *L. innocua*, *L. ivanovii*, and *L. seeligeri* elaborated a natural resistance to the fluoroquinolones, enoxacin, and sparfloxacin (Table 4) (68).

Listeria species are rarely reported to develop acquired resistance to antimicrobial compounds. Nonetheless, selective pressure imposed in the past following the overuse use of various antimicrobial agents has resulted in members of this genus acquiring target gene mutations and resistance-encoding genes on mobile genetic elements (69). Transfer of resistance genes

Table 4 Intrinsic or natural antibiotic susceptibility and resistance of *Listeria* species

Listeria spp.	Naturally susceptible	Naturally resistant
L. monocytogenes	Trimethoprim	Fosfomycin
	Co-trimoxazole	Fusidic acid
L. innocua	Trimethoprim	Fosfomycin
	Co-trimoxazole	Fusidic acid
		Enoxacin
		Sparfloxacin
L. welshimeri	Trimethoprim	Fusidic acid
	Co-trimoxazole	
L. ivanovii	Fosfomycin	Enoxacin
	Fusidic acid*a*	Fusidic acid*a*
	Trimethoprim	Fleroxacin
	Co-trimoxazole	Pefloxacin
		Sparfloxacin
L. seeligeri	Trimethoprim	Enoxacin
	Co-trimoxazole	Fleroxacin
		Pefloxacin
		Sparfloxacin
		Fusidic acid
L. grayi	All Fluoroquinolones	Fusidic acid
		Trimethoprim
		Co-trimoxazole

*a*Both fusidic acid-susceptible and -resistant *L. ivanovii* isolates occur naturally in the environment.

between *Listeria* species and other bacteria, such as *Enterococcus* and *Streptococcus*, by self-transferable plasmids has also been demonstrated (70).

Multidrug resistance was first documented in *L. monocytogenes* in 1988 in France (71). Since then, other *Listeria* species that are resistant to one or more compounds have been isolated, and several antimicrobial-resistance genes have been identified and characterized (62).

The following section provides a summary of the resistance-encoding genes that have been identified and mutations known to be associated with resistance to different classes of antibiotics, biocides, and heavy metals in *Listeria* species.

Antibiotics

Since the discovery of penicillin in 1929, antibiotics have been commercially used for the treatment of a wide variety of clinical diseases and have also been used for animal production purposes as additives in animal feed (72, 73). Over this period of time, selective pressure arising from the overuse of antimicrobial compounds has led to the emergence of bacteria expressing resistance to one or more of these agents. Similarly, members of the genus *Listeria* have developed mutations in the chromosome and/or acquired resistance genes carried on mobile genetic elements. In contrast and in comparison to other foodborne pathogens of human health importance, *Listeria* species do not exhibit these same features. Thus, data describing antimicrobial resistance in *Listeria* species is limited. Similar to other bacteria, *Listeria* species can express innate resistance to certain classes of antimicrobial compounds. In addition, several resistance genes have been reported to be located on mobile genetic elements such as conjugative transposons and plasmids. Therefore, members of the genus *Listeria* may play a role in the dissemination of resistance genes among bacteria.

Multidrug resistance has been documented in various isolates of *Listeria*, and several antimicrobial-resistance-encoding genes have been identified by means of molecular-based approaches. In the subsections below, a summary of the known mutations and genes associated with resistance to the different classes of antimicrobial agents is provided. The location of resistance genes on mobile genetic elements and the colocation of other markers is discussed.

Resistance to quinolones and fluoroquinolones

Quinolones and fluoroquinolones represent a class of antimicrobial agent which is important for the treatment of severe and invasive infections in animals and humans, with special interest for public and animal health. Quinolones were introduced into clinical use in 1962 in the form of nalidixic acid, and fluoroquinolones were first licensed for veterinary use in several countries in the 1980s (74). Subsequently, their use was followed by the reported emergence of antimicrobial resistance in bacteria. These bacteria were isolated from humans and food-producing animals (69, 75). Resistance to ciprofloxacin is mainly attributed to target gene mutations within the quinolone-resistance-determining regions of genes encoding the bacterial topoisomerase enzymes (76). The presence of plasmid-mediated quinolone-resistance (PMQR)-encoding genes can also contribute to the ciprofloxacin-resistance phenotype (77). Although these PMQR genes confer only low-level resistance to fluoroquinolones, the presence of PMQR (particularly *qnr* genes) may provide a selective advantage for bacteria exposed to fluoroquinolones and facilitate the subsequent development of high-level chromosomal quinolone resistance. In some *Listeria* isolates, the quinolone-resistance-determining region of DNA gyrase subunit A was altered; the deduced amino acid sequences revealed substitutions including Ser84 → Thr and Asp/Glu88 → Phe, both representing amino acid changes at hot spots commonly associated with resistance to these agents (78, 79). Another mechanism, involving efflux pumps such as Lde, MdrL, and FepA (see "Concluding Remarks"), has also been associated with resistance to fluoroquinolones in *Listeria* species (67, 80, 81). Macrolide-based antibiotics and cefotaxime, as well as heavy metals and ethidium bromide, are also exported by MdrL (80).

Resistance to penicillins and cephalosporins

Penicillins and cephalosporins are β-lactam-based antibiotics that inhibit bacterial cell wall synthesis. *Listeria* species are usually susceptible to penicillins, with the exception of oxacillin, monobactams, and broad-spectrum cephalosporins including cefetamet, cefixime, ceftibuten, ceftazidime, cefdinir, cefpodoxime, cefotaxime, ceftriaxone, and cefuroxime, to which this bacterium is naturally resistant (68). Only, the *penA*-encoding gene, a known PBP first identified from *Neisseria meningitides*, has been associated with resistance to penicillin G in *L. monocytogenes* (82). Some of the previously described mechanisms associated with the innate or natural resistance to cephalosporins most often include cell wall-acting gene products, two-component systems, and efflux pumps. The PBPs are enzymes that are responsible for extending the glycan chains in peptidoglycan and cross-linking the peptides between chains. Several PBPs were identified in *Listeria* and function to confer a natural resistance phenotype to modern cephalosporins (83). The gene *oatA* encodes an *O*-acetyltransferase, which catalyzes the acetylation of muramic acid in peptidoglycan, thus conferring resistance to cefotaxime and gallidermin. OatA is important for pathogenesis in mice, probably via protection from macrophage killing (84). Other mechanisms also confer reduced susceptibility to cephalosporins, including the two-component systems CesR and LiaSR, and efflux pumps (MdrL and AnrAB) (85).

Resistance to aminoglycosides

Aminoglycosides inhibit protein synthesis by binding to the 30S ribosomal subunit. Although more than 170 aminoglycoside-resistance-encoding genes have been described in bacteria, these can be grouped into three major classes: acetyltransferase-acting modifying enzymes, nucleotidyltransferases, and phosphotransferases (86). The streptomycin-resistance gene, *aad6*, which encodes for 6-*N*-streptomycin adenylyltransferase, has been identified in *L. monocytogenes* and *L. innocua* (69, 70). To date, no other aminoglycoside-resistance genes have been described in *Listeria* species.

Resistance to tetracyclines

Tetracycline resistance is the most frequent resistance phenotype detected in *Listeria* species. Tetracyclines inhibit protein synthesis by binding to the 30S ribosomal subunit. More than 50 tetracycline-resistance-encoding genes have been described, and five of these—*tet*(A), *tet*(K), *tet*(L), *tet*(M), and *tet*(S)—have been reported in *Listeria* species. Two known mechanisms of resistance to tetracyclines have been reported in *Listeria* species. These are mechanisms that involve efflux of the drug mediated by proton antiporters, conferring resistance to tetracycline only [including the genes *tet*(A), *tet*(K), and *tet*(L)] and ribosome protection proteins, conferring resistance to both tetracycline and minocycline [encoded by *tet*(M) and *tet*(S)]. Two types of mobile genetic elements, conjugative plasmids and transposons originating from *Enterococcus-Streptococcus*, are thought to be responsible for the emergence of resistance to tetracycline in *Listeria*. The *tet*(M) gene is often associated with the conjugative transposon Tn*916*, while *tet*(S) and *tet*(L) are more often carried on plasmids (87).

Resistance to phenicols

The molecular basis of bacterial resistance to chloramphenicol and its fluorinated derivative florfenicol has been reviewed by van Hoek et al. and Schwarz et al. (88, 89). In *Listeria* species, enzymatic inactivation of this drug by type A chloramphenicol acetyltransferases

(Cat) and the export of chloramphenicol/florfenicol by specific efflux proteins are the dominant resistance mechanisms. A *cat* gene (type A-8) has been detected in *Listeria*, located on a plasmid (89, 90). The *floR* gene is associated with the export of florfenicol in *L. monocytogenes*, and 50% of *floR*-positive isolates may also confer resistance to chloramphenicol (82). Florfenicol and chloramphenicol coresistance conferred by *floR* has also been reported in Gram-negative bacteria such as *Pasteurella piscicida* and *E. coli* (82).

Resistance to macrolides (macrolides-lincosamides-streptogramin)

The macrolides (macrolides-lincosamides-streptogramin B [MLS$_B$]) inhibit protein synthesis through binding to the 50S ribosomal subunit of bacteria. The resistance determinants responsible include rRNA methylases that modify the 23S ribosomal target sites, ATP-binding cassette (ABC) transporters, and efflux proteins of the major facilitator superfamily (MFS), as well as factors such as the *ere*-encoding genes that function as inactivating enzymes. The most common mechanism of MLS$_B$ resistance is due to the presence of rRNA methylases, encoded by the *erm* genes. These enzymes methylate an adenine base, which prevents drug binding to the 50S ribosomal subunit, resulting in MLS$_B$ resistance. There are currently 92 MLS$_B$ resistance genes recognized in bacteria (88), but only *erm*(A), *erm*(B), and *erm*(C) have been reported in *Listeria* species (91, 92). Plasmid pDB2011 from *L. innocua*, isolated from prepackaged sprouts in Switzerland, contained three antibiotic genes: *spc* (spectinomycin-adenyltransferase), *erm*(A) (erythromycin-methylase), and *dfrD* (trimethoprim-dihydrofolate); *spc* was located together with *erm*(A) on the transposon Tn*554* (93). In Gram-positive bacteria, resistance to 14- and 15-membered-ring macrolides, such as erythromycin, can also be mediated by efflux pumps belonging to the ABC transporter family, such as *msr*(A) found in *Staphylococcus* species, or to the MFS *mef*(A) found in *Streptococcus pneumoniae* (69, 92). Although several studies have investigated the possible presence of *mef*(A) and *msr*(A) in *Listeria* species, further studies are necessary to extend our knowledge of the possible role of these efflux pumps in *Listeria*.

Resistance to trimethoprim

Trimethoprim is a folate pathway inhibitor, and folic acid is essential for the synthesis of adenine and thymine, two of the four bases that are involved as structural components of nucleic acids. Trimethoprim resistance has been described in *L. monocytogenes* due to the *dfrD* resistance-encoding gene. High-level trimethoprim resistance in *Listeria* is mainly due to the replacement of a trimethoprim-sensitive dihydrofolate reductase by a plasmid-, transposon-, or cassette-borne version. To date, more than 40 trimethoprim-resistant dihydrofolate resistance-mediating reductase (*dfr*) genes have been identified (94). Initially, the *dfr* genes were classified into two major families according to their amino acid structure, *dfrA* and *dfrB*, and currently, six plasmid-mediated families can be distinguished in Gram-positive bacteria, including *dfrC*, *dfrD*, *dfrG*, and *dfrK* (88).

In *Listeria*, only two of these—*dfrG* and *dfrD*—have been reported. The *dfrD* gene was found to be encoded on the plasmid pIP823 (95), while the *dfrG* gene was recently found in Tn*6198*, a Tn*916*-like element associated with a trimethoprim-resistance gene (96).

Biocides

Biocides have been widely used to control the microbial ecology of various niches for centuries. European Union regulation no. 528/2102, covering biocidal products (97), divides biocides into four categories: disinfectants, preservatives, pest control agents, and other biocidal products. These compounds are used in a wide variety of settings including the food and cosmetic industries, for personal hygiene, and for applications in veterinary practice and farming (98). Currently, there is a diverse range of chemicals including alcohols, biguanides, bisphenols, chlorine-releasing agents, iodophors, peroxides, and quaternary ammonium compounds (QACs), among others, that constitute biocides. Reduced susceptibility to these agents has been recognized for decades and is increasing (98, 99).

This section provides a summary of the known mechanisms of resistance or tolerance of *Listeria* species.

Quaternary ammonium compounds

QACs are amphoteric surfactants with a broad spectrum of antimicrobial activity and are widely used as disinfectants in clinical, domestic, and environmental settings (100). The most commonly used QAC is benzalkonium chloride (BC), also known as alkyl dimethyl benzyl ammonium chloride, which targets cytoplasmic membrane permeability functions, causing potassium leakage, osmoregulation disruption, enzyme inactivation, and protein denaturation (101, 102). Tolerance to BC was first described in *L. monocytogenes* and *L. innocua* isolates in 1998. BC tolerance may be conferred by transposons or efflux pumps encoded on the chromosome or on plasmids. One such tolerance mechanism previously described in *L. monocytogenes* was associated with the *bcrABC* operon, which can be

encoded in the chromosome or on a putative IS*1216* composite transposon harbored by the large plasmid pLM80 (103, 104). The *bcrABC* cassette is composed of a TetR-like transcriptional regulator (*bcrA*) and two small multidrug resistance (SMR) efflux pump-encoding genes (*bcrB* and *bcrC*) (103, 104). Another resistance mechanism identified in *L. monocytogenes* is the chromosomally integrated transposon Tn*6188*, which is related to other Tn*554*-like transposons. Transposon Tn*6188* is a 5,117-bp structure found integrated within the *radC* gene, and it consists of three transposase genes (*tnpABC*), along with genes encoding a putative transcriptional regulator and QacH, an SMR transmembrane protein associated with the export of BC (105, 106). The *qacH* gene also confers tolerance to a wide range of QACs including BC, benzethonium chloride, cetylpyridinium chloride monohydrate, cetyltrimethylammonium bromide, domiphen bromide, dodecyltrimethylammonium bromide, ethidium bromide, and the sanitizer Weiquat, resulting in higher MIC values being recorded as well as in increased expression of the transporter (106). Although Tn*6188* has been widely identified in *L. monocytogenes*, Tn*6188* has not been identified in other *Listeria* species to date. The putative EmrE SMR-related efflux pump located within Listeria genomic island 1 (LGI1) in *L. monocytogenes* can also confer tolerance to BC and QAC-based sanitizers (107). There are two MFS efflux pumps, MdrL and Lde, that have also been reported to be partially responsible for BC tolerance in *L. monocytogenes* (108–110).

Triclosan

Triclosan is a chlorinated aromatic compound with a broad spectrum of antibacterial and antifungal activity, which has been used for over 40 years as an antiseptic, disinfectant, and preservative in clinical and cosmetics settings (111, 112). It is bacteriostatic in nature at low or sublethal concentrations, acting to inhibit a specific enzyme, FabI, an enoyl-acyl carrier protein reductase linked to fatty acid biosynthesis, (113–116). Inhibition of FabI results in reductions in lipid biosynthesis (117). At high or bactericidal concentrations, triclosan has a more general membrane-disrupting action, consistent with potassium leakage from the cell (118, 119). It has been shown that point mutations and overexpression of the *fabI*-encoding gene conferred tolerance to triclosan in some bacteria, but not in *Listeria* species (116, 120, 121). Exposure of *L. monocytogenes* to sublethal concentrations of triclosan can cause cross-resistance to several aminoglycosides and exhibit two types of colony morphology: normal-size and pinpoint colonies.

This study demonstrated that adaptation to triclosan may be due to point mutations in several genes including ferrochelatase (*hemH*) or glutamyl tRNA reductase (*hemA*) (122).

Heavy Metals

From a saprophytic bacterium (all *Listeria* species) to intracellular pathogen (*L. monocytogenes* and *L. ivanovii*), maintaining heavy metal homeostasis is central to the survival of *Listeria* species across a broad range of environmental niches. Many heavy metals, such as iron and zinc, are an essential component of cellular function, and bacteria compete to sequester them using a variety of mechanisms such as siderophores and ATP-transporters. As heavy metal concentrations increase, associated toxicity can lead to cell death. Many factors can lead to an increase in heavy metal concentration in niches associated with *Listeria* species. The use of fertilizers or industrial processing can contaminate soil or water environments with heavy metals to levels which can be toxic to bacteria. Similarly, for pathogenic *Listeria* species, both heavy metal scavenging and resistance are necessary for survival and infection. It is becoming clear that heavy metals are an integral part of the host immune defense, either through host sequestering to deny availability or by exploiting their toxicity to kill invading pathogens (123–125).

Balancing the intracellular concentration of heavy metals is thus a matter of life or death for bacteria such as *Listeria* species. Studies investigating heavy metal resistance (HMR) in *Listeria* largely focus on *L. monocytogenes*, although these resistance mechanisms are often found in other *Listeria* species (126, 127). While much progress has been made in identifying mechanisms utilized by *Listeria* in resistance to certain heavy metals (e.g., cadmium and arsenic), less is known about many others (e.g., mercury and lead).

Many genes for HMR in bacteria are contained on mobile genetic elements such as plasmids and transposons (127–129), and as such, they are often found in association with a variety of other genetic markers, some of which may confer resistance to other antimicrobial agents or environmental stressors. Perhaps the most significant implication of this is the possibility of one resistance phenotype coselecting for another (130). Although mobile genetic element-mediated antibiotic resistance has not been frequently reported in *Listeria*, the potential coselection of *Listeria* plasmids containing multiple resistance markers has been reported (127, 131). In particular, heavy metal-mediated coselection of environmental stress resistance markers may contribute to survival and persistence of *Listeria* species in various

environmental niches. Coselection of HMR plasmids may be elicited by a number of factors, including the use of heavy metals in agriculture in fertilizers or supplemented into animal diets as growth promoters or therapeutics (132, 133), heavy metal discharge in industrial wastewater effluent (134), and global mining activities (135). In addition, genetic markers of HMR may be associated with genes coding for disinfectant-resistance determinants (136); as a result, the use of disinfectants in food processing environments, which are frequently colonized by *Listeria* species (137, 138), may also serve to coselect for HMR (139). A multipronged approach will thus be necessary in any effort designed to limit the maintenance and spread of HMR-mediating mobile genetic elements in bacterial populations including *Listeria* species and others.

Cadmium resistance

Cadmium is not essential for the growth or survival of *Listeria* species, and it can be toxic to bacteria at low levels (140). Of all the heavy metals, cadmium-resistance phenotypes and mechanisms are among the most extensively studied in *L. monocytogenes* (136, 139, 141, 142). Resistance to cadmium was first correlated with plasmid carriage, with a *cadAC* operon being subsequently identified as the resistance determinant (143, 144). Efflux of Cd^{2+} is driven by the *cadA*-encoded energy-dependent pump, while *cadC* serves as a negatively acting regulatory protein of the operon (145, 146). The *Listeria cadAC* genes were first identified in a plasmid-borne Tn*5422* transposon and were initially thought to be more prevalent among serotype 1/2 isolates (147). Recent studies have shown a more uniform distribution across serotype 1/2 and 4 isolates (148). Based on the frequency of plasmid carriage, plasmid profiling along with cadmium and arsenic-resistance phenotyping and serotyping has been suggested as a simpler means of subtyping *L. monocytogenes* isolates with acceptable discriminatory power (147). Variations of *cadA* described in *Listeria* include *cadA1*, the Tn*5422* determinant described above, the *cadA2* gene identified on plasmid pLM80 (149), *cadA3* harbored by the EGD-e strain (3, 150), and *cadA4* located on the chromosome of the outbreak strain ScottA (Fig. 4) (151).

Arsenic resistance

Like cadmium, arsenic is also a nonessential heavy metal for bacterial growth and metabolism but becomes toxic as concentrations increase. Arsenic contamination of soil and water environments can arise from a number of sources including mining, industrial processing, and geothermal activity (152). Organic

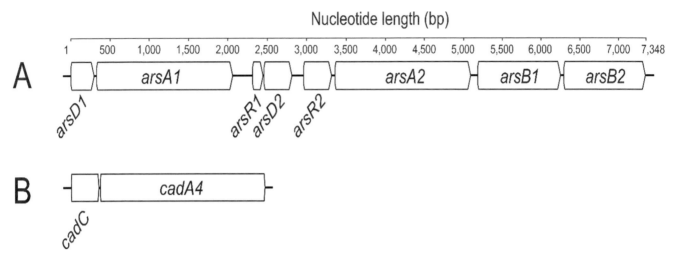

Figure 4   Heavy metal resistance operons in the *L. monocytogenes* strain ScottA. (A) Arsenic resistance operon. (B) *cadAC* cadmium resistance operon.

arsenic is less toxic than the inorganic form, and the use of arsenic has applications in medicine, pest control, and organic arsenic-based drugs. Organoarsenates have also been used as growth enhancers in food production systems (153, 154). Arsenic resistance in *Listeria* has been well characterized, and an arsenic-resistance cassette initially identified in *L. innocua* CLIP11262 on plasmid pLI100 has subsequently been identified in a number of *L. monocytogenes* isolates (Fig. 4) (127, 141, 151). Although harbored on plasmid pLI100, arsenic resistance in *L. monocytogenes* isolates to date typically show chromosomal association (141, 147). In contrast to cadmium resistance, which does not appear to have serotype-specific association, arsenic resistance has been primarily associated with serotype 4b isolates (139, 147). The use of organoarsenates in intensive poultry food production systems has also been implicated in selecting for arsenic resistance in *Listeria* species (139).

Zinc resistance

Unlike cadmium and arsenic, zinc is an essential micronutrient for *Listeria* species and is involved in diverse functions such as metabolism, cell division, and stress resistance (155). Two principle transport mechanisms responsible for sequestering zinc have been characterized in *Listeria*: the *zurLAM* and the *zinABC* operons (155). As with other heavy metals, however, zinc becomes toxic to *Listeria* species as the concentration increases. Elevated zinc levels are utilized in the host response to pathogen infection, and previous work has shown that this is associated with a bacteriostatic effect on *L. monocytogenes* (124, 156). Unlike other bacteria,

cadA has not been shown to contribute to zinc resistance in *Listeria* species (128, 144).

Copper resistance

Although copper plays an important role in cellular function, *Listeria* species must maintain copper homeostasis to combat cytotoxic effects due to elevated concentrations (155). The *csoR-copA-copZ* operon confers copper resistance in *L. monocytogenes* (157). Other genetic markers implicated in copper resistance include the copper transporter CptA and a CutC homolog encoded by *lmo1018* (155, 157). Copper is used as a growth promoter in food animals and, as such, has implications for selection of copper-resistant *Listeria* species; future work should address the implications of this selection pressure on coselection of other resistance markers.

MOBILE GENETIC ELEMENTS ASSOCIATED WITH ANTIMICROBIAL RESISTANCE IN *LISTERIA* SPECIES

DNA elements that can transfer within a genome or to another genome are generally referred to as mobile genetic elements. Transposons and plasmids are among the most commonly described mobile genetic elements in *Listeria* species and have been identified as one of the most important driving forces underlying the evolution of the species (158). As knowledge of the diversity of these mobile genetic elements increases, it is becoming apparent that they are frequently associated with a plethora of resistance phenotypes. Their dissemination through the *Listeria* population raises a number of concerns for food safety and public health; mobile genetic elements contributing to resistance of *Listeria* strains to disinfection regimes utilized in food processing have already been described, and reports are now emerging of resistance to clinically relevant antibiotics (96, 103, 105).

Transposons

Transposons are an important mechanism for the transfer of resistance markers through bacterial populations. A number of transposons and their insert sites (both chromosomal and plasmid) have been identified among *Listeria* species (129, 158), harboring resistance markers to different classes of antimicrobial agents, some of which include the transposon Tn*917*, which is implicated in cadmium resistance and is closely related to another plasmid-borne Tn*5422* cadmium-resistance transposon (144, 159), the Tn*554*-like transposon, which carries an arsenic-resistance operon (158), a Tn*6188* transposon (also a Tn*554*-like transposon), which carries the *qacH* gene and confers increased resistance to QACs, a *bcrABC* resistance cassette, which harbors an IS*1216* composite transposon, a Tn*916* to Tn*1545* family conjugative transposon associated with tetracycline resistance and which contains *tet*(M) (160), and a Tn*6198* multidrug-resistance transposon that confers resistance to tetracycline and trimethoprim (96).

Previous studies have noted the capacity for the transfer of chromosomal-located resistance determinants between *Listeria* species as well as other genera (96, 161), highlighting the potential for proliferation of antimicrobial resistance in *Listeria* species populations. The recent increase in whole-genome sequencing of *Listeria* genomes will undoubtedly expand our understanding of the repertoire of transposable elements present in *Listeria* species and provide insights into their putative transfer patterns. Such knowledge will be crucial in directing future control strategies aimed at tackling the issue of horizontal gene transfers among *Listeria* species.

Plasmids

Maintaining plasmids can impose a fitness cost on the host bacterium, which could lead to that host being outcompeted by other bacteria, in the absence of a selective pressure (162). However, resistance plasmid carriage is widespread in bacterial species, including subgroups of *Listeria* species (147, 163). Recent advances in understanding the factors underlying their ubiquity among bacterial populations have shown that very low levels of antimicrobial agent, often significantly below the MIC, can select for their carriage (164). This is further exacerbated by coselection, because plasmids often confer resistance to many different antimicrobial compounds, such as antibiotics, heavy metals, or biocides, and thus are maintained in bacterial populations by a multitude of selective pressures (103, 165).

Plasmids sharing replication mechanisms generally cannot exist together in the same host, which is often referred to as plasmid incomparability, and this feature forms the basis of incompatibility (Inc) grouping. Although commonly used for classification of Gram-negative plasmids, its use is less common among Gram-positive bacteria (166, 167). Studies relating to *Listeria* species plasmids suggest two distinct groupings based on their associated replicon and genetic diversity (127). Few instances of *Listeria* species harboring more than one plasmid have been reported (168), but more research is needed to understand the dynamics of plasmid carriage and incompatibility in *Listeria* species.

HMR markers are among the most commonly described with regard to *Listeria* plasmids, particularly cadmium-resistance genes (129, 144, 169). These plasmids frequently harbor other resistance markers associated with biocide and/or stress resistance, as well as efflux systems (127, 129, 136). These markers may contribute to the survival and persistence of *Listeria* species in food processing environments and, as such, present a significant concern for food safety and public health (127, 131). Another intriguing observation is the conservation of identical or similar plasmids among isolates from geographically diverse locations, suggesting that strong selective pressures are maintaining plasmid carriage among *Listeria* species (131).

Although the frequency of antibiotic resistance among *Listeria* species has been reported to be low (69, 170), plasmid carriage of resistance-encoding mechanisms to antibiotics including chloramphenicol, erythromycin, and tetracycline has been reported (71, 171, 172). In addition, a recently identified multidrug-resistance plasmid in *L. innocua* conferring resistance to both trimethoprim and spectinomycin exhibited a broad host range (93). The emergence of such resistance mechanisms highlights the need for increased surveillance efforts to attempt to minimize the risk of emergence of clinically relevant antimicrobial resistance in *Listeria* species and in *L. monocytogenes* in particular.

EFFLUX PUMPS ASSOCIATED WITH ANTIMICROBIAL RESISTANCE IN *LISTERIA* SPECIES

Efflux pumps are transmembrane-spanning protein complexes capable of transporting a broad range of chemically and structurally unrelated substrate molecules from inside the bacterial cell to the extracellular matrix

(173). Bacterial efflux pumps have been classified into five families: the ABC superfamily, the multidrug and toxic compound extrusion family (MATE), the MFS, the SMR family, and the resistance-nodulation-division superfamily (174). The most commonly identified efflux pumps found in Gram-positive bacteria are those represented by the MFS family, in contrast to those of the resistance-nodulation-division family being found in Gram-negative bacteria. The latter family is rarely reported in Gram-positive bacteria. All of these systems harness the proton motive force as an energy source, with the exception of the ABC transporters, which use direct ATP hydrolysis to drive the transport of substrates (Fig. 5) (175). In the past few years, several efflux pumps have been described in *L. monocytogenes*.

The first efflux pump to be described in *L. monocytogenes* was *cadAC*. Shortly thereafter, an MFS efflux pump, denoted MdrL, was described in *L. monocytogenes*, and it was reported to export cefotaxime, ethidium bromide, heavy metals, and macrolides (Table 5) (80). Several subsequent studies have also reported on the role of MdrL in the adaptation of *L. monocytogenes* to BC (108, 109). *L. monocytogenes* encodes two efflux pumps that are highly similar to QacA in *Staphylococcus aureus*, and they were identified as MdrT and MdrM. Both MFS efflux pumps confer resistance to cholic acid (176, 177). MrdT and MdrM also play a role during bacterial replication within the cytosol of infected cells, by secreting cyclic-di-AMP, which triggers the production of type I interferons, including beta interferon, which promotes *L. monocytogenes* virulence (178).

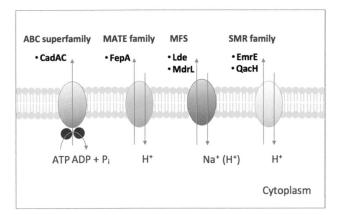

Figure 5 *Diagrammatic representation of the four families of efflux pumps in* L. monocytogenes. *The ATP-binding cassette (ABC) superfamily, the major facilitator superfamily (MFS), the multidrug and toxic-compound extrusion (MATE) family, and the small multidrug resistance (SMR) family. Common examples of the individual proteins that form each class of efflux pump are shown.*

Table 5 Multidrug efflux transporters characterzsed in *L. monocytogenes*

Gene	Efflux pump	Regulator	Substrates
lmo1409	MdrL	LadR	Ethidium bromide
			Macrolides
			Cefotaxime
			Heavy metals
			Benzalkonium chloride
lmo1617	MdrM	MarR	Rhodamine 6 G
			Cholic acid
lmo2588	MdrT	BrtA*a*	Tetraphenylphosphonium
			Cholic acid
			Bile
lmo2741	Lde	Unknown	Ciprofloxacin
			Norfloxacin
			Ethidium bromide
			Acridine orange
			Benzalkonium chloride
lmo1851	EmrE	Unknown	Benzalkonium chloride
lmo2089	FepA	FepR*a*	Norfloxacin
			Ciprofloxacin
			Ethidium bromide
lmo2115	AnrB	VirR	Nisin
			Bacitracin
			Gallidermin
			Cefuroxime
			Cefotaxime
			Ampicillin
			Penicillin
cadAC	CadAC	CadC	Cadmium
			Benzalkonium chloride*a*
			Arsenic
bcrABC	BcrBC	BcrA*a*	Benzalkonium chloride
qacH	QacH	TetR	Benzalkonium chloride
			Benzethonium chloride
			Cetylpyridinium chloride monohydrate
			Cetyltrimethylammonium bromide
			Domiphen bromide
			Dodecyltrimethylammonium bromide
			Ethidium bromide

*a*Belongs to the TetR family.

Two efflux pumps that confer resistance to fluoro-quinolones have been characterized in *L. monocytogenes*, Lde and FepA. The former is encoded by the *lde* gene, whose protein product is a 12-segment trans-membrane-spanning putative MFS efflux pump with 44% amino acid identity with PmrA from *S. pneumoniae*. Lde was characterized in *L. monocytogenes* CLIP 21369 by insertional inactivation of the *lde* gene, and these data demonstrated that this pump conferred resistance to ciprofloxacin and norfloxacin together with a reduced susceptibility to the dyes acridine orange and ethidium bromide (Table 5) (67, 179). Other studies have also suggested that *lde* may be partly responsible for BC tolerance (110). Lde has other interesting functions, because it may also cooperate with a eukaryotic multidrug resistance-related protein (MRP)-like efflux transporter to reduce the activity of ciprofloxacin, a substrate for both pumps, in J774 macrophages infected with *L. monocytogenes* (174, 180). Furthermore, the *L. monocytogenes in vivo*-induced virulence factor Hpt mediates uptake of fosfomycin in *L. monocytogenes*, thereby conferring a resistant phenotype *in vitro* and thus constituting an antibacterial *in vitro-in vivo* paradox, since the bacteria are resistant *in vitro* but susceptible to the drug *in vivo* (174, 181).

Another mechanism that may confer resistance to fluoroquinolones in *L. monocytogenes* is linked with the overexpression of a multidrug and toxic compound extrusion efflux pump, FepA. It has been demonstrated that a single point mutation in the FepA transcriptional regulator *fepR*, which belongs to the TetR family, produces a frameshift mutation that causes the introduction of a premature stop codon, resulting in an inactive truncated protein. This single point mutation was responsible for the overexpression of *fepA*, which confers resistance to ciprofloxacin, ethidium bromide, and norfloxacin, thereby confirming the role of FepR as a local repressor of *fepA* (Table 5) (81).

AnrB, an ABC transporter, confers innate resistance of *L. monocytogenes* to the lantibiotic nisin. The AnrB function was demonstrated by a nonpolar deletion mutation in the *lmo2115* gene, and the loss of this multidrug transporter increased susceptibility to bacitracin, β-lactams, gallidermin, and nisin (Table 5) (182).

In 2015, a novel putative efflux pump, EmrE (324 bp), was described within LGI1 in *L. monocytogenes* (107). An *emrE* deletion mutant demonstrated an increase in the susceptibility to BC along with QAC-based sanitizers but exhibited no effect on the MICs for acriflavine, chloramphenicol, ciprofloxacin, erythromycin, gentamicin, tetracycline, and triclosan (Table 5) (107).

CONCLUDING REMARKS

Listeria species are ubiquitous throughout the food chain and the natural environment, and these microorganisms have been isolated from a wide variety of domestic and wild animals. Since 2009, nine new *Listeria* species have been discovered, and these remain to be further characterized.

Listeriosis may manifest in a mild form, presenting with gastroenteritis-like symptoms, or in a more severe form where *Listeria* crosses the blood-brain barrier and placenta, invading the CNS and the fetus. Antibiotic treatment strategies for listeriosis vary according to the infection type and the nature of the infected host. In humans, ampicillin or penicillin G in combination with an aminoglycoside is regarded as the front-line treatment (63). The primary antibiotics used to treat listeriosis in animals are chlortetracycline, penicillin, tetracycline, erythromycin, gentamicin, and trimethoprim/sulfamethoxazole (61). Although the incidence of antibiotic resistance in *Listeria* species remains low, multidrug-resistant *Listeria* species strains have been isolated from numerous sources including clinical isolates, retail foods, and the environment (69, 92, 183). Furthermore, the range of antibiotics to which resistance has been acquired is broad and includes compounds currently used to treat listeriosis, such as ampicillin, penicillin, trimethoprim, tetracycline, and erythromycin, among others (88, 183). Resistance to erythromycin, rifampicin, trimethoprim, and especially, to tetracycline has been commonly reported in *Listeria* species from Europe and North America and is consistent with the identification of *tet-*, *erm-*, *aad-*, and *dfr*-encoding genes (79). This development may be problematic for patients who are allergic to penicillin because the combination of trimethoprim and sulfamethoxazole is used for the treatment of listeriosis (63).

Multidrug resistance in *Listeria* species has also been linked to the presence of efflux pumps, which confer resistance to a wide variety of antimicrobials, including antibiotics, biocides, heavy metals, and other antimicrobial compounds. Lde and AnrB confer resistance to fluoroquinolones, whereas EmrE, BcrABC, and QacH confer tolerance to BC. Tolerance to biocides is of special concern in food-producing plants and farms, because these agents are used as sanitizers and their decreasing efficacy hinders the elimination of *Listeria* from these environments, increasing the risk of cross-contamination to the final product or animals. Efflux pumps and antimicrobial-resistance genes can be encoded chromosomally or on mobile genetic elements, e.g., plasmid pDB2011 from *L. innocua*, which contains three antibiotic resistant genes, *spc*, *erm*(A), and *dfrD*, and confers resistance to spectinomycin, erythromycin, and trimethoprim, and Tn*6188*, which encodes for the *qacH* gene and confers resistance to QACs. Furthermore, *Listeria* can acquire antimicrobial genes from foreign sources by self-transferable plasmids or conjugative transposons from other bacterial species such as *Enterococcus* and *Streptococcus* (62, 170, 183).

Despite the ever-increasing threat of antimicrobial resistance to human health and the fact that *Listeria* is widespread in the environment and agriculture, relatively little research has been focused on this topic to date.

Acknowledgments. This work was supported by grant 11/F/008 from the Irish Department of Agriculture and Food and the Marine (DAFM) under the Food Institutional Research Measure (FIRM) Network.

Citation. Luque-Sastre L, Arroyo C, Fox EM, McMahon BJ, Bai L, Li F, Fanning S. 2018. Antimicrobial resistance in *Listeria* species. Microbiol Spectrum 6(4):ARBA-0031-2017.

References

1. Orsi RH, Wiedmann M. 2016. Characteristics and distribution of *Listeria* spp., including *Listeria* species newly described since 2009. *Appl Microbiol Biotechnol* 100:5273–5287.

2. Feresu SB, Jones D. 1988. Taxonomic studies on *Brochothrix*, *Erysipelothrix*, *Listeria* and atypical lactobacilli. *J Gen Microbiol* 134:1165–1183.

3. Glaser P, Frangeul L, Buchrieser C, Rusniok C, Amend A, Baquero F, Berche P, Bloecker H, Brandt P, Chakraborty T, Charbit A, Chetouani F, Couvé E, de Daruvar A, Dehoux P, Domann E, Domínguez-Bernal G, Duchaud E, Durant L, Dussurget O, Entian KD, Fsihi H, García-del Portillo F, Garrido P, Gautier L, Goebel W, Gómez-López N, Hain T, Hauf J, Jackson D, Jones LM, Kaerst U, Kreft J, Kuhn M, Kunst F, Kurapkat G, Madueno E, Maitournam A, Vicente JM, Ng E, Nedjari H, Nordsiek G, Novella S, de Pablos B, Pérez-Diaz JC, Purcell R, Remmel B, Rose M, Schlueter T, Simoes N, et al. 2001. Comparative genomics of *Listeria* species. *Science* 294:849–852.

4. Orsi RH, den Bakker HC, Wiedmann M. 2011. *Listeria monocytogenes* lineages: genomics, evolution, ecology, and phenotypic characteristics. *Int J Med Microbiol* 301:79–96.

5. Piffaretti JC, Kressebuch H, Aeschbacher M, Bille J, Bannerman E, Musser JM, Selander RK, Rocourt J. 1989. Genetic characterization of clones of the bacterium *Listeria monocytogenes* causing epidemic disease. *Proc Natl Acad Sci USA* 86:3818–3822.

6. Roberts A, Nightingale K, Jeffers G, Fortes E, Kongo JM, Wiedmann M. 2006. Genetic and phenotypic characterization of *Listeria monocytogenes* lineage III. *Microbiology* 152:685–693.

7. Ward TJ, Ducey TF, Usgaard T, Dunn KA, Bielawski JP. 2008. Multilocus genotyping assays for single nucleotide polymorphism-based subtyping of *Listeria monocytogenes* isolates. *Appl Environ Microbiol* 74:7629–7642.

8. Scallan E, Hoekstra RM, Angulo FJ, Tauxe RV, Widdowson M-A, Roy SL, Jones JL, Griffin PM. 2011. Foodborne illness acquired in the United States: major pathogens. *Emerg Infect Dis* 17:7–15.

9. Murray EGD, Webb RA, Swann MBR. 1926. A disease of rabbits characterised by a large mononuclear leucocytosis, caused by a hitherto undescribed bacillus *Bacterium monocytogenes* (n.sp.). *J Pathol Bacteriol* 29:407–439.

10. Walland J, Lauper J, Frey J, Imhof R, Stephan R, Seuberlich T, Oevermann A. 2015. *Listeria monocytogenes* infection in ruminants: is there a link to the environment, food and human health? A review. *Schweiz Arch Tierheilkd* 157:319–328.

11. Lyautey E, Hartmann A, Pagotto F, Tyler K, Lapen DR, Wilkes G, Piveteau P, Rieu A, Robertson WJ, Medeiros DT, Edge TA, Gannon V, Topp E. 2007. Characteristics and frequency of detection of fecal *Listeria monocytogenes* shed by livestock, wildlife, and humans. *Can J Microbiol* 53:1158–1167.

12. Lopez J. 2008. *Listeria monocytogenes*, p. 1238–1254. *In* OIE Biological Standards Commission (ed), *Manual of Diagnostic Tests and Vaccines for Terrestrial Animals*, vol 2, 6th ed. World Organisation for Animal Health (OIE), Paris, France.

13. Dhama K, Karthik K, Tiwari R, Shabbir MZ, Barbuddhe S, Malik SVS, Singh RK. 2015. Listeriosis in animals, its public health significance (food-borne zoonosis) and advances in diagnosis and control: a comprehensive review. *Vet Q* 35:211–235.

14. Gray ML. 1958. Listeriosis in fowls: a review. *Avian Dis* 2:296.

15. Loncarevic A, Artursson, Johansson. 1999. A case of canine cutaneous listeriosis. *Vet Dermatol* 10:69–71.

16. Revold T, Abayneh T, Brun-Hansen H, Kleppe SL, Ropstad E-O, Hellings RA, Sørum H. 2015. *Listeria monocytogenes* associated kerato-conjunctivitis in four horses in Norway. *Acta Vet Scand* 57:76.

17. Weber A, Prell A, Potel J, Schäfer R. 1993. Occurrence of *Listeria monocytogenes* in snakes, tortoises, lizards and amphibians raised as pets. *Berl Munch Tierarztl Wochenschr* 106:293–295. (In German.)

18. Arumugaswamy R, Gibson LF. 1999. *Listeria* in zoo animals and rivers. *Aust Vet J* 77:819–820.

19. Bauwens L, Vercammen F, Hertsens A. 2003. Detection of pathogenic *Listeria* spp. in zoo animal faeces: use of immunomagnetic separation and a chromogenic isolation medium. *Vet Microbiol* 91:115–123.

20. Yoshida T, Sugimoto T, Sato M, Hirai K. 2000. Incidence of *Listeria monocytogenes* in wild animals in Japan. *J Vet Med Sci* 62:673–675.

21. Nowakiewicz A, Zięba P, Ziółkowska G, Gnat S, Muszyńska M, Tomczuk K, Majer Dziedzic B, Ulbrych Ł, Trościańczyk A. 2016. Free-living species of carnivorous mammals in Poland: red fox, beech marten, and raccoon as a potential reservoir of *Salmonella*, *Yersinia*,

Listeria spp. and coagulase-positive *Staphylococcus*. *PLoS One* **11**:e0155533.

22. **Fenlon DR, Wilson J, Donachie W.** 1996. The incidence and level of *Listeria monocytogenes* contamination of food sources at primary production and initial processing. *J Appl Bacteriol* **81**:641–650.

23. **Fieseler L, Doyscher D, Loessner MJ, Schuppler M.** 2014. Acanthamoeba release compounds which promote growth of *Listeria monocytogenes* and other bacteria. *Appl Microbiol Biotechnol* **98**:3091–3097.

24. **Freitag NE, Port GC, Miner MD.** 2009. *Listeria monocytogenes*: from saprophyte to intracellular pathogen. *Nat Rev Microbiol* **7**:623–628.

25. **Nightingale KK, Schukken YH, Nightingale CR, Fortes ED, Ho AJ, Her Z, Grohn YT, McDonough PL, Wiedmann M.** 2004. Ecology and transmission of *Listeria monocytogenes* infecting ruminants and in the farm environment. *Appl Environ Microbiol* **70**:4458–4467.

26. **Oliver SP, Jayarao BM, Almeida RA.** 2005. Foodborne pathogens in milk and the dairy farm environment: food safety and public health implications. *Foodborne Pathog Dis* **2**:115–129.

27. **Wilkes G, Edge TA, Gannon VPJ, Jokinen C, Lyautey E, Neumann NF, Ruecker N, Scott A, Sunohara M, Topp E, Lapen DR.** 2011. Associations among pathogenic bacteria, parasites, and environmental and land use factors in multiple mixed-use watersheds. *Water Res* **45**:5807–5825.

28. **Esteban JI, Oporto B, Aduriz G, Juste RA, Hurtado A, Roberts A, Wiedmann M, Buncic S, Iida T, Kanzaki M, Nakama A, Kokubo Y, Maruyama T, Kaneuchi C, Skovgaard N, Norrung B, de Valk H, Vaillant V, Jacquet C, Rocourt J, Le Querrec F, Stainer F, Quelquejeu N, Pierre O, Pierre V, Desenclos J, Goulet V, McLauchlin J, Hall S, Velani S, Gilbert R, Giovannacci I, Ragimbeau C, Queguiner S, Salvat G, Vendeuvre J, Carlier V, Ermel G, Nightingale K, Schukken Y, Nightingale C, Fortes E, Ho A, Her Z, Grohn Y, McDonough P, Wiedmann M, Gandhi M, Chikindas M, Fenlon D, et al.** 2009. Faecal shedding and strain diversity of *Listeria monocytogenes* in healthy ruminants and swine in Northern Spain. *BMC Vet Res* **5**:2.

29. **Weber A, Potel J, Schäfer-Schmidt R, Prell A, Datzmann C.** 1995. Studies on the occurrence of *Listeria monocytogenes* in fecal samples of domestic and companion animals. *Zentralbl Hyg Umweltmed* **198**:117–123. (In German.)

30. **Walland J, Lauper J, Frey J, Imhof R, Stephan R, Seuberlich T, Oevermann A.** 2015. *Listeria monocytogenes* infection in ruminants: is there a link to the environment, food and human health? A review. *Schweiz Arch Tierheilkd* **157**:319–328.

31. **Rocourt J, Hof H, Schrettenbrunner A, Malinverni R, Bille J.** 1986. Acute purulent *Listeria seelingeri* meningitis in an immunocompetent adult. *Schweiz Med Wochenschr* **116**:248–251. (In French.)

32. **Perrin M, Bemer M, Delamare C.** 2003. Fatal case of *Listeria innocua* bacteremia. *J Clin Microbiol* **41**:5308–5309.

33. **Vázquez-Boland JA, Kuhn M, Berche P, Chakraborty T, Domínguez-Bernal G, Goebel W, González-Zorn B, Wehland J, Kreft J.** 2001. *Listeria* pathogenesis and molecular virulence determinants. *Clin Microbiol Rev* **14**:584–640.

34. **Cossart P, Lebreton A.** 2014. A trip in the "New Microbiology" with the bacterial pathogen *Listeria monocytogenes*. *FEBS Lett* **588**:2437–2445.

35. **Appelberg R, Castro AG, Silva MT.** 1994. Neutrophils as effector cells of T-cell–mediated, acquired immunity in murine listeriosis. *Immunology* **83**:302–307.

36. **Carvalho F, Sousa S, Cabanes D.** 2014. How *Listeria monocytogenes* organizes its surface for virulence. *Front Cell Infect Microbiol* **4**:48.

37. **Cossart P, Lecuit M.** 1998. Interactions of *Listeria monocytogenes* with mammalian cells during entry and actin-based movement: bacterial factors, cellular ligands and signaling. *EMBO J* **17**:3797–3806.

38. **Pizarro-Cerdá J, Kühbacher A, Cossart P.** 2012. Entry of *Listeria monocytogenes* in mammalian epithelial cells: an updated view. *Cold Spring Harb Perspect Med* **2**:a010009.

39. **Camejo A, Carvalho F, Reis O, Leitão E, Sousa S, Cabanes D.** 2011. The arsenal of virulence factors deployed by *Listeria monocytogenes* to promote its cell infection cycle. *Virulence* **2**:379–394.

40. **Mohammed HO, Stipetic K, McDonough PL, Gonzalez RN, Nydam DV, Atwill ER.** 2009. Identification of potential on-farm sources of *Listeria monocytogenes* in herds of dairy cattle. *Am J Vet Res* **70**:383–388.

41. **Walker JK, Morgan JH, McLauchlin J, Grant KA, Shallcross JA.** 1994. *Listeria innocua* isolated from a case of ovine meningoencephalitis. *Vet Microbiol* **42**:245–253.

42. **Oevermann A, Di Palma S, Doherr MG, Abril C, Zurbriggen A, Vandevelde M.** 2010. Neuropathogenesis of naturally occurring encephalitis caused by *Listeria monocytogenes* in ruminants. *Brain Pathol* **20**:378–390.

43. **Hird DW, Genigeorgis C.** 1990. Listeriosis in food animals: clinical signs and livestock as a potential source of direct (nonfoodborne) infection for humans, p 31–39. *In* Miller AJ, Smith JL, Somkuti GA (ed), *Foodborne Listeriosis: Topics in Industrial Microbiology*. Elsevier, Amsterdam, The Netherlands.

44. **Clark RG, Gill JM, Swanney S.** 2004. *Listeria monocytogenes* gastroenteritis in sheep. *N Z Vet J* **52**:46–47.

45. **Starič J, Križanec F, Zadnik T.** 2008. *Listeria monocytogenes* keratoconjunctivitis and uveitis in dairy cattle. *Bull Vet Inst Pulawy* **52**:351–355.

46. **Ivanek R, Gröhn YT, Wiedmann M.** 2006. *Listeria monocytogenes* in multiple habitats and host populations: review of available data for mathematical modeling. *Foodborne Pathog Dis* **3**:319–336.

47. **Kahn CM.** 2005. Listeriosis, p. 2240–2241. *In* Kahn CN, Line Scott (ed), *The Merck Veterinary Manual*, 9th ed. Merck Publishing Group, Rahway, NJ.

48. **Jeckel S, Wood A, Grant K, Amar C, King SA, Whatmore AM, Koylass M, Anjum M, James J, Welchman DB.**

2015. Outbreak of encephalitic listeriosis in red-legged partridges (*Alectoris rufa*). *Avian Pathol* 44:269–277.

49. Kurazono M, Nakamura K, Yamada M, Yonemaru T, Sakoda T. 2003. Pathology of listerial encephalitis in chickens in Japan. *Avian Dis* 47:1496–1502.

50. Guillet C, Join-Lambert O, Le Monnier A, Leclercq A, Mechaï F, Mamzer-Bruneel M-F, Bielecka MK, Scortti M, Disson O, Berche P, Vazquez-Boland J, Lortholary O, Lecuit M. 2010. Human listeriosis caused by *Listeria ivanovii*. *Emerg Infect Dis* 16:136–138.

51. Lecuit M, Nelson DM, Smith SD, Khun H, Huerre M, Vacher-Lavenu M-C, Gordon JI, Cossart P. 2004. Targeting and crossing of the human maternofetal barrier by *Listeria monocytogenes*: role of internalin interaction with trophoblast E-cadherin. *Proc Natl Acad Sci USA* 101:6152–6157.

52. McLauchlin J. 1992. Listeriosis. *BMJ* 304:1583–1584.

53. Goulet V, King LA, Vaillant V, de Valk H. 2013. What is the incubation period for listeriosis? *BMC Infect Dis* 13:11.

54. Wesley IV. 1999. Listeriosis in animals, p. 39–73. *In* Ryser ET, Marth EH (ed), *Listeria, Listeriosis, and Food Safety*, 2nd ed. Marcel Dekker Inc., New York, NY.

55. Portnoy DA, Auerbuch V, Glomski IJ. 2002. The cell biology of *Listeria monocytogenes* infection: the intersection of bacterial pathogenesis and cell-mediated immunity. *J Cell Biol* 158:409–414.

56. Edelson BT, Cossart P, Unanue ER. 1999. Cutting edge: paradigm revisited: antibody provides resistance to *Listeria* infection. *J Immunol* 163:4087–4090.

57. Berche P, Bonnichon M, Beretti JL, Raveneau J, Gaillard JL, Veron M, Kreis H, Reich KA, Cossart P, Geoffroy C, Geslin P. 1990. Detection of anti-listeriolysin O for serodiagnosis of human listeriosis. *Lancet* 335:624–627.

58. Low JC, Davies RC, Donachie W. 1992. Purification of listeriolysin O and development of an immunoassay for diagnosis of listeric infections in sheep. *J Clin Microbiol* 30:2705–2708.

59. Baetz AL, Wesley IV, Stevens MG. 1996. The use of listeriolysin O in an ELISA, a skin test and a lymphocyte blastogenesis assay on sheep experimentally infected with *Listeria monocytogenes*, *Listeria ivanovii*, or *Listeria innocua*. *Vet Microbiol* 51:151–159.

60. Hof H, Nichterlein T, Kretschmar M. 1997. Management of listeriosis. *Clin Microbiol Rev* 10:345–357.

61. Chopra S, Sharma V, Shukla S, Nayak A. 2015. Antibiogram of *Listeria* spp. isolated from reproductive disorders and livestock products of ruminants. *J Anim Res* 2:187–190.

62. Charpentier E, Courvalin P. 1999. Antibiotic resistance in *Listeria* spp. *Antimicrob Agents Chemother* 43:2103–2108.

63. Janakiraman V. 2008. Listeriosis in pregnancy: diagnosis, treatment, and prevention. *Rev Obstet Gynecol* 1:179–185.

64. Wright GD. 2010. Q&A: Antibiotic resistance: where does it come from and what can we do about it? *BMC Biol* 8:123.

65. Blair JMA, Webber MA, Baylay AJ, Ogbolu DO, Piddock LJV. 2015. Molecular mechanisms of antibiotic resistance. *Nat Rev Microbiol* 13:42–51.

66. Charpentier E, Gerbaud G, Courvalin P. 1999. Conjugative mobilization of the rolling-circle plasmid pIP823 from *Listeria monocytogenes* BM4293 among Gram-positive and Gram-negative bacteria. *J Bacteriol* 181:3368–3374.

67. Godreuil S, Galimand M, Gerbaud G, Jacquet C, Courvalin P. 2003. Efflux pump Lde is associated with fluoroquinolone resistance in *Listeria monocytogenes*. *Antimicrob Agents Chemother* 47:704–708.

68. Troxler R, von Graevenitz A, Funke G, Wiedemann B, Stock I. 2000. Natural antibiotic susceptibility of *Listeria* species: *L. grayi*, *L. innocua*, *L. ivanovii*, *L. monocytogenes*, *L. seeligeri* and *L. welshimeri* strains. *Clin Microbiol Infect* 6:525–535.

69. Morvan A, Moubareck C, Leclercq A, Hervé-Bazin M, Bremont S, Lecuit M, Courvalin P, Le Monnier A. 2010. Antimicrobial resistance of *Listeria monocytogenes* strains isolated from humans in France. *Antimicrob Agents Chemother* 54:2728–2731.

70. Lungu B, O'Bryan CA, Muthaiyan A, Milillo SR, Johnson MG, Crandall PG, Ricke SC. 2011. *Listeria monocytogenes*: antibiotic resistance in food production. *Foodborne Pathog Dis* 8:569–578.

71. Poyart-Salmeron C, Carlier C, Trieu-Cuot P, Courtieu AL, Courvalin P. 1990. Transferable plasmid-mediated antibiotic resistance in *Listeria monocytogenes*. *Lancet* 335:1422–1426.

72. Jones FT, Ricke SC. 2003. Observations on the history of the development of antimicrobials and their use in poultry feeds. *Poult Sci* 82:613–617.

73. Castanon JIR. 2007. History of the use of antibiotic as growth promoters in European poultry feeds. *Poult Sci* 86:2466–2471.

74. Robicsek A, Jacoby GA, Hooper DC. 2006. The worldwide emergence of plasmid-mediated quinolone resistance. *Lancet Infect Dis* 6:629–640.

75. Lyon SA, Berrang ME, Fedorka-Cray PJ, Fletcher DL, Meinersmann RJ. 2008. Antimicrobial resistance of *Listeria monocytogenes* isolated from a poultry further processing plant. *Foodborne Pathog Dis* 5:253–259.

76. Chen S, Cui S, McDermott PF, Zhao S, White DG, Paulsen I, Meng J. 2007. Contribution of target gene mutations and efflux to decreased susceptibility of *Salmonella enterica* serovar typhimurium to fluoroquinolones and other antimicrobials. *Antimicrob Agents Chemother* 51:535–542.

77. Liu J-H, Deng Y-T, Zeng Z-L, Gao J-H, Chen L, Arakawa Y, Chen Z-L. 2008. Coprevalence of plasmid-mediated quinolone resistance determinants QepA, Qnr, and AAC(6′)-Ib-cr among 16S rRNA methylase RmtB-producing *Escherichia coli* isolates from pigs. *Antimicrob Agents Chemother* 52:2992–2993.

78. Lampidis R, Kostrewa D, Hof H. 2002. Molecular characterization of the genes encoding DNA gyrase and topoisomerase IV of *Listeria monocytogenes*. *J Antimicrob Chemother* 49:917–924.

79. Moreno LZ, Paixão R, Gobbi DDS, Raimundo DC, Ferreira TP, Moreno AM, Hofer E, Reis CMF, Matté GR, Matté MH. 2014. Characterization of antibiotic resistance in *Listeria* spp. isolated from slaughterhouse environments, pork and human infections. *J Infect Dev Ctries* 8:416–423.

80. Mata MT, Baquero F, Pérez-Díaz JC. 2000. A multidrug efflux transporter in *Listeria monocytogenes*. *FEMS Microbiol Lett* 187:185–188.

81. Guérin F, Galimand M, Tuambilangana F, Courvalin P, Cattoir V. 2014. Overexpression of the novel MATE fluoroquinolone efflux pump FepA in *Listeria monocytogenes* is driven by inactivation of its local repressor FepR. *PLoS One* 9:e106340.

82. Srinivasan V, Nam HM, Nguyen LT, Tamilselvam B, Murinda SE, Oliver SP. 2005. Prevalence of antimicrobial resistance genes in *Listeria monocytogenes* isolated from dairy farms. *Foodborne Pathog Dis* 2:201–211.

83. Zawadzka-Skomial J, Markiewicz Z, Nguyen-Distèche M, Devreese B, Frère J-M, Terrak M. 2006. Characterization of the bifunctional glycosyltransferase/acyltransferase penicillin-binding protein 4 of *Listeria monocytogenes*. *J Bacteriol* 188:1875–1881.

84. Aubry C, Goulard C, Nahori M-A, Cayet N, Decalf J, Sachse M, Boneca IG, Cossart P, Dussurget O. 2011. OatA, a peptidoglycan O-acetyltransferase involved in *Listeria monocytogenes* immune escape, is critical for virulence. *J Infect Dis* 204:731–740.

85. Allen KJ, Wałecka-Zacharska E, Chen JC, Katarzyna K-P, Devlieghere F, Van Meervenne E, Osek J, Wieczorek K, Bania J. 2016. *Listeria monocytogenes*: an examination of food chain factors potentially contributing to antimicrobial resistance. *Food Microbiol* 54:178–189.

86. Shaw KJ, Rather PN, Hare RS, Miller GH. 1993. Molecular genetics of aminoglycoside resistance genes and familial relationships of the aminoglycoside-modifying enzymes. *Microbiol Rev* 57:138–163.

87. Lancaster H, Roberts AP, Bedi R, Wilson M, Mullany P. 2004. Characterization of Tn916S, a Tn916-like element containing the tetracycline resistance determinant *tet*(S). *J Bacteriol* 186:4395–4398.

88. van Hoek AHAM, Mevius D, Guerra B, Mullany P, Roberts AP, Aarts HJM. 2011. Acquired antibiotic resistance genes: an overview. *Front Microbiol* 2:203.

89. Schwarz S, Kehrenberg C, Doublet B, Cloeckaert A. 2004. Molecular basis of bacterial resistance to chloramphenicol and florfenicol. *FEMS Microbiol Rev* 28:519–542.

90. Li L, Olsen RH, Shi L, Ye L, He J, Meng H. 2016. Characterization of a plasmid carrying *cat*, *ermB* and *tetS* genes in a foodborne *Listeria monocytogenes* strain and uptake of the plasmid by cariogenic *Streptococcus mutans*. *Int J Food Microbiol* 238:68–71.

91. Roberts MC, Facinelli B, Giovanetti E, Varaldo PE. 1996. Transferable erythromycin resistance in *Listeria* spp. isolated from food. *Appl Environ Microbiol* 62:269–270.

92. Granier SA, Moubareck C, Colaneri C, Lemire A, Roussel S, Dao T-T, Courvalin P, Brisabois A. 2011. Antimicrobial resistance of *Listeria monocytogenes* isolates from food and the environment in France over a 10-year period. *Appl Environ Microbiol* 77:2788–2790.

93. Bertsch D, Anderegg J, Lacroix C, Meile L, Stevens MJA. 2013. pDB2011, a 7.6 kb multidrug resistance plasmid from *Listeria innocua* replicating in Gram-positive and Gram-negative hosts. *Plasmid* 70:284–287.

94. Huovinen P, Huovinen P. 2001. Resistance to trimethoprim-sulfamethoxazole. *Clin Infect Dis* 32:1608–1614.

95. Charpentier E, Courvalin P. 1997. Emergence of the trimethoprim resistance gene *dfrD* in *Listeria monocytogenes* BM4293. *Antimicrob Agents Chemother* 41:1134–1136.

96. Bertsch D, Uruty A, Anderegg J, Lacroix C, Perreten V, Meile L. 2013. Tn6198, a novel transposon containing the trimethoprim resistance gene *dfrG* embedded into a Tn916 element in *Listeria monocytogenes*. *J Antimicrob Chemother* 68:986–991.

97. European Union. 2012. Regulation (EU) 528/2012 of 22 May 2012 concerning the making available on the market and use of biocidal products. European Union Regul.

98. Harbarth S, Tuan Soh S, Horner C, Wilcox MH. 2014. Is reduced susceptibility to disinfectants and antiseptics a risk in healthcare settings? A point/counterpoint review. *J Hosp Infect* 87:194–202.

99. Ortega Morente E, Fernández-Fuentes MA, Grande Burgos MJ, Abriouel H, Pérez Pulido R, Gálvez A. 2013. Biocide tolerance in bacteria. *Int J Food Microbiol* 162:13–25.

100. McBain AJ, Ledder RG, Moore LE, Catrenich CE, Gilbert P. 2004. Effects of quaternary-ammonium-based formulations on bacterial community dynamics and antimicrobial susceptibility. *Appl Environ Microbiol* 70:3449–3456.

101. McDonnell G, Russell AD. 1999. Antiseptics and disinfectants: activity, action, and resistance. *Clin Microbiol Rev* 12:147–179.

102. Goddard P, McCue K. 2001. *Disinfectants and Antiseptics. Disinfection, Sterilization, and Preservation*. Lippincott Williams & Wilkins, Philadelphia, PA.

103. Elhanafi D, Dutta V, Kathariou S. 2010. Genetic characterization of plasmid-associated benzalkonium chloride resistance determinants in a *Listeria monocytogenes* strain from the 1998–1999 outbreak. *Appl Environ Microbiol* 76:8231–8238.

104. Dutta V, Elhanafi D, Kathariou S. 2013. Conservation and distribution of the benzalkonium chloride resistance cassette *bcrABC* in *Listeria monocytogenes*. *Appl Environ Microbiol* 79:6067–6074.

105. Müller A, Rychli K, Muhterem-Uyar M, Zaiser A, Stessl B, Guinane CM, Cotter PD, Wagner M, Schmitz-Esser S. 2013. Tn6188: a novel transposon in *Listeria monocytogenes* responsible for tolerance to benzalkonium chloride. *PLoS One* 8:e76835.

106. Müller A, Rychli K, Zaiser A, Wieser C, Wagner M, Schmitz-Esser S. 2014. The *Listeria monocytogenes* transposon Tn6188 provides increased tolerance to var-

ious quaternary ammonium compounds and ethidium bromide. *FEMS Microbiol Lett* 361:166–173.

107. Kovacevic J, Ziegler J, Wałecka-Zacharska E, Reimer A, Kitts DD, Gilmour MW. 2015. Tolerance of *Listeria monocytogenes* to quaternary ammonium sanitizers is mediated by a novel efflux pump encoded by *emrE*. *Appl Environ Microbiol* 82:939–953.

108. Tamburro M, Ripabelli G, Vitullo M, Dallman TJ, Pontello M, Amar CFL, Sammarco ML. 2015. Gene expression in *Listeria monocytogenes* exposed to sublethal concentration of benzalkonium chloride. *Comp Immunol Microbiol Infect Dis* 40:31–39.

109. Mereghetti L, Quentin R, Marquet-Van Der Mee N, Audurier A. 2000. Low sensitivity of *Listeria monocytogenes* to quaternary ammonium compounds. *Appl Environ Microbiol* 66:5083–5086.

110. Romanova NA, Wolffs PFG, Brovko LY, Griffiths MW. 2006. Role of efflux pumps in adaptation and resistance of *Listeria monocytogenes* to benzalkonium chloride. *Appl Environ Microbiol* 72:3498–3503.

111. Jones RD, Jampani HB, Newman JL, Lee AS. 2000. Triclosan: a review of effectiveness and safety in health care settings. *Am J Infect Control* 28:184–196.

112. Schweizer HP. 2001. Triclosan: a widely used biocide and its link to antibiotics. *FEMS Microbiol Lett* 202:1–7.

113. Heath RJ, Yu YT, Shapiro MA, Olson E, Rock CO. 1998. Broad spectrum antimicrobial biocides target the FabI component of fatty acid synthesis. *J Biol Chem* 273:30316–30320.

114. Heath RJ, Rubin JR, Holland DR, Zhang E, Snow ME, Rock CO. 1999. Mechanism of triclosan inhibition of bacterial fatty acid synthesis. *J Biol Chem* 274: 11110–11114.

115. Slater-Radosti C, Van Aller G, Greenwood R, Nicholas R, Keller PM, DeWolf WE Jr, Fan F, Payne DJ, Jaworski DD. 2001. Biochemical and genetic characterization of the action of triclosan on *Staphylococcus aureus*. *J Antimicrob Chemother* 48:1–6.

116. Fan F, Yan K, Wallis NG, Reed S, Moore TD, Rittenhouse SF, DeWolf WE Jr, Huang J, McDevitt D, Miller WH, Seefeld MA, Newlander KA, Jakas DR, Head MS, Payne DJ. 2002. Defining and combating the mechanisms of triclosan resistance in clinical isolates of *Staphylococcus aureus*. *Antimicrob Agents Chemother* 46:3343–3347.

117. Kampf G, Kramer A. 2004. Epidemiologic background of hand hygiene and evaluation of the most important agents for scrubs and rubs. *Clin Microbiol Rev* 17: 863–893.

118. Villalaín J, Mateo CR, Aranda FJ, Shapiro S, Micol V. 2001. Membranotropic effects of the antibacterial agent triclosan. *Arch Biochem Biophys* 390:128–136.

119. Escalada MG, Russell AD, Maillard J-Y, Ochs D. 2005. Triclosan-bacteria interactions: single or multiple target sites? *Lett Appl Microbiol* 41:476–481.

120. Bailey AM, Constantinidou C, Ivens A, Garvey MI, Webber MA, Coldham N, Hobman JL, Wain J, Woodward MJ, Piddock LJV. 2009. Exposure of *Escherichia coli* and *Salmonella enterica* serovar Typhimu-

rium to triclosan induces a species-specific response, including drug detoxification. *J Antimicrob Chemother* 64:973–985.

121. Nielsen LN, Larsen MH, Skovgaard S, Kastbjerg V, Westh H, Gram L, Ingmer H. 2013. *Staphylococcus aureus* but not *Listeria monocytogenes* adapt to triclosan and adaptation correlates with increased *fabI* expression and *agr* deficiency. *BMC Microbiol* 13:177.

122. Kastbjerg VG, Hein-Kristensen L, Gram L. 2014. Triclosan-induced aminoglycoside-tolerant *Listeria monocytogenes* isolates can appear as small-colony variants. *Antimicrob Agents Chemother* 58:3124–3132.

123. Appelberg R. 2006. Macrophage nutriprive antimicrobial mechanisms. *J Leukoc Biol* 79:1117–1128.

124. Botella H, Peyron P, Levillain F, Poincloux R, Poquet Y, Brandli I, Wang C, Tailleux L, Tilleul S, Charrière GM, Waddell SJ, Foti M, Lugo-Villarino G, Gao Q, Maridonneau-Parini I, Butcher PD, Castagnoli PR, Gicquel B, de Chastellier C, Neyrolles O. 2011. Mycobacterial p(1)-type ATPases mediate resistance to zinc poisoning in human macrophages. *Cell Host Microbe* 10:248–259.

125. White C, Lee J, Kambe T, Fritsche K, Petris MJ. 2009. A role for the ATP7A copper-transporting ATPase in macrophage bactericidal activity. *J Biol Chem* 284: 33949–33956.

126. den Bakker HC, Cummings CA, Ferreira V, Vatta P, Orsi RH, Degoricija L, Barker M, Petrauskene O, Furtado MR, Wiedmann M. 2010. Comparative genomics of the bacterial genus *Listeria*: genome evolution is characterized by limited gene acquisition and limited gene loss. *BMC Genomics* 11:688.

127. Kuenne C, Voget S, Pischimarov J, Oehm S, Goesmann A, Daniel R, Hain T, Chakraborty T. 2010. Comparative analysis of plasmids in the genus *Listeria*. *PLoS One* 5:5.

128. Yoon KP, Silver S. 1991. A second gene in the *Staphylococcus aureus cadA* cadmium resistance determinant of plasmid pI258. *J Bacteriol* 173:7636–7642.

129. Allnutt TR, Bradbury MI, Fanning S, Chandry PS, Fox EM. 2016. Draft genome sequences of 15 isolates of *Listeria monocytogenes* serotype 1/2a, subgroup ST204. *Genome Announc* 4:4.

130. Wales AD, Davies RH. 2015. Co-selection of resistance to antibiotics, biocides and heavy metals, and its relevance to foodborne pathogens. *Antibiotics (Basel)* 4: 567–604.

131. Schmitz-Esser S, Müller A, Stessl B, Wagner M. 2015. Genomes of sequence type 121 *Listeria monocytogenes* strains harbor highly conserved plasmids and prophages. *Front Microbiol* 6:380.

132. Mortvedt JJ. 1996. Heavy metal contaminants in inorganic and organic fertilizers. *Fert Res* 43:55–61.

133. Yazdankhah S, Rudi K, Bernhoft A. 2014. Zinc and copper in animal feed: development of resistance and co-resistance to antimicrobial agents in bacteria of animal origin. *Microb Ecol Health Dis* 25:25.

134. Barakat MA. 2011. New trends in removing heavy metals from industrial wastewater. *Arab J Chem* 4: 361–377.

135. Guan Y, Shao C, Ju M. 2014. Heavy metal contamination assessment and partition for industrial and mining gathering areas. *Int J Environ Res Public Health* 11:7286–7303.

136. Xu D, Nie Q, Wang W, Shi L, Yan H. 2016. Characterization of a transferable *bcrABC* and *cadAC* genes-harboring plasmid in *Listeria monocytogenes* strain isolated from food products of animal origin. *Int J Food Microbiol* 217:117–122.

137. Pritchard TJ, Flanders KJ, Donnelly CW. 1995. Comparison of the incidence of *Listeria* on equipment versus environmental sites within dairy processing plants. *Int J Food Microbiol* 26:375–384.

138. Fox EM, Wall PG, Fanning S. 2015. Control of *Listeria* species food safety at a poultry food production facility. *Food Microbiol* 51:81–86.

139. Mullapudi S, Siletzky RM, Kathariou S. 2008. Heavy-metal and benzalkonium chloride resistance of *Listeria monocytogenes* isolates from the environment of turkey-processing plants. *Appl Environ Microbiol* 74:1464–1468.

140. Khan Z, Rehman A, Hussain SZ, Nisar MA, Zulfiqar S, Shakoori AR. 2016. Cadmium resistance and uptake by bacterium, *Salmonella enterica* 43C, isolated from industrial effluent. *AMB Express* 6:54.

141. Lee S, Rakic-Martinez M, Graves LM, Ward TJ, Siletzky RM, Kathariou S. 2013. Genetic determinants for cadmium and arsenic resistance among *Listeria monocytogenes* serotype 4b isolates from sporadic human listeriosis patients. *Appl Environ Microbiol* 79:2471–2476.

142. Xu D, Li Y, Zahid MSH, Yamasaki S, Shi L, Li JR, Yan H. 2014. Benzalkonium chloride and heavy-metal tolerance in *Listeria monocytogenes* from retail foods. *Int J Food Microbiol* 190:24–30.

143. Lebrun M, Loulergue J, Chaslus-Dancla E, Audurier A. 1992. Plasmids in *Listeria monocytogenes* in relation to cadmium resistance. *Appl Environ Microbiol* 58:3183–3186.

144. Lebrun M, Audurier A, Cossart P. 1994. Plasmid-borne cadmium resistance genes in *Listeria monocytogenes* are similar to *cadA* and *cadC* of *Staphylococcus aureus* and are induced by cadmium. *J Bacteriol* 176:3040–3048.

145. Tynecka Z, Gos Z, Zajac J. 1981. Energy-dependent efflux of cadmium coded by a plasmid resistance determinant in *Staphylococcus aureus*. *J Bacteriol* 147:313–319.

146. Endo G, Silver S. 1995. CadC, the transcriptional regulatory protein of the cadmium resistance system of *Staphylococcus aureus* plasmid pI258. *J Bacteriol* 177:4437–4441.

147. McLauchlin J, Hampton MD, Shah S, Threlfall EJ, Wieneke AA, Curtis GD. 1997. Subtyping of *Listeria monocytogenes* on the basis of plasmid profiles and arsenic and cadmium susceptibility. *J Appl Microbiol* 83:381–388.

148. Ratani SS, Siletzky RM, Dutta V, Yildirim S, Osborne JA, Lin W, Hitchins AD, Ward TJ, Kathariou S. 2012. Heavy metal and disinfectant resistance of *Listeria monocytogenes* from foods and food processing plants. *Appl Environ Microbiol* 78:6938–6945.

149. Nelson KE, Fouts DE, Mongodin EF, Ravel J, DeBoy RT, Kolonay JF, Rasko DA, Angiuoli SV, Gill SR, Paulsen IT, Peterson J, White O, Nelson WC, Nierman W, Beanan MJ, Brinkac LM, Daugherty SC, Dodson RJ, Durkin AS, Madupu R, Haft DH, Selengut J, Van Aken S, Khouri H, Fedorova N, Forberger H, Tran B, Kathariou S, Wonderling LD, Uhlich GA, Bayles DO, Luchansky JB, Fraser CM. 2004. Whole genome comparisons of serotype 4b and 1/2a strains of the food-borne pathogen *Listeria monocytogenes* reveal new insights into the core genome components of this species. *Nucleic Acids Res* 32:2386–2395.

150. Mullapudi S, Siletzky RM, Kathariou S. 2010. Diverse cadmium resistance determinants in *Listeria monocytogenes* isolates from the turkey processing plant environment. *Appl Environ Microbiol* 76:627–630.

151. Briers Y, Klumpp J, Schuppler M, Loessner MJ. 2011. Genome sequence of *Listeria monocytogenes* Scott A, a clinical isolate from a food-borne listeriosis outbreak. *J Bacteriol* 193:4284–4285.

152. Sarkar A, Paul B. 2016. The global menace of arsenic and its conventional remediation: a critical review. *Chemosphere* 158:37–49.

153. Henke KR, Atwood DA. Arsenic in human history and modern societies, p 277–302. *In* Arsenic. John Wiley & Sons, Ltd., Chichester, United Kingdom.

154. Chapman HD, Johnson ZB. 2002. Use of antibiotics and roxarsone in broiler chickens in the USA: analysis for the years 1995 to 2000. *Poult Sci* 81:356–364.

155. Jesse HE, Roberts IS, Cavet JS. 2014. Metal ion homeostasis in *Listeria monocytogenes* and importance in host-pathogen interactions. *Adv Microb Physiol* 65:83–123.

156. Castillo Y, Tachibana M, Nakatsu Y, Watanabe K, Shimizu T, Watarai M. 2015. Combination of zinc and all-trans retinoic acid promotes protection against *Listeria monocytogenes* infection. *PLoS One* 10:e0137463.

157. Corbett D, Schuler S, Glenn S, Andrew PW, Cavet JS, Roberts IS. 2011. The combined actions of the copper-responsive repressor CsoR and copper-metallochaperone CopZ modulate CopA-mediated copper efflux in the intracellular pathogen *Listeria monocytogenes*. *Mol Microbiol* 81:457–472.

158. Kuenne C, Billion A, Mraheil MA, Strittmatter A, Daniel R, Goesmann A, Barbuddhe S, Hain T, Chakraborty T. 2013. Reassessment of the *Listeria monocytogenes* pan-genome reveals dynamic integration hotspots and mobile genetic elements as major components of the accessory genome. *BMC Genomics* 14:47.

159. Camejo A, Buchrieser C, Couvé E, Carvalho F, Reis O, Ferreira P, Sousa S, Cossart P, Cabanes D. 2009. *In vivo* transcriptional profiling of *Listeria monocytogenes* and mutagenesis identify new virulence factors involved in infection. *PLoS Pathog* 5:e1000449.

160. Bertrand S, Huys G, Yde M, D'Haene K, Tardy F, Vrints M, Swings J, Collard J-M. 2005. Detection and characterization of *tet*(M) in tetracycline-resistant

Listeria strains from human and food-processing origins in Belgium and France. *J Med Microbiol* **54**:1151–1156.

161. **Pourshaban M, Ferrini AM, Mannoni V, Oliva B, Aureli P.** 2002. Transferable tetracycline resistance in *Listeria monocytogenes* from food in Italy. *J Med Microbiol* **51**: 564–566.

162. **Humphrey B, Thomson NR, Thomas CM, Brooks K, Sanders M, Delsol AA, Roe JM, Bennett PM, Enne VI.** 2012. Fitness of *Escherichia coli* strains carrying expressed and partially silent IncN and IncP1 plasmids. *BMC Microbiol* **12**:53.

163. **Clewell DB, Weaver KE, Dunny GM, Coque TM, Francia MV, Hayes F.** 2014. Extrachromosomal and mobile elements in enterococci: transmission, maintenance, and epidemiology. *In* Gilmore MS, Clewell DB, Ike Y, Shankar N (ed), *Enterococci: From Commensals to Leading Causes of Drug Resistant Infection.* Massachusetts Eye and Ear Infirmary, Boston, MA. Available from https://www.ncbi.nlm.nih.gov/books/NBK190430/.

164. **Gullberg E, Cao S, Berg OG, Ilbäck C, Sandegren L, Hughes D, Andersson DI.** 2011. Selection of resistant bacteria at very low antibiotic concentrations. *PLoS Pathog* **7**:e1002158.

165. **Gullberg E, Albrecht LM, Karlsson C, Sandegren L, Andersson DI.** 2014. Selection of a multidrug resistance plasmid by sublethal levels of antibiotics and heavy metals. *MBio* **5**:e01918–e14.

166. **Jensen LB, Garcia-Migura L, Valenzuela AJS, Løhr M, Hasman H, Aarestrup FM.** 2010. A classification system for plasmids from enterococci and other Gram-positive bacteria. *J Microbiol Methods* **80**:25–43.

167. **Carattoli A.** 2009. Resistance plasmid families in *Enterobacteriaceae*. *Antimicrob Agents Chemother* **53**: 2227–2238.

168. **Romanova N, Favrin S, Griffiths MW.** 2002. Sensitivity of *Listeria monocytogenes* to sanitizers used in the meat processing industry. *Appl Environ Microbiol* **68**: 6405–6409.

169. **Zhang H, Zhou Y, Bao H, Zhang L, Wang R, Zhou X.** 2015. Plasmid-borne cadmium resistant determinants are associated with the susceptibility of *Listeria monocytogenes* to bacteriophage. *Microbiol Res* **172**:1–6.

170. **Bertsch D, Muelli M, Weller M, Uruty A, Lacroix C, Meile L.** 2014. Antimicrobial susceptibility and antibiotic resistance gene transfer analysis of foodborne, clinical, and environmental *Listeria* spp. isolates including *Listeria monocytogenes*. *MicrobiologyOpen* **3**: 118–127.

171. **Poyart-Salmeron C, Trieu-Cuot P, Carlier C, MacGowan A, McLauchlin J, Courvalin P.** 1992. Genetic basis of tetracycline resistance in clinical isolates of *Listeria monocytogenes*. *Antimicrob Agents Chemother* **36**: 463–466.

172. **Hadorn K, Hächler H, Schaffner A, Kayser FH.** 1993. Genetic characterization of plasmid-encoded multiple antibiotic resistance in a strain of *Listeria monocytogenes* causing endocarditis. *Eur J Clin Microbiol Infect Dis* **12**:928–937.

173. **Piddock LJV.** 2006. Multidrug-resistance efflux pumps: not just for resistance. *Nat Rev Microbiol* **4**:629–636.

174. **Li X-Z, Nikaido H.** 2009. Efflux-mediated drug resistance in bacteria: an update. *Drugs* **69**:1555–1623.

175. **Webber MA, Piddock LJV.** 2003. The importance of efflux pumps in bacterial antibiotic resistance. *J Antimicrob Chemother* **51**:9–11.

176. **Crimmins GT, Herskovits AA, Rehder K, Sivick KE, Lauer P, Dubensky TW Jr, Portnoy DA.** 2008. *Listeria monocytogenes* multidrug resistance transporters activate a cytosolic surveillance pathway of innate immunity. *Proc Natl Acad Sci USA* **105**:10191–10196.

177. **Kaplan Zeevi M, Shafir NS, Shaham S, Friedman S, Sigal N, Nir Paz R, Boneca IG, Herskovits AA.** 2013. *Listeria monocytogenes* multidrug resistance transporters and cyclic di-AMP, which contribute to type I interferon induction, play a role in cell wall stress. *J Bacteriol* **195**:5250–5261.

178. **Schwartz KT, Carleton JD, Quillin SJ, Rollins SD, Portnoy DA, Leber JH.** 2012. Hyperinduction of host beta interferon by a *Listeria monocytogenes* strain naturally overexpressing the multidrug efflux pump MdrT. *Infect Immun* **80**:1537–1545.

179. **Marquez B, Pourcelle V, Vallet CM, Mingeot-Leclercq M-P, Tulkens PM, Marchand-Bruynaert J, Van Bambeke F.** 2014. Pharmacological characterization of 7-(4-(Piperazin-1-yl)) ciprofloxacin derivatives: antibacterial activity, cellular accumulation, susceptibility to efflux transporters, and intracellular activity. *Pharm Res* **31**:1290–1301.

180. **Lismond A, Tulkens PM, Mingeot-Leclercq M-P, Courvalin P, Van Bambeke F.** 2008. Cooperation between prokaryotic (Lde) and eukaryotic (MRP) efflux transporters in J774 macrophages infected with *Listeria monocytogenes*: studies with ciprofloxacin and moxifloxacin. *Antimicrob Agents Chemother* **52**:3040–3046.

181. **Scortti M, Lacharme-Lora L, Wagner M, Chico-Calero I, Losito P, Vázquez-Boland JA.** 2006. Coexpression of virulence and fosfomycin susceptibility in *Listeria*: molecular basis of an antimicrobial *in vitro-in vivo* paradox. *Nat Med* **12**:515–517.

182. **Collins B, Curtis N, Cotter PD, Hill C, Ross RP.** 2010. The ABC transporter AnrAB contributes to the innate resistance of *Listeria monocytogenes* to nisin, bacitracin, and various beta-lactam antibiotics. *Antimicrob Agents Chemother* **54**:4416–4423.

183. **Walsh D, Duffy G, Sheridan JJ, Blair IS, McDowell DA.** 2001. Antibiotic resistance among *Listeria*, including *Listeria monocytogenes*, in retail foods. *J Appl Microbiol* **90**:517–522.

Antimicrobial Resistance in Bacteria from Livestock and Companion Animals
Edited by Frank Møller Aarestrup, Stefan Schwarz, Jianzhong Shen, and Lina Cavaco
© 2018 American Society for Microbiology, Washington, DC
doi:10.1128/microbiolspec.ARBA-0014-2017

Antimicrobial Resistance in Nontyphoidal *Salmonella*

12

Patrick F. McDermott[1], Shaohua Zhao[1], and Heather Tate[1]

BACKGROUND

Nontyphoidal *Salmonella enterica* (NTS) is a ubiquitous, motile, Gram-negative bacillus that is one of the most common bacterial causes of gastrointestinal disease worldwide. Salmonellae colonize the intestinal tract of a wide range of animal hosts, including pigs, cattle, poultry (1), and wildlife, as well as companion animals such as dogs, cats, birds, and reptiles (2). Humans acquire infection from the ingestion of contaminated foods. In the United States, most illnesses are associated with seeded vegetables, eggs, poultry, beef, and pork. Other sources include dairy, fruits, sprouts, and fish (3). Its ubiquity in nature and the variety of vectors mediating fecal-oral spread have made salmonellosis the most important foodborne bacterial zoonosis. For many decades, the cornerstone of *Salmonella* epidemiology has been the Kaufmann-White serotyping scheme (4). Based on antibodies to the three major surface antigens (somatic O, flagellar H, and capsular Vi antigens), over 2,500 distinct serovars are currently recognized. A comprehensive body of scientific information on *Salmonella* developed over the years makes it one of the best-understood bacterial pathogens. A great deal is known about *Salmonella* epidemiology and genetics, the various virulence factors, interaction of the bacterium with host cells, the host range of serovars, and the causes of antibiotic resistance.

Most human cases of acute NTS diarrhea are self-limiting and do not require treatment with antibiotics unless they are severe, invasive, or occur in the elderly, children, or those with underlying comorbidities (5). Cases that become invasive may result in life-threatening bloodstream infections. Antimicrobial resistance is especially problematic in these systemic infections, where antibiotic therapy can be life-saving. Efforts to limit the public health burden of salmonellosis, and the pressures leading to antibiotic resistance, have focused on farm practices, interventions in processing facilities, and consumer education on safe food handling practices.

In animals, *Salmonella* may cause overt signs of disease or may be carried asymptomatically and be shed into the environment (6). In food-producing animals, *Salmonella* is a continuous threat to animal health, especially in cattle, where infection typically presents as diarrhea with fever, anorexia, and dehydration (2). Less commonly, infection results in respiratory disease and death. *Salmonella* infections in dairy herds, where they may become endemic (7), result in decreased milk production and increased production costs, including the use of antibiotics. In addition to overt salmonellosis, a chronic asymptomatic carrier state may exist in food-producing animals. In both the carrier state and in cases of overt infection, exposure to antimicrobials promotes the evolution of resistant serovars that may be transmitted to humans. In the case of foodborne zoonotic bacteria, resistance spreads from food-producing animals to humans via the consumption of meat products derived either from treated animals or from foods cross-contaminated at processing or retail (8). Resistance also can spread by direct animal contact (as with pets) or environmental routes such as water or wildlife. The U.S. Centers for Disease Control and Prevention (CDC) classifies antibiotic-resistant *Salmonella* as a serious public health threat (9).

Bacterial resistance to antibiotics is a naturally occurring phenomenon that can be accelerated by selection pressures exerted through the use of antibiotics in medical and veterinary practice (10). Resistance is mediated by a limited number of mechanisms common to other pathogens. These include enzymatic modification, target protection, energy-dependent efflux, and permeability changes in the cell wall. The use and

---

[1]U.S. Food & Drug Administration, Center for Veterinary Medicine, Office of Research Laurel, MD 20708.

misuse of antimicrobials in both humans and animals result in antimicrobial resistance in both pathogenic and commensal bacteria within the treated host. Many classes of antimicrobial agents used in food-producing and companion animals are the same as those used in human medicine (11). Therefore, resistance developing in one drug use environment can compromise the efficacy of drugs used in other settings. For this reason, many countries are attempting to implement antimicrobial drug use monitoring.

The relationship between resistances in food animal bacteria and antibiotic use in animal agriculture is poorly defined. Very few countries can collect detailed information on the amounts and indications of antimicrobial compounds in different animal species over time. Only in Denmark is it mandatory for veterinarians to report (via VetStat) medicines used in their own practices. Like most countries, the United States and Japan collect data on total annual sales (in kilograms of active ingredient) by drug class. Japan collects sales data only for drugs used therapeutically (12). Most European Union countries also mandate collection of sales data (13). While usually the only practicable approach, bulk annual amounts of active ingredient sold is of limited utility and is not a reliable surrogate for actual drug use in the production environment (14). In July 2016, the U.S. FDA mandated that pharmaceutical companies report antimicrobial sales by the four major animal species: cattle, chickens, turkey, and swine, along with a combined "other" category (15). The goal of this provision is to better monitor drug use and better understand the drivers of antimicrobial resistance in *Salmonella* and other foodborne microorganisms.

While there are numerous small targeted surveys in the scientific literature describing antimicrobial resistance in *Salmonella* from different places and sources, an ongoing integrated national surveillance system is necessary to combat antibiotic resistance (16). The WHO defines integrated surveillance as "the coordinated sampling and testing of bacteria from food animals, foods, and clinically ill humans; and the subsequent evaluation of antimicrobial resistance trends throughout the food production and supply chain using harmonized methods" (1). It provides necessary data to identify emerging hazards, assess risks, monitor trends, measure interventions, and inform mitigation policies. The generation of robust and consistent data is important to the development and assessment of response measures used to combat antimicrobial resistance. In the United States, this work is conducted by the National Antimicrobial Resistance Monitoring System (NARMS). Similar systems are in place across the European Union, in Canada, across

Latin America, and in some Asian and African countries. Most of these programs are focused on susceptibility surveillance of human clinical isolates. Active surveillance of animal and retail meat isolates operates to varying degrees in different countries (1). This article will review the latest available information on resistance in *Salmonella* (through test year 2014), with an emphasis on the situation in the United States and Europe.

THE BURDEN OF SALMONELLOSIS

NTS is recognized as one of the most common bacterial causes of foodborne diarrheal disease worldwide. Foodborne NTS is estimated to cause over 93 million cases of gastroenteritis annually and 155,000 deaths globally (8), resulting in about 4 million disability-adjusted life years (17). At-risk populations include children <1 year of age and adults ≥60, who are most vulnerable to infection and tend to have more severe disease (18). Extraintestinal or invasive NTS infections, often associated with certain serovars or phylogenetic clades, add to the global burden of illness, especially in resource-poor countries and immunocompromised patients (19). An estimated 3.4 million invasive infections occur annually, resulting in 681,000 deaths, with the young and old in Africa being most affected (20). The relatively high prevalence of highly invasive strain subtypes, such as those that have been identified among *S. enterica* serovars Enteritidis (21), Typhimurium (22), and Kentucky (23) may be expected to drive different antibiotic use practices to control disease in countries where invasive subtypes are endemic (24).

Despite sustained efforts to control NTS in animals and to educate the public on safe food-handling practices, the incidence of human salmonellosis has not changed significantly in the United States (25). The latest data from the CDC on microbial causes of zoonotic foodborne diseases ranked *Salmonella* first in incidence, at 15.5 cases per 100,000 inhabitants, resulting in over 2,100 hospitalizations and 32 deaths (18). In the European Union in 2014, the incidence of *Salmonella* infections (23 per 100,000) ranked well behind *Campylobacter* (71 per 100,000). In 2014, a total of 88,715 confirmed cases of salmonellosis were reported by 28 European Union member states and 4 nonmember states (26). In both the United States and the European Union (and in many other countries), *S. enterica* serovars Typhimurium and Enteritidis are consistently the most frequently isolated among confirmed human cases of disease (18, 26). In the United States and the European Union, poultry meat is the most commonly contaminated animal-derived food commodity (26, 27).

TREATMENT OF SALMONELLOSIS

The extent of antibiotic resistance in *Salmonella* varies by country and is influenced by antimicrobial use practices in humans and animals, as well as geographical differences in the epidemiology of *Salmonella* and regional serovar differences. In developed countries, drug resistance in *Salmonella* is driven largely by the use of antimicrobials in food-producing animals (28). In general, resistance profiles reflect the length of time an agent has been in use. Thus, irrespective of isolation source (humans, foods, food animals), the most frequent types of resistances are usually for older antimicrobials such as tetracycline, sulfamethoxazole, and streptomycin (26, 27, 29, 30).

Antimicrobial therapy is usually not indicated for uncomplicated infection. Therapy should be considered for populations at increased risk for invasive infection such as people >50 years of age with atherosclerosis, the immunocompromised, and those with cardiac disease. In these patients, the recommended antimicrobials include a fluoroquinolone such as ciprofloxacin, a third-generation cephalosporin such as ceftriaxone, trimethoprim/sulfamethoxazole, or amoxicillin. The recommended empiric antimicrobial therapy for bloody diarrhea in immunocompetent adults is either a fluoroquinolone or azithromycin, both of which show potent *in vitro* activity against *Salmonella* in the United States and the European Union. Additionally, most highly resistant strains of *Salmonella* are susceptible to carbapenem drugs (31, 32), making it a drug of last resort. Recommended empiric therapy for children includes a third-generation cephalosporin for those <3 months of age or azithromycin. Because fluoroquinolones, extended-spectrum cephalosporins, azithromycin, and carbapenems are critically important antibiotics for the management of salmonellosis, emerging resistance to these drug classes is a paramount concern (33).

ANTIMICROBIAL RESISTANCE IN *SALMONELLA* FROM THE UNITED STATES

The United States has extensive data back to 1996 on antimicrobial resistance in *Salmonella*, which is collected through NARMS (34). The NARMS program generates susceptibility data on *Salmonella* representing 5% of the nationally reported human clinical cases. These results are compared with data on *Salmonella* from 13 other sources that include (i) samples of retail chicken, turkey, pork, and beef collected in 14 states; (ii) cecal specimens from chickens, turkeys, cattle (dairy and beef), and pigs (hogs and sows) at slaughter; and (iii) carcass swabs, carcass rinses, and ground product

from chickens, turkeys, cattle, and pigs at slaughter. A line listing of these data is freely available online (35), where information on nearly 160,000 isolates dating back to the start of NARMS can be downloaded and analyzed using standard spreadsheet and database software programs.

Few data are available from before 1996 to document the historical trends in *Salmonella* resistance. To address this gap, Tadesse et al. (36) conducted a retrospective study of 2,149 banked human clinical *Salmonella* strains and documented changing resistance patterns in strains dating back to 1948. Comparing data from pre-1960 with those from post-1989 for *S.* Typhimurium (which constituted most of the banked isolates) showed that resistance rose from 0% to 33% for ampicillin, 0% to 26% for chloramphenicol, 0% to 43% for streptomycin, 20% to 43% for tetracycline, and 0% to 37% for sulfamethoxazole. While recognizing the inherent limitations in directly comparing two disparate data sets, it is striking how the historical and modern data in juxtaposition show a monotonic increasing trend in resistance to older antimicrobial compounds (ampicillin, chloramphenicol, streptomycin, sulfonamide, tetracycline) from pre-1960s up until the 1990s, followed by a decline to current levels approximating those of the 1970s (Fig. 1). This study examined just over 2,100 human clinical isolates collected over 6 decades, a number now tested annually in NARMS.

In NARMS, antimicrobial susceptibility testing is centralized at government laboratories of the FDA, the CDC, and the U.S. Department of Agriculture. All three laboratories employ identical media, methods, quality control parameters, and repeat testing criteria, along with a common drug panel from a single manufacturer. The compounds tested have many commonalities with the European Union testing design (see below) except that ceftriaxone is used in the United States as a class representative for extended-spectrum cephalosporins (Table 1), while in Europe either ceftazidime or cefotaxime is used. The United States currently also includes amoxicillin-clavulanate, cefoxitin, streptomycin, and trimethoprim/sulfamethoxazole, while the European Union member states test trimethoprim alone. Some European Union countries report resistance data for tigecycline and colistin.

Different breakpoints are used that result in more conservative interpretations in the European Union compared with the United States (Table 1). The European Union uses EUCAST epidemiological cutoff values (ECOFFs) as breakpoints where available (37), which are based on the highest MIC of the wild-type population. In contrast, the United States currently interprets

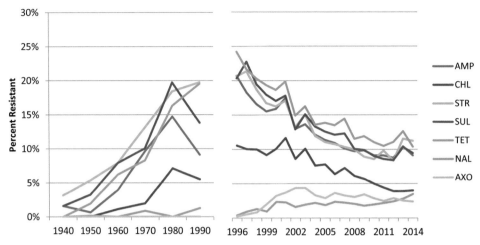

Figure 1   Temporal changes in resistance of clinical nontyphoidal *Salmonella* from the 1940s to 2014. AMP, ampicillin; CHL, chloramphenicol; STR, streptomycin; SUL, sulfonamides; TET, tetracycline; NAL, nalidixic acid; AXO, ceftriaxone.

susceptibility results in *Salmonella* based on the Clinical and Laboratory Standards Institute (CLSI) clinical breakpoints (for all agents except streptomycin). Clinical breakpoints also rely on data from MIC distributions, which are combined with pharmacological information and clinical outcome trials to set clinical

Table 1   Antimicrobials tested in the European Union and United States and criteria used to interpret microbiological and clinical resistance

	Breakpoints (µg/ml)		
	European Union[a]		U.S.[a]
Antimicrobial	Microbiological	Clinical	Clinical
Tetracycline (TET)	>8	>4[b]	>8
Sulfonamide (SUL)	>256	>256[b]	>256
Ampicillin (AMP)	>8	>8	>16
Chloramphenicol (CHL)	>16	>8	>16
Nalidixic acid (NAL)	>16	>16[b]	>16
Third-generation cephalosporin (CEP)[c]	>0.5	>1	>2
Gentamicin (GEN)	>2	>2	>8
Trimethoprim-sulfa (COT)[d]	>2	>2	>2
Ciprofloxacin (CIP)	>0.064	>0.064	>0.5
Azithromycin (AZI)	>16[e]	>16[e]	>16[f]
Colistin (COL)	>2		N/A

[a]European Union breakpoints are from EUCAST, and U.S. breakpoints are from CLSI unless otherwise noted.
[b]Derived from CLSI.
[c]In the European Union, isolates are tested against ceftazidime and cefotaxime.
[d]In the European Union, non-human isolates are tested against trimethoprim and sulfonamide separately. In the United States, isolates are tested against trimethoprim-sulfamethoxazole and sulfamethoxazole.
[e]Reference 150, 151.
[f]Reference 149.

breakpoints. In accord with WHO recommendations (1), NARMS MIC data are also presented as MIC distributions so that other interpretive criteria can be applied to allow direct comparisons (27). The presentation of MIC data also allows for increased power in detecting slight shifts in bacterial susceptibility to some antibiotics, giving users of the data increased ability to create predictive models of resistance based on policy interventions (38).

The latest U.S. surveillance data (test year 2014) from NARMS comprised antimicrobial susceptibility results for 5,043 NTS isolates, including 2,127 from humans, 262 from retail meats, 1,579 from hazard analysis and critical control point samples (39), and 1,075 from animal cecal samples (27). The prevalence of *Salmonella* in U.S. retail meats in 2014 was 9.1% in chicken, 5.5% in ground turkey, 1.3% in pork, and 0.8% in beef.

A general overview of key antibiotic resistance trends in U.S. clinical isolates of *Salmonella* is shown in Fig. 2. Approximately 82% of *Salmonella* isolated from humans in 2014 had no resistance to any of the antimicrobial drugs tested, a trend that has improved since NARMS testing began in 1996. Multidrug resistance (MDR, resistant to ≥3 antimicrobial classes) was present in around 10% of isolates on average, appearing in 9.3% of human isolates in 2014. In 2014, resistance in human strains was most frequent to streptomycin (11.2%), tetracycline (10.4%), sulfamethoxazole (9.4%), and ampicillin (9.1%), followed by lower levels of resistance to chloramphenicol (4.0%), nalidixic acid (3.5%), ceftriaxone (2.4%), cefoxitin (2.2%), amoxicillin-clavulanate (2.1%), gentamicin (1.4%), trimethoprim-

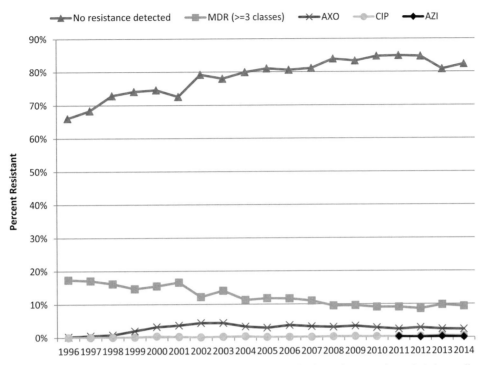

Figure 2 Resistances to critically important antimicrobials in human clinical *Salmonella* isolates from the United States. MDR, multidrug resistant; AXO, ceftriaxone; AZI, azithromycin; CIP, ciprofloxacin.

sulfamethoxazole (1.3%), ciprofloxacin (0.4%), and azithromycin (<0.1%) (27). Resistance to the three critically important drugs ceftriaxone, azithromycin, and ciprofloxacin was below 3% (Fig. 2). These three major findings were largely unchanged from the previous 10 years. The most common *Salmonella* serovars infecting humans in the United States in 2014 were Enteritidis (21%), Typhimurium (12%), and Newport (11%), followed by Javiana (6%), I 4,[5],12:i:– (5%), and Infantis (3.4%) (27).

Multidrug resistance

In general, resistance in human isolates of *Salmonella* has been fairly low and stable over the past decade in the United States. Because a substantial proportion of human infections are acquired from non-food-animal sources (3), however, it is not unexpected that resistance in animal isolates tends to be higher. By animal species, resistance to any of the 14 tested compounds was most frequent in turkey sources (approximately 60% to 80% resistant to ≥1 agent), followed by broilers (about 30% to 60%), and cattle (30% to 40%). These findings are consistent with other studies that show that *Salmonella* from poultry sources tend to be more resistant than *Salmonella* from cattle sources (38) and that swine isolates tend to be more resistant than those from cattle (40).

In human clinical strains, MDR is most frequent in *S. enterica* serovars Typhimurium (28.9%), I 4,[5],12: i:– (27.9%), and Heidelberg (7.6%). While MDR is declining in *S.* Typhimurium (see below), it has risen in *S.* 4,[5],12:i:–, from 5.5% in 2007 to 50% in 2014, with 47.3% exhibiting resistance to more than four drug classes. In animals at slaughter, MDR was most frequent in isolates from turkeys (47%) and hogs (20%), followed by broilers (15%), dairy cattle (10%), beef cattle (6%), and sows (6%) (27). In 2014, MDR was detected in 36% of retail ground turkey isolates and 20% of retail chicken meat. MDR is disproportionately high in broilers among serovars Kentucky (33% hazard analysis and critical control point to 58% cecal isolates) and Typhimurium (16% to 53% among hazard analysis and critical control point and cecal isolates, respectively).

Measuring MDR by the number of resistance phenotypes without regard to the importance of the drug classes involved is of limited value. To help overcome this limitation, NARMS has published new tools online that allow the user to investigate any combination of specific MDR patterns and their changes over time (31). This permits a more refined analysis of MDR patterns in assessing risks, for identifying specific resistance trends of higher public health importance, and to better understand the specific drivers of resistance where coresistances are involved.

The percentage of *Salmonella* strains that are resistant to ampicillin, chloramphenicol, streptomycin, sulfonamide, and tetracycline (the ACSSuT penta-resistant phenotype) has been tracked as a hallmark of the globally disseminated *Salmonella* Typhimurium DT104 for decades. The ACSSuT resistance pattern has declined steadily in all U.S. salmonellae from 34% in 1996 to 14.5% in 2014. Declining levels of both *S.* Typhimurium (27) and MDR *S.* Typhimurium (41) are the main drivers behind overall declining levels of MDR *Salmonella* in human isolates. The ACSSuT resistance in cattle isolates of *S.* Typhimurium declined sharply from 67% in 2009 to 7% in 2014. This highlights an important feature of *Salmonella* resistance, namely, the serovar-specific nature of some resistance patterns whose ascendancy and decline may be temporally associated with the prevalence of specific strains.

In the United States in recent years, the ASSuT (ampicillin, streptomycin, sulfonamide, tetracycline) MDR pattern has increased among human isolates of *S.* I 4,[5],12:i:–, where it climbed from 1.4% in 2009 to 43% in 2014. Outbreak investigations of this strain have pointed to swine as a possible source (42), backed by findings of increased *S.* I 4,[5],12:i:– in diseased pigs in Minnesota (40), one of the top five pig-producing states in the United States.

While MDR is not common in *S.* Enteritidis, it is driven by a higher resistance to nalidixic acid compared with other serovars. MDR is common in *S.* Newport, where the MDR-AmpC phenotype on an IncA/C or IncI backbone is a common feature of resistance (43).

Quinolone Resistance

Overall, fluoroquinolone resistance has been consistently low among *Salmonella* isolated from all U.S. surveillance sources. In human isolates, it predominantly presents in serovar Enteritidis (47%) and is associated with travel (44). Since 2007, ciprofloxacin resistance has been detected in a total of only four cattle and six swine isolates in the United States. Ciprofloxacin resistance is not present (using CLSI breakpoints) in isolates from U.S. poultry *Salmonella*, where fluoroquinolones have not been used since 2005. In 2014, the first instance of ciprofloxacin-resistant *Salmonella* in meat was a single isolate from a retail pork sample which carried the *qnrS* gene. This was the first report of *qnr* genes present in retail meat *Salmonella* isolated in the United States (27).

While ciprofloxacin resistance is rare in U.S. salmonellae in general, decreased susceptibility to ciprofloxa-

cin (DSC, MIC ≥ 0.125 µg/ml) has increased in humans and cattle strains as well as in swine strains. (Strains with this MIC would be considered microbiologically resistant according to EUCAST breakpoints.) Studies have reported extremely low quinolone resistance among *Salmonella* isolated from feedlot and beef cows as well as dairy cows (45, 46). However, decreased susceptibility is rarely assessed. Distribution of extrachromosomal *qnr* genes is thought to be the main reason why this phenotype is increasing in frequency. Because fluoroquinolones are widely, and often repeatedly, used to treat bovine respiratory disease, a common illness in cattle herds, there is a possibility that fluoroquinolone use may help to propagate an acquired resistance gene. Particularly concerning is the emergence of DSC in *S. enterica* serovar Dublin isolates from humans and cattle, where increasing cephalosporin resistance is also occurring. The incidence of human *S.* Dublin infections is relatively low, but it can cause invasive disease with more severe outcomes. *S.* Dublin also causes severe disease in cattle, mainly respiratory infections, and ranks among the top four serovars isolated from retail ground beef and cattle samples in NARMS and the top serovar among isolates derived from clinical specimens (40). As of the 2014 NARMS testing year, 57% (4/7) of DSC *S.* Dublin isolates from humans and 40% (18/42) of DSC *S.* Dublin isolates from cattle were also resistant to ceftriaxone. This combination of DSC and ceftriaxone resistance puts significant limitations on possible treatment options for human illness.

Cephalosporin Resistance

Among critically important human antibiotics, the temporal association of ceftiofur use in food animals and the emergence of ceftriaxone resistance in both animals and humans has been an area of concern in the United States, the European Union, and elsewhere. In the United States, ceftriaxone resistance was not detected in *Salmonella* prior to the approval of ceftiofur (36) and rose following its approval for use in the United States in livestock and poultry (Fig. 3). From 1996 through 2009, the percentage of NTS human isolates resistant to ceftriaxone increased from 0.2% to 3.4% (41). These rising trends have caused several countries, including the United States, to limit certain uses of cephalosporins in animal agriculture, with positive effects. A well-known example occurred in Canada when voluntary restrictions on ceftiofur use were followed by a rapid and significant decline in ceftriaxone-resistant *S.* Heidelberg (and *Escherichia coli*) in chickens, retail chicken meats, and human clinical isolates (47). In the United States, the FDA announced plans in 2008 to

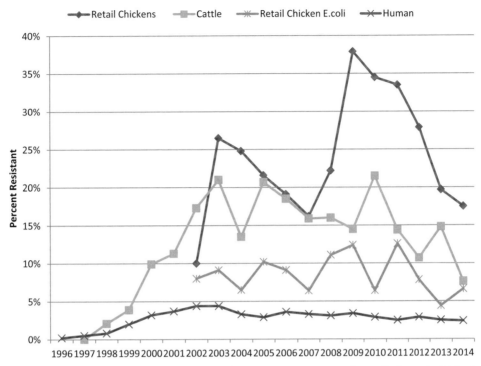

Figure 3 Trends in third-generation cephalosporin resistance in *Salmonella* from the United States.

restrict the use of some cephalosporins, which went into effect in 2012 (48). As of 2014, it appears that the restrictions may be producing the desired effect of reducing cephalosporin resistance in humans and select animal species. Ceftriaxone resistance has declined since 2009 in human (3.4% to 2.4%) and retail chicken (38% to 18%) *Salmonella* isolates (Fig. 3).

Changes in ceftriaxone resistance were most notable for *S.* Heidelberg, where resistance in human isolates declined to 8.5% in 2014, down from a peak of 24% in 2010 (27). Ceftriaxone resistance in retail chicken *S.* Heidelberg remained at 0% from 2011 to 2013 (down from a peak of 32% in 2009), but reappeared in 3/24 isolates in 2014. In retail ground turkey isolates in 2014, resistance continued to decline to 7% after peaking at 22% in 2011. In cattle *Salmonella* isolates in 2014, ceftriaxone resistance reached its lowest level (7.6%) since 1999 (31). Studies of diagnostic cattle isolates show varied results. While some studies show demonstrable decreases in cephalosporin resistance among dairy cattle since 2012 (46), others show continued increases (40) or even no resistance at all among healthy feedlot cattle (49). Many of these disparities are due to regionalization of serovar frequencies, as well as the types of samples analyzed (diseased versus healthy animals).

Ceftriaxone resistance in human strains is most common in the same serovars in which MDR prevails,

namely, Typhimurium, Newport, Heidelberg, and I 4,[5],12:i:–, with the addition of Dublin, 11.5% of which were ceftriaxone resistant. Ceftriaxone resistance was also high in *S.* Dublin from cattle (34.6%) and ground beef (60%). In other nonhuman sources, ceftriaxone was disproportionately high in serovars Newport from cattle (66.7%), Kentucky from broilers (66%), Typhimurium from broiler meat (72%), and Heidelberg from fattening turkeys (60%).

NARMS data show that extended-spectrum cephalosporin resistance among U.S. isolates of *Salmonella* (and *E. coli*) is usually mediated by bla_{CMY} genes, whereas extended-spectrum beta-lactamases (ESBLs) have been rare (50). This appears to be changing. Examining NARMS strains from 2012 to 2014, 26 instances of ESBLs occurred, mainly conferred by members of the CTX-M family, along with 3 instances of bla_{SHV-12} and one case of bla_{SHV-30}. Finding $bla_{CTX-M-65}$ in a 2014 retail chicken sample led to an expanded examination of U.S. human and animal strains and revealed that the gene had become widespread in a strain of serovar Infantis previously identified in Europe and South America (51).

ANTIMICROBIAL RESISTANCE IN EUROPE

Denmark established the world's first integrated antimicrobial resistance surveillance program in 1995, and other members of the European Union have followed with their own national programs. In the European Union, antimicrobial resistance in *Salmonella* is tracked in data submitted by European Union member states and Norway and is reported jointly by the European Food Safety Authority (EFSA) and the European Centre for Disease Prevention and Control (ECDC).

The latest European Union data are from 2014 (26), when for the first time, all 28 member states along with Iceland and Norway submitted isolate-level data on poultry and poultry meat products. Therefore, the European Union report focuses on resistance in human and poultry sources of isolates. Countries submit both MIC data, which is interpreted using published ECOFFS, and susceptibility categories interpreted from disk diffusion. In 2014, 21 member states and Norway provided data on human *Salmonella* isolates. Twelve countries (Austria, Denmark, Estonia, Finland, Greece, Ireland, Italy, Luxembourg, the Netherlands, Norway, Portugal, and Romania) reported isolate-level results in the form of inhibition zone diameters or MICs, which allows for improved comparability between human and animal/food isolates. Ten countries reported categorical interpretations of susceptible (S), intermediate (I), or resistant (R) according to the clinical breakpoints. The number and types of antimicrobials reported varied by country, from 2 countries testing only three antimicrobials to 13 countries testing all 10 antimicrobials in the priority panel. This mixture of breakpoints and testing methods, sampling strategies, differences in serovar by country, and the incomplete nature of the isolate-level data mean that the results must be interpreted, and the country differences compared, with caution.

In 2014 in the European Union, a total of 14,412 *Salmonella* isolates from human infections were tested, constituting 16% of all confirmed human cases of illness. When examining all serovars (*n* = 247) and countries (*n* = 22) combined, the most common resistances in human *Salmonella* isolates were to tetracyclines (30.3%), sulfonamides (28.6%), and ampicillin (28.2%), followed by lower levels of resistance to trimethoprim-sulfamethoxazole (9.2%), ciprofloxacin (8.8%), chloramphenicol (6%), gentamicin (2.7%), and cefotaxime (1.1%) (26). The top three resistances mirror the order of resistance profiles in the United States (except for streptomycin, which is not reported by EFSA).

Although the United States and the European Union employ different criteria for surveillance reporting, these differences are absent or minor for most drugs. Small discrepancies are evident for extended-spectrum cephalosporins and gentamicin that have nugatory effect on reported rates of resistance. Breakpoints for ciprofloxacin have the largest affect, where application of the EUCAST criteria changes the U.S. resistance percentage in human isolate data from 0.4% to 4.3%. The EUCAST breakpoints were applied for the purposes of comparison below.

Monitoring data from food sources show some commonalities with the U.S. situation. An overall comparison between the European Union and the United States of resistance to the "older" antimicrobials of chloramphenicol, tetracycline, gentamicin, and ampicillin is shown for human isolates (Fig. 4) and broiler isolates (Fig. 5) of *Salmonella* spp. For human data, the U.S. surveillance data are comparable to Slovenia, which reports the lowest resistance levels for these drugs among the member states. Resistance data for broiler strains of *Salmonella* spp. show that the United States is slightly below the European Union average.

Other general features of resistance in both the European Union and the United States are evident. With some exceptions, *Salmonella* recovered from poultry meats is generally more resistant than isolates from human infections in both regions (26, 31). Among poultry isolates, resistance levels in the European Union were generally higher in turkeys than chickens. This is comparable to what was observed in the United States, where turkey isolates tended to be the most resistant, followed by those from chicken, swine, and cattle (27). One might presume that this pattern is the result of higher antimicrobial use in turkeys than in broilers, but there have been no on-farm studies that confirm a causal relationship (52). In general, fluoroquinolone resistance is higher in the European Union, and third-generation cephalosporin resistance is higher in the United States. Other resistance patterns are compared below.

Multidrug Resistance

In 2014, 10 member states tested *Salmonella* against 9 classes of antimicrobials (26). Overall, only 54.8% of human isolates were susceptible to all agents tested. MDR was high overall (26.0%) in human isolates from the European Union, with very high prevalence in some countries. Among poultry sources, MDR was low in laying hens; high in broiler meat, turkey meat, and broilers; and very high in turkeys. As with other types of resistance, MDR tends to be associated with certain serovars, generally being rare in *S.* Enteritidis. In Europe, MDR variants of *S.* Kentucky (74.6%), along with monophasic *S.* Typhimurium I 4,[5],12:i:– (69.4%) and *S.* Infantis (61.9%), are especially problematic in humans. As noted above, the United States also is witnessing a rise in MDR *S.* Typhimurium I 4,[5],12:i:–.

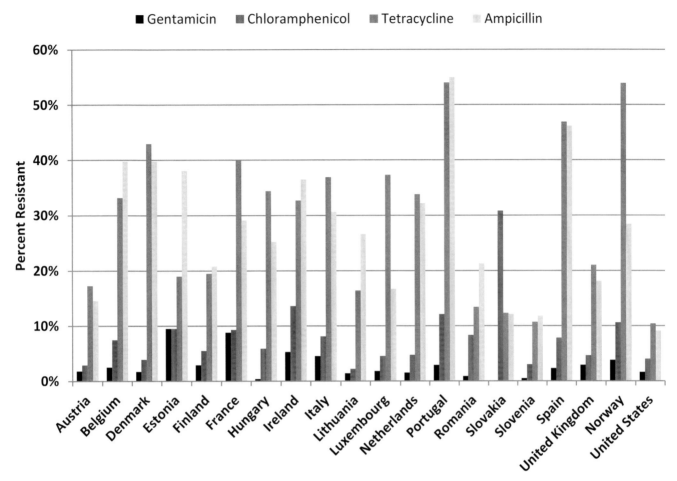

Figure 4   Resistance to gentamicin, chloramphenicol, tetracycline, and ampicillin in human *Salmonella* isolates from select European Union countries, Norway, and the United States. Breakpoints used for interpreting MICs were derived from the EUCAST.

While *S.* Kentucky rarely causes human disease in the United States, it commonly exhibits MDR.

Extended-spectrum cephalosporin-resistant *S.* Infantis (carrying the *bla*CTX-M65 gene) has emerged in the United States as a public health concern. The circulating clone is similar to an Italian strain of *S.* Infantis carrying the *bla*CTX-M65 gene (53). While MDR *S.* Infantis has not increased in poultry isolates collected for NARMS surveillance, EFSA reports that *S.* Infantis isolates from European Union broiler meat express very high levels of MDR (>70.0%). Isolates from Italian broilers exhibit exceptionally high levels of resistance to third-generation cephalosporins, which may be characteristic of the CTX-M clone. Particularly concerning was the detection of high-level resistance to ciprofloxacin in these isolates. The clone may be limited to chickens, because no resistance to third-generation cephalosporin was detected in fattening turkeys (26).

Much of the difference in resistance among poultry isolates from the United States and the European Union is likely due to the variation in serovar profiles of poultry isolates between the two regions. *S.* Infantis and *S.* Enteritidis are among the top three serovars in chickens and chicken meats in the European Union, but in the United States, serovar Kentucky predominates. Likewise, in European Union fattening turkeys, serovars Derby, Kentucky, and Newport account for 30% of *Salmonella* isolates, but in the United States, serovars Hadar and Reading round out the top two in turkeys and turkey meats (31).

Quinolone Resistance

A comparison of human isolates from European countries that reported data for both fluoroquinolones and extended-spectrum cephalosporins is shown alongside the U.S. data in Fig. 6. The average resistance to

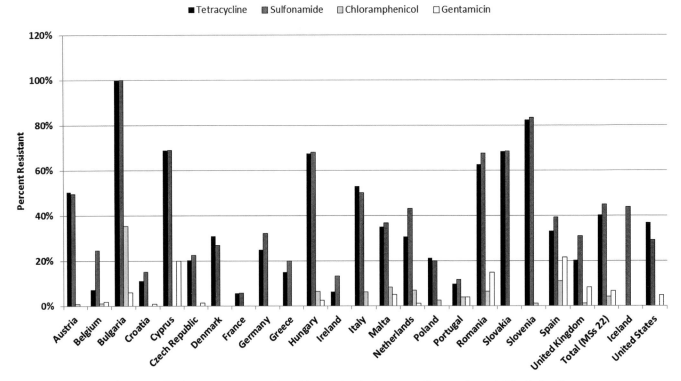

Figure 5 Resistance to gentamicin, chloramphenicol, tetracycline, and ampicillin in broiler *Salmonella* isolates from select European Union countries, Iceland, and the United States. Breakpoints used for interpreting MICs were derived from the EUCAST.

extended-spectrum cephalosporins is low (1.1%) in the European Union data, while ciprofloxacin resistance was found in 8.8% of all human isolates, ranging from 0% to 19% among reporting countries compared with 4.3% in the United States. The European Union resistance to ciprofloxacin is driven in part by a high prevalence of ciprofloxacin resistance in serovar Kentucky, where 84% were resistant to ciprofloxacin. This aligns with previous findings on the establishment of ST198 *S.* Kentucky in humans and poultry flocks throughout Europe and other areas (23). While this strain has been found in the United States, it has predominated in travelers and imported foods (54).

Differences between Europe and the United States for critically important resistances are evident in isolates from poultry and poultry meat (Fig. 7). In the European Union, a very high proportion of *Salmonella* from broilers (average = 53.5%; *n* = 23 countries) was resistant to ciprofloxacin, ranging from 0% (Denmark and Ireland) to over 80% (Bulgaria, Hungary, and Slovenia). Similarly, ciprofloxacin resistance in broiler meats (average = 42.6%; *n* = 11 countries) ranged from 0% (Ireland) to 97.9% (Hungary). In meat from fattening turkeys, for which only three European Union

countries reported, ciprofloxacin resistance rates varied from 6.9% in France to 74.2% in Germany and 91% in Hungary. Some of the ciprofloxacin-resistant isolates were not resistant to nalidixic acid, which is common for plasmid-mediated quinolone-resistance (PMQR) mechanisms (55). In contrast, the U.S. data show that 1/143 retail chicken meat isolates in 2014 was nonsusceptible to ciprofloxacin (MIC = 0.125 µg/ml), and no other ciprofloxacin resistance was detected from any poultry sources.

Cephalosporin Resistance

Resistance to third-generation cephalosporins ranged from 0% to 10.8% in the European Union (26) and was present in 2.4% of U.S. human clinical isolates (31). Among broiler isolates, the European Union averaged 2.3% resistance to third-generation cephalosporin (cefotaxime), with resistance entirely absent from 14 of the 23 reporting countries. Resistance was higher in the United States, where ceftriaxone resistance was detected in 8.7% of broiler isolates collected at slaughter. Only Italy (27.3%) and Cyprus (8.9%) were higher. Among the 11 member states that monitor meat derived from broilers, rare resistance was reported from

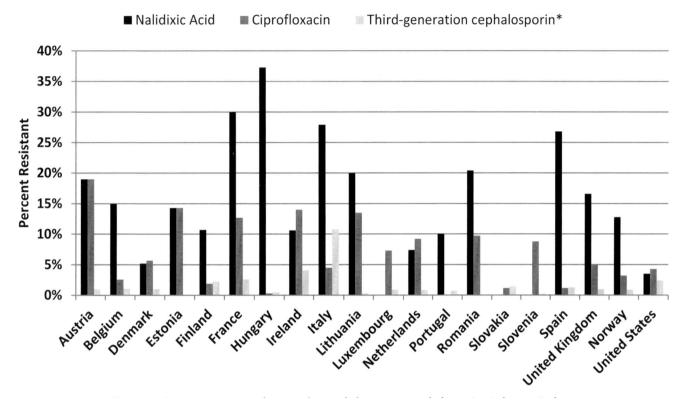

Figure 6 Resistance to quinolones and extended-spectrum cephalosporins in human isolates of *Salmonella* from select European Union countries, Norway, and the United States. Breakpoints used for interpreting MICs were derived from the EUCAST. Among critically important drugs (defined here as macrolides, fluoroquinolones, extended-spectrum cephalosporins, and carbapenems), azithromycin, meropenem, and colistin resistances were very rare and not reported in most countries. *Percentage based on reporting of either cefotaxime or ceftazidime resistance from the European Union or ceftriaxone from the United States.

Belgium (3.7%) and Spain (0.8%), compared with NARMS data which showed 17.5% resistance in 2014 isolates, down from a peak of 37.9% in 2009 (Fig. 7).

CTX-M is just one of several ESBL enzymes that can confer resistance to extended-spectrum cephalosporins and most other beta-lactam antimicrobials. In 2014, EFSA reported that serovar Infantis comprised the highest proportion of broiler isolates exhibiting an ESBL phenotype (18/30, 60%), followed by serovar Paratyphi B L(+) tartrate positive (6/30, 20%). Member states did not report molecular characterization of isolates, so the determination of ESBL positivity is presumptive; however, other studies do show that CTX-M is the most prevalent ESBL in Europe (56), dominating over the TEM and SHV enzyme families. Though they predominate in the United States, AmpC enzymes, which confer resistance to most beta-lactams and beta-lactamase inhibitors, are less frequently encountered in Europe. Genes encoding AmpC enzymes are typically carried on large plasmids that harbor other antimicrobial resistance genes but can also be chromosomally

located (57). Of the 18 broiler isolates with an AmpC phenotype, 9 (50%) were serovar Heidelberg. Eleven of the eighteen isolates were from the Netherlands.

Colistin Resistance

Following the discovery of transmissible colistin resistance mediated by the *mcr-1* gene in *E. coli* in China, (58) colistin-resistant *Salmonella* isolates were found in several countries (59). Colistin resistance was reported in The Netherlands (21.5%) and Denmark (5.9%) in 2014 (26). Overall, EFSA reports colistin resistance in *Salmonella* recovered from broilers (8.3%), laying hens (13.5%), and turkeys (1.8%) (Fig. 7). Most of these (72% of broilers and 80% of laying hens) were serovar Enteritidis, which may reflect a level of intrinsic resistance. Numerous separate studies have detected the *mcr-1* gene in food animal and human *Salmonella* strains from several European countries (60–62) and from human strains in the United States (63). Additionally, *mcr-1* has been found in multidrug-resistant isolates, raising the possibility of coselection (64). While

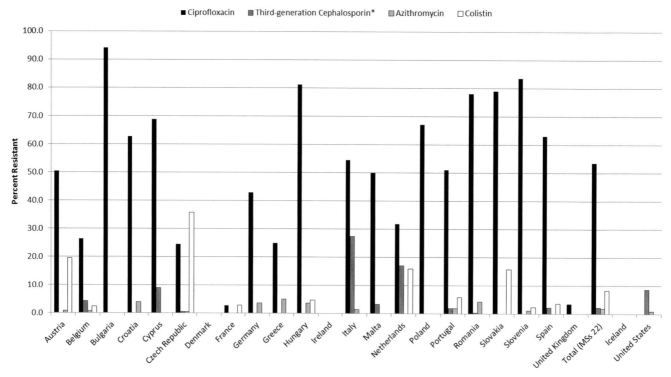

Figure 7 Resistance to quinolones, extended-spectrum cephalosporins, macrolides, and colistin in broiler strains of *Salmonella* from select European Union countries, Iceland, and the United States. Breakpoints used for interpreting MICs were derived from the EUCAST. Among critically important drugs (defined here as macrolides, fluoroquinolones, extended-spectrum cephalosporins, and carbapenems), azithromycin, meropenem, and colistin resistances were very rare and not reported in most countries. *Percentage based on reporting of either cefotaxime or ceftazidime resistance from the European Union or ceftriaxone from United States.

colistin has been used routinely in livestock in several countries, it is not marketed or available for use in food animals in the United States. Therefore, NARMS does not test for phenotypic colistin resistance in routine surveillance. In addition, the *mcr-1* gene was not found in whole-genome sequence data on over 6,500 U.S. *Salmonella* genomes, mostly from retail meats (65).

Other Resistances

In regard to other critically important antibiotics, azithromycin resistance remains rare in *Salmonella* from both continents, ranging in detection from <0.1% of U.S. isolates to 1.7% of strains from Denmark. Similarly, azithromycin resistance in *Salmonella* from chickens and turkeys was identified but was not frequent (Fig. 7).

Very few cases of carbapenem-resistant *Salmonella* infections have been reported in humans in the European Union and the United States (66–69), and resistance has only occasionally been found in *Salmonella* and other Gram-negative bacteria from food animals (70, 71).

The impact of these sporadic findings on public health is of paramount concern. While currently, this impact appears to be small, there is speculation that carbapenemase genes can transfer between humans, animals, and the environment and that the use of third-generation cephalosporins may maintain bacterial populations that express these genes (70). Regardless, as of the writing of this article, carbapenem resistance had not been reported in any retail meat or food isolates of *Salmonella*.

Tigecycline also is not licensed for veterinary use, is not targeted in NARMS, and is an optional drug for susceptibility testing in the European Union. The 2014 EFSA data show microbiological resistance to tigecycline in 9.3% of all *Salmonella* spp. from broilers and 8% from turkeys. Most tigecycline resistance was associated with serovar Infantis in poultry, and most resistant strains had MICs just above the ECOFF breakpoint at 2 or 4 µg/ml. Resistance to tigecycline in *Salmonella* is thought to be mediated by regulatory gene mutations leading to increased efflux.

RESISTANCE IN OTHER REGIONS

Few countries have ongoing surveillance of antimicrobial susceptibility in *Salmonella* from food-producing or companion animals. Most data on antimicrobial resistance in *Salmonella* is derived from cases of human clinical illness. Sustained integrated surveillance of the food chain exists to different degrees outside the European Union and North America. In South America, for example, the Colombian Integrated Program for Antimicrobial Resistance Surveillance (COIPARS) monitors *Salmonella* from poultry farms, slaughterhouses, and retail poultry for resistance (72). In Southeast Asia, some *Salmonella* resistance data are systematically collected and published in periodic summary reports. The Japanese Veterinary Antimicrobial Resistance Monitoring System (JVARM) (73) began in 2000 and tracks antimicrobial resistance in food animal *Salmonella* throughout Japan.

In 2013, JVARM reported *Salmonella* resistance data collected from 2008 to 2011 on isolates from diagnostic samples from livestock and poultry infections (73). MICs were determined for a total of 688 *Salmonella* isolates: 301 from cattle, 236 from pigs, and 151 from chickens. Most were serovars Typhimurium (244 isolates, 35.5%), Choleraesuis (85 isolates, 12.4%), and Infantis (48 isolates, 7%).

JVARM reports that resistance rates against most antimicrobials studied were largely unchanged during the 2008 to 2011 sampling interval, with some slight declines (73). For compounds tested in both 2008 and 2011, resistances were as follows: tetracycline, 61% and 46%; ampicillin, 37% and 24%; kanamycin, 19% and 13%; chloramphenicol, 19% and 11%; nalidixic acid, 11% and 9%; gentamicin, 6% and 3%; cefazolin, 1.8% and 3.6%. Among critically important antimicrobial agents, resistance to cefotaxime was found in 1.7% of pig strains and 3% of chicken strains in 2010. In 2011, cefotaxime resistance was present in 10% of cattle isolates. Resistance to nalidixic acid was most common in pig isolates (16% to 21%). No resistance to colistin or ciprofloxacin was detected (73).

In 2012, JVARM added sampling of bacteria from animals at slaughter (12). The top serovars again were Typhimurium (37.5%), Choleraesuis (12.6%), and Infantis (6%). Between 2012 and 2013, a total of 365 *Salmonella* isolates (140 from cattle, 143 from pigs, and 82 from chickens) were subjected to antimicrobial susceptibility testing (12). Resistance was most frequent in *Salmonella* from cattle and swine for streptomycin (67.9% and 70.0% respectively), tetracycline (34.5% to 66.1% and 53.0% to 66.7%, respectively), and ampicillin (34.5% to 60.7% and 25.3% to 45.0%, respec-

tively). Resistance to cefazolin and cefotaxime was rare in *Salmonella* isolates from cattle and chickens (0% to 8.9%). Resistance to colistin was found in a few isolates from pigs and chickens (0% to 8.9%). When comparing resistance between 2008 and 2009 with data from 2012 to 2013, overall resistance to most antimicrobials was stable in Japan except for nalidixic acid, which increased significantly (0.6% to 5.0%) in *Salmonella* from cattle, and kanamycin, tetracycline, and chloramphenicol resistance, which decreased significantly in isolates from pigs. Among the 212 *Salmonella* isolates tested between 2012 and 2013 from broilers at slaughter, resistance was common for streptomycin (77.7% to 84.7%), tetracycline (74.5% to 82.2%), ampicillin (22.9% to 31.9%), kanamycin (31.9% to 42.4%), and trimethoprim-sulfamethoxazole (31.9% to 48.3%). Resistance to nalidixic acid was high (29.8% to 19.5%), but resistance was infrequent for cefazolin (5.9% to 7.4%), cefotaxime (5.1% to 7.4%), and chloramphenicol (0% to 0.8%) (12). The JVARM program is planning to add retail meat testing in the near future.

China has one of the largest food animal production economies of any country. It is estimated that there are about 30 million annual cases of salmonellosis in China (74). One study estimated that between 1994 and 2005, about 22% of foodborne diseases in China were caused by *Salmonella* (75). While China works to implement an integrated national antimicrobial resistance monitoring system suited to its annual production volume, the status of resistance in *Salmonella* can be assessed only from a limited number of targeted studies, most of which target retail meats or human cases of salmonellosis or focus on specific resistance traits.

A 2005 survey by Yan et al. (76) examined raw retail samples of pork (*n* = 45), chicken (*n* =120), beef (*n* = 45), mutton (*n* = 45), seafood (*n* = 96), and milk powder (*n* = 36) in nine cities in Hebei province in northern China. The most common serovars were Agona (13.6%), Senftenberg (9.9%), Meleagridis (8.6%), and Derby (8.6%). MDR was most common in serovars Derby, Indiana, and Saintpaul. Among critical antimicrobial agents, nalidixic acid resistance was found in 31% of isolates, most commonly in isolates recovered from chicken (14/16, 74%). Ceftriaxone resistance was found in two (2.5%) isolates, and ciprofloxacin resistance was detected in eight (9.9%) isolates. Two years later, a study by Yang et al. (77) examined retail meats consisting of 515 chicken, 91 pork, 78 beef, and 80 lamb samples from nearby Shanxi Province in 2007 to 2008. The most common serovars were Enteritidis (31.5%), Typhimurium (13.4%), Shubra (10.0%), Indiana (9.7%), and Derby

(9.5%). In addition to the common resistance to sulfamethoxazole (67%), trimethoprim/sulfamethoxazole (58%), and tetracycline (56%), a very high proportion of isolates were resistant to nalidixic acid (35%), ciprofloxacin (21%), and ceftriaxone (16%). Of particular interest, nearly all isolates of serovars Shubra (89%) and Indiana (88%) were resistant to more than antimicrobials, much higher than in other serovars (77).

A 2011 study by Bai et al. (78) examined resistance in *Salmonella* from large-scale chicken and swine abattoirs in Henan, China, where 128/283 (45.2%) chicken samples and 70/240 (29.2%) pig samples yielded *Salmonella* isolates for antimicrobial susceptibility. The most common resistance was to nalidixic acid (91%), followed by ampicillin (66%) and tetracycline (47%). Ciprofloxacin resistance was detected in 11 (8.6%) poultry strains, all of which were serovar Indiana and 6 of which also carried an ESBL. In the pig strains, the most common resistance was to tetracycline (67%), followed by nalidixic acid (64%) and chloramphenicol (60%). Ciprofloxacin resistance was found in 10% (7/70) of the isolates, 5 of which also carried an ESBL. This study shed light on the nature of MDR in serovar Indiana in China, where 11 of 198 isolates were coresistant to ciprofloxacin and cefotaxime and harbored $bla_{CTX-M-65}$ and *aac(6′)-Ib-cr* genes, typically carried by plasmids and conferring resistance to the front-line drugs for salmonellosis. Another important study, by Lai et al., examined resistance in *Salmonella* in the Shandong province of China from 2009 to 2012. This survey showed a general rise in resistance during the sampling interval, with ciprofloxacin resistance appearing in 42% of salmonellae in 2012 (79).

Various later reports described the MDR traits found in serovar Indiana in China (77, 80, 81). In a study of ESBL-producing *Salmonella* from production environments in China, Zhang et al. (82) explored the genetic constituents of resistance in CTX-M-producing *Salmonella* isolates from chickens and pig facilities. They found that serovars Typhimurium and Indiana most commonly carried various transmissible CTX-M alleles, which in some cases was coupled to PMQR along with other resistance determinants. Serovar Indiana showed higher resistance levels than serovar Typhimurium. This combination of ESBL and PMQR in *Salmonella* has been noted in other studies from China (83, 84).

Despite that fact that *Salmonella* serovars and resistance can display distinct geographic characteristics, *Salmonella* clones have shown a remarkable ability to spread worldwide. This presents a perpetual public health issue concerning the international spread of new resistant clones as has been seen in the past. The

striking example of global dissemination illustrated by MDR DT104 is a case in point. This strain spread to almost all countries and became a major driver of resistance reported in many regions (85–87). However, there has been a decrease in reported MDR DT104 in the past 10 years (41). Recent phylogenetic analysis indicates that the strain may have initially emerged in Europe in the early 1970s, followed by multiple transmission events between countries and hosts (88), likely related to the trade in breeding animals, human travel, and international sales of food products. The case of DT104 exemplifies the need to consider salmonellosis in the context of a global One Health paradigm, where resistance gaining ascendancy in animals can gain a foothold and spread around the world to become a major cause of resistant human infections.

ANTIMICROBIAL-RESISTANT *SALMONELLA* FROM COMPANION ANIMALS

Companion animals pose a public health risk for human salmonellosis in many countries (2, 89, 90). Although the prevalence of *Salmonella* in companion animals, especially in dogs and cats, varies greatly (ranging from 0% and 70% [2, 91, 92]), a number of serovars important to human health have been found in pet animals. Hoelzer (2) reported that among the top 20 most common human *Salmonella* serovars, 15 have been isolated from domestic dogs and cats, including Typhimurium, Enteritidis, Newport, Heidelberg, Montevideo, Muenchen, Oranienburg, Braederup, Agona, Infantis, Thompson, Paratpyhi B, Stanley, Tennessee, and Hadar. According to a 2006 annual report of the National Veterinary Services Laboratories of the U.S. Department of Agriculture (USDA), serovars Newport, Typhimurium, Montevideo, and Enteritidis were the most common serovars isolated from sick dogs and cats in the United States (93).

Because companion animals, especially dogs and cats, are considered family members, many antimicrobials that are important to human health have been used in veterinary practice to treat infections of dogs and cats, including category I antimicrobial agents, such as third/fourth-generation cephalosporins, fluoroquinolones, nitroimidazoles, penicillin beta-lactam inhibitors; category II agents, such as first/second-generation cephalosporins, penicillin, lincosamides, macrolides, and trimethoprim-sulfonamides; and category III agents, such as chloramphenicol, sulfonamides, and tetracycline (94–97). There is an increased concern about the rapid emergence and spread of MDR bacteria from pets to humans due to the extensive use of antimicrobial agents in these animals and their close contact with humans (98). Various MDR bacteria such as *E. coli*, *Salmonella*, *Staphylococcus*, *Pseudomonas*, *Streptococcus*, *Klebsiella*, *Proteus*, and *Enterococcus* have been isolated from diseased dogs and cats (95–100).

Currently, there is no surveillance program in the United States for antimicrobial resistance in bacteria from companion animals, and antimicrobial use in these animals is not routinely monitored. Therefore, no reliable data are available to assess the trend of antimicrobial resistance in bacteria isolated from companion animals. Several reports have shown that the increased use of antimicrobials to treat diseased dogs and cats is associated with the emergence of antimicrobial resistance in *Salmonella*. Among these reports are early U.S. NARMS Animal Arm reports (1997 to 2004), which feature data on antimicrobial resistance in *Salmonella* isolated from sick dogs and cats. The *Salmonella* isolates were submitted to the USDA National Veterinary Services Laboratory in Ames, IA, and tested for susceptibilities to 16 antimicrobials. *Salmonella* isolated from diseased dogs and cats had varied rates of resistance to different antimicrobials: ampicillin (24.6% to 58.8%), streptomycin (23.7% to 58.8%), tetracycline (22.7% to 53.8%), sulfamethoxazole (6.3% to 58.8%), and chloramphenicol (9.4% to 43.8%) (101). When surveillance first began in 1997, *Salmonella* isolates from sick dogs (*n* = 38) were susceptible to amoxicillin/clavulanic acid, ceftiofur, ceftriaxone, cephalothin, gentamicin, nalidixic acid, and trimethoprim/sulfamethoxazole, but 1 year later, isolates appeared resistant to all of these drugs except nalidixic acid. By 2002, resistance to amoxicillin/clavulanic reached 30.3%, ceftiofur 29.5%, ceftriaxone 29.5%, cephalothin 31.2%, and trimethoprim/sulfamethoxazole 12.3%. While dog isolates from 1997 were susceptible to most drugs tested, cat isolates (*n* = 28) from that same year were resistant to amoxicillin/clavulanic acid (10.7%) and ceftiofur, ceftriaxone, and cephalothin (10.7%) but were susceptible to gentamicin, nalidixic acid, and trimethoprim/sulfamethoxazole. All *Salmonella* isolates from sick dogs and cats from 1997 to 2004 were susceptible to amikacin and ciprofloxacin (Table 2). Overall, these NARMS data show that *Salmonella* isolates from sick dogs and cats have increased in their resistance to amoxicillin/clavulanic acid, ceftiofur, gentamicin, and nalidixic acid over the years, with nalidixic acid resistance first appearing in dog isolates in 2000 and in cat isolates in 2004. Analysis of all 5,709 *Salmonella* isolates from domestic food and companion animals collected for NARMS in 1997 and 1998 showed that extended-spectrum cephalosporin-resistance levels differed significantly among host animal species, with higher resistances found in isolates from turkeys, horses, cats, and dogs. All *Salmonella* isolates resistant to extended-spectrum cephalosporins carried the bla_{CMY} gene (102).

Other countries have also reported antimicrobial resistance in *Salmonella* from companion animals. A 2005 to 2006 Canadian survey of pet dog feces showed that 23.2% of the dogs carried *Salmonella*, and 20% of the *Salmonella* isolates were resistant to at least one antimicrobial, while 14% were resistant to multiple antimicrobials. The most common pattern, found in 13.3% of isolates, was resistance to amoxicillin/clavulanic acid, ampicillin, cefoxitin, ceftiofur, and ceftriaxone (103). Among the resistant *Salmonella* isolates, 79.2% were *S.* Heidelberg, 12.5% were *S.* Kentucky, and 8.3% were *S.* Indiana (103). A Belgian study by Van Immerseel et al. (104) showed that the prevalence of *Salmonella* in different cat groups (healthy house cats, group-housed cats, and sick cats) ranged from 0.36% to 51.4%. In this study, *S.* Typhimurium, *S.* Enteritidis, *S.* Bovismorbificans, and *S.* 4:i:– were identified. Most *S.* Typhimurium isolates from group-housed cats were resistant to ampicillin, chloramphenicol, and tetracycline; *S.* 4:i:– from diseased cats was resistant to ampicillin, chloramphenicol, sulfonamides, tetracycline, and trimethoprim/sulfamethoxazole. The resistance genes bla_{TEM}, *cat*, *sul2*, *tet*(A), and *dfrA* were identified in this *S.* 4:i:– isolate. Another study in the Netherlands found that 1% of diarrheic dogs were positive for *Salmonella* and that 53% of the *Salmonella* isolates were resistant to cephalexin, 37% to tetracycline, 14% to amoxicillin/clavulanic acid, 6% to trimethoprim/sulfonamides, and 4% to enrofloxacin (98).

S. Typhimurium DT104 with the ACSSuT resistance profile was first isolated in the United Kingdom from sea gulls in the mid-1980s, but not from humans until 1989. During the past 30 years, the strain has become prevalent in humans, food animals, and companion animals in many countries (98, 105). *S.* Typhimurium DT104 in humans significantly increased in England and Wales from 1991 to 1995, from 259 in 1990 to 2,873 in 1994 and 3,837 in 1995. Most of the human *S.* Typhimurium DT104 isolates had R-type ACSSuT. Further epidemiologic studies indicated that cats played an important role in the epidemic spread of this organism through many populations (106). A similar report from Scotland during the same time period showed that *S.* Typhimurium DT104 was isolated in 1% to 2% of cat fecal samples, and the cats shed the organism for at least 7 to 14 weeks (107). MDR Typhimurium var. Copenhagen DT104 also was isolated from horses,

Table 2   Percentage resistance of *Salmonella* isolated from clinical companion animals[a]

Antimicrobials[b]	1997 Dog	1997 Cat	1998 Dog	1998 Cat	1999 Dog	1999 Cat	2000 Dog	2000 Cat	2001[c] Dog	2002 Dog	2002 Cat	2003 Dog	2003 Cat	2004 Dog	2004 Cat
	n = 38	n = 28	n = 57	n = 29	n = 57	n = 25	n = 44	n = 17	n = 64	n = 92	n = 19	n = 68	n = 32	n = 53	n = 22
Amoxicillin/clavulanic acid	0	10.7	7.0	6.9	10.5	8.0	13.6	17.6	29.7	38.0	10.5	20.6	3.1	26.4	18.2
Ampicillin	31.6	53.6	24.6	48.3	26.3	40.0	34.1	58.8	35.9	43.5	26.3	29.4	25.0	30.2	31.8
Apramycin	0	3.6	1.8	0	0	4.0	4.5	0	1.6						
Cefoxitin	0	10.7	7.0	6.9	8.8	8.0	11.4	17.6	29.7	37.0	10.5	20.6	3.1	22.6	13.6
Ceftiofur	0	10.7	8.8	13.8	14.0	8.0	11.4	17.6	29.7	37.0	10.5	20.6	3.1	22.6	13.6
Cephalothin	13.2	28.6	21.1	20.7	17.5	36.0	25.0	23.5	29.7	39.1	10.5	26.5	9.4		
Chloramphenicol	0	0	10.5	6.9	1.8	12.0	6.8	35.3	29.7	43.5	18.5	26.5	9.4	28.3	22.7
Gentamicin								11.8	9.4	5.4	5.3	17.6	3.1	1.9	9.1
Kanamycin	18.4	32.2	12.3	27.6	12.3	24.0	9.1	35.3	10.9	20.7	5.3	19.1	12.5	9.4	0
Nalidixic acid	0	0	0	0	0	0	4.5	0	1.6	15.2	0	4.4	0	5.7	4.5
Streptomycin	23.7	35.7	33.3	51.7	31.6	48.0	31.8	58.8	39.1	44.6	21.1	32.4	21.9	32.1	27.3
Sulfisoxazole	31.6	50	31.6	48.3	29.8	44.0	34.1	58.8	40.6	38.0	21.1	30.9	6.3	30.2	31.8
Tetracycline	36.8	57.1	31.6	44.8	33.3	48.0	31.8	52.9	45.3	45.7	26.3	38.2	25.0	30.2	22.7
Trimethoprim/sulfamethoxazole	0	0	5.3	3.4	10.5	4.0	2.3	11.8	1.6	16.3	5.3	7.4	3.1	0	0

[a]The data were obtained from the animal arm of NARMS report (http://www.ars.usda.gov/Main/docs.htm?docid=18034). All isolates were obtained from the National Veterinary Services Laboratories.
[b]The resistant breakpoints were adopted from early CLSI guidelines as described in the NARMS 1997 to 2004 reports. All isolates were susceptible to amikacin, ceftriaxone, and ciprofloxacin (resistant breakpoints of 64 ug/ml and 4 ug/ml were used for ceftriaxone and ciprofloxacin, respectively).
[c]No cat isolates were tested in 2001.

dogs, and cats in Germany (108). The dog and cat isolates had R-type ACSSuT. Two horse isolates showed additional resistance to florfenicol, gentamicin, kanamycin, and trimethoprim. In the United States, several human outbreaks of MDR *S.* Typhimurium DT104 with R-type ACSSuT or ACKSSuT were associated with small-animal veterinary clinics and animal shelters in Idaho, Minnesota, and Washington in 1999 to 2000. During these outbreaks, cats were confirmed as a source of infections (109, 110). A number of MDR *S.* Typhimurium outbreaks associated with pet rodents were also reported in the United States from 2003 to 2004 (111). The *S.* Typhimurium isolated from patients and pet hamsters showed the same R-type ACSSuT resistance profile and an indistinguishable pulsed field gel electrophoresis profile.

Multidrug-resistant *S.* Typhimurium with high-level fluoroquinolone resistance has been isolated from dogs and cats in Japan (112). These isolates had MICs of >256 μg/ml for nalidixic acid, 24 to 32 μg/ml for ciprofloxacin, and 24 to 32 μg/ml for norfloxacin. Two of the isolates had R-type ACSSuT in addition to resistance to nalidixic acid and ciprofloxacin (ACSSuTNCp). Another isolate from a dog showed additional resistance to trimethoprim/sulfamethoxazole, trimethoprim, and gentamicin (112).

Contaminated dog and cat foods are increasingly recognized as a risk factor for *Salmonella* infections in pets. Several surveys conducted in the United States and Canada showed that the prevalence of *Salmonella* in pet foods and treats ranged from 21% to 50% (2). A survey was conducted by the U.S. FDA to investigate the prevalence and antimicrobial resistance of *Salmonella* in dog treats sold in the U.S. market (113). Investigators found that 41% of animal-derived pet treats were contaminated with *Salmonella* and 26% of the isolates were resistant to tetracycline, 23% to streptomycin, 19% to sulfamethoxazole, 8% to chloramphenicol, and 8% to ampicillin. More than one third (36%) of the *Salmonella* isolates were resistant to at least one antimicrobial, and 13% of isolates displayed resistance to four or more antimicrobials. Two isolates were identified as *S.* Typhimurium DT104, with the characteristic R-type ACSSuT. One *S.* Typhimurium isolate was resistant to kanamycin in addition to the above five antimicrobials. One *S.* Brandenburg isolate was resistant to eight antimicrobials, including ampicillin, chloramphenicol, streptomycin, sulfamethoxazole, tetracycline, gentamicin, apramycin, and cephalothin. Pet foods are also a risk factor for human infections. A multistate outbreak of tetracycline-resistant *Salmonella* serovar I 4,[5],12:i– was attributed to frozen feeder rodents. This outbreak caused over 500 clinical illnesses between 2008 and 2010 (114).

Salmonella has also been isolated from other types of pets, such as lizards, snakes, turtles, birds, and fish. Unfortunately, most reports do not contain antimicrobial resistance information for these isolates (115–117). Reptiles are considered a natural reservoir of *Salmonella* and constitute a significant source of human salmonellosis (2, 89, 90). The U.S. NARMS animal testing component reports from 1997 to 2004 feature antimicrobial susceptibility data on *Salmonella* isolated from exotic animals, including lizard, snakes, iguanas, and other reptiles and turtles. Those isolates showed low levels of resistance to most antimicrobials tested: a little over 10% resistance to ampicillin, streptomycin, sulfamethoxazole, and tetracycline but <10% resistance to amoxicillin/clavulanic acid, cefoxitin, ceftiofur, ceftriaxone, cephalothin, chloramphenicol, gentamicin, kanamycin, nalidixic acid, and trimethoprim/sulfamethoxazole. They were all susceptible to amikacin and ciprofloxacin (101).

These data indicate that companion animals are important reservoirs of *Salmonella* and that many *Salmonella* strains isolated from companion animals have developed resistance. Furthermore, some *Salmonella* isolates showed high resistance to medically important antimicrobials. To protect public health, there is a need to establish an antimicrobial resistance surveillance program for companion animals. There are ongoing discussions on how existing U.S. surveillance programs can fill this void.

ANTIMICROBIAL RESISTANCE GENES
To fully interpret the antimicrobial resistance data, it is important to characterize the underlying genetic mechanisms in bacteria from humans, animals, and food (16). Acquired resistance in *Salmonella* results from mutations in chromosomal genes (both structural and regulatory sequences) and by acquisition of preformed, exogenous genes transmitted on mobile elements such as plasmids, integrons, and transposons. While both mechanisms can lead to rapid changes in bacterial populations, horizontal gene transfer is more consequential in the evolution of resistance in *Salmonella*, where a single plasmid conjugation event can confer resistance to seven or more agents (118). Following conjugative transfer, mobile DNA elements can be maintained as extrachromosomal plasmids or be incorporated wholly or partially into the chromosome as genomic islands. Detailed information on the genes and their context provides insights into the evolution of resistance and its sources.

THE IMPACT OF ROUTINE WHOLE-GENOME SEQUENCING

The DNA sequence information on the number and types of different resistance genes in *Salmonella* is growing at a very rapid rate, perhaps faster than for any other pathogen at this time. This is due to a push in the public health arena for early adoption of whole-genome sequencing (WGS) as a tool for food safety monitoring and outbreak investigations. Specialists in food safety have spearheaded initiatives to set data quality standards, provide proficiency testing, explore analytical approaches, and foster data sharing arrangements to deploy WGS globally to combat infectious diseases (119). As of this writing, the National Center for Biotechnology Information (NCBI) pathogen detection web portal (https://www.ncbi.nlm.nih.gov/pathogens/) lists *Salmonella* first among genera with completed genomic sequence (>100,000 genomes), followed by *E. coli/Shigella* (>37,000), *Listeria* (>16,000), and *Campylobacter* (>14,000), with the majority of each belonging to environmental (including food) isolates and with several hundred new genomes being uploaded weekly. Currently, most of the *Salmonella* genomes are generated by the U.S. FDA's GenomeTrakr program, which submitted an average of 2,400 *Salmonella* genomic sequences per month in 2015 (120). The unprecedented stream of WGS data on current strains of *Salmonella* will soon expand greatly when the CDC PulseNet program and other food safety monitoring systems worldwide shift away from pulsed field gel electrophoresis to WGS for routine surveillance and outbreak investigations. Based on past PuslNet testing volumes in the United States alone, this will add approximately 45,000 more *Salmonella* genomic sequences annually to public databases.

Beginning in test year 2014, the U.S. NARMS program began including WGS analysis of *Salmonella* in annual reports and uploading the raw WGS data to the NCBI. In addition, the WGS has been determined for all the historical *Salmonella* (currently over 6,500 isolates) recovered from retail meat sources since testing began in 2002. These genomes also are available in the public domain at NCBI and have accompanying susceptibility phenotypes (Bioproject number PRJNA290865). As WGS data accumulate in NARMS and other surveillance programs, methods for analyzing and reporting changes in the resistome will augment traditional susceptibility information (see Chapter 28). Studies show a very high correlation between the presence of known resistance genes and clinical resistance in *Salmonella* (121, 122) and other foodborne bacteria (123, 124). Thus, it is a simple process to predict resistance in *Sal-*

monella with a high degree of accuracy for most major drug classes based on WGS data alone. The NARMS web page (35) provides simple and powerful tools to explore the *Salmonella* resistome in U.S. national surveillance. Resistome Tracker (125) is one publicly available tool that provides visually informative displays of antibiotic resistance genes in *Salmonella*. Similar tools to quickly identify the resistance (and other) genes in sequence reads have been incorporated into automated analytical processes at NCBI (https://www.ncbi.nlm.nih.gov/pathogens/) or can be applied locally using software applications and resistance gene databases freely available on the web (e.g., ResFinder, CARD). The development of simple bioinformatics tools will enable a comprehensive, near-real-time monitoring of the resistome in *Salmonella* from foods, the environment, animals, and human infections that will be accessible by all interested parties.

After many years of surveillance and research, and especially with the large amounts of WGS data now being generated through surveillance programs, much is known about the specific alleles underlying resistance in different *Salmonella* serovars. Michael and Schwarz (126–128) have published three comprehensive reviews on this topic since 2006. Table 3 shows the WGS-based resistome of the U.S. *Salmonella* isolates that are deposited at NCBI. While the canon of resistance genes is changing very rapidly, the current status in *Salmonella* is summarized below.

Fluoroquinolone Resistance

Fluoroquinolone resistance has been well characterized in *Salmonella* and other bacterial pathogens. It has long been known that a combination of mutations in specific regions of the topoisomerase genes encoded by *gyrA*, *gyrB*, *parC*, and *parE* confers resistance to fluoroquinolones in *Salmonella* and other enterics. More recently, PMQR determinants have been identified including multiple alleles of *qnrA*, *qnrB*, *qnrD*, and *qnrS*, which function by protecting the topoisomerase targets from inhibition resulting in decreased fluoroquinolone susceptibility (129). A total of 32 *qnr* genes have been identified in *Salmonella* (Table 3). The *qnrB19* allele has emerged to become the predominant one in *Salmonella* in the United States, where it is present in 0.5% of resistant human strains. The quinolone efflux pump encoded by *qepA* (130, 131), a bifuntional enzyme encoded by *aac(60)-Ib-cr* (132), and the *oqxA* gene (133) are known also to affect quinolone MICs in *Salmonella* isolates. The PMQR gene, *oqxAB*, also mediates resistance to nalidixic acid and chloramphenicol, as well as olaquindox. It has been found in multiple serovars in

Table 3 Acquired antimicrobial resistance genes in nontyphoidal *Salmonella*[a]

Antimicrobial class	Resistance genes
Rifampicin	*arr-2, arr-3*
Fluoroquinolone	*qnrA1, qnrA2, qnrB1, qnrB11, qnrB12, qnrB17, qnrB19, qnrB2, qnrB25, qnrB26, qnrB3, qnrB32, qnrB34, qnrB35, qnrB37, qnrB38, qnrB4, qnrB40, qnrB4, qnrB47, qnrB48, qnrB51, qnrB6, qnrB69, qnrB7, qnrB9, qnrD, qnrS1, qnrS2, qnrS3, qnrS4, qnrVC4, aac(6′)Ib-cr, norA, oqxA, oqxB, qepA*
Aminoglycoside	*aac(2′)-Ia, aac(2′)-Ib, aac(2′)-Ic, aac(3)-IIa, aac(3)-IId, aac(3)-IIe, aac(3)-IVa, aac(3)-Ia, aac(3)-Id, aac(3)-Ik, aac(3)-VIa, aac(6′)-33, aac(6′)-IIa, aac(6′)-IIc, aac(6′)-Ib, aac(6′)-Ic, aac(6′)-If, aac(6′)-Ii, aac(6′)-Im, aac(6′)-Iz, aac(6′)-aph(2′′), aacA4, aadA1, aadA10, aadA11, aadA12, aadA13, aadA14, aadA15, aadA16, aadA17, aadA2, aadA22, aadA23, aadA24, aadA3, aadA4, aadA5, aadA6, aadA7, aadA8, aadA8b, aadB, aadD, ant(6)-Ia, aph(2′′)-Ib, aph(3′)-III, aph(3′)-IIa, aph(3′)-IIb, aph(3′)-IIc, aph(3′)-Ia, aph(3′)-Ic, aph(3′)-Id, aph(3′)-VIa, aph(4)-Ia, aph(6)-Ic, armA, rmtB, rmtE, spc, sph, strA, strB*
Beta-lactam (*bla* genes)	ACT-4, ACT-5, ACT-6, ACT-7, CARB-1, CARB-2, CARB-3, CARB-5, CARB-6, CEPH-A, CKO-1, CMG, CMY-15, CMY-16, CMY-17, CMY-18, CMY-2, CMY- 20, CMY-22, CMY-23, CMY-24, CMY-3, CMY-30, CMY-32, CMY-33, CMY-36, CMY-4, CMY-41, CMY-42, CMY-44, CMY-46, CMY-47, CMY-48, CMY-5, CMY-53, CMY-54, CMY-56, CMY-58, CMY-59, CMY-6, CMY-61, CMY-64, CMY-68 ,CMY-70, CMY-83, CMY-87, CMY-98, CTX-M-1, CTX-M-11, CTX-M-14, CTX-M-14b, CTX-M-15, CTX-M-2, CTX-M-24, CTX-M-27, CTX-M-3, CTX-M-5, CTX-M-55, CTX-M-65, CTX-M-8, CTX-M-9, DHA-1, DHA-2, DHA- 3, DHA-5, HERA-3, HERA-5, HERA-6, KPC-2, LEN1, LEN11, LEN9, MAL-1, MIR-3, MIR-5, MOR-1, MOR-2, NDM-1, OKP-B-12, OXA-1, OXA-10, OXA- 114, OXA-129, OXA-134, OXA-17, OXA-2, OXA-21, OXA-23, OXA-27, OXA-278, OXA-335, OXA-34, OXA-36, OXA-4, OXA-48, OXA-50, OXA-58, OXA-61, OXA-66, OXA-9, OXA-90, OXY-1-4, OXY-1-5, OXY-2, OXY-2-7, OXY-2-8, OXY-5-1, OXY-6, OXY-6-1, OXY-6-2, PAO, PER-2, SED1, SHV-1, SHV-100, SHV-105, SHV-11, SHV-12, SHV-122, SHV-129, SHV-2, SHV-25, SHV-28, SHV-39, SHV-45, SHV-99, TEM-1, TEM-10, TEM-104, TEM-105, TEM-106, TEM-116, TEM-12 , TEM-123, TEM-124, TEM-126, TEM-127, TEM-135, TEM- 141 ,TEM-143, TEM-144, TEM-148, TEM-154, TEM-155, TEM-156, TEM-157, TEM-159, TEM-162, TEM-166, TEM-169, TEM-171, TEM-176, TEM-183, TEM-199, TEM-1A, TEM-1B, TEM-1C, TEM-1D, TEM-2 ,TEM-205, TEM-213, TEM-22, TEM-30, TEM-33, TEM-42, TEM-52, TEM-52B, TEM-57, TEM-59, TEM-63, TEM-67, TEM-7, TEM-70, TEM-76, TEM-79, TEM-90, TEM-95, VEB- 5, VIM-1, Z, ZEG-1
Beta-lactam (other)	*cepA-29, cfxA, cfxA3, cphA1, mecA, hugA*
Phenicol	*cat(pC221), catA1, catA2, catA3, catB2, catB3, catB7, catQ, cml, cmlA1, fexA, floR*
Trimethoprim	*dfrA10, dfrA12, dfrA14, dfrA15, dfrA16, dfrA17, dfrA18, dfrA21, dfrA23, dfrA24, dfrA25, dfrA27, dfrA29, dfrA31, dfrA32, dfrA5, dfrA7, dfrA8, dfrB1, dfrB3, dfrB5, dfrG*
Macrolides/ lincosamides	*ere*(A), *erm*(42), *erm*(A), *erm*(B), *erm*(C), *erm*(D), *erm*(F), *erm*(G), *lnu*(A), *lnu*(C), *lnu*(F), *lsa*(A), *mef*(A), *mef*(B), *mph*(A), *mph*(B), *mph*(C), *mph*(E), *msr*(A), *msr*(C), *msr*(D), *msr*(E), *vga*(A)
Polymyxin	*mcr-1*
Sulfonamide	*sul1, sul2, sul3*
Tetracycline	*tet*(32), *tet*(38), *tet*(39), *tet*(41), *tet*(A), *tet*(B), *tet*(C), *tet*(D), *tet*(E), *tet*(G), *tet*(H), *tet*(J), *tet*(K), *tet*(L), *tet*(M), *tet*(O), *tet*(P), *tet*(Q), *tet*(W), *tet*(X)
Fosfomycin	*fosA*
Fusidic acid	*fusA, fusB3*

[a]NCBI last accessed 4 March 2017. Total number of genomes, N = 81,936: U.S., *n* = 38,725; non-U.S., *n* = 27,095; unknown origin, *n* = 16,116.

China (134) and in *S.* Typhimurium strains in Europe (135). It appears to augment the development of fluoroquinolone resistance in *Salmonella* (136) and can be selected by florfenicol exposure (137).

Beta-lactamase Resistance

Resistance to the β-lactam class of compounds is conferred by at least 1,177 beta-lactamase genes. Michael and Schwarz report that 13 beta-lactamase families have been identified in *Salmonella*, including ACC,

CMY, CTX-M, DHA, PER, PSE, SCO, SHV, and TEM, as well as 4 carbapenemases of types KPC, NDM, OXA, and VIM (126). To this list can be added FOX (in a U.S. clinical strain of serovar Newport), multiple HERA alleles (prevalent in U.S. turkey isolates), and LAP (in a U.S. clinical strain of *S.* Saintpaul) (121), as well as HUGA and CEP (in United Kingdom clinical isolates), VEB (linked to *armA* in a U.S. clinical isolate), and ZEG (in a U.S. riverine isolate) (NCBI Bioproject number PRJNA290865). In the United States, the bla_{CMY} gene is present in most strains exhibiting resistance to extended-spectrum cephalosporins. Carbapenems are not used in U.S. agriculture, nor are they approved for food-producing animals in any country. No carbapenemases producing salmonellae have been found in NARMS testing, and two cases have been associated with travel (66, 69).

Macrolide Resistance

Among the critically important macrolide class of drugs, only azithromycin has been explored as a treatment for salmonellosis, mainly for *S.* Typhi. Resistance to azithromycin (MIC, ≥16 µg/ml) in NTS has been associated with the presence of *mphA* (121, 138) and *mphE* (unpublished data), although other macrolide resistance genes have been found in *Salmonella*, including *ere*(A), *lnu*(F), *mef*(B), and *msr*(E) (121, 126, 138). The full complement of known macrolide-lincosamide resistance genes in *Salmonella* is shown in Table 3.

Trimethoprim-Sulfonamide Resistance

Trimethoprim-sulfonamide has long been a recommended treatment for salmonellosis. At least 42 trimethoprim resistance genes have been identified in bacteria, 19 of which have been detected in *Salmonella*. These include *dfrA1*, *dfrA3*, *dfrA5*, *dfrA7*, *dfrA8*, *dfrA10*, *dfrA12*, *dfrA13*, *dfrA14*, *dfrA15*, *dfrA16*, *dfrA17*, *dfrA18*, *dfrA19*, *dfrA21*, *dfrA23*, *dfrA24*, *dfrA25*, *dfrA27*, *dfrA29*, *dfrA31*, and *dfrA32*, along with *dfrB1*, *dfrB3*, *dfrB5*, *dfrB6*, and *dfrG*. At least eight of these have been found in U.S. isolates (*dfrA1*, *dfrA5*, *dfrA7*, *dfrA8*, *dfrA12*, *dfrA14*, *dfrA15*, *dfrA17*, and *dfrA18*). Sulfonamide resistance mediated by *sul1*, *sul2*, and *sul3* are common in *Salmonella*.

Tetracycline Resistance

Among the 46 tetracycline resistance genes identified in bacteria to date (139), 20 have been reported in *Salmonella*. These include energy efflux pumps encoded by *tet*(A), *tet*(B), *tet*(C), *tet*(D), *tet*(E), *tet*(G), *tet*(H), *tet*(J), *tet*(K), and *tet*(L). The *tet*(A) and *tet*(B) genes are consistently the most common ones identified. Ribosomal protection mechanisms conferred by *tet*(M) and *tet*(O), as well as rare instances of *tet*(X), which encodes a tetracycline-degrading enzyme, have been found in U.S. isolates of *Salmonella* (121), usually along with other *tet* genes.

Aminoglycoside Resistance

Aminoglycoside resistance is coded by a wide range of alleles, which is complicated by the use of two different naming systems in the literature. More than 146 alleles

have been found in bacteria. Resistance occurs by ribosomal modification, efflux, and enzymatic inactivation. Among these mechanisms, those based on enzymatic modification of the drug are most common in the clinical setting. These enzymes function through three general reactions resulting in phosphorylation, adenylation, or acelylation. The streptomycin phosphotransferases encoded by *strA* and *strB* (also designated *aph*) are the most common overall, present in about 27% of resistant U.S. strains (Table 3) (121). A total of 23 3′ O-adenyltransferase (*aad*) genes have been identified in *Salmonella*, including *aadA1*, *aadA2*, *aadA3*, *aadA4*, *aadA5*, *aadA6*, *aadA7*, *aadA8*, *aadA8b*, *aadA10*, *aadA11*, *aadA12*, *aadA13*, *aadA14*, *aadA15*, *aadA16*, *aadA17*, *aadA21*, *aadA22*, *aadA23*, *aadA24*, *aadA26*, and *aadA27* (126). At least 10 of these have been found in U.S. isolates. Various forms of the *aac* gene family conferring gentamicin resistance are present in *Salmonella*. These include *aac(2′)-Ia*, *aac(2′)-Ib*, *aac(2′)-Ic*, *aac(3)-IIa*, *aac(3)-IId*, *aac(3)-IIe*, *aac(3)-Iva*, *aac(3)-Ia*, *aac(3)-Id*, *aac(3)-Ik*, *aac(3)-Via*, *aac(6′)-33*, *aac(6′)-IIa*, *aac(6′)-IIc*, *aac(6′)-Ib*, *aac(6′)-Ic*, *aac(6′)-If*, *aac(6′)-Ii*, *aac(6′)-Im*, *aac(6′)-Iz*, *aac(6′)-aph(2′′)* (bifunctional enzyme conferring coresistance to low levels of fluoroquinolones), and *aacA4*.

At least six RNA methylase enzymes (ArmA, RmtA, RmtB, RmtC, RmtD, and NpmA) are known, which reside on mobile elements, often with other resistance genes, and confer very high levels of resistance to various aminoglycosides (140). Among the *Enterobacteriaceae*, ArmA is the most frequently identified, and both *armA* and *rmtC* have been found in *Salmonella* (141, 142). An interesting feature of aminoglycoside resistance revealed by WGS is the propensity for *Salmonella* to harbor numerous aminoglycoside resistance genes (and often other resistance gene classes) within a single bacterium (121). In fact, a small minority of aminoglycoside-resistant strains sequenced to date in the United States was found to carry just one resistance gene, and many carry five or more alleles. For example, one U.S. isolate of *S.* I 4,5,12:i:– has the aminoglycoside genotype *aph(3′)-Ic*, *aac(6′)-IIc*, *rmtE*, *aph(3′)-Ia*, *strA*, *strB*, *aph(3′)-Ic* along with unrelated resistance determinants coded by bla_{SHV-12}, bla_{TEM-1B}, *ere*(A), *anrB19*, *sul1*, *sul2*, *tet*(B), *tet*(A), and *tet*(M). The advantage of carrying so many resistance determinants all conferring resistance to the same drug class is not obvious but may partly reflect the fact that aminoglycosides have been used longer than most drug classes in food animal production and that individual strains have adapted to accommodate the array of genes enriched by decades of selective pressures.

Phenicol Resistance

Chloramphenicol was the first broad-spectrum antibiotic to be used both orally and systemically, and it has been used around the world to treat *Salmonella* infections. Resistance in *Salmonella* is associated with the presence of chloramphenicol acetyltransferase genes encoded by a small number of variants of *catA* (*catA1*, *catA2*, *catA3*) and *catB* (*catB2*, *catB3*, *catB7*, *catB8*), as well as efflux by *cmlA* (*cmlA1*, *cmlA4*, *cmlA9*) and *floR*. Acetylation blocks binding of the drug to the ribosome target. The fluorine atom of florfenicol prevents acetylation, circumventing modification by the *cat* genes. Florfenicol efflux resistance also results from expression of *floR* and *fexA*.

Colistin Resistance

Colistin (polymyxin E) is now considered a reserve drug for treating MDR Gram-negative bacteria, including carbapenem-resistant strains. The first report of mobile colistin resistance gene *mcr-1* was reported in late 2015 in *E. coli* in China (58). Soon thereafter, several instances of *mcr-1* in *Salmonella* were reported (143–148). In the NCBI database, there are now at least five alleles of *mcr* designated *mcr-1* through *mcr-5*.

CONCLUDING REMARKS

The global challenge of antimicrobial resistance is being addressed on many fronts. The nature and magnitude of resistance in the agriculture/food sector is perhaps best evaluated by examining resistance in the principal foodborne bacterial pathogen *Salmonella*. The situations in North America and Europe, where surveillance data are extensive, provide a good backdrop to a global understanding of resistance in this important pathogen, including resistance data to measure the impact of drug use restrictions designed to limit resistance.

Overall, antimicrobial resistance surveillance data for *Salmonella* show common and unique features in different regions, where resistance to older drugs is generally highest and serovar differences impact overall trends. Differences in resistance by serovar often illustrate the most salient trends, as demonstrated by fluoroquinolone-resistant *S.* Kentucky in Europe or MDR *S.* Dublin in the United States.

The contribution of zoonotic infections from companion animals is not well understood or adequately addressed by surveillance programs. However, the relative ease with which the resistome of *Salmonella* can be evaluated by examination of WGS data heralds a new era in antimicrobial resistance monitoring where the resistance allele will become more prominent as the hazard under surveillance. As more is learned about the array of resistant strain types infecting humans, the range of sources causing human infections will become clearer, including the proportion of those arising from companion animals and other sources. Along with more detailed drug use information, this will lead to a better understanding of the sources and drivers of resistance and better interventions to protect public health.

Acknowledgments. We acknowledge our FDA colleagues Claudine Kabera and Chih-Hao Hsu for help with the tables and graphs, and John Graham and Adrienne Ivory for review of the manuscript.

Citation. McDermott PF, Zhao S, Tate H. 2018. Antimicrobial resistance in nontyphoidal *Salmonella*. Microbiol Spectrum 6(4):ARBA-0014-2017.

References

1. **WHO.** 2013. *Integrated Surveillance of Antimicrobial Resistance: Guidance from a WHO Advisory Group.* World Health Organization, Geneva, Switzerland.

2. **Hoelzer K, Moreno Switt AI, Wiedmann M.** 2011. Animal contact as a source of human non-typhoidal salmonellosis. *Vet Res (Faisalabad)* 42:34.

3. **Interagency Food Safety Analytics Collaboration (IFSAC).** 2015. *Foodborne illness source attribution estimates for* Salmonella, Escherichia coli O157 *(E. coli O157),* Listeria monocytogenes *(Lm), and* Campylobacter *using outbreak surveillance data.* U.S. Department of Health and Human Services, CDC, FDA, USDA-FSIS.

4. **CDC.** 2014. *National Enteric Disease Surveillance:* Salmonella *Annual Report, 2014.* CDC, Atlanta, GA.

5. **Rabsch W, Tschäpe H, Bäumler AJ.** 2001. Non-typhoidal salmonellosis: emerging problems. *Microbes Infect* 3:237–247.

6. **Patterson SK, Kim HB, Borewicz K, Isaacson RE.** 2016. Towards an understanding of *Salmonella enterica* serovar Typhimurium persistence in swine. *Anim Health Res Rev* 17:159–168.

7. **Cobbold RN, Rice DH, Davis MA, Besser TE, Hancock DD.** 2006. Long-term persistence of multi-drug-resistant *Salmonella enterica* serovar Newport in two dairy herds. *J Am Vet Med Assoc* 228:585–591.

8. **Majowicz SE, Musto J, Scallan E, Angulo FJ, Kirk M, O'Brien SJ, Jones TF, Fazil A, Hoekstra RM, International Collaboration on Enteric Disease 'Burden of Illness' Studies.** 2010. The global burden of nontyphoidal *Salmonella* gastroenteritis. *Clin Infect Dis* 50:882–889.

9. **CDC.** 2013. Antibiotic resistance threats in the United States, 2013. http://www.cdc.gov/drugresistance/threat-report-2013/pdf/ar-threats-2013-508.pdf#page=112.

10. **McDermott PF, Zhao S, Wagner DD, Simjee S, Walker RD, White DG.** 2002. The food safety perspective of antibiotic resistance. *Anim Biotechnol* 13:71–84.

11. **FDA.** 2012. Guidance for Industry No. 209: The judicious use of medically important antimicrobials drugs in food-producing animals. HHS, Food and Drug

Administration, Rockville, MD. https://www.fda.gov/downloads/AnimalVeterinary/GuidanceCompliance Enforcement/GuidanceforIndustry/UCM216936.pdf.

12. **Ministry of Agriculture FaF, National Veterinary Assay Laboratory.** 2016. *JVARM: Report on the Japanese Veterinary Antimicrobial Resistance Monitoring System, 2012–2013.* Ministry of Agriculture, Forestry, and Fisheries, Tokyo, Japan.

13. **EMA.** 2016. Sales of veterinary antimicrobial agents in 29 European countries in 2014. Sixth ESVAC Report. European Medicines Agency, Agency EM, London, United Kingdom.

14. **Bondt N, Jensen VF, Puister-Jansen LF, van Geijlswijk IM.** 2013. Comparing antimicrobial exposure based on sales data. *Prev Vet Med* **108:**10–20.

15. **Federal Register.** 2016. Antimicrobial animal drug sales and distribution reporting. Docket no. FDA-2012-N-0447.

16. **WHO.** 2014. *Antimicrobial Resistance Global Report on Surveillance.* WHO, Geneva, Switzerland.

17. **Havelaar AH, Kirk MD, Torgerson PR, Gibb HJ, Hald T, Lake RJ, Praet N, Bellinger DC, de Silva NR, Gargouri N, Speybroeck N, Cawthorne A, Mathers C, Stein C, Angulo FJ, Devleesschauwer B, World Health Organization Foodborne Disease Burden Epidemiology Reference Group.** 2015. World Health Organization global estimates and regional comparisons of the burden of foodborne disease in 2010. *PLoS Med* **12:**e1001923.

18. **CDC.** 2014. *Foodborne Diseases Active Surveillance Network (FoodNet): FoodNet Surveillance Report for 2014 (Final Report).* U.S. Department of Health and Human Services, CDC, Atlanta, GA.

19. **Reddy EA, Shaw AV, Crump JA.** 2010. Community-acquired bloodstream infections in Africa: a systematic review and meta-analysis. *Lancet Infect Dis* **10:**417–432.

20. **Ao TT, Feasey NA, Gordon MA, Keddy KH, Angulo FJ, Crump JA.** 2015. Global burden of invasive nontyphoidal *Salmonella* disease, 2010(1). *Emerg Infect Dis* **21:**21.

21. **Feasey NA, Hadfield J, Keddy KH, Dallman TJ, Jacobs J, Deng X, Wigley P, Barquist L, Langridge GC, Feltwell T, Harris SR, Mather AE, Fookes M, Aslett M, Msefula C, Kariuki S, Maclennan CA, Onsare RS, Weill FX, Le Hello S, Smith AM, McClelland M, Desai P, Parry CM, Cheesbrough J, French N, Campos J, Chabalgoity JA, Betancor L, Hopkins KL, Nair S, Humphrey TJ, Lunguya O, Cogan TA, Tapia MD, Sow SO, Tennant SM, Bornstein K, Levine MM, Lacharme-Lora L, Everett DB, Kingsley RA, Parkhill J, Heyderman RS, Dougan G, Gordon MA, Thomson NR.** 2016. Distinct *Salmonella* Enteritidis lineages associated with enterocolitis in high-income settings and invasive disease in low-income settings. *Nat Genet* **48:**1211–1217.

22. **Kingsley RA, Msefula CL, Thomson NR, Kariuki S, Holt KE, Gordon MA, Harris D, Clarke L, Whitehead S, Sangal V, Marsh K, Achtman M, Molyneux ME, Cormican M, Parkhill J, MacLennan CA, Heyderman RS, Dougan G.** 2009. Epidemic multiple drug resistant *Salmonella* Typhimurium causing invasive disease in sub-Saharan Africa have a distinct genotype. *Genome Res* **19:**2279–2287.

23. **Le Hello S, Bekhit A, Granier SA, Barua H, Beutlich J, Zając M, Münch S, Sintchenko V, Bouchrif B, Fashae K, Pinsard JL, Sontag L, Fabre L, Garnier M, Guibert V, Howard P, Hendriksen RS, Christensen JP, Biswas PK, Cloeckaert A, Rabsch W, Wasyl D, Doublet B, Weill FX.** 2013. The global establishment of a highly-fluoroquinolone resistant *Salmonella enterica* serotype Kentucky ST198 strain. *Front Microbiol* **4:**395.

24. **Kariuki S, Gordon MA, Feasey N, Parry CM.** 2015. Antimicrobial resistance and management of invasive *Salmonella* disease. *Vaccine* **33**(Suppl 3):C21–C29.

25. **Marder EPC, Cieslak PR, Cronquist AB, Dunn J, Lathrop S, Rabatsky-Ehr T, Ryan P, Smith K, Tobin-D'Angelo M, Vugia DJ, Zansky S, Holt KG, Wolpert BJ, Lynch M, Tauxe R, Geissler AL.** 2017. Incidence and trends of infections with pathogens transmitted commonly through food and the effect of increasing use of culture-independent diagnostic tests on surveillance: Foodborne Diseases Active Surveillance Network, 10 U.S. sites, 2013–2016. *MMWR Morb Mortal Wkly Rep* **66:**397–403.

26. **EFSA-ECDC.** 2016. EFSA (European Food Safety Authority) and ECDC (European Centre for Disease Prevention and Control), 2016. The European Union summary report on antimicrobial resistance in zoonotic and indicator bacteria from humans, animals, and food in 2014. *EFSA J* **14:**207.

27. **FDA.** 2016. National Antimicrobial Resistance Monitoring System - Enteric Bacteria (NARMS): NARMS Integrated Report 2014. U.S. Department of Health and Human Services, Food & Drug Administration, Rockville, MD. http://www.fda.gov/AnimalVeterinary/SafetyHealth/AntimicrobialResistance/NationalAntimicrobialResistanceMonitoringSystem/default.htm.

28. **Anderson AD, Nelson JM, Rossiter S, Angulo FJ.** 2003. Public health consequences of use of antimicrobial agents in food animals in the United States. *Microb Drug Resist* **9:**373–379.

29. **CIPARS.** 2016. Canadian Integrated Program for Antimicrobial Resistance Surveillance (CIPARS), Annual Report, 2014.

30. **DANMAP.** 2015. DANMAP 2015: use of antimicrobial agents and occurrence of antimicrobial resistance in bacteria from food animals, foods and humans in Denmark. http://www.danmap.org.

31. **FDA.** 2017. *The 2015 NARMS Integrated Report.* U.S. Department of Health and Human Services, FDA, Rockville, MD.

32. **Miriagou V, Carattoli A, Fanning S.** 2006. Antimicrobial resistance islands: resistance gene clusters in *Salmonella* chromosome and plasmids. *Microbes Infect* **8:**1923–1930.

33. **WHO.** 2017. *WHO Guidelines on Use of Medically Important Antimicrobials in Food-Producing Animals.* World Health Organization, Geneva, Switzerland.

34. **Karp BE, Tate H, Plumblee JR, Dessai U, Whichard JM, Thacker EL, Hale KR, Wilson W, Friedman CR,**

Griffin PM, McDermott PF. 2017. National Antimicrobial Resistance Monitoring System: two decades of advancing public health through integrated surveillance of antimicrobial resistance. *Foodborne Pathog Dis* 14: 545–557.

35. FDA. 2016. NARMS now: integrated data. http://www.fda.gov/AnimalVeterinary/SafetyHealth/AntimicrobialResistance/NationalAntimicrobialResistanceMonitoringSystem/ucm416741.htm. Accessed 24 November 2017.

36. Tadesse DA, Singh A, Zhao S, Bartholomew M, Womack N, Ayers S, Fields PI, McDermott PF. 2016. Antimicrobial resistance in *Salmonella* in the United States from 1948 to 1995. *Antimicrob Agents Chemother* 60:2567–2571.

37. EUCAST. European Committee on Antimicrobial Susceptibility Testing. http://www.eucast.org. Accessed 25 January 2017.

38. Bjork KE, Kopral CA, Wagner BA, Dargatz DA. 2015. Comparison of mixed effects models of antimicrobial resistance metrics of livestock and poultry *Salmonella* isolates from a national monitoring system. *Prev Vet Med* 122:265–272.

39. Billy TJ, Wachsmuth IK. 1997. Hazard analysis and critical control point systems in the United States Department of Agriculture regulatory policy. *Rev Sci Tech* 16:342–348.

40. Hong S, Rovira A, Davies P, Ahlstrom C, Muellner P, Rendahl A, Olsen K, Bender JB, Wells S, Perez A, Alvarez J. 2016. Serotypes and antimicrobial resistance in *Salmonella enterica* recovered from clinical samples from cattle and swine in Minnesota, 2006 to 2015. *PLoS One* 11:e0168016.

41. Medalla F, Hoekstra RM, Whichard JM, Barzilay EJ, Chiller TM, Joyce K, Rickert R, Krueger A, Stuart A, Griffin PM. 2013. Increase in resistance to ceftriaxone and nonsusceptibility to ciprofloxacin and decrease in multidrug resistance among *Salmonella* strains, United States, 1996–2009. *Foodborne Pathog Dis* 10:302–309.

42. Kawakami VM, Bottichio L, Angelo K, Linton N, Kissler B, Basler C, Lloyd J, Inouye W, Gonzales E, Rietberg K, Melius B, Oltean H, Wise M, Sinatra J, Marsland P, Li Z, Meek R, Kay M, Duchin J, Lindquist S. 2016. Notes from the field: outbreak of multidrug-resistant *Salmonella* infections linked to pork–Washington, 2015. *MMWR Morb Mortal Wkly Rep* 65:379–381.

43. Folster JP, Grass JE, Bicknese A, Taylor J, Friedman CR, Whichard JM. 2016. Characterization of resistance genes and plasmids from outbreaks and illness clusters caused by *Salmonella* resistant to ceftriaxone in the United States, 2011–2012. *Microb Drug Resist*.

44. O'Donnell AT, Vieira AR, Huang JY, Whichard J, Cole D, Karp BE. 2014. Quinolone-resistant *Salmonella enterica* serotype Enteritidis infections associated with international travel. *Clin Infect Dis* 59:e139–e141.

45. Smith AB, Renter DG, Cernicchiaro N, Shi X, Nagaraja TG. 2016. Prevalence and quinolone susceptibilities of *Salmonella* isolated from the feces of preharvest cattle within feedlots that used a fluoroquinolone to treat bovine respiratory disease. *Foodborne Pathog Dis* 13:303–308.

46. Valenzuela JR, Sethi AK, Aulik NA, Poulsen KP. 2017. Antimicrobial resistance patterns of bovine *Salmonella enterica* isolates submitted to the Wisconsin Veterinary Diagnostic Laboratory: 2006–2015. *J Dairy Sci* 100:1319–1330.

47. Government of Canada. 2016. *Canadian Integrated Program for Antimicrobial Resistance Surveillance (CIPARS) 2014 Annual Report Summary*. Public Health Agency of Canada, Guelph, ON.

48. Federal Register. 2008. Cephalosporin Drugs; Extralabel Animal Drug Use; Order of Prohibition. https://www.federalregister.gov/documents/2012/01/06/2012-35/new-animal-drugs-cephalosporin-drugs-extralabel-animal-drug-use-order-of-prohibition

49. Khaitsa ML, Kegode RB, Bauer ML, Gibbs PS, Lardy GP, Doetkott DK. 2007. A longitudinal study of *Salmonella* shedding and antimicrobial resistance patterns in North Dakota feedlot cattle. *J Food Prot* 70:476–481.

50. Sjölund-Karlsson M, Howie RL, Blickenstaff K, Boerlin P, Ball T, Chalmers G, Duval B, Haro J, Rickert R, Zhao S, Fedorka-Cray PJ, Whichard JM. 2013. Occurrence of β-lactamase genes among non-Typhi *Salmonella enterica* isolated from humans, food animals, and retail meats in the United States and Canada. *Microb Drug Resist* 19:191–197.

51. Tate H, Folster JP, Hsu CH, Chen J, Hoffmann M, Li C, Morales C, Tyson GH, Mukherjee S, Brown AC, Green A, Wilson W, Dessai U, Abbott J, Joseph L, Haro J, Ayers S, McDermott PF, Zhao S. 2017. Comparative analysis of extended-spectrum-β-lactamase CTX-M-65-producing *Salmonella enterica* serovar Infantis isolates from humans, food animals, and retail chickens in the United States. *Antimicrob Agents Chemother* 61:61.

52. Helke KL, McCrackin MA, Galloway AM, Poole AZ, Salgado CD, Marriott BP. 2017. Effects of antimicrobial use in agricultural animals on drug-resistant foodborne salmonellosis in humans: a systematic literature review. *Crit Rev Food Sci Nutr* 57:472–488.

53. Franco A, Leekitcharoenphon P, Feltrin F, Alba P, Cordaro G, Iurescia M, Tolli R, D'Incau M, Staffolani M, Di Giannatale E, Hendriksen RS, Battisti A. 2015. Emergence of a clonal lineage of multidrug-resistant ESBL-producing *Salmonella* Infantis transmitted from broilers and broiler meat to humans in Italy between 2011 and 2014. *PLoS One* 10:e0144802.

54. Rickert-Hartman R, Folster JP. 2014. Ciprofloxacin-resistant *Salmonella enterica* serotype Kentucky sequence type 198. *Emerg Infect Dis* 20:910–911.

55. Jacoby GA, Strahilevitz J, Hooper DC. 2014. Plasmid-mediated quinolone resistance. *Microbiol Spectr* 2: PLAS-0006-2013.

56. Cantón R, González-Alba JM, Galán JC. 2012. CTX-M enzymes: origin and diffusion. *Front Microbiol* 3:110.

57. Fey PD, Safranek TJ, Rupp ME, Dunne EF, Ribot E, Iwen PC, Bradford PA, Angulo FJ, Hinrichs SH. 2000. Ceftriaxone-resistant *Salmonella* infection acquired by a child from cattle. *N Engl J Med* 342:1242–1249.

58. Liu YY, Wang Y, Walsh TR, Yi LX, Zhang R, Spencer J, Doi Y, Tian G, Dong B, Huang X, Yu LF, Gu D, Ren

H, Chen X, Lv L, He D, Zhou H, Liang Z, Liu JH, Shen J. 2016. Emergence of plasmid-mediated colistin resistance mechanism MCR-1 in animals and human beings in China: a microbiological and molecular biological study. *Lancet Infect Dis* **16**:161–168.

59. Liakopoulos A, Mevius DJ, Olsen B, Bonnedahl J. 2016. The colistin resistance *mcr-1* gene is going wild. *J Antimicrob Chemother* **71**:2335–2336.

60. Arcilla MS, van Hattem JM, Matamoros S, Melles DC, Penders J, de Jong MD, Schultsz C, COMBAT Consortium. 2016. Dissemination of the *mcr-1* colistin resistance gene. *Lancet Infect Dis* **16**:147–149.

61. Olaitan AO, Chabou S, Okdah L, Morand S, Rolain JM. 2016. Dissemination of the *mcr-1* colistin resistance gene. *Lancet Infect Dis* **16**:147.

62. Hasman H, Hammerum AM, Hansen F, Hendriksen RS, Olesen B, Agersø Y, Zankari E, Leekitcharoenphon P, Stegger M, Kaas RS, Cavaco LM, Hansen DS, Aarestrup FM, Skov RL. 2015. Detection of *mcr-1* encoding plasmid-mediated colistin-resistant *Escherichia coli* isolates from human bloodstream infection and imported chicken meat, Denmark 2015. *Euro Surveill* **20**:pii=30085.

63. Watkins LF, Folster J, Chen J, Karlsson MS, Boyd S, Leung V, McNutt A, Medus C, Wang X, Hanna S, Smith N, Colón A, Barringer A, Dunbar-Manley C, Balk J, Friedman C. 2017. Emergence of *mcr-1* among nontyphoidal *Salmonella* isolates in the United States. *Open Forum Infect Dis* **4**(suppl_1):S129–S130.

64. Anjum MF, Duggett NA, AbuOun M, Randall L, Nunez-Garcia J, Ellis RJ, Rogers J, Horton R, Brena C, Williamson S, Martelli F, Davies R, Teale C. 2016. Colistin resistance in *Salmonella* and *Escherichia coli* isolates from a pig farm in Great Britain. *J Antimicrob Chemother* **71**:2306–2313.

65. CDC. 2016. Newly reported gene, *mcr* -1, threatens last-resort antibiotics. https://www.cdc.gov/drugresistance/mcr1.html.

66. Savard P, Gopinath R, Zhu W, Kitchel B, Rasheed JK, Tekle T, Roberts A, Ross T, Razeq J, Landrum BM, Wilson LE, Limbago B, Perl TM, Carroll KC. 2011. First NDM-positive *Salmonella* sp. strain identified in the United States. *Antimicrob Agents Chemother* **55**:5957–5958.

67. Rasheed JK, Kitchel B, Zhu W, Anderson KF, Clark NC, Ferraro MJ, Savard P, Humphries RM, Kallen AJ, Limbago BM. 2013. New Delhi metallo-β-lactamase-producing *Enterobacteriaceae*, United States. *Emerg Infect Dis* **19**:870–878.

68. Day MR, Meunier D, Doumith M, de Pinna E, Woodford N, Hopkins KL. 2015. Carbapenemase-producing *Salmonella enterica* isolates in the UK. *J Antimicrob Chemother* **70**:2165–2167.

69. Miriagou V, Tzouvelekis LS, Rossiter S, Tzelepi E, Angulo FJ, Whichard JM. 2003. Imipenem resistance in a *Salmonella* clinical strain due to plasmid-mediated class A carbapenemase KPC-2. *Antimicrob Agents Chemother* **47**:1297–1300.

70. Mollenkopf DF, Stull JW, Mathys DA, Bowman AS, Feicht SM, Grooters SV, Daniels JB, Wittum TE. 2016. Carbapenemase-producing *Enterobacteriaceae* recovered from the environment of a swine farrow-to-finish operation in the United States. *Antimicrob Agents Chemother* AAC.01298-16.

71. Woodford N, Wareham DW, Guerra B, Teale C. 2014. Carbapenemase-producing *Enterobacteriaceae* and non-*Enterobacteriaceae* from animals and the environment: an emerging public health risk of our own making? *J Antimicrob Chemother* **69**:287–291.

72. Donado-Godoy P, Castellanos R, León M, Arevalo A, Clavijo V, Bernal J, León D, Tafur MA, Byrne BA, Smith WA, Perez-Gutierrez E. 2015. The establishment of the Colombian Integrated Program for Antimicrobial Resistance Surveillance (COIPARS): a pilot project on poultry farms, slaughterhouses and retail market. *Zoonoses Public Health* **62**(Suppl 1):58–69.

73. Ministry of Agriculture, Forestry and Fisheries, National Veterinary Assay Laboratory. 2013. *JVARM: A Report on the Japanese Veterinary Antimicrobial Resistance Monitoring System, 2008–2011*. Ministry of Agriculture, Forestry and Fisheries, Tokyo, Japan.

74. Wu H, Xia X, Cui Y, Hu Y, Xi M, Wang X, Shi X, Wang D, Meng J, Yang B. 2013. Prevalence of extended-spectrum β-lactamase-producing *Salmonella* on retail chicken in six provinces and two national cities in the People's Republic of China. *J Food Prot* **76**:2040–2044.

75. Wang S, Duan H, Zhang W, Li JW. 2007. Analysis of bacterial foodborne disease outbreaks in China between 1994 and 2005. *FEMS Immunol Med Microbiol* **51**:8–13.

76. Yan H, Li L, Alam MJ, Shinoda S, Miyoshi S, Shi L. 2010. Prevalence and antimicrobial resistance of *Salmonella* in retail foods in northern China. *Int J Food Microbiol* **143**:230–234.

77. Yang B, Qu D, Zhang X, Shen J, Cui S, Shi Y, Xi M, Sheng M, Zhi S, Meng J. 2010. Prevalence and characterization of *Salmonella* serovars in retail meats of marketplace in Shaanxi, China. *Int J Food Microbiol* **141**:63–72.

78. Bai L, Lan R, Zhang X, Cui S, Xu J, Guo Y, Li F, Zhang D. 2015. Prevalence of *Salmonella* isolates from chicken and pig slaughterhouses and emergence of ciprofloxacin and cefotaxime co-resistant *S. enterica* serovar Indiana in Henan, China. *PLoS One* **10**:e0144532.

79. Lai J, Wu C, Wu C, Qi J, Wang Y, Wang H, Liu Y, Shen J. 2014. Serotype distribution and antibiotic resistance of *Salmonella* in food-producing animals in Shandong province of China, 2009 and 2012. *Int J Food Microbiol* **180**:30–38.

80. Xia S, Hendriksen RS, Xie Z, Huang L, Zhang J, Guo W, Xu B, Ran L, Aarestrup FM. 2009. Molecular characterization and antimicrobial susceptibility of *Salmonella* isolates from infections in humans in Henan Province, China. *J Clin Microbiol* **47**:401–409.

81. Lu Y, Zhao H, Liu Y, Zhou X, Wang J, Liu T, Beier RC, Hou X. 2015. Characterization of quinolone resistance in *Salmonella enterica* serovar Indiana from chickens in China. *Poult Sci* **94**:454–460.

82. Zhang WH, Lin XY, Xu L, Gu XX, Yang L, Li W, Ren SQ, Liu YH, Zeng ZL, Jiang HX. 2016. CTX-M-27

producing *Salmonella enterica* serotypes Typhimurium and Indiana are prevalent among food-producing animals in China. *Front Microbiol* 7:436.

83. Jiang HX, Song L, Liu J, Zhang XH, Ren YN, Zhang WH, Zhang JY, Liu YH, Webber MA, Ogbolu DO, Zeng ZL, Piddock LJ. 2014. Multiple transmissible genes encoding fluoroquinolone and third-generation cephalosporin resistance co-located in non-typhoidal *Salmonella* isolated from food-producing animals in China. *Int J Antimicrob Agents* 43:242–247.

84. Li L, Liao XP, Liu ZZ, Huang T, Li X, Sun J, Liu BT, Zhang Q, Liu YH. 2014. Co-spread of oqxAB and blaCTX-M-9G in non-Typhi *Salmonella enterica* isolates mediated by ST2-IncHI2 plasmids. *Int J Antimicrob Agents* 44:263–268.

85. Baggesen DL, Sandvang D, Aarestrup FM. 2000. Characterization of *Salmonella enterica* serovar Typhimurium DT104 isolated from Denmark and comparison with isolates from Europe and the United States. *J Clin Microbiol* 38:1581–1586.

86. Davis MA, Hancock DD, Besser TE. 2002. Multiresistant clones of *Salmonella enterica*: the importance of dissemination. *J Lab Clin Med* 140:135–141.

87. Threlfall EJ, Ward LR, Hampton MD, Ridley AM, Rowe B, Roberts D, Gilbert RJ, Van Someren P, Wall PG, Grimont P. 1998. Molecular fingerprinting defines a strain of *Salmonella enterica* serotype Anatum responsible for an international outbreak associated with formula-dried milk. *Epidemiol Infect* 121:289–293.

88. Leekitcharoenphon P, Hendriksen RS, Le Hello S, Weill FX, Baggesen DL, Jun SR, Ussery DW, Lund O, Crook DW, Wilson DJ, Aarestrup FM. 2016. Global genomic epidemiology of *Salmonella enterica* serovar Typhimurium DT104. *Appl Environ Microbiol* 82:2516–2526.

89. Damborg P, Broens EM, Chomel BB, Guenther S, Pasmans F, Wagenaar JA, Weese JS, Wieler LH, Windahl U, Vanrompay D, Guardabassi L. 2015. Bacterial zoonoses transmitted by household pets: state-of-the-art and future perspectives for targeted research and policy actions. *J Comp Pathol* 155(1 Suppl 1):S27–S40.

90. Rijks JM, Cito F, Cunningham AA, Rantsios AT, Giovannini A. 2015. Disease risk assessments involving companion animals: an overview for 15 selected pathogens taking a European perspective. *J Comp Pathol* 155(1 Suppl 1):S75–S97.

91. Jay-Russell MT, Hake AF, Bengson Y, Thiptara A, Nguyen T. 2014. Prevalence and characterization of *Escherichia coli* and *Salmonella* strains isolated from stray dog and coyote feces in a major leafy greens production region at the United States-Mexico border. *PLoS One* 9:e113433.

92. Lowden P, Wallis C, Gee N, Hilton A. 2015. Investigating the prevalence of *Salmonella* in dogs within the Midlands region of the United Kingdom. *BMC Vet Res* 11:239.

93. USAHA. 2006. Report of the Committee on *Salmonella*. http://www.usaha.org/upload/Committee/Salmonella/report-sal-2008.pdf.

94. Anholt RM, Berezowski J, Ribble CS, Russell ML, Stephen C. 2014. Using informatics and the electronic medical record to describe antimicrobial use in the clinical management of diarrhea cases at 12 companion animal practices. *PLoS One* 9:e103190.

95. Summers JF, Hendricks A, Brodbelt DC. 2014. Prescribing practices of primary-care veterinary practitioners in dogs diagnosed with bacterial pyoderma. *BMC Vet Res* 10:240.

96. Prescott JF, Hanna WJ, Reid-Smith R, Drost K. 2002. Antimicrobial drug use and resistance in dogs. *Can Vet J* 43:107–116.

97. Hölsö K, Rantala M, Lillas A, Eerikäinen S, Huovinen P, Kaartinen L. 2005. Prescribing antimicrobial agents for dogs and cats via university pharmacies in Finland: patterns and quality of information. *Acta Vet Scand* 46:87–93.

98. Guardabassi L, Schwarz S, Lloyd DH. 2004. Pet animals as reservoirs of antimicrobial-resistant bacteria. *J Antimicrob Chemother* 54:321–332.

99. Rzewuska M, Czopowicz M, Kizerwetter-Świda M, Chrobak D, Błaszczak B, Binek M. 2015. Multidrug resistance in *Escherichia coli* strains isolated from infections in dogs and cats in Poland (2007–2013). *Sci World J* 2015:408205.

100. Cummings KJ, Aprea VA, Altier C. 2015. Antimicrobial resistance trends among canine *Escherichia coli* isolates obtained from clinical samples in the northeastern USA, 2004–2011. *Can Vet J* 56:393–398.

101. USDA-ARS. NARMS animal arm summary tables and reports. http://www.ars.usda.gov/Main/docs.htm?docid=18034. Accessed 17 October 2017.

102. Eaves DJ, Randall L, Gray DT, Buckley A, Woodward MJ, White AP, Piddock LJ. 2004. Prevalence of mutations within the quinolone resistance-determining region of *gyrA*, *gyrB*, *parC*, and *parE* and association with antibiotic resistance in quinolone-resistant *Salmonella enterica*. *Antimicrob Agents Chemother* 48:4012–4015.

103. Leonard EK, Pearl DL, Finley RL, Janecko N, Reid-Smith RJ, Peregrine AS, Weese JS. 2012. Comparison of antimicrobial resistance patterns of *Salmonella* spp. and *Escherichia coli* recovered from pet dogs from volunteer households in Ontario (2005–06). *J Antimicrob Chemother* 67:174–181.

104. Van Immerseel F, Pasmans F, De Buck J, Rychlik I, Hradecka H, Collard JM, Wildemauwe C, Heyndrickx M, Ducatelle R, Haesebrouck F. 2004. Cats as a risk for transmission of antimicrobial drug-resistant *Salmonella*. *Emerg Infect Dis* 10:2169–2174.

105. Poppe C, Smart N, Khakhria R, Johnson W, Spika J, Prescott J. 1998. *Salmonella typhimurium* DT104: a virulent and drug-resistant pathogen. *Can Vet J* 39:559–565.

106. Wall PG, Threlfall EJ, Ward LR, Rowe B. 1996. Multiresistant *Salmonella* Typhimurium DT104 in cats: a public health risk. *Lancet* 348:471.

107. Low JC, Tennant B, Munro D. 1996. Multiple-resistant *Salmonella* Typhimurium DT104 in cats. *Lancet* 348:1391.

108. Frech G, Kehrenberg C, Schwarz S. 2003. Resistance phenotypes and genotypes of multiresistant *Salmonella*

enterica subsp. *enterica* serovar Typhimurium var. Copenhagen isolates from animal sources. *J Antimicrob Chemother* 51:180–182.

109. Centers for Disease Control and Prevention (CDC). 2001. Outbreaks of multidrug-resistant *Salmonella* Typhimurium associated with veterinary facilities: Idaho, Minnesota, and Washington, 1999. *MMWR Morb Mortal Wkly Rep* 50:701–704.

110. Wright JG, Tengelsen LA, Smith KE, Bender JB, Frank RK, Grendon JH, Rice DH, Thiessen AM, Gilbertson CJ, Sivapalasingam S, Barrett TJ, Besser TE, Hancock DD, Angulo FJ. 2005. Multidrug-resistant *Salmonella* Typhimurium in four animal facilities. *Emerg Infect Dis* 11:1235–1241.

111. Swanson SJ, Snider C, Braden CR, Boxrud D, Wünschmann A, Rudroff JA, Lockett J, Smith KE. 2007. Multidrug-resistant *Salmonella enterica* serotype Typhimurium associated with pet rodents. *N Engl J Med* 356:21–28.

112. Izumiya H, Mori K, Kurazono T, Yamaguchi M, Higashide M, Konishi N, Kai A, Morita K, Terajima J, Watanabe H. 2005. Characterization of isolates of *Salmonella enterica* serovar Typhimurium displaying high-level fluoroquinolone resistance in Japan. *J Clin Microbiol* 43:5074–5079.

113. White DG, Datta A, McDermott P, Friedman S, Qaiyumi S, Ayers S, English L, McDermott S, Wagner DD, Zhao S. 2003. Antimicrobial susceptibility and genetic relatedness of *Salmonella* serovars isolated from animal-derived dog treats in the USA. *J Antimicrob Chemother* 52:860–863.

114. Cartwright EJ, Nguyen T, Melluso C, Ayers T, Lane C, Hodges A, Li X, Quammen J, Yendell SJ, Adams J, Mitchell J, Rickert R, Klos R, Williams IT, Barton Behravesh C, Wright J. 2016. A multistate investigation of antibiotic-resistant *Salmonella enterica* serotype I 4, [5],12:i:- infections as part of an international outbreak associated with frozen feeder rodents. *Zoonoses Public Health* 63:62–71.

115. Centers for Disease Control and Prevention (CDC). 2003. Reptile-associated salmonellosis: selected states, 1998–2002. *MMWR Morb Mortal Wkly Rep* 52:1206–1209.

116. Centers for Disease Control and Prevention (CDC). 2005. Salmonellosis associated with pet turtles: Wisconsin and Wyoming, 2004. *MMWR Morb Mortal Wkly Rep* 54:223–226.

117. Centers for Disease Control and Prevention (CDC). 2007. Turtle-associated salmonellosis in humans:United States, 2006–2007. *MMWR Morb Mortal Wkly Rep* 56:649–652.

118. Welch TJ, Fricke WF, McDermott PF, White DG, Rosso ML, Rasko DA, Mammel MK, Eppinger M, Rosovitz MJ, Wagner D, Rahalison L, Leclerc JE, Hinshaw JM, Lindler LE, Cebula TA, Carniel E, Ravel J. 2007. Multiple antimicrobial resistance in plague: an emerging public health risk. *PLoS One* 2:e309.

119. GMI. The Global Microbial Identifier. http://www.globalmicrobialidentifier.org/.

120. FDA. 2017. GenomeTrakr Network. https://www.fda.gov/Food/FoodScienceResearch/WholeGenomeSequencing ProgramWGS/ucm363134.htm. Accessed 24 November 2017.

121. McDermott PF, Tyson GH, Kabera C, Chen Y, Li C, Folster JP, Ayers SL, Lam C, Tate HP, Zhao S. 2016. Whole-genome sequencing for detecting antimicrobial resistance in nontyphoidal *Salmonella*. *Antimicrob Agents Chemother* 60:5515–5520.

122. Zankari E, Hasman H, Kaas RS, Seyfarth AM, Agersø Y, Lund O, Larsen MV, Aarestrup FM. 2013. Genotyping using whole-genome sequencing is a realistic alternative to surveillance based on phenotypic antimicrobial susceptibility testing. *J Antimicrob Chemother* 68:771–777.

123. Tyson GH, McDermott PF, Li C, Chen Y, Tadesse DA, Mukherjee S, Bodeis-Jones S, Kabera C, Gaines SA, Loneragan GH, Edrington TS, Torrence M, Harhay DM, Zhao S. 2015. WGS accurately predicts antimicrobial resistance in *Escherichia coli*. *J Antimicrob Chemother* 70:2763–2769.

124. Zhao S, Tyson GH, Chen Y, Li C, Mukherjee S, Young S, Lam C, Folster JP, Whichard JM, McDermott PF. 2015. Whole-genome sequencing analysis accurately predicts antimicrobial resistance phenotypes in *Campylobacter* spp. *Appl Environ Microbiol* 82:459–466.

125. FDA. 2017. Resistome Trakcer. https://www.fda.gov/AnimalVeterinary/SafetyHealth/AntimicrobialResistance/NationalAntimicrobialResistanceMonitoringSystem/ucm 570694.htm.

126. Michael GB, Schwarz S. 2016. Antimicrobial resistance in zoonotic nontyphoidal *Salmonella*: an alarming trend? *Clin Microbiol Infect* 22:968–974.

127. Michael GB, Butaye P, Cloeckaert A, Schwarz S. 2006. Genes and mutations conferring antimicrobial resistance in *Salmonella*: an update. *Microbes Infect* 8:1898–1914.

128. Michael GB, Schwarz S. 2013. Antimicrobial resistance in *Salmonella*, p 120–135. *In* Methner U (ed), *Salmonella in Domestic Animals*. CAB eBooks, Barrow, PA.

129. Tran JH, Jacoby GA. 2002. Mechanism of plasmid-mediated quinolone resistance. *Proc Natl Acad Sci USA* 99:5638–5642.

130. Périchon B, Courvalin P, Galimand M. 2007. Transferable resistance to aminoglycosides by methylation of G1405 in 16S rRNA and to hydrophilic fluoroquinolones by QepA-mediated efflux in *Escherichia coli*. *Antimicrob Agents Chemother* 51:2464–2469.

131. Yamane K, Wachino J, Suzuki S, Kimura K, Shibata N, Kato H, Shibayama K, Konda T, Arakawa Y. 2007. New plasmid-mediated fluoroquinolone efflux pump, QepA, found in an *Escherichia coli* clinical isolate. *Antimicrob Agents Chemother* 51:3354–3360.

132. Robicsek A, Strahilevitz J, Jacoby GA, Macielag M, Abbanat D, Park CH, Bush K, Hooper DC. 2006. Fluoroquinolone-modifying enzyme: a new adaptation of a common aminoglycoside acetyltransferase. *Nat Med* 12:83–88.

133. Hansen LH, Johannesen E, Burmølle M, Sørensen AH, Sørensen SJ. 2004. Plasmid-encoded multidrug efflux pump conferring resistance to olaquindox in *Escherichia coli*. *Antimicrob Agents Chemother* 48:3332–3337.

134. Bai L, Zhao J, Gan X, Wang J, Zhang X, Cui S, Xia S, Hu Y, Yan S, Wang J, Li F, Fanning S, Xu J. 2016. Emergence and diversity of *Salmonella enterica* serovar Indiana isolates with concurrent resistance to ciprofloxacin and cefotaxime from patients and food-producing animals in China. *Antimicrob Agents Chemother* 60: 3365–3371.

135. Campos J, Mourão J, Marçal S, Machado J, Novais C, Peixe L, Antunes P. 2016. Clinical *Salmonella* Typhimurium ST34 with metal tolerance genes and an IncHI2 plasmid carrying *oqxAB-aac(6′)-Ib-cr* from Europe. *J Antimicrob Chemother* 71:843–845.

136. Wong MH, Chan EW, Liu LZ, Chen S. 2014. PMQR genes *oqxAB* and *aac(6′)Ib-cr* accelerate the development of fluoroquinolone resistance in *Salmonella* typhimurium. *Front Microbiol* 5:521.

137. Chen Y, Sun J, Liao XP, Shao Y, Li L, Fang LX, Liu YH. 2016. Impact of enrofloxacin and florfenicol therapy on the spread of OqxAB gene and intestinal microbiota in chickens. *Vet Microbiol* 192:1–9.

138. Nair S, Ashton P, Doumith M, Connell S, Painset A, Mwaigwisya S, Langridge G, de Pinna E, Godbole G, Day M. 2016. WGS for surveillance of antimicrobial resistance: a pilot study to detect the prevalence and mechanism of resistance to azithromycin in a UK population of non-typhoidal *Salmonella*. *J Antimicrob Chemother* 71:3400–3408.

139. Nguyen F, Starosta AL, Arenz S, Sohmen D, Dönhöfer A, Wilson DN. 2014. Tetracycline antibiotics and resistance mechanisms. *Biol Chem* 395:559–575.

140. Wachino J, Arakawa Y. 2012. Exogenously acquired 16S rRNA methyltransferases found in aminoglycoside-resistant pathogenic Gram-negative bacteria: an update. *Drug Resist Updat* 15:133–148.

141. Folster JP, Rickert R, Barzilay EJ, Whichard JM. 2009. Identification of the aminoglycoside resistance determinants *armA* and *rmtC* among non-Typhi *Salmonella* isolates from humans in the United States. *Antimicrob Agents Chemother* 53:4563–4564.

142. Naas T, Bentchouala C, Lima S, Lezzar A, Smati F, Scheftel JM, Nordmann P. 2009. Plasmid-mediated 16S rRNA methylases among extended-spectrum-beta-lactamase-producing *Salmonella enterica* Senftenberg isolates from Algeria. *J Antimicrob Chemother* 64: 866–868.

143. Campos J, Cristino L, Peixe L, Antunes P. 2016. MCR-1 in multidrug-resistant and copper-tolerant clinically relevant *Salmonella* 1,4,[5],12:i:- and S. Rissen clones in Portugal, 2011 to 2015. *Euro Surveill* 21:pii=30270.

144. Carnevali C, Morganti M, Scaltriti E, Bolzoni L, Pongolini S, Casadei G. 2016. Occurrence of *mcr-1* in colistin-resistant *Salmonella enterica* isolates recovered from humans and animals in Italy, 2012 to 2015. *Antimicrob Agents Chemother* 60:7532–7534.

145. Doumith M, Godbole G, Ashton P, Larkin L, Dallman T, Day M, Day M, Muller-Pebody B, Ellington MJ, de Pinna E, Johnson AP, Hopkins KL, Woodford N. 2016. Detection of the plasmid-mediated *mcr-1* gene conferring colistin resistance in human and food isolates of *Salmonella enterica* and *Escherichia coli* in England and Wales. *J Antimicrob Chemother* 71:2300–2305.

146. Quesada A, Ugarte-Ruiz M, Iglesias MR, Porrero MC, Martínez R, Florez-Cuadrado D, Campos MJ, García M, Píriz S, Sáez JL, Domínguez L. 2016. Detection of plasmid mediated colistin resistance (MCR-1) in *Escherichia coli* and *Salmonella enterica* isolated from poultry and swine in Spain. *Res Vet Sci* 105:134–135.

147. Rau RB, de Lima-Morales D, Wink PL, Ribeiro AR, Martins AF, Barth AL. 2017. Emergence of *mcr-1* producing *Salmonella enterica* serovar Typhimurium from retail meat first detection in Brazil. *Foodborne Pathog Dis* 15(1):58–59.

148. Torpdahl M, Hasman H, Litrup E, Skov RL, Nielsen EM, Hammerum AM. 2017. Detection of mcr-1-encoding plasmid-mediated colistin-resistant *Salmonella* isolates from human infection in Denmark. *Int J Antimicrob Agents* 49:261–262.

149. Sjölund-Karlsson M, Joyce K, Blickenstaff K, Ball T, Haro J, Medalla FM, Fedorka-Cray P, Zhao S, Crump JA, Whichard JM. 2011. Antimicrobial susceptibility to azithromycin among *Salmonella enterica* isolates from the United States. *Antimicrob Agents Chemother* 55(9): 3985–3989.

150. Seidman JC, Coles CL, Silbergeld EK, Levens J, Mkocha H, Johnson LB, Muñoz B, West SK. 2014. Increased carriage of macrolide-resistant fecal *E. coli* following mass distribution of azithromycin for trachoma control. *Int J Epidemiol* 43(4):1105–1113.

151. Schmidt JW, Agga GE, Bosilevac JM, Brichta-Harhay DM, Shackelford SD, Wang R, Wheeler TL, Arthur TM. 2015. Occurrence of Antimicrobial-Resistant *Escherichia coli* and *Salmonella enterica* in the Beef Cattle Production and Processing Continuum. *Appl Environ Microbiol* 81(2):713–725.

Antimicrobial Resistance in Bacteria from Livestock and Companion Animals
Edited by Frank Møller Aarestrup, Stefan Schwarz, Jianzhong Shen, and Lina Cavaco
© 2018 American Society for Microbiology, Washington, DC
doi:10.1128/microbiolspec.ARBA-0026-2017

Antimicrobial Resistance in *Escherichia coli*

13

Laurent Poirel,[1,2,3] Jean-Yves Madec,[4] Agnese Lupo,[4] Anne-Kathrin Schink,[5] Nicolas Kieffer,[1] Patrice Nordmann,[1,2,3] and Stefan Schwarz[5]

INTRODUCTION

Escherichia coli is a bacterium with a special place in the microbiological world since it can cause severe infections in humans and animals but also represents a significant part of the autochthonous microbiota of the different hosts. Of major concern is a possible transmission of virulent and/or resistant *E. coli* between animals and humans through numerous pathways, such as direct contact, contact with animal excretions, or via the food chain. *E. coli* also represents a major reservoir of resistance genes that may be responsible for treatment failures in both human and veterinary medicine. An increasing number of resistance genes has been identified in *E. coli* isolates during the last decades, and many of these resistance genes were acquired by horizontal gene transfer. In the enterobacterial gene pool, *E. coli* acts as a donor and as a recipient of resistance genes and thereby can acquire resistance genes from other bacteria but can also pass on its resistance genes to other bacteria. In general, antimicrobial resistance in *E. coli* is considered one of the major challenges in both humans and animals at a worldwide scale and needs to be considered as a real public health concern.

This chapter gives an update of antimicrobial resistance in *E. coli* of animal origin by focusing on resistance to those classes of antimicrobial agents mainly used in veterinary medicine and to which *E. coli* isolates of animal origin are known to exhibit resistance.

E. COLI IN ANIMALS: A PATHOGENIC AND A COMMENSAL BACTERIUM

"Colibacillosis" is a general term for a disease caused by the bacterium *E. coli*, which normally resides in the lower intestines of most warm-blooded mammals. Hence, *E. coli* is a versatile microorganism with a number of pathogenic isolates prone to cause intestinal and extra-intestinal infections, while most others are harmless for their host and refer to commensalism. The pathogenic *E. coli* isolates can be classified into different pathotypes, or pathovars, where each pathotype causes a different disease (1). The intestinal pathogenic *E. coli* pathovars are responsible for disorders in the gut ranging from mild diarrhea to severe colitis, while the extra-intestinal pathogenic *E. coli* pathovars are mostly asymptomatic inhabitants of the intestinal tract that cause extra-intestinal diseases after migrating to other parts of the body, such as the urinary tract or the blood stream (2). Animal diseases due to *E. coli* can also be caused by *E. coli* isolates originating from the environmental reservoir or other infected individuals. Pathogenic and nonpathogenic *E. coli* differ by the acquisition or loss of virulence-associated traits associated with *E. coli* pathogenicity. The number of genes present in the *E. coli* genome varies from 4,000 to 5,000 genes, with approximately 3,000 genes shared by the different isolates, whereas the others mostly correspond to colonization or virulence determinants.

[1]Emerging Antibiotic Resistance Unit, Medical and Molecular Microbiology, Department of Medicine, University of Fribourg, Fribourg, Switzerland; [2]French INSERM European Unit, University of Fribourg (LEA-IAME), Fribourg, Switzerland; [3]National Reference Center for Emerging Antibiotic Resistance (NARA), Fribourg, Switzerland; [4]Université de Lyon – Agence Nationale de Sécurité Sanitaire (ANSES), Unité Antibiorésistance et Virulence Bactériennes, Lyon, France; [5]Institute of Microbiology and Epizootics, Centre of Infection Medicine, Department of Veterinary Medicine, Freie Universität Berlin, Berlin, Germany.

Advanced insights in the genomic plasticity of *E. coli* have been possible by the use of whole-genome sequencing, providing a better understanding of the core and accessory genomes of pathogenic and commensal *E. coli* isolates (3).

In animals, *E. coli* is one of the leading causes of diarrhea, together with other pathogens such as rotavirus, coronavirus, *Cryptosporidium parvum*, or a combination of these (4). These enterotoxigenic *E. coli* (ETEC) strains bind and colonize the intestinal epithelium through adhesins expressed in the context of fimbriae, such as the F4 (formerly designated K88), F5 (K99), F6 (987P), F17, and F18 fimbriae (5). ETEC also produces various enterotoxins, of which heat-labile and heat-stable toxins and/or enteroaggregative heat-stable toxin 1 (EAST1) lead to diarrhea. ETEC affects various animal species, mostly young animals, particularly food-producing animals (piglets, newborn calves, chickens) but also companion animals such as dogs. In livestock, diarrhea is considered one of the major diseases, which can propagate among animals with possibly significant consequences at the herd/flock level. Diarrhea is observed in pigs and calves during the first 3 to 5 days of life and in pigs 3 to 10 days after weaning. The trend toward early weaning in several countries and continents may have played a significant role in the rising occurrence of postweaning diarrhea in the pig sector. As a consequence, lethal ETEC infections in animals can also occur as a result of severe dehydration and electrolyte imbalance.

E. coli infections in animals are not restricted to young individuals but occur in adults as well. As mentioned above, extra-intestinal pathogenic *E. coli* is responsible for infections of the lower and upper urinary tract, particularly in companion animals (6, 7). In poultry, avian-pathogenic *E. coli* causes colibacillosis initiated in the respiratory tract by inhalation of fecal dust before spreading further in the whole body, causing septicemia, pericarditis, and mortality (8). In dairy cattle, mastitis is a common inflammatory response of the mammary gland, significantly decreasing milk production and causing dramatic economic losses, with *E. coli* being one of the major causes—together with *Staphylococcus aureus*, *Streptococcus uberis*, *Streptococcus agalactiae*, and *Streptococcus dysgalactiae* (9, 10). In particular, *E. coli* is responsible for more than 80% of cases of acute mastitis where the severe clinical signs are induced by the lipopolysaccharide (LPS) as a primary virulence factor followed by the subsequent release of inflammatory mediators (11). Nonetheless, it is broadly considered that mastitis in dairy cattle due to *E. coli* is neither associated with specific *E. coli* serovars nor involves a common set of virulence factors shared among *E. coli* isolates.

E. coli infections in animals are subjected to various pharmaceutical treatments including antimicrobials. For instance, ampicillin, streptomycin, sulfonamides, or oxytetracyclines are commonly used to treat bovine mastitis, but broad-spectrum cephalosporins and fluoroquinolones also have indications through systemic or local administration depending on the severity of the clinical symptoms (12) and the resistance properties of the causative *E. coli* isolates. Nonetheless, the role of antimicrobials in the treatment of coliform mastitis is becoming more and more open to debate. Recommendations provided for veterinarians refer to the preferable use of first-line antimicrobial agents and avoidance of antimicrobial therapy during the dry-off period of dairy cattle. Global data and trends on the antimicrobial resistance of *E. coli* in mastitis have been highlighted in several national reports and vary among countries even though relevant comparisons are difficult. To date, the global picture indicates that antimicrobial susceptibility of *E. coli* in mastitis remains high. In particular, extended-spectrum β-lactamases (ESBLs) or overexpressed cephalosporinases (AmpCs) produced by *E. coli* and conferring resistance to broad-spectrum cephalosporins have been sporadically isolated from milk samples (13–16). Those families of antimicrobial agents may also be prescribed in newborns affected by diarrhea. Again, action plans against antimicrobial resistance in the animal sector constantly advise veterinarians to use antimicrobials prudently and emphasize the need to consider all other preventive and therapeutic options and restrict the use of antimicrobial agents to those situations where it is indispensable (17). For instance, strategies to prevent and treat neonatal diarrhea should include not only the prescription of antimicrobials but also good colostrum management practices to ensure adequate passive immunity and appropriate oral or intravenous fluid therapy to compensate for dehydration, acidosis, and electrolyte imbalance (18). Global hygiene procedures at the farm level and vaccinations are also essential measures for improvement in antimicrobial stewardship. In contrast to mastitis, ESBL/AmpC genes have been abundantly reported in *E. coli* originating from the digestive tract in animals. This includes pathogenic *E. coli* recovered from diarrheic samples of young animals, yet it remains highly difficult to confirm that a specific *E. coli* isolate is responsible for the intestinal disease. More importantly, ESBL/AmpC genes have been widely recognized in commensal *E. coli* isolated from fecal samples of various food-producing and companion animals through selective screenings using cephalosporin-containing media (19–21). High prevalence rates of ESBL/AmpC-producing *E. coli* were found in certain settings and countries, such as in the veal calves sector in Europe and in broiler production worldwide. In those cases, it more likely reflects the selective impact of the use of antimicrobials—and particularly of broad-spectrum cephalosporins such as ceftiofur—on the commensal *E. coli* microbiota. In broilers, such a situation has become a point of major concern on a global scale since broad-spectrum cephalosporins are both of critical importance in human medicine and not authorized for use in poultry. In addition to national actions taken, mostly in Europe, to restrict the use of critically important antimicrobial agents in animals, the use of antimicrobial agents as growth promoters has been banned in animals in Europe since 2006, but it is still common practice in most countries. Altogether, since antimicrobial agents have a major impact on the gut microbiota where *E. coli* resides, multidrug-resistant *E. coli*, such as ESBL/AmpC-producing *E. coli*, has become one of the main indicators to estimate the burden of antimicrobial resistance in animals and other sectors in a One Health perspective.

RESISTANCE TO β-LACTAMS

There are numerous genes in *E. coli* of human and animal origin that confer resistance to β-lactams. Some of them, such as bla_{TEM-1}, are widespread in *E. coli* from animals but code only for narrow-spectrum β-lactamases that can inactivate penicillins and aminopenicillins. However, in recent years, genes that code for ESBLs/AmpCs have emerged in *E. coli* from humans and animals. Most recently, genes coding for carbapenemases have also been detected occasionally in *E. coli* of animal origin. Because of the relevance of these latter two groups of β-lactamases, the following subsections provide more detailed information on ESBLs, AmpCs, and carbapenemases.

Clavulanic-Acid Inhibited Class A ESBLs

ESBLs belong mostly to class A of the Ambler classification (22) and group 2be according to the updated functional classification of β-lactamases by Bush and Jacoby (23). ESBL-producing strains of *E. coli* are clinically relevant in veterinary medicine since they confer resistance to penicillins, aminopenicillins, and cephalosporins, including the third-generation cephalosporins ceftiofur and cefovecin and the fourth-generation cephalosporin cefquinome, which are approved veterinary drugs. Thus, ESBLs may be the cause of treatment failures and limit the therapeutic options of veterinar-

ians, because they have been identified in increasing numbers in *E. coli* of food-producing and companion animals worldwide (24, 25). ESBL-producing *E. coli* from animals has been isolated not only from infection sites, but also from the feces of healthy individuals (26–29). Moreover, ESBL-producing *E. coli* has also been detected in wild animals, emphasizing the wide distribution of these resistance determinants (30).

TEM- and SHV-ESBLs were among the first described ESBLs in the 1980s, and they were predominant until 2000. Since then, CTX-M-ESBLs emerged and have been predominantly identified in commensal and pathogenic ESBL-producing *E. coli* isolates of human and animal origin around the world (31, 32). The reason for this shift remains unknown, despite many investigations and surveillance studies. It is difficult to compare prevalence data of ESBL-producing *E. coli* isolates because several resistance-monitoring programs register the resistance rates for cephalosporins in *E. coli* isolates of animal origin but do not necessarily confirm whether this resistance is based on ESBL production or another β-lactamase. Moreover, the molecular identification of ESBL genes in monitoring programs is not systematic. The nonharmonized methodology is also reflected in sampling plans and therefore in the origin of the *E. coli* isolates, e.g., healthy or diseased animals (33). Nevertheless, the European Food Safety Authority compiled a scientific opinion which states that the prevalence of resistance to cefotaxime in food-producing animals varies by country and animal species. In addition, the ESBL genes $bla_{CTX-M-1}$, $bla_{CTX-M-14}$, bla_{TEM-52}, and bla_{SHV-12} were identified as the most common ones along with a wide range of other bla_{CTX-M}, bla_{TEM}, and bla_{SHV} variant genes (34) (Table 1).

A large study conducted in Germany analyzed ESBL-producing *E. coli* isolates collected from diseased food-producing animals in the GERM-Vet monitoring program from 2008 to 2014 (35). This study detected the gene $bla_{CTX-M-1}$ in 69.9% of the ESBL producers, followed by $bla_{CTX-M-15}$ in 13.6%, $bla_{CTX-M-14}$ in 11.7%, bla_{TEM-52} in 1.9%, and bla_{SHV-12} in 1.4%. The genes $bla_{CTX-M-3}$ and $bla_{CTX-M-2}$ were identified in 1.0% and 0.5%, respectively. The distribution of ESBL genes varies with regard to the different animal hosts and the isolation sites; for example, ESBL-producing *E. coli* were isolated more frequently from cases of enteritis in calves than from cases of bovine mastitis (35). Moreover, the geographical location also plays a role. For instance, the study by Day and co-workers identified the gene $bla_{CTX-M-1}$ as the most common among bovine ESBL-producing *E. coli* from Germany, while the gene $bla_{CTX-M-15}$ was most frequent in *E. coli*

Table 1 Examples of acquired ESBL genes in *E. coli* of animal origin from Europe, the U.S., Latin America, Africa, and Asia

ESBL gene	Geographical origin	Source	Sequence type(s)	Reference
$bla_{\text{CTX-M-1}}$	Denmark	Pig	10, 189, 206, 453, 542, 744, 910, 1406, 1684 2739, 4048, 4052, 4053, 4056,	257
	Sweden	Poultry	57, 135, 155, 219, 602, 752, 1594, 1640	258
	Great Britain	Poultry	4, 10, 57, 88, 155, 371, 1515, 1517, 1518, 1549, 1550	259
	Switzerland	Poultry, cattle, pig	48, 83, 305, 525, 528, 529, 533, 534, 536, 540	260
	The Netherlands	Veal calves	10, 58, 88, 117, 162, 224, 354, 448, 617, 648, 744, 973	21
	France	Dairy cattle	23, 58	13
	Germany	Dairy cattle	10, 117, 540, 1431, 5447	14
	Germany	Swine, cattle, poultry, horse	10, 23, 83, 100, 131, 167, 362, 453, 648, 925, 973, 1684, 2699	43
	Germany	Dog	10, 23, 69, 160, 224	28
	U.S.	Dog, cat	23, 38, 44, 68, 69, 131, 167, 405, 410, 443, 648, 1011, 1088, 5174, 5206, 5220	261
$bla_{\text{CTX-M-14}}$	The Netherlands	Veal calves	10, 57, 952	21
	France	Dairy cattle	10, 23, 45, 58	13
	China	Pig, poultry	10, 155, 206, 224, 359, 405, 602, 648, 2929, 2930, 2962	262
	China	Dog	10, 38, 104, 131, 167, 405, 648, 146, 3630	97
$bla_{\text{CTX-M-15}}$	UK	Poultry	57, 156	259
	UK	Dog	131, 410, 1284, 2348, 4184	99
	The Netherlands	Veal calves	58, 59, 88, 361, 410, 648	21
	Germany	Livestock	10, 88, 90, 167, 410, 617, 648	263
	Germany	Dairy cattle	10, 361, 1508	14
	Germany, Denmark, Spain, France, the Netherlands	Dog, horse	131	264
	Germany, Italy	Dog, cat, cattle, horse	648	96
	Germany	Dog	410, 3018	28
	U.S.	Dog, cat	23, 38, 44, 68, 69, 131, 167, 405, 410, 443, 617, 648, 1011, 1088, 5174, 5206, 5220	261
	Mexico	Dog	410, 617	138
	China	Dog	10, 38, 44, 69, 73, 75, 131, 302, 405, 648, 1700, 2375	97
	Nigeria	Poultry	10, 405	221
$bla_{\text{SHV-12}}$	Spain, Germany	Wild bird, dog, poultry	23, 57, 117, 155, 362, 371, 453, 616, 1564, 2001	39
	China	Dog	10, 75, 131, 167, 405, 648, 2375, 3058	97

isolates of bovine origin from the United Kingdom (36). In ESBL-producing *E. coli* isolates from European companion animals, the gene $bla_{\text{CTX-M-1}}$ was most common, but the gene $bla_{\text{CTX-M-15}}$ was also frequently identified (24, 37). In the United States, the gene $bla_{\text{CTX-M-15}}$ was predominant among ESBL-producing *E. coli* from urinary tract infections of companion animals (38). The gene $bla_{\text{CTX-M-14}}$ was less frequent in Europe, but in Asia among the most common ESBL genes in poultry, companion animals, and humans (24). The ESBL gene $bla_{\text{SHV-12}}$ was not frequently reported but was identified in ESBL-producing *E. coli* from poultry, dogs, and wild birds in Spain and Germany (39).

Worldwide, the most common ESBL gene in *E. coli* isolates of human origin is $bla_{\text{CTX-M-15}}$, which is mainly

associated with the pandemic *E. coli* clone O25:H4-ST131 (40). This clone has been rarely identified in animals and if so, mostly in companion animals (24, 25, 41, 42). The production of various ESBLs has been demonstrated in animal *E. coli* isolates of a wide variety of multilocus sequence types (24, 35, 36, 43) (Table 1). According to Ewers and colleagues, an exclusive linkage of a specific *bla* gene or a distinct host with a certain sequence type (ST) is not evident (24). Nevertheless, ESBL-producing *E. coli* belonging to certain STs have been more frequently detected among animals and humans than others, namely ST10, ST23, ST38, ST88, ST131, ST167, ST410, and ST648, which are supposed to facilitate the spread of ESBL genes (25, 36, 43, 44).

The dissemination of ESBL genes among *E. coli* from animals is mainly driven by horizontal gene transfer. ESBL genes are associated with several insertion sequences (ISs), such as IS*Ecp1*, IS*CR1*, IS*26*, and IS*10*, transposons such as Tn*2*, and integrons (43, 45, 46). The majority of ESBL genes are plasmid-located, whereas the integration of ESBL genes in the chromosomal DNA of *E. coli* of animal origin has been rarely described (47–49). The most prevalent replicon types identified among ESBL-carrying plasmids from *E. coli* are IncF, IncI1, IncN, IncHI1, and IncHI2, but plasmids of other replicon types also play a role in the dissemination of ESBL genes (47). The study by Day and co-workers identified 16 ESBL genes on 341 transferable plasmids, belonging to 19 replicon types (36). Despite this complexity, some plasmids that carry ESBL genes seem to be more successful than others. Plasmids carrying $bla_{CTX-M-15}$ and belonging to the IncF family had been detected in the pandemic *E. coli* clone O25:H4-ST131 (47). The ESBL gene $bla_{CTX-M-1}$ was frequently identified on plasmids belonging to the IncN or IncI1 families, while $bla_{CTX-M-14}$ was detected on IncK plasmids, and $bla_{CTX-M-3}$ on IncL/M plasmids (47). IncI1, IncK, and IncX plasmids carried the ESBL gene bla_{SHV-12} (39). A plasmid multilocus sequence typing scheme assigns members of the most common plasmid families to pSTs to trace epidemic plasmids (47). Some plasmids harbor additional resistance genes besides the ESBL gene, which may facilitate the coselection and persistence of ESBL gene-carrying plasmids even without the selective pressure of β-lactams, when the respective antimicrobial agents are used (14, 43).

Many studies have tried to figure out whether ESBL-producing *E. coli* identified in humans might originate from animal reservoirs. Most of those studies could not find an obvious link, and most often, it was clearly shown that there was no link at all, animals and humans representing reservoirs of different clonal lineages that possessed various ESBL determinants (50, 51). Nevertheless, a Dutch study showed that a significant number of either human- or poultry-associated ESBL-producing *E. coli* isolates harbored genetically indistinguishable ESBL-encoding plasmids, suggesting that plasmids might be common vehicles that are likely transmitted through the food chain (52). Indeed, numerous studies have pointed out that chickens may represent a significant reservoir of ESBLs, which has become a considerable concern worldwide, although broad-spectrum cephalosporins are not approved for use in the poultry sector. ESBL-producing *E. coli* has been reported as a cause of infections in broilers and laying hens but also as a colonizer of living chickens and a contaminant of chicken meat at retail in several European and non-European countries, including countries in which the use of antimicrobial agents has been reduced following national action plans in veterinary medicine (53).

Acquired AmpC Cephalosporinases

Although class A ESBL enzymes are the most common sources of acquired resistance to broad-spectrum cephalosporins in *E. coli*, class C β-lactamases, also known as AmpC-type enzymes, confer high-level resistance to those antimicrobial agents (54). The main plasmid-encoded AmpC enzymes are CMY-, DHA-, and ACC-type β-lactamases, with a higher prevalence of CMY-type enzymes worldwide (55). In animals, the majority of identified AmpC enzymes have been of the CMY type (Table 2) (25, 56). A recent study performed in Denmark identified CMY-2-producing *E. coli* isolates from poultry meat, poultry, and dogs (57). The study showed that the dissemination of bla_{CMY-2} was mainly due to the spread of IncI1-γ and IncK plasmids. In Sweden, though there are, in general, low rates of resistance to broad-spectrum cephalosporins, the occurrence of CMY-2-producing *E. coli* was demonstrated when Swedish chicken meat, Swedish poultry, and imported chicken meat were examined (58). The occurrence of CMY-2-producing *E. coli* in the Swedish broiler sector has been attributed to importation of 1-day old chicks from the United Kingdom, where broad-spectrum cephalosporins had been administered prophylactically to the young birds before exportation (59). It has also been shown that migratory birds may be colonized with CMY-2-positive *E. coli* (60). In a study conducted in Florida, a series of clonally unrelated CMY-2-producing *E. coli* isolates were recovered from feces of seagulls (61). They belong mainly to phylogroup D, corresponding to human commensal isolates, but some STs had previously been identified from human bacteremia. The bla_{CMY-2} gene was mainly found on IncI1 plasmids, as reported with human isolates. Therefore, there was a significant correlation between the genetic features of those isolates and those known for human isolates in the United States, showing that seagulls were likely colonized by human isolates. This is an example showing that migratory birds crossing long distances, such as along the eastern United States coastline, may be reservoirs and therefore sources of such multidrug-resistant isolates, as is also exemplified in South America and Europe (62, 63).

Acquired Carbapenemases

Carbapenemases have been rarely identified in animal *E. coli*. This is likely the consequence of a very weak

Table 2 Examples of acquired bla_{CMY-2} genes in *E. coli* of animal origin from Europe, the North and South America, Asia, and Africa

Geographical origin	Source	Sequence type(s)	Reference
Germany	Pig	625	265
Spain	Wild bird (yellow-legged gull)	10	266
Denmark, Germany, France	Poultry and poultry meat, dog	10, 23, 38, 48, 68, 69, 88, 93, 115, 117, 131, 206, 212, 219, 297, 350, 361, 372, 405, 410, 428, 448, 457, 546, 616, 746, 754, 919, 963, 1196, 1056, 1303, 1518, 1585, 1594, 1640, 1775, 2040, 2144, 2168, 2196, 2558, 3272, 3574, 4048, 4124, 4125, 4240, 4243	57
Portugal	Poultry	57, 117, 429, 2451	267
Switzerland	Poultry meat	38, 1564	268
Switzerland	Poultry	3, 9, 61, 527, 530, 535, 539	
Austria	Wild bird (rook)	224	60
U.S.	Poultry meat	131	269
Brazil	Poultry	453, 457, 1706	270
China	Pig, poultry	10, 48, 69, 101, 155, 156, 354, 359, 362, 457, 648, 1114, 1431, 2294, 2690, 3014, 3244, 3245, 3269, 3376, 3402, 3403, 3404	271
Japan	Cattle	1284, 2438	272
Japan	Dog	10, 354, 493, 648, 3557	273
Tunisia	Poultry	117, 155, 2197	274

selective pressure (if any) by carbapenems, since those antimicrobial agents are not (or only in rare cases for individual non-food-producing animals) prescribed in veterinary medicine. Nevertheless, there has been some concern in recent years since carbapenemase-producing bacteria, including *E. coli*, have been isolated from animals worldwide (64–66).

The first carbapenemase determinant identified in an animal *E. coli* isolate was VIM-1, which was recovered from a pig in Germany (67) (Table 3). Since then, other VIM-1-producing *E. coli* isolates have been identified in different pig farms in the same country (68, 69). This carbapenemase has so far never been found elsewhere in animal isolates. Other identified carbapenemases in *E. coli* are NDM-1 and NDM-5. NDM-1 has been identified in the United States and in China, in isolates re-

covered from dogs, cats, and pigs (70, 71). NDM-5 has been detected in China, India, and Algeria, from cattle, poultry, dogs, cats, and fish (72–75). The gene encoding IMP-4 has been identified in *E. coli* isolates recovered from silver gulls in Australia (76). Interestingly, the OXA-48 carbapenemase, which is the most prevalent carbapenemase in human enterobacterial isolates in Europe, has been found in *E. coli* isolates recovered from dogs, cats, and chickens in Germany, France, Lebanon, Algeria, and the United States (37, 77–79). Finally, the OXA-181 enzyme, which is a variant of OXA-48 increasingly reported in humans, has recently been identified in animals as well, being found in clonally unrelated *E. coli* isolates recovered from pigs in Italy (80). Even though the class A β-lactamase KPC is one of the most commonly identified carbapenemases

Table 3 Examples of acquired carbapenemase genes in *E. coli* of animal origin from Europe, North and South America, Africa, Australia, and Asia

Carbapenemase gene	Geographical origin	Source	Sequence types	Reference
bla_{NDM-1}	China, U.S.	Dog, cat, pig	167, 1695, 1585, 1721, 359	70, 275, 276
bla_{NDM-5}	China, Algeria, India	Dog, pig, cow, duck	48, 54, 90, 156, 165, 167, 410, 648, 1114, 1178, 1234, 1437, 2439, 3331, 4429, 4463, 4656	74, 75, 277–279
bla_{VIM-1}	Germany	Seafood, pig	10, 88	67, 68, 280, 281
bla_{IMP-4}	Australia	Silver gull	48, 58, 167, 189, 216, 224, 345, 354, 541, 542, 744, 746, 1114, 1139, 1178, 1421, 2178, 4657, 4658,	76
bla_{OXA-48}	Germany, U.S., France, Lebanon, Algeria	Dog, cat, chicken	38, 372, 648, 1196, 1431	77–79, 261
$bla_{OXA-181}$	Italy	Pig	359, 641	80
bla_{KPC-2}	Brazil	Dog	648	287

in human isolates in some parts of the world, including in North America, China, and some European countries (Italy, Greece, Poland), it has not yet been identified in animal *E. coli* isolates so far (81, 82), except for a single *bla*$_{KPC-2}$-carrying isolate from a dog in Brazil that suffered from a urinary tract infection (287).

Overall, and notably, the different carbapenemase genes that have been identified among animals in different countries reflect the types of carbapenemases known to be the most prevalent in human isolates in those countries. Considering that carbapenems are not used in veterinary medicine, it remains to be determined which antimicrobial selective pressure is responsible for the selection of such carbapenemase producers in animals. Penicillins, however, are excellent substrates for any kind of β-lactamases, including carbapenemases, and therefore their use might correspond to a selective pressure anyhow. In addition, it remains to be evaluated whether animals may act as potential sources of transmission of those resistance traits toward humans or if, conversely, this epidemiology just reflects the consequence of a higher prevalence in humans that may eventually target animals through an environmental dissemination. Since the occurrence of carbapenemase-producing *Enterobacteriaceae* in animals is marginal, it therefore does not correspond to a significant threat to human medicine (65).

RESISTANCE TO QUINOLONES AND FLUOROQUINOLONES

Quinolones and fluoroquinolones are important antimicrobial agents for treating various types of infections in both humans and animals. They are known to be bactericidal against virtually all bacteria. Resistance to these antimicrobial agents is usually due to mutations in the drug targets, namely, the genes for DNA gyrase and topoisomerase IV, but other mechanisms such as reduced permeability of the outer membrane, protection of the target structures, or upregulated efflux pumps may also play a role (83).

Resistance to (Fluoro)Quinolones by Chromosomal Target Site Mutations

The primary target of (fluoro)quinolones in *E. coli* is the gyrase, which consists of two GyrA subunits and two GyrB subunits. Topoisomerase IV constitutes a secondary target in Gram-negative bacteria. This enzyme consists of two ParC and two ParE subunits. Most mutations were found within the quinolone resistance-determining region, which is between Ala67 and Gln107

in GyrA, and most frequently mutations occur at codons 83 and 87 (83). Single mutations in the gene *gyrA* may confer resistance to quinolones, but for resistance to fluoroquinolones, further mutations within *gyrA* and/or *parC* are needed. Most *parC* mutations occur at codons 80 and 84 (83). In clinical *E. coli* isolates from companion animals, different combinations of mutations were detected at codons 83 and 87 in *gyrA* and at codons 80 and 84 in *parC* (84, 85). Mutations within *gyrA* and *parC* were also described in *E. coli* isolates originating from diseased food-producing animals (86, 87).

Resistance to (Fluoro)Quinolones by Plasmid-Borne Resistance Mechanisms

Since the identification of the first plasmid-mediated quinolone resistance (PMQR) determinant, *qnrA1*, in 1997, there is serious concern about the global dissemination of PMQR genes (88, 89). Several plasmid-encoded resistance mechanisms have been identified, including (i) Qnr-like proteins (QnrA, QnrB, QnrC, QnrD, and QnrS) which protect DNA from quinolone binding, (ii) the AAC(6′)-Ib-cr acetyltransferase that modifies certain fluoroquinolones such as ciprofloxacin and enrofloxacin, and (iii) active efflux pumps (QepA and OqxAB). Overall, these resistance determinants do not confer a high level of resistance to quinolones (or fluoroquinolones), but rather, confer reduced susceptibility to those antimicrobial agents. However, they might contribute to the selection of isolates exhibiting higher levels of resistance through additional chromosomally encoded mechanisms (89).

PMQRs have been identified widely among human isolates but also among animal isolates. Especially in China, numerous studies have shown high prevalences of Qnr, AAC(6′)-Ib-cr, and QepA determinants among food-producing animals (86, 90), and some studies highlighted an increased prevalence through the years (91). A Europe-wide retrospective study identified the genes *qnrS1* and *qnrB19* in *E. coli* isolates from food-producing animals, namely, poultry, cattle, and pigs (92). PMQRs were detected not only in food-producing animals, but also in companion animals. In *E. coli* isolates from diseased companion animals, the genes *qnrS1*, *qnrB1*, *qnrB4*, and *qnrB10* were identified (84). The gene *qnrB19* was described in equine *E. coli* isolates (93, 94). The replicon types often associated with plasmids that carried the PMQR genes *qnrS1* and *qnrB19* are IncN and IncX but also include several others (47, 94, 95).

In *E. coli* belonging to several STs of companion animal origin, the gene *aac(6′)Ib-cr* was identified

(96–99). This gene was located on plasmids of the IncF family, and a *bla*~CTX-M~ ESBL gene, usually *bla*~CTX-M-15~, was often colocated (96, 98). Furthermore, *aac(6′)Ib-cr* was described in *E. coli* isolates from the feces of French cattle, where it was also colocated with *bla*~CTX-M-15~ on plasmids belonging to the IncF family (100). The gene *qepA* was identified in *E. coli* of companion animal origin belonging to different STs (97). Plasmids of the IncF family harbored *qepA* in *E. coli* from food-producing and companion animals (101). The PMQR gene *oqxAB* was identified in unrelated *E. coli* isolates from food-producing animals and located on different plasmids belonging to the IncF and IncHI2 families (102). The case of OqxAB is peculiar since this resistance determinant confers reduced susceptibility not only to quinolones (such as flumequine), but also to other drugs such as trimethoprim and chloramphenicol that are also used in veterinary medicine. Therefore, this resistance determinant encompasses different families of antimicrobial agents to which resistance (or reduced susceptibility) can be coselected (103).

RESISTANCE TO AMINOGLYCOSIDES

Aminoglycosides are drugs of natural origins whose producers can be found in the genus *Streptomyces* (104, 105) and *Micromonospora*, and they are often used in combination with another antimicrobial (mostly a β-lactam) to exploit their rapid bactericidal action for treating complicated infections such as sepsis, pneumonia, meningitis, and urinary tract/abdominal infections, both in humans and animals, including food-producing animals and companion animals (106). The most frequently used molecules in veterinary medicine are neomycin and derivatives of streptomycin. Gentamicin, kanamycin, and paromomycin are used as well. Amikacin is reserved for the treatment of infections in pets and horses (106).

Aminoglycosides affect a broad spectrum of pathogens among Gram-negative and -positive bacterial species, interfering with translation (107). Two major issues could limit the therapeutic power of these important molecules: the first is linked to their toxicity. Nevertheless, this issue is managed by opportune therapeutic regimens based on recent advances in the understanding of aminoglycoside pharmacodynamics (108). The second issue is the emergence of bacterial resistance linked to the usage of aminoglycosides, which has disseminated globally. The following subsections provide an overview of mechanisms of resistance toward aminoglycosides and their epidemiology in *E. coli* of animal origin.

Resistance to Aminoglycosides by Target Modifications

Resistance to aminoglycosides can develop by target mutations involving the 16S RNA and/or the S5 and S12 ribosomal proteins (107, 109, 110). However, this strategy is successful in conferring high-level resistance only in bacterial species with a limited number of copies of 16S RNA encoding operons. *E. coli* harbors seven copies of such operons, making the establishment of aminoglycoside resistance by point mutations rather improbable.

Modification of the target site of aminoglycosides can be achieved also by methylation of residues G1405 and A1408 of site A of the 16S RNA, resulting in high-level resistance to amikacin, tobramycin, gentamicin, and netilmicin (109). The 16S RNA methylases, including ArmA, RmtA/B/C/D/E/F/G/H, and NmpA, originated from natural aminoglycoside producers as self-defense against antimicrobial production (104). The first detection of ArmA dates back to 2003, when Galimand and colleagues reported the enzyme in a *Klebsiella pneumoniae* isolate from a human and the respective gene on a conjugative plasmid (111). Since then, the *armA* gene has been reported in several enterobacteria, *Acinetobacter baumannii*, and *Pseudomonas aeruginosa* isolates (112–116). The dissemination of the *armA* gene is favored by its location on the composite transposon Tn*1548*, which also carries genes coding for sulfonamide resistance, which in turn is located on self-transmissible plasmids belonging to several incompatibility groups (117). Emergence of ArmA in *E. coli* from animals was reported in 2005 in Spain in one pig (118), whereas the first report of *E. coli* producing RmtB was in 2007 in China by Chen and co-workers who reported a prevalence of 32% (*n* = 49/152) among healthy pigs in farms (119). In an investigation conducted in China in 2008, Du et al. reported the presence of ArmA and RmtB in *E. coli* from diseased poultry, with an occurrence of 10% (*n* = 12/120) (120). Later, Liu et al. reported the presence of *E. coli* ArmA and RmtB producers among various food-producing animals in 2009 to 2010, with an occurrence of 1.27% and 11.5% for ArmA and RmtB, respectively (*n* = 2 and 18/157) (121). RmtB was found in *E. coli* isolates associated with bovine mastitis in China in 2013 to 2014, with an occurrence of 5.3% (*n* = 13/245) (122). Yang and colleagues reported the presence of *E. coli* producing RmtD in diseased chickens in 2012 to 2014 in China. The enzyme co-occurred with RmtB with a prevalence of 8.3% (*n* = 3/36). In the same study, other methylases were found, namely, RmtB together with ArmA in 8.3% of isolates (*n* = 3/36), RmtB alone in

72.2% of isolates (n = 26/36), and ArmA in 11.1% of isolates (n = 4/36) (123).

More recently, a scattered porcine *E. coli* isolate harboring the *armA* gene was detected in Italy. The isolate was multidrug-resistant, notably harboring the *bla*$_{CMY-2}$, *bla*$_{OXA-181}$, and *mcr-1* genes (80). Recently, two *E. coli* isolates producing RmtB were reported from diseased bovines in France. The gene colocalized on an IncF33:A1:B1 plasmid with *bla*$_{CTX-M-55}$ and in one isolate also with the *fosA3* gene (124). The RmtD variant has been found less frequently. Other than the report from Yang et al. (123), another recent report has been published from Brazil, on one *E. coli* isolate from a diseased horse producing RmtD and harboring the *bla*$_{CTX-M-15}$ and *aac(6′)-Ib-cr* genes (125). The RmtE methylase was reported for the first time from commensal *E. coli* isolates from healthy calves in the United States (126). Later, two *E. coli* isolates were identified as RmtE producers in diseased food-producing animals in China, from 2002 to 2012 (127). Reports on RmtA are also quite infrequent, with a recent one from Zou et al., who found a frequency of 10% of *rmtA* gene occurrence among 89 *E. coli* isolates from giant pandas in China (128). To the best of our knowledge, RmtF/G/H enzymes have not yet emerged in *E. coli*, and NmpA has never been reported from animals. Overall, it can be stated that methylases have not widely disseminated since their discovery, probably for reasons related to fitness (129, 130). An exception is in China, where probably the antimicrobial usage, not only relative to aminoglycosides, may play a role in the emergence and dissemination of these enzymes. On the contrary, aminoglycoside-modifying enzymes have disseminated globally, and an overview of those most frequently encountered in animals is provided in the next subsection.

Resistance to Aminoglycosides by Enzymatic Inactivation

The inactivation of aminoglycosides is conducted by enzymes which modify the molecules so that they become unable to reach or bind to the target site. Currently, three types of aminoglycoside-modifying enzymes are known, and according to the modifying group that is linked to the aminoglycosides, they are classified as acetyltransferases, nucleotidyltransferases, and phosphotransferases.

The aminoglycoside acetyltransferases catalyze the addition of an acetyl group (CH_3CO) to an amine group ($-NH_2$) at positions 1, 2, 3, or 6 of the aminoglycoside structure, which determines the subgroup of the enzyme (131). For each enzyme, several variants have been reported, and they are usually defined by a roman number. AAC(3)-II/IV and AAC(6)-Ib are the most frequently encountered acetyltransferases among *E. coli* of human and animal origins. They have been globally reported from several hosts (128, 132–140).

Among aminoglycosides, the nucleotidyltransferases ANT(2″) and ANT(3″) are most commonly found in Gram-negative bacteria. ANT(2″) and ANT(3″) are encoded by the genes *aadB* and *aadA*, respectively (131), which are both frequently located on gene cassettes in class 1 integrons. These genes have also spread globally, and they have been found in *E. coli* from animals including pets, wild animals, and food-producing animals (134, 141–148).

Among the aminoglycoside phosphotransferases, APH(6)-Ia and APH(6)-Id encoded by the *strA* and *strB* genes, respectively, are most commonly encountered in *E. coli* worldwide. They mediate resistance to streptomycin and are frequently associated with a unique mobile element, sometimes together with the *aph(3″)-I/II* genes mediating kanamycin resistance. These resistance mechanisms have been found in several hosts including wild rabbits (145), cattle (149–152), poultry (153, 154), and swine (155–157).

RESISTANCE TO FOSFOMYCIN

Fosfomycin inhibits the MurA enzyme, which is involved in peptidoglycan synthesis. The use of fosfomycin in veterinary medicine is limited to the treatment of infections caused by a number of Gram-positive and Gram-negative pathogens, including *E. coli*, mainly in piglets and broiler chickens (158, 159). Two major fosfomycin resistance mechanisms have been described: (i) mutations in the *glpT* and *uhpA/T* genes encoding proteins involved in the fosfomycin uptake system and (ii) the acquisition of fosfomycin-modifying enzymes such as the metalloenzymes FosA, FosB, and FosX or the kinases FomA and FomB (160). Most of the *fos*-like genes are plasmid-borne, and plasmids carrying the *fos* genes commonly carry additional resistance genes (124, 161, 162) that increase the risk of coselection of fosfomycin resistance under the selective pressure by other antimicrobial agents.

A considerable number of studies report acquired fosfomycin resistance among *E. coli* of animal origin. Isolates carrying the plasmid-mediated *fosA* gene have been reported from companion animals. The first cases were reported in China in 2012 and 2013 from dogs and cats (163). Another study described a high prevalence of FosA3-producing *E. coli* in pets and their owners, highlighting the transmission of fosfomycin-resistant *E. coli* isolates between humans and animals

(164). Another Chinese study described the *fosA3* gene in *E. coli* from fresh pork and chicken meat (165). In that study, the *fosA3* gene was often found together with ESBL genes (*bla*$_{CTX-M-55}$, *bla*$_{CTX-M-15}$, or *bla*$_{CTX-M-123}$) on plasmids of 78 to 138 kb in size. In a recent French study, the emergence of plasmids carrying multiple resistance determinants including *fosA3*, *bla*$_{CTX-M-55}$, *rmtB*, and *mcr-1* was reported in various animal species (124). In that study, it was speculated that this plasmid could have an Asian origin since *bla*$_{CTX-M-55}$ is the second most prevalent ESBL gene in that part of the world. In 2013, the complete sequence of the 76,878-bp plasmid pHN7A8 from a dog in China was determined. This plasmid represents a F33:A⁻:B⁻-type epidemic plasmid that carried the resistance genes *bla*$_{CTX-M-65}$, *fosA3*, and *rmtB* (166). Plasmids with similar *fosA3* regions were reported from *E. coli* isolates of pig (167), duck (168), and chicken origin (169). The widespread occurrence of the *fosA3* gene in China was demonstrated in a study that identified 12/892 *E. coli* isolates as *fosA3*-positive. These isolates originated from pigs, chickens, ducks, a goose, and a pigeon (170). Furthermore, the analysis of 1,693 *E. coli* isolates from various animal species identified 97 *fosA3*-positive isolates from beef cattle, pigs, broiler chickens, stray cats, stray dogs, and wild rodents in China (171). Recently, several epidemic *fosA3*-carrying multiresistance plasmids of diverse incompatibility groups have been identified to be disseminated among *E. coli* from pigs, dairy cattle, and chickens in northeast China (162). Some of these plasmids have been sequenced completely, including the plasmids pECM13 from cattle (113,006 bp, IncI1, and coharboring *bla*$_{CTX-M-14}$, *rmtB*, *aadA2*, and *bla*$_{TEM-1}$), pECB11 from chicken [92,545 bp, F33:A⁻:B⁻, and coharboring *bla*$_{CTX-M-55}$, *floR*, *cfr*, *bla*$_{TEM-1}$, *tet*(A), *strA*, and *strB*], and pECF12 from chicken [77,822 bp, F33:A⁻:B⁻, and coharboring *bla*$_{CTX-M-3}$, *rmtB*, *tet*(A), *strA*, and *strB*]. *E. coli* isolates from pigs harboring the *fosA3* gene were also detected in Taiwan (172).

RESISTANCE TO TETRACYCLINES

Tetracyclines are widely used in veterinary medicine. A summary of sales data in the 25 European Union and European Economic Area countries revealed that tetracyclines accounted for 37% of the total sales of veterinary antimicrobial agents, followed by penicillins (23%) (173). As a consequence of the selective pressure imposed by the widespread use of tetracyclines, many bacteria—including *E. coli*—have developed tetracycline resistance. According to the tetracycline resistance gene nomenclature center (https://faculty.washington.edu/marilynr/), nine tetracycline efflux genes [*tet*(A), *tet*(B), *tet*(C), *tet*(D), *tet*(E), *tet*(G), *tet*(J), *tet*(L), and *tet*(Y)], two tetracycline resistance genes encoding ribosome protective proteins [*tet*(M) and *tet*(W)], and one gene coding for an oxidoreductase that inactivates tetracyclines [*tet*(X)] have been identified in *E. coli*. The major mechanisms of tetracycline resistance encountered in *E. coli* of animal origin include (i) the active efflux by proteins of the major facilitator superfamily and (ii) ribosome protection. A PubMed search for tetracycline resistance genes in *E. coli* of animal origin revealed that not all of these 12 *tet* genes occur in *E. coli* from animal sources. The following examples provide an overview of the distribution of *tet* genes among *E. coli* from various animal sources.

Among 155 *E. coli* isolates from fecal samples of cattle in Korea, the genes *tet*(A), *tet*(B), and *tet*(C) were detected in 72, 70, and nine isolates, respectively. Two isolates each carried *tet*(A) + *tet*(B) or *tet*(B) + *tet*(C) (174). In 99 *E. coli* isolates from bovine mastitis in the United States collected from 1985 to 1987 and in 2009, the genes *tet*(A), *tet*(B), and *tet*(C) were detected, with *tet*(C) being present in more than half of the investigated isolates in each of the two time periods (175). Of 129 *E. coli* isolates from cases of bovine mastitis in the United States, 68 carried the gene *tet*(C), while another 14 isolates harbored *tet*(C) + *tet*(A) (176). A study in Switzerland identified the genes *tet*(A), *tet*(B), and *tet*(A) + *tet*(B) in 24, 16, and two *E. coli* isolates from bovine mastitis (177). In the same study, the genes *tet*(A), *tet*(B), *tet*(C), and *tet*(A) + *tet*(B) were detected in 60, five, one, and two *E. coli* isolates, respectively, from diarrhea and enterotoxemia in pigs (177). In 99 tetracycline-resistant *E. coli* isolates from pigs in Spain, the genes *tet*(A) (*n* = 46), *tet*(B) (*n* = 12), and *tet*(A) + *tet*(B) (*n* = 28) but also *tet*(A) + *tet*(M) (*n* = 11) and *tet*(A) + *tet*(B) + *tet*(M) (*n* = 2) were detected (178). The *tet*(M) gene was shown by Southern blot hybridization to be located on plasmids. In a study in Germany, either the genes *tet*(A) (*n* = 71), *tet*(B) (*n* = 46), and *tet*(C) (*n* = 3) alone or the combinations of the genes *tet*(A) + *tet*(B) (*n* = 2), *tet*(A) + *tet*(C) (*n* = 2), *tet*(A) + *tet*(D) (*n* = 3), *tet*(A) + *tet*(M) (*n* = 1), *tet*(B) + *tet*(M) (*n* = 2), *tet*(B) + *tet*(C) (*n* = 2), and *tet*(B) + *tet*(D) + *tet*(M) (*n* = 1) were detected in *E. coli* from pigs (179). Among 283 tetracycline-resistant extra-intestinal pathogenic *E. coli* isolates from pigs in China, the genes *tet*(A) (*n* = 68), *tet*(B) (*n* = 141), *tet*(C) (*n* = 3), *tet*(D) (*n* = 1), and *tet*(G) (*n* = 108) were identified (156). A wide variety of *tet* genes was also seen among 73 tetracycline-resistant *E. coli* isolates from broilers in Iran, including the gene *tet*(E) alone (*n* = 1) or in the combinations *tet*(E) +

tet(C) (*n* = 4), *tet*(E) + *tet*(D) + *tet*(M) (*n* = 2), *tet*(E) + *tet*(D) + *tet*(A) + *tet*(G) (*n* = 3), and *tet*(E) + *tet*(M) + *tet*(A) + *tet*(B) + *tet*(C) (*n* = 1) (180). In 33 *E. coli* isolates from cases of septicemia among laying hens in Switzerland, the genes *tet*(A) and *tet*(B) were found in 21 and 10 isolates, respectively, while two isolates carried neither *tet*(A), *tet*(B), nor *tet*(C) (177). In the same study, the genes *tet*(A) and *tet*(B) were detected in eight and nine *E. coli* isolates from urinary tract infections in dogs and cats, respectively. The same two *tet* genes were also found in *E. coli* isolates from healthy dogs and cats in Spain (181). A large-scale study of *tet* genes in 325 nonclinical *E. coli* isolates from various animal sources in the United States identified the gene *tet*(B) in isolates from a goose, a duck, and a deer; the genes *tet*(A) and *tet*(B) in isolates from turkeys, cats, goats, and cows; *tet*(A), *tet*(B), and *tet*(C) in isolates from dogs, sheep, and horses; and *tet*(A), *tet*(B), *tet*(C), and *tet*(M) in isolates from pigs and chickens (182). However, in that study neither *tet*(E) nor *tet*(G), *tet*(L), or *tet*t(X) were detected in the 325 *E. coli* isolates. Among 58 tetracycline-resistant *E. coli* isolates from giant pandas, the genes *tet*(A), *tet*(E), and/or *tet*(C) were detected in 33, 24, and four isolates, respectively (128).

These examples show that different *tet* genes—alone or in combination with others—occur at different frequencies in *E. coli* isolates from different animal sources and/or geographic regions. In general, the genes *tet*(A) and *tet*(B) were the most prevalent tetracycline resistance genes in *E. coli* of animal origin. Both of these genes are part of small nonconjugative transposons, Tn*1721* [*tet*(A)] (183) and Tn*10* [*tet*(B)] (184), which are often integrated into conjugative and nonconjugative plasmids. Several of the aforementioned examples revealed the presence of more than a single *tet* gene in the same isolate. This might be explained by the observation that several *tet* genes are frequently found on plasmids or other mobile genetic elements which may have been acquired by the respective *E. coli* isolates at different times and under different conditions. When other resistance genes are colocated with a *tet* gene on the same plasmid, such a plasmid can be acquired under the selective pressure imposed by the use of antimicrobial agents other than tetracyclines. Multidrug resistance plasmids that also carry *tet* genes have been detected in *E. coli* from bovine mastitis in Germany. Here, the gene *tet*(A) was located on IncHI2/IncP plasmids of ca. 225 kb, which also harbored the resistance genes *bla*CTX-M-2, *bla*TEM-1, *sul1*, *sul2*, *dfrA1*, and *aadA1* (14). IncI1 plasmids that range in size from 90 to 120 kb and carry the resistance gene *tet*(A) along with the genes *bla*SHV-12, *aadA1*, *cmlA1*, and *aadA2* or

the genes *bla*SHV-12, *qacG*, and *aadA6* were identified in *E. coli* isolates from wild birds, dogs, and poultry in Spain or Germany (39). In canine *E. coli* isolates from Brazil, several multiresistance plasmids were identified. These included (i) a ca. 250-kb IncFIB/IncHI2 plasmid that carried the gene *tet*(B) together with the resistance genes *bla*CTX-M-2, *sul1*, *aadA29*, *strA*, and *strB*; (ii) a ca. 240-kb IncFIC plasmid that harbored the *tet*(A) gene together with the resistance genes *bla*CMY-2, *cmlA*, *floR*, *strA*, *strB*, *sul1*, *sul3*, and *aadA7*; (iii) a 240-kb IncHI2 plasmid with the resistance genes *bla*CTX-M-2, *sul1*, *aadA29*, *strA*, and *strB*; and (iv) a 40-kb IncFIB/IncN plasmid with the resistance genes *tet*(A), *sul1*, *dfrA16*, and *dfrA29* (185). Lastly, an 81-kb plasmid that carried the resistance genes *qnrS1*, *bla*CTX-M-14, *bla*TEM-1, *floR*, and *tet*(A) was found in an *E. coli* isolate from a pig in China (186). These few examples illustrate that *tet* gene-carrying multiresistance plasmids occur in *E. coli* of different animal species in different parts of the world. Given the widespread use of tetracyclines in veterinary medicine, such plasmids not only facilitate the dissemination of certain *tet* genes, but also support the coselection and persistence of other resistance genes.

RESISTANCE TO PHENICOLS

Phenicols are broad-spectrum antimicrobial agents of which nonfluorinated (e.g., chloramphenicol) and fluorinated (e.g., florfenicol) derivatives are used in veterinary medicine. Due to its toxicity and important adverse effects in humans, such as dose-unrelated irreversible aplastic anemia, dose-related reversible bone marrow suppression, and Gray syndrome in neonates, chloramphenicol and its derivatives thiamphenicol and azidamfenicol were banned in 1994 in the European Union from use in food-producing animals (187). Currently, the use of nonfluorinated phenicols in animals is limited to the treatment of companion animals and pets. However, the fluorinated derivative florfenicol is licensed for the treatment of bacterial infections in food-producing animals (187).

Phenicol resistance in *E. coli* of animal origin is mediated by three major mechanisms: (i) enzymatic inactivation of nonfluorinated phenicols by chloramphenicol acetyltransferases encoded by *cat* genes, (ii) active efflux of nonfluorinated phenicols (*cmlA* genes) or fluorinated and nonfluorinated phenicols (*floR* genes) by major facilitator superfamily proteins, and (iii) target site methylation by an rRNA methylase encoded by the multiresistance gene *cfr*, which confers resistance to five classes of antimicrobial agents, including fluorinated and nonfluorinated phenicols (187).

Among 102 *E. coli* isolates from pigs in China, 91 (89%) were resistant to chloramphenicol. The genes *catA1* and *catA2* but also the cassette-borne gene *cmlA* were detected in 58%, 49%, and 65%, respectively, of the chloramphenicol-resistant isolates. In addition, the gene *floR* was detected in 57% of the florfenicol-resistant isolates and in 52% of chloramphenicol-resistant isolates (188). In a study of 318 ETEC, non-ETEC from cases of diarrhea, and commensal *E. coli* isolates from healthy pigs in Canada, the genes *catA1*, *cmlA*, and *floR* were detected among the chloramphenicol-resistant isolates. The gene *catA1* was significantly more frequent in ETEC than in non-ETEC and commensal *E. coli* (189). The genes *floR* and *cmlA* were detected among 48 *E. coli* isolates from calves with diarrhea. Of the 44 isolates for which florfenicol MICs were ≥16 mg/liter, 42 carried the *floR* gene. Twelve *E. coli* isolates were positive for *cmlA*, and their corresponding chloramphenicol MICs were ≥32 mg/liter. In addition, eight isolates were positive for *floR* and *cmlA*, and their florfenicol and chloramphenicol MICs were ≥64 mg/liter (190). In a study of antimicrobial resistance in German *E. coli* isolates from cattle, pigs, and poultry, not further specified *catA* genes were found in seven isolates from cattle and six isolates each from pigs and poultry. Moreover, *cmlA1*-like genes were detected in a single isolate from cattle, six isolates from pigs, and three isolates from poultry. The *floR* gene was not detected (191). Among 116 avian-pathogenic *E. coli* isolates from chickens in Egypt, 98 (84.5%) were resistant to chloramphenicol. The resistance genes *catA1*, *catA2*, and *cmlA* were found in 86, four, and eight isolates, respectively, while the genes *catA3* and *cmlB* were not detected (192). Among 102 chloramphenicol-resistant *E. coli* isolates from horses in the UK, 75 harbored the gene *catA1*. The remaining 27 isolates were PCR negative for the genes *catA2*, *catA3*, and *cmlA*, while the presence of the genes *floR* and *cfr* was not tested (193). The cassette-borne chloramphenicol resistance genes *catB3* and *cmlA6* were identified in four and two canine *E. coli* isolates, respectively, all from the United States. The gene *catB3* was located together with the resistance genes *aacA4* and *dfrA1*, and the gene *cmlA6* was located together with the genes *aadB* and *aadA1* in class 1 integrons of different sizes (194). In a study of 62 *E. coli* isolates from dogs in Iran, three isolates harbored the *cmlA* gene, whereas six isolates were positive for the *floR* gene (195). Among 36 chloramphenicol- and florfenicol-resistant *E. coli* isolates from dogs suffering from urinary tract infections in Taiwan, all isolates harbored the *cmlA* gene and 18 carried the *floR* gene (196). The *cmlA* gene was also detected in two

chloramphenicol-resistant *E. coli* isolates from fecal samples of free-range Iberian lynx (143). Of 89 *E. coli* isolates from giant pandas, 28 and 23 were resistant to chloramphenicol and florfenicol, respectively. The *floR* gene was detected in 23 isolates and the *cmlA* gene in nine isolates, with two isolates carrying both genes. The *cfr* gene was not detected in any of the isolates, and *cat* genes were not tested (128). The genes *catA1* and *cmlA* were also detected in two and one multiresistant *E. coli* isolates, respectively, from shellfish in Vietnam (197).

The genes *catA1*, *cmlA*, and *floR* are often found on plasmids. In bovine *E. coli* from the United States, the *floR* gene was located on large plasmids of 225 kb (190), which were larger than those found in *E. coli* from sick chickens (198). Southern blot analysis confirmed the presence of the *cmlA* gene on plasmids of >100 kb in *E. coli* from pigs (199). Conjugation assays identified two distinct class 1 integrons that linked *cmlA* to the streptomycin/spectinomycin resistance genes *aadA1* and *aadA2* and to the sulfonamide resistance genes *sul1* or *sul3* (199). Transformation experiments conducted with Canadian *E. coli* from pigs revealed that *aadA* and *sul1* were located together with *catA1* on a large ETEC plasmid (189). Plasmids that harbored the gene *cmlA* also carried the resistance genes *aadA* and *sul3*. Moreover, plasmids that harbored the genes *aadB* and *floR* also carried *sul2*, *tet*(A), *bla*_{CMY-2}, *strA*, and *strB* but occasionally also *aac(3)-IV* (189). Among Brazilian *E. coli* from dogs, a 35-kb IncF/IncFIB plasmid was identified that harbored the genes *strA* and *strB*, and an unusual class 1 integron with the genes *dfrA12*, *aadA2*, *cmlA1*, and *aadA1* linked to a *sul3* gene (185). The ca. 35-kb plasmid pMBSF1 from porcine *E. coli* in Germany carried the *floR* gene together with the genes *strA* and *strB* (200). The *floR* gene was also detected on conjugative plasmids ranging in size from 110 to 125 kb from bovine *E. coli* in France. All these plasmids mediated additional resistances to sulfonamides, streptomycin, ampicillin, and/or trimethoprim (201). These examples show that phenicol resistance genes can also be coselected under the selective pressure imposed by nonphenicol antimicrobial agents.

The multiresistance gene *cfr*—originally identified in staphylococci of animal origin—was also found to be functionally active in *E. coli* (202). The gene *cfr* was first reported in *E. coli* from a nasal swab of a pig in China (203). Later, it was identified on the 135,615-bp IncA/C multiresistance plasmid pSCEC2 from a pig in China. This plasmid also harbored the resistance genes *sul2*, *tet*(A), *floR*, *strA*, and *strB* (157). In another study in China, the *cfr* gene was detected on plasmids of ca. 30 kb in *E. coli* isolates from pigs (204). The complete sequence of the 37,672-bp plasmid pSD11, again from *E. coli* of porcine origin in China, was reported by Sun and colleagues (205). The colocation of *cfr* with the ESBL gene *bla*CTX-M-14b on the 41,646-bp plasmid pGXEC3 from a porcine *E. coli* isolate was reported in 2015 (206). In the same year, another *cfr*-carrying plasmid, the conjugative 33,885-bp plasmid pFSEC-01, was reported (207). Although this plasmid was found in a porcine *E. coli* isolate, it closely resembled in its structure the plasmid pEA3 from the plant pathogen *Erwinia amylovora*. Most recently, another six *cfr*-carrying *E. coli* isolates—five from pigs and one from a chicken—were identified. In all cases, the *cfr* gene was located as the only resistance gene on plasmids of either 37 or 67 kb. Two of these plasmids were completely sequenced: the 37,663-bp IncX4 plasmid pEC14cfr and the 67,077-bp F14: A⁻: B⁻ plasmid pEC29cfr (161).

RESISTANCE TO SULFONAMIDES AND TRIMETHOPRIM

Sulfonamides and trimethoprim are synthetic antimicrobial agents that inhibit different steps in the folic acid synthesis pathway. Each of these agents acts in a bacteriostatic manner, whereas the combination of a sulfonamide with trimethoprim results in synergistic bactericidal actions on susceptible organisms; as such, the combination is referred to as a "potentiated" sulfonamide. Sulfonamides and trimethoprim have been used for decades in animals and humans. Acquired resistance mechanisms have been frequently identified, mainly due to (i) mutational modifications in the genes encoding the target enzymes, namely, the dihydropteroate synthase or dihydrofolate reductase, respectively, or (ii) the acquisition of *sul* genes encoding dihydropteorate synthetases that are insensitive to sulfonamides or *dfr* genes encoding dihydrofolate reductases that are insensitive to trimethoprim (208).

Resistance to Sulfonamides

In *E. coli* from food-producing and companion animals, sulfonamide resistance is mediated by any of the following three *sul* genes: *sul1*, *sul2*, or *sul3*. The *sul1* gene is particularly widespread because it is part of the 3′-conserved segment of class 1 integrons (209). As such, the *sul1* gene is often found together with other antimicrobial resistance genes that are located on gene cassettes in the variable part of class 1 integrons (209). Class 1 integrons are present in *E. coli* from healthy and diseased food-producing animals, companion

animals, and wildlife all over the world as illustrated in the following examples. In Germany, 58 of 417 *E. coli* isolates from diseased swine, horses, dogs, and cats, collected in the BfT-GermVet monitoring study, harbored class 1 integrons (210). Other studies identified class 1 integrons in *E. coli* from healthy and diseased dogs in Brazil (185), in clinical avian *E. coli* isolates in the United States (211), in *E. coli* from lizards in Indonesia (212), in Shiga toxin-producing *E. coli* from cattle in the United States (213), in *E. coli* from free-range reindeer in Norway (214), in calf-pathogenic *E. coli* in China (215), in *E. coli* from pigs in Denmark (216), and even in *E. coli* from giant pandas in China (128). Class 1 integrons including the *sul1* gene are often located on plasmids, including ESBL-gene-carrying multi-resistance plasmids (14, 216–218).

The gene *sul2* is also widely disseminated among *E. coli* of various animal species in different parts of the world. It has been found in *E. coli* from pigs in Canada (219) and Denmark (216), in food-producing animals in Kenya (220), in poultry in Nigeria (221) and Germany (222), and in horses in the Czech Republic (93). The *sul2* gene is often linked to the streptomycin resistance genes *strA-strB*. Similarly to *sul1*, the *sul2* gene is commonly found on plasmids that also harbor other antimicrobial resistance genes (93, 157, 220, 221, 223).

The gene *sul3* was first described in 2003 in *E. coli* isolates from pigs in Switzerland (224). Since then, this gene has been identified mostly on plasmids in *E. coli* from pigs in the United States (199), Canada (219), and Denmark (216); from poultry in Germany (222); and from dogs in Spain (138) and Brazil (185). Several reports described the *sul3* gene to be linked to other resistance genes, such as the macrolide resistance gene *mef*(B) (225), and to unusual class 1 integrons (39, 185, 199, 226).

Resistance to Trimethoprim

Numerous *dfr* genes that confer trimethoprim resistance have been detected in *Enterobacteriaceae* and other Gram-negative bacteria. Based on their sizes and structures, they have been divided into two major groups, *dfrA* and *dfrB* (227). The *dfrA* genes code for proteins of 152 to 189 amino acids, while the *dfrB*-encoded proteins are only 78 amino acids in size. Most of the *dfrA* and *dfrB* genes found in *E. coli* of animal origin are located on gene cassettes that are inserted into class 1 or class 2 integrons. Some examples are given for *dfrA* genes that have been identified in *E. coli* from dogs (*dfrA1*, *dfrA12*, *dfrA17*, *dfrA29*) (138, 185, 210), cats (*dfrA1*, *dfrA12*) (210), horses (*dfrA1*, *dfrA9*, *dfrA12, dfrA17*) (193, 210), pigs (*dfrA1, dfrA5, dfrA8, dfrA12, dfrA13, dfrA14, dfrA16, dfrA17*) (144, 156, 210, 228, 229), cattle (*dfrA1, dfrA8, dfrA12, dfrA17*) (14, 215, 229), chickens (*dfrA1, dfrA5, dfrA12, dfrA14, dfrA16*) (144, 229), and giant pandas (*dfrA1, dfrA7, dfrA12, dfrA17*) (128). In contrast to *dfrA* genes, *dfrB* genes have rarely been detected in *E. coli* from animals. A *dfrB4* gene and a *dfrA17* gene were detected in class 1 integrons from sea lions (230). In the study by Seputiené et al. (229), the *dfrA8* gene was located in neither class 1 nor in class 2 integrons. Moreover, only seven of the 13 *dfrA14* genes in *E. coli* isolates of animal origin were integron-associated. In previous studies of *E. coli* from food-producing animals, a functionally active *dfrA14* gene was found outside an integron but inserted into a plasmid-borne *strA* gene (220, 231).

RESISTANCE TO POLYMYXINS

Colistin (also known as polymyxin E) is a polypeptide antimicrobial agent that targets the LPS in the outer membrane of Gram-negative bacteria (232). Colistin is widely used in veterinary medicine, mainly for the treatment or prevention of intestinal infections, particularly neonatal and postweaning diarrhea in pigs and intestinal infections in poultry and cattle (233). Very recently, due to the considerable concerns that colistin resistance might be transferable from animals to humans, specific regulations on the use of colistin have been set up in Europe under the umbrella of the European Medicines Agency (234). In April 2017, a ban of colistin as a growth promoter also became effective in China (235). Colistin is active against various species of *Enterobacteriaceae*, including *E. coli*, whereas others such as *Proteus* spp. and *Serratia* spp. are intrinsically resistant (232). Resistance to colistin can be due to mutations in chromosomal genes or to acquired resistance genes.

Chromosome-Encoded Polymyxin Resistance

Polymyxin resistance in *E. coli* isolates may be related to genes encoding LPS-modifying enzymes. The operon *pmrCAB* codes for three proteins, namely, a phosphoethanolamine phosphotransferase PmrC, a response regulator PmrA (also called BasR), and a sensor kinase protein PmrB (also called BasS) (232). Mutations either in PmrA or in PmrB have been found to be responsible for polymyxin resistance in *E. coli* isolates recovered from poultry in Spain (236). However, most of the mutations leading to polymyxin resistance in that operon or in others, such as the PhoPQ two-component system or its regulator MgrB, have been identified in human

E. coli isolates. Ongoing studies are being conducted to evaluate whether the same mechanisms might be responsible for polymyxin resistance in animal isolates. In one such study, mutations in the genes *pmrA, pmrB, mgrB, phoP,* and *phoQ* of *E. coli* isolates from pigs were identified (237).

Plasmid-Mediated Polymyxin Resistance

In November 2016, the first plasmid-borne polymyxin resistance gene was identified. This gene was designated *mcr-1*, and it encodes the MCR-1 phosphoethanolamine transferase (238). Production of MCR-1 leads to the modification of the lipid A moiety of the LPS, resulting in a more cationic LPS and, consequently, to resistance to polymyxins. Production of MCR-1 in *E. coli* leads to a 4- to 8-fold increase in the MICs of polymyxins (232).

The *mcr-1* gene has been detected mainly in *E. coli* isolates but also in other *Enterobacteriaceae* genera, such as *Salmonella, Shigella, Klebsiella,* and *Enterobacter* (239). This gene has now been identified worldwide, in both animal and human isolates. The *mcr-1* gene has been found to be located on plasmids of various incompatibility groups (IncI2, IncHI2, IncP, IncX4, IncY, IncFI, and IncFIB) and variable sizes (58 to 251 kb) (232). A few reports showed that it may be colocated with ESBL-encoding genes and/or other resistance genes (71, 240–244); nonetheless, most of the reports identified *mcr-1* as the sole resistance gene on the respective plasmids. This may suggest that a polymyxin-related selective pressure is responsible for the *mcr-1* acquisition, with corresponding plasmids providing no other obvious selective advantage. Upstream of the *mcr-1* gene, the IS*Apl1* insertion sequence element is frequently identified, although it is often, but not always, also identified downstream of it. Recent studies demonstrated that the *mcr-1* gene is mobilized by transposition when bracketed by two copies of IS*Apl1* that form a composite transposon structure (242, 245). So far, 11 variants of the *mcr-1* gene, designated *mcr-1.2* to *mcr-1.12* have been identified, with *mcr-1.3* being found in *E. coli* from chickens in China (246), *mcr-1.8* in *E. coli* from poultry in Brunei (GenBank accession no. KY683842.1), *mcr-1.9* in *E. coli* from swine in Portugal (KY964067.1), and *mcr-1.12* in *E. coli* from pork in Japan (LC337668.1).

Recently, the plasmid-mediated colistin-resistance *mcr-2* gene was identified in *E. coli* isolates recovered from piglets in Belgium (247). It shared 77% nucleotide sequence identity with *mcr-1* and was located on an IncX4 plasmid. The *mcr-2* gene has been sporadically identified so far (248). In addition, further *mcr* genes—

mcr-3 to *mcr-7*—and variants thereof have been described. Among them, the *mcr-3* gene was initially identified together with 18 additional resistance genes on the 261-kb IncHI2-type plasmid pWJ1 from porcine *E. coli* (249). The *mcr-3* gene showed 45.0% and 47.0% nucleotide sequence identity to *mcr-1* and *mcr-2*, respectively. So far, ten variants of *mcr-3*, designated *mcr-3.2* to *mcr-3.11*, have been identified, with the *mcr-3.2* gene being originally detected in *E. coli* from cattle in Spain (250). A recent study in France reported the spread of a single *E. coli* clone harboring *mcr-3* in the veal calves sector from 2011 to 2016 (251). The combination in those isolates of *mcr-3* and *bla*$_{CTX-M-55}$, an ESBL gene that is highly prevalent in Asian countries and rarely detected in Europe, may suggest the introduction and further dissemination of *mcr-3* in that specific animal setting due to international trade. The *mcr-4* gene was detected among *E. coli* from pigs in Spain and Belgium that suffered from postweaning diarrhea (252). The gene *mcr-5* and a variant, designated *mcr-5.2*, have recently been found in *E. coli* from pigs (253).

Epidemiology of *mcr-1*

The *mcr-1* gene is a resistance gene identified in human and animal *E. coli* isolates. Its occurrence in animal isolates is quite elevated (232), and it has been identified worldwide. MCR-1-producing *E. coli* isolates have been identified in several food-producing animals and meat, including chickens and chicken meat, pigs and piglets, cattle, calves, and turkeys (254, 255) (Table 4). Those isolates are from many Asian countries (Cambodia, China, Japan, Laos, Malaysia, Taiwan, Singapore, Vietnam, India, Pakistan, South Korea), from Europe (Belgium, Denmark, France, Germany, Portugal, Italy, the Netherlands, Spain, Sweden, Switzerland, the UK), the Americas (Argentina, Brazil, Canada, the U.S., Ecuador, Bolivia, Venezuela), Australia, and Africa (Algeria, Egypt, South Africa, Tunisia). Worryingly, a recent study performed in China identified a series

Table 4 Examples of acquired *mcr* genes in *E. coli* of animal origin from Europe, North and South America, and Asia

mcr gene	Geographical origin	Source	Sequence type(s)	Reference
mcr-1	China	Pig		238
	China	Pig		242
	China	Pig	48, 54, 90, 156, 165, 167, 410, 1114, 1178, 1437, 2439, 3331, 4429, 4463, 4656	277
	China	Poultry	10, 48, 58, 77, 88, 101, 117, 178, 215, 361, 501, 542, 616, 617, 648, 744, 761, 870, 873, 952, 971, 1290, 1431, 1642, 2345, 2491, 2599, 3044, 3133, 3481, 3944, 5542, 5815, 5865, 5879, 5909, 6050,	246
	Vietnam	Reptiles	117, 1011	282
	South Korea	Poultry, pig	1, 10, 88, 101, 156, 162, 226, 410, 1141, 2732	283
	Germany	Pig	1, 10, 846	240
	Germany	Pig (manure), fly, dog	10, 342, 1011, 5281	256
	France	Cattle		241
	Italy	Poultry (meat)	602	243
	U.S.	Pig	132, 3234	284
	Venezuela	Pig	452	285
	Brazil	Magellanic penguin	10	286
mcr-1.3	China	Poultry	155	246
mcr-1.8	Brunei	Poultry	101	KY683842.1[a]
mcr-1.9	Portugal	Pig		KY964067.1[a]
mcr-1.12	Japan	Pig		LC337668.1[a]
mcr-2	Belgium	Pig, cattle	10, 167	247
mcr-3	China	Pig	1642	249
	France	Cattle	744	251
mcr-3.2	Spain	Cattle	533	250
mcr-4	Spain, Belgium	Pig	10, 7029	252
mcr-5	Germany	Pig	29, 349	253
mcr-5.2	Germany	Pig	1494	253

[a]GenBank accession number.

of MCR-1-producing *E. coli* isolates recovered from poultry, with many of the isolates coproducing the carbapenemase NDM-1 (71). In addition, such multidrug-resistant isolates were recovered from flies and dogs present in the same farm environment, thus highlighting that those latter animals might also constitute sources of transmission (71). Additionally, some studies highlighted that *mcr-1*-positive *E. coli* may be also present in the environment or in food, being, for instance, identified in rivers but also in Asian imported vegetables in Switzerland (243). The environmental emission of MCR-1-producing and multiresistant *E. coli* isolates was recently stressed by studying the close surroundings of pig farms in Germany (256).

Dating the emergence of *mcr-1*-positive *E. coli* isolates remains difficult, although a Chinese study retrospectively identified *mcr-1*-positive isolates from chickens in the 1980s (255) and as early as 2005 in veal calves in France (254). It seems, therefore, that the emergence of *mcr*-positive isolates, at least in animals, is not a recent event. Very likely, there has been some silent dissemination of *mcr* genes through the past decades, and the current situation shows ongoing further dissemination rather than an emerging phenomenon.

CONCLUSIONS

Antimicrobial resistance in *E. coli* is an issue of the utmost importance since it occurs in both the human and animal sectors in a One Health perspective. In animals, multidrug resistance in *E. coli* may lead to difficult-to-treat infections, but even more importantly, it constitutes a major and shared reservoir of resistance determinants to most families of antimicrobial agents across a vast number of animal species, including humans. Even though the different transmission pathways of resistant *E. coli* isolates from animals to humans remain to be clarified and their relative importance quantified, some data may support the role of the food chain since those bacteria have been demonstrated as common colonizers of foodstuffs at retail in many countries and continents. Other routes of transmission may include direct contacts with animals or indirect transfers through the environment. Since *E. coli* is a bacterium that is widely spread in all sectors, antimicrobial resistance in *E. coli* in animals has led to numerous cross-sectorial and joint initiatives, encompassing translational research, epidemiology, and surveillance in both human and veterinary medicine. It is now considered that the battle against the increased occurrence of antimicrobial resistance in *E. coli* from humans cannot be won without acting on a very large scale. To tone down some

current and alarming speculations, and in view of all the studies that have been conducted during recent years, it is, however, likely that the occurrence of carbapenemase-producing *E. coli* in animals does not represent a significant threat for human health (31). In contrast, recent data have demonstrated that animals are very significant reservoirs of plasmid-mediated colistin resistance genes—mostly present in *E. coli* isolates—which may represent a further risk for humans.

Acknowledgments. This work was supported by the Swiss National Science Foundation (projects FNS-407240_177381 and 40AR40_173686) and by the University of Fribourg.

Citation. Poirel L, Madec J-Y, Lupo A, Schink A-K, Kieffer N, Nordmann P, and Schwarz S. 2018. Antimicrobial resistance in *Escherichia coli*. Microbiol Spectrum 6(1):ARBA-0026-2017.

References

1. **Kaper JB, Nataro JP, Mobley HL.** 2004. Pathogenic *Escherichia coli*. *Nat Rev Microbiol* 2:123–140.
2. **Köhler CD, Dobrindt U.** 2011. What defines extraintestinal pathogenic *Escherichia coli*? *Int J Med Microbiol* 301:642–647.
3. **Johnson JR, Russo TA.** 2005. Molecular epidemiology of extraintestinal pathogenic (uropathogenic) *Escherichia coli*. *Int J Med Microbiol* 295:383–404.
4. **Izzo MM, Kirkland PD, Mohler VL, Perkins NR, Gunn AA, House JK.** 2011. Prevalence of major enteric pathogens in Australian dairy calves with diarrhoea. *Aust Vet J* 89:167–173.
5. **Kolenda R, Burdukiewicz M, Schierack P.** 2015. A systematic review and meta-analysis of the epidemiology of pathogenic *Escherichia coli* of calves and the role of calves as reservoirs for human pathogenic *E. coli*. *Front Cell Infect Microbiol* 5:23.
6. **Bouillon J, Snead E, Caswell J, Feng C, Hélie P, Lemetayer J.** 2018. Pyelonephritis in dogs: retrospective study of 47 histologically diagnosed cases (2005–2015). *J Vet Intern Med* 32:249–259.
7. **Hutton TA, Innes GK, Harel J, Garneau P, Cucchiara A, Schifferli DM, Rankin SC.** 2018. Phylogroup and virulence gene association with clinical characteristics of *Escherichia coli* urinary tract infections from dogs and cats. *J Vet Diagn Invest* 30:64–70.
8. **Antão EM, Glodde S, Li G, Sharifi R, Homeier T, Laturnus C, Diehl I, Bethe A, Philipp HC, Preisinger R, Wieler LH, Ewers C.** 2008. The chicken as a natural model for extraintestinal infections caused by avian pathogenic *Escherichia coli* (APEC). *Microb Pathog* 45:361–369.
9. **Ruegg PL.** 2017. A 100-year review: mastitis detection, management, and prevention. *J Dairy Sci* 100:10381–10397.
10. **Taponen S, Liski E, Heikkilä AM, Pyörälä S.** 2017. Factors associated with intramammary infection in dairy cows caused by coagulase-negative staphylococci, *Staphylococcus aureus*, *Streptococcus uberis*, *Strepto-*

coccus dysgalactiae, Corynebacterium bovis, or *Escherichia coli. J Dairy Sci* **100:**493–503.

11. Shpigel NY, Elazar S, Rosenshine I. 2008. Mammary pathogenic *Escherichia coli. Curr Opin Microbiol* **11:**60–65.

12. Suojala L, Kaartinen L, Pyörälä S. 2013. Treatment for bovine *Escherichia coli* mastitis: an evidence-based approach. *J Vet Pharmacol Ther* **36:**521–531.

13. Dahmen S, Métayer V, Gay E, Madec JY, Haenni M. 2013. Characterization of extended-spectrum β-lactamase (ESBL)-carrying plasmids and clones of *Enterobacteriaceae* causing cattle mastitis in France. *Vet Microbiol* **162:**793–799.

14. Freitag C, Michael GB, Kadlec K, Hassel M, Schwarz S. 2017. Detection of plasmid-borne extended-spectrum β-lactamase (ESBL) genes in *Escherichia coli* isolates from bovine mastitis. *Vet Microbiol* **200:**151–156.

15. Su Y, Yu CY, Tsai Y, Wang SH, Lee C, Chu C. 2016. Fluoroquinolone-resistant and extended-spectrum β-lactamase-producing *Escherichia coli* from the milk of cows with clinical mastitis in southern Taiwan. *J Microbiol Immunol Infect* **49:**892–901.

16. Timofte D, Maciuca IE, Evans NJ, Williams H, Wattret A, Fick JC, Williams NJ. 2014. Detection and molecular characterization of *Escherichia coli* CTX-M-15 and *Klebsiella pneumoniae* SHV-12 β-lactamases from bovine mastitis isolates in the United Kingdom. *Antimicrob Agents Chemother* **58:**789–794.

17. Pempek JA, Holder E, Proudfoot KL, Masterson M, Habing G. 2018. Short communication: investigation of antibiotic alternatives to improve health and growth of veal calves. *J Dairy Sci* **101:**4473–4478.

18. Meganck V, Hoflack G, Opsomer G. 2014. Advances in prevention and therapy of neonatal dairy calf diarrhoea: a systematical review with emphasis on colostrum management and fluid therapy. *Acta Vet Scand* **56:**75.

19. Dierikx CM, van der Goot JA, Smith HE, Kant A, Mevius DJ. 2013. Presence of ESBL/AmpC-producing *Escherichia coli* in the broiler production pyramid: a descriptive study. *PLoS One* **8:**e79005.

20. Haenni M, Châtre P, Métayer V, Bour M, Signol E, Madec JY, Gay E. 2014. Comparative prevalence and characterization of ESBL-producing *Enterobacteriaceae* in dominant versus subdominant enteric flora in veal calves at slaughterhouse, France. *Vet Microbiol* **171:**321–327.

21. Hordijk J, Mevius DJ, Kant A, Bos ME, Graveland H, Bosman AB, Hartskeerl CM, Heederik DJ, Wagenaar JA. 2013. Within-farm dynamics of ESBL/AmpC-producing *Escherichia coli* in veal calves: a longitudinal approach. *J Antimicrob Chemother* **68:**2468–2476.

22. Ambler RP. 1980. The structure of β-lactamases. *Philos Trans R Soc Lond B Biol Sci* **289:**321–331.

23. Bush K, Jacoby GA. 2010. Updated functional classification of β-lactamases. *Antimicrob Agents Chemother* **54:**969–976.

24. Ewers C, Bethe A, Semmler T, Guenther S, Wieler LH. 2012. Extended-spectrum β-lactamase-producing and AmpC-producing *Escherichia coli* from livestock and companion animals, and their putative impact on public health: a global perspective. *Clin Microbiol Infect* **18:**646–655.

25. Madec JY, Haenni M, Nordmann P, Poirel L. 2017. Extended-spectrum β-lactamase/AmpC- and carbapenemase-producing *Enterobacteriaceae* in animals: a threat for humans? *Clin Microbiol Infect* **23:**826–833.

26. Hordijk J, Schoormans A, Kwakernaak M, Duim B, Broens E, Dierikx C, Mevius D, Wagenaar JA. 2013. High prevalence of fecal carriage of extended spectrum β-lactamase/AmpC-producing *Enterobacteriaceae* in cats and dogs. *Front Microbiol* **4:**242–247.

27. Lalak A, Wasyl D, Zając M, Skarżyńska M, Hoszowski A, Samcik I, Woźniakowski G, Szulowski K. 2016. Mechanisms of cephalosporin resistance in indicator *Escherichia coli* isolated from food animals. *Vet Microbiol* **194:**69–73.

28. Schaufler K, Bethe A, Lübke-Becker A, Ewers C, Kohn B, Wieler LH, Guenther S. 2015. Putative connection between zoonotic multiresistant extended-spectrum β-lactamase (ESBL)-producing *Escherichia coli* in dog feces from a veterinary campus and clinical isolates from dogs. *Infect Ecol Epidemiol* **5:**25334–25339.

29. Tian GB, Wang HN, Zhang AY, Zhang Y, Fan WQ, Xu CW, Zeng B, Guan ZB, Zou LK. 2012. Detection of clinically important β-lactamases in commensal *Escherichia coli* of human and swine origin in western China. *J Med Microbiol* **61:**233–238.

30. Guenther S, Ewers C, Wieler LH. 2011. Extended-spectrum β-lactamases producing *E. coli* in wildlife, yet another form of environmental pollution? *Front Microbiol* **2:**246–259.

31. Karim A, Poirel L, Nagarajan S, Nordmann P. 2001. Plasmid-mediated extended-spectrum β-lactamase (CTX-M-3 like) from India and gene association with insertion sequence IS*Ecp1*. *FEMS Microbiol Lett* **201:**237–241.

32. Pitout JD, Nordmann P, Laupland KB, Poirel L. 2005. Emergence of *Enterobacteriaceae* producing extended-spectrum β-lactamases (ESBLs) in the community. *J Antimicrob Chemother* **56:**52–59.

33. Michael GB, Freitag C, Wendlandt S, Eidam C, Feßler AT, Lopes GV, Kadlec K, Schwarz S. 2015. Emerging issues in antimicrobial resistance of bacteria from food-producing animals. *Future Microbiol* **10:**427–443.

34. EFSA. 2011. Panel on Biological Hazards (BIOHAZ); scientific opinion on the public health risks of bacterial strains producing extended-spectrum β-lactamases and/or AmpC β-lactamases in food and food-producing animals. *EFSA J* **9:**2322–2417.

35. Michael GB, Kaspar H, Siqueira AK, de Freitas Costa E, Corbellini LG, Kadlec K, Schwarz S. 2017. Extended-spectrum β-lactamase (ESBL)-producing *Escherichia coli* isolates collected from diseased food-producing animals in the GERM-Vet monitoring program 2008–2014. *Vet Microbiol* **200:**142–150.

36. Day MJ, Rodríguez I, van Essen-Zandbergen A, Dierikx C, Kadlec K, Schink AK, Wu G, Chattaway MA, DoNascimento V, Wain J, Helmuth R, Guerra B, Schwarz S, Threlfall J, Woodward MJ, Coldham N,

Mevius D, Woodford N. 2016. Diversity of STs, plasmids and ESBL genes among *Escherichia coli* from humans, animals and food in Germany, the Netherlands and the UK. *J Antimicrob Chemother* 71:1178–1182.

37. Schmiedel J, Falgenhauer L, Domann E, Bauerfeind R, Prenger-Berninghoff E, Imirzalioglu C, Chakraborty T. 2014. Multiresistant extended-spectrum β-lactamase-producing *Enterobacteriaceae* from humans, companion animals and horses in central Hesse, Germany. *BMC Microbiol* 14:187–200.

38. Shaheen BW, Nayak R, Foley SL, Kweon O, Deck J, Park M, Rafii F, Boothe DM. 2011. Molecular characterization of resistance to extended-spectrum cephalosporins in clinical *Escherichia coli* isolates from companion animals in the United States. *Antimicrob Agents Chemother* 55:5666–5675.

39. Alonso CA, Michael GB, Li J, Somalo S, Simón C, Wang Y, Kaspar H, Kadlec K, Torres C, Schwarz S. 2017. Analysis of *bla*SHV-12-carrying *Escherichia coli* clones and plasmids from human, animal and food sources. *J Antimicrob Chemother* 72:1589–1596.

40. Peirano G, Pitout JD. 2010. Molecular epidemiology of *Escherichia coli* producing CTX-M beta-lactamases: the worldwide emergence of clone ST131 O25:H4. *Int J Antimicrob Agents* 35:316–321.

41. Albrechtova K, Dolejska M, Cizek A, Tausova D, Klimes J, Bebora L, Literak I. 2012. Dogs of nomadic pastoralists in northern Kenya are reservoirs of plasmid-mediated cephalosporin- and quinolone-resistant *Escherichia coli*, including pandemic clone B2-O25-ST131. *Antimicrob Agents Chemother* 56:4013–4017.

42. Marques C, Belas A, Franco A, Aboim C, Gama LT, Pomba C. 2018. Increase in antimicrobial resistance and emergence of major international high-risk clonal lineages in dogs and cats with urinary tract infection: 16 year retrospective study. *J Antimicrob Chemother* 73:377–384.

43. Schink AK, Kadlec K, Kaspar H, Mankertz J, Schwarz S. 2013. Analysis of extended-spectrum-β-lactamase-producing *Escherichia coli* isolates collected in the GERM-Vet monitoring programme. *J Antimicrob Chemother* 68:1741–1749.

44. Wieler LH, Ewers C, Guenther S, Walther B, Lübke-Becker A. 2011. Methicillin-resistant staphylococci (MRS) and extended-spectrum β-lactamases (ESBL)-producing *Enterobacteriaceae* in companion animals: nosocomial infections as one reason for the rising prevalence of these potential zoonotic pathogens in clinical samples. *Int J Med Microbiol* 301:635–641.

45. Cantón R, González-Alba JM, Galán JC. 2012. CTX-M enzymes: origin and diffusion. *Front Microbiol* 3:110–129.

46. Poirel L, Naas T, Nordmann P. 2008. Genetic support of extended-spectrum β-lactamases. *Clin Microbiol Infect* 14(Suppl 1):75–81.

47. Carattoli A. 2013. Plasmids and the spread of resistance. *Int J Med Microbiol* 303:298–304.

48. Ferreira JC, Penha Filho RA, Andrade LN, Berchieri A Jr, Darini AL. 2014. Detection of chromosomal *bla*(CTX-M-2) in diverse *Escherichia coli* isolates

from healthy broiler chickens. *Clin Microbiol Infect* 20:O623–O626.

49. Guenther S, Semmler T, Stubbe A, Stubbe M, Wieler LH, Schaufler K. 2017. Chromosomally encoded ESBL genes in *Escherichia coli* of ST38 from Mongolian wild birds. *J Antimicrob Chemother* 72:1310–1313.

50. Valentin L, Sharp H, Hille K, Seibt U, Fischer J, Pfeifer Y, Michael GB, Nickel S, Schmiedel J, Falgenhauer L, Friese A, Bauerfeind R, Roesler U, Imirzalioglu C, Chakraborty T, Helmuth R, Valenza G, Werner G, Schwarz S, Guerra B, Appel B, Kreienbrock L, Käsbohrer A. 2014. Subgrouping of ESBL-producing *Escherichia coli* from animal and human sources: an approach to quantify the distribution of ESBL types between different reservoirs. *Int J Med Microbiol* 304:805–816.

51. Wu G, Day MJ, Mafura MT, Nunez-Garcia J, Fenner JJ, Sharma M, van Essen-Zandbergen A, Rodríguez I, Dierikx C, Kadlec K, Schink AK, Chattaway M, Wain J, Helmuth R, Guerra B, Schwarz S, Threlfall J, Woodward MJ, Woodford N, Coldham N, Mevius D. 2013. Comparative analysis of ESBL-positive *Escherichia coli* isolates from animals and humans from the UK, The Netherlands and Germany. *PLoS One* 8:e75392–e75402.

52. Leverstein-van Hall MA, Dierikx CM, Cohen Stuart J, Voets GM, van den Munckhof MP, van Essen-Zandbergen A, Platteel T, Fluit AC, van de Sande-Bruinsma N, Scharinga J, Bonten MJ, Mevius DJ, National ESBL Surveillance Group. 2011. Dutch patients, retail chicken meat and poultry share the same ESBL genes, plasmids and strains. *Clin Microbiol Infect* 17:873–880.

53. Casella T, Nogueira MCL, Saras E, Haenni M, Madec JY. 2017. High prevalence of ESBLs in retail chicken meat despite reduced use of antimicrobials in chicken production, France. *Int J Food Microbiol* 257:271–275.

54. Jacoby GA. 2009. AmpC β-lactamases. *Clin Microbiol Rev* 22:161–182.

55. Philippon A, Arlet G, Jacoby GA. 2002. Plasmid-determined AmpC-type β-lactamases. *Antimicrob Agents Chemother* 46:1–11.

56. Liebana E, Carattoli A, Coque TM, Hasman H, Magiorakos AP, Mevius D, Peixe L, Poirel L, Schuepbach-Regula G, Torneke K, Torren-Edo J, Torres C, Threlfall J. 2013. Public health risks of enterobacterial isolates producing extended-spectrum β-lactamases or AmpC β-lactamases in food and food-producing animals: an EU perspective of epidemiology, analytical methods, risk factors, and control options. *Clin Infect Dis* 56:1030–1037.

57. Hansen KH, Bortolaia V, Nielsen CA, Nielsen JB, Schønning K, Agersø Y, Guardabassi L. 2016. Host-specific patterns of genetic diversity among IncI1-Igamma and IncK plasmids encoding CMY-2 β-lactamase in *Escherichia coli* isolates from humans, poultry meat, poultry, and dogs in Denmark. *Appl Environ Microbiol* 82:4705–4714.

58. Börjesson S, Ny S, Egervärn M, Bergström J, Rosengren Å, Englund S, Löfmark S, Byfors S. 2016. Limited dissemination of extended-spectrum β-lactamase- and plasmid-encoded AmpC-producing *Escherichia coli*

from food and farm animals, Sweden. *Emerg Infect Dis* 22:634–640.

59. Nilsson O, Börjesson S, Landén A, Bengtsson B. 2014. Vertical transmission of *Escherichia coli* carrying plasmid-mediated AmpC (pAmpC) through the broiler production pyramid. *J Antimicrob Chemother* 69: 1497–1500.

60. Loncaric I, Stalder GL, Mehinagic K, Rosengarten R, Hoelzl F, Knauer F, Walzer C. 2013. Comparison of ESBL–and AmpC producing *Enterobacteriaceae* and methicillin-resistant *Staphylococcus aureus* (MRSA) isolated from migratory and resident population of rooks (*Corvus frugilegus*) in Austria. *PLoS One* 8:e84048.

61. Poirel L, Potron A, De La Cuesta C, Cleary T, Nordmann P, Munoz-Price LS. 2012. Wild coastline birds as reservoirs of broad-spectrum-β-lactamase-producing *Enterobacteriaceae* in Miami Beach, Florida. *Antimicrob Agents Chemother* 56:2756–2758.

62. Báez J, Hernández-García M, Guamparito C, Díaz S, Olave A, Guerrero K, Cantón R, Baquero F, Gahona J, Valenzuela N, Del Campo R, Silva J. 2015. Molecular characterization and genetic diversity of ESBL-producing *Escherichia coli* colonizing the migratory Franklin's gulls (*Leucophaeus pipixcan*) in Antofagasta, North of Chile. *Microb Drug Resist* 21:111–116.

63. Simões RR, Poirel L, Da Costa PM, Nordmann P. 2010. Seagulls and beaches as reservoirs for multidrug-resistant *Escherichia coli*. *Emerg Infect Dis* 16:110–112.

64. Köck R, Daniels-Haardt I, Becker K, Mellmann A, Friedrich AW, Mevius D, Schwarz S, Jurke A. 2018. Carbapenem-resistant *Enterobacteriaceae* in wildlife, food-producing, and companion animals: a systematic review. *Clin Microbiol Infect*. Epub ahead of print.

65. Poirel L, Stephan R, Perreten V, Nordmann P. 2014. The carbapenemase threat in the animal world: the wrong culprit. *J Antimicrob Chemother* 69:2007–2008.

66. Woodford N, Wareham DW, Guerra B, Teale C. 2014. Carbapenemase-producing *Enterobacteriaceae* and non-*Enterobacteriaceae* from animals and the environment: an emerging public health risk of our own making? *J Antimicrob Chemother* 69:287–291.

67. Fischer J, San José M, Roschanski N, Schmoger S, Baumann B, Irrgang A, Friese A, Roesler U, Helmuth R, Guerra B. 2017. Spread and persistence of VIM-1 carbapenemase-producing *Enterobacteriaceae* in three German swine farms in 2011 and 2012. *Vet Microbiol* 200:118–123.

68. Fischer J, Rodríguez I, Schmoger S, Friese A, Roesler U, Helmuth R, Guerra B. 2012. *Escherichia coli* producing VIM-1 carbapenemase isolated on a pig farm. *J Antimicrob Chemother* 67:1793–1795.

69. Guerra B, Fischer J, Helmuth R. 2014. An emerging public health problem: acquired carbapenemase-producing microorganisms are present in food-producing animals, their environment, companion animals and wild birds. *Vet Microbiol* 171:290–297.

70. Shaheen BW, Nayak R, Boothe DM. 2013. Emergence of a New Delhi metallo-β-lactamase (NDM-1)-encoding gene in clinical *Escherichia coli* isolates recovered from companion animals in the United States. *Antimicrob Agents Chemother* 57:2902–2903.

71. Wang Y, Zhang R, Li J, Wu Z, Yin W, Schwarz S, Tyrrell JM, Zheng Y, Wang S, Shen Z, Liu Z, Liu J, Lei L, Li M, Zhang Q, Wu C, Zhang Q, Wu Y, Walsh TR, Shen J. 2017. Comprehensive resistome analysis reveals the prevalence of NDM and MCR-1 in Chinese poultry production. *Nat Microbiol* 2:16260.

72. Liu Z, Wang Y, Walsh TR, Liu D, Shen Z, Zhang R, Yin W, Yao H, Li J, Shen J. 2017. Plasmid-mediated novel bla_{NDM-17} gene encoding a carbapenemase with enhanced activity in a sequence type 48 *Escherichia coli* strain. *Antimicrob Agents Chemother* 61:e02233-16.

73. Singh AS, Lekshmi M, Nayak BB, Kumar SH. 2016. Isolation of *Escherichia coli* harboring bla_{NDM-5} from fresh fish in India. *J Microbiol Immunol Infect* 49: 822–823.

74. Yang RS, Feng Y, Lv XY, Duan JH, Chen J, Fang LX, Xia J, Liao XP, Sun J, Liu YH. 2016. Emergence of NDM-5- and MCR-1-producing *Escherichia coli* clones ST648 and ST156 from a single Muscovy duck (*Cairina moschata*). *Antimicrob Agents Chemother* 60:6899–6902.

75. Yousfi M, Touati A, Mairi A, Brasme L, Gharout-Sait A, Guillard T, De Champs C. 2016. Emergence of carbapenemase-producing *Escherichia coli* isolated from companion animals in Algeria. *Microb Drug Resist* 22:342–346.

76. Dolejska M, Masarikova M, Dobiasova H, Jamborova I, Karpiskova R, Havlicek M, Carlile N, Priddel D, Cizek A, Literak I. 2016. High prevalence of *Salmonella* and IMP-4-producing *Enterobacteriaceae* in the silver gull on Five Islands, Australia. *J Antimicrob Chemother* 71:63–70.

77. Al Bayssari C, Olaitan AO, Dabboussi F, Hamze M, Rolain JM. 2015. Emergence of OXA-48-producing *Escherichia coli* clone ST38 in fowl. *Antimicrob Agents Chemother* 59:745–746.

78. Melo LC, Boisson MN, Saras E, Médaille C, Boulouis HJ, Madec JY, Haenni M. 2017. OXA-48-producing ST372 *Escherichia coli* in a French dog. *J Antimicrob Chemother* 72:1256–1258.

79. Stolle I, Prenger-Berninghoff E, Stamm I, Scheufen S, Hassdenteufel E, Guenther S, Bethe A, Pfeifer Y, Ewers C. 2013. Emergence of OXA-48 carbapenemase-producing *Escherichia coli* and *Klebsiella pneumoniae* in dogs. *J Antimicrob Chemother* 68:2802–2808.

80. Pulss S, Semmler T, Prenger-Berninghoff E, Bauerfeind R, Ewers C. 2017. First report of an *Escherichia coli* strain from swine carrying an OXA-181 carbapenemase and the colistin resistance determinant MCR-1. *Int J Antimicrob Agents* 50:232–236.

81. Mollenkopf DF, Stull JW, Mathys DA, Bowman AS, Feicht SM, Grooters SV, Daniels JB, Wittum TE. 2017. Carbapenemase-producing *Enterobacteriaceae* recovered from the environment of a swine farrow-to-finish operation in the United States. *Antimicrob Agents Chemother* 61:e01298-16.

82. Munoz-Price LS, Poirel L, Bonomo RA, Schwaber MJ, Daikos GL, Cormican M, Cornaglia G, Garau J,

Gniadkowski M, Hayden MK, Kumarasamy K, Livermore DM, Maya JJ, Nordmann P, Patel JB, Paterson DL, Pitout J, Villegas MV, Wang H, Woodford N, Quinn JP. 2013. Clinical epidemiology of the global expansion of *Klebsiella pneumoniae* carbapenemases. *Lancet Infect Dis* 13:785–796.

83. Hopkins KL, Davies RH, Threlfall EJ. 2005. Mechanisms of quinolone resistance in *Escherichia coli* and *Salmonella*: recent developments. *Int J Antimicrob Agents* 25:358–373.

84. de Jong A, Muggeo A, El Garch F, Moyaert H, de Champs C, Guillard T. 2018. Characterization of quinolone resistance mechanisms in *Enterobacteriaceae* isolated from companion animals in Europe (ComPath II study). *Vet Microbiol* 216:159–167.

85. Schink AK, Kadlec K, Hauschild T, Brenner Michael G, Dörner JC, Ludwig C, Werckenthin C, Hehnen HR, Stephan B, Schwarz S. 2013. Susceptibility of canine and feline bacterial pathogens to pradofloxacin and comparison with other fluoroquinolones approved for companion animals. *Vet Microbiol* 162:119–126.

86. Liu BT, Liao XP, Yang SS, Wang XM, Li LL, Sun J, Yang YR, Fang LX, Li L, Zhao DH, Liu YH. 2012. Detection of mutations in the *gyrA* and *parC* genes in *Escherichia coli* isolates carrying plasmid-mediated quinolone resistance genes from diseased food-producing animals. *J Med Microbiol* 61:1591–1599.

87. Redgrave LS, Sutton SB, Webber MA, Piddock LJ. 2014. Fluoroquinolone resistance: mechanisms, impact on bacteria, and role in evolutionary success. *Trends Microbiol* 22:438–445.

88. Cattoir V, Nordmann P. 2009. Plasmid-mediated quinolone resistance in Gram-negative bacterial species: an update. *Curr Med Chem* 16:1028–1046.

89. Rodríguez-Martínez JM, Machuca J, Cano ME, Calvo J, Martínez-Martínez L, Pascual A. 2016. Plasmid-mediated quinolone resistance: two decades on. *Drug Resist Updat* 29:13–29.

90. Ma J, Zeng Z, Chen Z, Xu X, Wang X, Deng Y, Lü D, Huang L, Zhang Y, Liu J, Wang M. 2009. High prevalence of plasmid-mediated quinolone resistance determinants *qnr*, *aac(6′)-Ib-cr*, and *qepA* among ceftiofur-resistant *Enterobacteriaceae* isolates from companion and food-producing animals. *Antimicrob Agents Chemother* 53:519–524.

91. Huang SY, Dai L, Xia LN, Du XD, Qi YH, Liu HB, Wu CM, Shen JZ. 2009. Increased prevalence of plasmid-mediated quinolone resistance determinants in chicken *Escherichia coli* isolates from 2001 to 2007. *Foodborne Pathog Dis* 6:1203–1209.

92. Veldman K, Cavaco LM, Mevius D, Battisti A, Franco A, Botteldoorn N, Bruneau M, Perrin-Guyomard A, Cerny T, De Frutos Escobar C, Guerra B, Schroeter A, Gutierrez M, Hopkins K, Myllyniemi AL, Sunde M, Wasyl D, Aarestrup FM. 2011. International collaborative study on the occurrence of plasmid-mediated quinolone resistance in *Salmonella enterica* and *Escherichia coli* isolated from animals, humans, food and the environment in 13 European countries. *J Antimicrob Chemother* 66:1278–1286.

93. Dolejska M, Duskova E, Rybarikova J, Janoszowska D, Roubalova E, Dibdakova K, Maceckova G, Kohoutova L, Literak I, Smola J, Cizek A. 2011. Plasmids carrying *bla*CTX-M-1 and *qnr* genes in *Escherichia coli* isolates from an equine clinic and a horseback riding centre. *J Antimicrob Chemother* 66:757–764.

94. Schink AK, Kadlec K, Schwarz S. 2012. Detection of *qnr* genes among *Escherichia coli* isolates of animal origin and complete sequence of the conjugative *qnrB19*-carrying plasmid pQNR2078. *J Antimicrob Chemother* 67:1099–1102.

95. Hordijk J, Bosman AB, van Essen-Zandbergen A, Veldman K, Dierikx C, Wagenaar JA, Mevius D. 2011. *qnrB19* gene bracketed by IS26 on a 40-kilobase IncR plasmid from an *Escherichia coli* isolate from a veal calf. *Antimicrob Agents Chemother* 55:453–454.

96. Ewers C, Bethe A, Stamm I, Grobbel M, Kopp PA, Guerra B, Stubbe M, Doi Y, Zong Z, Kola A, Schaufler K, Semmler T, Fruth A, Wieler LH, Guenther S. 2014. CTX-M-15-D-ST648 *Escherichia coli* from companion animals and horses: another pandemic clone combining multiresistance and extraintestinal virulence? *J Antimicrob Chemother* 69:1224–1230.

97. Liu X, Liu H, Li Y, Hao C. 2016. High prevalence of β-lactamase and plasmid-mediated quinolone resistance genes in extended-spectrum cephalosporin-resistant *Escherichia coli* from dogs in Shaanxi, China. *Front Microbiol* 7:1843–1852.

98. Pomba C, da Fonseca JD, Baptista BC, Correia JD, Martínez-Martínez L. 2009. Detection of the pandemic O25-ST131 human virulent *Escherichia coli* CTX-M-15-producing clone harboring the *qnrB2* and *aac(6′)-Ib-cr* genes in a dog. *Antimicrob Agents Chemother* 53:327–328.

99. Timofte D, Maciuca IE, Williams NJ, Wattret A, Schmidt V. 2016. Veterinary hospital dissemination of CTX-M-15 extended-spectrum β-lactamase-producing *Escherichia coli* ST410 in the United Kingdom. *Microb Drug Resist* 22:609–615.

100. Madec JY, Poirel L, Saras E, Gourguechon A, Girlich D, Nordmann P, Haenni M. 2012. Non-ST131 *Escherichia coli* from cattle harbouring human-like *bla*(CTX-M-15)-carrying plasmids. *J Antimicrob Chemother* 67:578–581.

101. Chen X, He L, Li Y, Zeng Z, Deng Y, Liu Y, Liu JH. 2014. Complete sequence of a F2:A-:B- plasmid pHN3A11 carrying *rmtB* and *qepA*, and its dissemination in China. *Vet Microbiol* 174:267–271.

102. Liu BT, Yang QE, Li L, Sun J, Liao XP, Fang LX, Yang SS, Deng H, Liu YH. 2013. Dissemination and characterization of plasmids carrying *oqxAB-bla*CTX-M genes in *Escherichia coli* isolates from food-producing animals. *PLoS One* 8:e73947.

103. Hansen LH, Jensen LB, Sørensen HI, Sørensen SJ. 2007. Substrate specificity of the OqxAB multidrug resistance pump in *Escherichia coli* and selected enteric bacteria. *J Antimicrob Chemother* 60:145–147.

104. Davies J, Wright GD. 1997. Bacterial resistance to aminoglycoside antibiotics. *Trends Microbiol* 5:234–240.

105. Doi Y, Wachino JI, Arakawa Y. 2016. Aminoglycoside resistance: the emergence of acquired 16S ribosomal RNA methyltransferases. *Infect Dis Clin North Am* 30: 523–537.

106. Anonymous. 2014. Concept paper on the of aminoglycosides in animals in the European Union: development of resistance and impact on human and animal health. EMA/CVMP/AWP/158821/2014 1-4.

107. Fourmy D, Yoshizawa S, Puglisi JD. 1998. Paromomycin binding induces a local conformational change in the A-site of 16 S rRNA. *J Mol Biol* 277:333–345.

108. Bowers DR SAN, Tam VH. 2016. Aminoglycoside pharmacodynamics, p 199–220. *In* Rotschafer J, Andes D, Rodvold K (ed), *Antibiotic Pharmacodynamics. Methods in Pharmacology and Toxicology.* Humana Press, New York, NY.

109. Griffey RH, Hofstadler SA, Sannes-Lowery KA, Ecker DJ, Crooke ST. 1999. Determinants of aminoglycoside-binding specificity for rRNA by using mass spectrometry. *Proc Natl Acad Sci USA* 96:10129–10133.

110. Llano-Sotelo B, Hickerson RP, Lancaster L, Noller HF, Mankin AS. 2009. Fluorescently labeled ribosomes as a tool for analyzing antibiotic binding. *RNA* 15:1597–1604.

111. Galimand M, Courvalin P, Lambert T. 2003. Plasmid-mediated high-level resistance to aminoglycosides in *Enterobacteriaceae* due to 16S rRNA methylation. *Antimicrob Agents Chemother* 47:2565–2571.

112. Batah R, Loucif L, Olaitan AO, Boutefnouchet N, Allag H, Rolain JM. 2015. Outbreak of *Serratia marcescens* coproducing ArmA and CTX-M-15 mediated high levels of resistance to aminoglycoside and extended-spectrum β-lactamases, Algeria. *Microb Drug Resist* 21: 470–476.

113. Dolejska M, Villa L, Poirel L, Nordmann P, Carattoli A. 2013. Complete sequencing of an IncHI1 plasmid encoding the carbapenemase NDM-1, the ArmA 16S RNA methylase and a resistance-nodulation-cell division/multidrug efflux pump. *J Antimicrob Chemother* 68: 34–39.

114. Gurung M, Moon DC, Tamang MD, Kim J, Lee YC, Seol SY, Cho DT, Lee JC. 2010. Emergence of 16S rRNA methylase gene *armA* and cocarriage of *bla*(IMP-1) in *Pseudomonas aeruginosa* isolates from South Korea. *Diagn Microbiol Infect Dis* 68:468–470.

115. Wachino J, Yamane K, Shibayama K, Kurokawa H, Shibata N, Suzuki S, Doi Y, Kimura K, Ike Y, Arakawa Y. 2006. Novel plasmid-mediated 16S rRNA methylase, RmtC, found in a *Proteus mirabilis* isolate demonstrating extraordinary high-level resistance against various aminoglycosides. *Antimicrob Agents Chemother* 50: 178–184.

116. Yu YS, Zhou H, Yang Q, Chen YG, Li LJ. 2007. Widespread occurrence of aminoglycoside resistance due to ArmA methylase in imipenem-resistant *Acinetobacter baumannii* isolates in China. *J Antimicrob Chemother* 60:454–455.

117. Galimand M, Sabtcheva S, Courvalin P, Lambert T. 2005. Worldwide disseminated *armA* aminoglycoside resistance methylase gene is borne by composite transposon Tn*1548*. *Antimicrob Agents Chemother* 49: 2949–2953.

118. González-Zorn B, Teshager T, Casas M, Porrero MC, Moreno MA, Courvalin P, Domínguez L. 2005. *armA* and aminoglycoside resistance in *Escherichia coli*. *Emerg Infect Dis* 11:954–956.

119. Chen L, Chen ZL, Liu JH, Zeng ZL, Ma JY, Jiang HX. 2007. Emergence of RmtB methylase-producing *Escherichia coli* and *Enterobacter cloacae* isolates from pigs in China. *J Antimicrob Chemother* 59:880–885.

120. Du XD, Wu CM, Liu HB, Li XS, Beier RC, Xiao F, Qin SS, Huang SY, Shen JZ. 2009. Plasmid-mediated ArmA and RmtB 16S rRNA methylases in *Escherichia coli* isolated from chickens. *J Antimicrob Chemother* 64:1328–1330.

121. Liu BT, Liao XP, Yue L, Chen XY, Li L, Yang SS, Sun J, Zhang S, Liao SD, Liu YH. 2013. Prevalence of β-lactamase and 16S rRNA methylase genes among clinical *Escherichia coli* isolates carrying plasmid-mediated quinolone resistance genes from animals. *Microb Drug Resist* 19:237–245.

122. Yu T, He T, Yao H, Zhang JB, Li XN, Zhang RM, Wang GQ. 2015. Prevalence of 16S rRNA methylase gene *rmtB* among *Escherichia coli* isolated from bovine mastitis in Ningxia, China. *Foodborne Pathog Dis* 12: 770–777.

123. Yang Y, Zhang A, Lei C, Wang H, Guan Z, Xu C, Liu B, Zhang D, Li Q, Jiang W, Pan Y, Yang C. 2015. Characteristics of plasmids coharboring 16S rRNA methylases, CTX-M, and virulence factors in *Escherichia coli* and *Klebsiella pneumoniae* isolates from chickens in China. *Foodborne Pathog Dis* 12:873–880.

124. Lupo A, Saras E, Madec JY, Haenni M. 2018. Emergence of *bla*CTX-M-55 associated with *fosA*, *rmtB* and *mcr* gene variants in *Escherichia coli* from various animal species in France. *J Antimicrob Chemother* 73:867–872.

125. Leigue L, Warth JF, Melo LC, Silva KC, Moura RA, Barbato L, Silva LC, Santos AC, Silva RM, Lincopan N. 2015. MDR ST2179-CTX-M-15 *Escherichia coli* co-producing RmtD and AAC(6′)-Ib-cr in a horse with extraintestinal infection, Brazil. *J Antimicrob Chemother* 70:1263–1265.

126. Lee CS, Hu F, Rivera JI, Doi Y. 2014. *Escherichia coli* sequence type 354 coproducing CMY-2 cephalosporinase and RmtE 16S rRNA methyltransferase. *Antimicrob Agents Chemother* 58:4246–4247.

127. Xia J, Sun J, Li L, Fang LX, Deng H, Yang RS, Li XP, Liao XP, Liu YH. 2015. First report of the IncI1/ST898 conjugative plasmid carrying *rmtE2* 16S rRNA methyltransferase gene in *Escherichia coli*. *Antimicrob Agents Chemother* 59:7921–7922.

128. Zou W, Li C, Yang X, Wang Y, Cheng G, Zeng J, Zhang X, Chen Y, Cai R, Huang Q, Feng L, Wang H, Li D, Zhang G, Chen Y, Zhang Z, Zhang H. 2018. Frequency of antimicrobial resistance and integron gene cassettes in *Escherichia coli* isolated from giant pandas (*Ailuropoda melanoleuca*) in China. *Microb Pathog* 116:173–179.

129. Gutierrez B, Escudero JA, San Millan A, Hidalgo L, Carrilero L, Ovejero CM, Santos-Lopez A, Thomas-Lopez D, Gonzalez-Zorn B. 2012. Fitness cost and interference of Arm/Rmt aminoglycoside resistance with the RsmF housekeeping methyltransferases. *Antimicrob Agents Chemother* 56:2335–2341.

130. Lioy VS, Goussard S, Guerineau V, Yoon EJ, Courvalin P, Galimand M, Grillot-Courvalin C. 2014. Aminoglycoside resistance 16S rRNA methyltransferases block endogenous methylation, affect translation efficiency and fitness of the host. *RNA* 20:382–391.

131. Ramirez MS, Tolmasky ME. 2010. Aminoglycoside modifying enzymes. *Drug Resist Updat* 13:151–171.

132. Choi MJ, Lim SK, Nam HM, Kim AR, Jung SC, Kim MN. 2011. Apramycin and gentamicin resistances in indicator and clinical *Escherichia coli* isolates from farm animals in Korea. *Foodborne Pathog Dis* 8:119–123.

133. Costa D, Poeta P, Sáenz Y, Vinué L, Coelho AC, Matos M, Rojo-Bezares B, Rodrigues J, Torres C. 2008. Mechanisms of antibiotic resistance in *Escherichia coli* isolates recovered from wild animals. *Microb Drug Resist* 14:71–77.

134. Haldorsen BC, Simonsen GS, Sundsfjord A, Samuelsen O, Norwegian Study Group on Aminoglycoside Resistance. 2014. Increased prevalence of aminoglycoside resistance in clinical isolates of *Escherichia coli* and *Klebsiella* spp. in Norway is associated with the acquisition of AAC(3)-II and AAC(6′)-Ib. *Diagn Microbiol Infect Dis* 78:66–69.

135. Medina A, Horcajo P, Jurado S, De la Fuente R, Ruiz-Santa-Quiteria JA, Domínguez-Bernal G, Orden JA. 2011. Phenotypic and genotypic characterization of antimicrobial resistance in enterohemorrhagic *Escherichia coli* and atypical enteropathogenic *E. coli* strains from ruminants. *J Vet Diagn Invest* 23:91–95.

136. Radhouani H, Poeta P, Gonçalves A, Pacheco R, Sargo R, Igrejas G. 2012. Wild birds as biological indicators of environmental pollution: antimicrobial resistance patterns of *Escherichia coli* and enterococci isolated from common buzzards (*Buteo buteo*). *J Med Microbiol* 61:837–843.

137. Radhouani H, Poeta P, Igrejas G, Gonçalves A, Vinué L, Torres C. 2009. Antimicrobial resistance and phylogenetic groups in isolates of *Escherichia coli* from seagulls at the Berlengas nature reserve. *Vet Rec* 165:138–142.

138. Rocha-Gracia RC, Cortés-Cortés G, Lozano-Zarain P, Bello F, Martínez-Laguna Y, Torres C. 2015. Faecal *Escherichia coli* isolates from healthy dogs harbour CTX-M-15 and CMY-2 β-lactamases. *Vet J* 203:315–319.

139. Silva N, Igrejas G, Figueiredo N, Gonçalves A, Radhouani H, Rodrigues J, Poeta P. 2010. Molecular characterization of antimicrobial resistance in enterococci and *Escherichia coli* isolates from European wild rabbit (*Oryctolagus cuniculus*). *Sci Total Environ* 408:4871–4876.

140. Xiao Y, Hu Y. 2012. The major aminoglycoside-modifying enzyme AAC(3)-II found in *Escherichia coli* determines a significant disparity in its resistance to gentamicin and amikacin in China. *Microb Drug Resist* 18:42–46.

141. Allen SE, Boerlin P, Janecko N, Lumsden JS, Barker IK, Pearl DL, Reid-Smith RJ, Jardine C. 2011. Antimicrobial resistance in generic *Escherichia coli* isolates from wild small mammals living in swine farm, residential, landfill, and natural environments in southern Ontario, Canada. *Appl Environ Microbiol* 77:882–888.

142. Gonçalves A, Igrejas G, Radhouani H, Correia S, Pacheco R, Santos T, Monteiro R, Guerra A, Petrucci-Fonseca F, Brito F, Torres C, Poeta P. 2013. Antimicrobial resistance in faecal enterococci and *Escherichia coli* isolates recovered from Iberian wolf. *Lett Appl Microbiol* 56:268–274.

143. Gonçalves A, Igrejas G, Radhouani H, Santos T, Monteiro R, Pacheco R, Alcaide E, Zorrilla I, Serra R, Torres C, Poeta P. 2013. Detection of antibiotic resistant enterococci and *Escherichia coli* in free range Iberian Lynx (*Lynx pardinus*). *Sci Total Environ* 456-457:115–119.

144. Marchant M, Vinué L, Torres C, Moreno MA. 2013. Change of integrons over time in *Escherichia coli* isolates recovered from healthy pigs and chickens. *Vet Microbiol* 163:124–132.

145. Marinho C, Igrejas G, Gonçalves A, Silva N, Santos T, Monteiro R, Gonçalves D, Rodrigues T, Poeta P. 2014. Azorean wild rabbits as reservoirs of antimicrobial resistant *Escherichia coli*. *Anaerobe* 30:116–119.

146. Radhouani H, Igrejas G, Gonçalves A, Pacheco R, Monteiro R, Sargo R, Brito F, Torres C, Poeta P. 2013. Antimicrobial resistance and virulence genes in *Escherichia coli* and enterococci from red foxes (*Vulpes vulpes*). *Anaerobe* 23:82–86.

147. Sacristán C, Esperón F, Herrera-León S, Iglesias I, Neves E, Nogal V, Muñoz MJ, de la Torre A. 2014. Virulence genes, antibiotic resistance and integrons in *Escherichia coli* strains isolated from synanthropic birds from Spain. *Avian Pathol* 43:172–175.

148. Santos T, Silva N, Igrejas G, Rodrigues P, Micael J, Rodrigues T, Resendes R, Gonçalves A, Marinho C, Gonçalves D, Cunha R, Poeta P. 2013. Dissemination of antibiotic resistant *Enterococcus* spp. and *Escherichia coli* from wild birds of Azores Archipelago. *Anaerobe* 24:25–31.

149. Karczmarczyk M, Abbott Y, Walsh C, Leonard N, Fanning S. 2011. Characterization of multidrug-resistant *Escherichia coli* isolates from animals presenting at a university veterinary hospital. *Appl Environ Microbiol* 77:7104–7112.

150. Shin SW, Byun JW, Jung M, Shin MK, Yoo HS. 2014. Antimicrobial resistance, virulence genes and PFGE-profiling of *Escherichia coli* isolates from South Korean cattle farms. *J Microbiol* 52:785–793.

151. Toszeghy M, Phillips N, Reeves H, Wu G, Teale C, Coldham N, Randall L. 2012. Molecular and phenotypic characterisation of extended spectrum β-lactamase CTX-M *Escherichia coli* from farm animals in Great Britain. *Res Vet Sci* 93:1142–1150.

152. Yamamoto S, Iwabuchi E, Hasegawa M, Esaki H, Muramatsu M, Hirayama N, Hirai K. 2013. Prevalence

and molecular epidemiological characterization of antimicrobial-resistant *Escherichia coli* isolates from Japanese black beef cattle. *J Food Prot* 76:394–404.

153. Adelowo OO, Fagade OE, Agersø Y. 2014. Antibiotic resistance and resistance genes in *Escherichia coli* from poultry farms, southwest Nigeria. *J Infect Dev Ctries* 8: 1103–1112.

154. Zhang FY, Huo SY, Li YR, Xie R, Wu XJ, Chen LG, Gao YH. 2014. A survey of the frequency of aminoglycoside antibiotic-resistant genotypes and phenotypes in *Escherichia coli* in broilers with septicaemia in Hebei, China. *Br Poult Sci* 55:305–310.

155. Gonçalves A, Torres C, Silva N, Carneiro C, Radhouani H, Coelho C, Araújo C, Rodrigues J, Vinué L, Somalo S, Poeta P, Igrejas G. 2010. Genetic characterization of extended-spectrum β-lactamases in *Escherichia coli* isolates of pigs from a Portuguese intensive swine farm. *Foodborne Pathog Dis* 7:1569–1573.

156. Tang X, Tan C, Zhang X, Zhao Z, Xia X, Wu B, Guo A, Zhou R, Chen H. 2011. Antimicrobial resistances of extraintestinal pathogenic *Escherichia coli* isolates from swine in China. *Microb Pathog* 50:207–212.

157. Zhang WJ, Xu XR, Schwarz S, Wang XM, Dai L, Zheng HJ, Liu S. 2014. Characterization of the IncA/C plasmid pSCEC2 from *Escherichia coli* of swine origin that harbours the multiresistance gene *cfr*. *J Antimicrob Chemother* 69:385–389.

158. Falagas ME, Vouloumanou EK, Samonis G, Vardakas KZ. 2016. Fosfomycin. *Clin Microbiol Rev* 29:321–347.

159. Pérez DS, Tapia MO, Soraci AL. 2014. Fosfomycin: uses and potentialities in veterinary medicine. *Open Vet J* 4:26–43.

160. Silver LL. 2017. Fosfomycin: mechanism and resistance. *Cold Spring Harb Perspect Med* 7:7.

161. Wang X, Zhu Y, Hua X, Chen F, Wang C, Zhang Y, Liu S, Zhang W. 2018. F14:A-:B- and IncX4 Inc group *cfr*-positive plasmids circulating in *Escherichia coli* of animal origin in Northeast China. *Vet Microbiol* 217: 53–57.

162. Wang XM, Dong Z, Schwarz S, Zhu Y, Hua X, Zhang Y, Liu S, Zhang WJ. 2017. Plasmids of diverse Inc groups disseminate the fosfomycin resistance gene *fosA3* among *Escherichia coli* isolates from pigs, chickens, and dairy cows in Northeast China. *Antimicrob Agents Chemother* 61:e00859–e00817.

163. Hou J, Huang X, Deng Y, He L, Yang T, Zeng Z, Chen Z, Liu JH. 2012. Dissemination of the fosfomycin resistance gene *fosA3* with CTX-M β-lactamase genes and *rmtB* carried on IncFII plasmids among *Escherichia coli* isolates from pets in China. *Antimicrob Agents Chemother* 56:2135–2138.

164. Yao H, Wu D, Lei L, Shen Z, Wang Y, Liao K. 2016. The detection of fosfomycin resistance genes in *Enterobacteriaceae* from pets and their owners. *Vet Microbiol* 193:67–71.

165. Xie M, Lin D, Chen K, Chan EW, Yao W, Chen S. 2016. Molecular characterization of *Escherichia coli* strains isolated from retail meat that harbor *bla*CTX-M

and *fosA3* genes. *Antimicrob Agents Chemother* 60: 2450–2455.

166. He L, Partridge SR, Yang X, Hou J, Deng Y, Yao Q, Zeng Z, Chen Z, Liu JH. 2013. Complete nucleotide sequence of pHN7A8, an F33:A-:B-type epidemic plasmid carrying *bla*CTX-M-65, *fosA3* and *rmtB* from China. *J Antimicrob Chemother* 68:46–50.

167. Ho PL, Chan J, Lo WU, Law PY, Chow KH. 2013. Plasmid-mediated fosfomycin resistance in *Escherichia coli* isolated from pig. *Vet Microbiol* 162:964–967.

168. Sun H, Li S, Xie Z, Yang F, Sun Y, Zhu Y, Zhao X, Jiang S. 2012. A novel multidrug resistance plasmid isolated from an *Escherichia coli* strain resistant to aminoglycosides. *J Antimicrob Chemother* 67:1635–1638.

169. Pan YS, Yuan L, Zong ZY, Liu JH, Wang LF, Hu GZ. 2014. A multidrug-resistance region containing *bla*CTX-M-65, *fosA3* and *rmtB* on conjugative IncFII plasmids in *Escherichia coli* ST117 isolates from chicken. *J Med Microbiol* 63:485–488.

170. Hou J, Yang X, Zeng Z, Lv L, Yang T, Lin D, Liu JH. 2013. Detection of the plasmid-encoded fosfomycin resistance gene *fosA3* in *Escherichia coli* of food-animal origin. *J Antimicrob Chemother* 68:766–770.

171. Ho PL, Chan J, Lo WU, Law PY, Li Z, Lai EL, Chow KH. 2013. Dissemination of plasmid-mediated fosfomycin resistance *fosA3* among multidrug-resistant *Escherichia coli* from livestock and other animals. *J Appl Microbiol* 114:695–702.

172. Tseng SP, Wang SF, Kuo CY, Huang JW, Hung WC, Ke GM, Lu PL. 2015. Characterization of fosfomycin resistant extended-spectrum β-lactamase-producing *Escherichia coli* isolates from human and pig in Taiwan. *PLoS One* 10:e0135864.

173. Grave K, Torren-Edo J, Muller A, Greko C, Moulin G, Mackay D, Group E, ESVAC Group. 2014. Variations in the sales and sales patterns of veterinary antimicrobial agents in 25 European countries. *J Antimicrob Chemother* 69:2284–2291.

174. Shin SW, Shin MK, Jung M, Belaynehe KM, Yoo HS. 2015. Prevalence of antimicrobial resistance and transfer of tetracycline resistance genes in *Escherichia coli* isolates from beef cattle. *Appl Environ Microbiol* 81: 5560–5566.

175. Metzger SA, Hogan JS. 2013. Short communication: antimicrobial susceptibility and frequency of resistance genes in *Escherichia coli* isolated from bovine mastitis. *J Dairy Sci* 96:3044–3049.

176. Srinivasan V, Gillespie BE, Lewis MJ, Nguyen LT, Headrick SI, Schukken YH, Oliver SP. 2007. Phenotypic and genotypic antimicrobial resistance patterns of *Escherichia coli* isolated from dairy cows with mastitis. *Vet Microbiol* 124:319–328.

177. Lanz R, Kuhnert P, Boerlin P. 2003. Antimicrobial resistance and resistance gene determinants in clinical *Escherichia coli* from different animal species in Switzerland. *Vet Microbiol* 91:73–84.

178. Jurado-Rabadán S, de la Fuente R, Ruiz-Santa-Quiteria JA, Orden JA, de Vries LE, Agersø Y. 2014. Detection and linkage to mobile genetic elements of tetracycline

resistance gene *tet*(M) in *Escherichia coli* isolates from pigs. *BMC Vet Res* 10:155–162.

179. Hölzel CS, Harms KS, Bauer J, Bauer-Unkauf I, Hörmansdorfer S, Kämpf P, Mölle G, Oehme C, Preikschat P, Schwaiger K. 2012. Diversity of antimicrobial resistance genes and class-1-integrons in phylogenetically related porcine and human *Escherichia coli*. *Vet Microbiol* 160:403–412.

180. Seifi S, Khoshbakht R. 2016. Prevalence of tetracycline resistance determinants in broiler isolated *Escherichia coli* in Iran. *Br Poult Sci* 57:729–733.

181. Costa D, Poeta P, Sáenz Y, Coelho AC, Matos M, Vinué L, Rodrigues J, Torres C. 2008. Prevalence of antimicrobial resistance and resistance genes in faecal *Escherichia coli* isolates recovered from healthy pets. *Vet Microbiol* 127:97–105.

182. Bryan A, Shapir N, Sadowsky MJ. 2004. Frequency and distribution of tetracycline resistance genes in genetically diverse, nonselected, and nonclinical *Escherichia coli* strains isolated from diverse human and animal sources. *Appl Environ Microbiol* 70:2503–2507.

183. Allmeier H, Cresnar B, Greck M, Schmitt R. 1992. Complete nucleotide sequence of Tn*1721*: gene organization and a novel gene product with features of a chemotaxis protein. *Gene* 111:11–20.

184. Chalmers R, Sewitz S, Lipkow K, Crellin P. 2000. Complete nucleotide sequence of Tn*10*. *J Bacteriol* 182:2970–2972.

185. Siqueira AK, Michael GB, Domingos DF, Ferraz MM, Ribeiro MG, Schwarz S, Leite DS. 2016. Diversity of class 1 and 2 integrons detected in *Escherichia coli* isolates from diseased and apparently healthy dogs. *Vet Microbiol* 194:79–83.

186. Huang SY, Zhu XQ, Wang Y, Liu HB, Dai L, He JK, Li BB, Wu CM, Shen JZ. 2012. Co-carriage of *qnrS1*, *floR*, and *bla*(CTX-M-14) on a multidrug-resistant plasmid in *Escherichia coli* isolated from pigs. *Foodborne Pathog Dis* 9:896–901.

187. Schwarz S, Kehrenberg C, Doublet B, Cloeckaert A. 2004. Molecular basis of bacterial resistance to chloramphenicol and florfenicol. *FEMS Microbiol Rev* 28:519–542.

188. Wang XM, Liao XP, Liu SG, Zhang WJ, Jiang HX, Zhang MJ, Zhu HQ, Sun Y, Sun J, Li AX, Liu YH. 2011. Serotypes, virulence genes, and antimicrobial susceptibility of *Escherichia coli* isolates from pigs. *Foodborne Pathog Dis* 8:687–692.

189. Travis RM, Gyles CL, Reid-Smith R, Poppe C, McEwen SA, Friendship R, Janecko N, Boerlin P. 2006. Chloramphenicol and kanamycin resistance among porcine *Escherichia coli* in Ontario. *J Antimicrob Chemother* 58:173–177.

190. White DG, Hudson C, Maurer JJ, Ayers S, Zhao S, Lee MD, Bolton L, Foley T, Sherwood J. 2000. Characterization of chloramphenicol and florfenicol resistance in *Escherichia coli* associated with bovine diarrhea. *J Clin Microbiol* 38:4593–4598.

191. Guerra B, Junker E, Schroeter A, Malorny B, Lehmann S, Helmuth R. 2003. Phenotypic and genotypic characterization of antimicrobial resistance in German *Escherichia coli* isolates from cattle, swine and poultry. *J Antimicrob Chemother* 52:489–492.

192. Awad A, Arafat N, Elhadidy M. 2016. Genetic elements associated with antimicrobial resistance among avian pathogenic *Escherichia coli*. *Ann Clin Microbiol Antimicrob* 15:59–67.

193. Ahmed MO, Clegg PD, Williams NJ, Baptiste KE, Bennett M. 2010. Antimicrobial resistance in equine faecal *Escherichia coli* isolates from North West England. *Ann Clin Microbiol Antimicrob* 9:12–19.

194. Shaheen BW, Oyarzabal OA, Boothe DM. 2010. The role of class 1 and 2 integrons in mediating antimicrobial resistance among canine and feline clinical *E. coli* isolates from the US. *Vet Microbiol* 144:363–370.

195. Derakhshandeh A, Eraghi V, Boroojeni AM, Niaki MA, Zare S, Naziri Z. 2018. Virulence factors, antibiotic resistance genes and genetic relatedness of commensal *Escherichia coli* isolates from dogs and their owners. *Microb Pathog* 116:241–245.

196. Chang SK, Lo DY, Wei HW, Kuo HC. 2015. Antimicrobial resistance of *Escherichia coli* isolates from canine urinary tract infections. *J Vet Med Sci* 77:59–65.

197. Van TT, Chin J, Chapman T, Tran LT, Coloe PJ. 2008. Safety of raw meat and shellfish in Vietnam: an analysis of *Escherichia coli* isolations for antibiotic resistance and virulence genes. *Int J Food Microbiol* 124:217–223.

198. Keyes K, Hudson C, Maurer JJ, Thayer S, White DG, Lee MD. 2000. Detection of florfenicol resistance genes in *Escherichia coli* isolated from sick chickens. *Antimicrob Agents Chemother* 44:421–424.

199. Bischoff KM, White DG, Hume ME, Poole TL, Nisbet DJ. 2005. The chloramphenicol resistance gene *cmlA* is disseminated on transferable plasmids that confer multiple-drug resistance in swine *Escherichia coli*. *FEMS Microbiol Lett* 243:285–291.

200. Blickwede M, Schwarz S. 2004. Molecular analysis of florfenicol-resistant *Escherichia coli* isolates from pigs. *J Antimicrob Chemother* 53:58–64.

201. Cloeckaert A, Baucheron S, Flaujac G, Schwarz S, Kehrenberg C, Martel JL, Chaslus-Dancla E. 2000. Plasmid-mediated florfenicol resistance encoded by the *floR* gene in *Escherichia coli* isolated from cattle. *Antimicrob Agents Chemother* 44:2858–2860.

202. Shen J, Wang Y, Schwarz S. 2013. Presence and dissemination of the multiresistance gene *cfr* in Gram-positive and Gram-negative bacteria. *J Antimicrob Chemother* 68:1697–1706.

203. Wang Y, He T, Schwarz S, Zhou D, Shen Z, Wu C, Wang Y, Ma L, Zhang Q, Shen J. 2012. Detection of the staphylococcal multiresistance gene *cfr* in *Escherichia coli* of domestic-animal origin. *J Antimicrob Chemother* 67:1094–1098.

204. Deng H, Sun J, Ma J, Li L, Fang LX, Zhang Q, Liu YH, Liao XP. 2014. Identification of the multi-resistance gene *cfr* in *Escherichia coli* isolates of animal origin. *PLoS One* 9:e102378.

205. Sun J, Deng H, Li L, Chen MY, Fang LX, Yang QE, Liu YH, Liao XP. 2015. Complete nucleotide sequence of

cfr-carrying IncX4 plasmid pSD11 from *Escherichia coli*. *Antimicrob Agents Chemother* 59:738–741.

206. Zhang WJ, Wang XM, Dai L, Hua X, Dong Z, Schwarz S, Liu S. 2015. Novel conjugative plasmid from *Escherichia coli* of swine origin that coharbors the multiresistance gene *cfr* and the extended-spectrum-β-lactamase gene *bla*CTX-M-14b. *Antimicrob Agents Chemother* 59:1337–1340.

207. Zhang R, Sun B, Wang Y, Lei L, Schwarz S, Wu C. 2015. Characterization of a *cfr*-carrying plasmid from porcine *Escherichia coli* that closely resembles plasmid pEA3 from the plant pathogen *Erwinia amylovora*. *Antimicrob Agents Chemother* 60:658–661.

208. van Duijkeren E, Schink AK, Roberts MC, Wang Y, Schwarz S. 2018. Mechanisms of bacterial resistance to antimicrobial agents. *Microbiol Spectr* 6.

209. Recchia GD, Hall RM. 1995. Gene cassettes: a new class of mobile element. *Microbiology* 141:3015–3027.

210. Kadlec K, Schwarz S. 2008. Analysis and distribution of class 1 and class 2 integrons and associated gene cassettes among *Escherichia coli* isolates from swine, horses, cats and dogs collected in the BfT-GermVet monitoring study. *J Antimicrob Chemother* 62:469–473.

211. Bass L, Liebert CA, Lee MD, Summers AO, White DG, Thayer SG, Maurer JJ. 1999. Incidence and characterization of integrons, genetic elements mediating multiple-drug resistance, in avian *Escherichia coli*. *Antimicrob Agents Chemother* 43:2925–2929.

212. Waturangi DE, Suwanto A, Schwarz S, Erdelen W. 2003. Identification of class 1 integrons-associated gene cassettes in *Escherichia coli* isolated from *Varanus* spp. in Indonesia. *J Antimicrob Chemother* 51:175–177.

213. Zhao S, White DG, Ge B, Ayers S, Friedman S, English L, Wagner D, Gaines S, Meng J. 2001. Identification and characterization of integron-mediated antibiotic resistance among Shiga toxin-producing *Escherichia coli* isolates. *Appl Environ Microbiol* 67:1558–1564.

214. Sunde M. 2005. Class I integron with a group II intron detected in an *Escherichia coli* strain from a free-range reindeer. *Antimicrob Agents Chemother* 49:2512–2514.

215. Du X, Shen Z, Wu B, Xia S, Shen J. 2005. Characterization of class 1 integrons-mediated antibiotic resistance among calf pathogenic *Escherichia coli*. *FEMS Microbiol Lett* 245:295–298.

216. Wu S, Dalsgaard A, Hammerum AM, Porsbo LJ, Jensen LB. 2010. Prevalence and characterization of plasmids carrying sulfonamide resistance genes among *Escherichia coli* from pigs, pig carcasses and human. *Acta Vet Scand* 52:47.

217. Sidjabat HE, Townsend KM, Hanson ND, Bell JM, Stokes HW, Gobius KS, Moss SM, Trott DJ. 2006. Identification of *bla*(CMY-7) and associated plasmid-mediated resistance genes in multidrug-resistant *Escherichia coli* isolated from dogs at a veterinary teaching hospital in Australia. *J Antimicrob Chemother* 57:840–848.

218. van Essen-Zandbergen A, Smith H, Veldman K, Mevius D. 2009. *In vivo* transfer of an incFIB plasmid

harbouring a class 1 integron with gene cassettes *dfrA1-aadA1*. *Vet Microbiol* 137:402–407.

219. Boerlin P, Travis R, Gyles CL, Reid-Smith R, Janecko N, Lim H, Nicholson V, McEwen SA, Friendship R, Archambault M. 2005. Antimicrobial resistance and virulence genes of *Escherichia coli* isolates from swine in Ontario. *Appl Environ Microbiol* 71:6753–6761.

220. Kikuvi GM, Schwarz S, Ombui JN, Mitema ES, Kehrenberg C. 2007. Streptomycin and chloramphenicol resistance genes in *Escherichia coli* isolates from cattle, pigs, and chicken in Kenya. *Microb Drug Resist* 13:62–68.

221. Ojo OE, Schwarz S, Michael GB. 2016. Detection and characterization of extended-spectrum β-lactamase-producing *Escherichia coli* from chicken production chains in Nigeria. *Vet Microbiol* 194:62–68.

222. Schwaiger K, Bauer J, Hölzel CS. 2013. Selection and persistence of antimicrobial-resistant *Escherichia coli* including extended-spectrum β-lactamase producers in different poultry flocks on one chicken farm. *Microb Drug Resist* 19:498–506.

223. Touzain F, Le Devendec L, de Boisséson C, Baron S, Jouy E, Perrin-Guyomard A, Blanchard Y, Kempf I. 2018. Characterization of plasmids harboring *bla*CTX-M and *bla*CMY genes in *E. coli* from French broilers. *PLoS One* 13:e0188768.

224. Perreten V, Boerlin P. 2003. A new sulfonamide resistance gene (*sul3*) in *Escherichia coli* is widespread in the pig population of Switzerland. *Antimicrob Agents Chemother* 47:1169–1172.

225. Liu J, Keelan P, Bennett PM, Enne VI. 2009. Characterization of a novel macrolide efflux gene, *mef*(B), found linked to *sul3* in porcine *Escherichia coli*. *J Antimicrob Chemother* 63:423–426.

226. Sunde M, Solheim H, Slettemeås JS. 2008. Genetic linkage between class 1 integrons with the *dfrA12-orfF-aadA2* cassette array and *sul3* in *Escherichia coli*. *Vet Microbiol* 130:422–425.

227. Pattishall KH, Acar J, Burchall JJ, Goldstein FW, Harvey RJ. 1977. Two distinct types of trimethoprim-resistant dihydrofolate reductase specified by R-plasmids of different compatibility groups. *J Biol Chem* 252:2319–2323.

228. Reid CJ, Wyrsch ER, Roy Chowdhury P, Zingali T, Liu M, Darling AE, Chapman TA, Djordjevic SP. 2017. Porcine commensal *Escherichia coli*: a reservoir for class 1 integrons associated with IS26. *Microb Genom* 3:3.

229. Seputiené V, Povilonis J, Ruzauskas M, Pavilonis A, Suziedéliené E. 2010. Prevalence of trimethoprim resistance genes in *Escherichia coli* isolates of human and animal origin in Lithuania. *J Med Microbiol* 59:315–322.

230. Delport TC, Harcourt RG, Beaumont LJ, Webster KN, Power ML. 2015. Molecular detection of antibiotic-resistance determinants in *Escherichia coli* isolated from the endangered Australian sea lion (*Neophoca Cinerea*). *J Wildl Dis* 51:555–563.

231. Ojo KK, Kehrenberg C, Schwarz S, Odelola HA. 2002. Identification of a complete *dfrA14* gene cassette inte-

grated at a secondary site in a resistance plasmid of uropathogenic *Escherichia coli* from Nigeria. *Antimicrob Agents Chemother* **46**:2054–2055.

232. Poirel L, Jayol A, Nordmann P. 2017. Polymyxins: antibacterial activity, susceptibility testing, and resistance mechanisms encoded by plasmids or chromosomes. *Clin Microbiol Rev* **30**:557–596.

233. Rhouma M, Beaudry F, Thériault W, Letellier A. 2016. Colistin in pig production: chemistry, mechanism of antibacterial action, microbial resistance emergence, and One Health perspectives. *Front Microbiol* **7**:1789.

234. Anonymous. 2016. European Medicines Agency. Updated advice on the use of colistin products in animals within the European Union: development of resistance and possible impact on human and animal health. EMA/CVMP/CHMP/231573.1-56.

235. Walsh TR, Wu Y. 2016. China bans colistin as a feed additive for animals. *Lancet Infect Dis* **16**:1102–1103.

236. Quesada A, Porrero MC, Téllez S, Palomo G, García M, Domínguez L. 2015. Polymorphism of genes encoding PmrAB in colistin-resistant strains of *Escherichia coli* and *Salmonella enterica* isolated from poultry and swine. *J Antimicrob Chemother* **70**:71–74.

237. Delannoy S, Le Devendec L, Jouy E, Fach P, Drider D, Kempf I. 2017. Characterization of colistin-resistant *Escherichia coli* isolated from diseased pigs in France. *Front Microbiol* **8**:2278.

238. Liu YY, Wang Y, Walsh TR, Yi LX, Zhang R, Spencer J, Doi Y, Tian G, Dong B, Huang X, Yu LF, Gu D, Ren H, Chen X, Lv L, He D, Zhou H, Liang Z, Liu JH, Shen J. 2016. Emergence of plasmid-mediated colistin resistance mechanism MCR-1 in animals and human beings in China: a microbiological and molecular biological study. *Lancet Infect Dis* **16**:161–168.

239. Schwarz S, Johnson AP. 2016. Transferable resistance to colistin: a new but old threat. *J Antimicrob Chemother* **71**:2066–2070.

240. Falgenhauer L, Waezsada SE, Yao Y, Imirzalioglu C, Käsbohrer A, Roesler U, Michael GB, Schwarz S, Werner G, Kreienbrock L, Chakraborty T, RESET consortium. 2016. Colistin resistance gene *mcr-1* in extended-spectrum β-lactamase-producing and carbapenemase-producing Gram-negative bacteria in Germany. *Lancet Infect Dis* **16**:282–283.

241. Haenni M, Poirel L, Kieffer N, Châtre P, Saras E, Métayer V, Dumoulin R, Nordmann P, Madec JY. 2016. Co-occurrence of extended spectrum β lactamase and MCR-1 encoding genes on plasmids. *Lancet Infect Dis* **16**:281–282.

242. Li R, Xie M, Zhang J, Yang Z, Liu L, Liu X, Zheng Z, Chan EW, Chen S. 2017. Genetic characterization of *mcr-1*-bearing plasmids to depict molecular mechanisms underlying dissemination of the colistin resistance determinant. *J Antimicrob Chemother* **72**:393–401.

243. Zurfluh K, Klumpp J, Nüesch-Inderbinen M, Stephan R. 2016. Full-length nucleotide sequences of *mcr-1*-harboring plasmids isolated from extended-spectrum-β-lactamase-producing *Escherichia coli* isolates of different origins. *Antimicrob Agents Chemother* **60**:5589–5591.

244. Zurfuh K, Poirel L, Nordmann P, Nüesch-Inderbinen M, Hächler H, Stephan R. 2016. Occurrence of the plasmid-borne *mcr-1* colistin resistance gene in extended-spectrum-β-lactamase-producing *Enterobacteriaceae* in river water and imported vegetable samples in Switzerland. *Antimicrob Agents Chemother* **60**:2594–2595.

245. Poirel L, Kieffer N, Nordmann P. 2017. *In vitro* study of IS*Apl1*-mediated mobilization of the colistin resistance gene *mcr-1*. *Antimicrob Agents Chemother* **61**:61.

246. Yang YQ, Li YX, Song T, Yang YX, Jiang W, Zhang AY, Guo XY, Liu BH, Wang YX, Lei CW, Xiang R, Wang HN. 2017. Colistin resistance gene *mcr-1* and its variant in *Escherichia coli* isolates from chickens in China. *Antimicrob Agents Chemother* **61**:e01204-16.

247. Xavier BB, Lammens C, Ruhal R, Kumar-Singh S, Butaye P, Goossens H, Malhotra-Kumar S. 2016. Identification of a novel plasmid-mediated colistin-resistance gene, *mcr-2*, in *Escherichia coli*, Belgium, June 2016. *Euro Surveill* **21**:30280.

248. Zhang J, Chen L, Wang J, Yassin AK, Butaye P, Kelly P, Gong J, Guo W, Li J, Li M, Yang F, Feng Z, Jiang P, Song C, Wang Y, You J, Yang Y, Price S, Qi K, Kang Y, Wang C. 2018. Molecular detection of colistin resistance genes (*mcr-1*, *mcr-2* and *mcr-3*) in nasal/oropharyngeal and anal/cloacal swabs from pigs and poultry. *Sci Rep* **8**:3705.

249. Yin W, Li H, Shen Y, Liu Z, Wang S, Shen Z, Zhang R, Walsh TR, Shen J, Wang Y. 2017. Novel plasmid-mediated colistin resistance gene *mcr-3* in *Escherichia coli*. *MBio* **8**:e00543-17.

250. Hernández M, Iglesias MR, Rodríguez-Lázaro D, Gallardo A, Quijada N, Miguela-Villoldo P, Campos MJ, Píriz S, López-Orozco G, de Frutos C, Sáez JL, Ugarte-Ruiz M, Domínguez L, Quesada A. 2017. Co-occurrence of colistin-resistance genes *mcr-1* and *mcr-3* among multidrug-resistant *Escherichia coli* isolated from cattle, Spain, September 2015. *Euro Surveill* **22**:30586.

251. Haenni M, Beyrouthy R, Lupo A, Châtre P, Madec JY, Bonnet R. 2018. Epidemic spread of *Escherichia coli* ST744 isolates carrying *mcr-3* and bla_CTX-M-55 in cattle in France. *J Antimicrob Chemother* **73**:533–536.

252. Carattoli A, Villa L, Feudi C, Curcio L, Orsini S, Luppi A, Pezzotti G, Magistrali CF. 2017. Novel plasmid-mediated colistin resistance *mcr-4* gene in *Salmonella* and *Escherichia coli*, Italy 2013, Spain and Belgium, 2015 to 2016. *Euro Surveill* **22**:30589.

253. Hammerl JA, Borowiak M, Schmoger S, Shamoun D, Grobbel M, Malorny B, Tenhagen BA, Käsbohrer A. 2018. *mcr-5* and a novel *mcr-5.2* variant in *Escherichia coli* isolates from food and food-producing animals, Germany, 2010 to 2017. *J Antimicrob Chemother* **73**:1433–1435.

254. Haenni M, Métayer V, Gay E, Madec JY. 2016. Increasing trends in *mcr-1* prevalence among extended-spectrum-β-lactamase-producing *Escherichia coli* isolates from French calves despite decreasing exposure to colistin. *Antimicrob Agents Chemother* **60**:6433–6434.

255. Shen Z, Wang Y, Shen Y, Shen J, Wu C. 2016. Early emergence of *mcr-1* in *Escherichia coli* from food-producing animals. *Lancet Infect Dis* **16**:293.

256. **Guenther S, Falgenhauer L, Semmler T, Imirzalioglu C, Chakraborty T, Roesler U, Roschanski N.** 2017. Environmental emission of multiresistant *Escherichia coli* carrying the colistin resistance gene *mcr-1* from German swine farms. *J Antimicrob Chemother* 72:1289–1292.

257. **Hammerum AM, Larsen J, Andersen VD, Lester CH, Skovgaard Skytte TS, Hansen F, Olsen SS, Mordhorst H, Skov RL, Aarestrup FM, Agersø Y.** 2014. Characterization of extended-spectrum β-lactamase (ESBL)-producing *Escherichia coli* obtained from Danish pigs, pig farmers and their families from farms with high or no consumption of third- or fourth-generation cephalosporins. *J Antimicrob Chemother* 69:2650–2657.

258. **Börjesson S, Bengtsson B, Jernberg C, Englund S.** 2013. Spread of extended-spectrum β-lactamase producing *Escherichia coli* isolates in Swedish broilers mediated by an incI plasmid carrying *bla*(CTX-M-1). *Acta Vet Scand* 55:3.

259. **Randall LP, Clouting C, Horton RA, Coldham NG, Wu G, Clifton-Hadley FA, Davies RH, Teale CJ.** 2011. Prevalence of *Escherichia coli* carrying extended-spectrum β-lactamases (CTX-M and TEM-52) from broiler chickens and turkeys in Great Britain between 2006 and 2009. *J Antimicrob Chemother* 66:86–95.

260. **Endimiani A, Rossano A, Kunz D, Overesch G, Perreten V.** 2012. First countrywide survey of third-generation cephalosporin-resistant *Escherichia coli* from broilers, swine, and cattle in Switzerland. *Diagn Microbiol Infect Dis* 73:31–38.

261. **Liu X, Thungrat K, Boothe DM.** 2016. Occurrence of OXA-48 carbapenemase and other β-lactamase genes in ESBL-producing multidrug resistant *Escherichia coli* from dogs and cats in the United States, 2009–2013. *Front Microbiol* 7:1057.

262. **Liao XP, Xia J, Yang L, Li L, Sun J, Liu YH, Jiang HX.** 2015. Characterization of CTX-M-14-producing *Escherichia coli* from food-producing animals. *Front Microbiol* 6:1136.

263. **Falgenhauer L, Imirzalioglu C, Ghosh H, Gwozdzinski K, Schmiedel J, Gentil K, Bauerfeind R, Kämpfer P, Seifert H, Michael GB, Schwarz S, Pfeifer Y, Werner G, Pietsch M, Roesler U, Guerra B, Fischer J, Sharp H, Käsbohrer A, Goesmann A, Hille K, Kreienbrock L, Chakraborty T.** 2016. Circulation of clonal populations of fluoroquinolone-resistant CTX-M-15-producing *Escherichia coli* ST410 in humans and animals in Germany. *Int J Antimicrob Agents* 47:457–465.

264. **Ewers C, Grobbel M, Stamm I, Kopp PA, Diehl I, Semmler T, Fruth A, Beutlich J, Guerra B, Wieler LH, Guenther S.** 2010. Emergence of human pandemic O25:H4-ST131 CTX-M-15 extended-spectrum-β-lactamase-producing *Escherichia coli* among companion animals. *J Antimicrob Chemother* 65:651–660.

265. **Schill F, Abdulmawjood A, Klein G, Reich F.** 2017. Prevalence and characterization of extended-spectrum β-lactamase (ESBL) and AmpC β-lactamase producing *Enterobacteriaceae* in fresh pork meat at processing level in Germany. *Int J Food Microbiol* 257:58–66.

266. **Alcalá L, Alonso CA, Simón C, González-Esteban C, Orós J, Rezusta A, Ortega C, Torres C.** 2016.

267. **Jones-Dias D, Manageiro V, Martins AP, Ferreira E, Caniça M.** 2016. New class 2 integron In2-4 among IncI1-positive *Escherichia coli* isolates carrying ESBL and PMAβ genes from food animals in Portugal. *Foodborne Pathog Dis* 13:36–39.

268. **Vogt D, Overesch G, Endimiani A, Collaud A, Thomann A, Perreten V.** 2014. Occurrence and genetic characteristics of third-generation cephalosporin-resistant *Escherichia coli* in Swiss retail meat. *Microb Drug Resist* 20:485–494.

269. **Park YS, Adams-Haduch JM, Rivera JI, Curry SR, Harrison LH, Doi Y.** 2012. *Escherichia coli* producing CMY-2 β-lactamase in retail chicken, Pittsburgh, Pennsylvania, USA. *Emerg Infect Dis* 18:515–516.

270. **Cunha MP, Lincopan N, Cerdeira L, Esposito F, Dropa M, Franco LS, Moreno AM, Knobl T.** 2017. Coexistence of CTX-M-2, CTX-M-55, CMY-2, FosA3, and QnrB19 in extraintestinal pathogenic *Escherichia coli* from poultry in Brazil. *Antimicrob Agents Chemother* 61:e02474-16.

271. **Guo YF, Zhang WH, Ren SQ, Yang L, Lü DH, Zeng ZL, Liu YH, Jiang HX.** 2014. IncA/C plasmid-mediated spread of CMY-2 in multidrug-resistant *Escherichia coli* from food animals in China. *PLoS One* 9:e96738.

272. **Ohnishi M, Okatani AT, Esaki H, Harada K, Sawada T, Murakami M, Marumo K, Kato Y, Sato R, Shimura K, Hatanaka N, Takahashi T.** 2013. Herd prevalence of *Enterobacteriaceae* producing CTX-M-type and CMY-2 β-lactamases among Japanese dairy farms. *J Appl Microbiol* 115:282–289.

273. **Sato T, Yokota S, Okubo T, Usui M, Fujii N, Tamura Y.** 2014. Phylogenetic association of fluoroquinolone and cephalosporin resistance of D-O1-ST648 *Escherichia coli* carrying *bla*CMY-2 from faecal samples of dogs in Japan. *J Med Microbiol* 63:263–270.

274. **Maamar E, Hammami S, Alonso CA, Dakhli N, Abbassi MS, Ferjani S, Hamzaoui Z, Saidani M, Torres C, Boutiba-Ben Boubaker I.** 2016. High prevalence of extended-spectrum and plasmidic AmpC β-lactamase-producing *Escherichia coli* from poultry in Tunisia. *Int J Food Microbiol* 231:69–75.

275. **Cui L, Lei L, Lv Y, Zhang R, Liu X, Li M, Zhang F, Wang Y.** 2017. bla NDM-1-producing multidrug-resistant *Escherichia coli* isolated from a companion dog in China. *J Glob Antimicrob Resist* 13:24–27.

276. **Lin D, Xie M, Li R, Chen K, Chan EW, Chen S.** 2016. IncFII conjugative plasmid-mediated transmission of *bla*NDM-1 elements among animal-borne *Escherichia coli* strains. *Antimicrob Agents Chemother* 61:e02285-16.

277. **Kong LH, Lei CW, Ma SZ, Jiang W, Liu BH, Wang YX, Guan R, Men S, Yuan QW, Cheng GY, Zhou WC, Wang HN.** 2017. Various sequence types of *Escherichia coli* isolates coharboring *bla*NDM-5 and *mcr-1* genes from a commercial swine farm in China. *Antimicrob Agents Chemother* 61:e02167-16.

267. (Wild birds, frequent carriers of extended-spectrum β-lactamase (ESBL) producing *Escherichia coli* of CTX-M and SHV-12 types. *Microb Ecol* 72:861–869.)

278. **Purkait D, Ahuja A, Bhattacharjee U, Singha A, Rhetso K, Dey TK, Das S, Sanjukta RK, Puro K, Shakuntala I, Sen A, Banerjee A, Sharma I, Bhatta RS, Mawlong M, Guha C, Pradhan NR, Ghatak S.** 2016. Molecular characterization and computational modelling of New Delhi metallo-β-lactamase-5 from an *Escherichia coli* isolate (KOEC3) of bovine origin. *Indian J Microbiol* **56:**182–189.

279. **Yaici L, Haenni M, Saras E, Boudehouche W, Touati A, Madec JY.** 2016. *bla*_{NDM-5}-carrying IncX3 plasmid in *Escherichia coli* ST1284 isolated from raw milk collected in a dairy farm in Algeria. *J Antimicrob Chemother* **71:**2671–2672.

280. **Roschanski N, Friese A, von Salviati-Claudius C, Hering J, Kaesbohrer A, Kreienbrock L, Roesler U.** 2017. Prevalence of carbapenemase producing *Enterobacteriaceae* isolated from German pig-fattening farms during the years 2011–2013. *Vet Microbiol* **200:**124–129.

281. **Roschanski N, Guenther S, Vu TTT, Fischer J, Semmler T, Huehn S, Alter T, Roesler U.** 2017. VIM-1 carbapenemase-producing *Escherichia coli* isolated from retail seafood, Germany 2016. *Euro Surveill* **22:** 17-00032.

282. **Unger F, Eisenberg T, Prenger-Berninghoff E, Leidner U, Ludwig ML, Rothe M, Semmler T, Ewers C.** 2017. Imported reptiles as a risk factor for the global distribution of *Escherichia coli* harbouring the colistin resistance gene *mcr-1*. *Int J Antimicrob Agents* **49:**122–123.

283. **Lim SK, Kang HY, Lee K, Moon DC, Lee HS, Jung SC.** 2016. First detection of the *mcr-1* gene in *Escherichia coli* isolated from livestock between 2013 and 2015 in South Korea. *Antimicrob Agents Chemother* **60:**6991–6993.

284. **Meinersmann RJ, Ladely SR, Plumblee JR, Cook KL, Thacker E.** 2017. Prevalence of *mcr-1* in the cecal contents of food animals in the United States. *Antimicrob Agents Chemother* **61:**e02244-16.

285. **Delgado-Blas JF, Ovejero CM, Abadia-Patiño L, Gonzalez-Zorn B.** 2016. Coexistence of *mcr-1* and *bla*_{NDM-1} in *Escherichia coli* from Venezuela. *Antimicrob Agents Chemother* **60:**6356–6358.

286. **Sellera FP, Fernandes MR, Sartori L, Carvalho MP, Esposito F, Nascimento CL, Dutra GH, Mamizuka EM, Pérez-Chaparro PJ, McCulloch JA, Lincopan N.** 2017. *Escherichia coli* carrying IncX4 plasmid-mediated *mcr-1* and *bla*_{CTX-M} genes in infected migratory Magellanic penguins (*Spheniscus magellanicus*). *J Antimicrob Chemother* **72:**1255–1256.

287. **Sellera FP, Fernandes MR, Ruiz R, Falleiros ACM, Rodrigues FP, Cerdeira L, Lincopan N.** 2018. Identification of KPC-2-producing *Escherichia coli* in a companion animal: a new challenge for veterinary clinicians. *J Antimicrob Chemother* [Epub ahead of print].

Antimicrobial Resistance in Bacteria from Livestock and Companion Animals
Edited by Frank Møller Aarestrup, Stefan Schwarz, Jianzhong Shen, and Lina Cavaco
© 2018 American Society for Microbiology, Washington, DC
doi:10.1128/microbiolspec.ARBA-0013-2017

Antimicrobial Resistance in *Campylobacter* spp.

14

Zhangqi Shen,[1] Yang Wang,[1] Qijing Zhang,[2] and Jianzhong Shen[1]

INTRODUCTION

Campylobacter, a foodborne bacterial pathogen, is the leading cause of human gastroenteritis worldwide. According to data from the World Health Organization, the estimated incidence of gastroenteritis due to *Campylobacter* spp. in high-income countries is between 4.4 and 9.3 per 1,000 people (1). Most *Campylobacter* infections are mild and self-limiting and may not require antimicrobial therapy; however, antibiotic treatment is required for severe or prolonged infections. In clinical settings, fluoroquinolones and macrolides are the drugs of choice to treat campylobacteriosis (2–6), but in some cases, tetracyclines and gentamicin are used to treat systemic infection with *Campylobacter* (5, 6). In a report from the Centers for Disease Control and Prevention (CDC) on antibiotic resistance threats in the United States in 2013, drug-resistant *Campylobacter* was listed under "microorganisms with a threat level of serious" (http://www.cdc.gov/drugresistance/threat-report-2013/pdf/ar-threats-2013-508.pdf). The CDC indicated that almost 24% of *Campylobacter* strains tested were resistant to ciprofloxacin (fluoroquinolone) or azithromycin (macrolide), indicating that approximately 310,000 *Campylobacter* infections are caused by drug-resistant *Campylobacter* each year in the United States. Although contaminated undercooked poultry meat is a main source of infection for human campylobacteriosis (2, 7), ruminant *Campylobacter* is also a significant contributor for foodborne illnesses (8–15).

As a foodborne pathogen transmitted via foodborne routes, *Campylobacter* is constantly exposed to antimicrobials used for food production. In dealing with antimicrobial selection, *Campylobacter* has evolved various mechanisms of resistance to antimicrobials. Some of the mechanisms confer resistance to a specific class of antimicrobials, while others may confer multidrug resistance. Previous publications have provided excellent reviews on antibiotic resistance in *Campylobacter* (5, 16–19). However, several new antibiotic resistance mechanisms have emerged in *Campylobacter* in recent years. Examples include the rRNA methylase Erm(B) (mediating macrolide resistance), a functionally enhanced multidrug efflux pump variant (RE-CmeABC), methylarsenite efflux permease ArsP conferring resistance to organoarsenicals, a novel *fosX*^{CC} gene conferring fosfomycin resistance, and the rRNA methyltransferase Cfr(C) mediating multidrug resistance. In this review, we will summarize the current state of antibiotic resistance in *Campylobacter*, with an emphasis on the newly emerged mechanisms.

RESISTANCE TO FLUOROQUINOLONES

The fluoroquinolones (e.g., ciprofloxacin, enrofloxacin, etc.) are a family of synthetic broad-spectrum antibacterial agents that are active against a wide range of Gram-positive and Gram-negative organisms (20, 21). To date, they are one of the drugs of choice to treat campylobacteriosis in humans as well as other bacterial diseases in both animals and humans (21–23). Fluoroquinolones target two essential enzymes, DNA gyrase and topoisomerase IV, and impair DNA replication (21, 24). Generally, mutations in the genes encoding the subunits of DNA gyrase (GyrA and GyrB), topoisomerase IV (ParC and ParE), or both are responsible for the resistance of bacteria to fluoroquinolones (25, 26). In *Campylobacter*, the main resistance mechanism to fluoroquinolones is mediated by point mutations in

[1]Beijing Advanced Innovation Center for Food Nutrition and Human Health, College of Veterinary Medicine, China Agricultural University, Beijing, 100193, China; [2]Department of Veterinary Microbiology and Preventive Medicine, College of Veterinary Medicine, Iowa State University, Ames, IA 50011.

the quinolone resistance-determining region of GyrA (4, 5). To date, mutations in GyrB have not been associated with fluoroquinolone resistance in *Campylobacter* (27–29). The absence of genes encoding ParC and ParE implies that they are not involved in fluoroquinolone action and resistance in *Campylobacter* (27–32). Notably, a single point mutation in the quinolone resistance-determining region of *gyrA* is sufficient to substantially reduce the susceptibility of *Campylobacter* to fluoroquinolone antimicrobials (5, 30, 33, 34). Multiple resistance-associated mutations, including T86I, T86K, A70T, and D90N, have been reported in *Campylobacter* (4, 5, 33, 35). The C257T change in the *gyrA* gene, which leads to the T86I substitution in gyrase, is the most frequently observed mutation conferring resistance to fluoroquinolones in *Campylobacter* (4, 5, 36). In addition to mutations in GyrA, the functional multidrug efflux pump, CmeABC, is also required for fluoroquinolone resistance in *Campylobacter*. Inactivation of *cmeABC* in fluoroquinolone-resistant mutants (carrying specific GyrA mutations) made the resistant mutants susceptible to fluoroquinolones (30). Until now, mutations in GyrA together with CmeABC have been the only identified mechanisms of fluoroquinolone resistance in *Campylobacter*. Plasmid-mediated quinolone-resistance determinants, such as *qnr*, *aac(6′)-Ib-cr*, and *qepA*, have not been reported in *Campylobacter*.

RESISTANCE TO MACROLIDES

The macrolide antibiotics (azithromycin, clarithromycin, erythromycin, telithromycin, etc.) are a class of drugs for the treatment of gastric diseases caused by *Helicobacter pylori* and *Campylobacter* and for respiratory tract infections in humans (37). Antibiotics in this class, including erythromycin, tylosin, spiramycin, tilmicosin, and roxithromycin, are also approved for growth promotion and therapeutic purposes in animals (38). Macrolides target the 50S subunit of the bacterial ribosome and inhibit protein synthesis through interference with the peptide translocation step (39, 40). Generally, bacterial resistance to macrolides is mediated by three mechanisms: enzymatic inactivation of macrolides, modification or point mutations in the target, and enhanced drug efflux (5, 41). In *Campylobacter*, modification of the ribosomal target, leading to macrolide resistance, can occur either by enzyme-mediated methylation or by point mutation in the 23S rRNA and/or ribosomal proteins L4 and L22 (4, 5, 41). Although an early report suggested the presence of rRNA methylation genes in *Campylobacter rectus* isolates based on the result of Southern hybridization (42), an rRNA

methylating enzyme was not formally identified until recently, when Erm(B) was identified in both *Campylobacter jejuni* and *Campylobacter coli* from various sources, including swine, chicken, ducks, and humans (43–45). The *erm*(B) gene was either located in the chromosomal DNA or carried by a plasmid (43). This gene alone is able to confer high-level resistance to macrolides (44). It is worth noting that the *erm*(B) gene is associated with multidrug resistance genomic islands (MDRGIs), which include several resistance genes [*aacA-aphD*, *sat4*, *aphA-3*, *fosX*^{CC}, *aad9*, and *tet*(O)] and mediate resistance to multiple classes of antibiotics (43, 44) (Fig. 1). Generally, MDRGIs are located in the region between *cadF* and *CCO1582*, *nfsB* and *cinA*, or *cj0168c* and *sodB* (43–45) and are transferrable among different *Campylobacter* spp. by natural transformation under laboratory conditions (43).

Point mutations in domain V of the 23S rRNA have been recognized as the most common mechanism for macrolide resistance in *Campylobacter* (4, 5, 41, 46). These point mutations occur at positions 2074 and 2075 of the 23S rRNA in *Campylobacter*, which correspond to positions 2058 and 2059, respectively, in *Escherichia coli*. Among the reported resistance-associated mutations, the A2074C, A2074G, and A2075G mutations confer high-level resistance to macrolide antibiotics (erythromycin MIC >128 g/ml) in *Campylobacter* (46–50), with A2075G being the predominant mutation in clinical and field isolates (4, 5, 41, 46). *Campylobacter* contains three copies of 23S rRNA genes (51), and usually, macrolide resistance-associated mutations occur in all three copies for most *Campylobacter* isolates with high-level resistance (47, 48, 52).

In addition to target modification, active efflux also contributes to macrolide resistance in *Campylobacter* (48–50, 53–56). The CmeABC efflux system functions synergistically with target mutations, and inactivation of CmeABC significantly reduces the resistance to macrolide antibiotics in isolates with high-, intermediate-, or low-level macrolide resistance (19). Additionally, the synergy between the CmeABC efflux pump and mutations in the ribosomal proteins L4 (G74D) and L22 (inserted at position 86 or 98) also confers macrolide resistance in *Campylobacter* (50, 53).

RESISTANCE TO TETRACYCLINES

Tetracyclines, discovered in the 1940s, are an important class of antibiotics that are widely used in both human and animal medicine. Tetracyclines have broad-spectrum activity against Gram-positive and Gram-

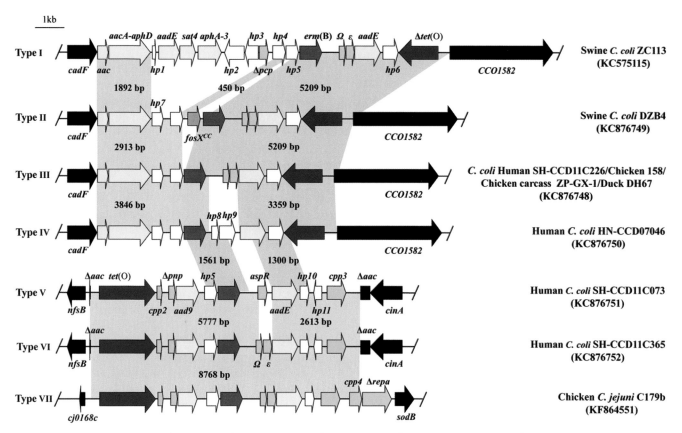

Figure 1 Chromosomal organization and comparison of seven types (I to VII) of MDRGIs containing the *erm*(B) gene (modified from references 43–45). *erm*(B) is in red, aminoglycoside resistance genes are in yellow, the streptothricin resistance gene (*sat4*) is in blue, the tetracycline resistance gene [*tet*(O)] is in purple, genes with predicted functions are in green, and genes coding hypothetical proteins are in white. The *tet*(O) gene is intact in types V and VI but is truncated in other types. The border genes of the MDRGIs are depicted by black box arrows. The gray shading indicates regions sharing more than 98% DNA identity. A representative strain for each type of MDRGI is indicated on the right side of the panel.

negative bacteria, as well as chlamydiae, mycoplasmas, rickettsiae, and protozoan parasites (57). It is well established that tetracyclines inhibit bacterial protein synthesis by preventing the attachment of aminoacyl-tRNA to the ribosomal acceptor (A) site (58, 59). Because of the long history and widespread use of tetracyclines, a number of resistance determinants to this class of drugs have been observed in a variety of bacteria (60, 61). Generally, the resistance to tetracyclines is mediated by one of four mechanisms: efflux pumps, chemical modification of tetracyclines, ribosomal protection proteins, and mutations in rRNA (60).

To date, resistance to tetracyclines in *Campylobacter* is conferred by the ribosomal protection protein Tet(O) and efflux pumps (CmeABC and CmeG). Tet(O) belongs to one of the characterized ribosomal protection proteins (61), several of which are paralogs of the

translational GTPase EF-G and actively remove tetracycline from the ribosome in a GTP hydrolysis-dependent fashion (62–64). The well-documented action mode is that Tet(O) recognizes and binds to an open A site on the bacterial ribosome and then induces a conformational change that results in the sequential release of the bound tetracycline molecule (60, 64). This conformational change is able to persist and allows the A site to function in protein elongation (60, 64). A recent study indicated that several critical residues located in the three loops of Tet(O) disrupt the binding of tetracycline to the ribosome complex (59). The *tet*(O) gene, which is widely present in *C. jejuni* and *C. coli* (65, 66), can be located either in the chromosomal DNA or on a plasmid (e.g., pTet and pCC31) (67–69). Based on the G-C content, sequence homology, codon usage, and hybridization analysis, it appears that the *Campylobacter* tet(O) gene was probably acquired from a Gram-positive origin by horizontal gene transfer (66, 68). The CmeABC and CmeG multidrug efflux pumps contribute to both intrinsic and acquired resistance to tetracycline in *Campylobacter* (55, 70–72). CmeABC functions synergistically with Tet(O) to confer high-level resistance to tetracycline (70). Inactivation of either CmeABC or CmeG increases the susceptibility of *Campylobacter* to tetracyclines (70, 72).

RESISTANCE TO AMINOGLYCOSIDES

Aminoglycosides are bactericidal antibiotics that bind to ribosomes and inhibit protein synthesis (73). They are structurally characterized by an aminocyclitol ring bound to one or more amino sugars by pseudoglycosidic bonds (74–76). This class of antimicrobials is generally considered to have broad-spectrum bacteriocidal activity and is clinically used to treat acute and systemic *Campylobacter* infections (77, 78), although they have limited activity in anaerobic environment. On the basis of the *in vitro* susceptibility of many *Campylobacter* strains to aminoglycosides (79, 80), oxygen levels in the microaerophilic environments preferred by *Campylobacter* are sufficient to allow the transport of compounds into the intracellular environment (18). A total of five mechanisms of aminoglycoside resistance in bacteria have been described (74, 76, 81): (i) reduced accumulation of the drug in the intracellular environment, conferred by a multidrug efflux pump that transports the drug back into the extracellular environment or due to decreased permeability of the bacterial cellular membrane to the drug (74), (ii) methylation of 16S rRNA in sites that interfere with drug binding (75, 82), (iii) mutations in the binding sites of rRNA, especially in *Mycobacterium* spp. with a single copy of the ribosomal operon (75), (iv) active swarming, a nonspecific mechanism in *P. aeruginosa* cells that exhibits adaptive antibiotic resistance against several antibiotics, including gentamicin (83), and (v) enzymatic modification at the -OH or -NH$_2$ groups of the 2-deoxystreptamine nucleus or sugar moieties of the antibiotic, which is considered the most important mechanism (81). Among the known mechanisms of aminoglycoside resistance, modification of the aminoglycoside structure by enzymes such as aminoglycoside acetyltransferases, aminoglycoside phosphotransferases, and aminoglycoside nucleotidyltransferases is the most significant and prevalent in several bacterial species, including *Campylobacter* spp. (16, 78, 84). In *Campylobacter*, each of the above-mentioned aminoglycoside-modifying enzymes has been detected.

Aminoglycoside phosphotransferases constitute the majority of aminoglycoside-modifying enzymes identified in *Campylobacter* spp. and are responsible for phosphorylation of the 3′ hydroxyl group of aminoglycosides. They also mediate kanamycin and neomycin resistance. Aminoglycoside phosphotransferases are divided into eight groups according to the resistance of additional specific aminoglycosides (I to VIII) (76, 81). To date, only types I, III, IV, and VII, which mainly mediate kanamycin resistance, have been detected in *Campylobacter*. The *aphA-1* gene, also known as *aph (3′)-Ia*, was identified adjacent to the insertion sequence IS*15*-delta commonly found in Gram-negative bacteria, suggesting that it may have originated from the *Enterobacteriaceae* family of organisms (85). Sequence analysis showed identical homology to the kanamycin resistance gene of the Tn*903* transposon in *E. coli* (85). The *aphA-1* gene is also commonly used as a resistance marker gene in cloning vehicles (81). Different from *aphA-1*, the *aphA-3* gene is commonly detected in Gram-positive bacteria, such as *Staphylococcus*, and has been identified in clinical *Campylobacter* isolates. It is located on plasmids or chromosomes (80, 84). Some plasmids in *C. jejuni* harbor the *aphA-3* gene as part of the resistance cluster that includes the *aadE* and *sat4* genes, which originated from Gram-positive bacteria (86). Subsequently, the *aadE-sat4-aphA-3* cluster together with additional aminoglycoside resistance genes, including *aacA-aphD* and *aac*, was identified in a genomic island on a chromosome of *C. coli* (87). Clonal expansion and horizontal transmission have been involved in dissemination of this novel aminoglycoside resistance genomic island (87). The identification of the *aphA-3* gene in *Campylobacter* provides another piece of evidence suggesting the transfer of antibiotic resistance genes from Gram-positive bacteria to Gram-negative bacteria. The plasmid-encoded *aphA-7* gene, mediating kanamycin resistance, may be an indigenous gene of *Campylobacter* based on its G+C content at 32.8%, which is similar to that of the *Campylobacter* genome (88). The *aphA-7* gene was found on small plasmids of 9.5 and 11.5 kb in *C. jejuni* (89), and the presence of this gene in *C. coli* has also been documented (87).

The *aacA4* gene encodes aminoglycoside 6′-N-acetyltransferase, AAC(6′)-Ib7, conferring resistance to tobramycin, kanamycin, and neomycin (90). Additionally, the *aacA4* gene was associated with class 1 integron and found in *C. jejuni* isolated from the water lines of a broiler chicken house environment (91). The plasmid-borne gene *aac(6′)-Ie/aph(2″)-Ia* (also named *aacA/aphD* and encoding a bifunctional enzyme) was described in a clinical isolate of *C. jejuni* from a U.S. soldier deployed to Thailand. It was found to encode phosphotransferase activity and was named *aph(2″)-If* (92). Gentamicin resistance, conferred by *aacA/aphD* that is associated with an aminoglycoside resistance genomic island, was reported in *C. coli* from China, and clonal expansion may be involved in dissemination of this entire resistance island (87). Subsequently, the gentamicin resistance-related gene *aph(2″)-Ig* (encoding a phosphotransferase) was detected in a *C. coli* isolate from retail chicken meat (93). Recently, several variants of gentamicin resistance genes [*aph(2″)-Ib, Ic, If1, If3, Ih*, and *aac(6′)-Ie/aph(2″)-If2*] were identified in *Campylobacter* isolates from humans and retail meats in the United States. The same resistance profile and similar pulsed-field gel electrophoresis patterns shared by isolates from human and retail chicken indicated that retail chicken is a potential source for gentamicin-resistant *C. coli* that causes infections in humans (94). The increasing prevalence and emergence of novel genes of gentamicin resistance has led to an increasing number of studies on gentamicin resistance mechanisms.

The *sat4* gene encoding a streptothricin acetyltransferase is present either as a single gene or in the *aadE-sat4-aphA-3* cluster in streptothricin-resistant *Campylobacter* spp. (87, 95). The aminoglycoside 3-adenyltransferase gene (*aadA*) confers resistance to streptomycin and spectinomycin, while the aminoglycoside 6-adenyltransferase gene (*aadE*) only confers resistance to streptomycin. The *aadA* gene was identified in the multidrug resistance plasmid pCG8245, which contains various aminoglycoside resistance genes in *C. jejuni* (95). In contrast, *aadE* was commonly associated with the *aadE-sat4-aphA-3* gene cluster that was detected on the plasmid or chromosome of *C. jejuni* and *C. coli* (87, 94, 95). The 286-amino-acid streptomycin resistance protein, ANT(6)-Ib, encoded by *ant(6)-Ib*, belongs to a family of aminoglycoside nucleotidyltransferases and was identified in *Campylobacter fetus* subsp. *fetus* (96). Recently, a novel streptomycin resistance gene was described, and its widespread presence among *C. coli* isolates may partly account for the prevalence of streptomycin resistance in *C. coli* (97).

RESISTANCE TO β-LACTAMS

β-Lactam antibiotics are a class of broad-spectrum antibiotics that inhibit bacterial cell wall biosynthesis. This class of antibiotic agents contains a β-lactam ring in their molecular structures. β-lactam antibiotics are the most widely used antibiotics and account for more than half of the total antibiotic market worldwide (98). For

the past decades, the prevalence of β-lactam-resistant bacteria has greatly increased (99, 100). To date, three mechanisms contributing to β-lactam resistance in *Campylobacter* have been identified: enzymatic inactivation, reduced uptake, and efflux pump. A previous study showed that β-lactamase-positive *Campylobacter* were more resistant than β-lactamase-negative *Campylobacter* to amoxicillin, ampicillin, and ticarcillin (101). OXA-61 (Cj0299) is the only identified and characterized β-lactamase in *C. jejuni* (102–104). Notably, almost half of OXA-61-carrying *Campylobacter* are susceptible to ampicillin, suggesting that the expression level of OXA-61 modulates the resistance phenotype (102). Indeed, a recent study indicated that a G → T transversion in the OXA-61 promoter enhances the expression of β-lactamase and is linked to high-level β-lactam resistance in *C. jejuni* isolates (104). The porins of *C. jejuni* and *C. coli* form a relatively small cation-selective pore that may contribute to intrinsic resistance to antimicrobial agents. These cation-selective pores in *C. jejuni* and *C. coli* are able to exclude most β-lactams with a molecular weight greater than 360 or that are anionic (105). The CmeABC and CmeDEF efflux pumps may also contribute to β-lactam resistance. Inactivation of these efflux pumps results in increased susceptibility to ampicillin (70, 106, 107).

RESISTANCE TO PHENICOLS

Nonfluorinated (chloramphenicol) or fluorinated phenicols (florfenicol) are highly effective against a wide variety of Gram-positive and Gram-negative bacteria. Phenicols were once widely applied in both human and veterinary practices for the prevention and treatment of many bacterial infections. Resistance to phenicols in *Campylobacter* is mediated by enzymatic inactivation via chloramphenicol acetyltransferases, target site mutations in 23S rRNA, target site modification in 23S rRNA via the rRNA methyltransferase Cfr(C), or enhanced extrusion by efflux pumps. Acetylation of the drug by chloramphenicol acetyltransferases (encoded by *cat*) confers resistance to chloramphenicol but not to florfenicol (108). The G2073A mutation in the 23S rRNA gene of *Campylobacter* (corresponding to position 2057 in the 23S rRNA gene of *E. coli*) is associated with chloramphenicol and florfenicol resistance (109). The first *cfr* gene was discovered in a bovine *Staphylococcus sciuri* isolate in 2000 (110). It encodes an rRNA methyltransferase that methylates the adenine at position 2503 in the 23S rRNA, resulting in resistance to five chemically unrelated antimicrobial classes: phenicols, lincosamides, oxazolidinones, pleuromutilins, and streptogramin A (known as the PhLOPSA phenotype) (111). Since its discovery, the *cfr* gene has been detected in a variety of Gram-positive and Gram-negative bacteria (110, 112–116). A recent study identified a novel plasmid-borne *cfr*-like gene, designated *cfr*(C), in multidrug-resistant *C. coli* isolates of cattle origin. Similar to *cfr* and *cfr*(B), the *cfr*(C) gene was found to confer transferable resistance to phenicols and oxazolidinones (linezolid) as well as lincosamides and pleuromutilins (*Campylobacter* is naturally resistant to streptogramin) in both *C. jejuni and C. coli* (117). Additionally, the recently identified multidrug efflux pump variant RE-CmeABC alone can confer elevated resistance to phenicols (see details in "CmeABC" below) (118).

RESISTANCE TO FOSFOMYCIN

Fosfomycin is a broad-spectrum antibiotic with bactericidal activity against both Gram-positive and Gram-negative bacteria (119). Fosfomycin inhibits bacterial cell wall synthesis by inactivating the essential enzyme for the catalysis of bacterial peptidoglycan biosynthesis (120). *Campylobacter* resistance to fosfomycin is rare, and the resistance rate has remained low (121, 122). To date, the only mechanism of fosfomycin resistance identified in *Campylobacter* is the *fosX^{CC}* gene, which encodes a protein that shares 63.9% identity to fosfomycin resistance determinant FosX, found in *Listeria monocytogenes*. FosX inactivates fosfomycin by catalyzing the addition of groups to its epoxide (120, 123). The *fosX^{CC}* gene is contained in the MDRGI in *C. coli*, and is transferrable to *C. jejuni* by natural transformation (43, 123).

RESISTANCE TO ARSENICS

Arsenic compounds have been commonly used in the poultry industry for promoting growth and controlling diseases. Due to their potential risk to human health and the environment, they were recently withdrawn from poultry use in the United States. However, the organic form of arsenic, roxarsone, is still used as a feed additive in other countries. To survive in the poultry production environment, *Campylobacter* has developed ways to resist the action of arsenic compounds. *Campylobacter* isolates from conventional poultry products showed significantly higher levels of arsenic resistance than those from antimicrobial-free poultry products (124). Recently, several arsenic detoxification mechanisms have been identified in *C. jejuni*, including arsenate reductase ArsC, arsenite efflux transporters Acr3 and ArsB, and methylarsenite efflux permease ArsP

(125–128). The two arsenite transporters (Acr3 and ArsB) belong to different families (129) and extrude toxic AS(III) out of bacterial cells. The ArsB family has been found only in bacteria and archaea, while the Acr3 family exists in prokaryotes and fungi, as well as in plant genomes (129–132). As an arsenate reductase, ArsC converts As(V) to AS(III) in the cytoplasm (130, 133), which is subsequently extruded by Acr3 or ArsB transporters (125, 130). Acr3 in *C. jejuni* consists of 347 amino acids and contains 10 predicted transmembrane helices. The presence of the *acr3*-containing operon is significantly associated with elevated resistance to arsenite and arsenate in *Campylobacter*. Furthermore, inactivation of *acr3* leads to reductions in the MICs of both arsenite and arsenate. Acr3 is not involved in the resistance to other classes of antibiotics in *Campylobacter* (125). ArsB in *C. jejuni* consists of 428 amino acids and contains 11 probable transmembrane helices. The amino acid sequence of ArsB is homologous to ArsB in *Shewanella* sp. ANA-3 (134), *S. aureus* (135), *E. coli* (136–138), and *Acidithiobacillus caldus* (139). Inactivation of *arsB* resulted in increased susceptibility of *Campylobacter* to both arsenite and arsenate, but not to other heavy metals and antibiotics (126). Interestingly, analysis of various *Campylobacter* isolates of different animal origins for the distribution of *arsB* and *acr3* genes indicated that all of the tested strains contained at least one of the two genes (126). ArsP in *C. jejuni* consists of 315 amino acids and contains 8 probable transmembrane helices. *arsP* is the first gene in the four-gene *ars* operon, which contains *arsP*, *arsR*, *arsC*, and *acr3*. The presence of ArsP is associated with elevated MIC of roxarsone. Inactivation of *arsP* results in reduced resistance to several organic arsenics including arsanilic acid, nitarsone, and roxarsone (127). It was also revealed that ArsP is an efflux permease for trivalent organoarsenicals including methylarsenite and trivalent forms of aromatic arsenicals (128). ArsP does not play a role in the resistance to inorganic arsenic.

MULTIDRUG EFFLUX PUMPS

The antibiotic efflux transporters play an essential role in the intrinsic and acquired resistance to structurally diverse antimicrobials. In *Campylobacter*, several multidrug efflux pumps (CmeABC, CmeDEF, and CmeG) have been functionally characterized for their contributions to antimicrobial resistance.

CmeABC

CmeABC is the predominant antibiotic efflux system in *C. jejuni* and belongs to the resistance-nodulation-cell division superfamily of multidrug efflux transporters. This efflux system is encoded by a three-gene operon comprising cmeA, cmeB, and cmeC (70) and consists of a membrane fusion protein (CmeA), an inner membrane transporter (CmeB), and an outer membrane protein (CmeC) (70). CmeABC extrudes toxic compounds and contributes to Campylobacter resistance to structurally diverse antimicrobials (70, 71). It should be noted that every component of the CmeABC system is required for its full function as an efflux pump. As mentioned above, CmeABC functions synergistically with other mechanisms in conferring high-level resistance to antibiotics (30, 48, 50, 53, 55, 70, 140, 141). These examples illustrate the important role of CmeABC in conferring resistance to clinically important antibiotics such as macrolide and fluoroquinolone. Interestingly, CmeABC also contributes to resistance to bacteriocins, antimicrobial peptides produced by bacteria (142, 143). As the predominant efflux system in Campylobacter, cmeABC is conserved among different Campylobacter spp. and is widely distributed in Campylobacter isolates (144). This efflux system has been functionally characterized in C. jejuni (70, 71, 145), C. coli (33, 141), Campylobacter lari, C. fetus, and Campylobacter hyointestinals (144) and has been shown to contribute to antibiotic resistance in all examined species. In general, the sequences of cmeABC are highly conserved within a species, but significant sequence polymorphisms are observed in the cmeABC genes among different Campylobacter spp. (144, 146–148). The expression of cmeABC is modulated by a transcriptional regulator called CmeR (149) that functions as a repressor for cmeABC. The cmeABC operon is inducible by bile salts and salicylate (150, 151), and the induction by bile is due to conformational changes in the DNA binding motif of CmeR, releasing its repression on the cmeABC promoter (152–154).

Notably, a potent variant of CmeABC, named RE-CmeABC, has recently emerged in C. jejuni (118). This variant CmeABC is much more powerful in conferring multidrug resistance and is especially potent to florfenicol and chloramphenicol. The RE-CmeABC operon has a unique CmeB sequence that shows only ~80% amino acid sequence identity to CmeB in other C. jejuni strains. The sequence variation in CmeB contributed mostly to the enhanced function of RE-CmeABC. In addition to the enhanced resistance to various antibiotics, RE-CmeABC also promotes the emergence of fluoroquinolone-resistant mutants under selection pressure. In the presence of GyrA mutations, RE-CmeABC confers exceedingly high-level resistance (ciprofloxacin MIC $\geq$ 128 g/ml) to fluoroquinolone

(118). Additionally, Re-CmeABC is increasingly prevalent in C. jejuni isolates in China, suggesting that it facilitates the adaptation of Campylobacter to antibiotic selection pressure.

CmeDEF

CmeDEF is another resistance-nodulation-cell division-type efflux pump identified in C. jejuni. CmeD (Cj1031) is an outer membrane protein of 424 amino acids which shares low but significant sequence homology to HefA of H. pylori and TolC of E. coli, the outer membrane components of antibiotic efflux systems (1). CmeE (Cj1032) is a membrane fusion protein composed of 246 amino acids, which shares significant homology with the membrane fusion protein of HefB in H. pylori. CmeF is an inner membrane transporter and is predicted to contain a 12-transmembrane helical domain structure. The sequence of CmeF (1,005 amino acids) shares certain homology with many other resistance-nodulation-cell division-type efflux transporters such as HefC of H. pylori and AcrB, AcrD, and AcrF of E. coli (1, 155). The low sequence identity between CmeDEF and CmeABC suggests that these two efflux systems may have different functions and abilities to extrude antibiotics and other toxic compounds. Several studies have determined the contribution of cmeDEF to antimicrobial resistance. Pumbwe et al. (106) reported that the insertional mutation of cmeF in Campylobacter resulted in increased susceptibility to structurally unrelated antimicrobial compounds, including ampicillin, ethidium bromide, acridine orange, SDS, sodium deoxycholate, bile, detrimide, and triclosan. Akiba et al. (107) also reported that the cmeF mutant of C. jejuni NCTC 11168 showed a 2-fold decrease in resistance to ampicillin and ethidium bromide, but the authors did not observe any changes in the susceptibility to other tested antimicrobials, including bile salts. Another study, by Ge et al. (33), found that inactivation of cmeF in C. jejuni 81-176 had no effects on susceptibility to ciprofloxaxin, erythromycin, tetracycline, and chloramphenicol. In general, CmeDEF appears to play a modest role in antibiotic resistance in a strain-dependent manner, and its natural function in Campylobacter physiology remains unknown.

CmeG

CmeG (Cj1375) is one of the predicted MFS (major facilitator superfamily) transporters and is present in all the C. jejuni strains sequenced to date. Analysis of its amino acid sequence revealed that CmeG is a homolog of Bmr of B. subtilis and NorA of S. aureus (72), both of which contribute to multidrug resistance in bacteria

(72). In addition, CmeG is predicated to be an inner membrane protein and possesses 12 transmembrane domains. Inactivation of *cmeG* significantly reduced resistance to various classes of antimicrobials, including ciprofloxacin, erythromycin, tetracycline, gentamicin, ethidium bromide, and cholic acid, while overexpression of *cmeG* enhanced the resistance to various fluoroquinolone antimicrobials, including ciprofloxacin, enrofloxacin, norfloxacin, and moxifloxacin but not to the other antibiotics tested in the study (72). Accumulation assays demonstrated that the *cmeG* mutant accumulated more ethidium bromide and ciprofloxacin than the wild-type strain (72). These results indicate that CmeG is a functional efflux transporter in *Campylobacter*. The expression of *cmeG* appears to be regulated by the Fur protein and iron concentrations, because inactivation of Fur or iron depletion resulted in the upregulation of *cmeG* (156–158). The detailed mechanism underlying *cmeG* regulation remains to be determined.

SUMMARY AND PERSPECTIVES

Campylobacter is a major foodborne pathogen, and its resistance to clinically important antibiotics is increasingly prevalent. Particularly, rising fluoroquinolone resistance in *Campylobacter* has been reported in many countries (6), limiting its usage for the treatment of campylobacteriosis. *Campylobacter* is highly mutable to fluoroquinolone treatment, and acquisition of resistance does not incur a fitness cost, contributing to the rapid development and persistence of fluoroquinolone-resistant *Campylobacter* (159). In contrast, development of macrolide resistance in *Campylobacter* occurs slowly and incurs a significant fitness cost in the absence of selection pressure, contributing to the overall low prevalence of macrolide-resistant *Campylobacter*. However, a horizontally transferable *erm*(B) has recently emerged in *Campylobacter* (43–45), which may significantly influence the epidemiology of macrolide-resistant *Campylobacter*. This possibility warrants enhanced efforts to monitor its further spread in *Campylobacter* isolates. Importantly, several new multidrug resistance mechanisms, including MDRGIs, Cfr(C), and RE-CmeABC, have been detected in *Campylobacter*, which greatly increases its ability to cope with selection pressure from multiple antibiotics. These examples illustrate the extraordinary ability of *Campylobacter* to acquire new mechanisms for adaptation to antimicrobial usage. With that said, it is likely that new antibiotic resistance mechanisms will continue to emerge in *Campylobacter*. Thus, innovative strategies are needed to curb the rise and spread of antibiotic-resistant *Campylobacter*.

Acknowledgments. *We apologize to all the investigators whose research could not be appropriately cited owing to space limitations. The work of Zhangqi Shen, Yang Wang, and Jianzhong Shen on antimicrobial resistance genes in* Campylobacter *during 2013–2017 was financially supported by the National Basic Research Program of China (2013CB127200). The work of Qijing Zhang is supported by grant R01AI118283 from the National Institute of Allergy and Infectious Diseases.*

Citation. Shen Z, Wang Y, Zhang Q, Shen J. 2017. Antimicrobial resistance in *Campylobacter* spp. Microbiol Spectrum 6(2):ARBA-0013-2017.

References

1. **WHO.** 2013. The global view of campylobacteriosis. Report of an expert consultation. World Health Organization, Utrecht, The Netherlands, 9–11 July 2012.

2. **Allos BM.** 2001. *Campylobacter jejuni* infections: update on emerging issues and trends. *Clin Infect Dis* 32: 1201–1206.

3. **Engberg J, Aarestrup FM, Taylor DE, Gerner-Smidt P, Nachamkin I.** 2001. Quinolone and macrolide resistance in *Campylobacter jejuni* and C. *coli*: resistance mechanisms and trends in human isolates. *Emerg Infect Dis* 7:24–34.

4. **Payot S, Bolla JM, Corcoran D, Fanning S, Mégraud F, Zhang Q.** 2006. Mechanisms of fluoroquinolone and macrolide resistance in *Campylobacter* spp. *Microbes Infect* 8:1967–1971.

5. **Luangtongkum T, Jeon B, Han J, Plummer P, Logue CM, Zhang Q.** 2009. Antibiotic resistance in *Campylobacter*: emergence, transmission and persistence. *Future Microbiol* 4:189–200.

6. **Blaser M, Engberg J.** 2008. Clinical aspects of *Campylobacter jejuni* and *Campylobacter coli* infections, p 99–121. *In* Nachamkin I, Szymanski CM, Blaser MJ (eds), *Campylobacter*, 3rd ed. ASM Press, Washington, DC.

7. **Altekruse SF, Tollefson LK.** 2003. Human campylobacteriosis: a challenge for the veterinary profession. *J Am Vet Med Assoc* 223:445–452.

8. **Wieczorek K, Denis E, Lynch O, Osek J.** 2013. Molecular characterization and antibiotic resistance profiling of *Campylobacter* isolated from cattle in Polish slaughterhouses. *Food Microbiol* 34:130–136.

9. **Sanad YM, Closs G Jr, Kumar A, LeJeune JT, Rajashekara G.** 2013. Molecular epidemiology and public health relevance of *Campylobacter* isolated from dairy cattle and European starlings in Ohio, USA. *Foodborne Pathog Dis* 10:229–236.

10. **Châtre P, Haenni M, Meunier D, Botrel MA, Calavas D, Madec JY.** 2010. Prevalence and antimicrobial resistance of *Campylobacter jejuni* and *Campylobacter coli* isolated from cattle between 2002 and 2006 inFrance. *J Food Prot* 73:825–831.

11. **Hakkinen M, Heiska H, Hänninen ML.** 2007. Prevalence of *Campylobacter* spp. in cattle in Finland and

antimicrobial susceptibilities of bovine *Campylobacter jejuni* strains. *Appl Environ Microbiol* 73:3232–3238.

12. Englen MD, Hill AE, Dargatz DA, Ladely SR, Fedorka-Cray PJ. 2007. Prevalence and antimicrobial resistance of *Campylobacter* in US dairy cattle. *J Appl Microbiol* 102:1570–1577.

13. Jesse TW, Englen MD, Pittenger-Alley LG, Fedorka-Cray PJ. 2006. Two distinct mutations in *gyrA* lead to ciprofloxacin and nalidixic acid resistance in *Campylobacter coli* and *Campylobacter jejuni* isolated from chickens and beef cattle. *J Appl Microbiol* 100:682–688.

14. Inglis GD, Morck DW, McAllister TA, Entz T, Olson ME, Yanke LJ, Read RR. 2006. Temporal prevalence of antimicrobial resistance in *Campylobacter* spp. from beef cattle in Alberta feedlots. *Appl Environ Microbiol* 72:4088–4095.

15. Bae W, Kaya KN, Hancock DD, Call DR, Park YH, Besser TE. 2005. Prevalence and antimicrobial resistance of thermophilic *Campylobacter* spp. from cattle farms in Washington State. *Appl Environ Microbiol* 71:169–174.

16. Iovine NM. 2013. Resistance mechanisms in *Campylobacter jejuni*. *Virulence* 4:230–240.

17. Wieczorek K, Osek J. 2013. Antimicrobial resistance mechanisms among *Campylobacter*. *BioMed Res Int* 2013:1.

18. Zhang Q, Plummer P. 2008. Mechanisms of antibiotic resistance in *Campylobacter*, p 263–276. *In* Nachamkin I, Szymanski CM, Blaser MJ (eds), *Campylobacter*, 3rd ed. ASM Press, Washington, DC.

19. Shen Z, Su C, Yu E, Zhang Q. 2013. Multidrug efflux transporters in *Campylobacter*, p 223–235. *In* Yu EW, Zhang Q, Brown MH (eds), *Microbial Efflux Pumps: Current Research*. Caister Academic Press, Norfolk, United Kingdom.

20. Appelbaum PC, Hunter PA. 2000. The fluoroquinolone antibacterials: past, present and future perspectives. *Int J Antimicrob Agents* 16:5–15.

21. Hooper DC. 1998. Clinical applications of quinolones. *Biochim Biophys Acta* 1400:45–61.

22. Martinez M, McDermott P, Walker R. 2006. Pharmacology of the fluoroquinolones: a perspective for the use in domestic animals. *Vet J* 172:10–28.

23. Oliphant CM, Green GM. 2002. Quinolones: a comprehensive review. *Am Fam Physician* 65:455–464.

24. Redgrave LS, Sutton SB, Webber MA, Piddock LJ. 2014. Fluoroquinolone resistance: mechanisms, impact on bacteria, and role in evolutionary success. *Trends Microbiol* 22:438–445.

25. Hooper DC. 1999. Mechanisms of fluoroquinolone resistance. *Drug Resist Updat* 2:38–55.

26. Hooper DC. 2001. Emerging mechanisms of fluoroquinolone resistance. *Emerg Infect Dis* 7:337–341.

27. Payot S, Cloeckaert A, Chaslus-Dancla E. 2002. Selection and characterization of fluoroquinolone-resistant mutants of *Campylobacter jejuni* using enrofloxacin. *Microb Drug Resist* 8:335–343.

28. Piddock LJ, Ricci V, Pumbwe L, Everett MJ, Griggs DJ. 2003. Fluoroquinolone resistance in *Campylobacter*

species from man and animals: detection of mutations in topoisomerase genes. *J Antimicrob Chemother* 51:19–26.

29. Bachoual R, Ouabdesselam S, Mory F, Lascols C, Soussy CJ, Tankovic J. 2001. Single or double mutational alterations of *gyrA* associated with fluoroquinolone resistance in *Campylobacter jejuni* and *Campylobacter coli*. *Microb Drug Resist* 7:257–261.

30. Luo N, Sahin O, Lin J, Michel LO, Zhang Q. 2003. *In vivo* selection of *Campylobacter* isolates with high levels of fluoroquinolone resistance associated with *gyrA* mutations and the function of the CmeABC efflux pump. *Antimicrob Agents Chemother* 47:390–394.

31. Cooper R, Segal H, Lastovica AJ, Elisha BG. 2002. Genetic basis of quinolone resistance and epidemiology of resistant and susceptible isolates of porcine *Campylobacter coli* strains. *J Appl Microbiol* 93:241–249.

32. Parkhill J, Wren BW, Mungall K, Ketley JM, Churcher C, Basham D, Chillingworth T, Davies RM, Feltwell T, Holroyd S, Jagels K, Karlyshev AV, Moule S, Pallen MJ, Penn CW, Quail MA, Rajandream MA, Rutherford KM, van Vliet AH, Whitehead S, Barrell BG. 2000. The genome sequence of the food-borne pathogen *Campylobacter jejuni* reveals hypervariable sequences. *Nature* 403:665–668.

33. Ge B, McDermott PF, White DG, Meng J. 2005. Role of efflux pumps and topoisomerase mutations in fluoroquinolone resistance in *Campylobacter jejuni* and *Campylobacter coli*. *Antimicrob Agents Chemother* 49:3347–3354.

34. Zhang Q, Lin J, Pereira S. 2003. Fluoroquinolone-resistant *Campylobacter* in animal reservoirs: dynamics of development, resistance mechanisms and ecological fitness. *Anim Health Res Rev* 4:63–71.

35. Hänninen ML, Hannula M. 2007. Spontaneous mutation frequency and emergence of ciprofloxacin resistance in *Campylobacter jejuni* and *Campylobacter coli*. *J Antimicrob Chemother* 60:1251–1257.

36. Smith JL, Fratamico PM. 2010. Fluoroquinolone resistance in *campylobacter*. *J Food Prot* 73:1141–1152.

37. Chu DT. 1999. Recent developments in macrolides and ketolides. *Curr Opin Microbiol* 2:467–474.

38. McEwen SA, Fedorka-Cray PJ. 2002. Antimicrobial use and resistance in animals. *Clin Infect Dis* 34(Suppl 3):S93–S106.

39. Brisson-Noel A, Trieu-Cuot P, Courvalin P. 1988. Mechanism of action of spiramycin and other macrolides. *J Antimicrob Chemother* 22(Suppl B):13–23.

40. Poehlsgaard J, Douthwaite S. 2005. The bacterial ribosome as a target for antibiotics. *Nat Rev Microbiol* 3:870–881.

41. Gibreel A, Taylor DE. 2006. Macrolide resistance in *Campylobacter jejuni* and *Campylobacter coli*. *J Antimicrob Chemother* 58:243–255.

42. Roe DE, Weinberg A, Roberts MC. 1995. Mobile rRNA methylase genes in *Campylobacter* (Wolinella) rectus. *J Antimicrob Chemother* 36:738–740.

43. Wang Y, Zhang M, Deng F, Shen Z, Wu C, Zhang J, Zhang Q, Shen J. 2014. Emergence of multidrug-

resistant *Campylobacter* species isolates with a horizontally acquired rRNA methylase. *Antimicrob Agents Chemother* 58:5405–5412.

44. Qin S, Wang Y, Zhang Q, Zhang M, Deng F, Shen Z, Wu C, Wang S, Zhang J, Shen J. 2014. Report of ribosomal RNA methylase gene *erm*(B) in multidrug-resistant *Campylobacter coli*. *J Antimicrob Chemother* 69:964–968.

45. Deng F, Wang Y, Zhang Y, Shen Z. 2015. Characterization of the genetic environment of the ribosomal RNA methylase gene *erm*(B) in *Campylobacter jejuni*. *J Antimicrob Chemother* 70:613–615.

46. Corcoran D, Quinn T, Cotter L, Fanning S. 2006. An investigation of the molecular mechanisms contributing to high-level erythromycin resistance in *Campylobacter*. *Int J Antimicrob Agents* 27:40–45.

47. Gibreel A, Kos VN, Keelan M, Trieber CA, Levesque S, Michaud S, Taylor DE. 2005. Macrolide resistance in *Campylobacter jejuni* and *Campylobacter coli*: molecular mechanism and stability of the resistance phenotype. *Antimicrob Agents Chemother* 49:2753–2759.

48. Lin J, Yan M, Sahin O, Pereira S, Chang YJ, Zhang Q. 2007. Effect of macrolide usage on emergence of erythromycin-resistant *Campylobacter* isolates in chickens. *Antimicrob Agents Chemother* 51:1678–1686.

49. Mamelli L, Prouzet-Mauléon V, Pagès JM, Mégraud F, Bolla JM. 2005. Molecular basis of macrolide resistance in *Campylobacter*: role of efflux pumps and target mutations. *J Antimicrob Chemother* 56:491–497.

50. Caldwell DB, Wang Y, Lin J. 2008. Development, stability, and molecular mechanisms of macrolide resistance in *Campylobacter jejuni*. *Antimicrob Agents Chemother* 52:3947–3954.

51. Fouts DE, Mongodin EF, Mandrell RE, Miller WG, Rasko DA, Ravel J, Brinkac LM, DeBoy RT, Parker CT, Daugherty SC, Dodson RJ, Durkin AS, Madupu R, Sullivan SA, Shetty JU, Ayodeji MA, Shvartsbeyn A, Schatz MC, Badger JH, Fraser CM, Nelson KE. 2005. Major structural differences and novel potential virulence mechanisms from the genomes of multiple *Campylobacter* species. *PLoS Biol* 3:e15.

52. Vacher S, Menard A, Bernard E, Santos A, Megraud F. 2005. Detection of mutations associated with macrolide resistance in thermophilic *Campylobacter* spp. by real-time PCR. *Microb Drug Resist* 11:40–47.

53. Cagliero C, Mouline C, Cloeckaert A, Payot S. 2006. Synergy between efflux pump CmeABC and modifications in ribosomal proteins L4 and L22 in conferring macrolide resistance in *Campylobacter jejuni* and *Campylobacter coli*. *Antimicrob Agents Chemother* 50:3893–3896.

54. Kurincic M, Botteldoorn N, Herman L, Smole Mozina S. 2007. Mechanisms of erythromycin resistance of *Campylobacter* spp. isolated from food, animals and humans. *Int J Food Microbiol* 120:186–190.

55. Gibreel A, Wetsch NM, Taylor DE. 2007. Contribution of the CmeABC efflux pump to macrolide and tetracycline resistance in *Campylobacter jejuni*. *Antimicrob Agents Chemother* 51:3212–3216.

56. Payot S, Avrain L, Magras C, Praud K, Cloeckaert A, Chaslus-Dancla E. 2004. Relative contribution of target gene mutation and efflux to fluoroquinolone and erythromycin resistance, in French poultry and pig isolates of *Campylobacter coli*. *Int J Antimicrob Agents* 23:468–472.

57. Chopra I, Roberts M. 2001. Tetracycline antibiotics: mode of action, applications, molecular biology, and epidemiology of bacterial resistance. *Microbiol Mol Biol Rev* 65:232–260.

58. Epe B, Woolley P, Hornig H. 1987. Competition between tetracycline and tRNA at both P and A sites of the ribosome of *Escherichia coli*. *FEBS Lett* 213:443–447.

59. Li W, Atkinson GC, Thakor NS, Allas U, Lu CC, Chan KY, Tenson T, Schulten K, Wilson KS, Hauryliuk V, Frank J. 2013. Mechanism of tetracycline resistance by ribosomal protection protein Tet(O). *Nat Commun* 4:1477.

60. Connell SR, Tracz DM, Nierhaus KH, Taylor DE. 2003. Ribosomal protection proteins and their mechanism of tetracycline resistance. *Antimicrob Agents Chemother* 47:3675–3681.

61. Roberts MC. 2005. Update on acquired tetracycline resistance genes. *FEMS Microbiol Lett* 245:195–203.

62. Dönhöfer A, Franckenberg S, Wickles S, Berninghausen O, Beckmann R, Wilson DN. 2012. Structural basis for TetM-mediated tetracycline resistance. *Proc Natl Acad Sci USA* 109:16900–16905.

63. Margus T, Remm M, Tenson T. 2007. Phylogenetic distribution of translational GTPases in bacteria. *BMC Genomics* 8:15.

64. Connell SR, Trieber CA, Dinos GP, Einfeldt E, Taylor DE, Nierhaus KH. 2003. Mechanism of Tet(O)-mediated tetracycline resistance. *EMBO J* 22:945–953.

65. Taylor DE, Courvalin P. 1988. Mechanisms of antibiotic resistance in *Campylobacter* species. *Antimicrob Agents Chemother* 32:1107–1112.

66. Taylor DE, Garner RS, Allan BJ. 1983. Characterization of tetracycline resistance plasmids from *Campylobacter jejuni* and *Campylobacter coli*. *Antimicrob Agents Chemother* 24:930–935.

67. Taylor DE. 1986. Plasmid-mediated tetracycline resistance in *Campylobacter jejuni*: expression in *Escherichia coli* and identification of homology with streptococcal class M determinant. *J Bacteriol* 165:1037–1039.

68. Batchelor RA, Pearson BM, Friis LM, Guerry P, Wells JM. 2004. Nucleotide sequences and comparison of two large conjugative plasmids from different *Campylobacter* species. *Microbiology* 150:3507–3517.

69. Sahin O, Plummer PJ, Jordan DM, Sulaj K, Pereira S, Robbe-Austerman S, Wang L, Yaeger MJ, Hoffman LJ, Zhang Q. 2008. Emergence of a tetracycline-resistant *Campylobacter jejuni* clone associated with outbreaks of ovine abortion in the United States. *J Clin Microbiol* 46:1663–1671.

70. Lin J, Michel LO, Zhang Q. 2002. CmeABC functions as a multidrug efflux system in *Campylobacter jejuni*. *Antimicrob Agents Chemother* 46:2124–2131.

71. Pumbwe L, Piddock LJ. 2002. Identification and molecular characterisation of CmeB, a *Campylobacter jejuni* multidrug efflux pump. *FEMS Microbiol Lett* **206:**185–189.

72. Jeon B, Wang Y, Hao H, Barton YW, Zhang Q. 2011. Contribution of CmeG to antibiotic and oxidative stress resistance in *Campylobacter jejuni*. *J Antimicrob Chemother* **66:**79–85.

73. Spahn CM, Schäfer MA, Krayevsky AA, Nierhaus KH. 1996. Conserved nucleotides of 23 S rRNA located at the ribosomal peptidyltransferase center. *J Biol Chem* **271:**32857–32862.

74. Jana S, Deb JK. 2006. Molecular understanding of aminoglycoside action and resistance. *Appl Microbiol Biotechnol* **70:**140–150.

75. Magnet S, Blanchard JS. 2005. Molecular insights into aminoglycoside action and resistance. *Chem Rev* **105:**477–498.

76. Smith CA, Baker EN. 2002. Aminoglycoside antibiotic resistance by enzymatic deactivation. *Curr Drug Targets Infect Disord* **2:**143–160.

77. Lawrence PK, Kittichotirat W, McDermott JE, Bumgarner RE. 2010. A three-way comparative genomic analysis of *Mannheimia haemolytica* isolates. *BMC Genomics* **11:**535.

78. Vakulenko SB, Mobashery S. 2003. Versatility of aminoglycosides and prospects for their future. *Clin Microbiol Rev* **16:**430–450.

79. Tenover FC, Elvrum PM. 1988. Detection of two different kanamycin resistance genes in naturally occurring isolates of *Campylobacter jejuni* and *Campylobacter coli*. *Antimicrob Agents Chemother* **32:**1170–1173.

80. Gibreel A, Sköld O, Taylor DE. 2004. Characterization of plasmid-mediated *aphA-3* kanamycin resistance in *Campylobacter jejuni*. *Microb Drug Resist* **10:**98–105.

81. Ramirez MS, Tolmasky ME. 2010. Aminoglycoside modifying enzymes. *Drug Resist Updat* **13:**151–171.

82. Doi Y, Arakawa Y. 2007. 16S ribosomal RNA methylation: emerging resistance mechanism against aminoglycosides. *Clin Infect Dis* **45:**88–94.

83. Overhage J, Bains M, Brazas MD, Hancock RE. 2008. Swarming of *Pseudomonas aeruginosa* is a complex adaptation leading to increased production of virulence factors and antibiotic resistance. *J Bacteriol* **190:**2671–2679.

84. Lambert T, Gerbaud G, Trieu-Cuot P, Courvalin P. 1985. Structural relationship between the genes encoding 3′-aminoglycoside phosphotransferases in *Campylobacter* and in Gram-positive cocci. *Ann Inst Pasteur Microbiol 1985* **136B:**135–150.

85. Ouellette M, Gerbaud G, Lambert T, Courvalin P. 1987. Acquisition by a *Campylobacter*-like strain of *aphA-1*, a kanamycin resistance determinant from members of the family *Enterobacteriaceae*. *Antimicrob Agents Chemother* **31:**1021–1026.

86. Gibreel A, Tracz DM, Nonaka L, Ngo TM, Connell SR, Taylor DE. 2004. Incidence of antibiotic resistance in *Campylobacter jejuni* isolated in Alberta, Canada, from 1999 to 2002, with special reference to *tet*(O)-mediated tetracycline resistance. *Antimicrob Agents Chemother* **48:**3442–3450.

87. Qin S, Wang Y, Zhang Q, Chen X, Shen Z, Deng F, Wu C, Shen J. 2012. Identification of a novel genomic island conferring resistance to multiple aminoglycoside antibiotics in *Campylobacter coli*. *Antimicrob Agents Chemother* **56:**5332–5339.

88. Tenover FC, Gilbert T, O'Hara P. 1989. Nucleotide sequence of a novel kanamycin resistance gene, *aphA-7*, from *Campylobacter jejuni* and comparison to other kanamycin phosphotransferase genes. *Plasmid* **22:**52–58.

89. Tenover FC, Fennell CL, Lee L, LeBlanc DJ. 1992. Characterization of two plasmids from *Campylobacter jejuni* isolates that carry the *aphA-7* kanamycin resistance determinant. *Antimicrob Agents Chemother* **36:**712–716.

90. Rather PN, Munayyer H, Mann PA, Hare RS, Miller GH, Shaw KJ. 1992. Genetic analysis of bacterial acetyltransferases: identification of amino acids determining the specificities of the aminoglycoside 6′-N-acetyltransferase Ib and IIa proteins. *J Bacteriol* **174:**3196–3203.

91. Lee MD, Sanchez S, Zimmer M, Idris U, Berrang ME, McDermott PF. 2002. Class 1 integron-associated tobramycin-gentamicin resistance in *Campylobacter jejuni* isolated from the broiler chicken house environment. *Antimicrob Agents Chemother* **46:**3660–3664.

92. Toth M, Frase H, Antunes NT, Vakulenko SB. 2013. Novel aminoglycoside 2″ phosphotransferase identified in a Gram-negative pathogen. *Antimicrob Agents Chemother* **57:**452–457.

93. Chen Y, Mukherjee S, Hoffmann M, Kotewicz ML, Young S, Abbott J, Luo Y, Davidson MK, Allard M, McDermott P, Zhao S. 2013. Whole-genome sequencing of gentamicin-resistant *Campylobacter coli* isolated from U.S. retail meats reveals novel plasmid-mediated aminoglycoside resistance genes. *Antimicrob Agents Chemother* **57:**5398–5405.

94. Zhao S, Mukherjee S, Chen Y, Li C, Young S, Warren M, Abbott J, Friedman S, Kabera C, Karlsson M, McDermott PF. 2015. Novel gentamicin resistance genes in *Campylobacter* isolated from humans and retail meats in the USA. *J Antimicrob Chemother* **70:**1314–1321.

95. Nirdnoy W, Mason CJ, Guerry P. 2005. Mosaic structure of a multiple-drug-resistant, conjugative plasmid from *Campylobacter jejuni*. *Antimicrob Agents Chemother* **49:**2454–2459.

96. Abril C, Brodard I, Perreten V. 2010. Two novel antibiotic resistance genes, *tet*(44) and *ant(6)-Ib*, are located within a transferable pathogenicity island in *Campylobacter fetus* subsp. *fetus*. *Antimicrob Agents Chemother* **54:**3052–3055.

97. Olkkola S, Culebro A, Juntunen P, Hänninen ML, Rossi M. 2016. Functional genomics in *Campylobacter coli* identified a novel streptomycin resistance gene located in a hypervariable genomic region. *Microbiology* **162:**1157–1166.

98. Hamad B. 2010. The antibiotics market. *Nat Rev Drug Discov* **9:**675–676.

99. Wise R. 2002. Antimicrobial resistance: priorities for action. *J Antimicrob Chemother* 49:585–586.

100. Jovetic S, Zhu Y, Marcone GL, Marinelli F, Tramper J. 2010. β-Lactam and glycopeptide antibiotics: first and last line of defense? *Trends Biotechnol* 28:596–604.

101. Lachance N, Gaudreau C, Lamothe F, Larivière LA. 1991. Role of the beta-lactamase of *Campylobacter jejuni* in resistance to beta-lactam agents. *Antimicrob Agents Chemother* 35:813–818.

102. Griggs DJ, Peake L, Johnson MM, Ghori S, Mott A, Piddock LJ. 2009. Beta-lactamase-mediated beta-lactam resistance in *Campylobacter* species: prevalence of Cj0299 (*bla*OXA-61) and evidence for a novel beta-lactamase in *C. jejuni*. *Antimicrob Agents Chemother* 53:3357–3364.

103. Alfredson DA, Korolik V. 2005. Isolation and expression of a novel molecular class D beta-lactamase, OXA-61, from *Campylobacter jejuni*. *Antimicrob Agents Chemother* 49:2515–2518.

104. Zeng X, Brown S, Gillespie B, Lin J. 2014. A single nucleotide in the promoter region modulates the expression of the β-lactamase OXA-61 in *Campylobacter jejuni*. *J Antimicrob Chemother* 69:1215–1223.

105. Page WJ, Huyer G, Huyer M, Worobec EA. 1989. Characterization of the porins of *Campylobacter jejuni* and *Campylobacter coli* and implications for antibiotic susceptibility. *Antimicrob Agents Chemother* 33:297–303.

106. Pumbwe L, Randall LP, Woodward MJ, Piddock LJ. 2004. Expression of the efflux pump genes *cmeB*, *cmeF* and the porin gene *porA* in multiple-antibiotic-resistant *Campylobacter jejuni*. *J Antimicrob Chemother* 54:341–347.

107. Akiba M, Lin J, Barton YW, Zhang Q. 2006. Interaction of CmeABC and CmeDEF in conferring antimicrobial resistance and maintaining cell viability in *Campylobacter jejuni*. *J Antimicrob Chemother* 57:52–60.

108. Wang Y, Taylor DE. 1990. Chloramphenicol resistance in *Campylobacter coli*: nucleotide sequence, expression, and cloning vector construction. *Gene* 94:23–28.

109. Ma L, Shen Z, Naren G, Li H, Xia X, Wu C, Shen J, Zhang Q, Wang Y. 2014. Identification of a novel G2073A mutation in 23S rRNA in amphenicol-selected mutants of *Campylobacter jejuni*. *PLoS One* 9:e94503.

110. Schwarz S, Werckenthin C, Kehrenberg C. 2000. Identification of a plasmid-borne chloramphenicol-florfenicol resistance gene in *Staphylococcus sciuri*. *Antimicrob Agents Chemother* 44:2530–2533.

111. Long KS, Poehlsgaard J, Kehrenberg C, Schwarz S, Vester B. 2006. The Cfr rRNA methyltransferase confers resistance to phenicols, lincosamides, oxazolidinones, pleuromutilins, and streptogramin A antibiotics. *Antimicrob Agents Chemother* 50:2500–2505.

112. Liu Y, Wang Y, Schwarz S, Li Y, Shen Z, Zhang Q, Wu C, Shen J. 2013. Transferable multiresistance plasmids carrying *cfr* in *Enterococcus* spp. from swine and farm environment. *Antimicrob Agents Chemother* 57:42–48.

113. Dai L, Wu CM, Wang MG, Wang Y, Wang Y, Huang SY, Xia LN, Li BB, Shen JZ. 2010. First report of the multidrug resistance gene *cfr* and the phenicol resistance gene *fexA* in a *Bacillus* strain from swine feces. *Antimicrob Agents Chemother* 54:3953–3955.

114. Wang Y, Wang Y, Schwarz S, Shen Z, Zhou N, Lin J, Wu C, Shen J. 2012. Detection of the staphylococcal multiresistance gene *cfr* in *Macrococcus caseolyticus* and *Jeotgalicoccus pinnipedialis*. *J Antimicrob Chemother* 67:1824–1827.

115. Wang Y, He T, Schwarz S, Zhou D, Shen Z, Wu C, Wang Y, Ma L, Zhang Q, Shen J. 2012. Detection of the staphylococcal multiresistance gene *cfr* in *Escherichia coli* of domestic-animal origin. *J Antimicrob Chemother* 67:1094–1098.

116. Shen J, Wang Y, Schwarz S. 2013. Presence and dissemination of the multiresistance gene *cfr* in Gram-positive and Gram-negative bacteria. *J Antimicrob Chemother* 68:1697–1706.

117. Tang Y, Dai L, Sahin O, Wu Z, Liu M, Zhang Q. 2017. Emergence of a plasmid-borne multidrug resistance gene *cfr*(C) in foodborne pathogen *Campylobacter*. *J Antimicrob Chemother* 72:1581–1588.

118. Yao H, Shen Z, Wang Y, Deng F, Liu D, Naren G, Dai L, Su CC, Wang B, Wang S, Wu C, Yu EW, Zhang Q, Shen J. 2016. Emergence of a potent multidrug efflux pump variant that enhances *Campylobacter* resistance to multiple antibiotics. *MBio* 7:e01543–e16.

119. Forsgren A, Walder M. 1983. Antimicrobial activity of fosfomycin *in vitro*. *J Antimicrob Chemother* 11:467–471.

120. Fillgrove KL, Pakhomova S, Newcomer ME, Armstrong RN. 2003. Mechanistic diversity of fosfomycin resistance in pathogenic microorganisms. *J Am Chem Soc* 125:15730–15731.

121. Schwaiger K, Schmied EM, Bauer J. 2008. Comparative analysis of antibiotic resistance characteristics of Gram-negative bacteria isolated from laying hens and eggs in conventional and organic keeping systems in Bavaria, Germany. *Zoonoses Public Health* 55:331–341.

122. Gomez-Garces JL, Cogollos R, Alos JL. 1995. Susceptibilities of fluoroquinolone-resistant strains of *Campylobacter jejuni* to 11 oral antimicrobial agents. *Antimicrob Agents Chemother* 39:542–544.

123. Wang Y, Yao H, Deng F, Liu D, Zhang Y, Shen Z. 2015. Identification of a novel *fosX*^{CC} gene conferring fosfomycin resistance in *Campylobacter*. *J Antimicrob Chemother* 70:1261–1263.

124. Sapkota AR, Price LB, Silbergeld EK, Schwab KJ. 2006. Arsenic resistance in *Campylobacter* spp. isolated from retail poultry products. *Appl Environ Microbiol* 72:3069–3071.

125. Wang L, Jeon B, Sahin O, Zhang Q. 2009. Identification of an arsenic resistance and arsenic-sensing system in *Campylobacter jejuni*. *Appl Environ Microbiol* 75:5064–5073.

126. Shen Z, Han J, Wang Y, Sahin O, Zhang Q. 2013. The contribution of ArsB to arsenic resistance in *Campylobacter jejuni*. *PLoS One* 8:e58894.

127. Shen Z, Luangtongkum T, Qiang Z, Jeon B, Wang L, Zhang Q. 2014. Identification of a novel membrane transporter mediating resistance to organic arsenic in *Campylobacter jejuni*. *Antimicrob Agents Chemother* 58:2021–2029.

128. Chen J, Madegowda M, Bhattacharjee H, Rosen BP. 2015. ArsP: a methylarsenite efflux permease. *Mol Microbiol* 98:625–635.

129. Rosen BP. 1999. Families of arsenic transporters. *Trends Microbiol* 7:207–212.

130. Rosen BP. 2002. Biochemistry of arsenic detoxification. *FEBS Lett* 529:86–92.

131. Indriolo E, Na G, Ellis D, Salt DE, Banks JA. 2010. A vacuolar arsenite transporter necessary for arsenic tolerance in the arsenic hyperaccumulating fern *Pteris vittata* is missing in flowering plants. *Plant Cell* 22:2045–2057.

132. Fu HL, Meng Y, Ordóñez E, Villadangos AF, Bhattacharjee H, Gil JA, Mateos LM, Rosen BP. 2009. Properties of arsenic efflux permeases (Acr3) from *Alkaliphilus metalliredigens* and *Corynebacterium glutamicum*. *J Biol Chem* 284:19887–19895.

133. Ji G, Silver S. 1992. Reduction of arsenate to arsenite by the ArsC protein of the arsenic resistance operon of *Staphylococcus aureus* plasmid pI258. *Proc Natl Acad Sci USA* 89:9474–9478.

134. Saltikov CW, Cifuentes A, Venkateswaran K, Newman DK. 2003. The *ars* detoxification system is advantageous but not required for As(V) respiration by the genetically tractable *Shewanella* species strain ANA-3. *Appl Environ Microbiol* 69:2800–2809.

135. Ji G, Silver S. 1992. Regulation and expression of the arsenic resistance operon from *Staphylococcus aureus* plasmid pI258. *J Bacteriol* 174:3684–3694.

136. Chen CM, Misra TK, Silver S, Rosen BP. 1986. Nucleotide sequence of the structural genes for an anion pump. The plasmid-encoded arsenical resistance operon. *J Biol Chem* 261:15030–15038.

137. San Francisco MJ, Tisa LS, Rosen BP. 1989. Identification of the membrane component of the anion pump encoded by the arsenical resistance operon of R-factor R773. *Mol Microbiol* 3:15–21.

138. Tisa LS, Rosen BP. 1990. Molecular characterization of an anion pump. The ArsB protein is the membrane anchor for the ArsA protein. *J Biol Chem* 265:190–194.

139. Tuffin IM, de Groot P, Deane SM, Rawlings DE. 2005. An unusual Tn21-like transposon containing an ars operon is present in highly arsenic-resistant strains of the biomining bacterium *Acidithiobacillus caldus*. *Microbiology* 151:3027–3039.

140. Piddock LJ, Griggs D, Johnson MM, Ricci V, Elviss NC, Williams LK, Jørgensen F, Chisholm SA, Lawson AJ, Swift C, Humphrey TJ, Owen RJ. 2008. Persistence of *Campylobacter* species, strain types, antibiotic resistance and mechanisms of tetracycline resistance in poultry flocks treated with chlortetracycline. *J Antimicrob Chemother* 62:303–315.

141. Cagliero C, Mouline C, Payot S, Cloeckaert A. 2005. Involvement of the CmeABC efflux pump in the macrolide resistance of *Campylobacter coli*. *J Antimicrob Chemother* 56:948–950.

142. Hoang KV, Stern NJ, Lin J. 2011. Development and stability of bacteriocin resistance in *Campylobacter* spp. *J Appl Microbiol* 111:1544–1550.

143. Hoang KV, Stern NJ, Saxton AM, Xu F, Zeng X, Lin J. 2011. Prevalence, development, and molecular mechanisms of bacteriocin resistance in *Campylobacter*. *Appl Environ Microbiol* 77:2309–2316.

144. Guo B, Lin J, Reynolds DL, Zhang Q. 2010. Contribution of the multidrug efflux transporter CmeABC to antibiotic resistance in different *Campylobacter* species. *Foodborne Pathog Dis* 7:77–83.

145. Lin J, Sahin O, Michel LO, Zhang Q. 2003. Critical role of multidrug efflux pump CmeABC in bile resistance and *in vivo* colonization of *Campylobacter jejuni*. *Infect Immun* 71:4250–4259.

146. Olah PA, Doetkott C, Fakhr MK, Logue CM. 2006. Prevalence of the *Campylobacter* multi-drug efflux pump (CmeABC) in *Campylobacter* spp. Isolated from freshly processed turkeys. *Food Microbiol* 23:453–460.

147. Cagliero C, Cloix L, Cloeckaert A, Payot S. 2006. High genetic variation in the multidrug transporter *cmeB* gene in *Campylobacter jejuni* and *Campylobacter coli*. *J Antimicrob Chemother* 58:168–172.

148. Fakhr MK, Logue CM. 2007. Sequence variation in the outer membrane protein-encoding gene *cmeC*, conferring multidrug resistance among *Campylobacter jejuni* and *Campylobacter coli* strains isolated from different hosts. *J Clin Microbiol* 45:3381–3383.

149. Lin J, Akiba M, Sahin O, Zhang Q. 2005. CmeR functions as a transcriptional repressor for the multidrug efflux pump CmeABC in *Campylobacter jejuni*. *Antimicrob Agents Chemother* 49:1067–1075.

150. Lin J, Cagliero C, Guo B, Barton YW, Maurel MC, Payot S, Zhang Q. 2005. Bile salts modulate expression of the CmeABC multidrug efflux pump in *Campylobacter jejuni*. *J Bacteriol* 187:7417–7424.

151. Shen Z, Pu XY, Zhang Q. 2011. Salicylate functions as an efflux pump inducer and promotes the emergence of fluoroquinolone-resistant *Campylobacter jejuni* mutants. *Appl Environ Microbiol* 77:7128–7133.

152. Gu R, Su CC, Shi F, Li M, McDermott G, Zhang Q, Yu EW. 2007. Crystal structure of the transcriptional regulator CmeR from *Campylobacter jejuni*. *J Mol Biol* 372:583–593.

153. Lei HT, Shen Z, Surana P, Routh MD, Su CC, Zhang Q, Yu EW. 2011. Crystal structures of CmeR-bile acid complexes from *Campylobacter jejuni*. *Protein Sci* 20:712–723.

154. Routh MD, Su CC, Zhang Q, Yu EW. 2009. Structures of AcrR and CmeR: insight into the mechanisms of transcriptional repression and multi-drug recognition in the TetR family of regulators. *Biochim Biophys Acta* 1794:844–851.

155. Pumbwe L, Randall LP, Woodward MJ, Piddock LJ. 2005. Evidence for multiple-antibiotic resistance in *Campylobacter jejuni* not mediated by CmeB or CmeF. *Antimicrob Agents Chemother* 49:1289–1293.

156. Palyada K, Sun YQ, Flint A, Butcher J, Naikare H, Stintzi A. 2009. Characterization of the oxidative stress stimulon and PerR regulon of *Campylobacter jejuni*. *BMC Genomics* **10**:481.

157. Holmes K, Mulholland F, Pearson BM, Pin C, McNicholl-Kennedy J, Ketley JM, Wells JM. 2005. *Campylobacter jejuni* gene expression in response to iron limitation and the role of Fur. *Microbiology* **151**:243–257.

158. Palyada K, Threadgill D, Stintzi A. 2004. Iron acquisition and regulation in *Campylobacter jejuni*. *J Bacteriol* **186**:4714–4729.

159. Luo N, Pereira S, Sahin O, Lin J, Huang S, Michel L, Zhang Q. 2005. Enhanced *in vivo* fitness of fluoroquinolone-resistant *Campylobacter jejuni* in the absence of antibiotic selection pressure. *Proc Natl Acad Sci USA* **102**:541–546.

Antimicrobial Resistance in Bacteria from Livestock and Companion Animals
Edited by Frank Møller Aarestrup, Stefan Schwarz, Jianzhong Shen, and Lina Cavaco
© 2018 American Society for Microbiology, Washington, DC
doi:10.1128/microbiolspec.ARBA-0022-2017

Antimicrobial Resistance in *Pasteurellaceae* of Veterinary Origin

15

Geovana B. Michael[1], Janine T. Bossé[2], and Stefan Schwarz[1]

THE FAMILY *PASTEURELLACEAE* AND ITS ROLE IN ANIMAL INFECTIONS

The family *Pasteurellaceae* (order *Pasteurellales*, class *Gammaproteobacteria*) comprises a highly heterogeneous group of Gram-negative bacteria. Evaluation by sequence comparison of housekeeping genes, 16s rRNA gene sequence-based phylogenetic analysis, DNA-DNA hybridization, and analysis of the biochemical and physiological capacities has identified a number of distinct genetic and phenotypic groups (1, 2). As a consequence, the family *Pasteurellaceae* has undergone numerous reclassifications during the past years and currently (late 2017) contains 25 genera: *Actinobacillus, Aggregatibacter, Avibacterium, Basfia, Bibersteinia, Bisgaardia, Chelonobacter, Cricetibacter, Frederiksenia, Gallibacterium, Haemophilus, Histophilus, Lonepinella, Mannheimia, Mesocricetibacter, Muribacter, Necropsobacter, Nicoletella, Otariodibacter, Pasteurella, Phocoenobacter, Testudinibacter, Ursidibacter, Vespertiliibacter,* and *Volucribacter* (International Committee on Sytematics of Prokaryotes, http://www.the-icsp.org/taxa-covered-family-pasteurellaceae). A new genus, *Rodentibacter*, has recently been proposed. *Rodentibacter pneumotropicus combinatio nova* (comb. nov.), which will be reclassified from [*Pasteurella*] *pneumotropica*, with NCTC 8141T (also designated CCUG 12398T) as the type strain (3). The use of square brackets enclosing the genus name indicates that there is a proposal to reclassify the species to another genus or that the species has been shown not to be a member of the genus *sensu stricto*, as is the case for [*Pasteurella*] *aerogenes*, which is now excluded from *Pasteurella sensu stricto* based on genetic analysis (4). Additional information related to reclassification of genera may be found in references 1, 2, and 5. The use of quotation

marks around "*Actinobacillus porcitonsillarum*" denotes that this is currently not a validated species name (5).

Whole-genome sequencing has become an important tool for the classification of members of the family *Pasteurellaceae*, providing a better understanding of the molecular evolution of isolates and their host specificities, niche preferences, pathogenic potential, and mechanisms of transfer and uptake of mobile genetic elements involved in antimicrobial (multi)resistance. Such knowledge can also be applied to improve/develop vaccines, diagnostic tests, disease control measures, and intervention strategies (2, 6–10).

This article deals with the genera which include pathogens of veterinary importance and will focus on the genera *Pasteurella, Mannheimia, Actinobacillus, Haemophilus,* and *Histophilus*, for which sufficient data on antimicrobial susceptibility and the detection of resistance genes are currently available. This article compiles the latest information on antimicrobial resistance, associated with the aforementioned genera, and the data published in previous book chapters (10, 11).

Many isolates of the genera *Pasteurella, Mannheimia, Actinobacillus, Haemophilus,* and *Histophilus* are commonly found on the mucous membranes of the respiratory tract and/or genital tract of reptiles, birds, and numerous mammals, including a wide variety of food-producing animals. Some species, e.g., *Pasteurella multocida*, may be found in many different hosts, including in humans, while others, such as *Actinobacillus pleuropneumoniae* and *Mannheimia haemolytica* (formerly [*Pasteurella*] *haemolytica*), have a narrow host range, being found primarily in pigs and ruminants, respectively (5).

P. multocida is the most relevant animal-pathogenic *Pasteurella* species. Various capsular types of *P. multo-*

[1]Institute of Microbiology and Epizootics, Freie Universität Berlin, Berlin, D-14163 Germany; [2]Section of Pediatrics, Department of Medicine London, Imperial College London, London W2 1PG, United Kingdom.

cida are known, some of which preferentially occur in connection with specific diseases in animals. For example, (i) capsular type A is the causative agent of pneumonia in several animal species including, but not limited to, cattle, sheep, and pigs; mastitis in sheep; snuffles in rabbits; and fowl cholera in poultry. (ii) Capsular types B and E are the causative agents of hemorrhagic septicemia of cattle and water buffaloes in Asia and Africa, respectively. (iii) Capsular type D isolates are mainly involved in atrophic rhinitis and pneumonia in swine (12, 13). (iv) Capsular type F isolates are mainly seen in poultry but may also be involved in fatal peritonitis in calves (14).

M. haemolytica comprises 12 capsular serotypes (A1, A2, A5 to A9, A12 to A14, A16, and A17). Serotypes A1 and A6 have been the ones most commonly associated with respiratory diseases in cattle (15) or in sheep (16), respectively.

A. pleuropneumoniae is the causative agent of porcine pleuropneumonia (13), which causes huge economic losses in the swine industry worldwide. Currently, two biovars (the NAD-dependent biovar 1 and the NAD-independent biovar 2) and 16 serovars of *A. pleuropneumoniae* are distinguished (17–19). Serovars 1, 5, 9, and 11 are considered to be more virulent than other serovars (20).

Several species of the genus *Haemophilus* also represent animal pathogens, with [*Haemophilus*] *parasuis* being of major economic importance. [*H.*] *parasuis* causes Glässer's disease (also known as porcine polyserositis or infectious polyarthritis) in pigs, which is characterized by high fevers, polyserositis, polysynovitis, respiratory distress, and meningitis. More than 15 serotypes have been identified, with serotypes 1, 5, 12, 13, and 14 being thought to be the most virulent (21).

Histophilus somni (formerly [*Haemophilus*] *somnus*), *Histophilus ovis*, and *Histophilus agni* are also pathogens of cattle and sheep. *H. somni* is the etiological agent of thromboembolic meningoencephalitis in cattle. It has also been associated with various other diseases in sheep and diseases such as bronchopneumonia, necrotic laryngitis, myocarditis, arthritis, conjunctivitis, myositis, mastitis, and abortion (10).

All diseases in which *Pasteurella*, *Mannheimia*, *Actinobacillus*, *Haemophilus*, or *Histophilus* isolates act as primary pathogens commonly occur as peracute or acute forms and are accompanied by a high mortality rate, although subacute and chronic forms are also observed. As secondary pathogens, *P. multocida* and *M. haemolytica* play a major role in the final progression to severe bronchopneumonia and pleuropneumonia in cattle, sheep, and goats (22), as well as in

enzootic pneumonia in calves (23) and progressive atrophic rhinitis of swine (24). Respiratory tract infections, in which bacteria such as *P. multocida* and *M. haemolytica* isolates are involved, are often multifactorial and polymicrobial diseases, with viruses and other bacteria, such as *Mycoplasma* spp. representing the primary pathogens (13, 22–24). Under certain environmental and/or management conditions (such as transport, marketing, change of feed, climate, or ventilation) which result in stress to the animals, especially in the presence of viruses and/or *Mycoplasma* spp. which may initiate damage to the host mucosal membranes, the bacterial pathogens can rapidly proliferate, resulting in high morbidity. Under conditions of low stress, the mortality rate may be low. As the amount of stress increases, however, the mortality rate also increases. Economic losses associated with acute pneumonic episodes are primarily due to increased costs in medications and retarded growth rates rather than mortality of the affected animals. Besides these major pathogens, various other members of the family *Pasteurellaceae* have been reported to be less frequently associated with diseases in humans and animals (10).

As seen for many other bacteria, members of the family *Pasteurellaceae* also respond to the selective pressure imposed by the use of antimicrobial agents by developing or acquiring resistance genes or resistance-mediating mutations. In this regard, mobile genetic elements, such as plasmids, transposons, or integrative and conjugative elements (ICEs) that carry resistance genes, play an important role in the dissemination of antimicrobial resistance, with members of the family *Pasteurellaceae* acting as donors and/or recipients. This article provides a brief description of the most recent data on the susceptibility status of selected members of the family *Pasteurellaceae* and an update on the current knowledge regarding genes and mutations conferring antimicrobial resistance among *Pasteurellaceae* of veterinary concern and on the dissemination, coselection, and persistence of such resistance genes.

ANTIMICROBIAL SUSCEPTIBILITY OF *PASTEURELLA, MANNHEIMIA, ACTINOBACILLUS, HAEMOPHILUS,* AND *HISTOPHILUS*

Although prudent use guidelines request identification of the causative pathogen and determination of its *in vitro* susceptibility prior to the onset of antimicrobial therapy, the generally acute nature of the diseases—and in veterinary medicine, the rapid spread of the causative pathogens within animal herds—often requires an immediate therapeutic intervention in which the initial choice of the antimicrobial agents may be revised on the basis of the results of the diagnostic tests. In this regard, two major aspects need to be considered: (i) the correct performance of *in vitro* susceptibility tests and (ii) representative data on the susceptibility status of members of the *Pasteurellaceae*.

Susceptibility Testing

In vitro antimicrobial susceptibility testing (AST) is performed to predict how a bacterium may respond to an antimicrobial agent *in vivo* (clinical response) or to monitor changes in susceptibility in relation to time and geographic location. In both instances, results may be reported qualitatively, e.g., susceptible, intermediate, or resistant (S-I-R), or quantitatively, e.g., as the minimal inhibitory concentration (MIC). When performing AST for surveillance purposes, the interpretive criteria are based on the bacterial population distributions relative to inhibition zone sizes and/or MIC values. Interpretive criteria for clinical consideration require the generation of a bacterium's antibiogram in addition to knowledge of the pharmacokinetic parameters of the chosen drug in the target animal species and the pharmacodynamic parameters associated with the *in vivo* bacterium-antimicrobial agent-host interactions. In either situation, to ensure intra- and interlaboratory reproducibility, it is essential that standardized AST methods be used (25). Recently, it has been suggested that whole-genome sequencing for identification of resistance genes may be a useful adjunct to phenotypic testing, because it not only provides a reproducible means of analysis, but can provide added data for epidemiological purposes (9, 26, 27).

The results of *in vitro* AST ensure the most efficacious antimicrobial therapy by excluding antimicrobial agents to which the causative bacterial pathogen already shows resistance, or reduced susceptibility, under *in vitro* conditions. Correct performance of the tests is essential to most accurately predict the clinical response of the bacterium. Several members of the family *Pasteurellaceae* are classified as "fastidious organisms" since they require specific growth conditions, e.g., supplementation of the media with components essential for the growth of the bacteria. In this regard, performance of *in vitro* AST should follow standardized and internationally accepted rules. The *in vitro* AST of *Pasteurella*, *Mannheimia*, *Actinobacillus*, *Haemophilus*, and *Histophilus* is no exception. While many studies have reported *in vitro* susceptibility data for isolates of the these genera, obtained from animal sources in various parts of the world, there has been a notable

absence of standardization in testing methods. In most cases, it is difficult to compare the results because of the use of different methods and breakpoints. The Clinical and Laboratory Standards Institute (CLSI) has published three documents, VET01-A4 (28), VET01-S (29), and VET06 (30), which provide the latest information on methods for *in vitro* susceptibility testing of *P. multocida*, *Pasteurella* spp. other than *P. multocida*, *M. haemolytica*, *A. pleuropneumoniae*, and *H. somni*. Because there is no CLSI-approved method for antimicrobial susceptibility testing of [*H.*] *parasuis*, methods recently developed and published should be followed when testing this organism (31, 32).

The CLSI documents VET01-S (29) and VET06 (30) also contain clinical breakpoints on the basis of which isolates are classified as susceptible, intermediate, or resistant. In contrast to epidemiological cutoff values, clinical breakpoints may predict the clinical outcome when the antimicrobial agent in question is dosed and administered as recommended (25, 33). Veterinary-specific clinical breakpoints applicable to bovine, canine, equine, feline, or porcine *P. multocida*, *M. haemolytica*, *H. somni*, and/or *A. pleuropneumoniae* are currently available for a number of antimicrobial agents, including ampicillin/amoxicillin, cefazolin, cefpodoxime, ceftiofur, chloramphenicol, danofloxacin, enrofloxacin, gamithromycin, florfenicol, gentamicin, penicillin G, pradofloxacin, spectinomycin, tetracycline, tiamulin, tildipirosin, tilmicosin, and/or tulathromycin (29, 34).

Susceptibility Status of Selected Pathogens of the Family *Pasteurellaceae*

In veterinary medicine, bacteria belonging to the family *Pasteurellaceae* are currently not included in most national antimicrobial susceptibility monitoring and surveillance programs. Only the German GERM-Vet program, which uses CLSI AST methodology and CLSI clinical breakpoints, included *P. multocida* and *A. pleuropneumoniae* from respiratory tract infections of swine (piglets, weaners, and adult swine), as well as *P. multocida* and *M. haemolytica* from cattle (calves and adult cattle) and *M. haemolytica* from sheep and goats (35) (Table 1). Moreover, *P. multocida* from dogs and cats suffering from either respiratory tract infections or infections of mouth, ear, or skin were collected between 2004 and 2006 in the BfT-GermVet monitoring program and analyzed for their *in vitro* susceptibility (36) (Table 1). In addition, Portis and coworkers (37) published susceptibility data collected in a large-scale surveillance program over a 10-year period (2000 to 2009) from the bovine respiratory disease pathogens *M. haemolytica*, *P. multocida*, and *H. somni* in the United

Table 1 Percentages of resistance of *P. multocida*, *M. haemolytica*, *H. somni*, and *A. pleuropneumoniae* isolates from different animal sources against selected antimicrobial agents

Bacteria	Origin	Year(s) of isolation	No. of isolates	% resistant isolates[a]							Reference
				PEN	XNL	FLO	ENR	TET	TIL	TUL	
P. multocida	Cattle/USA, Canada	2009	328	3.3	0.0	11.6	2.1	40.8	23.8	4.6	37
	Cattle/Germany	2013	48	2.1	0.0	0.0	0.0	10.4	2.1	0.0	35
	Adult swine/Germany	2013	90	5.6	0.0	0.0	0.0	11.1	0.0	0.0	35
	Weaner/Germany	2013	25	0.0	0.0	0.0	0.0	8.0	0.0	0.0	35
	Piglet/Germany	2013	35	2.9	0.0	2.9	0.0	2.9	0.0	0.0	35
	Dogs, cats/Germany	2004–2006	72	0.0	0.0	0.0	0.0	0.0	0.0	0.0	36
M. haemolytica	Cattle/USA, Canada	2009	304	27.3	0.0	8.6	6.6	43.7	27.3	8.9	37
	Calf/Germany	2012–2013	63	11.1	0.0	1.6	0.0	22.2	1.6	0.0	35
	Adult cattle/Germany	2012–2013	35	8.8	0.0	0.0	0.0	0.0	2.9	2.9	35
	Sheep, goat/Germany	2012–2013	42	4.8	0.0	0.0	0.0	2.4	0.0	0.0	35
H. somni	Cattle/USA, Canada	2009	174	4.5	0.0	1.7	7.4	42.5	18.4	10.9	37
A. pleuropneumoniae	Swine/Germany	2012	102	5.9	0.0	0.0	0.0	13.7	1.0	7.8	35

[a]PEN, penicillin G; XNL, ceftiofur; FLO, florfenicol; ENR, enrofloxacin; TET, tetracycline; TIL, tilmicosin; TUL, tulathromycin.

States and Canada (Table 1). A comparison of the percentages of resistance between the respective *P. multocida* and *M. haemolytica* isolates from North America and Germany showed that among the German isolates resistance to newer antimicrobial agents, such as ceftiofur, florfenicol, enrofloxacin, and tulathromycin, is rarely detected, if at all. In contrast, the isolates from North America showed low levels of resistance (up to 11.6%) to florfenicol, enrofloxacin, and tulathromycin. However, all isolates were susceptible to ceftiofur. It should also be noted that none of the 72 *P. multocida* isolates from respiratory tract infections of dogs and cats investigated in the BfT-GermVet program exhibited resistance to any of the antimicrobial agents shown in Table 1. Only sulfonamide resistance was seen in 31 (43%) isolates (36).

In addition to these data from GERM-Vet (35), Bft-GermVet (36), and the aforementioned large-scale surveillance program (37), numerous other studies have dealt with the *in vitro* susceptibility of bovine, porcine, and avian *Pasteurellaceae* in different countries (e.g., 31, 38–43). Major problems arising from a comparison of the results of these studies are that (i) isolates have not been selected according to a defined sampling plan, (ii) different AST methods have been used, (iii) different interpretive criteria have been used for the evaluation of the results, and/or (iv) isolates may have not been investigated for their relatedness to prevent the inclusion of multiple members of the same clone in the test collection.

Additional studies that have determined the susceptibility to antimicrobial agents of *Pasteurellaceae* isolates from animal sources in different countries include the following. VetPath is a pan-European antibiotic susceptibility monitoring program collecting pathogens from diseased (but not antimicrobial-treated) cattle, pigs, and poultry. Two studies dealing with respiratory tract pathogens, including *P. multocida* and *M. haemolytica* from cattle and *P. multocida* and *A. pleuropneumoniae* from pigs, and covering the years 2002 to 2006 (38) and 2009 to 2012 (39) have been published. The results of these studies showed that, for most antimicrobial agents and pathogens, the percentages of resistance remained largely unchanged in the period from 2009 to 2012 compared to those of the period from 2002 to 2006. Moreover, these data also showed that resistance to amoxicillin/clavulanic acid, ceftiofur, enrofloxacin, florfenicol, tulathromycin, tiamulin, and tilmicosin was absent or <2%. A study conducted in Australia investigated *P. multocida* and *A. pleuropneumoniae* isolates from pigs with respiratory tract infections for their antimicrobial susceptibility (40). This study illustrated that Australian isolates of swine bacterial respiratory pathogens also exhibited low levels of resistance to antimicrobial agents commonly used in the pig industry. A study from Canada in which *A. pleuropneumoniae* isolates were tested for their resistance pheno- and genotypes revealed that all isolates were susceptible to ceftiofur, florfenicol, enrofloxacin, erythromycin, clindamycin, trimethoprim/sulfamethoxazole, and tilmicosin. A low level of resistance was observed toward tiamulin, penicillin, and ampicillin as well as danofloxacin, whereas the majority of the tested isolates were resistant to chlortetracycline (88.4%) and oxytetracycline (90.7%) (41). A large-scale study of 2,989 *M. haemolytica* isolates from feedlot cattle in Canada revealed that 87.8% of the isolates were pan-susceptible, whereas the percentages of resistant isolates varied between 0.0 and 4.5% for the antimicrobial agents tested (42). It should also be noted that a literature review of antimicrobial resistance in pathogens associated with bovine respiratory disease has recently been published (43).

MOLECULAR MECHANISMS OF ANTIMICROBIAL RESISTANCE IN *PASTEURELLA, MANNHEIMIA, ACTINOBACILLUS, HAEMOPHILUS,* AND *HISTOPHILUS*

The following subsections provide an update of the current status of resistance genes and resistance-mediating mutations known to occur in *Pasteurellaceae*. The focus will be on members of the genera *Pasteurella, Mannheimia, Actinobacillus, Haemophilus,* and *Histophilus,* which infect animals and for which data on the genetic basis of resistance are available (Table 2). As far as information is available, the association of the resistance genes with mobile genetic elements and their potential to spread across species and genus borders will be discussed.

Resistance to Tetracyclines

Tetracycline resistance is a highly heterogeneous property with more than 40 resistance genes known to date (http://faculty.washington.edu/marilynr/). In bacteria of the genera *Pasteurella, Mannheimia, Actinobacillus,* and *Haemophilus,* at least nine tetracycline resistance genes (*tet* genes), representing two resistance mechanisms (tetracycline exporters and ribosome protective proteins) have been detected (Table 2).

Tetracycline resistance mediated by specific exporters

Among the *tet* genes coding for membrane-associated proteins of the major facilitator superfamily which specifically export tetracyclines from the bacterial cell, the genes *tet*(A), *tet*(B), *tet*(C), *tet*(G), *tet*(H), *tet*(L), and *tet*(K) have been identified in bacteria of the aforementioned five genera, but *tet*(K) is commonly found on small plasmids only in human pathogens. Studies from the late 1970s and 1980s reported transferable tetracycline resistance among *P. multocida* and *M. haemolytica* isolates of animal origin (44–47), although the type of *tet* gene involved was not determined in any of these studies. In 1993, Hansen and coworkers identified a novel type of *tet* gene, designated *tet*(H) (48). The *tet*(H) gene was first detected on plasmid pVM111, which originated from a *P. multocida* isolate

obtained from a turkey in the late 1970s in the United States. (44). In a subsequent study, Hansen et al. found the *tet*(H) gene to be the predominant *tet* gene among *P. multocida* and *M. haemolytica* from infections of cattle and pigs in North America (49). Since the *tet*(H) gene was located either in chromosomal DNA or on plasmids, they speculated about the involvement of a transposable element in the spread of *tet*(H) (49). The corresponding transposon, Tn*5706*, was identified in 1998 on plasmid pPMT1 from a bovine *P. multocida* isolate (50). Tn*5706* is a small, nonconjugative composite transposon of 4,378 bp and represents the first known resistance-mediating transposon identified among members of the genus *Pasteurella* (51). The *tetR*-*tet*(H) gene region in Tn*5706* is bracketed by inverted copies of the two closely related insertion sequences, IS*1596* and IS*1597* (50) (Fig. 1). Truncated Tn*5706* elements, in which these insertion sequences were deleted in part or completely, have been found on small plasmids in isolates of *M. haemolytica, P. multocida,* and [*P.*] *aerogenes* (52, 53) and more recently as part of ICEs in isolates of *P. multocida, H. somni,* and *M. haemolytica* (54–57). The *tet*(H) gene has also been found in bacteria outside of the family *Pasteurellaceae,* namely in *Moraxella* spp. and *Acinetobacter radioresistens* (58), both obtained from salmon farms in Chile. The *A. radioresistens* isolate also harbored the insertion sequence IS*1599* (58), which is closely related to the Tn*5706*-associated insertion sequences IS*1596* and IS*1597*.

The *tetR*-*tet*(H) gene region of the *P. multocida* plasmid pVM111 is bracketed by the *sul2* sulfonamide resistance gene and the *strA* and *strB* streptomycin resistance genes and thus represents part of a novel resistance gene cluster (59) (Fig. 1). The *tet*(H) gene is occasionally present in tetracycline-resistant *A. pleuropneumoniae* (9, 41, 60–63). Two *tet*(H)-carrying plasmids, p9956 and p12494 (5,674 bp and 14,393 bp, respectively), have been isolated from porcine *A. pleuropneumoniae* and sequenced completely (61). Structural analysis showed that they differed distinctly from one another and from the *tet*(H)-carrying plasmids previously found in *Pasteurella* spp. and *Mannheimia* spp. (Fig. 1). In plasmid p12494, a 100-bp insertion in the *tetR* gene was detected which resulted in the loss of 60 amino acids at the C-terminus. MIC determination of the corresponding *A. pleuropneumoniae* isolate, in the presence and absence of tetracycline, suggested that this *tet*(H) gene was constitutively expressed (61).

The *tet*(B) gene has been identified as the dominant *tet* gene among porcine [*P.*] *aerogenes* isolates (53) and has also been detected in porcine *P. multocida* isolates from the United States and Germany (64) and Spain

Table 2 Antimicrobial resistance genes and mutations identified in *Pasteurella*, *Mannheimia*, *Actinobacillus*, *Haemophilus*, and *Histophilus* isolates of veterinary importance

Antimicrobial agent	Resistance gene or resistance-mediating mutation(s)	Protein specified by the resistance gene or mutation position	Detected in[a]					Reference[b]/Accession number[c]
			Pas	Man	Act	Hae	His	
Tetracycline	*tet*(A)	12-TMS efflux protein	–	–	+	–	–	72, 81
	tet(B)	12-TMS efflux protein	+	+	+	+	–	53, 66, 75, 81
	tet(C)	12-TMS efflux protein	–	–	+	+	–	81
	tet(G)	12-TMS efflux protein	+	+	+	–	–	64, 76, 81
	tet(H)	12-TMS efflux protein	+	+	+	–	+	48, 49, 57, 61
	tet(L)	14-TMS efflux protein	+	+	+	–	–	79, 81
	tet(M)	Ribosome protective protein	+	–	+	–	–	49, 81
	tet(O)	Ribosome protective protein	+	–	+	–	–	65, 81
Penicillins	*bla*$_{CMY-2}$	β-Lactmase	+	–	–	–	–	90
	bla$_{OXA-2}$	β-Lactmase	+	+	–	–	+	55, 57
	bla$_{PSE-1}$	β-Lactmase	+	–	–	–	–	76
	bla$_{ROB-1}$	β-Lactmase	+	+	+	+	+	85, 87, 88, 93
	bla$_{TEM-1}$	β-Lactmase	+	–	–	–	+	89
Streptomycin	*strA*	Aminoglycoside-3″-phosphotransferase	+	+	+	+	+	55–57, 121, 194
	strB	Aminoglycoside-6-phosphotransferase	+	+	+	–	+	55–57, 121
Streptomycin/spectinomycin	*aadA1*	aminoglycoside-3″-adenyltransferase	+	–	–	–	–	76
	aadA14	aminoglycoside-3″-adenyltransferase	+	–	–	–	–	132
	aadA25	aminoglycoside-3″-adenyltransferase	+	+	–	–	+	55, 57
Spectinomycin	Mutation in 16S rRNA	C1192G	+	–	–	–	–	143
	Mutation in *rpsE* coding for ribosomal protein S5	3-bp deletions resulting in S32I and loss of F33 or loss of K33	+	–	–	–	–	143
Kanamycin/neomycin	*aphA1*	Aminoglycoside-3′-phosphotransferase	+	+	–	+	+	55–57, 123; JN202624
	aphA3	Aminoglycoside-3′-phosphotransferase	+	–	–	–	–	135
Gentamicin	*aacC2*	Aminoglycoside 3-N-acetyltransferase	–	–	+	+	–	95; JN202624
	aacC4	Aminoglycoside 3-N-acetyltransferase	–	–	+	–	–	81
	aadB	Aminoglycoside-2″-adenyltransferase	+	+	+	–	+	55, 57, 81

			Pas	Man	Act	Hae	His	Reference[b]
Sulfonamides	sul2	Sulfonamide-resistant dihydropteroate synthase	+	+	+	+	+	55–57, 95; JN202624
Trimethoprim	dfrA1	Trimethoprim-resistant DHFR	+	–	–	–	–	76
	dfrA14	Trimethoprim-resistant DHFR	–	–	+	–	–	122
	dfrA20	Trimethoprim-resistant DHFR	+	–	–	–	–	62
Macrolides	erm(T)	rRNA methylase	–	–	+	–	–	154
	erm(A)	rRNA methylase	–	–	+	–	–	70
	erm(C)	rRNA methylase	–	–	+	–	–	70
	erm(42)	rRNA methylase	+	+	–	–	+	57, 155, 157
	Mutation in 23S rRNA	A2058G, A2059G	+	+	–	–	+	153, 159
	mrs(E)-mph(E)	Macrolide efflux protein and phospotransferase	+	+	–	–	+	57, 155, 157
Lincosamides	lnu(C)	O-nucleotidyltransferase	–	–	+	–	–	161
Chloramphenicol	catA1	Type A chloramphenicol acetyltransferase	+	+	–	–	–	163
	catA3	Type A chloramphenicol acetyltransferase	+	+	+	+	–	95, 163; JN202624
	catB2	Type B chloramphenicol acetyltransferase	+	–	–	–	–	76
Chloramphenicol/ florfenicol	floR	12-TMS efflux protein	+	+	+	+	+	57, 73, 174, 179, 180
(Fluoro)quinolones	Mutation in gyrA	G75S, S83F, S83I, S83R, S83V, S83Y, A84P, D87G, D87H, D87N, D87Y, D492G, D492V, G627E	+	+	+	+	–	9, 55, 187, 189–192
	Mutation in gyrB	V211I, D254G	+[d]	–	–	–	–	192
	Mutation in parC	S73I, S73R, S80L, G83C, I84S, S85R, S85Y, E89K, Q227H, L379I, C578Y	+	+	+	+	–	55, 187, 189, 190, 192
	Mutation in parE	P440S, S459F, E461D, E461K, D479E, T551A	–	+	+	+	–	190, 192
	qnrA1	Quinolone resistance protein	–	–	–	+	–	191
	qnrB6	Quinolone resistance protein	–	–	–	+	–	191
	aac(6′)-Ib-cr	Quinolone resistance protein	–	–	–	+	–	191
Streptothricin	sat2	Streptothricin-acetyl-transferase	+	–	–	–	–	130

[a]Pas, Pasteurella; Man, Mannheimia; Act, Actinobacillus; Hae, Haemophilus; His, Histophilus; +, present; –, absent. Additional information and references may be found in the text of this chapter.
[b]At least a reference or an accession number is included for each genus in which a specific gene or mutation is found.
[c]Accession number was provided in case of unpublished data.
[d]The mutations in gyrB were detected in Pasteurella isolates after passage on subinhibitory concentrations of fluoroquinolones.

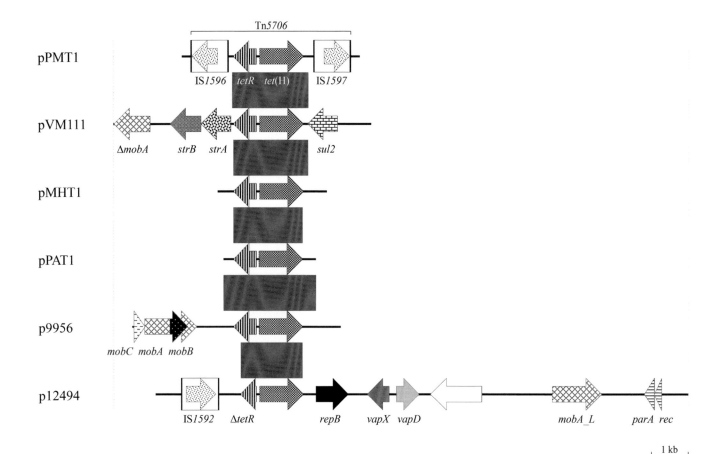

Figure 1 Schematic representation of the structure and organization of genes found in *tet*(H)-carrying plasmids from *P. multocida*, *M. haemolytica*, [*P.*] *aerogenes*, and *A. pleuropneumoniae*. Comparison of the maps of the partially sequenced plasmids pPMT1 (accession no. Y15510) and pVM111 (accession nos. AJ514834 and U00792), both from *P. multocida*, pMHT1 (accession no. Y16103) from *M. haemolytica*, and pPAT1 (accession no. AJ245947) from [*P.*] *aerogenes* (accession no. Z21724) and the completely sequenced plasmids p9956 (accession no. AY362554; 5,674 bp) and p12494 (accession no. DQ517426; 14,393 bp), both from *A. pleuropneumoniae*. Genes are shown as arrows, with the arrowhead indicating the direction of transcription. The following genes are involved in antimicrobial resistance: *tetR-tet*(H) (tetracycline resistance), *sul2* (sulfonamide resistance), and *strA* and *strB* (streptomycin resistance); plasmid replication: *repB*; mobilization functions: *mobA*, *mobB*, *mobC*, and *mobA_L*; recombination functions: *rec*; DNA partition: *par*; virulence: *vapD* and *vapX*; unknown function: the open reading frame indicated by the white arrow. The Δ symbol indicates a truncated functionally inactive gene. The white boxes in the maps of pPMT1 and p12494 indicate the limits of the insertion sequences IS*1592*, IS*1596*, and IS*1597*; the arrows within these boxes indicate the reading frames of the corresponding transposase genes. Gray shaded areas indicate the *tetR-tet*(H) gene region common to all these plasmids with ≥95% nucleotide sequence identity. A distance scale in kilobases is shown at the bottom of the figure.

(65), as well as in a bovine *M. haemolytica* isolate from France (66). In all but two cases, the *tet*(B) gene was located in one or two copies in the chromosome. The gene *tet*(B) is part of the nonconjugative transposon Tn*10* (67, 68) and represents the most widely spread *tet* gene among *Enterobacteriaceae* (69). Hybridiza-

tion studies using SfuI-digested whole cellular DNA of *tet*(B)-carrying *P. multocida* and [*P.*] *aerogenes* isolates suggested that there are complete copies of Tn*10* in the majority of the isolates investigated (53, 64). In the 4.8-kb plasmid pPAT2, recovered from [*P.*] *aerogenes* in Germany, the *tetR-tet*(B) genes proved to be part of a largely truncated Tn*10* element (53), whereas in the 5.1-kb *P. multocida* plasmid from Spain, pB1001, the *tet*(B) gene was found without *tetR* (65).

Studies of tetracycline-resistant *A. pleuropneumoniae* from pigs (9, 60, 70, 71) also revealed the presence of the gene *tet*(B), which appears to be the predominant *tet* gene in isolates, including those from Spain, Switzerland, Japan, Korea, Australia, and the United Kingdom (9, 60, 62, 63, 72, 73). This gene was also detected in the "*A. porcitonsillarum*" reference strain CCUG46996, and a single field isolate of this bacterium (62). Recently, whole-genome sequencing revealed that some United Kingdom isolates of *A. pleuropneumoniae* carry *tet*(B) in their chromosome as part of a transposon insertion disrupting the *comM* gene, whereas other isolates have Tn*10* insertions carrying *tet*(B) as part of the 56-kb ICE*Apl1*, located in a copy of tRNA-Leu (9, 74). Neither of the ICEs so far identified in *P. multocida* (ICE*Pmu1*) and *M. haemolytica* (ICE*Mh1*) carry *tet*(B) (54–56). It would be interesting to determine if the previously reported chromosomally encoded *tet*(B) genes in these species are part of ICEs related to ICE*Apl1* or other distinct ICEs. As more whole-genome sequences become available, it is likely that more ICEs will be identified in isolates of the *Pasteurellaceae*.

Among the Spanish *A. pleuropneumoniae* isolates, the *tet*(B) gene was found mainly on small plasmids, which were indistinguishable by their HindIII and DraI restriction patterns (60). One of these, p11745, a 5,486-bp plasmid, was sequenced completely. Again, as with pB1001 from *P. multocida*, neither the *tetR* repressor gene nor other parts of Tn*10* were detectable in p11745 (60) (Fig. 2). Although both of these plasmids, isolated in Spain, encode a replication gene, *rep*, upstream of the *tet*(B) gene, there is little sequence similarity outside of the *tet*(B) gene (Fig. 2). In addition, genes for mobilization, *mobC* and *mobA/L*, are found in p11745, but not in pB1001. The 4,597-bp plasmid pHPS1019, isolated from [*H.*] *parasuis* in China (accession number HQ622101), encodes the same *rep* and *tet*(B) genes as pB1001 and also shares an extended region of identity downstream of the *tet*(B) gene (Fig. 2). In these two plasmids, there are direct repeats flanking the *tet*(B) gene, extending from within the 3′ terminus of *rep* for 484 bp in pB1001 and 198 bp in in pHPS1019. Another distinct *tet*(B) plasmid, pHS-Tet, was isolated from [*H.*] *parasuis* in Australia (75). This 5,147-bp plasmid, also without an accompanying *tetR* repressor gene, carries different mobilization genes than those in p11745 (Fig. 2).

The gene *tet*(G) has been found on the chromosome of six epidemiologically related *M. haemolytica* isolates from cattle (64) and on plasmid pJR1 from avian *P. multocida* (76). Surprisingly, the *tet*(G) structural gene in plasmid pJR1 was found in the absence of a corresponding *tetR* repressor gene, which is considered to be essential for the tetracycline-inducible expression of *tet*(G). It should be noted that plasmid pJR1 has not been transferred into susceptible recipient strains for phenotypic confirmation of the activity of the resistance genes found on this plasmid (76). Previously, *tet*(G) was shown to be part of the multiresistance gene cluster present in *Salmonella enterica* serovar Typhimurium DT104 (77), which has since been shown to be part of an integrative mobilizable element, SGI1 (78). It is currently not known whether a related integrative mobilizable element is present in the chromosomes of the six *M. haemolytica* isolates carrying *tet*(G).

The *tet*(L) gene, which is commonly found in Gram-positive cocci and *Bacillus* spp., was detected on small plasmids of *M. haemolytica* and *Mannheimia glucosida*, but also in the chromosomal DNA of single *M. haemolytica* and *P. multocida* isolates, all originating from cattle in Belgium (79). One such plasmid of 5,317 bp from *M. haemolytica*, designated pCCK3259, was sequenced completely (Fig. 2). Besides the *tet*(L) gene, it contains only the *mobABC* operon responsible for mobilization of the plasmid (79). In Gram-positive bacteria, the *tet*(L) gene is inducibly expressed via translational attenuation (80). The corresponding regulatory region, however, was absent in plasmid pCCK3259, whereas all elements required for constitutive expression of the *tet*(L) gene were detected in the upstream sequence (79). Two different-sized *tet*(L)-carrying plasmids (5.6 and >12 kb) have also been identified in porcine *A. pleuropneumoniae* (60). The smaller one of these plasmids, p9555, was sequenced completely and revealed striking structural similarities to plasmid pCCK3259 from *M. haemolytica* (60). Again, the regulatory region of the *tet*(L) gene was missing in plasmid p9555. While plasmid p9555 could be transferred into *Escherichia coli*, where it expressed tetracycline resistance (60), plasmid pCCK3259 did not replicate in *E. coli* but did in a *P. multocida* host (79).

More recently, isolates of *A. pleuropneumoniae* from Japan and South Korea were shown to harbor the *tet*(A) gene, as well as other tetracycline resistance genes (72, 81). In both reports, detection of resistance genes was by PCR, and localization to plasmid or chromosome was not determined. Of the 65 isolates tested by Kim et al. (81), 62 were resistant to tetracycline, with 21 of them carrying *tet*(A). Eleven of these isolates harboured two or more tetracycline resistance genes, as for example one isolate with *tet*(A), *tet*(B), *tet*(C),

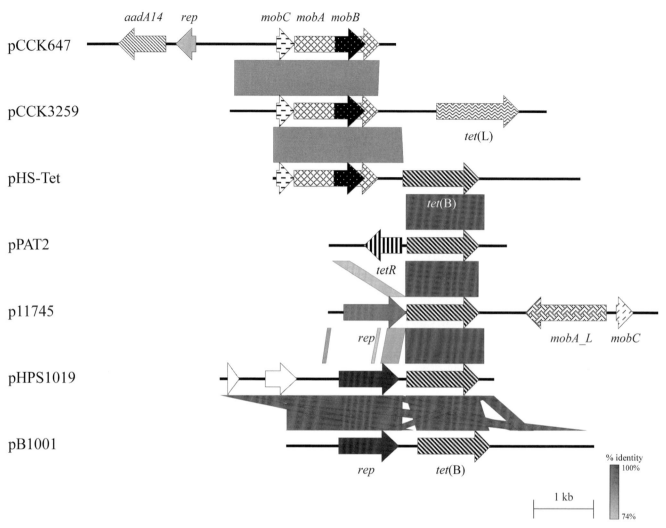

Figure 2 Schematic representation of the structure and organization of *aadA14*-, *tet*(L)-, and *tet*(B)-carrying plasmids from *P. multocida*, *M. haemolytica*, [*H.*] *parasuis*, [*P.*] *aerogenes*, and *A. pleuropneumoniae*. Comparison of the maps of the *aadA14*-carrying strepto-mycin/spectinomycin resistance plasmid pCCK647 (accession no. AJ884726; 5,198 bp) from *P. multocida*, the *tet*(L)-carrying tetracycline resistance plasmid pCCK3259 (accession no. AJ966516; 5,317 bp) from *M. haemolytica*, and the *tet*(B)-carrying tetracycline resistance plasmids pHS-Tet (accession no. AY862435; 5,147 bp) from [*H.*] *parasuis*, pPAT2 (accession no. AJ278685; partially sequenced) from [*P.*] *aerogenes*, p11745 (accession no. DQ176855; 5,486 bp) from *A. pleuropneumoniae*, pHPS1019 (accession no. HQ622101; 4,597 bp) from [*H.*] *parasuis*, and pB1001 (accession no. EU252517; 5,128 bp) from *P. multocida*. Genes are shown as arrows, with the arrowhead indicating the direction of transcription. The fol-lowing genes are involved in antimicrobial resistance: *tetR-tet*(B), *tet*(B), and *tet*(L) (tetracy-cline resistance) and *aadA14* (streptomycin/spectinomycin resistance); plasmid replication: *rep*; mobilization functions: *mobA*, *mobB*, and *mobC*; unknown function: the open reading frames indicated by white arrows. Gray-shaded areas indicate the regions common to plas-mids, and the different shades of gray illustrate the percentages of nucleotide sequence iden-tity between the plasmids, as indicated by the scale at the bottom of the figure. A distance scale in kilobases is shown.

tet(G), and *tet*(L); another with *tet*(A), *tet*(B), *tet*(C), and *tet*(G); and another with *tet*(A), *tet*(B), and *tet*(M)/*tet*(O) (81).

Tetracycline resistance mediated by ribosome protective proteins

Another two tetracycline resistance genes, *tet*(M) and *tet*(O), both coding for ribosome protective proteins, have been identified in *P. multocida* and *A. pleuropneumoniae*. The gene *tet*(M) is associated with the conjugative transposon Tn*916* (82). It is considered to be the most widespread *tet* gene among Gram-positive and Gram-negative bacteria (69; http://faculty.washington. edu/marilynr/). It has been detected by hybridization in the chromosomal DNA of two bovine *P. multocida* isolates (49, 66). The gene *tet*(O), previously identified in *Campylobacter* spp. and streptococci, was detected in chromosomal DNA of a porcine *A. pleuropneumoniae* isolate in 2004 (71). More recently, the *tet*(O) gene was also detected in eight porcine *A. pleuropneumoniae* isolates from Spain (60), five from Japan (72), four from Korea (73), and seven from Canada (41). In the isolates from Spain, the *tet*(O) gene was located on small plasmids of ca. 6 kb. Sequencing of a 2,489-bp region, including the complete *tet*(O) gene, of one of these plasmids (p13142) revealed 99% sequence identity to the *tet*(O) gene of *Campylobacter jejuni* (60).

Resistance to β-Lactam Antibiotics

In general, resistance of *Pasteurellaceae* to β-lactam antibiotics is based on the production of a β-lactamase or the presence of penicillin-binding proteins with low affinity to β-lactams (10, 11, 83). However, the latter mechanism has only been reported for the human pathogen *Haemophilus influenzae* (10, 11, 83). Other mechanisms, such as reduced outer membrane permeability or multidrug efflux systems that can efficiently export β-lactams from the bacterial cell (10, 11, 83), have rarely—if at all—been identified in *Pasteurellaceae*.

So far, five β-lactamase (*bla*) genes have been identified among *Pasteurellaceae*: *bla*ROB-1 (84–88), *bla*TEM-1 (89), *bla*PSE-1 (76), *bla*CMY-2 (90), and *bla*OXA-2 (55, 57). It is interesting to note that the complete *bla*OXA-2 gene, identified as part of ICE*Pmu1*, was found to be nonfunctional in *P. multocida* but functional in *E. coli* (55). According to the existing classification schemes of β-lactamases, the ROB-1 and TEM enzymes are assigned to the Ambler class A because of their structure and to the Bush class 2b on the basis of their substrate profile (91). Members of this class can hydrolyze penicillins and first-generation cephalosporins (narrow spectrum of activity) but are sensitive to inhibition by

β-lactamase inhibitors such as clavulanic acid. The PSE-1 β-lactamase also belongs to the Ambler class A but to the Bush class 2c. This enzyme, also known as CARB-2 β-lactamase, can hydrolyze carbenicillin and is also inactivated by clavulanic acid.

Although initially identified in *H. influenzae* from a human infection (92), ROB-1 β-lactamases are widely distributed and have been detected in porcine *A. pleuropneumoniae* isolates (62, 93–95), porcine "*A. porcitonsillarum*" isolates (62), bovine and porcine *P. multocida*, [*P.*] *aerogenes*, and *M. haemolytica* isolates (84, 85, 96), as well as porcine [*H.*] *parasuis* isolates (88, 97). Comparisons confirmed that the similar sized *bla*ROB-1-carrying plasmids from *P. multocida* and *M. haemolytica* (85) were structurally closely related. The sequences of the small *bla*ROB-1-carrying plasmids pB1000 from [*H.*] *parasuis* and pB1002 from *P. multocida* (65, 88) are also structurally related to the *bla*ROB-1-carrying plasmid pAB2 from bovine *M. haemolytica* (98) and the APP7_A plasmid from *A. pleuropneumoniae* (accession number CP001094) (Fig. 3), as well as to the *tet*(B)-carrying tetracycline resistance plasmid pHS-Tet from [*H.*] *parasuis* (75). Comparative analysis confirmed that all so far sequenced *bla*ROB-1 genes from *M. haemolytica*, *A. pleuropneumoniae*, "*A. porcitonsillarum*," and [*H.*] *parasuis* code for an identical β-lactamase protein of 305 amino acids. Mutations in the *bla*ROB-1 gene, which resulted in resistance to extended-spectrum cephalosporins and β-lactamase inhibitors, have been produced *in vitro* (99). Only a single report has described the detection of a TEM-1 β-lactamase in a *P. multocida* isolate from a human dog-bite wound (89). Similarly, PSE-1 β-lactamase has been found in a single avian *P. multocida* isolate (76). In these studies, the TEM-1 β-lactamase was confirmed by isoelectric focusing and sequence analysis of part of the *bla*TEM-1 gene, whereas the *bla*PSE-1 gene was completely sequenced. The *bla*CMY-2 gene, detected by Chander and coworkers (90) in an apparently ceftiofur-resistant *P. multocida* isolate from a pig, was only detected by PCR. Since the *bla*CMY-2 gene was also detected in ceftiofur-susceptible isolates in the same study and no functional analysis has been conducted, the role of *bla*CMY-2 in ceftiofur resistance of *P. multocida* remains questionable.

β-Lactam resistance among *Pasteurellaceae* is often associated with small plasmids. These range in size between 4.1 and 5.7 kb in *P. multocida* (65, 84, 89), 4.1 and 5.2 kb in *M. haemolytica* (85, 87, 98, 100–104), 2.5 and 15.1 kb in *A. pleuropneumoniae* (93–95, 105–107), 8.7 and 13.4 kb in "*A. porcitonsillarum*" (62, 108), and 2.7 and 4.6 kb in [*H.*] *parasuis* (88, 97). Complete sequences indicate that *bla*ROB-1-carrying

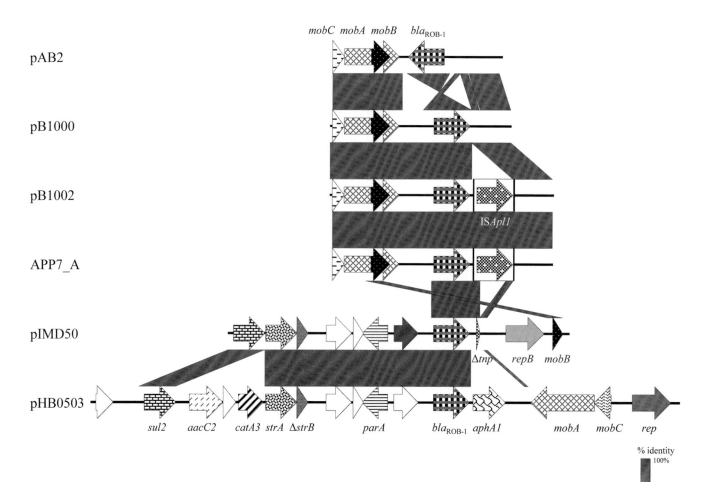

Figure 3 Schematic representation of the structure and organization of the bla_{ROB-1}-carrying resistance plasmids from *M. haemolytica*, [*H.*] *parasuis*, *P. multocida*, *A. pleuropneumoniae*, and "*A. porcitonsillarum*." Comparison of the maps of bla_{ROB-1}-carrying resistance plasmids pAB2 (accession no. Z21724; 4,316 bp) from *M. haemolytica*, pB1000 (accession no. DQ840517; 4,613 bp) from [*H.*] *parasuis*, pB1002 (accession no. EU283341; 5,685 bp) from *P. multocida*, APP7_A (accession no. CP001094; 5,685 bp) from *A. pleuropneumoniae*, pIMD50 (accession no. AJ830711; 8,751 bp) from "*A. porcitonsillarum*," and pHB0503 (accession no. EU715370; 15,079 bp) from *A. pleuropneumoniae*. It should be noted that another three pIMD50-related bla_{ROB-1}-carrying resistance plasmids from "*A. porcitonsillarum*" have been sequenced completely: pKMA5 (accession no. AM748705), pKMA202 (accession no. AM748706), and pKMA1467 (accession no. AJ830712). Genes are shown as arrows, with the arrowhead indicating the direction of transcription. The following genes are involved in antimicrobial resistance: *sul2* (sulfonamide resistance), *strA* and *strB* (streptomycin resistance), bla_{ROB-1} (β-lactam resistance), *aacC2* (gentamicin resistance), *catA3* (chloramphenicol resistance), and *aphA1* (kanamycin/neomycin resistance); plasmid replication: *rep*; mobilization functions: *mobA*, *mobB*, and *mobC*; resolvase function: *res*; DNA partition: *parA*; unknown function: open reading frames indicated by white arrows. The prefix Δ indicates a truncated functionally inactive gene. Gray-shaded areas indicate the regions common to plasmids, and the different shades of gray illustrate the percentages of nucleotide sequence identity between the plasmids, as indicated by the scale at the bottom of the figure. A distance scale in kilobases is shown.

plasmids of ≥6 kb encode additional resistance genes, as shown in Table 3. Most of the β-lactam resistance plasmids detected among *Pasteurellaceae* have been identified phenotypically by transformation or conjugation experiments. Recently, some β-lactam-resistant *A. pleuropneumoniae* isolates from South Korea were found to be negative by PCR for both *bla*ROB-1 and *bla*TEM-1 (73, 81). The mechanism of this resistance has not yet been investigated.

Resistance to Aminoglycosides and Aminocyclitols

Resistance to aminoglycoside and aminocyclitol antibiotics is usually mediated by enzymes that inactivate the drugs by adenylation, acetylation, or phosphorylation. Moreover, mutations in chromosomal genes have also been identified to mediate resistance to selected members of these classes of antimicrobial agents (109).

Resistance to aminoglycosides and aminocyclitols by enzymatic inactivation

Streptomycin and/or spectinomycin resistance mediated by enzymatic inactivation

The first aminoglycoside resistance genes detected in *Pasteurella* and *Mannheimia* were those mediating streptomycin resistance. In 1978, Berman and Hirsh published a report on plasmids coding for streptomycin resistance along with sulfonamide resistance, or sulfonamide and tetracycline resistance, in *P. multocida* from turkeys (44). Streptomycin resistance is commonly associated with small nonconjugative plasmids of less than 15 kb in *P. multocida* (44–47, 59, 65, 110–114), [*P.*] *aerogenes* (53), *M. haemolytica* (103, 115), *Mannheimia varigena* (116), "*A. porcitonsillarum*" (62), *A. pleuropneumoniae* (94, 95, 107, 117–122), and *Avibacterium paragallinarum* (123). In one case, streptomycin resistance was mediated by a conjugative multiresistance plasmid of approximately 113 kb in an avian *P. multocida* isolate, but the resistance genes were not investigated (47). Many of these plasmids carry additional resistance genes such as the sulfonamide resistance gene *sul2*, the kanamycin/neomycin resistance gene *aphA1*, the chloramphenicol resistance gene *catA3* (Fig. 4), and/or the ampicillin resistance gene *bla*ROB-1 (Fig. 3) (Table 3).

The predominant streptomycin resistance gene in bacteria of the genera *Pasteurella*, *Mannheimia*, and *Actinobacillus* is *strA*. It codes for an aminoglycoside-3″-phosphotransferase of 269 amino acids and is sometimes found together with the gene *strB*, which codes for an aminoglycoside-6-phosphotransferase of 278 amino acids. Both genes are part of transposon Tn5393 from *Erwinia amylovora* (124). In the streptomycin-resistant *Pasteurella*, *Mannheimia*, and *Actinobacillus* isolates, *strA* is usually complete, whereas various truncated *strB* genes have been identified (116, 121, 125). Isolates that carry a functionally active *strA* gene, but a largely truncated *strB* gene, have been shown to be highly resistant to streptomycin (125), suggesting that *strA* is the relevant gene for the expression of streptomycin resistance. Further support for this hypothesis comes from the observation that plasmid pSTOJO1, which carries an intact *strB* gene but a functionally inactive *strA* gene that is disrupted by the integration of a *dfrA14* gene cassette, does not express streptomycin resistance in *E. coli* (126). Studies of the prevalence and distribution of the *strA-strB* genes showed that the *strA* gene—in combination with a complete or truncated copy of *strB*—occurs on plasmids or in the chromosomal DNA of a wide range of commensal and pathogenic bacteria from humans, animals, and plants (127–129).

An *aadA1* gene coding for an aminoglycoside-3″-adenyltransferase that mediates resistance to both the aminoglycoside streptomycin and the aminocyclitol spectinomycin has been detected on the 5.2-kb plasmid pJR2 from avian *P. multocida* (76) and the 5.4-kb plasmid pCCK343 from porcine [*P.*] *aerogenes* (130). In pJR2, the *aadA1* gene is part of a gene cassette, along with *bla*PSE-1, that is inserted into a relic of a class 1 integron. The *intI1* gene coding for the integrase in the 5′-conserved segment of this integron is truncated, but without affecting the promotor, and the *sul1* gene in the 3′ conserved fragment is missing completely (76). In plasmid pCCK343, a gene cassette array comprised of *dfrA1-sat2-aadA1* is part of a truncated class 2 integron (130). In this case, the streptothricin acetyltransferase gene, *sat2*, conferred resistance to the streptothricin antibiotic nourseothricin (MIC, >256 mg/liter), in addition to the streptomycin and spectinomycin resistance (MICs of >256 mg/liter for both) conferred by the aminoglycoside adenyltransferase gene, *aadA1*. Attempts to identify the *aadA* genes in bovine isolates of *P. multocida* and *M. haemolytica* from Germany that are highly resistant to streptomycin and spectinomycin using PCR were unsuccessful (131). In all these isolates, streptomycin resistance was based on an *strA* gene, whereas a spectinomycin resistance gene could not be identified.

A novel streptomycin-spectinomycin resistance gene, designated *aadA14*, was identified on a small 5.2-kb plasmid from a bovine *P. multocida* capsular type F isolate from Belgium (132). The corresponding isolate was

Table 3 Subset of resistance plasmids identified in *Pasteurella*, *Mannheimia*, and *Actinobacillus* of veterinary importance

Plasmid designation	Plasmid size (kb)	Plasmid sequencing	Resistance genotype	Bacterial source	Accession number	Reference
pARD3079	4.0	Complete	*sul2*	*A. pleuropneumoniae*	AM748707	108
pKMA2425	3.1	Complete	*sul2*	*A. pleuropneumoniae*	AJ830714	108
pKMA757	4.5	Complete	*sul2*	"*A. porcitonsillarum*"	AJ830713	108
ABB7_B	4.2	Complete	*sul2, strA*	*A. pleuropneumoniae*	NC_010941	Unpublished
pFZG1012	Unknown	Partial	*sul2, strA*	[*H.*] *parasuis*	HQ015158	Unpublished
pYC93	4.2	Complete	*sul2, strA*	[*H.*] *parasuis*	HM486907	194
pB1005	4.2	Complete	*sul2, strA*	*P. multocida*	FJ197818	65
pHN06	5.4	Complete	*sul2, strA*	*P. multocida*	NC_017035	114
Unnamed	5.4	Complete	*sul2, strA*	*P. multocida*	CP003314	114
pCCK1900	10.2	Complete	*sul2, strA, strB, floR*	*P. multocida*	FM179941	178
pMS260	8.1	Complete	*sul2, strA, strB*	*A. pleuropneumoniae*	AB109805	121
pTYM1	4.2	Complete	*sul2, strA, ΔstrB*	*A. pleuropneumoniae*	AF303375	94
pPSAS1522	4.2	Complete	*sul2, strA, ΔstrB*	*A. pleuropneumoniae*	AJ877041	108
pYFC1	4.2	Complete	*sul2, strA, ΔstrB*	*M. haemolytica*	M83717	103
pPASS2	4.7	Partial	*sul2, strA, ΔstrB*	[*P.*] *aerogenes*	Not provided	125
pPASS1	5.5	Partial	*sul2, strA, ΔstrB*	[*P.*] *aerogenes*	Not provided	125
pIG1	5.4	Complete	*sul2, strA, ΔstrB*	*P. multocida*	U57647	150
pB1003	5.1	Complete	*sul2, strA, ΔstrB*	*P. multocida*	EU360945	65
pPMSS1	4.2	Partial	*sul2, strA, ΔstrB*	*P. multocida*	Not provided	125
pB1003	5.0	Complete	*sul2, strA, ΔstrB*	*P. multocida*	EU360945	65
pKMA505	8.6	Complete	*sul2, strA, ΔstrB*	"*A. porcitonsillarum*"	NC_007094	108
pYMH5	5.0	Complete	*sul2, Δsul2, strA, ΔstrB, aphA1*	*A. paragallinarum*	EF015636	123
pIMD50	8.8	Complete	*sul2, strA, ΔstrB, bla*$_{\text{ROB-1}}$	"*A. porcitonsillarum*"	NC_007095	108
pKMA5	9.5	Complete	*sul2, strA, ΔstrB, bla*$_{\text{ROB-1}}$	"*A. porcitonsillarum*"	NC_009623	108
pKMA1467	11.1	Complete	*sul2, strA, ΔstrB, bla*$_{\text{ROB-1}}$	"*A. porcitonsillarum*"	NC_007096	108
pOV	13.6	Complete	*sul2, strA, ΔstrB, bla*$_{\text{ROB-1}}$	*P. multocida*	JX827416	Unpublished
pKMA202	13.4	Complete	*sul2, strA, strB, bla*$_{\text{ROB-1}}$	"*A. porcitonsillarum*"	AM748706	108
pM3389T	6.1	Complete	*sul2, ΔstrA, dfrA14*	*A. pleuropneumoniae*	KP197005	122
pM3224T	6.1	Complete	*sul2, ΔstrA, dfrA14, strB*	*A. pleuropneumoniae*	KP197004	122
pMHSCS1	5.0	Complete	*sul2, catA3, strA, ΔstrB*	*Mannheimia* taxon 10[a]	AJ249249	125
pMVSCS1	5.6	Complete	*sul2, catA3, strA, ΔstrB*	*M. varigena*	NC_003411	116
pPASCS1	5.6	Partial	*sul2, catA3, strA, ΔstrB*	[*P.*] *aerogenes*	Not provided	125
pPASCS2	6.0	Partial	*sul2, catA3, strA, ΔstrB*	[*P.*] *aerogenes*	Not provided	125
pPASCS3	6.1	Partial	*sul2, catA3, strA, ΔstrB*	[*P.*] *aerogenes*	Not provided	125
pCCK13698	15.0	Complete	*sul2, catA3, ΔstrA, floR*	*B. trehalosi*	AM183225	183
pFZ51	15.7	Complete	*sul2, aacC2, catA3, strA, ΔstrB, bla*$_{\text{ROB-1}}$*, aphA1*	[*H.*] *parasuis*	JN202624	Unpublished
pHB0503	15.1	Complete	*sul2, aacC2, catA3, strA, strB, bla*$_{\text{ROB-1}}$*, aphA1*	*A. pleuropneumoniae*	EU715370	95
pVM111	9.8	Partial	*sul2, tetR-tet(H), strA, strB*	*P. multocida*	AJ514834	49, 59

Plasmid	Size (kb)	Status	Resistance gene(s)	Species	Accession no.	Reference
pCCK154	11.0	Partial	*sul2, dfrA20*	*P. multocida*	AJ605332	146
pJR1	6.8	Complete	*sul2, tet*(G), *catB2*	*P. multocida*	AY232670	76
p9956	5.7	Complete	*tetR-tet*(H)	*A. pleuropneumoniae*	AY362554	60
pMHT1	4.4	Partial	*tetR-tet*(H)	*M. haemolytica*	Y16103	64
pPAT1	5.5	Partial	*tetR-tet*(H)	[*P.*] *aerogenes*	AJ245947	52
pPMT1	6.8	Partial	*tetR-tet*(H)	*P. multocida*	Y15510	50
pB1018	6.0	Complete	*tetR-tet*(H)	*P. multocida*	JQ319774	Unpublished
p12494	14.4	Complete	Δ*tetR-tet*(H)	*A. pleuropneumoniae*	DQ517426	61
p9555	5.7	Complete	*tet*(L)	*A. pleuropneumoniae*	AY359464	60
pCCK3259	5.3	Complete	*tet*(L)	*M. haemolytica*	NC_006976	79
p11745	5.5	Complete	*tet*(B)	*A. pleuropneumoniae*	DQ176855	60
pHS-Tet	5.1	Complete	*tet*(B)	[*H.*] *parasuis*	AY862435	75
pTetHS016	3.4	Complete	*tet*(B)	[*H.*] *parasuis*	KC818265	195
pHPS1019	4.6	Complete	*tet*(B)	[*H.*] *parasuis*	HQ622101	Unpublished
pB1001	5.1	Complete	*tet*(B)	*P. multocida*	EU252517	65
pPAT2	4.8	Partial	*tetR-tet*(B)	[*P.*] *aerogenes*	AJ278685	53
p13142	6.0	Partial	*tet*(O)	*A. pleuropneumoniae*	AY987963	60
pB1006	6.0	Complete	*tet*(O)	*P. multocida*	FJ234438	65
pJR2	5.3	Complete	*aadA1, bla*$_{\text{PSE-1}}$	*P. multocida*	AY232671	76
pCCK343	5.4	Complete	*aadA1, dfrA1, sat2*	[*P.*] *aerogenes*	FR687372	130
pCCK647	5.2	Complete	*aadA14*	*P. multocida*	NC_006868	132
Unnamed	Unknown	Partial	*bla*$_{\text{ROB-1}}$	*A. pleuropneumoniae*	Not provided	105
APP7_A	5.7	Complete	*bla*$_{\text{ROB-1}}$	*A. pleuropneumoniae*	CP001094	Unpublished
pB1000	4.6	Complete	*bla*$_{\text{ROB-1}}$	[*H.*] *parasuis* *P. multocida*	DQ840517GU080062, GU080067	8865
pAB2	4.3	Complete	*bla*$_{\text{ROB-1}}$	*M. haemolytica*	Z21724	98
pPH51	4.1	Partial	*bla*$_{\text{ROB-1}}$	*M. haemolytica*	X52872	85
pYFC2	4.2	Partial	*bla*$_{\text{ROB-1}}$	*M. haemolytica*	Not provided	103
pB1002	5.7	Complete	*bla*$_{\text{ROB-1}}$	*P. multocida*	EU283341	65
pJMA-1	2.7	Complete	*bla*$_{\text{ROB-1}}$	[*H.*] *parasuis*	KP164834	97
pCCK411	5.3	Complete	*bla*$_{\text{ROB-1}}$, *aphA3*	*P. multocida*	FR798946.1	135
pFS39	7.6	Complete	*bla*$_{\text{ROB-1}}$, *erm*(T)	[*H.*] *parasuis*	KC405064	154
pFAB-1	4.3	Partial	*bla*$_{\text{TEM-1}}$	*P. multocida*	Not provided	89
pHPSF1	6.3	Complete	*floR*	[*H.*] *parasuis*	KR262062.1	180
pM3446F	7.7	Complete	*floR*	*A. pleuropneumoniae*	KP696484	181
pCCK381	10.8	Complete	*floR*	*P. multocida*	NC_006994	174
pMH1405	7.7	Complete	*floR*	*P. multocida*	NC_019260[1]	179
p518	3.9	Complete	*floR, strA, strB*	*A. pleuropneumoniae*	KT355773	182
pQY431	7.8	Complete	*aacA-aphD*	[*H.*] *parasuis*	KC405065	Unpublished
FJS5863	7.8	Complete	*aacA-aphD, bla*$_{\text{ROB-1}}$	[*H.*] *parasuis*	HQ015159	Unpublished
pHN61	6.3	Complete	*lnu*(C)	[*H.*] *parasuis*	FJ947048	161

[a]Initially identified as *M. haemolytica*.

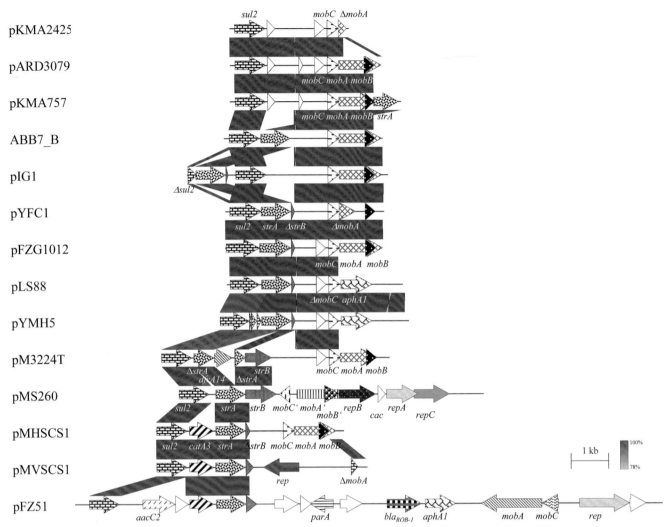

Figure 4 Schematic representation of the structure and organization of selected *sul2*-based (multi-)resistance plasmids from *A. pleuropneumoniae*, "*A. porcitonsillarum*," *A. paragallinarum*, *H. ducreyi*, [*H.*] *parasuis*, *M. haemolytica*, *Mannheimia* unnamed taxon 10, *M. varigena*, and *P. multocida*. Comparison of the maps of the plasmids pKMA2425 (accession no. AJ830714; 3,156 bp) from *A. pleuropneumoniae*, pARD3079 (accession no. AM748707; 4,065 bp) from *A. pleuropneumoniae*, pKMA757 (accession no. AJ830713; 4,556 bp) from "*A. porcitonsillarum*," ABB7_B (accession no. NC_010941; 4,236 bp) from *A. pleuropneumoniae*, pIG1 (accession no. U57647) from *P. multocida*, pYFC1 (accession no. M83717) from *M. haemolytica*, pFZG1012 (accession no. HQ015158; partially sequenced) from [*H.*] *parasuis*, pLS88 (accession no. L23118; 4,772 bp) from *H. ducreyi*, pYMH5 (accession no. EF015636; 4,772 bp) from *A. paragallinarum*, pM3224T (accession no. KP197004; 6,050 bp) from *A. pleuropneumoniae*, pMS260 (accession no. AB109805; 8,124 bp) from *A. pleuropneumoniae*, pMVSCS1 (accession no. AJ319822; 5,621 bp) from *M. varigena*, pMHSCS1 (accession no. AJ249249; 4,992 bp) from *Mannheimia* unnamed taxon 10, pFZ51 (accession no. JN202624; 15,672 bp) from [*H.*] *parasuis*, and pKMA757 (accession no. AJ830713; 4,556 bp) from "*A. porcitonsillarum*." The map of another *sul2*-based multiresistance plasmid, pIMD50 (accession no. AJ830711) from "*A. porcitonsillarum*," is displayed in Fig. 3. Genes are shown as arrows, with the arrowhead indicating the direction of transcription. The following genes are involved in antimicrobial resistance: *sul2* (sulfonamide resistance), *strA* and *strB* (streptomycin resistance), *catA3* (chloramphenicol resistance), *aphA1* (kanamycin/neomycin resistance), and *bla*$_{ROB-1}$ (β-lactam resistance); plasmid replication: *rep*, *repA*, *repB*, and *repC*; mobilization functions: *mobA*, *mobB*, *mobC*, *mobA´*, *mobB´*, and *mobC´*; unknown function: open reading frames indicated by white arrows. The prefix Δ indicates a truncated functionally inactive gene. Gray-shaded areas indicate the regions common to plasmids and the different shades of gray illustrate the percentages of nucleotide sequence identity between the plasmids, as indicated by the scale at the bottom of the figure. A distance scale in kilobases is shown.

obtained from a case of fatal peritonitis in a calf (14). The 261-amino acid AadA14 adenyltransferase protein exhibited only 51.4 to 56.0% identity to the so far known AadA proteins and hence proved to be only distantly related to AadA proteins previously found in other bacteria.

Two ICEs from *Pasteurellaceae*, ICE*Pmu*1 and ICE*Mh*1, have been shown to contain genes associated with resistance to streptomycin and other aminoglycosides and aminocyclitols (55, 56). In addition to other resistance genes, the 92-kb ICE*Mh*1 contains *strA* and *strB*, conferring resistance to streptomycin (MIC, 256 mg/liter), as well as *aphA1*, conferring resistance to kanamycin/neomycin (MICs, ≥512 mg/liter and 64 mg/liter, respectively) (56). The 82-kb ICE*Pmu*1 carries 12 resistance genes, including *strA* and *strB*, *aadA25*, *aadB*, and *aphA1*, with the latter three genes conferring resistance to streptomycin (MIC, ≥256 mg/liter) and spectinomycin (MIC, ≥512 mg/liter), gentamicin (MIC, 128 mg/liter), and kanamycin/neomycin (MICs, ≥128 mg/liter and ≥32 mg/liter), respectively, in *P. multocida* strain 36950 (54, 55).

Kanamycin and neomycin resistance mediated by enzymatic inactivation

Kanamycin/neomycin resistance has been associated with the gene *aphA1*, also known as *aph(3')-Ia*, which codes for an aminoglycoside-3'-phosphotransferase that mediates resistance to kanamycin and neomycin. This gene has been identified on transposon Tn*903* (133). Subsequently, it was detected together with the streptomycin resistance genes *strA-strB* and the sulfonamide resistance gene *sul2* on the broad-host-range plasmid pLS88 from human host-specific *Haemophilus ducreyi* (134). A pLS88-related plasmid has also been identified in the *A. paragallinarum* strain A14 (123) (Fig. 4). Further studies on kanamycin/neomycin-resistant [*P.*] *aerogenes*, *P. multocida*, and *M. glucosida* isolates identified the *aphA1* gene mostly in chromosomal DNA (135). In a single *P. multocida* isolate, this gene was found on the 5,955-bp plasmid pCCK3152, along with complete *strA* and *sul2* genes and a truncated *strB* gene (135). The 15.1-kb multiresistance plasmid pHB0503 (95) and the 15.7-kb plasmid pFZ51 (accession number JN202624), both carrying *sul2*, *aacC2*, *catA3*, *strA*, *strB*, and *bla*ROB-1, along with *aphA1*, have been identified in Chinese *A. pleuropneumoniae* and [*H.*] *parasuis* isolates, respectively. Kang et al. (95) reported that the *A. pleuropneumoniae* isolate harboring pHB0503 was resistant to streptomycin (MIC, 512 mg/liter), kanamycin (MIC, 256 mg/liter), and gentamicin (MIC, 512 mg/liter), as well as to penicillin (MIC, 256 mg/liter),

sulfadimidine (MIC, 1,024 mg/liter), and chloramphenicol (MIC, 16 mg/liter), whereas the [*H.*] *parasuis* isolate harboring pFZ51 has not been characterized (Fig. 4).

A second kanamycin/neomycin resistance gene, *aphA3* [also known as *aph(3')-III*], was detected on the 5.1-kb plasmid pCCK411 in single isolates of *P. multocida* and [*P.*] *aerogenes* (135). In addition to the *aphA3* gene, this plasmid also carried a *mobABC* operon for mobilization. A not further specified aminoglycoside-3'-phosphotransferase gene mediating kanamycin resistance was also found, together with a *bla*ROB-1 gene, on the 6-kb plasmid pTMY2 from *A. pleuropneumoniae* (94). Two virtually identical 7,777-bp plasmids from [*H.*] *parasuis*, FJS5863 (accession number HQ015159), and pQY431 (accession number KC405065) contain the *aacA-aphD* gene encoding a bifunctional aminoglycoside N-acetyltransferase and aminoglycoside phosphotransferase, in addition to the *bla*ROB-1 gene, but no functional studies of these plasmids have been published.

Gentamicin resistance mediated by enzymatic inactivation

Although *P. multocida*, *A. pleuropneumoniae*, and "*A. porcitonsillarum*" isolates with MICs of gentamicin of ≥32 mg/liter have been detected, most attempts to detect specific resistance genes, such as *aadB* [*ant (2'')-Ia*], *aacC2* [*aac(3)-IIc*], or *aacC4* [*aac(3)-IVa*], have failed (62; Kehrenberg and Schwarz, unpublished data). Moreover, attempts to transfer gentamicin resistance from *P. multocida* donors were also unsuccessful (Kehrenberg and Schwarz, unpublished data). Recently, PCR analysis revealed that among 12 gentamicin-resistant *A. pleuropneumoniae* isolates from South Korea, 11 produced amplicons specific for *aadB* [*ant (2'')-Ia*], and one for *aacC4* [*aac(3)-IVa*] (81). In addition, a 15.1-kb plasmid from *A. pleuropneumoniae* (pHB0503) has been found carrying *aacC2*, encoding an aminoglycoside-acetyltransferase (95). This plasmid conferred an MIC of gentamicin of 512 mg/liter in the original serovar 4 clinical isolate (from China) and an MIC of 256 mg/liter when transformed into M62, the reference strain of *A. pleuropneumoniae* serovar 4 (95). The 15.7-kb plasmid pFZ51 (accession number JN202624) from [*H.*] *parasuis* also carries *aacC2* but has not been functionally characterized (Fig. 4).

Resistance to aminocyclitols by mutations

Ribosomal mutations conferring spectinomycin resistance have been described in a variety of bacteria (136–140). All these mutations were present in a specific region of helix 34 in 16S rRNA. This region encompassed the cross-linked positions 1063 to 1066 and 1090 to

1093, which are known to be involved in the binding of spectinomycin to the ribosome. Moreover, the *rpsE* gene coding for the ribosomal protein S5 is also relevant for the drug binding, and mutations in *rpsE* have been described to affect spectinomycin binding (141, 142). The analysis of high-level spectinomycin-resistant *P. multocida* isolates (MICs of spectinomycin ≥4,096 mg/liter), in which no enzymatic inactivation of the drug could be detected, revealed four types of mutations: (i) a C1192G transversion (no additional mutations in positions which have been associated with spectinomycin resistance were found) in 16S rRNA in all six or (ii) in five of the six rRNA operons, (iii) the aforementioned transversion in only two of the six operons accompanied by a 3-bp deletion in *rpsE* that resulted in a change of the amino acids 32-SF-33 to 32-I, and (iv) a 3-bp deletion in *rpsE* that resulted in the loss of 23-K without additional rRNA mutations (143). Molecular modeling suggested that both types of mutations in the S5 protein have a negative impact on spectinomycin binding to the ribosome.

Resistance to Folate Pathway Inhibitors

Sulfonamides and trimethoprim are competitive inhibitors of different enzymatic steps in folic acid metabolism. Sulfonamides represent structural analogs of *p*-aminobenzoic acid and inhibit the enzyme dihydropteroate synthase (DHPS), which—in the initial step of folic acid metabolism—catalyzes the synthesis of dihydropteroic acid from dihydropteridin and *p*-aminobenzoic acid. Trimethoprim inhibits the enzyme dihydrofolate reductase (DHFR), which—in a later step of folic acid metabolism—reduces dihydrofolic acid to tetrahydrofolic acid. Resistance to both drugs is commonly mediated by replacement of susceptible DHPS or DHFR enzymes by those with reduced affinity to sulfonamides or trimethoprim, respectively. Moreover, overproduction of susceptible targets, or mutations in chromosomal DHPS or DHFR genes, which alter substrate specificity, may also cause resistance (109). However, overproduction of a trimethoprim-sensitive DHFR, encoded by the gene *folH* (144), or a short insertion into the chromosomal gene *folP* encoding a DHPS (145), have so far only been reported to confer resistance to trimethoprim or sulfonamides, respectively, in human host-specific *H. influenzae*.

Sulfonamide resistance mediated by altered DHPSs

Sulfonamide resistance among *Pasteurella*, *Mannheimia*, *Actinobacillus*, and *Haemophilus* isolates is commonly mediated by a type 2 DHPS with reduced affinity to sulfonamides. The corresponding gene, *sul2*, is frequently found on small plasmids with sizes ranging from 3.1 to 15.7 kb (Table 3). The *sul2*-encoded DHPS proteins commonly consist of 271 amino acids. However, several variants ranging in size between 263 and 289 amino acids have also been reported (11, 55, 56, 125, 134, 146). Sequence analysis showed that single-base pair insertions downstream of codon 225 in the DHPS of the *H. ducreyi* plasmid pLS88 (134) resulted in a shortened C-terminus that differs from all so far known DHPS variants. A mutation in the translational stop codon of the *sul2* gene from plasmids pYFC1 of *M. haemolytica* (103) and pTYM1 of *A. pleuropneumoniae* (94) led to an extension of 12 amino acids at the C-terminus. In plasmid pCCK154 from *P. multocida*, the loss of a single "A" at position 793 within the *sul2* gene caused a frame-shift mutation which led to the substitution of 6 codons and extended the reading frame by 18 codons (146). Finally, a recombination in the 3′ end of the *sul2* reading frame changed the final three codons and extended the *sul2* reading frame by one codon in plasmid pVM111 from *P. multocida* (59). Plasmids carrying *sul2* have also been identified in bacteria other than *Pasteurellaceae*, e.g., *E. coli* (147) and *Photobacterium damselae* subsp. *piscicida* (148). In addition to their location on small plasmids, *sul2* genes have also been detected on broad-host-range conjugative (e.g., pGS05) or nonconjugative (e.g., RSF1010, pLS88) plasmids (134, 147, 149) and on the ICE*Pmu1* (55).

Various studies revealed that the *sul2* gene is often linked to the *strA-strB* genes (65, 103, 108, 122, 125, 134, 150). PCR assays were developed to confirm the linkage of *sul2* and *strA* in both orientations (125). In some cases, the *strA* gene followed by a truncated Δ*strB* gene was detected upstream of *sul2* (125, 150). However, in most *P. multocida*, [*P.*] *aerogenes*, and *Mannheimia* isolates studied, these genes were found in the orientation *sul2-strA*, whereas a truncated Δ*strA* may also be found upstream of *sul2* (65, 103, 125, 134). Detailed studies of the noncoding spacer between *sul2* and *strA* revealed different lengths (121, 125) and showed that this region might represent a hot spot for recombination events. A *catA3* gene, coding for chloramphenicol resistance, was found to be inserted between *sul2* and *strA* via illegitimate recombination. Such *sul2-catA3-strA* clusters have been found on various plasmids as well as in the chromosomal DNA of [*P.*] *aerogenes*, *M. haemolytica*, *M. varigena*, and *Mannheimia* taxon 10 isolates (116, 125). Further insertion of *aacC2* between *sul2* and *catA3* was identified in pHB0503 from *A. pleuropneumoniae* (95). In plasmid pVM111 from an avian *P. multocida* isolate (44, 48), a

Tn*5706*-like *tetR-tet*(H) segment, responsible for tetracycline resistance, was also found to be inserted between *sul2* and *strA* via illegitimate recombination (59). The resulting *sul2-tetR-tet*(H)-*strA* cluster, however, has not yet been detected on plasmids other than pVM111 or in the chromosomal DNA of *Pasteurella*, *Mannheimia*, or *Actinobacillus* isolates (Fig. 1). In addition to insertions between *sul2* and *strA*, two recent *A. pleuropneumoniae* plasmids, pM3224T and pM3389T, were found to have insertions of *dfrA14* (encoding trimethoprim resistance) disrupting the *strA* gene, located either downstream (pM3224T) (Fig. 4) or upstream (pM3389T) of *sul2* (122).

Several small plasmids that carry only the sulfonamide resistance gene *sul2*, but no other resistance genes, have been sequenced completely. These include the plasmids pKMA2425 (3,156 bp) and pARD3079 (4,065 bp), both from *A. pleuropneumoniae*, as well as pKMA757 (4,556 bp) from "*A. porcitonsillarum*" (108) (Fig. 4). A 4,236-bp *A. pleuropneumoniae* plasmid, ABB7_B (accession number NC_010941), carries *sul2* and *strA*. All of these plasmids share the same mobilization genes (*mobABC*), except pKM2425, which contains only *mobC* and a truncated copy of *mobA* (Fig. 4).

Other *sul* genes, such as *sul1* and *sul3*, which also code for dihydropteroate synthetases with reduced affinity to sulfonamides, have not yet been detected among *Pasteurellaceae* species (62; Kehrenberg and Schwarz, unpublished data).

Trimethoprim Resistance Mediated by Altered DHFRs

A novel trimethoprim resistance gene was detected on the 11-kb plasmid pCCK154 from bovine *P. multocida* (146). This plasmid was transferable into *E. coli*, where it replicated and expressed high-level resistance to sulfonamides and trimethoprim. Sequence analysis identified the gene *sul2* for sulfonamide resistance and a novel gene, designated *dfrA20*, for trimethoprim resistance. The *dfrA20* gene codes for a trimethoprim-resistant DHFR of 169 amino acids, which is only distantly related to the DHFRs of Gram-negative bacteria, but upon cluster analysis appears to be related to those found in the Gram-positive genera *Staphylococcus*, *Bacillus*, and *Listeria* (146).

A different trimethoprim resistance gene, *dfrA1*, was identified on plasmid pCCK343 recovered from a porcine intestinal [*P.*] *aerogenes* isolate (130). This 5,415-bp plasmid contains a backbone sequence with homology to pHS-Tet, including the *mobC* gene (but not *mobAB*), with insertion of a partially truncated class 2 integron containing *dfrA1-sat2-aadA1*. In addition to conferring trimethoprim resistance (MIC, >256 mg/liter), the presence of the streptothricin acetyltransferase gene, *sat2*, and the aminoglycoside adenyltransferase gene, *aadA1*, conferred resistance to the streptothricin antibiotic nourseothricin (MIC, >256 mg/liter) and to streptomycin and spectinomycin (MICs of >256 mg/liter each), respectively. The truncated integron showed high identity with a sequence found in an *E. coli* ICE, AGI-5 (130).

Earlier studies of trimethoprim-resistant bovine *M. haemolytica* isolates from France revealed that this resistance was not associated with plasmids, and also was not transferable by conjugation. Hybridization experiments with gene probes specific for the genes *dfrA1* to *dfrA5* did not yield positive results (151). Similar negative PCR results were obtained for *A. pleuropneumoniae* and "*A. porcitonsillarum*" isolates in Switzerland, in which none of 27 different *dfrA* or *dfrB* genes—including *dfrA20*—could be identified using primers designed to detect groups of *dfr* genes (62). Recently, whole-genome sequencing was used to identify *dfrA14* in trimethoprim-resistant *A. pleuropneumoniae* isolates from the United Kingdom (122). This gene may have been responsible for trimethoprim resistance in the Swiss isolates of "*A. porcitonsillarum*" and *A. pleuropneumoniae* (62), if there was a failure to amplify a product using the primers designed to detect *dfrA5*/*dfrA14*/*dfrA25*. Alternatively, these isolates possess another mechanism for trimethoprim resistance that remains to be elucidated. The study by Bossé et al. (122) highlights the value of whole-genome sequencing for determination of the genetic basis of resistance, not only providing information regarding the presence of specific resistance genes and/or mutations, but also facilitating localization of the gene(s) within the chromosomal DNA or on plasmids.

In the United Kingdom isolates, two distinct mobilizable trimethoprim resistance plasmids were identified (122) in which the *dfrA14* gene was inserted into *strA*, as has been reported for enterobacterial plasmids pSTOJO1 and pCERC1 (126, 152). Differences in the gene order of flanking regions, with pM3224T carrying *sul2-strA-dfrA14-strA-strB* (Fig. 4) and pM3389T carrying *strA-dfrA14-strA-sul2*, suggest separate recombination of the *strA-dfrA14-strA* cassette (likely of enterobacterial origin) into different *Pasteurellaceae* plasmids.

Resistance to Macrolides

Many Gram-negative bacteria are believed to be innately resistant to macrolides due to permeability barriers or multidrug efflux pumps. However, chemical modification of the ribosomal target site by rRNA methylases or mutations in ribosomal proteins have also been described (109).

Macrolide Resistance Mediated by rRNA Methylases

Studies of the presence of macrolide resistance genes in bacteria of the genus *Actinobacillus* led to the identification of the rRNA methylase genes *erm*(A) and *erm*(C) in *A. pleuropneumoniae* (70). Mating experiments showed that these genes were transferred into *Moraxella catarrhalis* and/or *Enterococcus faecalis* (70). PCR-directed analysis of bovine *P. multocida* and *M. haemolytica* which exhibited MICs of erythromycin of ≥16 mg/liter did not detect any of the three genes *erm*(A), *erm*(B), or *erm*(C) (Kehrenberg and Schwarz, unpublished data). Matter and coworkers obtained similar results for *A. pleuropneumoniae* and "*A. porcitonsillarum*" isolates with MICs of tilmicosin of ≥32 mg/liter, in which none of the genes *erm*(A), *erm*(B), or *erm*(C) could be detected by PCR (62). Australian isolates of *A. pleuropneumoniae* with MICs of erythromycin of ≥16 mg/liter and/or MICs of tilmicosin of ≥32 mg/liter (40) also failed to amplify specific products for *erm*(A), *erm*(B), *erm*(C), *erm*(42), *mph*(E), *mef*(A), *msr*(A), or *msr*(E) (153). Furthermore, whole-genome sequencing of *A. pleuropneumoniae* HS 3572 (MIC of erythromycin of 16 mg/liter; MIC of tilmicosin of 32 mg/liter; MIC of tulathromycin of 16 mg/liter) revealed neither specific macrolide resistance genes nor any known point mutations previously associated with macrolide resistance (153). In [*H.*] *parasuis*, a 7,577-bp plasmid, pFS39, has been reported to carry the *erm*(T) gene, previously only identified in Gram-positive bacteria, along with *bla*_{ROB-1} (154). The [*H.*] *parasuis* isolate harboring pFS39 had MICs of 64 mg/liter for both erythromycin and lincomycin (154). A novel mono-methyltransferase gene, *erm*(42), has been identified in the chromosome of *M. haemolytica* and *P. multocida* isolates with high levels of resistance to multiple macrolides (155–157). The sequence of this monomethyltransferase gene was found to be divergent from previously reported *erm* genes and was only detected by whole-genome sequencing of the resistant isolates.

Macrolide Resistance Mediated by Mutations in Ribosomal Proteins and 23S rRNA

Mutations in ribosomal proteins L4 or L22 have been reported in human macrolide-resistant *H. influenzae* (158). In isolates of *P. multocida* and *M. haemolytica* reported to be highly resistant (MICs >64 mg/liter) to multiple macrolides including erythromycin, tilmicosin,

tildipirosin, tulathromycin, and gamithromycin, mutations were found in one of two locations (either A2058G or A2059G) in all six copies of the 23S rRNA (159). Similarly, genome sequencing revealed an A2059G transition in all six copies of the 23S rRNA gene in one isolate of [*H.*] *parasuis* (HS 315) with MICs of erythromycin of 64 mg/liter, tilmicosin of ≥128 mg/liter, and tulathromycin of 64 mg/liter; however, other isolates with MICs of erythromycin of 64 mg/liter, but lower MICs of tilmicosin and tulathromycin compared to HS 315, did not show this, or any other known, mutation associated with macrolide resistance (153).

Macrolide Resistance Mediated by Active Efflux or Inactivation by Phosphotransferases

It was shown that some isolates of *M. haemolytica*, *P. multocida*, and *H. somni* had genes, *mrs*(E) and *mph*(E), encoding macrolide efflux and phospotransferase proteins, respectively (57, 155–157). These two genes, found in tandem and expressed from the same promoter, were also predicted to be chromosomally encoded (155, 156). When found in combination with *erm*(42), the presence of the *mrs*(E)-*mph*(E) operon resulted in the highest level of resistance to all macrolides tested (tulathromycin, gamithromycin, tilmicosin, and clindamycin), whereas those with just the *mrs*(E)-*mph*(E) genes were not resistant to clindamycin and had lower MICs for tilmicosin but higher MICs for gamithromycin and tulathromycin compared to isolates with only the *erm*(42) gene (155, 156, 160). All three genes [*erm*(42), *mrs*(E), and *mph*(E)] were identified as part of ICE*Pmu*1 (55), which might explain their dissemination across strain, species, and genus boundaries.

Resistance to Lincosamides

Resistance mechanisms to lincosamides may involve 23S rRNA methyltransferase, efflux proteins, inactivation enzyme genes, and mutations (e.g., 23S rRNA, L4 and/or L22 genes). Lincosamide transferase genes have been commonly detected among Gram-positive bacteria, and the *lnu*(F) gene has been detected in *Salmonella* and *E. coli* (http://faculty.washington.edu/marilynr/ermweb4.pdf). However, an *lnu*(C) gene, located on the 6.3-kb plasmid pHN61, was identified in a porcine [*H.*] *parasuis* isolate from China (161). The high MICs of lincomycin (32 mg/liter) and clindamycin (8 mg/liter) and the low MIC of erythromycin (0.25 mg/liter) indicates that *lnu*(C) mediates resistance to lincosamides but not to macrolides. The replication and mobilization region of pHN61 shares sequence similarity with that in pHB0503 from an *A. pleuropneumoniae* isolate.

Resistance to Phenicols

Resistance to nonfluorinated phenicols may be due to enzymatic inactivation by chloramphenicol acetyltransferases, whereas resistance to fluorinated and/or nonfluorinated phenicols can be mediated by phenicol-specific exporters (109, 162). Other mechanisms, such as permeability barriers, have rarely been detected among *Pasteurellaceae*.

Chloramphenicol resistance mediated by enzymatic inactivation

Resistance to chloramphenicol is usually due to enzymatic inactivation of the drug by chloramphenicol acetyltransferases. Two types of chloramphenicol acetyltransferases, A and B, specified by a number of different *catA* and *catB* genes, are currently known (162). The *catA* and *catB* genes are often located on plasmids, transposons, or gene cassettes. Plasmids mediating chloramphenicol resistance have been identified in porcine *P. multocida* isolates (113), bovine *P. multocida* and *M. haemolytica* isolates (163), porcine [*P.*] *aerogenes* (125), bovine *Mannheimia* spp. (116, 125), and porcine *A. pleuropneumoniae* (95, 106, 117, 164, 165). As previously seen with other resistance plasmids, those mediating chloramphenicol resistance are commonly less than 15 kb in size and occasionally carry additional resistance genes (Table 3). Initial molecular studies of chloramphenicol resistance among *P. multocida* and *M. haemolytica* isolates included the detection of the three most frequently occurring *cat* genes among Gram-negative bacteria—*catA1*, *catA2*, and *catA3* (formerly known as *catI*, *catII*, and *catIII*)—by specific PCR assays (163). The *catA3* gene was detected on small plasmids of 5.1 kb, whereas the *catA1* gene was located on plasmids of either 17.1 or 5.5 kb (163). In porcine [*P.*] *aerogenes* and bovine *Mannheimia* isolates, *catA3* genes have been identified as parts of chromosomal or plasmid-borne resistance gene clusters (116, 125). In these gene clusters, the *catA3* gene was always inserted between the sulfonamide resistance gene *sul2* and the streptomycin resistance gene *strA* (116, 125) (Fig. 4). In pHB0503, a 15.1-kb plasmid isolated from *A. pleuropneumoniae*, this gene arrangement has been disrupted by insertion of *aacC2* and a truncated copy of an ATPase gene between *sul2* and *catA3* (95). A similar 15.7-kb plasmid from [*H.*] *parasuis*, pFZ51, contains the same resistance gene cluster as pHB0503 (accession number JN202624; Fig. 4, Table 3).

Although the *catA2* gene is commonly found in *H. influenzae* (166, 167), this gene has not yet been detected in chloramphenicol-resistant *Pasteurella*, *Mannheimia*, or *Actinobacillus*. However, a *catB2* gene, which codes for a different type of chloramphenicol acetyltransferase than the aforementioned *catA* genes (162), was found on plasmid pJR1 from avian *P. multocida* (76). The *catB2* gene is part of a gene cassette and thus needs the integron-associated promotor for its expression. In plasmid pJR1, the *catB2* cassette was located outside of an integron structure. Gene cassettes located at secondary sites outside of integrons may be expressed if a suitable promotor is available (126). However, such a promotor has not been identified in pJR1 (76).

Chloramphenicol and florfenicol resistance mediated by active efflux

So far, resistance to florfenicol, a structural analogue of thiamphenicol, has rarely been detected among *Pasteurellaceae*, except in Korea, where 34% of *A. pleuropneumoniae* isolates collected between 2006 and 2010 and 43% of isolates collected between 2010 and 2013 were resistant to florfenicol (73, 81). All of the isolates characterized by Yoo et al. (73) had MICs of florfenicol of between 8 and ≤64 mg/liter and carried the *floR* gene, which codes for an exporter of the major facilitator family that mediates the efflux of phenicols from the bacterial cell. Monitoring studies to specifically determine the MIC values of florfenicol among bovine and porcine respiratory tract pathogens showed that all *P. multocida*, *M. haemolytica*, and *A. pleuropneumoniae* isolates collected between 1994 and 2005 were susceptible to florfenicol (168–171; Schwarz, unpublished data). Data from the monitoring programs GERM-Vet and BfT-GermVet, conducted in Germany, also confirmed that all *P. multocida* from pigs, poultry, dogs, and cats were susceptible to florfenicol (36, 172, 173), whereas 8.6% of *M. haemolytica* and 11.6% of *P. multocida* isolated from cattle in Canada and United States in 2009 were resistant (37).

The first report of a florfenicol-resistant bovine *P. multocida* isolate was published in 2005 (174). This isolate of capsular type A originated from a calf that had died from pneumonia in the United Kingdom. Florfenicol resistance was based on the presence of the gene *floR*. This gene was located on the 10,874-bp plasmid pCCK381 (Fig. 5). Interestingly, a florfenicol-resistant *S. enterica* subsp. *enterica* serovar Dublin isolate recovered from the same calf carried a plasmid indistinguishable from pCCK381. This observation, and the fact that plasmid pCCK381 was able to replicate and express florfenicol resistance in different *E. coli* hosts (174), strongly suggested that the plasmid pCCK381 can be exchanged between bacteria of different genera. Sequence analysis confirmed that this plasmid consists of three segments that show extended similarity to plasmids pDN1 from *Dichelobacter nodosus* (175), pMBSF1 from *E. coli* (176), and pRVS1 from *Vibrio salmonicida* (177). All these plasmids have been found either in bacteria such as *E. coli* from cattle and pigs, which have previously been shown to carry the *floR* gene along with a variable length ORF with homology to a *lysR* regulator gene, or in bacteria which cause diseases in fish and ruminants, such as cold-water vibriosis (*V. salmonicida*) or infectious pododermatitis (*D. nodosus*), for the control of which florfenicol is approved in several non-European Union countries. Although it is not possible to determine in retrospect where and when plasmid pCCK381 evolved, structural analysis suggested that this plasmid is most likely the result of interplasmid recombination processes (174). It is also interesting to note that pCCK381 has been isolated from both porcine and bovine isolates of *P. multocida* in Germany (178).

More recently, a number of smaller plasmids with *floR* as the only resistance gene have been identified in [*H.*] *parasuis* (pHPSF1), *M. haemolytica* (pMH1405), and *A. pleuropneumoniae* (pM3446F and p518) (179–182). Plasmids pMH1405 and pM3446F, both 7.7 kb, share extensive regions of identity with pCCK381, including the mobilization and replication genes, whereas the 6.3-kb pHPSF1 contains different *mob* and *rep* genes. The smallest plasmid, the 3.9-kb p518, shares the *floR-lsyR* region (high sequence identity) with pMh1405, and the remaining region, containing ΔmobC and strA-ΔstrB sequences, with [*H.*] *parasuis* plasmid pFZG1012 (Fig. 5).

The *floR* gene has also been found on multiresistance plasmids pCCK13698 and pCCK1900 (178, 183), and it is part of ICE*Pmu1* and ICE*Pmu1*-related ICEs detected in *M. haemolytica* and *H. somni* (55). The 14,969-bp pCCK13698 plasmid was identified in a bovine isolate of *Bibersteinia trehalosi* (184) which originated from a calf that had died from a respiratory tract infection in France (183). The 10.2-kb pCCK1900 plasmid was recovered from a porcine *P. multocida* isolate in Germany (178). Both plasmids differ structurally from plasmid pCCK381 and from each other (Fig. 5). While in pCCK13698, the *floR-lysR* sequence is located downstream of the complete genes *sul2* and *catA3*, and a truncated *strA* streptomycin resistance gene (183), in plasmid pCCK1900, the *floR-lysR* genes are found downstream of (and in the opposite orientation to) complete *sul2*, *strA*, and *strB* genes (Fig. 5). Moreover, plasmid pCCK13698 shares almost 6.8 kb of identity with the [*H.*] *parasuis* plasmid pHS-Rec (75) and harbors two insertion sequences, IS1592 and IS26 (183).

In contrast, pCCK1900 appears to have arisen by insertion of the *floR-lysR* genes into the broad-host-range plasmid RSF1010 (178). Such analysis reveals a high level of involvement of the region *floR-lysR* in interplasmid recombination events. In ICE*Pmu1*, *floR* is found as part of "resistance region 1," a 15,711-bp sequence bracketed by copies of IS*Apl1*, an insertion sequence initially identified in *A. pleuropneumoniae* (185). This region carries *aphA1*, *strA*, *strB*, *sul2*, *floR*, and *erm*(42), with the *floR-lysR* genes found to be bracketed by a truncated and a complete ISCR2 element (55).

Resistance to (Fluoro)quinolones

Quinolones are broad-spectrum antimicrobial agents that inhibit bacterial DNA gyrase and topoisomerase IV. Resistance is commonly due to mutational alterations in the genes coding for the different subunits of both enzymes but is also due to active efflux or protection of the enzymes by Qnr proteins (109).

(Fluoro)quinolone resistance mediated by target site mutations

Very little is known about (fluoro)quinolone resistance in *Pasteurella*, *Mannheimia*, *Actinobacillus*, or *Haemophilus*. Studies of *Pasteurella* spp. from humans and animals (36, 172, 173, 186) and *A. pleuropneumoniae* (62) identified virtually all isolates to be highly susceptible to the fluoroquinolones tested. The first report describing the analysis of the quinolone resistance determining region (QRDR) of the proteins encoded by the genes *gyrA* and *parC* in *P. multocida* isolates identified a Ser83Ile alteration in GyrA in an isolate that had a nalidixic acid MIC of 256 mg/liter, whereas Asp87Gly alterations were detected in isolates with nalidixic acid MICs of 4 and 12 mg/liter (187). None of these isolates exhibited resistance to fluoroquinolones. Whole-genome sequencing of the multiresistant bovine *P. multocida* isolate 36950, exhibiting an enrofloxacin MIC of 2 mg/liter, led to the identification of two base pair exchanges in the QRDR of *gyrA*, which resulted in amino acid alterations GGT → AGT (Gly75Ser) and AGC → AGA (Ser83Arg). In addition, a single base pair exchange in the QRDR of *parC*, TCA → TTA, which resulted in a Ser80Leu exchange, was also seen (55).

More recently, fluoroquinolone-resistant clinical isolates of *P. multocida*, with MICs of 0.5 mg/liter for both enrofloxacin and ciprofloxacin, were found to have Asp87Asn or Ala84Pro mutations in GyrA (188). In isolates further selected for resistance by passage on subinhibitory concentrations of fluoroquinolones,

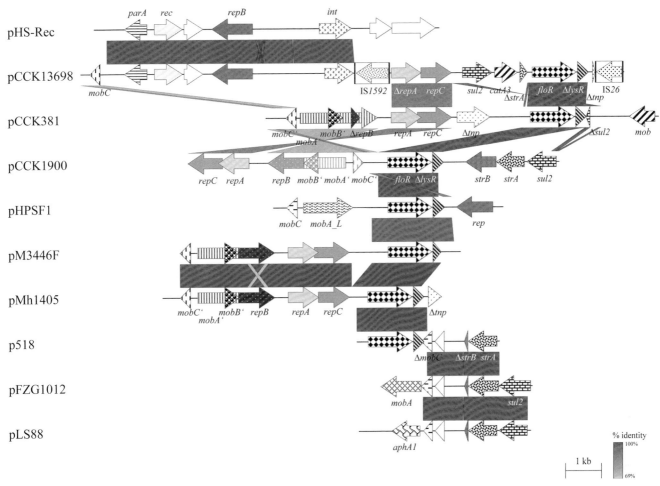

Figure 5 Schematic representation of the structure and organization of selected *floR*-based (multi-)resistance plasmids from *B. trehalosi* compared to an in-part-related plasmid from [*H.*] *parasuis*, and *A. pleuropneumoniae*, [*H.*] *parasuis*, *P. multocida*, and *sul2*-based (multi-)resistance plasmids from *H. ducreyi* and [*H.*] *parasuis*. Comparison of the maps of plasmids pCCK13698 (accession no. AM183225) from *B. trehalosi* and its in-part-related plasmid pHS-Rec (accession no. AY862436; 9,462 bp) from [*H.*] *parasuis*, pCCK381 (accession no. AJ871969; 10,874 bp) from *P. multocida*, pCCK1900 (accession no. FM179941; 10,226 bp) from *P. multocida*, pHPSF1 (accession no. KR262062; 6,328 bp) from [*H.*] *parasuis*, pM3446F (accession no. KP696484; 7,709 bp) from *A. pleuropneumoniae*, pMh1405 (accession no. NC_019260; 7,674 bp) from *M. haemolytica*, p518 (accession no. KT355773; 3,937 bp) from *A. pleuropneumoniae*, pFZG1012 (accession no. HQ015158; partially sequenced) from [*H.*] *parasuis*, and pLS88 (accession no. L23118; 4,772 bp) from *H. ducreyi*. Genes are shown as arrows, with the arrowhead indicating the direction of transcription. The following genes are involved in antimicrobial resistance: *sul2* (sulfonamide resistance), *strA* and *strB* (streptomycin resistance), *catA3* (chloramphenicol resistance), *floR* (chloramphenicol/florfenicol resistance), and *aphA1* (kanamycin/neomycin resistance); plasmid replication: *rep*, *repA*, *repB*, and *repC*; mobilization functions: *mobA*, *mobB*, *mobC*, and *mob*; transposition functions: *tnp*; recombinase or integrase functions: *rec* and *int*; DNA partition: *parA*; unknown function: open reading frames indicated by white arrows. The prefix Δ indicates a truncated functionally inactive gene. The boxes in the map of pCCK13698 indicate the limits of the insertion sequences IS*1592* and IS*26*; the arrows within these boxes indicate the reading frames of the corresponding transposase genes. Gray-shaded areas indicate the regions common to plasmids, and the different shades of gray illustrate the percentages of nucleotide sequence identity between the plasmids, as indicated by the scale at the bottom of the figure. A distance scale in kilobases is shown.

multiple mutations in *gyrA*, *gyrB*, and *parC*, but not *parE*, were found to be associated with high-level fluoroquinolone resistance (MICs, >4 mg/liter). Similarly, in M. *haemolytica*, resistance to nalidixic acid was associated with at least one amino acid substitution in one or both of GyrA and ParC, whereas all of the isolates with fluoroquinolone MICs ≥8.0 mg/liter had two mutations in GyrA and one additional change in ParC (189). A study of enrofloxacin-resistant *A. pleuropneumoniae* isolates in Taiwan (190) identified various mutations in *gyrA*, *parC*, and *parE*, with resistant isolates carrying at least one mutation in the QRDR of *gyrA*, resulting in amino acid changes at codon 83 or 87. Functional efflux pumps were also found to contribute to enrofloxacin resistance in these isolates, as demonstrated by addition of an efflux pump inhibitor (190). In a recent study comparing antimicrobial resistance profiles and the presence of resistance genes in whole-genome sequences of *A. pleuropneumoniae* (9), only a slightly elevated enrofloxacin MIC of 0.25 mg/liter was detected in a limited number of isolates, and in all cases this resistance was associated with the GyrA Ser83Phe substitution described by Wang et al. (190).

In a survey of 115 [H.] *parasuis* isolates collected from South China between 2008 and 2010, 20 were identified with high levels of resistance to nalidixic acid (MICs ≥128 mg/liter) as well as resistance to enrofloxacin and other fluoroquinolones (MICs ≥4 mg/liter), and these were shown to have at least one mutation in the *gyrA* gene causing changes at codon 83 or 87 (191). In another survey, of 138 [H.] *parasuis* isolates from China between 2002 and 2009, 60% were found to be resistant to enrofloxacin, and sequencing of PCR products demonstrated 10 point mutations in the quinolone QRDR regions of *gyrA*, *gyrB*, *parC*, and *parE* contributing to varying degrees of enrofloxacin resistance (192). However, the mutation causing the amino acid change Asp87Asn was common to all resistant isolates. This study further showed, by site-directed mutagenesis, that point mutations leading to three amino acid changes (Asp87Asn in GyrA, Ser73Arg in ParC, and Thr551Ala in ParE) were specifically involved in fluoroquinolone resistance (192).

(Fluoro)quinolone resistance mediated by other mechanisms

The AcrAB efflux pump has been shown in *Enterobacteriaceae* to be able to export fluoroquinolones from the cell (193). Although the use of efflux inhibitors has demonstrated a contribution of efflux pump(s) to fluoroquinolone resistance in *A. pleuropneumoniae* and *P. multocida* (188, 190), the specific proteins involved were not identified. A PCR survey of 115 Chinese [H.] *parasuis* isolates detected quinolone resistance genes *qnrA1*, *qnrB6*, and *aac(6′)-Ib-cr* in three, one, and three isolates, respectively (191). To date, this is the only report of acquired quinolone resistance genes in the *Pasteurellaceae*.

DISSEMINATION, COSELECTION, AND PERSISTENCE OF RESISTANCE GENES IN *PASTEURELLA*, *MANNHEIMIA*, *ACTINOBACILLUS*, *HAEMOPHILUS*, AND *HISTOPHILUS*

Molecular analysis of isolates of *Pasteurella*, *Mannheimia*, *Actinobacillus*, and *Haemophilus* revealed that, in many cases, antimicrobial resistance genes are associated with plasmids. Most of the resistance plasmids identified to date are <15 kb in size and are nonconjugative, though many carry *mob* genes (Table 3) (Fig. 1 to 5) and have been shown to be mobilizable. For these plasmids to be horizontally transferred by conjugation, the genes encoding the conjugation machinery must be supplied *in trans*. The only conjugative elements so far identified in members of the *Pasteurellaceae* are ICEs, including those recently described in *P. multocida*, *M. haemolytica*, *H. somni*, and *A. pleuropneumoniae* (55–57, 74). These ICEs are likely, along with others yet to be identified, be the source of the genes required for conjugal transfer of the smaller mobilizable plasmids identified in these species.

The number of plasmids for which complete sequences are available continues to grow. Currently, there are complete sequences for 60 plasmids carrying antimicrobial resistance genes (Table 3). In addition, the resistance gene regions of several other plasmids (also listed in Table 3) have been sequenced. Despite the relatively small size of these plasmids, many of them carry two or more resistance genes (Table 3, Fig. 3 to 5). To date, there are no sequences for resistance plasmids from *Histophilus* isolates in GenBank (last accessed October 27, 2017). Sequence analysis has provided insights into (i) the genes involved in antimicrobial resistance of *Pasteurella*, *Mannheimia*, *Actinobacillus*, and *Haemophilus* and their organization; (ii) the structural relationships between the resistance plasmids; and (iii) mechanisms resulting in the formation of multiresistance plasmids and plasmid-borne multiresistance gene clusters.

Some of the genes accounting for antimicrobial resistance in *Pasteurella*, *Mannheimia*, *Haemophilus*, and *Actinobacillus*, such as the tetracycline resistance gene *tet*(H) and the β-lactamase gene *bla*ROB-1, appear to be more commonly found among *Pasteurellaceae*. In contrast, other resistance genes, such as the streptomycin resistance genes *strA-strB*, have been detected in a wide range of Gram-negative bacteria. The fact that these genes are associated with the transposon Tn*5393* (124), and have also been found on two mobilizable broad-host-range plasmids, pLS88 (134) and RSF1010 (147), might explain their widespread occurrence, which is likely due to horizontal gene transfer.

The location of resistance genes on mobile genetic elements allows their spread into bacteria of other species and genera. This has been confirmed by the detection of highly similar plasmids in different host bacteria, such as the *tet*(H)-carrying plasmid pMHT1, which was found in *P. multocida*, *M. haemolytica*, *M. varigena*, and *M. glucosida* (64), and the *sul2-strA*-carrying plasmid pPMSS1, which was identified in *P. multocida*, [*P.*] *aerogenes*, and *M. haemolytica* (125). Several of these small plasmids carry *mob* genes which allow mobilization in the presence of a conjugative element. Mobilization has also been confirmed for the 8.1-kb *sul2-strA*-carrying plasmid pMS260 from *A. pleuropneumoniae* (121). This plasmid, which closely resembles the broad-host-range plasmid RSF1010 (147), proved to be mobilizable into a wide variety of respiratory tract pathogens including *P. multocida*, *Bordetella bronchiseptica*, and *Pseudomonas aeruginosa*, as well as other isolates of *A. pleuropneumoniae* (119). Moreover, most of the small resistance plasmids found in *Pasteurella*, *Mannheimia*, *Actinobacillus*, and *Haemophilus* are able to replicate and express their resistance properties in *E. coli*. On the other hand, most resistance plasmids originating from the *Enterobacteriaceae* and harboring either *catA3*, *strA-strB*, *tet*(B), or *sul2*, usually cannot replicate in *Pasteurella*, *Mannheimia*, *Actinobacillus*, or *Haemophilus* hosts. With the exception of the RSF1010-like plasmid pMS260 from *A. pleuropneumoniae* (121), analysis of the regions flanking the *sul2* and *strA-strB* genes in plasmids of *Pasteurella*, *Mannheimia*, *Actinobacillus*, and *Haemophilus* revealed sequences similar not to those of *Enterobacteriaceae* plasmids, but rather to those of plasmids known to occur in *Pasteurellaceae*. This observation suggests that, most likely, recombination events between endogenous plasmids of *Pasteurellaceae* and resistance plasmids from other bacterial sources, which may be replication-deficient in *Pasteurellaceae*, have occurred. As a result, the horizontally acquired resistance genes became inserted into new plasmidic replicons which then have been stably maintained in *Pasteurellaceae*. Studies of the plasmid-borne *sul2-strA* gene cluster in *Pasteurella* and *Mannheimia* showed that the non-

coding spacer region between the two resistance genes may represent the target site for further recombination events (116, 125). So far, a *catA3* gene and the entire *tetR-tet*(H) region, respectively, have been found to be integrated between the genes *sul2* and *strA* in different plasmids (59, 116).

Based on the observation that many of the resistance plasmids so far detected in *Pasteurella*, *Mannheimia*, and *Actinobacillus* carry more than one resistance gene, coselection of these resistance genes is likely. Once such a plasmid is transferred to a new host, all resistance genes located on it are also transferred. As a consequence, a new host bacterium gains resistance to two or more antimicrobial agents, or classes of antimicrobial agents, by the acquisition of a single small plasmid. In these cases, selective pressure imposed by the use of one such antimicrobial agent, e.g., tetracyclines, is sufficient to favor the exchange of the multiresistance plasmid. The location of different resistance genes on the same plasmid also enables their persistence, particularly if the resistance genes are organized in a cluster. A multiresistance gene cluster in which the genes *sul2*, *catA3*, and *strA* are organized as a transcriptional unit has been identified on several plasmids, as well as in chromosomal DNA of [*P.*] *aerogenes* and several *Mannheimia* spp. (116, 125). It is highly unlikely that individual genes from such a cluster are lost. A study of the location of chloramphenicol resistance genes in *Pasteurella* and *Mannheimia* isolates from Germany showed that the dominant chloramphenicol resistance gene *catA3* was located in a *sul2-catA3-strA* cluster in all cases, except for a single bovine *M. glucosida* isolate (125). Although chloramphenicol has been prohibited for use in food-producing animals in the European Union and the United States for many years, aminoglycosides, including streptomycin, as well as sulfonamides are still used. Thus, streptomycin and/or sulfonamides might present the selective pressure that ensures the maintenance of the entire cluster. Thus, clusters such as that containing the genes *sul2-catA3-strA* may play an important role in maintaining resistance genes without direct selective pressure.

Analysis of the resistance genes, their location, and their organization provides insight into (i) the gene pool to which bacteria of the genera *Pasteurella*, *Mannheimia*, *Actinobacillus*, and *Haemophilus* have access; (ii) horizontal transfer processes which play a key role in the dissemination of the resistance genes between and beyond bacteria of the four aforementioned genera; and (iii) integration and recombination events which are of major importance for the development of novel resistance plasmids and the formation of multiresistance gene clusters in *Pasteurella*, *Mannheimia*, *Actinobacillus*, and *Haemophilus* isolates.

CONCLUDING REMARKS

Isolates of several genera in the family *Pasteurellaceae* cause a number of economically important diseases in cattle, swine, and other food-producing animals. Due to the multifactorial and polymicrobial nature of some of the infections in which *Pasteurella*, *Mannheimia*, *Actinobacillus*, *Haemophilus*, and *Histophilus* isolates are involved, prevention is—except in confined production systems with high biosecurity—a cumbersome task that often yields unsatisfying results. Despite hygienic measures, improved management and the use of vaccines, antimicrobial agents are indispensable tools for the control of infections in which bacteria of the family *Pasteurellaceae* are involved. Increasing numbers of resistant, or multiresistant, isolates are reducing the efficacy of antimicrobial agents currently approved for use in animals. It is anticipated that in the near future, there will be no new classes of antimicrobial agents approved for use in veterinary medicine. Thus, veterinarians will have to rely on currently available antimicrobial agents. To retain their efficacy, prescription and administration of antimicrobial agents should be undertaken with discretion supported by an accurate diagnosis, a careful choice of the antimicrobial agent(s), and the most appropriate dosing regimen. Imprudent use of antimicrobials bears a high risk of selecting resistant bacteria.

Many of the resistance genes known to be present in *Pasteurella*, *Mannheimia*, *Actinobacillus*, and *Haemophilus* are associated with plasmids or transposons and thus may be exchanged horizontally, not only between bacteria of the family *Pasteurellaceae*, but also with other Gram-negative bacteria. This update on the molecular basis of antimicrobial resistance illustrates that *Pasteurella*, *Mannheimia*, *Actinobacillus*, and *Haemophilus* have obviously acquired a number of resistance genes from other Gram-negative, or maybe even Gram-positive, bacteria. Knowledge of the location and colocation of the resistance genes on mobile genetic elements, as well as the conditions for their coselection and persistence, will be valuable information for veterinarians and will assist them in selecting the most efficacious antimicrobial agents for control of isolates of the family *Pasteurellaceae*. Even though the current susceptibility status of *Pasteurellaceae* from infections in animals looks rather favorable, continuous monitoring of the antimicrobial susceptibility of *Pasteurellaceae* is required for early detection of changes in the susceptibility status and for analyzing the respective isolates for newly acquired/developed resistance genes and resistance-mediating mutations.

Acknowledgments. Funding for GBM and SS was provided by grant SCHW382/10-2 from the German Research Foundation (DFG). Funding for JB was provided by the Biotechnology and Biological Sciences Research Council (BB/K021109/1, BB/G018553, and BB/M023052/1), as well as through a CONFAP-the UK Academies Fellowship (FAPEMIG – APQ-00689-16).

Citation. Michael GB, Bossé JT, Schwarz S. 2017. Antimicrobial resistance in Pasteurellaceae of veterinary origin. Microbiol Spectrum 6(3):ARBA-0022-2017.

References

1. Christensen H, Kuhnert P, Busse HJ, Frederiksen WC, Bisgaard M. 2007. Proposed minimal standards for the description of genera, species and subspecies of the *Pasteurellaceae*. *Int J Syst Evol Microbiol* 57:166–178.

2. Christensen H, Kuhnert P, Nørskov-Lauritsen N, Planet PJ, Bisgaard M. 2014. The family *Pasteurellaceae*, p 535–564. *In* DeLong EF, Lory S, Stackebrandt E, Thompson F (ed), *The Prokaryotes*. Springer-Verlag, Berlin, Germany.

3. Adhikary S, Nicklas W, Bisgaard M, Boot R, Kuhnert P, Waberschek T, Aalbæk B, Korczak B, Christensen H. 2017. Rodentibacter gen. nov. including *Rodentibacter pneumotropicus* comb. nov., *Rodentibacter heylii* sp. nov., *Rodentibacter myodis* sp. nov., *Rodentibacter ratti* sp. nov., *Rodentibacter heidelbergensis* sp. nov., *Rodentibacter trehalosifermentans* sp. nov., *Rodentibacter rarus* sp. nov., *Rodentibacter mrazii* and two genomospecies. *Int J Syst Evol Microbiol* 67:1793–1806.

4. Christensen H, Kuhnert P, Bisgaard M, Mutters R, Dziva F, Olsen JE. 2005. Emended description of porcine [*Pasteurella*] aerogenes, [*Pasteurella*] mairii and [*Actinobacillus*] rossii. *Int J Syst Evol Microbiol* 55:209–223.

5. Christensen H, Bisgaard M. 2008. Taxonomy and biodiversity of members of *Pasteurellaceae*, p 1–25. *In* Kuhnert P, Christensen H (ed), *Pasteurellaceae: Biology, Genomics and Molecular Aspects*. Caister Academic Press, Norfolk, United Kingdom.

6. Bonaventura MP, Lee EK, Desalle R, Planet PJ. 2010. A whole-genome phylogeny of the family *Pasteurellaceae*. *Mol Phylogenet Evol* 54:950–956.

7. Moustafa AM, Seemann T, Gladman S, Adler B, Harper M, Boyce JD, Bennett MD. 2015. Comparative genomic analysis of Asian haemorrhagic septicaemia-associated strains of *Pasteurella multocida* identifies more than 90 haemorrhagic septicaemia-specific genes. *PLoS One* 10: e0130296.

8. Clawson ML, Murray RW, Sweeney MT, Apley MD, DeDonder KD, Capik SF, Larson RL, Lubbers BV, White BJ, Kalbfleisch TS, Schuller G, Dickey AM, Harhay GP, Heaton MP, Chitko-McKown CG, Brichta-Harhay DM, Bono JL, Smith TP. 2016. Genomic signatures of *Mannheimia haemolytica* that associate with the lungs of cattle with respiratory disease, an integrative conjugative

element, and antibiotic resistance genes. *BMC Genomics* **17**:982.

9. Bossé JT, Li Y, Rogers J, Fernandez Crespo R, Li Y, Chaudhuri RR, Holden MT, Maskell DJ, Tucker AW, Wren BW, Rycroft AN, Langford PR. 2017. Whole genome sequencing for surveillance of antimicrobial resistance in *Actinobacillus pleuropneumoniae*. *Front Microbiol* **8**:311.

10. Kehrenberg C, Walker RD, Wu CC, Schwarz S. 2006. Antimicrobial resistance in members of the family *Pasteurellaceae*, p 167–186. *In* Aarestrup FM (ed), *Antimicrobial Resistance in Bacteria of Animal Origin*. ASM Press, Washington, DC.

11. Schwarz S. 2008. Mechanisms of antimicrobial resistance in *Pasteurellaceae*, p 199–228. *In* Kuhnert P, Christensen H (ed), *Pasteurellaceae: Biology, Genomics and Molecular Aspects*. Caister Academic Press, Norfolk, United Kingdom.

12. Quinn PJ, Markey BK, Carter ME, Donnelly WJ, Leonard FC. 2002. *Veterinary Microbiology and Microbial Disease*, 2nd ed. Blackwell Publishing, Ames, IA.

13. Radostits OM, Gay C, Blood DC, Hinchcliff KW. 2000. Diseases caused by bacteria III, p 779–908. *In* Radostits OM, Gay C, Blood DC, Hinchcliff KW (eds), *Veterinary medicine: a textbook of the diseases of cattle, sheep, pigs, goats, and horses*. 9th ed. Saunders, Philadelphia, London.

14. Catry B, Chiers K, Schwarz S, Kehrenberg C, Decostere A, de Kruif A. 2005. A case of fatal peritonitis in calves caused by *Pasteurella multocida* capsular type F. *J Clin Microbiol* **43**:1480–1483.

15. Singh K, Ritchey JW, Confer AW. 2011. *Mannheimia haemolytica*: bacterial-host interactions in bovine pneumonia. *Vet Pathol* **48**:338–348.

16. Rice JA, Carrasco-Medina L, Hodgins DC, Shewen PE. 2007. *Mannheimia haemolytica* and bovine respiratory disease. *Anim Health Res Rev* **8**:117–128.

17. Maldonado J, Valls L, Martínez E, Riera P. 2009. Isolation rates, serovars, and toxin genotypes of nicotinamide adenine dinucleotide-independent *Actinobacillus pleuropneumoniae* among pigs suffering from pleuropneumonia in Spain. *J Vet Diagn Invest* **21**:854–857.

18. Sárközi R, Makrai L, Fodor L. 2015. Identification of a proposed new serovar of *Actinobacillus pleuropneumoniae*: serovar 16. *Acta Vet Hung* **63**:444–450.

19. Bossé JT, Li Y, Sárközi R, Gottschalk M, Angen Ø, Nedbalcova K, Rycroft AN, Fodor L, Langford PR. 2017. A unique capsule locus in the newly designated *Actinobacillus pleuropneumoniae* serovar 16 and development of a diagnostic PCR assay. *J Clin Microbiol* **55**:902–907.

20. Frey J. 1995. Virulence in *Actinobacillus pleuropneumoniae* and RTX toxins. *Trends Microbiol* **3**:257–261.

21. Oliveira S, Blackall PJ, Pijoan C. 2003. Characterization of the diversity of *Haemophilus parasuis* field isolates by use of serotyping and genotyping. *Am J Vet Res* **64**:435–442.

22. Hodgins DC, Conlon JA, Shewen PE. 2002. Respiratory viruses and bacteria in cattle, p 213–229. *In* Brogden KA, Guthmiller JM (ed), *Polymicrobial Diseases*. ASM Press, Washington, DC.

23. Brockmeier SL, Halbur PG, Thacker EL. 2002. Porcine respiratory disease complex, p 231–258. *In* Brogden KA, Guthmiller JM (ed), *Polymicrobial Diseases*. ASM Press, Washington, DC.

24. Magyar T, Lax AJ. 2002. Atrophic rhinitis, p 169–197. *In* Brogden KA, Guthmiller JM (ed), *Polymicrobial Diseases*. ASM Press, Washington, DC.

25. Watts J, Sweeney MT, Lubbers B. 2017. Antimicrobial susceptibility testing of bacteria of veterinary origin. *In* Aarestrup F, Schwarz S, Shen J, Cavaco L (ed), *Antimicrobial Resistance in Bacteria from Livestock and Companion Animals*, ASM Press, Washington, DC.

26. Zankari E, Hasman H, Kaas RS, Seyfarth AM, Agersø Y, Lund O, Larsen MV, Aarestrup FM. 2013. Genotyping using whole-genome sequencing is a realistic alternative to surveillance based on phenotypic antimicrobial susceptibility testing. *J Antimicrob Chemother* **68**:771–777.

27. Köser CU, Ellington MJ, Peacock SJ. 2014. Whole-genome sequencing to control antimicrobial resistance. *Trends Genet* **30**:401–407.

28. Clinical and Laboratory Standards Institute (CLSI). 2013. *Performance standards for antimicrobial disk and dilution susceptibility tests for bacteria isolated from animals; Approved standard*, 4th edition. CLSI document VET01-A4. Clinical and Laboratory Standards Institute; Wayne, PA.

29. Clinical and Laboratory Standards Institute (CLSI). 2015. *Performance standards for antimicrobial disk and dilution susceptibility tests for bacteria isolated from animals*, 3rd ed. CLSI suplement VET01S. Clinical and Laboratory Standards Institute, Wayne, PA.

30. Clinical and Laboratory Standards Institute (CLSI). 2017. *Methods for antimicrobial susceptibility testing of infrequently isolated or fastidious bacteria isolated from animals*, 1st ed. CLSI document VET06-Ed1. Clinical and Laboratory Standards Institute; Wayne, PA.

31. Dayao DA, Kienzle M, Gibson JS, Blackall PJ, Turni C. 2014. Use of a proposed antimicrobial susceptibility testing method for *Haemophilus parasuis*. *Vet Microbiol* **172**:586–589.

32. Prüller S, Turni C, Blackall PJ, Beyerbach M, Klein G, Kreienbrock L, Strutzberg-Minder K, Kaspar H, Meemken D, Kehrenberg C. 2016. Towards a standardized method for broth microdilution susceptibility testing of *Haemophilus parasuis*. *J Clin Microbiol* **55**:264–273.

33. Bywater R, Silley P, Simjee S. 2006. Antimicrobial breakpoints: definitions and conflicting requirements. *Vet Microbiol* **118**:158–159.

34. Schwarz S, Böttner A, Goossens L, Hafez HM, Hartmann K, Kaske M, Kehrenberg C, Kietzmann M, Klarmann D, Klein G, Krabisch P, Luhofer G, Richter A, Schulz B, Sigge C, Waldmann KH, Wallmann J, Werckenthin C. 2008. A proposal of clinical breakpoints for amoxicillin applicable to porcine respiratory tract pathogens. *Vet Microbiol* **126**:178–188.

35. Bundesamt für Verbraucherschutz und Lebensmittelsicherheit (BVL). 2016. *Berichte zur Resistenzmonitoringstudie 2012/2013 - Resistenzsituation bei klinisch wichtigen tierpathogenen Bakterien.* Springer Nature, Cham, Switzerland. http://www.bvl.bund.de/SharedDocs/Downloads/09_Untersuchungen/Archiv_berichte_Resistenzmonitoring/Bericht_Resistenzmonitoring_2012_2013.pdf;jsessionid=05577AB30DA96869657351B75EAE9267.2_cid350?__blob=publicationFile&v=5.

36. Schwarz S, Alesík E, Grobbel M, Lübke-Becker A, Werckenthin C, Wieler LH, Wallmann J. 2007. Antimicrobial susceptibility of *Pasteurella multocida* and *Bordetella bronchiseptica* from dogs and cats as determined in the BfT-GermVet monitoring program 2004–2006. *Berl Munch Tierarztl Wochenschr* 120:423–430.

37. Portis E, Lindeman C, Johansen L, Stoltman G. 2012. A ten-year (2000–2009) study of antimicrobial susceptibility of bacteria that cause bovine respiratory disease complex—*Mannheimia haemolytica, Pasteurella multocida,* and *Histophilus somni*—in the United States and Canada. *J Vet Diagn Invest* 24:932–944.

38. de Jong A, Thomas V, Simjee S, Moyaert H, El Garch F, Maher K, Morrissey I, Butty P, Klein U, Marion H, Rigaut D, Vallé M. 2014. Antimicrobial susceptibility monitoring of respiratory tract pathogens isolated from diseased cattle and pigs across Europe: the VetPath study. *Vet Microbiol* 172:202–215.

39. El Garch F, de Jong A, Simjee S, Moyaert H, Klein U, Ludwig C, Marion H, Haag-Diergarten S, Richard-Mazet A, Thomas V, Siegwart E. 2016. Monitoring of antimicrobial susceptibility of respiratory tract pathogens isolated from diseased cattle and pigs across Europe, 2009–2012: VetPath results. *Vet Microbiol* 194:11–22.

40. Dayao DA, Gibson JS, Blackall PJ, Turni C. 2014. Antimicrobial resistance in bacteria associated with porcine respiratory disease in Australia. *Vet Microbiol* 171:232–235.

41. Archambault M, Harel J, Gouré J, Tremblay YDN, Jacques M. 2012. Antimicrobial susceptibilities and resistance genes of Canadian isolates of *Actinobacillus pleuropneumoniae. Microb Drug Resist* 18:198–206.

42. Noyes NR, Benedict KM, Gow SP, Booker CW, Hannon SJ, McAllister TA, Morley PS. 2015. *Mannheimia haemolytica* in feedlot cattle: prevalence of recovery and associations with antimicrobial use, resistance, and health outcomes. *J Vet Intern Med* 29:705–713.

43. DeDonder KD, Apley MD. 2015. A literature review of antimicrobial resistance in pathogens associated with bovine respiratory disease. *Anim Health Res Rev* 16:125–134.

44. Berman SM, Hirsh DC. 1978. Partial characterization of R-plasmids from *Pasteurella multocida* isolated from turkeys. *Antimicrob Agents Chemother* 14:348–352.

45. Hirsh DC, Martin LD, Rhoades KR. 1981. Conjugal transfer of an R-plasmid in *Pasteurella multocida. Antimicrob Agents Chemother* 20:415–417.

46. Hirsh DC, Martin LD, Rhoades KR. 1985. Resistance plasmids of *Pasteurella multocida* isolated from turkeys. *Am J Vet Res* 46:1490–1493.

47. Hirsh DC, Hansen LM, Dorfman LC, Snipes KP, Carpenter TE, Hird DW, McCapes RH. 1989. Resistance to antimicrobial agents and prevalence of R plasmids in *Pasteurella multocida* from turkeys. *Antimicrob Agents Chemother* 33:670–673.

48. Hansen LM, McMurry LM, Levy SB, Hirsh DC. 1993. A new tetracycline resistance determinant, Tet H, from *Pasteurella multocida* specifying active efflux of tetracycline. *Antimicrob Agents Chemother* 37:2699–2705.

49. Hansen LM, Blanchard PC, Hirsh DC. 1996. Distribution of *tet*(H) among *Pasteurella* isolates from the United States and Canada. *Antimicrob Agents Chemother* 40:1558–1560.

50. Kehrenberg C, Werckenthin C, Schwarz S. 1998. Tn*5706*, a transposon-like element from *Pasteurella multocida* mediating tetracycline resistance. *Antimicrob Agents Chemother* 42:2116–2118.

51. Hunt ML, Adler B, Townsend KM. 2000. The molecular biology of *pasteurella multocida. Vet Microbiol* 72:3–25.

52. Kehrenberg C, Schwarz S. 2000. Identification of a truncated, but functionally active *tet*(H) tetracycline resistance gene in *Pasteurella aerogenes* and *Pasteurella multocida. FEMS Microbiol Lett* 188:191–195.

53. Kehrenberg C, Schwarz S. 2001. Molecular analysis of tetracycline resistance in *Pasteurella aerogenes. Antimicrob Agents Chemother* 45:2885–2890.

54. Michael GB, Kadlec K, Sweeney MT, Brzuszkiewicz E, Liesegang H, Daniel R, Murray RW, Watts JL, Schwarz S. 2012. ICE*Pmu1*, an integrative conjugative element (ICE) of *Pasteurella multocida*: structure and transfer. *J Antimicrob Chemother* 67:91–100.

55. Michael GB, Kadlec K, Sweeney MT, Brzuszkiewicz E, Liesegang H, Daniel R, Murray RW, Watts JL, Schwarz S. 2012. ICE*Pmu1*, an integrative conjugative element (ICE) of *Pasteurella multocida*: analysis of the regions that comprise 12 antimicrobial resistance genes. *J Antimicrob Chemother* 67:84–90.

56. Eidam C, Poehlein A, Leimbach A, Michael GB, Kadlec K, Liesegang H, Daniel R, Sweeney MT, Murray RW, Watts JL, Schwarz S. 2015. Analysis and comparative genomics of ICE*Mh1*, a novel integrative and conjugative element (ICE) of *Mannheimia haemolytica. J Antimicrob Chemother* 70:93–97.

57. Klima CL, Zaheer R, Cook SR, Booker CW, Hendrick S, Alexander TW, McAllister TA, Onderdonk AB. 2014. Pathogens of bovine respiratory disease in North American feedlots conferring multidrug resistance via integrative conjugative elements. *J Clin Microbiol* 52:438–448.

58. Miranda CD, Kehrenberg C, Ulep C, Schwarz S, Roberts MC. 2003. Diversity of tetracycline resistance genes in bacteria from Chilean salmon farms. *Antimicrob Agents Chemother* 47:883–888.

59. Kehrenberg C, Tham NTT, Schwarz S. 2003. New plasmid-borne antibiotic resistance gene cluster in *Pasteurella multocida. Antimicrob Agents Chemother* 47:2978–2980.

60. Blanco M, Gutiérrez-Martin CB, Rodríguez-Ferri EF, Roberts MC, Navas J. 2006. Distribution of tetracycline resistance genes in *Actinobacillus pleuropneumoniae* isolates from Spain. *Antimicrob Agents Chemother* 50:702–708.

61. Blanco M, Kadlec K, Gutiérrez Martín CB, de la Fuente AJ, Schwarz S, Navas J. 2007. Nucleotide sequence and transfer properties of two novel types of *Actinobacillus pleuropneumoniae* plasmids carrying the tetracycline resistance gene *tet*(H). *J Antimicrob Chemother* 60:864–867.

62. Matter D, Rossano A, Limat S, Vorlet-Fawer L, Brodard I, Perreten V. 2007. Antimicrobial resistance profile of *Actinobacillus pleuropneumoniae* and *Actinobacillus porcitonsillarum*. *Vet Microbiol* 122:146–156.

63. Dayao D, Gibson JS, Blackall PJ, Turni C. 2016. Antimicrobial resistance genes in *Actinobacillus pleuropneumoniae*, *Haemophilus parasuis* and *Pasteurella multocida* isolated from Australian pigs. *Aust Vet J* 94:227–231.

64. Kehrenberg C, Salmon SA, Watts JL, Schwarz S. 2001. Tetracycline resistance genes in isolates of *Pasteurella multocida*, *Mannheimia haemolytica*, *Mannheimia glucosida* and *Mannheimia varigena* from bovine and swine respiratory disease: intergeneric spread of the tet (H) plasmid pMHT1. *J Antimicrob Chemother* 48:631–640.

65. San Millan A, Escudero JA, Gutierrez B, Hidalgo L, Garcia N, Llagostera M, Dominguez L, Gonzalez-Zorn B. 2009. Multiresistance in *Pasteurella multocida* is mediated by coexistence of small plasmids. *Antimicrob Agents Chemother* 53:3399–3404.

66. Chaslus-Dancla E, Lesage-Descauses M-C, Leroy-Sétrin S, Martel J-L, Lafont J-P. 1995. Tetracycline resistance determinants, Tet B and Tet M, detected in *Pasteurella haemolytica* and *Pasteurella multocida* from bovine herds. *J Antimicrob Chemother* 36:815–819.

67. Chalmers R, Sewitz S, Lipkow K, Crellin P. 2000. Complete nucleotide sequence of Tn*10*. *J Bacteriol* 182:2970–2972.

68. Lawley TD, Burland V, Taylor DE. 2000. Analysis of the complete nucleotide sequence of the tetracycline-resistance transposon Tn*10*. *Plasmid* 43:235–239.

69. Chopra I, Roberts M. 2001. Tetracycline antibiotics: mode of action, applications, molecular biology, and epidemiology of bacterial resistance. *Microbiol Mol Biol Rev* 65:232–260.

70. Wasteson Y, Roe DE, Falk K, Roberts MC. 1996. Characterization of tetracycline and erythromycin resistance in *Actinobacillus pleuropneumoniae*. *Vet Microbiol* 48:41–50.

71. Ouellet V, Forest A, Nadeau M, Sirois M. 2004. Characterization of tetracycline resistance determinants in *Actinobacillus pleuropneumoniae*. Abstr A-113, 104th ASM General Meeting, p 22.

72. Morioka A, Asai T, Nitta H, Yamamoto K, Ogikubo Y, Takahashi T, Suzuki S. 2008. Recent trends in antimicrobial susceptibility and the presence of the tetracycline resistance gene in *Actinobacillus pleuropneumoniae* isolates in Japan. *J Vet Med Sci* 70:1261–1264.

73. Yoo AN, Cha SB, Shin MK, Won HK, Kim EH, Choi HW, Yoo HS. 2014. Serotypes and antimicrobial resistance patterns of the recent Korean *Actinobacillus pleuropneumoniae* isolates. *Vet Rec* 174:223.

74. Bossé JT, Li Y, Fernandez Crespo R, Chaudhuri RR, Rogers J, Holden MTG, Maskell DJ, Tucker AW, Wren BW, Rycroft AN, Langford PR, the BRaDP1T Consortium. 2016. ICE*Apl1*, an integrative conjugative element related to ICE*Hin1056*, identified in the pig pathogen *Actinobacillus pleuropneumoniae*. *Front Microbiol* 7:810.

75. Lancashire JF, Terry TD, Blackall PJ, Jennings MP. 2005. Plasmid-encoded Tet B tetracycline resistance in *Haemophilus parasuis*. *Antimicrob Agents Chemother* 49:1927–1931.

76. Wu J-R, Shieh HK, Shien J-H, Gong S-R, Chang P-C. 2003. Molecular characterization of plasmids with antimicrobial resistant genes in avian isolates of *Pasteurella multocida*. *Avian Dis* 47:1384–1392.

77. Briggs CE, Fratamico PM. 1999. Molecular characterization of an antibiotic resistance gene cluster of *Salmonella* typhimurium DT104. *Antimicrob Agents Chemother* 43:846–849.

78. Doublet B, Boyd D, Mulvey MR, Cloeckaert A. 2005. The *Salmonella* genomic island 1 is an integrative mobilizable element. *Mol Microbiol* 55:1911–1924.

79. Kehrenberg C, Catry B, Haesebrouck F, de Kruif A, Schwarz S. 2005. *tet*(L)-mediated tetracycline resistance in bovine *Mannheimia* and *Pasteurella* isolates. *J Antimicrob Chemother* 56:403–406.

80. Schwarz S, Cardoso M, Wegener HC. 1992. Nucleotide sequence and phylogeny of the *tet*(L) tetracycline resistance determinant encoded by plasmid pSTE1 from *Staphylococcus hyicus*. *Antimicrob Agents Chemother* 36:580–588.

81. Kim B, Hur J, Lee JY, Choi Y, Lee JH. 2016. Molecular serotyping and antimicrobial resistance profiles of *Actinobacillus pleuropneumoniae* isolated from pigs in South Korea. *Vet Q* 36:137–144.

82. Flannagan SE, Zitzow LA, Su YA, Clewell DB. 1994. Nucleotide sequence of the 18-kb conjugative transposon Tn*916* from *Enterococcus faecalis*. *Plasmid* 32:350–354.

83. Tristram S, Jacobs MR, Appelbaum PC. 2007. Antimicrobial resistance in *Haemophilus influenzae*. *Clin Microbiol Rev* 20:368–389.

84. Livrelli VO, Darfeuille-Richaud A, Rich CD, Joly BH, Martel J-L. 1988. Genetic determinant of the ROB-1 β-lactamase in bovine and porcine *Pasteurella* strains. *Antimicrob Agents Chemother* 32:1282–1284.

85. Livrelli V, Peduzzi J, Joly B. 1991. Sequence and molecular characterization of the ROB-1 β-lactamase gene from *Pasteurella haemolytica*. *Antimicrob Agents Chemother* 35:242–251.

86. Juteau J-M, Levesque RC. 1990. Sequence analysis and evolutionary perspectives of ROB-1 β-lactamase. *Antimicrob Agents Chemother* 34:1354–1359.

87. Azad AK, Coote JG, Parton R. 1992. Distinct plasmid profiles of *Pasteurella haemolytica* serotypes and the

characterization and amplification in *Escherichia coli* of ampicillin-resistance plasmids encoding ROB-1 β-lactamase. *J Gen Microbiol* **138**:1185–1196.

88. San Millan A, Escudero JA, Catalan A, Nieto S, Farelo F, Gibert M, Moreno MA, Dominguez L, Gonzalez-Zorn B. 2007. β-lactam resistance in *Haemophilus parasuis* is mediated by plasmid pB1000 bearing *bla*_{ROB-1}. *Antimicrob Agents Chemother* **51**:2260–2264.

89. Naas T, Benaoudia F, Lebrun L, Nordmann P. 2001. Molecular identification of TEM-1 β-lactamase in a *Pasteurella multocida* isolate of human origin. *Eur J Clin Microbiol Infect Dis* **20**:210–213.

90. Chander Y, Oliveira S, Goyal SM. 2011. Characterisation of ceftiofur resistance in swine bacterial pathogens. *Vet J* **187**:139–141.

91. Bush K, Jacoby GA, Medeiros AA. 1995. A functional classification scheme for β-lactamases and its correlation with molecular structure. *Antimicrob Agents Chemother* **39**:1211–1233.

92. Medeiros AA, Levesque R, Jacoby GA. 1986. An animal source for the ROB-1 β-lactamase of *Haemophilus influenzae* type b. *Antimicrob Agents Chemother* **29**:212–215.

93. Juteau J-M, Sirois M, Medeiros AA, Levesque RC. 1991. Molecular distribution of ROB-1 β-lactamase in *Actinobacillus pleuropneumoniae*. *Antimicrob Agents Chemother* **35**:1397–1402.

94. Chang C-F, Yeh T-M, Chou C-C, Chang Y-F, Chiang T-S. 2002. Antimicrobial susceptibility and plasmid analysis of *Actinobacillus pleuropneumoniae* isolated in Taiwan. *Vet Microbiol* **84**:169–177.

95. Kang M, Zhou R, Liu L, Langford PR, Chen H. 2009. Analysis of an *Actinobacillus pleuropneumoniae* multiresistance plasmid, pHB0503. *Plasmid* **61**:135–139.

96. Philippon A, Joly B, Reynaud D, Paul G, Martel J-L, Sirot D, Cluzel R, Névot P. 1986. Characterization of a β-lactamase from *Pasteurella multocida*. *Ann Inst Pasteur Microbiol 1985* **137A**:153–158.

97. Moleres J, Santos-López A, Lázaro I, Labairu J, Prat C, Ardanuy C, González-Zorn B, Aragon V, Garmendia J. 2015. Novel *bla*_{ROB-1}-bearing plasmid conferring resistance to β-lactams in *Haemophilus parasuis* isolates from healthy weaning pigs. *Appl Environ Microbiol* **81**:3255–3267.

98. Wood AR, Lainson FA, Wright F, Baird GD, Donachie W. 1995. A native plasmid of *Pasteurella haemolytica* serotype A1: DNA sequence analysis and investigation of its potential as a vector. *Res Vet Sci* **58**:163–168.

99. Galán JC, Morosini MI, Baquero MR, Reig M, Baquero F. 2003. *Haemophilus influenzae* bla(ROB-1) mutations in hypermutagenic deltaampC *Escherichia coli* conferring resistance to cefotaxime and β-lactamase inhibitors and increased susceptibility to cefaclor. *Antimicrob Agents Chemother* **47**:2551–2557.

100. Craig FF, Coote JG, Parton R, Freer JH, Gilmour NJ. 1989. A plasmid which can be transferred between *Escherichia coli* and *Pasteurella haemolytica* by electroporation and conjugation. *J Gen Microbiol* **135**:2885–2890.

101. Schwarz S, Spies U, Reitz B, Seyfert H-M, Lämmler C, Blobel H. 1989. Detection and interspecies-transformation of a β-lactamase-encoding plasmid from *Pasteurella haemolytica*. *Zentralbl Bakteriol Mikrobiol Hyg [A]* **270**:462–469.

102. Rossmanith SER, Wilt GR, Wu G. 1991. Characterization and comparison of antimicrobial susceptibilities and outer membrane protein and plasmid DNA profiles of *Pasteurella haemolytica* and certain other members of the genus *Pasteurella*. *Am J Vet Res* **52**:2016–2022.

103. Chang YF, Ma DP, Bai HQ, Young R, Struck DK, Shin SJ, Lein DH. 1992. Characterization of plasmids with antimicrobial resistant genes in *Pasteurella haemolytica* A1. *DNA Seq* **3**:89–97.

104. Murphy GL, Robinson LC, Burrows GE. 1993. Restriction endonuclease analysis and ribotyping differentiate *Pasteurella haemolytica* serotype A1 isolates from cattle within a feedlot. *J Clin Microbiol* **31**:2303–2308.

105. Chang YF, Shi J, Shin SJ, Lein DH. 1992. Sequence analysis of the ROB-1 β-lactamase gene from *Actinobacillus pleuropneumoniae*. *Vet Microbiol* **32**:319–325.

106. Lalonde G, Miller JF, Tompkins LS, O'Hanley P. 1989. Transformation of *Actinobacillus pleuropneumoniae* and analysis of R factors by electroporation. *Am J Vet Res* **50**:1957–1960.

107. Ishii H, Hayashi F, Iyobe S, Hashimoto H. 1991. Characterization and classification of *Actinobacillus (Haemophilus) pleuropneumoniae* plasmids. *Am J Vet Res* **52**:1816–1820.

108. Matter D, Rossano A, Sieber S, Perreten V. 2008. Small multidrug resistance plasmids in *Actinobacillus porcitonsillarum*. *Plasmid* **59**:144–152.

109. Schwarz S, Cloeckaert A, Roberts MC. 2006. Mechanisms and spread of bacterial resistance to antimicrobial agents, p 73–98. *In* Aarestrup FM (ed), *Antimicrobial Resistance in Bacteria of Animal Origin*. ASM Press, Washington, DC.

110. Schwarz S, Spies U, Schäfer F, Blobel H. 1989. Isolation and interspecies-transfer of a plasmid from *Pasteurella multocida* encoding for streptomycin resistance. *Med Microbiol Immunol (Berl)* **178**:121–125.

111. Silver RP, Leming B, Garon CF, Hjerpe CA. 1979. R-plasmids in *Pasteurella multocida*. *Plasmid* **2**:493–497.

112. Coté S, Harel J, Higgins R, Jacques M. 1991. Resistance to antimicrobial agents and prevalence of R plasmids in *Pasteurella multocida* from swine. *Am J Vet Res* **52**:1653–1657.

113. Yamamoto J, Sakano T, Shimizu M. 1990. Drug resistance and R plasmids in *Pasteurella multocida* isolates from swine. *Microbiol Immunol* **34**:715–721.

114. Liu W, Yang M, Xu Z, Zheng H, Liang W, Zhou R, Wu B, Chen H. 2012. Complete genome sequence of *Pasteurella multocida* HN06, a toxigenic strain of serogroup D. *J Bacteriol* **194**:3292–3293.

115. Zimmerman ML, Hirsh DC. 1980. Demonstration of an R plasmid in a strain of *Pasteurella haemolytica* isolated from feedlot cattle. *Am J Vet Res* **41**:166–169.

116. Kehrenberg C, Schwarz S. 2002. Nucleotide sequence and organization of plasmid pMVSCS1 from

Mannheimia varigena: identification of a multiresistance gene cluster. *J Antimicrob Chemother* 49:383–386.

117. Gilbride KA, Rosendal S, Brunton JL. 1989. Plasmid mediated antimicrobial resistance in Ontario isolates of *Actinobacillus* (*Haemophilus*) *pleuropneumoniae*. *Can J Vet Res* 53:38–42.

118. Willson PJ, Deneer HG, Potter A, Albritton W. 1989. Characterization of a streptomycin-sulfonamide resistance plasmid from *Actinobacillus pleuropneumoniae*. *Antimicrob Agents Chemother* 33:235–238.

119. Ishii H, Nakasone Y, Shigehara S, Honma K, Araki Y, Iyobe S, Hashimoto H. 1990. Drug-susceptibility and isolation of a plasmid in *Haemophilus* (*Actinobacillus*) *pleuropneumoniae*. *Nippon Juigaku Zasshi* 52:1–9.

120. Kiuchi A, Hara M, Tabuchi K. 1992. Drug resistant plasmid of *Actinobacillus pleuropneumoniae* isolated from swine pleuropneumonia in Thailand. *Kansenshogaku Zasshi* 66:1243–1247.

121. Ito H, Ishii H, Akiba M. 2004. Analysis of the complete nucleotide sequence of an *Actinobacillus pleuropneumoniae* streptomycin-sulfonamide resistance plasmid, pMS260. *Plasmid* 51:41–47.

122. Bossé JT, Li Y, Walker S, Atherton T, Fernandez Crespo R, Williamson SM, Rogers J, Chaudhuri RR, Weinert LA, Oshota O, Holden MTG, Maskell DJ, Tucker AW, Wren BW, Rycroft AN, Langford PR, BRaDP1T Consortium. 2015. Identification of *dfrA14* in two distinct plasmids conferring trimethoprim resistance in *Actinobacillus pleuropneumoniae*. *J Antimicrob Chemother* 70:2217–2222.

123. Hsu YM, Shieh HK, Chen WH, Sun TY, Shiang J-H. 2007. Antimicrobial susceptibility, plasmid profiles and haemocin activities of *Avibacterium paragallinarum* strains. *Vet Microbiol* 124:209–218.

124. Chiou C-S, Jones AL. 1993. Nucleotide sequence analysis of a transposon (Tn5393) carrying streptomycin resistance genes in *Erwinia amylovora* and other Gram-negative bacteria. *J Bacteriol* 175:732–740.

125. Kehrenberg C, Schwarz S. 2001. Occurrence and linkage of genes coding for resistance to sulfonamides, streptomycin and chloramphenicol in bacteria of the genera *Pasteurella* and *Mannheimia*. *FEMS Microbiol Lett* 205:283–290.

126. Ojo KK, Kehrenberg C, Schwarz S, Odelola HA. 2002. Identification of a complete *dfrA14* gene cassette integrated at a secondary site in a resistance plasmid of uropathogenic *Escherichia coli* from Nigeria. *Antimicrob Agents Chemother* 46:2054–2055.

127. Sundin GW. 2000. Examination of base pair variants of the *strA-strB* streptomycin resistance genes from bacterial pathogens of humans, animals and plants. *J Antimicrob Chemother* 46:848–849.

128. Sundin GW. 2002. Distinct recent lineages of the *strA-strB* streptomycin-resistance genes in clinical and environmental bacteria. *Curr Microbiol* 45:63–69.

129. Sundin GW, Bender CL. 1996. Dissemination of the *strA-strB* streptomycin-resistance genes among commensal and pathogenic bacteria from humans, animals, and plants. *Mol Ecol* 5:133–143.

130. Kehrenberg C, Schwarz S. 2011. Trimethoprim resistance in a porcine *Pasteurella aerogenes* isolate is based on a *dfrA1* gene cassette located in a partially truncated class 2 integron. *J Antimicrob Chemother* 66:450–452.

131. Schwarz S, Kehrenberg C, Salmon SA, Watts JL. 2004. *In vitro* activities of spectinomycin and comparator agents against *Pasteurella multocida* and *Mannheimia haemolytica* from respiratory tract infections of cattle. *J Antimicrob Chemother* 53:379–382.

132. Kehrenberg C, Catry B, Haesebrouck F, de Kruif A, Schwarz S. 2005. Novel spectinomycin/streptomycin resistance gene, *aadA14*, from *Pasteurella multocida*. *Antimicrob Agents Chemother* 49:3046–3049.

133. Oka A, Sugisaki H, Takanami M. 1981. Nucleotide sequence of the kanamycin resistance transposon Tn903. *J Mol Biol* 147:217–226.

134. Dixon LG, Albritton WL, Willson PJ. 1994. An analysis of the complete nucleotide sequence of the *Haemophilus ducreyi* broad-host-range plasmid pLS88. *Plasmid* 32:228–232.

135. Kehrenberg C, Schwarz S. 2005. Molecular basis of resistance to kanamycin and neomycin in *Pasteurella* and *Mannheimia* isolates of animal origin. Abstr A47, ASM Conference on *Pasteurellaceae* 2005, p. 55.

136. Makosky PC, Dahlberg AE. 1987. Spectinomycin resistance at site 1192 in 16S ribosomal RNA of *E. coli*: an analysis of three mutants. *Biochimie* 69:885–889.

137. De Stasio EA, Moazed D, Noller HF, Dahlberg AE. 1989. Mutations in 16S ribosomal RNA disrupt antibiotic-RNA interactions. *EMBO J* 8:1213–1216.

138. Brink MF, Brink G, Verbeet MP, de Boer HA. 1994. Spectinomycin interacts specifically with the residues G_{1064} and C_{1192} in 16S rRNA, thereby potentially freezing this molecule into an inactive conformation. *Nucleic Acids Res* 22:325–331.

139. Galimand M, Gerbaud G, Courvalin P. 2000. Spectinomycin resistance in *Neisseria* spp. due to mutations in 16S rRNA. *Antimicrob Agents Chemother* 44:1365–1366.

140. O'Connor M, Dahlberg AE. 2002. Isolation of spectinomycin resistance mutations in the 16S rRNA of *Salmonella enterica* serovar Typhimurium and expression in *Escherichia coli* and *Salmonella*. *Curr Microbiol* 45:429–433.

141. Funatsu G, Schiltz E, Wittmann HG. 1972. Ribosomal proteins. XXVII. Localization of the amino acid exchanges in protein S5 from two *Escherichia coli* mutants resistant to spectinomycin. *Mol Gen Genet* 114:106–111.

142. Davies C, Bussiere DE, Golden BL, Porter SJ, Ramakrishnan V, White SW. 1998. Ribosomal proteins S5 and L6: high-resolution crystal structures and roles in protein synthesis and antibiotic resistance. *J Mol Biol* 279:873–888.

143. Kehrenberg C, Schwarz S. 2007. Mutations in 16S rRNA and ribosomal protein S5 associated with high-level spectinomycin resistance in *Pasteurella multocida*. *Antimicrob Agents Chemother* 51:2244–2246.

144. de Groot R, Sluijter M, de Bruyn A, Campos J, Goessens WH, Smith AL, Hermans PW. 1996. Genetic characterization of trimethoprim resistance in *Haemophilus influenzae*. *Antimicrob Agents Chemother* **40:** 2131–2136.

145. Enne VI, King A, Livermore DM, Hall LM. 2002. Sulfonamide resistance in *Haemophilus influenzae* mediated by acquisition of *sul2* or a short insertion in chromosomal *folP*. *Antimicrob Agents Chemother* **46:** 1934–1939.

146. Kehrenberg C, Schwarz S. 2005. *dfrA20*, A novel trimethoprim resistance gene from *Pasteurella multocida*. *Antimicrob Agents Chemother* **49:**414–417.

147. Scholz P, Haring V, Wittmann-Liebold B, Ashman K, Bagdasarian M, Scherzinger E. 1989. Complete nucleotide sequence and gene organization of the broad-host-range plasmid RSF1010. *Gene* **75:**271–288.

148. Kim EH, Aoki T. 1996. Sulfonamide resistance gene in a transferable R plasmid of *Pasteurella piscicida*. *Microbiol Immunol* **40:**397–399.

149. Rådström P, Swedberg G. 1988. RSF1010 and a conjugative plasmid contain *sulII*, one of two known genes for plasmid-borne sulfonamide resistance dihydropteroate synthase. *Antimicrob Agents Chemother* **32:**1684–1692.

150. Wright CL, Strugnell RA, Hodgson ALM. 1997. Characterization of a *Pasteurella multocida* plasmid and its use to express recombinant proteins in *P. multocida*. *Plasmid* **37:**65–79.

151. Escande F, Gerbaud G, Martel J-L, Courvalin P. 1991. Resistance to trimethoprim and 2,4-diamino-6,7-diisopropyl-pteridine (0/129) in *Pasteurella haemolytica*. *Vet Microbiol* **26:**107–114.

152. Anantham S, Hall RM. 2012. pCERC1, a small, globally disseminated plasmid carrying the *dfrA14* cassette in the *strA* gene of the *sul2-strA-strB* gene cluster. *Microb Drug Resist* **18:**364–371.

153. Dayao DAE, Seddon JM, Gibson JS, Blackall PJ, Turni C. 2016. Whole genome sequence analysis of pig respiratory bacterial pathogens with elevated minimum inhibitory concentrations for macrolides. *Microb Drug Resist* **22:**531–537.

154. Yang SS, Sun J, Liao XP, Liu BT, Li LL, Li L, Fang LX, Huang T, Liu YH. 2013. Co-location of the *erm*(T) gene and *bla*ROB-1 gene on a small plasmid in *Haemophilus parasuis* of pig origin. *J Antimicrob Chemother* **68:**1930–1932.

155. Kadlec K, Brenner Michael G, Sweeney MT, Brzuszkiewicz E, Liesegang H, Daniel R, Watts JL, Schwarz S. 2011. Molecular basis of macrolide, triamilide, and lincosamide resistance in *Pasteurella multocida* from bovine respiratory disease. *Antimicrob Agents Chemother* **55:**2475–2477.

156. Desmolaize B, Rose S, Warrass R, Douthwaite S. 2011. A novel Erm monomethyltransferase in antibiotic-resistant isolates of *Mannheimia haemolytica* and *Pasteurella multocida*. *Mol Microbiol* **80:**184–194.

157. Michael GB, Eidam C, Kadlec K, Meyer K, Sweeney MT, Murray RW, Watts JL, Schwarz S. 2012. Increased

MICs of gamithromycin and tildipirosin in the presence of the genes *erm*(42) and *msr*(E)-*mph*(E) for bovine *Pasteurella multocida* and *Mannheimia haemolytica*. *J Antimicrob Chemother* **67:**1555–1557.

158. Peric M, Bozdogan B, Jacobs MR, Appelbaum PC. 2003. Effects of an efflux mechanism and ribosomal mutations on macrolide susceptibility of *Haemophilus influenzae* clinical isolates. *Antimicrob Agents Chemother* **47:**1017–1022.

159. Olsen AS, Warrass R, Douthwaite S. 2015. Macrolide resistance conferred by rRNA mutations in field isolates of *Mannheimia haemolytica* and *Pasteurella multocida*. *J Antimicrob Chemother* **70:**420–423.

160. Desmolaize B, Rose S, Wilhelm C, Warrass R, Douthwaite S. 2011. Combinations of macrolide resistance determinants in field isolates of *Mannheimia haemolytica* and *Pasteurella multocida*. *Antimicrob Agents Chemother* **55:**4128–4133.

161. Chen LP, Cai XW, Wang XR, Zhou XL, Wu DF, Xu XJ, Chen HC. 2010. Characterization of plasmid-mediated lincosamide resistance in a field isolate of *Haemophilus parasuis*. *J Antimicrob Chemother* **65:** 2256–2258.

162. Schwarz S, Kehrenberg C, Doublet B, Cloeckaert A. 2004. Molecular basis of bacterial resistance to chloramphenicol and florfenicol. *FEMS Microbiol Rev* **28:** 519–542.

163. Vassort-Bruneau C, Lesage-Descauses MC, Martel J-L, Lafont J-P, Chaslus-Dancla E. 1996. CAT III chloramphenicol resistance in *Pasteurella haemolytica* and *Pasteurella multocida* isolated from calves. *J Antimicrob Chemother* **38:**205–213.

164. Kawahara K, Kawase H, Nakai T, Kume K, Danbara H. 1990. Drug resistance plasmids of *Actinobacillus* (*Haemophilus*) *pleuropneumoniae* serotype 2 strains isolated from swine. *Kitasato Arch Exp Med* **63:**131–136.

165. Ishii H, Fukuyasu T, Iyobe S, Hashimoto H. 1993. Characterization of newly isolated plasmids from *Actinobacillus pleuropneumoniae*. *Am J Vet Res* **54:**701–708.

166. Powell M, Livermore DM. 1988. Mechanisms of chloramphenicol resistance in *Haemophilus influenzae* in the United Kingdom. *J Med Microbiol* **27:**89–93.

167. Murray IA, Martinez-Suarez JV, Close TJ, Shaw WV. 1990. Nucleotide sequences of genes encoding the type II chloramphenicol acetyltransferases of *Escherichia coli* and *Haemophilus influenzae*, which are sensitive to inhibition by thiol-reactive reagents. *Biochem J* **272:**505–510.

168. Hörmansdorfer S, Bauer J. 1996. Resistance pattern of bovine *Pasteurella*. *Berl Munch Tierarztl Wochenschr* **109:**168–171. (In German.)

169. Hörmansdorfer S, Bauer J. 1998. Resistance of bovine and porcine *Pasteurella* against florfenicol and other antibiotics. *Berl Munch Tierarztl Wochenschr* **111:**422–426. (In German.)

170. Priebe S, Schwarz S. 2003. *In vitro* activities of florfenicol against bovine and porcine respiratory tract pathogens. *Antimicrob Agents Chemother* **47:**2703–2705.

171. Kehrenberg C, Mumme J, Wallmann J, Verspohl J, Tegeler R, Kühn T, Schwarz S. 2004. Monitoring of florfenicol susceptibility among bovine and porcine respiratory tract pathogens collected in Germany during the years 2002 and 2003. *J Antimicrob Chemother* **54**: 572–574.

172. Kaspar H, Schröer U, Wallmann J. 2007. Quantitative resistance level (MIC) of *Pasteurella multocida* isolated from pigs between 2004 and 2006: national resistance monitoring by the BVL. *Berl Munch Tierarztl Wochenschr* **120**:442–451.

173. Wallmann J, Schröer U, Kaspar H. 2007. Quantitative resistance level (MIC) of bacterial pathogens (*Escherichia coli, Pasteurella multocida, Pseudomonas aeruginosa, Salmonella* sp., *Staphylococcus aureus*) isolated from chickens and turkeys: national resistance monitoring by the BVL 2004/2005. *Berl Munch Tierarztl Wochenschr* **120**:452–463.

174. Kehrenberg C, Schwarz S. 2005. Plasmid-borne florfenicol resistance in *Pasteurella multocida*. *J Antimicrob Chemother* **55**:773–775.

175. Whittle G, Katz ME, Clayton EH, Cheetham BF. 2000. Identification and characterization of a native *Dichelobacter nodosus* plasmid, pDN1. *Plasmid* **43**: 230–234.

176. Blickwede M, Schwarz S. 2004. Molecular analysis of florfenicol-resistant *Escherichia coli* isolates from pigs. *J Antimicrob Chemother* **53**:58–64.

177. Sørum H, Roberts MC, Crosa JH. 1992. Identification and cloning of a tetracycline resistance gene from the fish pathogen *Vibrio salmonicida*. *Antimicrob Agents Chemother* **36**:611–615.

178. Kehrenberg C, Wallmann J, Schwarz S. 2008. Molecular analysis of florfenicol-resistant *Pasteurella multocida* isolates in Germany. *J Antimicrob Chemother* **62**: 951–955.

179. Katsuda K, Kohmoto M, Mikami O, Tamamura Y, Uchida I. 2012. Plasmid-mediated florfenicol resistance in *Mannheimia haemolytica* isolated from cattle. *Vet Microbiol* **155**:444–447.

180. Li B, Zhang Y, Wei J, Shao D, Liu K, Shi Y, Qiu Y, Ma Z. 2015. Characterization of a novel small plasmid carrying the florfenicol resistance gene *floR* in *Haemophilus parasuis*. *J Antimicrob Chemother* **70**:3159–3161.

181. Bossé JT, Li Y, Atherton TG, Walker S, Williamson SM, Rogers J, Chaudhuri RR, Weinert LA, Holden MTG, Maskell DJ, Tucker AW, Wren BW, Rycroft AN, Langford PR, BRaDP1T Consortium. 2015. Characterisation of a mobilisable plasmid conferring florfenicol and chloramphenicol resistance in *Actinobacillus pleuropneumoniae*. *Vet Microbiol* **178**:279–282.

182. da Silva GC, Rossi CC, Santana MF, Langford PR, Bossé JT, Bazzolli DMS. 2017. p518, A small *floR* plasmid from a South American isolate of *Actinobacillus pleuropneumoniae*. *Vet Microbiol* **204**:129–132.

183. Kehrenberg C, Meunier D, Targant H, Cloeckaert A, Schwarz S, Madec J-Y. 2006. Plasmid-mediated flor-

fenicol resistance in *Pasteurella trehalosi*. *J Antimicrob Chemother* **58**:13–17.

184. Blackall PJ, Bojesen AM, Christensen H, Bisgaard M. 2007. Reclassification of [*Pasteurella*] *trehalosi* as *Bibersteinia trehalosi* gen. nov., comb. nov. *Int J Syst Evol Microbiol* **57**:666–674.

185. Tegetmeyer HE, Jones SC, Langford PR, Baltes N. 2008. IS*Apl1*, a novel insertion element of *Actinobacillus pleuropneumoniae*, prevents ApxIV-based serological detection of serotype 7 strain AP76. *Vet Microbiol* **128**: 342–353.

186. Goldstein EJC, Citron DM, Merriam CV, Warren YA, Tyrrell KL, Fernandez HT. 2002. *In vitro* activities of garenoxacin (BMS-284756) against 170 clinical isolates of nine *Pasteurella* species. *Antimicrob Agents Chemother* **46**:3068–3070.

187. Cárdenas M, Barbé J, Llagostera M, Miró E, Navarro F, Mirelis B, Prats G, Badiola I. 2001. Quinolone resistance-determining regions of *gyrA* and *parC* in *Pasteurella multocida* strains with different levels of nalidixic acid resistance. *Antimicrob Agents Chemother* **45**:990–991.

188. Kong LC, Gao D, Gao YH, Liu SM, Ma HX. 2014. Fluoroquinolone resistance mechanism of clinical isolates and selected mutants of *Pasteurella multocida* from bovine respiratory disease in China. *J Vet Med Sci* **76**:1655–1657.

189. Katsuda K, Kohmoto M, Mikami O, Uchida I. 2009. Antimicrobial resistance and genetic characterization of fluoroquinolone-resistant *Mannheimia haemolytica* isolates from cattle with bovine pneumonia. *Vet Microbiol* **139**:74–79.

190. Wang Y-C, Chan JP-W, Yeh K-S, Chang C-C, Hsuan S-L, Hsieh Y-M, Chang Y-C, Lai T-C, Lin W-H, Chen T-H. 2010. Molecular characterization of enrofloxacin resistant *Actinobacillus pleuropneumoniae* isolates. *Vet Microbiol* **142**:309–312.

191. Guo L, Zhang J, Xu C, Zhao Y, Ren T, Zhang B, Fan H, Liao M. 2011. Molecular characterization of fluoroquinolone resistance in *Haemophilus parasuis* isolated from pigs in South China. *J Antimicrob Chemother* **66**:539–542.

192. Zhang Q, Zhou M, Song D, Zhao J, Zhang A, Jin M. 2013. Molecular characterisation of resistance to fluoroquinolones in *Haemophilus parasuis* isolated from China. *Int J Antimicrob Agents* **42**:87–89.

193. Poole K. 2005. Efflux-mediated antimicrobial resistance. *J Antimicrob Chemother* **56**:20–51.

194. Chen L, Wu D, Cai X, Guo F, Blackall PJ, Xu X, Chen H. 2012. Electrotransformation of *Haemophilus parasuis* with *in vitro* modified DNA based on a novel shuttle vector. *Vet Microbiol* **155**:310–316.

195. Luan SL, Chaudhuri RR, Peters SE, Mayho M, Weinert LA, Crowther SA, Wang J, Langford PR, Rycroft A, Wren BW, Tucker AW, Maskell DJ, BRaDP1T Consortium. 2013. Generation of a Tn5 transposon library in *Haemophilus parasuis* and analysis by transposon-directed insertion-site sequencing (TraDIS). *Vet Microbiol* **166**:558–566.

Antimicrobial Resistance in Bacteria from Livestock and Companion Animals
Edited by Frank Møller Aarestrup, Stefan Schwarz, Jianzhong Shen, and Lina Cavaco
© 2018 American Society for Microbiology, Washington, DC
doi:10.1128/microbiolspec.ARBA-0024-2017

Antimicrobial Resistance in *Bordetella bronchiseptica*

16

Kristina Kadlec[1] and Stefan Schwarz[2]

BORDETELLA BRONCHISEPTICA

B. bronchiseptica is a bacterium within the phylum *Proteobacteria* and the class *Betaproteobacteria*. It belongs to the order *Burkholderiales* and the family *Alcaligenaceae*. In the genus *Bordetella*, *B. bronchiseptica* is one of 14 approved species (http://www.bacterio.net/bordetella.html). *B. bronchiseptica* is a small, coccoid-shaped Gram-negative bacterium with a size of about 0.2 to 0.5 m by 0.5 to 2 m. It is motile due to peritrichous flagella. In comparison to other *Bordetella* spp., its nutritional requirements are simple, and it grows on blood agar plates at 35 to 37°C overnight. The colonies are small, grayish-white, smooth, and shiny, usually without or only with a small zone of hemolysis.

B. bronchiseptica is a commensal of the upper respiratory tract of diverse animal species, including mammals and birds. In veterinary medicine, it also plays an important role as a primary and secondary pathogen of the upper respiratory tract in several mammals but is most important and best described in dogs and in pigs. In contrast, *Bordetella pertussis*, the causative agent of whooping cough in humans, has rarely been reported in other mammals. Experimental infections showed that rhesus macaques and baboons can develop clinical disease (1), and at least one case of an epizootic of whooping cough among chimpanzees in a zoo has been described (2). *Bordetella avium* is commonly identified in birds, although *B. avium* infections have also been described in single human patients with cystic fibrosis (3, 4).

Clinical Relevance

B. bronchiseptica is a facultative respiratory tract pathogen and causes respiratory tract infections in mammals (5). In general, clinical infections caused by *B. bronchiseptica* require additional factors (infectious or noninfectious stressors) and can be seen as multifactorial diseases (6). In addition to other bacteria or viruses, for example, transport and crowding are accompanying factors in the porcine respiratory disease complex. In the clinical scenario, *B. bronchiseptica* may be a primary pathogen and pave the way for other respiratory tract pathogens such as *Pasteurella multocida*. This is commonly the case in one of the major diseases associated with *B. bronchiseptica* in pigs: atrophic rhinitis. A mild form of atrophic rhinitis is seen when *B. bronchiseptica* is the only pathogen, whereas a progressive and much more severe form is seen when *P. multocida* is involved (7, 8). In dogs, *B. bronchiseptica* may also act as a secondary pathogen in the kennel cough complex, also known as canine infectious tracheobronchitis. In kennel cough, canine parainfluenza virus is considered the major pathogen and may pave the way for a subsequent *B. bronchiseptica* infection.

Zoonotic Potential

The vast majority of patients suffering from a clinical infection with *B. bronchiseptica* are either very young or old. Rarely, reports can be found with patients in the age group of 10 to 50 years; commonly, people in that age group and infected by *B. bronchiseptica* are immunocompromised, such as a 43-year-old man who was HIV-positive (9, 10) and an 11-year-old girl suffering from cystic fibrosis (11). However, contact with infected animals may also play a role in human *B. bronchiseptica* infections (12). The patients show respiratory symptoms, such as sinusitis, tracheobronchitis, or a pertussis-like cough (13). Septicemia and meningitis have been also described (14, 15).

[1]Institute of Farm Animal Genetics, Friedrich-Loeffler-Institut, 31535 Neustadt-Mariensee, Germany; [2]Institute of Microbiology and Epizootics, Freie Universität Berlin, 14163 Berlin, Germany.

Prophylaxis and Therapy

On the one hand, vaccination is available for small animals, especially for dogs. Kennel cough vaccines comprising either *B. bronchiseptica* alone or *B. bronchiseptica* and canine parainfluenza virus type 2 are commercially available, the former available as an injectable vaccine and the latter as an injectable vaccine or a vaccine for intranasal application. For cats, only an intranasal vaccine against *B. bronchiseptica* is available. For rabbits, an injectable vaccine against *B. bronchiseptica* and *P. multocida* is on the market. In pigs, autogenous vaccination is used.

On the other hand, in addition to symptomatic treatment, a treatment with antimicrobial agents is a good and successful option to treat *B. bronchiseptica* infections. This prevents additional complications or additional secondary bacterial infections but does not help against other components of the multifactorial disease complexes. Thus, it is important to also reduce viral and environmental stressors. Because these respiratory diseases are highly contagious, it is also helpful to avoid contact of diseased animals with healthy animals. Such a quarantine is likely possible for pets but difficult if not impossible for pigs and rabbit breeding units, because *B. bronchiseptica* has already spread between animals before they show the first clinical signs of disease.

In human patients also, *B. bronchiseptica* infections can be treated with antimicrobial agents. However, in human medicine, the correct identification of *B. bronchiseptica* is the major problem, because this bacterium is not a common human pathogen. Of note, the very common use of β-lactams as first-choice antibiotics does not lead to therapeutic success in *B. bronchiseptica* infections. In contrast, in combination with a β-lactamase inhibitor, this treatment was successful (16). However, most patients with clinical infections have other severe underlying diseases hampering the treatment and leading to the critical situations described in the few case reports available (13, 17).

ANTIMICROBIAL SUSCEPTIBILITY OF *B. BRONCHISEPTICA*

Antimicrobial susceptibility testing prior to the treatment of clinical *B. bronchiseptica* infections is of major relevance in both human and veterinary medicine. To predict the success or failure of an antimicrobial therapy, the correct *in vitro* determination of the antimicrobial susceptibility of the *B. bronchiseptica* isolates is of utmost importance.

Antimicrobial Susceptibility Testing Methods

An internationally accepted testing procedure is available from the Clinical and Laboratory Standards Institute (CLSI) (18, 19). *B. bronchiseptica* isolates can be tested by agar disk diffusion or by determining the MIC by agar dilution or by broth micro- or macrodilution. For this, the standard procedure as described for fast-growing aerobic bacteria in CLSI document VET01-S (19) should be applied. The inoculum can be prepared by either the growth method or the direct colony suspension method and should be equivalent to a 0.5 McFarland standard. Incubation should be for 16 to 20 h at 35°C ± 2°C in ambient air. The CLSI-approved media are Mueller-Hinton agar for disk diffusion and agar dilution as well as cation-adjusted Mueller-Hinton broth for broth dilution assays. *Escherichia coli* ATCC 25922 or *Staphylococcus aureus* ATCC 25923 (disk diffusion)/ATCC 29213 (MIC determination) are recommended as quality controls (19). However, it has been reported that an increase of the incubation time to 24 h may be advantageous. The authors of this study showed that the MIC values of ten isolates determined in five replicates were more stable when read after 24 h incubation time, although the classification of the isolates as susceptible, intermediate, or resistant did not change (20).

Clinical Breakpoints

CLSI document VET01-S is currently the only antimicrobial susceptibility testing document that contains approved clinical breakpoints specific to *B. bronchiseptica* (19). However, breakpoints are only available for a few agents, namely, for ampicillin (test result can be extrapolated to amoxicillin and hetacillin), florfenicol, tildipirosin, and tulathromycin. For tulathromycin, it is worthwhile to mention that it is absolutely essential to stick to the prescribed pH value to end up with correct results for *B. bronchiseptica* as well as for other bacteria. Breakpoints are available for disk diffusion and for MICs determined by broth dilution or agar dilution for florfenicol, tildipirosin, and tulathromycin (19). In contrast, there are only MIC breakpoints for ampicillin (19, 21). Since *B. bronchiseptica* is commonly resistant to ampicillin, these breakpoints serve the diagnostic laboratory mainly to exclude ampicillin and related antimicrobial agents of the β-lactam class from treatment recommendations.

Epidemiological Cutoff Values

An interpretation of the susceptibility testing results by using epidemiological cutoff values is even more difficult. Epidemiological cutoff values for *B. bronchiseptica* had been available solely for trimethoprim-sulfamethoxazole on the EUCAST homepage and have been removed in the meantime (https://mic.eucast.org/Eucast2/). The only data still shown on the website are tetracycline MICs without giving an epidemiological cutoff value (https://mic.eucast.org/Eucast2/SearchController/search.jsp?action=performSearch&BeginIndex=0&Micdif=mic&NumberIndex=50&Antib=-1&Specium=791). In contrast to other MIC values, the MICs for trimethoprim-sulfamethoxazole show a very wide range for *B. bronchiseptica* isolates, for example, comprising more than all 12 dilution steps tested from ≤0.03 mg/liter to ≥64 mg/liter (22). In comparison, tetracycline MICs of the same 349 isolates were distributed from ≤0.12 mg/liter to 2 mg/liter representing the wild-type population, with the vast majority of isolates (n = 227) having a MIC of 0.25 mg/liter (22). Three isolates showed a distinctly higher MIC of 64 mg/liter and were considered non-wild type and were later shown to harbor a specific tetracycline resistance gene (23). A very similar situation is seen on the EUCAST website, with 443 isolates distributed normally from 0.12 mg/liter to 4 mg/liter and 4 isolates showing higher MICs of 64 mg/liter (https://mic.eucast.org/Eucast2/SearchController/search.jsp?action=performSearch&BeginIndex=0&Micdif=mic&NumberIndex=50&Antib=-1&Specium=791). Tetracycline MIC distributions are compared in Table 1.

Published Monitoring Studies

Collected information about antimicrobial susceptibility testing studies in a PhD thesis (23) shows that a direct comparison of susceptibility data is very difficult to accomplish due to different methodologies used. In the corresponding study, MIC determination followed the CLSI-approved antimicrobial susceptibility testing protocol (22). This study showed an overall favorable situation with low MIC values and no change in MICs over a period of 4 years among 349 porcine *B. bronchiseptica* isolates from pigs. More recent publications, however, were performed basically—but not exactly—according to the CLSI standard (24, 25). Commonly, in routine diagnostics as well as in some publications, such as a study of *B. bronchiseptica* isolates from Poland (26), disk diffusion is performed. While in the case of MIC determination, MIC distributions are often shown, the distribution of inhibitory zone diameters is not provided, and results are only given as percentages of isolates classified as susceptible, resistant, or (if available) intermediate. Due to the lack of approved breakpoints, these results have to be used with caution. Distributions of MIC values for florfenicol are shown in Table 2. While clinical breakpoints are available for

Table 1 Tetracycline MIC distributions of *B. bronchiseptica* isolates

Origin	Country	Year of isolation	No. of isolates	No. of isolates with an MIC of ... mg/liter[a]												Reference
				0.03	0.06	0.12	0.25	0.5	1	2	4	8	16	32	64	128	
Pigs	Germany	2011/2012	90	n.t.	n.t.	0	1	52	27	5	3	0	0	0	2	0	27
Companion animals[b]	Germany	2010–2012	43	n.t.	n.t.	1	14	22	4	1	0	0	0	0	1	0	24
Pigs	Germany	2010-2012	107	n.t.	n.t.	2	51	37	4	5	0	0	0	1	4	3	24
Pigs	Europe[c]	2010–2012	118	n.t.	0	0	42	52	9	7	4	1	0	0	0	3	25
Pigs	Germany	2010	43	n.t.	n.t.	0	4	24	10	4	1	0	0	0	0	0	26
Dogs (n = 8), cats (n = 5)	Germany	2010	13	n.t.	n.t.	0	0	9	2	1	1	0	0	0	0	0	60
Pigs	Germany	2009	69	n.t.	n.t.	0	9	51	3	2	1	0	0	0	0	3	29
Pigs	Germany	2008	93	n.t.	n.t.	0	49	35	5	1	0	0	1	1	1	0	30
Dogs (n = 34), cats (= 8)	Germany	2004–2006	42	0	0	0	13	18	3	6	1	0	0	0	1	0	39
Pigs	Germany	2003	82	n.t.	n.t.	8	60	11	2	1	0	0	0	0	0	0	22
Pigs	Germany	2002/2003	138	n.t.	n.t.	9	99	23	3	2	0	0	0	0	2	0	58
Pigs	Germany	2002	91	n.t.	n.t.	6	63	17	1	1	0	0	0	0	3	0	22
Pigs	Germany	2001	98	n.t.	n.t.	5	65	27	1	0	0	0	0	0	0	0	22
Pigs	Germany	2000	78	n.t.	n.t.	29	39	7	3	0	0	0	0	0	0	0	22

[a]n.t., not tested.
[b]Horses (n = 24), dogs (n = 8), rabbits (n = 8), cats (n = 2), ferret (n = 1).
[c]Belgium (n = 24), Denmark (n = 9), France (n = 12), Germany (n = 14), The Netherlands (n = 22), Poland (n = 14), Spain (n = 21), United Kingdom (n = 2).

florfenicol and often the testing range is reduced to the dilution steps of clinical interest, for tetracycline, a wider test range is applied. The tetracycline MICs show a clear bimodal distribution, with most of the isolates having an MIC value around 0.25 or 0.5 mg/liter and single isolates showing MICs of 16 mg/liter or higher (Table 1). For the florfenicol MICs, a bimodal distribution is not so clear, which is not due to the shorter testing ranges (Table 2). Isolates with an MIC in the upper range of the normal distribution around the MIC values of 1 to 4 mg/liter have to be classified as intermediate or even as resistant according to the clinical breakpoints.

Another fact reducing the information on susceptibility of B. bronchiseptica is that often several agents of the same class are tested (24, 25, 27–30). Moreover, two classes licensed and used to treat respiratory tract infections are most commonly included in the panel for B. bronchiseptica: β-lactams and macrolides. Both classes are not useful against B. bronchiseptica, and in vitro susceptibility testing revealed high MIC values and—when breakpoints were available—100% resistant isolates (24, 25, 27–30). For other antimicrobial agents, the studies shown in Table 1 confirm the favorable situation with respect to susceptibility and resistance of B. bronchiseptica.

ANTIMICROBIAL RESISTANCE IN B. BRONCHISEPTICA

In general, little information concerning antimicrobial resistance in B. bronchiseptica is available from the published literature. As a facultative pathogen in a genus of bacteria that harbors human pathogens (B. pertussis) as well as apathogenic species (e.g., Bordetella tumbae), several publications focused on virulence factors and the pathogenicity of bordetellae including B. bronchiseptica (31). Other studies dealt with immunity and vaccination strategies (32). In fact, a B. bronchiseptica vaccine was one of the first antibacterial vaccines and started as a temperature-sensitive vaccine for intranasal application (33). Treatment of clinical B. bronchiseptica infections is easily possible with the appropriate antimicrobial agents licensed for food-producing animals. Commonly, tetracyclines are used, and more than 90% of all B. bronchiseptica isolates show low tetracycline MIC values (https://mic.eucast.org/Eucast2/Search Controller/search.jsp?action=performSearch&Begin Index=0&Micdif=mic&NumberIndex=50&Antib=-1& Specium=791; 22, 34, 35). Overall, due to the favorable situation in terms of antimicrobial susceptibility, treatment problems are rare, and a search for alternative agents is often not necessary.

All three antimicrobial resistance mechanisms—enzymatic inactivation of the antimicrobial agent, reduced intracellular accumulation, and target site modifications—have been identified and described in B. bronchiseptica isolates.

Tetracycline Resistance

High tetracycline MIC values are seen in single isolates of virtually all publications and throughout all years. In contrast to other respiratory tract pathogens, such as Pasteurellaceae with about 30% tetracycline-resistant isolates, only about 1% of the B. bronchiseptica isolates are tetracycline-resistant, e.g., 3 of 349 German porcine isolates (22) and 4 of 447 isolates (https://mic. eucast.org/Eucast2/SearchController/search.jsp?action= performSearch&BeginIndex=0&Micdif=mic&Number Index=50&Antib=-1&Specium=791). Isolates collected from pretreated animals, because tetracyclines are commonly used, might show a higher resistance rate.

The first two B. bronchiseptica isolates considered tetracycline-resistant were isolated in the United Kingdom from cats (35). The gene tet(C) was identified in these feline isolates. This gene codes for a specific efflux protein of the major facilitator superfamily (MFS) conferring resistance in various Gram-negative bacteria by active efflux of tetracyclines. To date, the tet(C) gene has been also identified in a porcine isolate (Kadlec and Schwarz, unpublished). Another MFS tet gene, tet(A), was identified for the first time in B. bronchiseptica in porcine isolates from Germany (23). Later, tet(A) was also identified in all eight tetracycline-resistant isolates from another study of German isolates (24). A third MFS gene, tet(31), has been confirmed in B. bronchiseptica (36). All three genes have also been described in other Gram-negative bacteria but not in other common respiratory tract pathogens, except tet(C) in Chlamydia suis (37).

Sulfonamide Resistance

Among the three sulfonamide resistance genes sul1, sul2, and sul3, so far only sul1 and sul2 have been identified in B. bronchiseptica. All sul genes code for an alternative dihydropteroate synthase that is insensitive to sulfonamides. As in other bacteria, sul1 was in B. bronchiseptica a part of the 3′-conserved segment of class 1 integrons that were located on plasmids (38). The gene sul2 has also been identified in B. bronchiseptica isolates obtained from dogs and cats in the BfT-GermVet study (39). This gene is commonly seen in close proximity to strA and strB (40). In a study by Prüller and coworkers (24), the sul2-positive B. bronchiseptica isolates were also strA and strB positive, but

Table 2 Florfenicol MIC distributions of *B. bronchiseptica* isolates

Origin	Country	Year of isolation	No. of isolates	No. of isolates with an MIC of ... mg/liter[a]												Isolates in %[b]			Reference
				0.03	0.06	0.12	0.25	0.5	1	2	4	8	16	32	64	S	I	R	
Companion animals[c]	Germany	2010–2012	43	n.t.	n.t.	0	0	1	16	11	12	2	1	0	0				24
Pigs	Germany	2010–2012	107	n.t.	n.t.	0	1	3	39	49	14	1	0	0	0	86.0	13.1	0.9	24
Pigs	Germany	2011/2012	90	n.t.	n.t.	0	0	0	1	8	79	2	0	0	0	10.0	87.8	2.2	27
Pigs	Europe[d]	2010–2012	118	n.t.	n.t.	n.t.	n.t.	n.t.	10	52	50	1	1	0	5	52.5	42.4	5.1	25
Pigs	Germany	2010	43	n.t.	n.t.	0	0	0	3	4	32	1	1	2	0	16.3	74.4	9.3	28
Pigs	Germany	2009	69	n.t.	n.t.	0	0	0	2	15	46	4	0	1	1	24.6	66.7	8.7	29
Pigs	Germany	2008	93	n.t.	n.t.	0	0	1	18	41	31	1	0	1	0	64.5	33.3	2.2	30
Dogs (n = 34), cats (n = 8)	Germany	2004–2006	42	0	0	0	0	0	0	9	32	0	0	1	0				39
Pigs	Germany	2003	82	n.t.	n.t.	n.t.	n.t.	n.t.	n.t.	67	11	0	0	4	n.t.	81.7	13.4	4.9	22
Pigs	Germany	2003	51	n.t.	n.t.	0	0	0	4	40	7	0	0	0	0	72.5	26.5	1.0	61
Pigs	Germany	2002/2003	138	n.t.	n.t.	n.t.	n.t.	n.t.	n.t.	111	25	0	0	2	n.t.	80.4	18.2	1.4	58
Pigs	Korea	1998–2003	70	n.t.	n.t.	0	0	0	remaining 67 isolates		3	0	0	0	0	95.7	4.3	0.0	59
Pigs	Germany	2002	91	n.t.	n.t.	n.t.	n.t.	n.t.	n.t.	73	17	0	1	0	n.t.	80.2	18.7	1.1	22
Pigs	Germany	2002	80	n.t.	n.t.	0	0	2	17	59	1	0	1	1	0	97.4	1.3	1.3	61
Pigs	Germany	2001	73	n.t.	n.t.	0	0	0	9	17	38	5	0	4	0	35.6	52.1	12.3	62
Pigs	Germany	2001	98	n.t.	n.t.	0	0	0	n.t.	71	26	0	0	0	n.t.	72.5	26.5	1.0	22
Pigs	Germany	2000	87	n.t.	n.t.	0	0	0	11	18	26	26	6	0	0	33.3	29.9	36.8	62
Pigs	Germany	2000	78	n.t.	n.t.	n.t.	n.t.	n.t.	n.t.	67	7	2	2	0	n.t.	85.9	9.0	5.1	22

[a]n.t., not tested.
[b]Given for the porcine isolates, for which clinical breakpoints are available from the CLSI: S, susceptible; I, intermediate; R, resistant.
[c]Horses (n = 24), dogs (n = 8), rabbits (n = 8), cats (n = 2), ferret (n = 1).
[d]Belgium (n = 24), Denmark (n = 24), France (n = 9), Germany (n = 14), The Netherlands (n = 22), Poland (n = 14), Spain (n = 21), United Kingdom (n = 2).

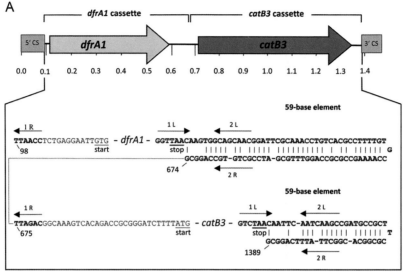

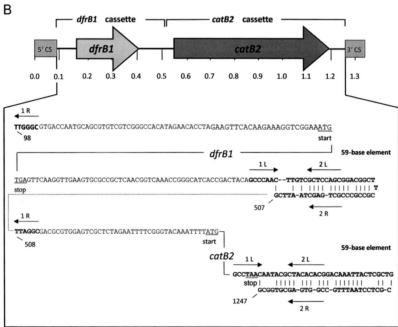

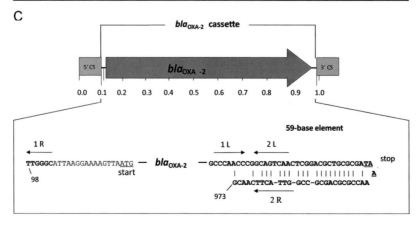

an analysis of the linkage of these genes was not performed. Complete class 1 integrons are common in other Gram-negative bacteria but have not been described in respiratory tract pathogens of the family *Pasteurellaceae* so far. In contrast, the gene cluster *sul2-strA-strB* has been seen in *Pasteurellaceae* and is also common in several other Gram-negative bacteria (40–42).

Trimethoprim Resistance

Up to now, three trimethoprim resistance genes have been described in *B. bronchiseptica* (24, 38). All three genes (*dfrA1*, *dfrA7*, and *dfrB1*) code for alternative dihydrofolate reductases. Among the various *dfr* genes that have been described in Gram-negative bacteria, about 30 genes code for class A dihydrofolate reductases, such as the genes *dfrA1* and *dfrA7*, and only seven code for class B dihydrofolate reductases, namely, *dfrB1*, *dfrB2*, *dfrB3*, *dfrB4*, *dfrB5*, *dfrB6*, and *dfrB7* (43). The acquisition of such a resistance gene and thereby the replacement of the naturally occurring trimethoprim-sensitive dihydrofolate reductase by an alternative trimethoprim-insensitive enzyme leads to very high trimethoprim MIC values (>256 mg/liter) compared to wild-type isolates with low MIC values of <0.12 mg/liter. This observation has also been made in *B. bronchiseptica* (38). However, trimethoprim alone is usually neither tested nor used for treatment. These *dfr* genes are commonly located on gene cassettes, a fact that has been also described for *dfrA1* and *dfrB1* in *B. bronchiseptica* (38). The *dfr*-carrying gene cassettes described in *B. bronchiseptica* are shown in Fig. 1. In the study that described the identification of *dfrA7*, the authors also detected a *sul1* gene, a hint about the presence of a class 1 integron, but did not confirm the location of *dfrA7* in a gene cassette (24).

Aminoglycoside and Aminocyclitol Resistance

In general, the streptomycin MIC values of *B. bronchiseptica* isolates are high, as described for 150 isolates, 132 of which had MICs of 32 to 128 mg/liter and the remaining 18 of which had distinctly higher MICs of ≥1,024 mg/liter. In 17/18 streptomycin-resistant isolates (tentatively classified as resistant by MICs of ≥1,024 mg/liter), the genes *strA* and *strB* were detected (24). These genes often occur together and code for phosphotransferases, namely for the aminoglycoside-3′-phosphotransferase and the aminoglycoside-6′-phosphotransferase, respectively. Thus, they confer resistance by the inactivation of streptomycin. For neomycin, the majority of *B. bronchiseptica* isolates showed MICs of 1 to 8 mg/liter (22, 24). In four isolates with distinctly higher MICs of ≥128 mg/liter, no resistance gene was detected (24). MICs of gentamicin are commonly around 2 mg/liter (22, 24), and isolates exhibiting high MICs have not yet been observed. For the aminocyclitol spectinomycin, data from the German BfT-GermVet study revealed that all 42 isolates from cats and dogs had very high MICs of ≥512 mg/liter (39).

Phenicol Resistance

B. bronchiseptica isolates resistant to florfenicol that also exhibited high MICs to chloramphenicol, but also isolates that were susceptible to florfenicol but had high chloramphenicol MIC values have been described (22, 44). Among the latter isolates, two phenicol resistance mechanisms were identified. The *catB1* and *catB3* genes code for class B chloramphenicol acetyltransferases which inactivate only nonfluorinated phenicols, such as chloramphenicol. As described for other Gram-negative bacteria, these genes were located on gene cassettes and integrated into class 1 integrons (Fig. 1) (38). Another chloramphenicol resistance mechanism was identified in one *B. bronchiseptica* isolate. The isolate harbored a novel gene, *cmlB1*, coding for an MFS exporter. Database searches revealed that the gene is still very rare. Only one additional database entry was found which described the *cmlB1* gene in the whole-genome sequence of an *Acinetobacter pittii* isolate (45). No phenotype was described for this *A. pittii* isolate. In contrast to *cmlA* genes, *cmlB1* was not part of a gene cassette. It was located on a large nonconjugative plasmid and also conferred chloramphenicol resistance after transfer to *E. coli* (44).

Most of the *B. bronchiseptica* isolates that were resistant to florfenicol and had high chloramphenicol

Figure 1 Schematic presentation of the class 1 integrons described so far in *B. bronchiseptica* isolates. The reading frames of the antimicrobial resistance genes are shown as arrows, and the conserved segments of the class 1 integron are shown as boxes. The beginning and the end of the integrated cassettes are shown in detail below. The translational start and stop codons are underlined. The 59-base elements are shown in bold type, and the putative IntI1 integrase binding domains 1L, 2L, 2R, and 1R are indicated by arrows. The numbers refer to the positions of the bases in the EMBL database entries with the following accession numbers: (a) AJ844287, (b) AJ879564, and (c) AJ877267 (41, 50).

MICs harbored the widely distributed resistance gene *floR*. This gene also codes for an MFS exporter and was located in the chromosomal DNA of 7/10 florfenicol-resistant *B. bronchiseptica* isolates (44). The remaining three isolates showed distinctly lower florfenicol and chloramphenicol MIC values and were no longer classified as florfenicol-resistant when an efflux inhibitor was added. The inhibitor PaβNA indicates the presence of a not further specified exporter of the resistance-nodulation-cell division type (44).

β-Lactam Resistance

In *B. bronchiseptica*, the species-specific β-lactamase gene bla_{BOR-1} has been described (46). Involvement of a β-lactam hydrolyzing enzyme in the decreased susceptibility of *B. bronchiseptica* to β-lactam antibiotics is underlined by the fact that β-lactam MICs are lower in the presence of the β-lactamase inhibitor clavulanic acid. Among 150 isolates from pigs, cats, and dogs, 147 were positive in a PCR for bla_{BOR-1} (24). In addition to this class A β-lactamase gene, the class D β-lactamase gene bla_{OXA-2} has been described in *B. bronchiseptica* (47). As previously reported in *Enterobacteriaceae*, bla_{OXA-2} was located on a gene cassette and integrated into a class 1 integron (Fig. 1). In

addition, it was shown that low membrane permeability could contribute to the β-lactam resistance of *B. bronchiseptica* (47).

Fluoroquinolone Resistance

Fluoroquinolones are usually highly active against *B. bronchiseptica*. An early study in which fluoroquinolones were evaluated for their activity against porcine respiratory bacterial pathogens revealed that ciprofloxacin was the most active quinolone against nine strains of *B. bronchiseptica* with mean MICs of 0.58 mg/liter (48). In another study, all 78 canine *B. bronchiseptica* isolates were reported to be susceptible to enrofloxacin (49). In a study of feline *B. bronchiseptica* isolates, all 43 strains tested were susceptible to marbofloxacin and enrofloxacin (MIC_{90}, 0.5 mg/liter), while 93% and 84% of the strains were susceptible, respectively, to ciprofloxacin and difloxacin, with MIC_{90} values of 1 and 8 mg/liter, respectively (50). Testing of 42 *B. bronchiseptica* isolates from dogs and cats for their susceptibility to pradofloxacin revealed MICs in the range between 0.12 mg/liter and 1 mg/liter with both MIC_{50} and MIC_{90} values of 0.25 mg/liter (51). Porcine *B. bronchiseptica* isolates ($n = 349$; 2000 to 2003) ranged in their MICs between

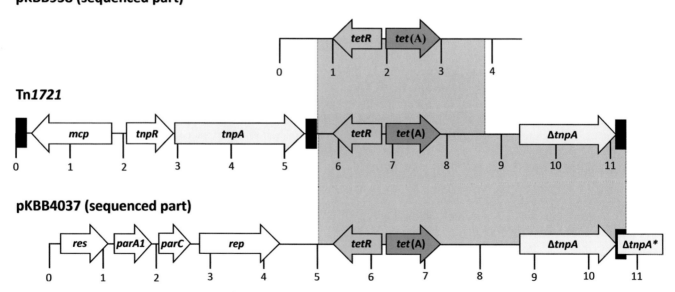

Figure 2 Comparison of Tn*1721* (GenBank accession no. X61367) and the sequenced parts of the resistance plasmids pKBB958 (GenBank accession no. AM183165) and pKBB4037 (GenBank accession no. AJ877266) from *B. bronchiseptica*. A distance scale in kb is given below each map. The genes *tetR*, *tet*(A), *mcp*, *tnpR*, *tnpA*, Δ*tnpA*, *res*, *parA1*, *parC*, and Δ*tnpA** are presented as arrows, with the arrowhead indicating the direction of transcription. The Δ symbol indicates a truncated, functionally inactive gene. The black boxes represent the terminal or internal 38-bp repeats of Tn*1721*. The gray shaded areas indicate the homologous parts between the *B. bronchiseptica* plasmids and Tn*1721* (26).

≤0.015 mg/liter and 2 mg/liter with MIC_{50} and MIC_{90} values of 0.25 and 0.5 mg/liter, respectively (22). The marbofloxacin MIC values of 504 *B. bronchiseptica* isolates collected in various European countries between 1994 and 2013 ranged between 0.06 mg/liter and 2 mg/liter with both MIC_{50} and MIC_{90} values of 0.5 mg/liter (52).

LOCATION OF RESISTANCE GENES ON MOBILE GENETIC ELEMENTS

Most of the resistance genes described so far were located on plasmids. In all cases, the corresponding resistance plasmid was the only plasmid harbored by the respective field isolates. Most of these plasmids were conjugative and could be successfully transferred to *E. coli* (23, 35, 38, 44). The easy transfer into *E. coli* and also the good maintenance in *E. coli* is in contrast to the transfer of plasmids isolated from other respiratory tract pathogens, namely *Pasteurellaceae*.

In addition to plasmids, *B. bronchiseptica* makes use of gene cassettes as mobile genetic elements. Trimethoprim, chloramphenicol, and β-lactam resistance genes have been already described as part of gene cassettes in *B. bronchiseptica* (Fig. 1). While very common in *Enterobacteriaceae*, other respiratory tract pathogens do not often carry class 1 integrons.

Moreover, for the tetracycline resistance gene *tet*(A), remnants of the small nonconjugative transposon Tn*1721* occurring commonly in *E. coli* and other *Enterobacteriaceae* were identified by sequence analysis (Fig. 2). The fact that different parts of transposon Tn*1721* were present on the two further analyzed plasmids indicates that different genetic events led to the final plasmid structure and that, very likely, a Tn*1721*-located gene *tet*(A) was acquired more than once by *B. bronchiseptica*. Tn*1721* has been described in *E. coli* but not in *Pasteurellaceae*. In *Pasteurella*, the genes *tet*(B) and *tet*(H) are the most common tetracycline resistance genes (41, 53). The streptomycin resistance genes *strA* and *strB* are often located on plasmids and are associated with the transposon Tn*5393* (54). Although not described so far, it is very likely that such a location is also present in *B. bronchiseptica*. The genes *strA* and *strB* are also found in *Pasteurellaceae*: plasmids and integrative and conjugative elements carrying *strA*, *strB*, and/or *sul2* have been described (41, 42, 53, 55, 56). However, these genes seem to be ancient and have also been found in streptomycin-resistant bacteria from permafrost (57). Thus, it is not astonishing that these genes are present in a wide variety of bacterial genera.

CONCLUDING REMARKS

B. bronchiseptica is in general susceptible to most antimicrobial agents, which therefore can be used to treat clinical infections. In addition to taxonomy and the identification of novel species, as well as pathogenicity and immunization, in which *B. bronchiseptica* offers a lot of lessons to learn, antimicrobial resistance in *B. bronchiseptica* appears to be of less interest judging from the number of published studies. *B. bronchiseptica* has proved to be able to acquire resistance genes from other bacterial genera, especially from *E. coli*. The future will show whether *B. bronchiseptica* will gain further resistance genes directed against important or critically important antimicrobial agents.

Acknowledgments. We acknowledge support for the work done on B. bronchiseptica from Heike Kaspar, Federal Office of Consumer Protection and Food Safety (BVL), Berlin, Germany.

Citation. Kadlec K, Schwarz S. 2018. Antimicrobial resistance in *Bordetella bronchiseptica*. Microbiol Spectrum 6(4): ARBA-0024-2017.

References

1. **Warfel JM, Beren J, Kelly VK, Lee G, Merkel TJ.** 2012. Nonhuman primate model of pertussis. *Infect Immun* **80:** 1530–1536.

2. **Gustavsson OE, Röken BO, Serrander R.** 1990. An epizootic of whooping cough among chimpanzees in a zoo. *Folia Primatol (Basel)* **55:**45–50.

3. **Spilker T, Liwienski AA, LiPuma JJ.** 2008. Identification of *Bordetella* spp. in respiratory specimens from individuals with cystic fibrosis. *Clin Microbiol Infect* **14:** 504–506.

4. **Harrington AT, Castellanos JA, Ziedalski TM, Clarridge JE III, Cookson BT.** 2009. Isolation of *Bordetella avium* and novel *Bordetella* strain from patients with respiratory disease. *Emerg Infect Dis* **15:**72–74.

5. **Goodnow RA.** 1980. Biology of *Bordetella bronchiseptica*. *Microbiol Rev* **44:**722–738.

6. **Brockmeier SL, Halbur PG, Thacker EL.** 2002. Porcine respiratory disease complex, p 231–258. *In* Brogden KA, Guthmiller JM (ed), *Polymicrobial Diseases*. ASM Press, Washington, DC.

7. **Magyar T, Lax AJ.** 2002. Atrophic rhinitis, p 169–197. *In* Brogden KA, Guthmiller JM (ed), *Polymicrobial Diseases*. ASM Press, Washington, DC.

8. **OIE.** 2012. Atrophic rhinitis of swine, chapter 2.8.2. *In Terrestrial Manual 2012*. OIE, Paris, France.

9. **Rampelotto RF, Hörner A, Hörner C, Righi R, Hörner R.** 2016. Pneumonia caused by *Bordetella bronchiseptica* in two HIV-positive patients. *Sao Paulo Med J* **134:** 268–272.

10. **Mazumder SA, Cleveland KO.** 2010. *Bordetella bronchiseptica* bacteremia in a patient with AIDS. *South Med J* **103:**934–935.

11. Register KB, Sukumar N, Palavecino EL, Rubin BK, Deora R. 2012. *Bordetella bronchiseptica* in a paediatric cystic fibrosis patient: possible transmission from a household cat. *Zoonoses Public Health* 59:246–250.

12. Gueirard P, Weber C, Le Coustumier A, Guiso N. 1995. Human *Bordetella bronchiseptica* infection related to contact with infected animals: persistence of bacteria in host. *J Clin Microbiol* 33:2002–2006.

13. Woolfrey BF, Moody JA. 1991. Human infections associated with *Bordetella bronchiseptica*. *Clin Microbiol Rev* 4:243–255.

14. Dworkin MS, Sullivan PS, Buskin SE, Harrington RD, Olliffe J, MacArthur RD, Lopez CE. 1999. *Bordetella bronchiseptica* infection in human immunodeficiency virus-infected patients. *Clin Infect Dis* 28:1095–1099.

15. Belen O, Campos JM, Cogen PH, Jantausch BA. 2003. Postsurgical meningitis caused by *Bordetella bronchiseptica*. *Pediatr Infect Dis J* 22:380–381.

16. Wernli D, Emonet S, Schrenzel J, Harbarth S. 2011. Evaluation of eight cases of confirmed *Bordetella bronchiseptica* infection and colonization over a 15-year period. *Clin Microbiol Infect* 17:201–203.

17. Mattoo S, Cherry JD. 2005. Molecular pathogenesis, epidemiology, and clinical manifestations of respiratory infections due to *Bordetella pertussis* and other *Bordetella* subspecies. *Clin Microbiol Rev* 18:326–382.

18. CLSI. 2013. Performance standards for antimicrobial disk and dilution susceptibility tests for bacteria isolated from animals; approved standard, 4th ed. CLSI document VET01-A4. Clinical and Laboratory Standards Institute, Wayne, PA.

19. CLSI. 2015. *Performance standards for antimicrobial disk and dilution susceptibility tests for bacteria isolated from animals*; CLSI supplement VET01-S3. Clinical and Laboratory Standards Institute, Wayne, PA.

20. Prüller S, Frömke C, Kaspar H, Klein G, Kreienbrock L, Kehrenberg C. 2015. Recommendation for a standardised method of broth microdilution susceptibility testing for porcine *Bordetella bronchiseptica*. *PLoS One* 10:e0123883.

21. Schwarz S, Böttner A, Goossens L, Hafez HM, Hartmann K, Kaske M, Kehrenberg C, Kietzmann M, Klarmann D, Klein G, Krabisch P, Luhofer G, Richter A, Schulz B, Sigge C, Waldmann KH, Wallmann J, Werckenthin C. 2008. A proposal of clinical breakpoints for amoxicillin applicable to porcine respiratory tract pathogens. *Vet Microbiol* 126:178–188.

22. Kadlec K, Kehrenberg C, Wallmann J, Schwarz S. 2004. Antimicrobial susceptibility of *Bordetella bronchiseptica* isolates from porcine respiratory tract infections. *Antimicrob Agents Chemother* 48:4903–4906.

23. Kadlec K, Kehrenberg C, Schwarz S. 2006. *tet*(A)-mediated tetracycline resistance in porcine *Bordetella bronchiseptica* isolates is based on plasmid-borne Tn*1721* relics. *J Antimicrob Chemother* 58:225–227.

24. Prüller S, Rensch U, Meemken D, Kaspar H, Kopp PA, Klein G, Kehrenberg C. 2015. Antimicrobial susceptibility of *Bordetella bronchiseptica* isolates from swine and companion animals and detection of resistance genes. *PLoS One* 10:e0135703.

25. El Garch F, de Jong A, Simjee S, Moyaert H, Klein U, Ludwig C, Marion H, Haag-Diergarten S, Richard-Mazet A, Thomas V, Siegwart E. 2016. Monitoring of antimicrobial susceptibility of respiratory tract pathogens isolated from diseased cattle and pigs across Europe, 2009-2012: VetPath results. *Vet Microbiol* 194:11–22.

26. Stepniewska K, Urbaniak K, Markowska-Daniel I. 2014. Phenotypic and genotypic characterization of *Bordetella bronchiseptica* strains isolated from pigs in Poland. *Pol J Vet Sci* 17:71–77.

27. GERM-Vet. 2016. *BVL-Report · 10.5 Berichte zur Resistenzmonitoringstudie*. ISBN 978-3-319-31696-3. Springer, Basel, Switzerland. (in German).

28. GERM-Vet. 2014. *BVL-Report · 8.6 Berichte zur Resistenzmonitoringstudie*. ISBN 978-3-319-05995-2. Springer, Basel, Switzerland. (in German).

29. GERM-Vet. 2012. *Berichte zur Resistenzmonitoringstudie* 2009. ISBN 978-3-0348-0504-9. Springer, Basel, Switzerland. (in German).

30. GERM-Vet. 2012. *Berichte zur Resistenzmonitoringstudie* 2008. ISBN 978-3-0348-0422-6. Springer, Basel, Switzerland. (in German).

31. Gerlach G, von Wintzingerode F, Middendorf B, Gross R. 2001. Evolutionary trends in the genus *Bordetella*. *Microbes Infect* 3:61–72.

32. Carbonetti NH, Wirsing von König CH, Lan R, Jacob-Dubuisson F, Cotter PA, Deora R, Merkel TJ, van Els CA, Locht C, Hozbor D, Rodriguez ME. 2016. Highlights of the 11th International *Bordetella* Symposium: from basic biology to vaccine development. *Clin Vaccine Immunol* 23:842–850.

33. Shimizu T. 1978. Prophylaxis of *Bordetella bronchiseptica* infection in guinea pigs by intranasal vaccination with live strain ts-S34. *Infect Immun* 22:318–321.

34. Mortensen JE, Brumbach A, Shryock TR. 1989. Antimicrobial susceptibility of *Bordetella avium* and *Bordetella bronchiseptica* isolates. *Antimicrob Agents Chemother* 33:771–772.

35. Speakman AJ, Binns SH, Osborn AM, Corkill JE, Kariuki S, Saunders JR, Dawson S, Gaskell RM, Hart CA. 1997. Characterization of antibiotic resistance plasmids from *Bordetella bronchiseptica*. *J Antimicrob Chemother* 40:811–816.

36. Kadlec K, Kaspar H, Mankertz J, Schwarz. 2012. First identification of *tet*(31) among tetracycline-resistant porcine *Bordetella bronchiseptica*. Interscience Conference on Antimicrobial Agents and Chemotherapy (ICAAC) 16–19 June 2012, San Francisco, CA.

37. Dugan J, Rockey DD, Jones L, Andersen AA. 2004. Tetracycline resistance in *Chlamydia suis* mediated by genomic islands inserted into the chlamydial *inv*-like gene. *Antimicrob Agents Chemother* 48:3989–3995.

38. Kadlec K, Kehrenberg C, Schwarz S. 2005. Molecular basis of resistance to trimethoprim, chloramphenicol and sulphonamides in *Bordetella bronchiseptica*. *J Antimicrob Chemother* 56:485–490.

39. Schwarz S, Alešík E, Grobbel M, Lübke-Becker A, Werckenthin C, Wieler LH, Wallmann J. 2007. Antimicrobial susceptibility of *Pasteurella multocida* and

Bordetella bronchiseptica from dogs and cats as determined in the BfT-GermVet monitoring program 2004-2006. *Berl Munch Tierarztl Wochenschr* 120:423–430.

40. Sundin GW, Bender CL. 1996. Dissemination of the *strA-strB* streptomycin-resistance genes among commensal and pathogenic bacteria from humans, animals, and plants. *Mol Ecol* 5:133–143.

41. Kehrenberg C, Tham NT, Schwarz S. 2003. New plasmid-borne antibiotic resistance gene cluster in *Pasteurella multocida*. *Antimicrob Agents Chemother* 47:2978–2980.

42. Michael GB, Kadlec K, Sweeney MT, Brzuszkiewicz E, Liesegang H, Daniel R, Murray RW, Watts JL, Schwarz S. 2012. ICEPmu1, an integrative conjugative element (ICE) of *Pasteurella multocida*: analysis of the regions that comprise 12 antimicrobial resistance genes. *J Antimicrob Chemother* 67:84–90.

43. Toulouse JL, Edens TJ, Alejaldre L, Manges AR, Pelletier JN. 2017. Integron-associated DfrB4, a previously uncharacterized member of the trimethoprim-resistant dihydrofolate reductase B family, is a clinically identified emergent source of antibiotic resistance. *Antimicrob Agents Chemother* 61:5.

44. Kadlec K, Kehrenberg C, Schwarz S. 2007. Efflux-mediated resistance to florfenicol and/or chloramphenicol in *Bordetella bronchiseptica*: identification of a novel chloramphenicol exporter. *J Antimicrob Chemother* 59:191–196.

45. Barreto-Hernández E, Falquet L, Reguero MT, Mantilla JR, Valenzuela EM, González E, Cepeda A, Escalante A. 2013. Draft genome sequences of multidrug-resistant *Acinetobacter* sp. strains from Colombian hospitals. *Genome Announc* 1:e00868-e13.

46. Lartigue MF, Poirel L, Fortineau N, Nordmann P. 2005. Chromosome-borne class A BOR-1 β-lactamase of *Bordetella bronchiseptica* and *Bordetella parapertussis*. *Antimicrob Agents Chemother* 49:2565–2567.

47. Kadlec K, Wiegand I, Kehrenberg C, Schwarz S. 2007. Studies on the mechanisms of β-lactam resistance in *Bordetella bronchiseptica*. *J Antimicrob Chemother* 59:396–402.

48. Hannan PC, O'Hanlon PJ, Rogers NH. 1989. *In vitro* evaluation of various quinolone antibacterial agents against veterinary mycoplasmas and porcine respiratory bacterial pathogens. *Res Vet Sci* 46:202–211.

49. Speakman AJ, Dawson S, Corkill JE, Binns SH, Hart CA, Gaskell RM. 2000. Antibiotic susceptibility of canine *Bordetella bronchiseptica* isolates. *Vet Microbiol* 71:193–200.

50. Carbone M, Pennisi MG, Masucci M, De Sarro A, Giannone M, Fera MT. 2001. Activity and postantibiotic effect of marbofloxacin, enrofloxacin, difloxacin and ciprofloxacin against feline *Bordetella bronchiseptica* isolates. *Vet Microbiol* 81:79–84.

51. Schink AK, Kadlec K, Hauschild T, Brenner Michael G, Dörner JC, Ludwig C, Werckenthin C, Hehnen HR, Stephan B, Schwarz S. 2013. Susceptibility of canine and feline bacterial pathogens to pradofloxacin and comparison with other fluoroquinolones approved for companion animals. *Vet Microbiol* 162:119–126.

52. El Garch F, Kroemer S, Galland D, Morrissey I, Woehrle F. 2017. Survey of susceptibility to marbofloxacin in bacteria isolated from diseased pigs in Europe. *Vet Rec* 180:591.

53. Kehrenberg C, Schwarz S. 2002. Nucleotide sequence and organization of plasmid pMVSCS1 from *Mannheimia varigena*: identification of a multiresistance gene cluster. *J Antimicrob Chemother* 49:383–386.

54. Chiou CS, Jones AL. 1993. Nucleotide sequence analysis of a transposon (Tn5393) carrying streptomycin resistance genes in *Erwinia amylovora* and other Gram-negative bacteria. *J Bacteriol* 175:732–740.

55. San Millan A, Escudero JA, Gutierrez B, Hidalgo L, Garcia N, Llagostera M, Dominguez L, Gonzalez-Zorn B. 2009. Multiresistance in *Pasteurella multocida* is mediated by coexistence of small plasmids. *Antimicrob Agents Chemother* 53:3399–3404.

56. Eidam C, Poehlein A, Leimbach A, Michael GB, Kadlec K, Liesegang H, Daniel R, Sweeney MT, Murray RW, Watts JL, Schwarz S. 2015. Analysis and comparative genomics of ICEMh1, a novel integrative and conjugative element (ICE) of *Mannheimia haemolytica*. *J Antimicrob Chemother* 70:93–97.

57. Petrova M, Kurakov A, Shcherbatova N, Mindlin S. 2014. Genetic structure and biological properties of the first ancient multiresistance plasmid pKLH80 isolated from a permafrost bacterium. *Microbiology* 160:2253–2263.

58. Wallmann J, Kaspar H, Kroker R. 2004. [The prevalence of antimicrobial susceptibility of veterinary pathogens isolated from cattle and pigs: national antibiotic resistance monitoring 2002/2003 of the BVL]. *Berl Munch Tierarztl Wochenschr* 117:480–492. The prevalence of antimicrobial susceptibility of veterinary pathogens isolated from cattle and pigs: national reistance monitoring 2002/2003 of the BVL.

59. Shin SJ, Kang SG, Nabin R, Kang ML, Yoo HS. 2005. Evaluation of the antimicrobial activity of florfenicol against bacteria isolated from bovine and porcine respiratory disease. *Vet Microbiol* 106:73–77.

60. Schwarz S, Kadlec K, Silley P. 2013. *Antimicrobial Resistance in Bacteria of Animal Origin*. ZETT-Verlag, Steinen, Germany.

61. Kehrenberg C, Mumme J, Wallmann J, Verspohl J, Tegeler R, Kühn T, Schwarz S. 2004. Monitoring of florfenicol susceptibility among bovine and porcine respiratory tract pathogens collected in Germany during the years 2002 and 2003. *J Antimicrob Chemother* 54:572–574.

62. Priebe S, Schwarz S. 2003. *In vitro* activities of florfenicol against bovine and porcine respiratory tract pathogens. *Antimicrob Agents Chemother* 47:2703–2705.

Antimicrobial Resistance in Bacteria from Livestock and Companion Animals
Edited by Frank Møller Aarestrup, Stefan Schwarz, Jianzhong Shen, and Lina Cavaco
© 2018 American Society for Microbiology, Washington, DC
doi:10.1128/microbiolspec.ARBA-0007-2017

Antimicrobial Resistance in *Acinetobacter* spp. and *Pseudomonas* spp.

17

Agnese Lupo[1], Marisa Haenni[1], and Jean-Yves Madec[1]

ACINETOBACTER SPP.

The *Acinetobacter* genus includes 50 species of non-motile Gram-negative rods that are strictly aerobic, adapted to a wide range of temperatures, and able to survive on abiotic surfaces. Many species belonging to the *Acinetobacter* genus are able to cause infections, favored by the presence of indwelling devices, inimmune-compromised human hosts (1). The lethality of *Acinetobacter* infections is elevated in more than 50% of cases (2). Among the *Acinetobacter* spp., *A. baumannii* is the most prevalent, responsible for 95% of infections and outbreaks in hospitals, followed by *A. nosocomialis* and *A. pittii*. The ability of *A. baumannii* to survive in the hospital environment promotes its diffusion by outbreaks and epidemics. To date, several global epidemics have occurred, sustained by a few strains belonging to successful lineages, namely, clonal complex I-III, as characterized by multilocussequence typing (3). Recently, another lineage with the potential for global diffusion, delineated as sequence type (ST) 25, has emerged (4). Preventing the introduction of *A. baumannii* into hospital settings could contribute to preventing the further spread of multidrug-resistant isolates. Although its reservoir remains unknown, this organism has been found in soil, water, and food, including fish, milk, raw vegetables, and meat, which has earned it the definition of "ubiquitous." The presence in retail meat samples of *A. baumannii* isolates belonging to a clonal complex commonly associated with multidrug-resistant clones invites the speculation that food may carry organisms into hospital settings. A highly selective pressure exerted by antimicrobial usage may positively select those isolates able to acquire and/or develop resistance mechanisms (5). Unfortunately,

Acinetobacter spp. can also be pathogenic for animals. In the following paragraphs, an overview of the infections, the principal mechanisms of antibiotic resistance, and their epidemiology in *Acinetobacter* spp. among animals will be presented.

Acinetobacter Infections in Animal Hosts

Acinetobacter species are commensals of several body sites in many animal hosts. *A. baumannii* is frequently isolated from the eyes of horses. It is also isolated from the fecal flora of cattle, equids, and rabbits; from lice and ked of cattle, sheep and dogs; and from the mouths of dogs and cats, with a reported prevalence of 6.5% (9/138) in Reunion Island (6–12). Besides commensalism, the pathogenic role of *Acinetobacter* in animals cannot be neglected, with infections occurring that are similar to those observed in humans. The presence of foreign bodies in critically ill animals represents a risk factor for developing *Acinetobacter* spp. infections (13, 14). Furthermore, propagation of multidrug-resistant isolates may occur that are similar to the outbreaks generated in human clinics (15, 16). In the effort to understand the relevance of *Acinetobacter* as an animal pathogen, Mathewson and Simpson analyzed 347 animal specimens. Although the analysis was conducted on a phenotypic basis, they found *Acinetobacter* to be prevalent in as many as 14.5% (50/347) of isolates, principally from equine hosts (27%) followed by canine (17%), feline (2%), bovine (2%), and various other hosts (2%) (17). *Acinetobacter* spp. have also been associated with wound and respiratory tract infections in horses (18, 19) and with urinary tract and respiratory infections and sepsis in dogs and cats (20, 21). Less frequently, *Acinetobacter* spp. have been found in

[1]Université de Lyon–ANSES, Unité Antibiorésistance et Virulence Bactériennes, Lyon, France.

association with other animal diseases such as bovine mastitis (22, 23) and skin and mucous diseases in birds.

Besides the veterinary relevance of *Acinetobacter* spp. and, in particular, *A. baumannii* as an infective agent, many investigations have been conducted with an anthropocentric perspective, studying animals as a reservoir of antimicrobial-resistant bacteria and a source of infections for humans. Indeed, sporadic investigations of animals infected by multidrug-resistant isolates of *Acinetobacter* spp. have been reported and their epidemiology discussed. In the following section, the most common antimicrobial resistance mechanisms detected in *Acinetobacter* spp. will be described.

Antimicrobial Resistance in *Acinetobacter* spp.

A. baumannii poses a public health concern because of its propensity to develop multidrug resistance. In particular, the acquisition of carbapenem resistance poses a serious threat of therapeutic failures (1). The occurrence of *Acinetobacter* spp. infections in animal hosts poses principally two issues: first, treating such infections is challenging because *Acinetobacter* spp. isolates are often naturally resistant to many of the antibiotics authorized for use in veterinary medicine; second, the presence and/or the development of multidrug-resistant isolates in animal hosts may serve as reservoir of multidrug-resistant isolates for humans.

Intrinsic resistance

A. baumannii exhibits an intrinsic reduced susceptibility to several antibiotic classes, including beta-lactams, macrolides, trimethoprim, and fosfomycin (24). The mechanisms underlying such intrinsic resistances consist of natural membrane impermeability, basal efflux activity, and the presence of two chromosomally encoded beta-lactamases, an ADC cephalosporinase and an OXA-51 oxacillinase (25). To date, three efflux systems belonging to the resistance-nodulation-division family have been characterized in *A. baumannii*, encoded by the *adeABC*, *adeFGH*, and *adeIJK* operons (26). Homologs of these operons have been recovered in other *Acinetobacter* spp. such as *A. calcoaceticus*, *A. nosocomialis*, and *A. pittii*, among others (27–29). The AdeIJK efflux system is constitutively expressed and contributes to a basal resistance to beta-lactams, tetracyclines, macrolides and lincosamides, phenicols, fusidic acid, and fluoroquinolones.

Acquired resistance

The development of acquired resistance can occur by two processes: mutation in chromosomal structures and the acquisition of exogenous genes by horizontal gene transfer. Mutations in the two-component regulatory system AdeRS and in the regulators AdeL and AdeN have been shown to lead to the overproduction of the efflux pumps AdeABC, AdeFGH, and AdeIJK, respectively, and consequently to an increase in resistance. In particular, overproduction of AdeABC contributes to an increase of resistance to beta-lactams, aminoglycosides, fluoroquinolones, tetracyclines and tigecycline, macrolides and lincosamides, and chloramphenicol, whereas overproduction of AdeFGH contributes to resistance to quinolones, antifolates, and chloramphenicol (27).

Resistance to beta-lactams in *A. baumannii*

Certain insertion sequences, including IS*Aba*I among others, can provide a strong promoter for the overexpression of the genes located downstream. This phenomenon can be responsible for the overproduction of ADC and OXA-51, leading to the development of high-level resistance to third- and fourth-generation cephalosporins in the first case and of carbapenem resistance in the second case (30, 31). Other insertion sequences, such as IS*Aba*125 and IS*Aba*825, are able to insert into porin-encoding genes, causing the inactivation of the porins and subsequent resistance to carbapenems (32).

Resistance to third- and/or fourth-generation cephalosporins, other than penicillins and their derivatives, can also be mediated by the acquisition of genes coding for exogenous enzymes such as the class A beta-lactamases TEM and SHV in the extended-spectrum variants CTX-M, PER, GES, and VEB (33, 34). Among *A. baumannii* isolates from human infections, the most common mechanism of carbapenem resistance is mediated by the acquisition of OXAs hydrolyzing carbapenems. The enzymes OXA-23 and OXA-58 are frequently identified in clinical isolates, whereas OXA-24/40 and OXA-143 are rarer. The insertion sequence IS*Aba*I can mediate the overexpression of the acquired bla_{OXAs}, leading to high-level resistance to carbapenems (35). The presence of class B metallo-beta-lactamases such as SIM, IMP, VIM, and NDM-1 has also been reported (36).

Resistance to aminoglycosides in *A. baumannii*

Frequently, resistance to carbapenems is associated with aminoglycoside resistance. This is classically mediated by aminoglycoside-modifying enzymes, which catalyze reactions of acetylation, phosphorylation, or O-nucleotidyl transfer. Among such enzymes,

AAC(6′)-I is cryptic in several *Acinetobacter* spp. and confers, when the relative gene is expressed, resistance to netilmicin, tobramycin, gentamicin, and amikacin. Acquired aminoglycoside-modifying enzymes have been frequently detected in *A. baumannii*, with AAC(3)-I, APH(3′)-VI, and ANT(2″)-I being the most prevalent (37). More recently, 16S rRNA methylases have been described as another mechanism conferring resistance to aminoglycosides (38, 39). This mechanism confers high-level resistance to amikacin, gentamicin, netilmicin, tobramycin, and kanamycin. Among the known methylases, ArmA is the only one to be reported in *A. baumannii* clinical human isolates, whereas no report exists from animals (40, 41).

Resistance to fluoroquinolones in *A. baumannii*

In contrast to beta-lactam and aminoglycoside resistances, which are mostly based on the acquisition of exogenous determinants, the development of fluoroquinolone resistances is mainly due to point mutations of the gyrase and topoisomerase enzymes. Of particular importance for high-level resistance are GyrA Ser83Leu together with ParC Ser80Leu and Glu84Lys amino acid substitutions (42, 43).

Resistance to other antibiotics in *A. baumannii*

Certain antibiotic classes are of limited therapeutic interest for the treatment of *A. baumannii* infections, mainly because of their toxicity in humans. However, in certain circumstances some of these antibiotics' properties are fundamental, as in the case of rifampicin, which is able to easily penetrate tissues. Resistance to this antibiotic occurs principally by mutation of the *rpoB* gene and acquisition of an enzyme that modifies the rifampicin, encoded by the *arr-2* gene, and that is usually located on class I integrons (44). The development of multidrug resistance has forced intensified usage of "old antibiotics" such as colistin. Resistance to colistin is mediated by mutation in the proteins PmrAB, a two-component system in *A. baumannii* (45). Colistin resistance in animal isolates has never been reported. Tigecycline is considered a last-resort treatment of infections caused by multidrug-resistant *Acinetobacter* spp. Emergence of resistant isolates, mainly overexpressing efflux pumps, has been reported among human patients (46). Furthermore, coselection of tigecycline resistance by usage of other antibiotics, including tetracycline, has been demonstrated in enterococci (47). This is a concern, considering that tigecycline is not allowed in veterinary practice, whereas tetracycline could contribute to the development of a potential reservoir for human contamination. Recently, Ewers et al. reported two tigecycline-resistant *A. baumannii* isolates from two dogs in Germany (48).

Most common mobile genetic elements in *A. baumannii*

All the described acquired resistance mechanisms can be located on the chromosome or on plasmids, eventually associated with transposons. For instance, bla_{OXA-23} has been found located on several transposon structures containing IS*Aba*I, such as Tn*2006*, Tn*2007*, Tn*2008*, Tn*2008B*, and Tn*2009* (49). A very successful strategy for *A. baumannii* to develop multidrug resistance is the acquisition of the so-called resistance islands, such as *AbaR*. The acquisition of such islands seems to be consecutive to a transposition event in a hot-spot sequence, the ATPase encoding gene. Several *AbaR* islands have been described, with *AbaR1* containing as many as 25 genes encoding mechanisms conferring resistance to several antimicrobial classes (50, 51). This brief overview of resistance mechanisms encountered in *A. baumannii* is far from exhaustive but highlights the potential and the propensity for multidrug resistance development. Therefore, understanding the epidemiology of this species and the intersection of its different habitats and hosts is a high priority. In the following section, we will focus on reports concerning resistance to carbapenems, aminoglycosides, and fluoroquinolones in *A. baumannii* from animal settings.

Antimicrobial Resistance in *Acinetobacter* spp. from Food-Producing Animals

The first evidence of carbapenemase-producing *Acinetobacter* spp. of animal origin dates back to 2010, when Poirel et al. (52) investigated the carriage of carbapenem-resistant Gram-negative organisms in a dairy farm in France. In this investigation, nine isolates sampled from 50 cows were identified as *Acinetobacter* genomospecies 15TU, a close relative of the species *Acinetobacter lwoffii*, and all isolates were resistant to carbapenems, harboring a bla_{OXA-23} gene located on a Tn*2008* transposon. The isolates demonstrated resistance not to fluoroquinolones but to kanamycin. Later, an *A. lwoffii* isolate producing NDM-1 was found in a chicken in China. The isolate was multidrug-resistant, and the bla_{NDM-1} gene was located on a conjugative plasmid (53). Later, a sporadic *A. baumannii* isolate was found in China in a survey conducted in 2011 to 2012 for carbapenem resistance in Gram-negative organisms from food-producing animals. The isolates harbored bla_{NDM-1} located on a plasmid that revealed similarity to plasmids found in isolates of human origin; furthermore, it demonstrated coresistance to aminoglycosides, with the exception of amikacin, and fluoroquinolones. Unfortunately, the sequence type of the isolate was not determined (54). The presence of *A. baumannii* isolates producing OXA-23 has been documented in wild fish from the Mediterranean Sea. In these isolates, also demonstrating multidrug resistance, the *aac(6′)-Ib* and *aac(3′)-I* genes coding for aminoglycoside-modifying enzymes were found. The isolates belonged to ST2, the most widely spread clone in human clinics with which multidrug-resistant isolates are associated. Further investigations revealed that the isolates found in fish were similar to the isolates found contemporaneously in human clinical infections (55). Most likely, the fish were colonized after exposure of water contaminated with clinical waste. Contemporaneously, Al Bayssari et al. (56) reported the presence of *A. baumannii* demonstrating high-level resistance to imipenem in livestock in Lebanon. The isolates (*n* = 5) were found in cattle, pigs, and fowls, and all of them harbored the bla_{OXA-23} gene. One isolate coharbored bla_{OXA-58}. Sequence type determination revealed that among the isolates, one belonged to ST2 and another to ST20, the first being globally spread in human clinics and the second also found in dogs in Switzerland (13). Recently, a report from Pailhoriès et al. (57) revealed the presence of bla_{OXA-24} in *A. baumannii* in healthy cattle in Reunion Island. The bla_{OXA-24} gene occurred in an ST that had never been reported before, suggesting that carbapenem resistance can emerge and disseminate among animals independently from human cross-contamination. The presence of OXA-23 in species other than *A. baumannii* is quite infrequent, but Klotz et al. (58) has reported the emergence of bla_{OXA-23} located on Tn2008 in two isolates identified as *Acinetobacter indicus* colonizing two calves in Germany.

Antimicrobial Resistance in *Acinetobacter* spp. from Companion Animals

In 2011, a study conducted in Switzerland demonstrated the presence of *A. baumannii* isolates (*n* = 19) in infections of pets and horses (13). The majority of these isolates (*n* = 12) were resistant to fluoroquinolones and harbored the GyrA Ser83Leu and ParC Ser80Leu mutations. Seventeen isolates were resistant to aminoglycosides, and among those the genes *aacC2*, *aacC1*, and *aadA1* were present. Three isolates in this study, identified in three diseased dogs, demonstrated reduced susceptibility to carbapenems and harbored an IS*AbaI* inserted upstream from the bla_{OXA-51} gene. These isolates belonged to ST12 and ST15, which are common among human isolates. An even more worrisome finding has been the detection of *Acinetobacter* spp. harboring bla_{OXA-23} in companion animals. The first report dates from 2012 from a screening of fecal carriage in hospitalized horses. On this occasion Smet et al. (59) found two multidrug-resistant *Acinetobacter* spp. harboring bla_{OXA-23} located on a Tn2008 transposon. The second report concerned a single isolate associated with a urinary tract infection in a cat in Portugal in 2009. In this isolate, bla_{OXA-23} was located on a Tn2006 transposon that was chromosomally located. Furthermore, an IS*AbaI* copy was located upstream from bla_{ADC}, and mutations conferring fluoroquinolone resistance were detected, as well (60). This isolate also belonged to ST2, reinforcing the hypothesis that a cross-transmission among humans and pets could be at the base of the animal colonization. In our recent study (21) conducted in the framework of Resapath, the French network for the surveillance of antimicrobial resistance in diseased animals, we analyzed 49 *Acinetobacter* spp. isolates collected from 2011 to 2015. Among those isolates, the majority were identified as *A. baumannii* (*n* = 41), three as *A. lwoffii*, and one each as *A. haemolyticus*, *A. radioresistens*, *A. schindleri*, *A. johnsonii*, and *A. junii*. Among the *A. baumannii* isolates, seven isolated from the urine of dogs and cats affected by urinary tract infections demonstrated multidrug resistance with high-level resistance to carbapenems. All these isolates harbored a bla_{OXA-23} located on a chromosomal Tn2008B-like transposon and belonged to ST25. This finding was quite surprising since all previously described *A. baumannii* isolates of animal origin that were resistant to carbapenems by OXA enzymes production have been reported as belonging to ST2. We also demonstrated that this clone was able to propagate in two regions of France and persist for at least two years among diseased pets. Our study was amplified by a contemporaneous report from the Nantes region, where two dogs were found to be colonized by ST25 *A. baumannii* harboring bla_{OXA-23} (61). During a 13-year (2000 to 2013) investigation conducted in Germany by Ewers et al. (48) on diagnostic veterinary samples, three out of 223 *A. baumannii* isolates harbored bla_{OXA-23} on a Tn2008 transposon located on a plasmid. These isolates belonged to ST10 and to ST1, two multidrug-resistant sequence types associated with isolates responsible for human infections. In Japan, two isolates of *A. radioresistens* have been isolated from a diseased cat and dog. The isolates were resistant to carbapenems and harbored a bla_{OXA-23}

gene, which *A. radioresistens* is considered to be the source of, and a *bla*$_{IMP-1}$ gene, together with genes encoding aminoglycoside-modifying enzymes (62). A summary of all the reports described at time of writing is provided in Figure 1.

Overall, recovering carbapenem-resistant *A. baumannii* in animal hosts continues to be surprising when considering that usage of carbapenems is not allowed in veterinary medicine. However, coselective pressure on OXA enzymes by the usage of other beta-lactams can be speculated, similalry to the role of other environmental factors.

PSEUDOMONAS spp.

Pseudomonas spp. are Gram-negative bacteria comprising more than 200 species at the time of writing (http://www.bacterio.net/pseudomonas.html) that can be ubiquitously found in humans, animals, soil, and plants (63, 64). *Pseudomonas* spp. were extensively studied for their beneficial or deleterious associations with plants (*P. putida*, *P. syringae*, *P. fluorescens*, etc.) but also for their roles in soil bioremediation due to specific biodegradation properties (*P. putida*, *P. stutzeri*, *P. alcaligenes*, etc.) (65–67). Only a few species are of clinical interest in either humans or animals, and *P. aeruginosa* is by far the most frequently reported pathogen. For this reason, this section will focus on this unique species, which is also the only one in which antibiotic resistance was reported in animal hosts.

P. aeruginosa Infections in Animal Hosts

P. aeruginosa is a ubiquitous bacterium normally found in water and soil, but also an opportunistic pathogen of humans, animals, and plants (68). In humans, *P. aeruginosa* is mostly nosocomial, causing severe infections in patients with underlying conditions. Immunosuppressed or intubated-ventilated patients presenting compromised host defenses are particularly vulnerable to this pathogen. It is primarily associated with burn victims and cystic fibrosis patients (69, 70).

P. aeruginosa has not been extensively studied in infections of animal origin since this bacterium is more often considered an environmental contaminant rather than a true pathogen. Apart from sporadic descriptions, it has mostly been reported in cats and dogs,

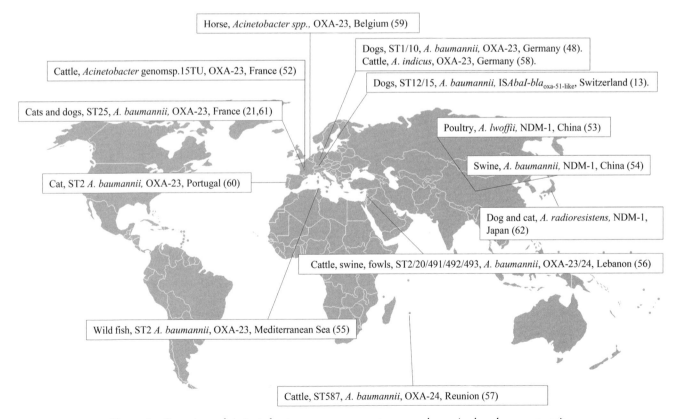

Figure 1 Overview of *Acinetobacter* spp., sequence types, and acquired carbapenem resistance mechanisms.

where it is an important pathogen causing otitis externa and otitis media (71–74). Together with *Staphylococcus pseudintermedius*, it is one of the two main ear pathogens, and its prevalence ranges from 6.5 to 27.8% depending on the study (71, 72, 75, 76). However, *P. aeruginosa* is also implicated in skin infections, including deep pyoderma, often in association with other bacterial pathogens (72, 77, 78).

More surprisingly, *P. aeruginosa* infections have been recurrently described in fur animals, where it seems to be particularly virulent (79, 80). The first victims are minks (*Neovison vison*). These mammalian carnivores of the *Mustelidae* family are raised for fur production, principally in Denmark, China, the Netherlands, Poland, and the United States. First described in 1953, the acute and fatal hemorrhagic pneumonia caused by *P. aeruginosa* can decimate farmed minks and lead to high economic losses (81). The second victims are chinchillas, a rodent species which is raised for both pets and laboratory animals—but not for fur. The infections, mainly otitis, are often due to uncleaned water and cage environment and are favored by a weak immunity of this animal species. Since *P. aeruginosa* has a particular capacity of dissemination between these animals, it is very important to rapidly isolate the diseased individuals.

P. aeruginosa is much less reported in livestock animals. It is an opportunistic pathogen that is very rarely reported in etiological surveys of bovine mastitis (82–86). However, several case reports suggest that, though unusual, outbreaks of *P. aeruginosa* can be severe and spread either clonally or nonclonally in different herds (87–90). The origin of the infection is often contaminated liquids, teat dips, or even a contaminated antibiotic preparation (91, 92). One study also reports its implication in 12% of the urinary tract infections in cattle in Israel (93).

Antimicrobial Resistance in *P. aeruginosa*

P. aeruginosa is one of the ESKAPE bacteria (*Enterococcus faecium*, *Staphylococcus aureus*, *Klebsiella pneumoniae*, *A. baumannii*, *P. aeruginosa*, and *Enterobacter* spp.), for which the therapeutic options are increasingly limited (94). In addition to its capacity to form biofilms, *P. aeruginosa* is intrinsically resistant to many antibiotics, including beta-lactams (penicillin G, aminopenicillins alone or in combination with inhibitors, first- and second-generation cephalosporins, cefixime, cefuroxime, cefotaxime, ceftriaxone, ertapenem), kanamycin, tetracycline, chloramphenicol, trimethoprim, and quinolones (95). *P. aeruginosa* is also known for its capacity to rapidly acquire additional resistances,

so that the combination of intrinsic and acquired resistances can lead to therapeutic failures (96).

Intrinsic resistance

It is commonly admitted that in *P. aeruginosa*, intrinsic resistance is mainly mediated by a combination of impermeability, production of the inducible AmpC cephalosporinase, and the presence of efflux pumps (97). On the one hand, the permeability of the outer membrane is up to 100-fold lower in *P. aeruginosa* than in *Escherichia coli* (97), and on the other hand, two constitutively expressed drug efflux systems, MexAB-OprM and MexXY-OprM, directly participate in intrinsic resistance. Both systems belong to the resistance-nodulation-division family and were identified in the laboratory strain PAO1 (98). MexAB-OprM confers resistance to beta-lactams (with the exception of imipenem), fluoroquinolones, trimethoprim-sulfonamides, chloramphenicol, and tetracyclines, while MexXY-OprM is involved in resistance to cefepime, aminoglycosides, fluoroquinolones, tetracyclines, chloramphenicol, trimethoprim-sulfonamides, and macrolides. Ten other efflux systems were also described in *P. aeruginosa*, none of which plays a role in intrinsic resistance. Finally, *P. aeruginosa* harbors two beta-lactamase encoding genes. The first one is the constitutively expressed bla_{OXA-50} oxacillinase, which only plays a minor role in beta-lactam resistance (99). The second is the inducible AmpC beta-lactamase, which confers resistance to beta-lactams, including cefuroxime and ceftriaxone, even though this mechanism may be redundant with the MexAB-OprM efflux system (100, 101).

Like many bacterial species, *P. aeruginosa* can live either as planktonic cells or as organized communities called biofilms (102). Quorum-sensing, the cell-to-cell communication mechanism involving the Las, Rhl, and PQS systems in *P. aeruginosa*, was shown to be involved in biofilm formation, particularly through the Rhl system (103, 104). An important characteristic of biofilms is their tolerance to different external stresses, including antibiotic treatment (105). Tolerance is a physiological state of the bacteria that does not involve any acquired mutation and cannot be transmitted to the progeny of a mother cell. For example, tolerance to aminoglycosides (gentamicin, tobramycin), tetracyclines, and colistin has been described (93, 106). Colistin targets different zones of the biofilm compared to other molecules, so that combined treatment with colistin/gentamicin or colistin/tetracycline is more appropriate to eradicate the majority of the cells composing the biofilm (106).

Acquired resistance

Besides intrinsic resistance, *P. aeruginosa* is capable of acquiring numerous additional resistances, either through point mutations in pre-existing genes or through horizontal transfer of resistance determinants (96). The use of specific antibiotics during treatment can readily select for point mutations which lead to the overexpression of one or another efflux system. Depending on the affected system (MexAB-OprM, MexXY-OprM, MexCD-OprJ, or MexEF-OprN), elevated resistance levels toward their specific antibiotic substrates are observed (98, 107). Overproduction of AmpC can also be obtained through mutations in regulatory genes. The porin OprD can also be modified, which is the preferential pathway toward carbapenem resistance in human clinical isolates of *P. aeruginosa*. And finally, mutations in the target genes *gyrA/gyrB* and *parC/parD* confer resistance to fluoroquinolones (see below).

In parallel, a large number of acquired enzymes conferring beta-lactam resistance were identified in *P. aeruginosa* (108). These include extended-spectrum beta-lactamases of the PER, SHV, PME, GES, and VEB families, as well as the CTX-M enzymes typically found in *Enterobacteriaceae*. Metallo-beta-lactamases conferring resistance to carbapenems were also reported, mainly IMP and VIM enzymes, even though carbapenem resistance in *P. aeruginosa* is mostly due to the *oprD* gene, which can be repressed, mutated, or deleted (108). These enzymes are increasingly found in human clinical isolates but have not been reported yet in animal isolates.

Antimicrobial Resistance in *Pseudomonas* spp. in Cats and Dogs

P. aeruginosa is one of the main pathogens causing otitis externa and otitis media (71–74) but is also implicated in skin infections (72, 77, 78). The treatment of such infections starts by a thorough cleaning (deep ear flush in the case of otitis) and a topical disinfection, which is often followed by an antibiotic treatment using mainly fluoroquinolones, aminoglycosides or polymyxins. In this respect, monitoring of antimicrobial resistance in *P. aeruginosa* is clearly needed. However, most of the clinically relevant antibiotics do not have referenced clinical breakpoints, which is a serious data gap for effective surveillance that will have to be filled in in the near future.

Resistance to fluoroquinolones

Ciprofloxacin is considered the most active fluoroquinolone against *P. aeruginosa* (109). The prevalence of resistance to this molecule in *P. aeruginosa* of animal origin ranges from very low to high rates (Table 1). Indeed, variable resistance rates have been reported, ranging from 3.7% in China in 2009 to 2010 and 8.7% in Croatia (2007 to 2009) to 16% in Canada (2003 to 2006), 4.8% and 20% in two Brazilian studies, and 21% in the United States (73, 74, 78, 110–113), and even reaching 63% in France between 2008 and 2011. These divergences may be due to the methodology (MICs versus disk diffusion), the levels of fluoroquinolone usage in the countries where strains were collected, or the type of sampling (otitis versus skin infection or mild versus severe infections).

The importance of resistance to ciprofloxacin also has to be put into perspective here since this molecule is not used in veterinary medicine. Nevertheless, among the three main fluoroquinolones prescribed in animals (enrofloxacin, marbofloxacin, and the more recent pradofloxacin), the most frequently tested is enrofloxacin, which presents high rates of resistance (Table 1). Indeed, 18.2% of isolates collected throughout Europe were resistant (and 81.8% presented an intermediate phenotype), as were 24% in Germany (49% intermediately resistant), 26.2% in Croatia, 31% and 38% in two Canadian studies, 49% in the United States, and 26.0% and 70% in two Brazilian studies (71, 73, 76, 111, 112, 114–116). On the other hand, even though ciprofloxacin is the major active metabolite of enrofloxacin, divergences in the prevalence of resistance are observed when both antibiotics are tested on the same collection of isolates (116). This may be because of the different *in vitro* activities of enrofloxacin, marbofloxacin, and ciprofloxacin. Globally, there is a lack of harmonized studies to clarify the clinical relevance of those discrepancies in the resistance of *P. aeruginosa* to the major fluoroquinolones used in routine veterinary practice.

The targets of quinolones and fluoroquinolones are the DNA gyrase and the DNA topoisomerase IV, which are both constituted of two subunits, named GyrA/GyrB and ParC/ParE, respectively (117). The main resistance mechanism in both Gram-positive and Gram-negative bacteria involves mutations in these targets. In *P. aeruginosa*, GyrA and ParC mutations were identified (though not systematically) in ciprofloxacin-resistant clinical isolates, while GyrB mutations are thought to confer only moderate resistance (118). Such point mutations were also reported in veterinary isolates, and the most frequent ones, namely Thr83Ile in GyrA and Ser87Leu in ParC, were also reported in human isolates (73, 110, 118, 119). Efflux pumps have also been identified as a key mechanism in fluoroquinolone resistance, notably through the MexAB-OprM or

Table 1 Antimicrobial susceptibility to fluoroquinolones and aminoglycosides in *P. aeruginosa* isolates of animal origin

Country	Year	Animal host	Pathology	No. of isolates	Method	Percentage (%) of resistance[d]				Reference
						CIP	ENR	GEN	AMI	
US.	1998–2003	Dogs/cats	Otitis	319	Sensititre	–[e]	38.0	15.0	11.0	71
U.S.	1992–2005	Dogs	Pyoderma	20	Disk diffusion	25.0	40.0	5.0	5.0	78
Europe[a]	2008–2010	Dogs	SSTI[f]	160	Agar dilution	–	16.9	18.8	–	114
		Cats	SSTI	11		–	18.2	9.0	–	
Croatia	2007–2009	Dogs	Otitis	104	Etest	8.7	51.9	43.3	–	74
Croatia	1998–2000	Dogs	Otitis	183	Agar dilution	3.8	26.2	10.9	7.6	116
Canada	2003–2006	Dogs	SSTI	106	Sensititre	16.0	31.0	7.0	3.0	73
China	2009–2010	Dogs	SSTI	27	Broth microdilution	14.8	–	14.8	11.1	110
Germany	2004–2006	Dogs/cats	SSTI	71	Broth microdilution	–	24.0	27.0	–	115
			Urinary/genital tract	28		–	11.0	11.0	–	
France	2008–2011	Dogs	SSTI	46	Agar dilution	63.0	–	56.5	15.2	124
		Horses	Diverse[b]	10		0.0	–	10.0	0.0	
		Cows	Diverse[c]	12		0.0	–	8.4	0.0	
Brazil	2010–2012	Dogs	Otitis, pyoderma	104	Disk diffusion	4.8	26.0	4.8	2.9	113
Japan	2005–2007	Cows	Mastitis	116	Broth microdilution	0.0	31.0	4.3	1.7	154
Japan	Unknown	Chinchillas	Healthy	22		4.5	81.0	0.0	0.0	150
Denmark	2002–2005	Minks	Hemorrhagic pneumonia	39	Sensititre	–	5.1	0.0	–	144
China	2010–2011	Minks	Hemorrhagic pneumonia	30	VITEK-2	13.3	–	0.0	0.0	146

[a]Czech Republic, France, Germany, Hungary, Italy, the Netherlands, Poland, Spain, Sweden, and the United Kingdom.
[b]Respiratory infections, skin or eye infections, metritis.
[c]Mastitis, digestive and respiratory infections.
[d]CIP, ciprofloxacin; ENR, enrofloxacin; GEN, gentamicin; AMI, amikacin.
[e]–, Not performed.
[f]SSTI, Skin and Soft Tissues Infections.

MexF-OprN systems (108, 120–122). Only one study reported the overexpression of these efflux systems in veterinary isolates (123). However, this subject should definitely be further explored in *P. aeruginosa* of animal origin, since overproduction of efflux pumps is easily selected by usage of veterinary-licensed antibiotics, conferring resistance to several antibiotics including aminoglycosides and even a few carbapenems due to their wide substrate specificity (98).

Resistance to aminoglycosides

Resistances to gentamicin and amikacin are often reported, probably because they are used as first- and second-line antibiotics for the treatment of otitis but also of pyoderma and corneal ulcers in cats and dogs. Precautions need to be taken with this family of antibiotics because of their nephro- and ototoxicity.

The prevalence of resistance to gentamicin is systematically higher than resistance to amikacin (Table 1). Gentamicin resistance was reported from dogs in two studies of soft tissue infections in the United States (5% and 7%), in ophthalmic infections in Brazil (10%), in otitis in Canada (15%), in diverse infectious contexts in Germany (11%) and Brazil (4.8%), in soft tissue infections in China and in Europe (14.8% and 18.8%), in otitis in Croatia (16.9% and 43.3% in two studies, respectively), and in otitis in France (56.5%) (71, 73, 74, 78, 110–112, 114–116, 124). On the other hand, amikacin resistance rates observed in the same studies (when available) ranged from 5% and 3% in the United States, 10% (ophthalmic infections) and 2.9% (otitis and pyoderma) in Brazil, 11% in Canada, 11.1% in China, 12.6% in Croatia, and 15.2% in France. The divergences between the two antibiotics may have the same causes as cited above for fluoroquinolones.

Aminoglycoside resistance in *P. aeruginosa* is principally mediated by the MexXY-OprM multidrug efflux system. This system is constitutively expressed and implicated in the intrinsic resistance of *P. aeruginosa* to aminoglycosides (112). However, its overexpression can easily be induced by the use of its substrate antibiotics, thus conferring an elevated resistance to these very same antibiotics, including aminoglycosides (98, 125). The role of MexXY-OprM in animal strains was studied by Chuanchuen et al. in pets and bovine mastitis (see below) (126, 127). The role of the MexXY efflux pump in aminoglycoside resistance was evidenced in cats and dogs sampled in Thailand and the United States (123, 127), in addition to the presence of aminoglycoside-modifying enzymes, which have also been reported in isolates from the United States and Canada (73, 110). Aminoglycoside resistance can be achieved by inactivation of these antibiotics through specific modifications mediated by enzymes of the AAC, APH, and ANT families (128). The nature of the modifications and the spectrum of inactivated molecules depend on the modifying enzyme implicated (128). Finally, three methylases—which bind to the target site of the aminoglycosides and confer high-resistance phenotypes to several molecules, including gentamicin and amikacin—have been described in *P. aeruginosa*, namely ArmA, RmtA, and RmtD (129–131), none of which have been reported yet in veterinary isolates.

Resistance to polymyxins

Polymyxin B is one of the first-line antibiotic treatments in cases of otitis and eye infections in cats and dogs (132). Antimicrobial susceptibility data on this molecule are still rare, but when data are available, polymyxin B is always the most efficient antibiotic. Indeed, no resistant isolate was described in the United States (78), in Canada (71), or in Brazil (112). Polymyxin-resistant veterinary isolates were nonetheless reported in Germany—where four isolates (4/71, 5.6%) from soft tissue infections and two isolates (2/28, 7.1%) from urinary/genital tract infections presented an MIC to colistin of >2 mg/liter—and recently in Brazil, where 3/10 isolates from ophthalmic infections showed polymyxin B resistance (111, 115). However, the molecular basis of these resistant phenotypes remains unknown.

The discovery of a plasmidic gene, *mcr-1*, conferring resistance to *Enterobacteriaceae* has shed new light on colistin resistance (133). Interestingly, this gene has been successfully transferred *in vitro* to *P. aeruginosa*, but no field strain of *mcr-1*-carrying *P. aeruginosa* has been reported yet. Colistin-resistance can also be achieved under laboratory conditions in a reversible manner by repeated exposure to subinhibitory concentrations of colistin (134). Colistin is a last-resort antibiotic in cases of multidrug-resistant strains, but colistin resistance is fortunately still very rare in human clinical isolates (135). When studied molecularly, these resistant isolates mostly present modifications in the lipopolysaccharide (136–138).

Resistance to carbapenems

Carbapenem use is forbidden in veterinary medicine, including in companion animals. Consequently, the occurrence of carbapenem-resistant pathogens in animals has only sporadically been described. In 2014, an IMP-45-producing *P. aeruginosa* strain was detected in a dog during routine surveillance for carbapenem resistance (139). Recently, a study was performed in France on 30 isolates from cats and dogs (including one cattle isolate) presenting a decreased susceptibility to imipenem and/or meropenem (140). No carbapenemase gene was detected, and only a few isolates showed an altered OprD (6/30), which is a major cause of carbapenem resistance in humans. On the contrary, most of the isolates displayed alterations in efflux pumps (MexAB-OprM [*n* = 12], MexEF-OprN [*n* = 4], MexXY [*n* = 8], and CzcCBA [*n* = 3]). Since these efflux pumps also confer resistances to antibiotics that are used in veterinary medicine (notably fluoroquinolones and aminoglycosides), the observed decreased susceptibility to carbapenems is thus probably a consequence of noncarbapenem antibiotic use. In Brazil, carbapenem-resistant isolates were also reported (7.7% of isolates resistant to imipenem, 1.0% to meropenem), but no molecular characterization was performed (112).

Antimicrobial Resistance in *Pseudomonas* spp. in Minks

P. aeruginosa is especially virulent in minks, where it is a major cause of hemorrhagic pneumonia. This infection is decimating farmed minks (*N. vison*) and causes high economic losses (81). *P. aeruginosa* dissemination is due to local outbreaks of clonal strains, but clones vary between outbreaks (79, 141, 142). The origin of the contamination is mostly environmental, and clones spread in farms due to contaminated water containers or food, standing water, and uncleaned cages (79). Prevention of hemorrhagic pneumonia mostly relies on multivalent vaccines, but their expensive price and short protection period leads to innovative research such as research in phages (79, 142, 143).

Antibiotics are used to treat minks. Penicillins, aminoglycosides, and macrolides are the main families of molecules used to treat fur animals in Denmark, independent of the pathology and the pathogen identified. Their use steadily increased between 2001 and 2006 (144) and increased significantly (102% increase) from 2007 to 2012 (145). However, data on antimicrobial resistance in *P. aeruginosa* from hemorrhagic pneumonia were only reported in three studies, which showed an overall high susceptibility of most of the isolates. The first study included 39 isolates collected in Denmark between 2000 and 2005 (144), the second one comprised 30 isolates originating from China from 2010 to 2011 (146), and the third one included 41 isolates collected in Denmark between 2014 and 2016 (147). Danish isolates from the first sampling period (2000 to 2005) were susceptible to gentamicin and colistin, while 5.1% were resistant to enrofloxacin. Resistance to aminoglycosides was suspected in both collections, but no proportions can be inferred because of the lack of referenced breakpoints. Isolates from the same country but the second sampling period (2014 to 2016) were also susceptible to gentamicin and ciprofloxacin, while 17% were resistant to colistin. Unfortunately, colistin resistance was only inferred by MIC results, but no molecular characterization was performed. Chinese isolates were more resistant to fluoroquinolones (13.3%) and also presented resistance to ticarcillin/clavulanic acid. However, no resistance was observed to aminoglycosides. The differences in resistance may reflect local specificities in terms of antibiotic treatment.

Antimicrobial Resistance in *Pseudomonas* spp. in Chinchillas

P. aeruginosa is the main cause of infections in chinchillas, often due to uncleaned water and cages. Chinchillas have been extensively studied as models of middle ear infections (148), but studies dedicated to otitis media in this animal species are scarce (149).

Antibiotic susceptibility has only been reported once, in 67 chinchillas in Japan (150), of which 23 were raised as pets and 21 as laboratory animals. A total of 22 *P. aeruginosa* isolates were identified, which clustered in seven pulsed-field gel electrophoresis patterns. No resistance phenotype was observed for aminoglycosides, even though nine isolates presented a decreased susceptibility to gentamicin and one to amikacin. One isolate was resistant to ciprofloxacin, while MICs for enrofloxacin—the major veterinary fluoroquinolone—were much higher than those to ciprofloxacin. Finally, six isolates showed intermediate resistance to ceftazidime and five to imipenem. The number of isolates presenting reduced susceptibilities should undoubtedly prompt further studies in these animals which are in close contact with humans.

Antimicrobial Resistance in *Pseudomonas* spp. in Food-Producing Animals

Cattle are the only food-producing animals for which substantial data on antimicrobial resistance in *P. aeruginosa* are available. Data for chickens and pigs are very scarce and mostly describe *Pseudomonas* spp. as environmental contaminants (151, 152). Only two studies specifically designed for the detection of carbapenem-resistant isolates reported the presence of VIM-2 in

P. aeruginosa in fowl in Lebanon and VIM-1 in *Pseudomonas putida* in chicken cloacal swabs as well as in their environment in China (56, 153).

In cattle, only three articles reported on resistance phenotypes in *P. aeruginosa* isolates from bovine mastitis. Ohnishi et al. studied 116 *P. aeruginosa* strains collected from the milk of 115 cows in Japan between 2005 and 2007 (154). *P. aeruginosa* was found in 0.65% of the milk isolates that had been under control and caused moderate to severe infections in half of the cases. Isolates presented high susceptibility rates toward piperacillin, ceftazidime, cefepime, imipenem, ciprofloxacin, amikacin, and tobramycin. Amikacin resistance was suspected in two isolates and carbapenem-resistance in two others, but this could not be confirmed molecularly. This is considerably different from what has been seen in Japan in human isolates, where multidrug-resistant and carbapenemase-producing strains were recurrently found. Haenni et al. also reported 12 isolates from cattle in France in 2010 (124), which all belonged to nonhuman clones. In parallel, *P. aeruginosa* was recovered in 0.61% of the bovine isolates collected the same year through the Resapath network (www.resapath.anses.fr). Isolates originated from mastitis and respiratory tract infections and were susceptible to the majority of antibiotics tested, except fosfomycin (9/12, 75%) and ticarcillin (3/12, 25%). Thus, these results confirm the low incidence of *P. aeruginosa* in bovine mastitis in both countries, suggest that clones circulating in animals differ from the ones isolated in humans, and prove their capacity to cause severe infections.

Chuanchuen et al. reported a molecular study of the MexXY efflux pumps in 18 *P. aeruginosa* isolates collected from bovine mastitis in Thailand (126). All of these field isolates presented decreased susceptibility to a variety of aminoglycosides, and three displayed an MIC to gentamicin higher than those of the PAO1 control strains. These decreased susceptibilities to aminoglycosides were partly attributed to overexpression of the MexXY efflux system but also to the presence of genes coding for aminoglycoside-modifying genes, such as *aph(3′)-IIb* and *aac(6′)-IIb*. Finally, two carbapenem-resistant isolates producing the VIM-2 enzyme were reported in Lebanon (56).

Antimicrobial Resistance in *Pseudomonas* spp. in Horses

P. aeruginosa is a rare pathogen in horses, sporadically causing skin or respiratory infections. It is more frequently associated with genital tract infections such as endometritis, which can lead to reduced fertility or even sterility. Horse-to-horse transmission is a potential source of transmission since nonpathogenic isolates may be incidentally introduced into the vagina of the mare during coitus (155). However, a wide variety of clones was identified in certain studies, suggesting transmission through contaminated material during artificial insemination or opportunistic growth of bacteria from environmental sources if conditions are favorable (156–158).

Only two limited studies from France and Brazil reported the antimicrobial susceptibility of *P. aeruginosa* isolates from horses (111, 124). No multi-resistant isolates were reported in France among the 10 animals sampled, and only fosfomycin resistance was prevalent (6/10, 60%). Interestingly, two strains belonged to clones ST155 and ST27, which are associated with human outbreaks and sometimes display multiresistance phenotypes. In Brazil, only three animals were included in the study, and two out of the three *P. aeruginosa* isolates studied presented multiple resistances to fluoroquinolones and aminoglycosides.

The paucity of infections due to *P. aeruginosa* in horses may explain the lack of information on antimicrobial resistance in such isolates. However, the spread of resistance in all reservoirs (human, animal, and environmental) and the need for data on all potential niches will probably prompt scientists to explore this field.

CONCLUSION

A. baumannii and *P. aeruginosa* are two major nosocomial pathogens in humans, and increasingly resistant strains are being characterized all over the world. In contrast, they are more rarely found in animals, as is evidenced by the low number of publications in the veterinary field. However, when considering taking measures to avoid further spread of antimicrobial-resistant organisms or emergence of further resistance, the intersections of all the ecological domains must be explored. The crossroads of humans and animals is especially important—on the one hand for protection of professionals, as in the case of breeders and livestock farmers, and on the other hand, for physical proximity, adoption of pets in Europe being a growing phenomenon with 75 million pet-owing households. In this context, the emergence of multidrug-resistant bacteria from animals is worrisome: first, because the therapeutic options for animals are dramatically diminishing and, second, because the animal reservoir of multidrug-resistant bacteria is gaining in prevalence and complexity. The process contributing to such development is articulated, consisting of cross-contamination between human and animals, selective and coselective pressure by antimicrobial usage, and the spread of multidrug-resistant organisms in intensive breeding frameworks. Considering this context, studies dedicated to *Acinetobacter* spp. and *Pseudomonas* spp. on farms or generally in animal hosts are both limited in number and quite sparse in their geographical distribution, thus impeding the elaboration of a general picture of the modality of the spread of certain clones and the emergence of resistance mechanisms. Ideally, concerted investigations between human and veterinary clinics would provide useful keys to understanding such phenomena. To this end, global and vigilant surveys are priorities to preserve public health.

Acknowledgments. *We thank Katy Jeannot for her helpful proofreading.*

Citation. Lupo A, Haenni M, Madec J-Y. 2018. Antimicrobial resistance in *Acinetobacter* spp. and *Pseudomonas* spp. Microbiol Spectrum 6(3):ARBA-0007-2017.

References

1. **Fishbain J, Peleg AY.** 2010. Treatment of *Acinetobacter* infections. *Clin Infect Dis* **51:**79–84.

2. **Karaiskos I, Giamarellou H.** 2014. Multidrug-resistant and extensively drug-resistant Gram-negative pathogens: current and emerging therapeutic approaches. *Expert Opin Pharmacother* **15:**1351–1370.

3. **Bartual SG, Seifert H, Hippler C, Luzon MA, Wisplinghoff H, Rodríguez-Valera F.** 2005. Development of a multilocus sequence typing scheme for characterization of clinical isolates of *Acinetobacter baumannii*. *J Clin Microbiol* **43:**4382–4390.

4. **Sahl JW, Del Franco M, Pournaras S, Colman RE, Karah N, Dijkshoorn L, Zarrilli R.** 2015. Phylogenetic and genomic diversity in isolates from the globally distributed *Acinetobacter baumannii* ST25 lineage. *Sci Rep* **5:**15188.

5. **Lupo A, Vogt D, Seiffert SN, Endimiani A, Perreten V.** 2014. Antibiotic resistance and phylogenetic characterization of *Acinetobacter baumannii* strains isolated from commercial raw meat in Switzerland. *J Food Prot* **77:** 1976–1981.

6. **Belmonte O, Pailhoriès H, Kempf M, Gaultier MP, Lemarié C, Ramont C, Joly-Guillou ML, Eveillard M.** 2014. High prevalence of closely-related *Acinetobacter baumannii* in pets according to a multicentre study in veterinary clinics, Reunion Island. *Vet Microbiol* **170:** 446–450.

7. **Cattabiani F, Cabassi E, Allodi C, Gianelli F.** 1976. Bacterial flora of the conjunctival sac of the horse. *Ann Sclavo* **18:**91–119. (In Italian.)

8. **Johns IC, Baxter K, Booler H, Hicks C, Menzies-Gow N.** 2011. Conjunctival bacterial and fungal flora in healthy horses in the UK. *Vet Ophthalmol* **14:**195–199.

9. **Kumsa B, Socolovschi C, Parola P, Rolain JM, Raoult D.** 2012. Molecular detection of *Acinetobacter* species in lice and keds of domestic animals in Oromia Regional State, Ethiopia. *PLoS One* **7:**e52377.

10. **Moore CP, Heller N, Majors LJ, Whitley RD, Burgess EC, Weber J.** 1988. Prevalence of ocular microorganisms in hospitalized and stabled horses. *Am J Vet Res* **49:**773–777.

11. **Rudi K, Moen B, Sekelja M, Frisli T, Lee MR.** 2012. An eight-year investigation of bovine livestock fecal microbiota. *Vet Microbiol* **160:**369–377.

12. **Saphir DA, Carter GR.** 1976. Gingival flora of the dog with special reference to bacteria associated with bites. *J Clin Microbiol* **3:**344–349.

13. **Endimiani A, Hujer KM, Hujer AM, Bertschy I, Rossano A, Koch C, Gerber V, Francey T, Bonomo RA, Perreten V.** 2011. *Acinetobacter baumannii* isolates from pets and horses in Switzerland: molecular characterization and clinical data. *J Antimicrob Chemother* **66:**2248–2254.

14. **Vaneechoutte M, Devriese LA, Dijkshoorn L, Lamote B, Deprez P, Verschraegen G, Haesebrouck F.** 2000. *Acinetobacter baumannii*-infected vascular catheters collected from horses in an equine clinic. *J Clin Microbiol* **38:**4280–4281.

15. **Boerlin P, Eugster S, Gaschen F, Straub R, Schawalder P.** 2001. Transmission of opportunistic pathogens in a veterinary teaching hospital. *Vet Microbiol* **82:**347–359.

16. **Zordan S, Prenger-Berninghoff E, Weiss R, van der Reijden T, van den Broek P, Baljer G, Dijkshoorn L.** 2011. Multidrug-resistant *Acinetobacter baumannii* in veterinary clinics, Germany. *Emerg Infect Dis* **17:**1751–1754.

17. **Mathewson JJ, Simpson RB.** 1982. Glucose-nonfermenting Gram-negative bacilli associated with clinical veterinary specimens. *J Clin Microbiol* **15:**1016–1018.

18. **Abbott Y, O'Mahony R, Leonard N, Quinn PJ, van der Reijden T, Dijkshoorn L, Fanning S.** 2005. Characterization of a 2.6 kbp variable region within a class 1 integron found in an *Acinetobacter baumannii* strain isolated from a horse. *J Antimicrob Chemother* **55:**367–370.

19. **Boguta L, Gradzki Z, Borges E, Maurin F, Kodjo A, Winiarczyk S.** 2002. Bacterial flora in foals with upper respiratory tract infections in Poland. *J Vet Med B Infect Dis Vet Public Health* **49:**294–297.

20. **Francey T, Gaschen F, Nicolet J, Burnens AP.** 2000. The role of *Acinetobacter baumannii* as a nosocomial pathogen for dogs and cats in an intensive care unit. *J Vet Intern Med* **14:**177–183.

21. **Lupo A, Châtre P, Ponsin C, Saras E, Boulouis HJ, Keck N, Haenni M, Madec JY.** 2016. Clonal spread of *Acinetobacter baumannii* sequence type 25 carrying *bla*OXA-23 in companion animals in France. *Antimicrob Agents Chemother* **61:**61.

22. **Malinowski E, Lassa H, Kłossowska A, Smulski S, Markiewicz H, Kaczmarowski M.** 2006. Etiological agents of dairy cows' mastitis in western part of Poland. *Pol J Vet Sci* **9:**191–194.

23. **Nam HM, Lim SK, Kang HM, Kim JM, Moon JS, Jang KC, Kim JM, Joo YS, Jung SC.** 2009. Prevalence and antimicrobial susceptibility of Gram-negative bacteria isolated from bovine mastitis between 2003 and 2008 in Korea. *J Dairy Sci* **92:**2020–2026.

24. **Ruppé É, Woerther PL, Barbier F.** 2015. Mechanisms of antimicrobial resistance in Gram-negative bacilli. *Ann Intensive Care* **5:**61.

25. **Bonomo RA, Szabo D.** 2006. Mechanisms of multidrug resistance in *Acinetobacter* species and *Pseudomonas* aeruginosa. *Clin Infect Dis* **43**(Suppl 2):S49–S56.

26. **Coyne S, Courvalin P, Périchon B.** 2011. Efflux-mediated antibiotic resistance in *Acinetobacter* spp. *Antimicrob Agents Chemother* **55:**947–953.

27. **Coyne S, Rosenfeld N, Lambert T, Courvalin P, Périchon B.** 2010. Overexpression of resistance-nodulation-cell division pump AdeFGH confers multidrug resistance in *Acinetobacter baumannii*. *Antimicrob Agents Chemother* **54:**4389–4393.

28. **Damier-Piolle L, Magnet S, Brémont S, Lambert T, Courvalin P.** 2008. AdeIJK, a resistance-nodulation-cell division pump effluxing multiple antibiotics in *Acinetobacter baumannii*. *Antimicrob Agents Chemother* **52:** 557–562.

29. **Rosenfeld N, Bouchier C, Courvalin P, Périchon B.** 2012. Expression of the resistance-nodulation-cell division pump AdeIJK in *Acinetobacter baumannii* is regulated by AdeN, a TetR-type regulator. *Antimicrob Agents Chemother* **56:**2504–2510.

30. **Corvec S, Caroff N, Espaze E, Giraudeau C, Drugeon H, Reynaud A.** 2003. AmpC cephalosporinase hyperproduction in *Acinetobacter baumannii* clinical strains. *J Antimicrob Chemother* **52:**629–635.

31. **Mugnier PD, Poirel L, Nordmann P.** 2009. Functional analysis of insertion sequence ISAba1, responsible for genomic plasticity of *Acinetobacter baumannii*. *J Bacteriol* **191:**2414–2418.

32. **Mussi MA, Relling VM, Limansky AS, Viale AM.** 2007. CarO, an *Acinetobacter baumannii* outer membrane protein involved in carbapenem resistance, is essential for L-ornithine uptake. *FEBS Lett* **581:**5573–5578.

33. **Bonnin RA, Potron A, Poirel L, Lecuyer H, Neri R, Nordmann P.** 2011. PER-7, an extended-spectrum beta-lactamase with increased activity toward broad-spectrum cephalosporins in *Acinetobacter baumannii*. *Antimicrob Agents Chemother* **55:**2424–2427.

34. **Naas T, Coignard B, Carbonne A, Blanckaert K, Bajolet O, Bernet C, Verdeil X, Astagneau P, Desenclos JC, Nordmann P, French Nosocomial Infection Early Warning Investigation and Surveillance Network.** 2006. VEB-1 Extended-spectrum beta-lactamase-producing *Acinetobacter baumannii*, France. *Emerg Infect Dis* **12:** 1214–1222.

35. **Evans BA, Amyes SG.** 2014. OXA β-lactamases. *Clin Microbiol Rev* **27:**241–263.

36. **Mathlouthi N, Al-Bayssari C, Bakour S, Rolain JM, Chouchani C.** 2017. Prevalence and emergence of carbapenemases-producing Gram-negative bacteria in Mediterranean basin. *Crit Rev Microbiol* **43:**43–61.

37. **Seward RJ, Lambert T, Towner KJ.** 1998. Molecular epidemiology of aminoglycoside resistance in *Acinetobacter* spp. *J Med Microbiol* **47:**455–462.

38. Liou GF, Yoshizawa S, Courvalin P, Galimand M. 2006. Aminoglycoside resistance by ArmA-mediated ribosomal 16S methylation in human bacterial pathogens. *J Mol Biol* 359:358–364.

39. Périchon B, Courvalin P, Galimand M. 2007. Transferable resistance to aminoglycosides by methylation of G1405 in 16S rRNA and to hydrophilic fluoroquinolones by QepA-mediated efflux in *Escherichia coli*. *Antimicrob Agents Chemother* 51:2464–2469.

40. Doi Y, Adams JM, Yamane K, Paterson DL. 2007. Identification of 16S rRNA methylase-producing *Acinetobacter baumannii* clinical strains in North America. *Antimicrob Agents Chemother* 51:4209–4210.

41. Yu YS, Zhou H, Yang Q, Chen YG, Li LJ. 2007. Widespread occurrence of aminoglycoside resistance due to ArmA methylase in imipenem-resistant *Acinetobacter baumannii* isolates in China. *J Antimicrob Chemother* 60:454–455.

42. Vila J, Ruiz J, Goñi P, Jimenez de Anta T. 1997. Quinolone-resistance mutations in the topoisomerase IV *parC* gene of *Acinetobacter baumannii*. *J Antimicrob Chemother* 39:757–762.

43. Vila J, Ruiz J, Goñi P, Marcos A, Jimenez de Anta T. 1995. Mutation in the *gyrA* gene of quinolone-resistant clinical isolates of *Acinetobacter baumannii*. *Antimicrob Agents Chemother* 39:1201–1203.

44. Houang ET, Chu YW, Lo WS, Chu KY, Cheng AF. 2003. Epidemiology of rifampin ADP-ribosyltransferase (*arr-2*) and metallo-beta-lactamase (*bla*IMP-4) gene cassettes in class 1 integrons in *Acinetobacter* strains isolated from blood cultures in 1997 to 2000. *Antimicrob Agents Chemother* 47:1382–1390.

45. Adams MD, Nickel GC, Bajaksouzian S, Lavender H, Murthy AR, Jacobs MR, Bonomo RA. 2009. Resistance to colistin in *Acinetobacter baumannii* associated with mutations in the PmrAB two-component system. *Antimicrob Agents Chemother* 53:3628–3634.

46. Peleg AY, Adams J, Paterson DL. 2007. Tigecycline efflux as a mechanism for nonsusceptibility in *Acinetobacter baumannii*. *Antimicrob Agents Chemother* 51:2065–2069.

47. Freitas AR, Novais C, Correia R, Monteiro M, Coque TM, Peixe L. 2011. Non-susceptibility to tigecycline in enterococci from hospitalised patients, food products and community sources. *Int J Antimicrob Agents* 38:174–176.

48. Ewers C, Klotz P, Leidner U, Stamm I, Prenger-Berninghoff E, Göttig S, Semmler T, Scheufen S. 2017. OXA-23 and ISAba1-OXA-66 class D β-lactamases in *Acinetobacter baumannii* isolates from companion animals. *Int J Antimicrob Agents* 49:37–44.

49. Nigro SJ, Hall RM. 2016. Structure and context of *Acinetobacter* transposons carrying the oxa23 carbapenemase gene. *J Antimicrob Chemother* 71:1135–1147.

50. Iacono M, Villa L, Fortini D, Bordoni R, Imperi F, Bonnal RJ, Sicheritz-Ponten T, De Bellis G, Visca P, Cassone A, Carattoli A. 2008. Whole-genome pyrosequencing of an epidemic multidrug-resistant *Acinetobacter baumannii* strain belonging to the European clone II group. *Antimicrob Agents Chemother* 52:2616–2625.

51. Shaikh F, Spence RP, Levi K, Ou HY, Deng Z, Towner KJ, Rajakumar K. 2009. ATPase genes of diverse multidrug-resistant *Acinetobacter baumannii* isolates frequently harbour integrated DNA. *J Antimicrob Chemother* 63:260–264.

52. Poirel L, Berçot B, Millemann Y, Bonnin RA, Pannaux G, Nordmann P. 2012. Carbapenemase-producing *Acinetobacter* spp. in cattle, France. *Emerg Infect Dis* 18:523–525.

53. Wang Y, Wu C, Zhang Q, Qi J, Liu H, Wang Y, He T, Ma L, Lai J, Shen Z, Liu Y, Shen J. 2012. Identification of New Delhi metallo-β-lactamase 1 in *Acinetobacter lwoffii* of food animal origin. *PLoS One* 7:e37152.

54. Zhang WJ, Lu Z, Schwarz S, Zhang RM, Wang XM, Si W, Yu S, Chen L, Liu S. 2013. Complete sequence of the *bla(NDM-1)*-carrying plasmid pNDM-AB from *Acinetobacter baumannii* of food animal origin. *J Antimicrob Chemother* 68:1681–1682.

55. Brahmi S, Touati A, Cadière A, Djahmi N, Pantel A, Sotto A, Lavigne JP, Dunyach-Remy C. 2016. First description of two sequence type 2 *Acinetobacter baumannii* isolates carrying OXA-23 carbapenemase in *Pagellus acarne* fished from the Mediterranean Sea near Bejaia, Algeria. *Antimicrob Agents Chemother* 60:2513–2515.

56. Al Bayssari C, Dabboussi F, Hamze M, Rolain JM. 2015. Emergence of carbapenemase-producing *Pseudomonas aeruginosa* and *Acinetobacter baumannii* in livestock animals in Lebanon. *J Antimicrob Chemother* 70:950–951.

57. Pailhoriès H, Kempf M, Belmonte O, Joly-Guillou ML, Eveillard M. 2016. First case of OXA-24-producing *Acinetobacter baumannii* in cattle from Reunion Island, France. *Int J Antimicrob Agents* 48:763–764.

58. Klotz P, Göttig S, Leidner U, Semmler T, Scheufen S, Ewers C. 2017. Carbapenem-resistance and pathogenicity of bovine *Acinetobacter indicus*-like isolates. *PLoS One* 12:e0171986.

59. Smet A, Boyen F, Pasmans F, Butaye P, Martens A, Nemec A, Deschaght P, Vaneechoutte M, Haesebrouck F. 2012. OXA-23-producing *Acinetobacter* species from horses: a public health hazard? *J Antimicrob Chemother* 67:3009–3010.

60. Pomba C, Endimiani A, Rossano A, Saial D, Couto N, Perreten V. 2014. First report of OXA-23-mediated carbapenem resistance in sequence type 2 multidrug-resistant *Acinetobacter baumannii* associated with urinary tract infection in a cat. *Antimicrob Agents Chemother* 58:1267–1268.

61. Hérivaux A, Pailhoriès H, Quinqueneau C, Lemarié C, Joly-Guillou ML, Ruvoen N, Eveillard M, Kempf M. 2016. First report of carbapenemase-producing *Acinetobacter baumannii* carriage in pets from the community in France. *Int J Antimicrob Agents* 48:220–221.

62. Kimura Y, Miyamoto T, Aoki K, Ishii Y, Harada K, Watarai M, Hatoya S. 2017. Analysis of IMP-1 type metallo-β-lactamase-producing *Acinetobacter radio-*

resistens isolated from companion animals. *J Infect Chemother* 23:655–657.

63. Silby MW, Winstanley C, Godfrey SAC, Levy SB, Jackson RW. 2011. *Pseudomonas* genomes: diverse and adaptable. *FEMS Microbiol Rev* 35:652–680.

64. Argudín MA, Deplano A, Meghraoui A, Dodémont M, Heinrichs A, Denis O, Nonhoff C, Roisin S. 2017. Bacteria from animals as a pool of antimicrobial resistance genes. *Antibiotics (Basel)* 6:6.

65. O'Brien HE, Desveaux D, Guttman DS. 2011. Next-generation genomics of *Pseudomonas syringae*. *Curr Opin Microbiol* 14:24–30.

66. Wu X, Monchy S, Taghavi S, Zhu W, Ramos J, van der Lelie D. 2011. Comparative genomics and functional analysis of niche-specific adaptation in *Pseudomonas putida*. *FEMS Microbiol Rev* 35:299–323.

67. Lalucat J, Bennasar A, Bosch R, García-Valdés E, Palleroni NJ. 2006. Biology of *Pseudomonas stutzeri*. *Microbiol Mol Biol Rev* 70:510–547.

68. Walker TS, Bais HP, Déziel E, Schweizer HP, Rahme LG, Fall R, Vivanco JM. 2004. *Pseudomonas aeruginosa*-plant root interactions: pathogenicity, biofilm formation, and root exudation. *Plant Physiol* 134:320–331.

69. Davies JC. 2002. *Pseudomonas aeruginosa* in cystic fibrosis: pathogenesis and persistence. *Paediatr Respir Rev* 3:128–134.

70. Lyczak JB, Cannon CL, Pier GB. 2000. Establishment of *Pseudomonas aeruginosa* infection: lessons from a versatile opportunist. *Microbes Infect* 2:1051–1060.

71. Hariharan H, Coles M, Poole D, Lund L, Page R. 2006. Update on antimicrobial susceptibilities of bacterial isolates from canine and feline otitis externa. *Can Vet J* 47:253–255.

72. Petersen AD, Walker RD, Bowman MM, Schott HC II, Rosser EJ Jr. 2002. Frequency of isolation and antimicrobial susceptibility patterns of *Staphylococcus intermedius* and *Pseudomonas aeruginosa* isolates from canine skin and ear samples over a 6-year period (1992–1997). *J Am Anim Hosp Assoc* 38:407–413.

73. Rubin J, Walker RD, Blickenstaff K, Bodeis-Jones S, Zhao S. 2008. Antimicrobial resistance and genetic characterization of fluoroquinolone resistance of *Pseudomonas aeruginosa* isolated from canine infections. *Vet Microbiol* 131:164–172.

74. Mekić S, Matanović K, Šeol B. 2011. Antimicrobial susceptibility of *Pseudomonas aeruginosa* isolates from dogs with otitis externa. *Vet Rec* 169:125.

75. ANSES. 2016. Résapath - Réseau d'épidémiosurveillance de l'antibiorésistance des bactéries pathogènes animales, bilan 2015, Lyon et Ploufragan-Plouzané, France, November 2016.

76. Colombini S, Merchant SR, Hosgood G. 2000. Microbial flora and antimicrobial susceptibility patterns from dogs with otitis media. *Vet Dermatol* 11:235–239.

77. Done SH. 1974. *Pseudomonas aeruginosa* infection in the skin of a dog: a case report. *Br Vet J* 130:lxviii–lxix.

78. Hillier A, Alcorn JR, Cole LK, Kowalski JJ. 2006. Pyoderma caused by *Pseudomonas aeruginosa* infection in dogs: 20 cases. *Vet Dermatol* 17:432–439.

79. Wilson DJ, Baldwin TJ, Whitehouse CH, Hullinger G. 2015. Causes of mortality in farmed mink in the Intermountain West, North America. *J Vet Diagn Invest* 27:470–475.

80. Shimizu T, Homma JY, Aoyama T, Onodera T, Noda H. 1974. Virulence of *Pseudomonas aeruginosa* and spontaneous spread of pseudomonas pneumonia in a mink ranch. *Infect Immun* 10:16–20.

81. Farrell RK, Leader RW, Gorham JR. 1958. An outbreak of hemorrhagic pneumonia in mink; a case report. *Cornell Vet* 48:378–384.

82. Daniel RC, O'Boyle D, Marek MS, Frost AJ. 1982. A survey of clinical mastitis in South-East Queensland dairy herds. *Aust Vet J* 58:143–147.

83. Bradley AJ, Leach KA, Breen JE, Green LE, Green MJ. 2007. Survey of the incidence and aetiology of mastitis on dairy farms in England and Wales. *Vet Rec* 160:253–257.

84. Persson Y, Nyman AK, Grönlund-Andersson U. 2011. Etiology and antimicrobial susceptibility of udder pathogens from cases of subclinical mastitis in dairy cows in Sweden. *Acta Vet Scand* 53:36.

85. Botrel MA, Haenni M, Morignat E, Sulpice P, Madec JY, Calavas D. 2010. Distribution and antimicrobial resistance of clinical and subclinical mastitis pathogens in dairy cows in Rhône-Alpes, France. *Foodborne Pathog Dis* 7:479–487.

86. Nam HM, Kim JM, Lim SK, Jang KC, Jung SC. 2010. Infectious aetiologies of mastitis on Korean dairy farms during 2008. *Res Vet Sci* 88:372–374.

87. Sela S, Hammer-Muntz O, Krifucks O, Pinto R, Weisblit L, Leitner G. 2007. Phenotypic and genotypic characterization of *Pseudomonas aeruginosa* strains isolated from mastitis outbreaks in dairy herds. *J Dairy Res* 74:425–429.

88. Daly M, Power E, Björkroth J, Sheehan P, O'Connell A, Colgan M, Korkeala H, Fanning S. 1999. Molecular analysis of *Pseudomonas aeruginosa*: epidemiological investigation of mastitis outbreaks in Irish dairy herds. *Appl Environ Microbiol* 65:2723–2729.

89. McLennan MW, Kelly WR, O'Boyle D. 1997. *Pseudomonas* mastitis in a dairy herd. *Aust Vet J* 75:790–792.

90. Osborne AD, Armstrong K, Catrysse NH, Butler G, Versavel L. 1981. An outbreak of *Pseudomonas mastitis* in dairy cows. *Can Vet J* 22:215–216.

91. Anderson B, Barton M, Corbould A, Dunford PJ, Elliott J, Leis T, Nicholls TJ, Sharman M, Stephenson GM. 1979. *Pseudomonas aeruginosa* mastitis due to contamination of an antibiotic preparation used in dry-cow therapy. *Aust Vet J* 55:90–91.

92. Kirk J, Mellenberger R. 2016. *Mastitis control program for* Pseudomonas *mastitis in dairy cows*. Purdue Dairy Page. https://www.extension.purdue.edu/dairy/health/hlthpub_mastitis.htm.

93. Yeruham I, Elad D, Avidar Y, Goshen T, Asis E. 2004. Four-year survey of urinary tract infections in calves in Israel. *Vet Rec* 154:204–206.

94. Rice LB. 2008. Federal funding for the study of antimicrobial resistance in nosocomial pathogens: no ESKAPE. *J Infect Dis* 197:1079–1081.

95. CA-SFM/EUCAST. 2016. Comité de l'antibiogramme de la Société Française de Microbiologie. http://www.sfm-microbiologie.org/page/page/showpage/page_id/90.html.

96. Breidenstein EB, de la Fuente-Núñez C, Hancock RE. 2011. *Pseudomonas aeruginosa*: all roads lead to resistance. *Trends Microbiol* 19:419–426.

97. Hancock RE. 1998. Resistance mechanisms in *Pseudomonas aeruginosa* and other nonfermentative Gram-negative bacteria. *Clin Infect Dis* 27(Suppl 1):S93–S99.

98. Li XZ, Plésiat P, Nikaido H. 2015. The challenge of efflux-mediated antibiotic resistance in Gram-negative bacteria. *Clin Microbiol Rev* 28:337–418.

99. Girlich D, Naas T, Nordmann P. 2004. Biochemical characterization of the naturally occurring oxacillinase OXA-50 of *Pseudomonas aeruginosa*. *Antimicrob Agents Chemother* 48:2043–2048.

100. Masuda N, Gotoh N, Ishii C, Sakagawa E, Ohya S, Nishino T. 1999. Interplay between chromosomal beta-lactamase and the MexAB-OprM efflux system in intrinsic resistance to beta-lactams in *Pseudomonas aeruginosa*. *Antimicrob Agents Chemother* 43:400–402.

101. Lodge JM, Minchin SD, Piddock LJ, Busby SJ. 1990. Cloning, sequencing and analysis of the structural gene and regulatory region of the *Pseudomonas aeruginosa* chromosomal ampC beta-lactamase. *Biochem J* 272:627–631.

102. Davey ME, O'toole GA. 2000. Microbial biofilms: from ecology to molecular genetics. *Microbiol Mol Biol Rev* 64:847–867.

103. de Kievit TR. 2009. Quorum sensing in *Pseudomonas aeruginosa* biofilms. *Environ Microbiol* 11:279–288.

104. Lequette Y, Greenberg EP. 2005. Timing and localization of rhamnolipid synthesis gene expression in *Pseudomonas aeruginosa* biofilms. *J Bacteriol* 187:37–44.

105. Harmsen M, Yang L, Pamp SJ, Tolker-Nielsen T. 2010. An update on *Pseudomonas aeruginosa* biofilm formation, tolerance, and dispersal. *FEMS Immunol Med Microbiol* 59:253–268.

106. Pamp SJ, Gjermansen M, Johansen HK, Tolker-Nielsen T. 2008. Tolerance to the antimicrobial peptide colistin in *Pseudomonas aeruginosa* biofilms is linked to metabolically active cells, and depends on the *pmr* and *mexAB-oprM* genes. *Mol Microbiol* 68:223–240.

107. Jeannot K, Elsen S, Köhler T, Attree I, van Delden C, Plésiat P. 2008. Resistance and virulence of *Pseudomonas aeruginosa* clinical strains overproducing the MexCD-OprJ efflux pump. *Antimicrob Agents Chemother* 52:2455–2462.

108. Potron A, Poirel L, Nordmann P. 2015. Emerging broad-spectrum resistance in *Pseudomonas aeruginosa* and *Acinetobacter baumannii*: mechanisms and epidemiology. *Int J Antimicrob Agents* 45:568–585.

109. Oliphant CM, Green GM. 2002. Quinolones: a comprehensive review. *Am Fam Physician* 65:455–464.

110. Lin D, Foley SL, Qi Y, Han J, Ji C, Li R, Wu C, Shen J, Wang Y. 2012. Characterization of antimicrobial resistance of *Pseudomonas aeruginosa* isolated from canine infections. *J Appl Microbiol* 113:16–23.

111. Leigue L, Montiani-Ferreira F, Moore BA. 2016. Antimicrobial susceptibility and minimal inhibitory concentration of *Pseudomonas aeruginosa* isolated from septic ocular surface disease in different animal species. *Open Vet J* 6:215–222.

112. Aires JR, Köhler T, Nikaido H, Plésiat P. 1999. Involvement of an active efflux system in the natural resistance of *Pseudomonas aeruginosa* to aminoglycosides. *Antimicrob Agents Chemother* 43:2624–2628.

113. Arais LR, Barbosa AV, Carvalho CA, Cerqueira AM. 2016. Antimicrobial resistance, integron carriage, and *gyrA* and *gyrB* mutations in *Pseudomonas aeruginosa* isolated from dogs with otitis externa and pyoderma in Brazil. *Vet Dermatol* 27:113-7e31.

114. Ludwig C, de Jong A, Moyaert H, El Garch F, Janes R, Klein U, Morrissey I, Thiry J, Youala M. 2016. Antimicrobial susceptibility monitoring of dermatological bacterial pathogens isolated from diseased dogs and cats across Europe (ComPath results). *J Appl Microbiol* 121:1254–1267.

115. Werckenthin C, Alesík E, Grobbel M, Lübke-Becker A, Schwarz S, Wieler LH, Wallmann J. 2007. Antimicrobial susceptibility of *Pseudomonas aeruginosa* from dogs and cats as well as *Arcanobacterium pyogenes* from cattle and swine as determined in the BfT-GermVet monitoring program 2004–2006. *Berl Munch Tierarztl Wochenschr* 120:412–422.

116. Seol B, Naglić T, Madić J, Bedeković M. 2002. In vitro antimicrobial susceptibility of 183 *Pseudomonas aeruginosa* strains isolated from dogs to selected antipseudomonal agents. *J Vet Med B Infect Dis Vet Public Health* 49:188–192.

117. Jacoby GA. 2005. Mechanisms of resistance to quinolones. *Clin Infect Dis* 41(Suppl 2):S120–S126.

118. Mouneimné H, Robert J, Jarlier V, Cambau E. 1999. Type II topoisomerase mutations in ciprofloxacin-resistant strains of *Pseudomonas aeruginosa*. *Antimicrob Agents Chemother* 43:62–66.

119. Matsumoto M, Shigemura K, Shirakawa T, Nakano Y, Miyake H, Tanaka K, Kinoshita S, Arakawa S, Kawabata M, Fujisawa M. 2012. Mutations in the *gyrA* and *parC* genes and in vitro activities of fluoroquinolones in 114 clinical isolates of *Pseudomonas aeruginosa* derived from urinary tract infections and their rapid detection by denaturing high-performance liquid chromatography. *Int J Antimicrob Agents* 40:440–444.

120. Li XZ, Nikaido H, Poole K. 1995. Role of mexA-mexB-oprM in antibiotic efflux in *Pseudomonas aeruginosa*. *Antimicrob Agents Chemother* 39:1948–1953.

121. Masuda N, Sakagawa E, Ohya S, Gotoh N, Tsujimoto H, Nishino T. 2000. Contribution of the MexX-MexY-oprM efflux system to intrinsic resistance in *Pseudomonas aeruginosa*. *Antimicrob Agents Chemother* 44:2242–2246.

122. Le Thomas I, Couetdic G, Clermont O, Brahimi N, Plésiat P, Bingen E. 2001. In vivo selection of a target/efflux double mutant of *Pseudomonas aeruginosa* by ciprofloxacin therapy. *J Antimicrob Chemother* 48:553–555.

123. Beinlich KL, Chuanchuen R, Schweizer HP. 2001. Contribution of multidrug efflux pumps to multiple antibiotic resistance in veterinary clinical isolates of *Pseudomonas aeruginosa*. *FEMS Microbiol Lett* 198:129–134.

124. Haenni M, Hocquet D, Ponsin C, Cholley P, Guyeux C, Madec JY, Bertrand X. 2015. Population structure and antimicrobial susceptibility of *Pseudomonas aeruginosa* from animal infections in France. *BMC Vet Res* 11:9.

125. Morita Y, Tomida J, Kawamura Y. 2012. MexXY multidrug efflux system of *Pseudomonas aeruginosa*. *Front Microbiol* 3:408.

126. Chuanchuen R, Wannaprasat W, Ajariyakhajorn K, Schweizer HP. 2008. Role of the MexXY multidrug efflux pump in moderate aminoglycoside resistance in *Pseudomonas aeruginosa* isolates from *Pseudomonas* mastitis. *Microbiol Immunol* 52:392–398.

127. Poonsuk K, Chuanchuen R. 2012. Contribution of the MexXY multidrug efflux pump and other chromosomal mechanisms on aminoglycoside resistance in *Pseudomonas aeruginosa* isolates from canine and feline infections. *J Vet Med Sci* 74:1575–1582.

128. Poole K. 2005. Aminoglycoside resistance in *Pseudomonas aeruginosa*. *Antimicrob Agents Chemother* 49:479–487.

129. Yokoyama K, Doi Y, Yamane K, Kurokawa H, Shibata N, Shibayama K, Yagi T, Kato H, Arakawa Y. 2003. Acquisition of 16S rRNA methylase gene in *Pseudomonas aeruginosa*. *Lancet* 362:1888–1893.

130. Doi Y, de Oliveira Garcia D, Adams J, Paterson DL. 2007. Coproduction of novel 16S rRNA methylase RmtD and metallo-beta-lactamase SPM-1 in a pan-resistant *Pseudomonas aeruginosa* isolate from Brazil. *Antimicrob Agents Chemother* 51:852–856.

131. Li J, Zou M, Dou Q, Hu Y, Wang H, Yan Q, Liu WE. 2016. Characterization of clinical extensively drug-resistant *Pseudomonas aeruginosa* in the Hunan province of China. *Ann Clin Microbiol Antimicrob* 15:35.

132. Jeannot K, Bolard A, Plésiat P. 2017. Resistance to polymyxins in Gram-negative organisms. *Int J Antimicrob Agents* 49:526–535.

133. Liu YY, Wang Y, Walsh TR, Yi LX, Zhang R, Spencer J, Doi Y, Tian G, Dong B, Huang X, Yu LF, Gu D, Ren H, Chen X, Lv L, He D, Zhou H, Liang Z, Liu JH, Shen J. 2016. Emergence of plasmid-mediated colistin resistance mechanism MCR-1 in animals and human beings in China: a microbiological and molecular biological study. *Lancet Infect Dis* 16:161–168.

134. Lee JY, Park YK, Chung ES, Na IY, Ko KS. 2016. Evolved resistance to colistin and its loss due to genetic reversion in *Pseudomonas aeruginosa*. *Sci Rep* 6:25543.

135. Martis N, Leroy S, Blanc V. 2014. Colistin in multidrug resistant *Pseudomonas aeruginosa* blood-stream infections: a narrative review for the clinician. *J Infect* 69:1–12.

136. Muller C, Plésiat P, Jeannot K. 2011. A two-component regulatory system interconnects resistance to polymyxins, aminoglycosides, fluoroquinolones, and β-lactams in *Pseudomonas aeruginosa*. *Antimicrob Agents Chemother* 55:1211–1221.

137. Moskowitz SM, Brannon MK, Dasgupta N, Pier M, Sgambati N, Miller AK, Selgrade SE, Miller SI, Denton M, Conway SP, Johansen HK, Høiby N. 2012. PmrB mutations promote polymyxin resistance of *Pseudomonas aeruginosa* isolated from colistin-treated cystic fibrosis patients. *Antimicrob Agents Chemother* 56:1019–1030.

138. Gutu AD, Sgambati N, Strasbourger P, Brannon MK, Jacobs MA, Haugen E, Kaul RK, Johansen HK, Høiby N, Moskowitz SM. 2013. Polymyxin resistance of *Pseudomonas aeruginosa phoQ* mutants is dependent on additional two-component regulatory systems. *Antimicrob Agents Chemother* 57:2204–2215.

139. Wang Y, Wang X, Schwarz S, Zhang R, Lei L, Liu X, Lin D, Shen J. 2014. IMP-45-producing multidrug-resistant *Pseudomonas aeruginosa* of canine origin. *J Antimicrob Chemother* 69:2579–2581.

140. Haenni M, Bour M, Châtre P, Madec JY, Plésiat P, Jeannot K. 2017. Resistance of animal strains of *Pseudomonas aeruginosa* to carbapenems. *Front Microbiol* 8:1847.

141. Salomonsen CM, Themudo GE, Jelsbak L, Molin S, Høiby N, Hammer AS. 2013. Typing of *Pseudomonas aeruginosa* from hemorrhagic pneumonia in mink (*Neovison vison*). *Vet Microbiol* 163:103–109.

142. Hammer AS, Pedersen K, Andersen TH, Jørgensen JC, Dietz HH. 2003. Comparison of *Pseudomonas aeruginosa* isolates from mink by serotyping and pulsed-field gel electrophoresis. *Vet Microbiol* 94:237–243.

143. Gu J, Li X, Yang M, Du C, Cui Z, Gong P, Xia F, Song J, Zhang L, Li J, Yu C, Sun C, Feng X, Lei L, Han W. 2016. Therapeutic effect of *Pseudomonas aeruginosa* phage YH30 on mink hemorrhagic pneumonia. *Vet Microbiol* 190:5–11.

144. Pedersen K, Hammer AS, Sørensen CM, Heuer OE. 2009. Usage of antimicrobials and occurrence of antimicrobial resistance among bacteria from mink. *Vet Microbiol* 133:115–122.

145. Jensen VF, Sommer HM, Struve T, Clausen J, Chriél M. 2016. Factors associated with usage of antimicrobials in commercial mink (*Neovison vison*) production in Denmark. *Prev Vet Med* 126:170–182.

146. Qi J, Li L, Du Y, Wang S, Wang J, Luo Y, Che J, Lu J, Liu H, Hu G, Li J, Gong Y, Wang G, Hu M, Shiganyan, Liu Y. 2014. The identification, typing, and antimicrobial susceptibility of *Pseudomonas aeruginosa* isolated from mink with hemorrhagic pneumonia. *Vet Microbiol* 170:456–461.

147. Nikolaisen NK, Lassen DCK, Chriél M, Larsen G, Jensen VF, Pedersen K. 2017. Antimicrobial resistance among pathogenic bacteria from mink (*Neovison vison*) in Denmark. *Acta Vet Scand* 59:60.

148. Giebink GS. 1999. Otitis media: the chinchilla model. *Microb Drug Resist* 5:57–72.

149. Wideman WL. 2006. *Pseudomonas aeruginosa* otitis media and interna in a chinchilla ranch. *Can Vet J* 47:799–800.

150. Hirakawa Y, Sasaki H, Kawamoto E, Ishikawa H, Matsumoto T, Aoyama N, Kawasumi K, Amao H.

2010. Prevalence and analysis of *Pseudomonas aeruginosa* in chinchillas. *BMC Vet Res* **6:**52.

151. **Agersø Y, Sandvang D.** 2005. Class 1 integrons and tetracycline resistance genes in alcaligenes, arthrobacter, and *Pseudomonas* spp. isolated from pigsties and manured soil. *Appl Environ Microbiol* **71:**7941–7947.

152. **de Oliveira KM, dos S Júlio PD, Grisolia AB.** 2013. Antimicrobial susceptibility profile of *Pseudomonas spp.* isolated from a swine slaughterhouse in Dourados, Mato Grosso do Sul State, Brazil. *Rev Argent Microbiol* **45:**57–60.

153. **Zhang R, Liu Z, Li J, Lei L, Yin W, Li M, Wu C, Walsh TR, Wang Y, Wang S, Wu Y.** 2017. Presence of VIM-positive *Pseudomonas* species in chickens and their surrounding environment. *Antimicrob Agents Chemother* **61:**61.

154. **Ohnishi M, Sawada T, Hirose K, Sato R, Hayashimoto M, Hata E, Yonezawa C, Kato H.** 2011. Antimicrobial susceptibilities and bacteriological characteristics of bovine *Pseudomonas aeruginosa* and *Serratia marcescens* isolates from mastitis. *Vet Microbiol* **154:**202–207.

155. **Metcalf ES.** 2001. The role of international transport of equine semen on disease transmission. *Anim Reprod Sci* **68:**229–237.

156. **Atherton JG, Pitt TL.** 1982. Types of *Pseudomonas aeruginosa* isolated from horses. *Equine Vet J* **14:**329–332.

157. **Tazumi A, Maeda Y, Buckley T, Millar B, Goldsmith C, Dooley J, Elborn J, Matsuda M, Moore J.** 2009. Molecular epidemiology of clinical isolates of *Pseudomonas aeruginosa* isolated from horses in Ireland. *Ir Vet J* **62:**456–459.

158. **Kidd TJ, Gibson JS, Moss S, Greer RM, Cobbold RN, Wright JD, Ramsay KA, Grimwood K, Bell SC.** 2011. Clonal complex *Pseudomonas aeruginosa* in horses. *Vet Microbiol* **149:**508–512.

Antimicrobial Resistance in Bacteria from Livestock and Companion Animals
Edited by Frank Møller Aarestrup, Stefan Schwarz, Jianzhong Shen, and Lina Cavaco
© 2018 American Society for Microbiology, Washington, DC
doi:10.1128/microbiolspec.ARBA-0021-2017

Antimicrobial Resistance in *Corynebacterium* spp., *Arcanobacterium* spp., and *Trueperella pyogenes*

18

Andrea T. Feßler[1] and Stefan Schwarz[1]

THE GENERA *CORYNEBACTERIUM*, *ARCANOBACTERIUM*, AND *TRUEPERELLA*

The genus *Corynebacterium* was introduced in 1896 by Lehmann and Neumann. It belongs to the family *Corynebacteriaceae* and was listed with 30 species in the "approved lists of bacterial names" from 1980 (1) including also later reclassified species. To date, the genus *Corynebacterium* includes more than 90 species (www.bacterio.net), some of which play a role as pathogens in veterinary medicine. Corynebacteria are Gram-positive, pleomorphic rods that grow as small white colonies on blood agar after 24 to 48 h of incubation (2). In veterinary medicine, *Corynebacterium pseudotuberculosis* and the *Corynebacterium renale* complex are the most widespread bacterial pathogens. *C. pseudotuberculosis* causes caseous lymphadenitis in goats and sheep; ulcerative lymphangitis in horses, cattle, and sheep; as well as mastitis in cattle (2, 3). *C. renale* is associated with urinary tract infections in ruminants and pigs (2).

The genus *Arcanobacterium* was introduced in 1982 by Collins et al. (4) and belongs to the family *Actinomycetaceae*, which includes eight species: *Arcanobacterium canis*, *Arcanobacterium haemolyticum*, *Arcanobacterium hippocoleae*, *Arcanobacterium phocae*, *Arcanobacterium phocisimile*, *Arcanobacterium pinnipediorum*, *Arcanobacterium pluranimalium* (www.bacterio.net), and the recently described *Arcanobacterium wilhelmae* sp. nov. (5). Arcanobacteria are facultatively anaerobic, and their growth is enhanced by blood or serum (4).

The comparatively new genus *Trueperella* also belongs to the family *Actinomycetaceae*. In 2011, Yassin et al. (6) published a comparative chemotaxonomic and phylogenetic study of the genus *Arcanobacterium* and showed that it is not monophyletic. As a consequence, the taxonomy was revised and the new genus *Trueperella* established. It currently comprises five species—namely, *Trueperella abortisuis*, *Trueperella bernardiae*, *Trueperella bialowiezensis*, *Trueperella bonasi*, and *Trueperella pyogenes* (www.bacterio.net). Bacteria of the genus *Trueperella* are Gram-positive, pleomorphic rods that grow under facultatively anaerobic conditions on blood agar and produce hemolytic colonies of 0.5 to 1 mm after 48 h (2). Among the genus *Trueperella*, *T. pyogenes* is the most important veterinary pathogen, being commonly involved in a wide variety of diseases in domestic animals, including mastitis, pneumonia, metritis, arthritis, lymphadenitis, otitis, peritonitis, pyodermatitis, endocarditis, abscesses, osteomyelitis, and urinary and genital tract infections, with bovine mastitis being the most common disease in livestock (7).

SUSCEPTIBILITY TESTING OF *CORYNEBACTERIUM*, *ARCANOBACTERIUM*, AND *TRUEPERELLA*

As outlined in reference 8, antimicrobial susceptibility testing (AST) has to follow an internationally accepted performance standard. For bacteria of animal origin, the standards of the Clinical and Laboratory Standards

[1]Institute of Microbiology and Epizootics, Centre of Infection Medicine, Department of Veterinary Medicine, Freie Universität Berlin, 14163 Berlin, Germany.

Institute (CLSI) are most frequently used worldwide. So far, there is only a standard broth microdilution method approved for "*Corynebacterium* spp. (including *Corynebacterium diptheriae*) and related coryneform genera" from humans, which is described in the human-specific CLSI document M45 (9). For isolates of "*Corynebacterium* spp. and Coryneforms" from animals, there is also only a broth microdilution method available in the recently published veterinary document VET06 (10). The "related coryneform genera" or "Coryneforms" include the genera *Arcanobacterium, Arthrobacter, Brevibacterium, Cellulomonas, Cellulosimicrobium, Dermabacter, Leifsonia, Microbacterium, Oerskovia, Rothia* (excluding *Rothia mucilaginosa*), *Trueperella,* and *Turicella* (9, 10). It should be noted that all clinical breakpoints listed for these bacteria in the aforementioned documents are from human medicine. Since pharmacological properties of antimicrobial agents may differ between humans and animals, the use of breakpoints adopted from human medicine may result in misclassifications of veterinary isolates (11). A specific method for AST of *T. pyogenes* of animal origin has been developed (12) and included in the VET06 document. Based on MIC distributions (12), breakpoints for the category "susceptible" have been proposed for penicillin, ampicillin, erythromycin, and trimethoprim-sulfamethoxazole (10).

Since studies of the susceptibility of coryneform bacteria date back to the 1960s, a variety of susceptibility testing methods and interpretive criteria has been used, making it difficult—if not impossible—to compare the results of the different studies (Table 1) (11). Another problem arises with studies that only report the classification as susceptible, intermediate, or resistant without indicating quantitative values or the interpretive criteria used. These studies were not included in the description of resistance properties given below. Moreover, an evaluation of data obtained by agar disk diffusion is not possible because no interpretive criteria for this method are available in the current CLSI documents M45 and VET06 (9, 10). Therefore, these studies have also been excluded from the analysis of the resistance properties.

RESISTANCE PROPERTIES OF *CORYNEBACTERIUM* SPP.

AST studies of *Corynebacterium* spp. are available for at least the past 50 years, but varying AST methods, test media, incubation times and conditions, as well as interpretive criteria have been used. Antimicrobial susceptibility data have been obtained by broth microdilution in six studies (13–18), with five of them

referring to a methodology approved by CLSI or its previous organization, the National Committee for Clinical Laboratory Standards (NCCLS) (Table 2) (13–15, 17, 18). One of these studies reported all 45 canine *Corynebacterium ulcerans* isolates as susceptible to 14 antimicrobial agents without giving exact MIC values (17). The same situation was seen in a study of equine *Corynebacterium pseudotuberculosis*, which described all isolates as susceptible to a panel of 16 antimicrobial agents (15). Agar dilution tests were performed in three studies, conducted by Adamson et al. (19) using Mueller-Hinton agar supplemented with 5% laked horse blood, Judson and Songer (3) using blood agar base supplemented with 3% citrated bovine blood, and Prescott and Yielding (20) using Mueller-Hinton agar supplemented with 0.001% NAD and 5% chocolatized calf blood. Moreover, Olson et al. (21) measured MICs and minimum bactericidal concentrations using the Calgary Biofilm Device. Ten studies (22–31) described the use of agar disk diffusion. Although five studies referred to NCCLS or CLSI methods (24, 28–31), to date there is no approved agar disk diffusion method for corynebacteria, resulting in a lack of approved interpretive criteria.

Resistance to β-Lactams

Rhodes et al. (18) determined a ceftiofur MIC_{90} of 2 mg/liter for equine *C. pseudotuberculosis* isolates, which the authors considered a poor choice for treatment since plasma concentrations of 2 mg/liter could not be achieved for >50% of the dosing interval using the labeled dosage. In comparison, ampicillin (MIC_{90}: 0.5 mg/liter) was considered a good choice for intravenous administration, but the abscess penetrability needs to be considered due to the low lipid solubility of ampicillin (18). For penicillin, Rhodes et al. (18) measured a MIC_{90} value of 0.25 mg/liter, which is below the plasma concentrations that can be reached via intramuscular injection for adequate duration. The current CLSI breakpoints classify isolates with MICs of 0.25 to 2 mg/liter as intermediate (10). Watts and Rossbach (13) determined MIC_{90} values for *Corynebacterium bovis* from bovine mastitis of 0.25 mg/liter (ampicillin), 4 mg/liter (oxacillin), 0.5 mg/liter (cephalothin), and 0.5 mg/liter (ceftiofur). Except for oxacillin with a slightly lower MIC_{90} of 2 mg/liter, *Corynebacterium amycolatum* isolates had the same values as the *C. bovis* isolates (13). Fernández et al. (14) investigated corynebacteria from mastitis in ewes including the species *Corynebacterium camporealensis, C. bovis, C. pseudotuberculosis, Corynebacterium pseudodiphtericum,* and *Corynebacterium mastitidis.* The penicillin MICs ranged

Table 1 Examples of different AST methods and test conditions

Method	Bacterial species	Medium	Temperature	Incubation time	Reference
Broth microdilution	*Arcanobacterium* spp., *Corynebacterium* spp., *Trueperella* spp. (except *T. pyogenes*)	Cation-adjusted Mueller-Hinton broth + 2.5 to 5% lysed horse blood	35 ± 2°C	24–48 h ambient air	9, 10
	T. pyogenes	Cation-adjusted Mueller-Hinton broth + 2.5 to 5% lysed horse blood	35 ± 2°C	20–24 h with 5% CO_2	10
	C. camporealensis, C. bovis, C. mastitidis. C. pseudotuberculosis, C. pseudodiptheriticum, T. pyogenes	Mueller-Hinton broth + 1% Tween 80	37°C	48 h	14
	T. pyogenes	Mueller-Hinton broth + TES biological buffer + lysed horse blood and 10% fetal calf serum	35–37°C	18–24 h	46
	T. pyogenes	Serum-free medium	39°C	36 h with 5% CO_2	38
	T. pyogenes	Modified chopped meat medium	37°C	24 h anaerobically	37
Agar dilution	*C. pseudotuberculosis*	Mueller-Hinton agar + 5% laked horse blood	37°C	Overnight	19
	T. pyogenes	Mueller-Hinton agar + 5% defibrinated horse blood	37°C	48 h	55
	T. pyogenes	Mueller-Hinton agar + 5% fetal calf serum	37°C	24 h with 5% CO_2	57
	C. pseudotuberculosis, T. pyogenes	Mueller-Hinton agar + 0.001% NAD + 5% chocolatized calf blood	37°C	24 or 48 h in air	20
Agar disk diffusion	*T. pyogenes*	Iso-Sensitest agar + 7% hemolyzed sheep blood	36°C	1–2 days	53
	A. haemolyticum, A. pluranimalium	Mueller-Hinton agar + 5% sheep blood	37°C	48 h (candle jar)	34, 35
	T. pyogenes	Mueller-Hinton agar with 0.5% sheep blood and 0.5% Tween 80	37°C	48 h	7
Calgary Biofilm Device	*T. pyogenes*	Columbia agar with 5% sheep blood	37°C	Overnight 5% CO_2	64
	C. ovis, T. pyogenes	Bacto tryptose blood agar plates	37°C	24 h	22
	C. renale, C. pseudotuberculosis, T. pyogenes	Tryptic soy broth + 2% fetal calf serum	37°C	24 h + 10% CO_2	21

Table 2 Corynebacterium spp. AST data determined by broth microdilution according to CLSI/NCCLS standards

Animal origin	Bacterial species	Disease	Years of isolation	Number of isolates tested	MICs (in mg/liter) of selected antimicrobial agents[a]									Reference
					PEN	AMP	ERY	CLI	TET	CHL	ENR	SXT	GEN	
Cattle	C. bovis	Mastitis		46		≤0.06–0.25	≤0.06–≥128	0.125–0.5	0.125–≥64		≤0.03–≥64			13
Cattle	C. amycolatum	Mastitis		13		≤0.06–0.25	≤0.06–≥128	0.25–≥64	0.125–32		0.06–0.25			13
Sheep	C. camporealensis	Mastitis		4	0.06		0.125		2	4			0.008–0.125	14
Sheep	C. bovis	Mastitis		4	0.05		0.06–4		1	4			0.008–0.125	14
Sheep	C. pseudotuberculosis	Mastitis		10	0.125		0.25–2		1	2			0.5	14
Sheep	C. pseudodiphtheriticum	Mastitis		13	0.5		0.06–1		0.5–8	2			0.07–0.5	14
Sheep	C. mastititis	Mastitis		14	0.06–0.5		0.06–16		1	0.03–2			0.008–0.125	14
Horses (n = 49), cattle (n = 4), sheep (n = 1)	C. pseudotuberculosis	Infections (internal, external abscesses)	2000–2003	54										15
Dogs	C. ulcerans	Throat swabs	2007–2008	45				2						17
Horses	C. pseudotuberculosis	Naturally infected	1996–2012[b]		≤0.06–4 (n = 178)	≤0.25–16 (n = 204)	≤0.12–2 (n = 146)		≤0.25–2 (n = 148)	≤0.25–4 (n = 203)	≤0.06–4 (n = 182)	≤0.25–4 (n = 203)	≤0.25–8 (n = 206)	18

[a]PEN, penicillin; AMP, ampicillin; ERY, erythromycin; CLI, clindamycin; TET, tetracycline; CHL, chloramphenicol; ENR, enrofloxacin; SXT, trimethoprim/sulfamethoxazole; GEN, gentamicin.
[b]In this study, not all isolates were tested for susceptibility to all antimicrobial agents; thus, the numbers of isolates tested are given for each antimicrobial agent.

from 0.06 to 0.5 mg/liter, resulting in C. pseudodiphteriticum and C. mastitidis isolates, with MICs of 0.5 mg/liter being classified as intermediate according to the CLSI (10, 14). The MIC values ranged from 0.03 to 8 mg/liter for amoxicillin and cephalothin, and from 8 to 16 mg/liter for ceftazidime (14).

Resistance to Macrolides and Lincosamides

In their study of equine C. pseudotuberculosis isolates, Rhodes et al. (18) determined MIC_{90} values of ≤0.25 mg/liter, ≤1 mg/liter, and ≤0.25 mg/liter for azithromycin, clarithromycin, and erythromycin, respectively. The use of macrolides for treatment was considered appropriate for Corynebacterium abscesses or lymphangitis due to the lipophilicity of the drugs (18). For C. bovis and C. amycolatum, macrolide and lincosamide MIC values are available for bovine mastitis isolates, ranging from ≤0.06 to 64 mg/liter (13). While the MIC_{90} values for erythromycin, clindamycin, and pirlimycin did not exceed 0.5 mg/liter, the MIC_{90} values for tilmicosin were ≥64 mg/liter for C. bovis and 32 mg/liter for C. amycolatum (13). In some of the isolates, Fernández et al. (14) found elevated MICs of up to 16 mg/liter and 128 mg/liter for erythromycin and lincomycin, respectively. When applying the CLSI breakpoints for erythromycin, isolates with MICs of ≥2 mg/liter are classified as resistant (10, 14).

Resistance to Tetracyclines

MIC_{90} values of 2 mg/liter for tetracycline and ≤2 mg/liter for doxycycline were determined for equine C. pseudotuberculosis isolates (18). Despite the lipophilic character of the drugs and the attainable plasma concentration, the authors recommend a treatment only for isolates with MICs of up to 0.25 mg/liter (18). Due to the different test panels used, only part of the collection from Rhodes et al. (18) (isolates from 2007 to 2012) was tested for lower doxycycline concentrations than 2 mg/liter. A MIC_{90} value of ≤0.25 mg/liter was determined for these isolates (18). For the C. bovis and C. amycolatum isolates from the strain collection investigated by Watts and Rossbach (13), tetracycline MIC_{50} values of 0.25 mg/liter were determined for both species, whereas tetracycline MIC_{90} values of 0.25 mg/liter and 16 mg/liter were seen for C. bovis and C. amycolatum, respectively. It should be noted that isolates with MICs of ≥32 mg/liter were seen in both species (13), suggesting the presence of resistant isolates (10). Fernández et al. (14) found a single Corynebacterium pseudodiphtheriticum isolate that was classified as intermediate to tetracycline when applying CLSI breakpoints (10).

Resistance to Aminoglycosides

For gentamicin, Rhodes et al. (18) found a MIC_{90} value of 2 mg/liter, while the MIC_{90} value for amikacin was 8 mg/liter. Since hydrophilic characteristics of the drugs complicate the treatment of abscesses, aminoglycosides are not a first choice for the treatment of corynebacterial infections (18). The corynebacterial isolates from mastitis in ewes had kanamycin MICs ranging from 0.06 to 16 mg/liter and gentamicin MICs from 0.008 to 0.5 mg/liter, suggesting a reduced susceptibility for kanamycin in a single C. mastitidis isolate with a kanamycin MIC of 16 mg/liter, whereas all isolates were gentamicin-susceptible when applying the CLSI breakpoints (10, 14).

Resistance to Phenicols

Equine C. pseudotuberculosis isolates had chloramphenicol MIC_{50} and MIC_{90} values of 2 mg/liter and ≤4 mg/liter, respectively (18). Among C. bovis isolates, florfenicol MIC_{50} and MIC_{90} values of 1 mg/liter and 2 mg/liter, respectively, have been detected (13). In comparison, the C. amycolatum isolates had MIC_{50} and MIC_{90} values of 32 mg/liter each for florfenicol (13). The chloramphenicol MICs of the corynebacteria from mastitis in ewes ranged from 0.03 to 4 mg/liter (14).

Resistance to Sulfonamides and Diaminopyrimidines

C. pseudotuberculosis from horses had a MIC_{90} value of 0.5/9.5 mg/liter for trimethoprim/sulfamethoxazole, and isolates with MICs of up to 4/76 mg/liter were also detected (18). According to the CLSI breakpoints, isolates with trimethoprim/sulfamethoxazole MICs of ≥4/76 mg/liter are classified as resistant (10). Fernández et al. (14) found trimethoprim MICs between 1 and 128 mg/liter, while the MICs for sulfisoxazole ranged from 0.03 to 64 mg/liter.

Resistance to Fluoroquinolones

For equine C. pseudotuberculosis isolates, the achievable plasma concentrations in horses were above the enrofloxacin MIC_{90} value of 0.25 mg/liter (18). Only 2 of the 92 isolates had MIC values of >0.5 mg/liter (18). Enrofloxacin MIC_{90} values of 0.25 mg/liter were detected for C. bovis and C. amycolatum isolates from bovine mastitis (13). For the other fluoroquinolones tested—namely, sarafloxacin, danofloxacin, and premafloxacin—the MIC_{90} values ranged from 0.015 to 0.5 mg/liter (13). Ciprofloxacin MICs of the corynebacterial isolates from ewes ranged between 0.03 and 3 mg/liter (14), indicating the presence of resistant isolates of C. camporealensis, C. bovis,

C. pseudotuberculosis, *C. pseudodiptheriticum*, and *C. mastitidis* when applying the breakpoints of the human-specific CLSI document M45 (9).

Resistance to Other Antimicrobial Agents

Vancomycin resistance could not be detected in corynebacteria from mastitis in ewes when using CLSI breakpoints (10, 14). Rifampicin resistance was not detected in corynebacteria from ewes with mastitis (14) when using the CLSI breakpoints (10). The rifampicin MIC_{90} value obtained by Rhodes et al. (18) was ≤1 mg/liter, which would also classify the respective isolates as susceptible (10).

RESISTANCE PROPERTIES OF *ARCANOBACTERIUM* SPP.

In veterinary medicine, arcanobacteria are of minor importance, and susceptibility data are limited to *A. phocae* isolates from marine mammals obtained from tissue sites with abnormal discharge or signs of inflammation (32), an odontogenic abscess from a rabbit (33), *A. pluranimalium* isolates from a dog with pyoderma (34), and *A. haemolyticum* isolates from diseased horses (35). While the study by Tyrrell and coworkers (33) used agar dilution as the AST method, the latter two studies (34, 35) used agar disk diffusion, another method currently not approved for *Arcanobacterium* spp. by the CLSI.

During 1994 to 2000, Johnson et al. (32) investigated *A. phocae* isolates from marine mammals, such as sea lions, harbor seals, elephant seals, sea otters, and a dolphin, from the central California coast and tested 18 *A. phocae* isolates for their antimicrobial susceptibility by broth microdilution. They followed document M31-A from the NCCLS. However, the breakpoints given in this document are for a variety of livestock and companion animals but not specifically for marine mammals. Consequently, the reliability of the classification of these isolates as being susceptible, intermediate, or resistant is questionable.

The *A. phocae* isolates from marine mammals were tested for their susceptibility to β-lactams including penicillin (MICs: ≤0.03 to 0.12 mg/liter), ampicillin (MICs: ≤0.25 mg/liter), amoxicillin/clavulanic acid (MICs: ≤2 mg/liter), ticarcillin/clavulanic acid (MICs: ≤8 mg/liter), oxacillin (MICs: ≤2 mg/liter), cefazolin (MICs: ≤2 mg/liter), ceftiofur (MICs: ≤0.06 to 0.5 mg/liter), and ceftizoxime (MICs: ≤0.5 to 4 mg/liter) (32). When re-evaluating the results using the clinical breakpoints for penicillin (10), the isolates would still be classified as susceptible. The erythromycin and tetracycline

MICs of all *A. phocae* isolates from marine mammals were ≤0.12 mg/liter and ≤0.5 mg/liter, respectively (32). They were classified as susceptible to erythromycin and tetracycline, which is in accordance with the current CLSI-approved breakpoints (10). Testing of the aminoglycosides amikacin and gentamicin yielded MIC values of ≤0.5 to 16 mg/liter and ≤0.25 to 4 mg/liter for the *A. phocae* isolates. All isolates were considered susceptible, based on the NCCLS breakpoints of ≤64 mg/liter for amikacin and ≤16 mg/liter for gentamicin. The recent CLSI document classifies isolates with gentamicin MICs of 8 mg/liter as intermediate and ≥16 mg/liter as resistant (10). The chloramphenicol MIC values of the *A. phocae* isolates from marine mammals ranged between ≤0.25 and 1 mg/liter, and thus, all isolates were classified as susceptible (32). The *A. phocae* isolates with MICs of ≤0.25/4.75 mg/liter were classified as susceptible to the combination trimethoprim/sulfamethoxazole (10, 32). The enrofloxacin MICs of the *A. phocae* isolates varied between ≤0.25 and 1 mg/liter (32). The rifampicin MICs were ≤0.12 mg/liter, which classified the isolates as susceptible (32). This is in accordance with the current clinical breakpoints for corynebacteria and related species (10).

RESISTANCE PROPERTIES OF *T. PYOGENES*

T. pyogenes is an important pathogen in veterinary medicine, commonly involved in various diseases of domestic animals (7). As already mentioned, the susceptibility testing method for corynebacteria and related species also includes *Trueperella* spp. (9, 10). However, a broth microdilution susceptibility testing method for *T. pyogenes* of animal origin has been developed (12) and has been included in CLSI document VET06 (10). Based on the MIC distributions shown (12), clinical breakpoints for penicillin, ampicillin, erythromycin, and trimethoprim/sulfamethoxazole have been proposed (10).

In 17 studies the antimicrobial susceptibility of *T. pyogenes* was tested using broth microdilution (12, 14, 36–50), with 14 of them referring to NCCLS or CLSI methodology (Table 3) (12, 14, 36, 40–50). Eight studies used agar dilution as the susceptibility testing method (20, 51–57), with three of them referring to NCCLS or CLSI (53, 54, 57), and in another two studies the MICs were determined by the Calgary Biofilm Device or E-test (21, 54). The agar disk diffusion method was used in 14 studies (7, 22, 58–69). Despite the lack of an accepted agar disk diffusion method and the respective interpretive criteria for *T. pyogenes*, five studies referred to CLSI or NCCLS methods (7, 63, 65, 66, 68).

Table 3 *T. pyogenes* AST data determined by broth microdilution according to CLSI/NCCLS standards

Animal origin	Disease	Years of isolation	Number of isolates tested	MICs (in mg/liter) of selected antimicrobial agents[a]										Reference
				PEN	AMP	ERY	CLI	TET	CHL	ENR	SXT	GEN	STR	
Cattle	Mastitis		1	0.125		0.5				0.25				36
Sheep	Mastitis		5	0.008–0.5		0.008–0.25		16	4			2		14
Cattle (n = 27), pigs (n = 17), dogs (n = 2), cat (n = 1), macaw (n = 1)			48		≤0.06–≥128	≤0.06–≥128	≤0.06–≥128	≤0.06–16						41
Cattle (n = 76), pigs (n = 24), birds (n = 5), dogs (n = 2), deer (n = 1), sheep (n = 1), cat (n = 1)			11			0.06–1,024								43
Cattle	Urinary, genital tract infections	2004–2006	43	≤0.015	≤0.03–0.06	≤0.015–≥64	≤0.03–≥128	0.12–64	1–2	0.25–8	≤0.015–0.25	0.25–32		12
Cattle	Umbilical cord infections, septicemia	2004–2006	35	≤0.015	≤0.03	≤0.015–≥64	≤0.03–≥128	0.12–64	1–2	0.5–1	≤0.015–0.12	0.5–2		12
Pigs	Infections of the central nervous system, musculoskeletal system	2004–2006	12	≤0.015	≤0.03	≤0.015	≤0.03–0.06	0.12–16	1–2	1	≤0.015–0.06	0.5		12
Cattle	Endometritis	2006	32	0.125–16	≤0.06–0.125	0.0625–≥32	0.125–≥32	0.5–32		0.25–1		0.25–≥32	1–≥64	44
Cattle	Infections of the uterus	2008	72	≤0.06–32	≤0.06–≥64			1–≥64	8–≥64				0.5–≥64	45
White-tailed deer	Infections of the lung	2009–2010	29	≤0.12–2	≤0.25–4		≤0.25–16			0.5–2	2			46
Cattle	Mastitis	2008–2011	55	≤0.06	≤0.06–0.125	≤0.125–≥4		≤0.5–≥8						47
Cattle	Endometritis			0.125–16	0.125–64									48
Cattle	Infections of the uterus		35	≤0.06–0.125	≤0.06–0.125		≤0.06–0.25			0.5–1				49

[a]PEN, penicillin; AMP, ampicillin; ERY, erythromycin; CLI, clindamycin; TET, tetracycline; CHL, chloramphenicol; ENR, enrofloxacin; SXT, trimethoprim/sulfamethoxazole; GEN, gentamicin; STR, steptomycin.

Resistance to β-Lactams

Using a breakpoint of ≥2 mg/liter, resistance to penicillin (MICs: 0.125 to 16 mg/liter), amoxicillin (MICs: 0.125 to 16 mg/liter), and oxacillin (MICs: 0.125 to 32 mg/liter) was determined in isolates from bovine uterine samples at dairy farms in Inner Mongolia (44). The finding of resistant isolates is in accordance with the lower CLSI breakpoints for coryneforms classifying isolates with MICs of ≤0.12 mg/liter and *T. pyogenes* with MICs of ≤0.03 mg/liter as susceptible (10). Cephalosporin resistance has been observed using the breakpoints of ≥16 mg/liter for cefazolin and 4 mg/liter for ceftiofur (44). In another study, de Boer et al. (49) found cloxacillin MICs of ≤0.06 to 4 mg/liter in *T. pyogenes* of bovine uterine samples, while the MIC values for ampicillin and ticarcillin/clavulanic acid were ≤0.013 mg/liter. For ceftiofur, the MIC values ranged between 0.25 and 4 mg/liter, while the MIC values for cefuroxime and cephapirin were ≤0.5 mg/liter (49). In a study by Santos et al. (45), *T. pyogenes* isolates from uterine secretions of postpartum dairy cows showed MIC distributions of ≤0.06 to 32 mg/liter for penicillin and amoxicillin, as well as ≤0.06 to ≥64 mg/liter for ampicillin and ceftiofur. With resistance breakpoints of ≥0.125 mg/liter for penicillin and ≥2 mg/liter for the other β-lactams tested, resistant isolates could be detected (45). Resistance would be also detected when applying the current CLSI breakpoints (10). Zastempowska and Lassa (47) described isolates from bovine mastitis being susceptible to the β-lactams, penicillin, ampicillin, ceftiofur, and cephalothin, with all isolates having MIC values of ≤1 mg/liter. For penicillin, all isolates had MICs of ≤0.06 mg/liter (47). Since the *T. pyogenes* breakpoint of penicillin or ampicillin is ≤0.03 mg/liter, isolates with a MIC of 0.06 mg/liter may be misclassified (10). MICs of up to 0.12 mg/liter result in the detection of ampicillin resistance (10).

In the German BfT-GermVet study, *T. pyogenes* isolates from bovine infections of the umbilical cord and the urinary and genital tract and septicemia, as well as porcine infections of the central nervous system and the musculoskeletal system revealed MIC$_{90}$ values of ≤0.015 to 0.5 mg/liter for the β-lactams tested (penicillin, ampicillin, oxacillin, amoxicillin/clavulanic acid, cephalothin, cefazolin, cefoperazone, ceftiofur, and cefquinome) (12). Tell et al. (46) identified *T. pyogenes* isolates from white-tailed deer with MICs of ≥0.5 mg/liter and ≥0.25 mg/liter as being resistant to ampicillin and penicillin, respectively, while resistance to ceftiofur was not detected (MICs: ≤1 mg/liter). Using the CLSI-proposed penicillin breakpoint (10) resistance would be seen among *T. pyogenes* from ewe's mastitis (14). The amoxicillin MIC was 0.25 mg/liter, while the MICs for ceftazidime and cephalothin were 8 mg/liter (14). A single *T. pyogenes* isolate from dairy heifers had MICs of 0.125 mg/liter, 0.5 mg/liter, 0.5 mg/liter, and 1 mg/liter for penicillin, cloxacillin, cefapirin, and ceftiofur, respectively (36). Applying CLSI breakpoints for penicillin would result in the classification as susceptible using the breakpoint for the coryneforms, but as resistant using the *T. pyogenes* breakpoints (10). Zhang et al. (48) found high MIC values of up to 64 mg/liter for ampicillin, up to 32 mg/liter for ceftiofur and oxacillin, and up to 16 mg/liter for penicillin, amoxicillin, and cefazolin in isolates from cattle with endometritis. Testing bovine *T. pyogenes* from mastitis samples in China identified isolates that were resistant to penicillin (MIC: ≥0.25 mg/liter), ampicillin (MIC: ≥0.5 mg/liter), and cefaclor (MIC: ≥32 mg/liter) (10, 50). Zhao et al. (57) investigated *T. pyogenes* isolates from forest musk deer by agar dilution and found 16 isolates that were resistant to cefazolin and 17 resistant to cefotaxime, based on a breakpoint of 16 mg/liter for both substances. The β-lactam resistance gene *blaP1* has been detected in only eight of the resistant isolates (57).

Resistance to Macrolides and Lincosamides

In *T. pyogenes* from bovine uterine samples, de Boer et al. (49) determined clindamycin MIC values of ≤0.25 mg/liter, which classify the isolates as susceptible according to the breakpoints for the coryneforms (susceptible: ≤0.5 mg/liter), whereas it cannot be interpreted by using breakpoints for *T. pyogenes* due to the lack of interpretive criteria for lincosamides (10). Liu et al. (44) found all bovine metritis and endometritis isolates from dairy farms in Inner Mongolia to be susceptible to tilmicosin (MICs: 0.25 mg/liter) and azithromycin (MICs: 0.5 to 2 mg/liter) using ≥2 mg/liter and ≥8 mg/liter as breakpoints for the two macrolides, respectively. Resistance to erythromycin (MICs: 0.0625 to 32 mg/liter) and clindamycin (MICs: 0.125 to 32 mg/liter) was seen when using 1 mg/liter and ≥2 mg/liter as breakpoints, respectively (44). Resistance to clindamycin (resistance breakpoint ≥4 mg/liter) was detected in isolates from white-tailed deer investigated by Tell et al. (46). The detection of erythromycin and clindamycin resistance in the latter two studies is in accordance with the current CLSI breakpoints (10). *T. pyogenes* isolates were classified as intermediate to tulathromycin (MIC: 64 mg/liter) and either resistant (MIC: ≥32 mg/liter) or intermediate (MIC: 16 mg/liter) to tilmicosin (46). The tylosin MICs of the corresponding isolates ranged from 0.5 to 64 mg/liter (46). AST of 48 *T. pyogenes* isolates of bovine and porcine origin revealed MIC_{50} and MIC_{90} values for erythromycin, tylosin, and clindamycin of ≤0.06 and ≥64 mg/liter, respectively, resulting in resistant isolates for all three antimicrobial agents, when using 8 mg/liter as the resistance breakpoint (41).

Induction tests were performed for isolates with erythromycin MICs of 1 to 8 mg/liter, and inducible macrolide/lincosamide resistance was seen in all isolates tested (41). Three isolates with tylosin MICs of 0.5 to 8 mg/liter were tested, and two showed an inducible phenotype, while the single isolate with a clindamycin MIC of 8 mg/liter was noninducible as confirmed by its tylosin and clindamycin MICs (41). While resistance to erythromycin, tylosin, and clindamycin might point towards a resistance mechanism due to a macrolide-, lincosamide-, and streptogramin B resistance gene, the single noninducible strain had an erythromycin MIC of ≥64 mg/liter and might be resistant via a different mechanism (41). Fernández et al. (14) found erythromycin MICs of 0.008 to 0.25 mg/liter, which indicates the presence of nonsusceptible isolates when using the CLSI-proposed breakpoint for *T. pyogenes* of ≤0.03 mg/liter (10). The lincomycin MICs were up to 16 mg/liter (14). Watts et al. (36) found an erythromycin MIC of 0.5 mg/liter for the bovine mastitis isolate, which would classify it as susceptible by the breakpoints for coryneforms but as nonsusceptible by the *T. pyogenes* breakpoints (10). The corresponding pirlimycin MIC was 0.25 mg/liter (36). In bovine *T. pyogenes* isolates from China, resistance to azithromycin (MICs: ≥8 mg/liter), erythromycin (MICs: ≥8 mg/liter), and clindamycin (MICs: ≥4 mg/liter) was detected (50).

Jost et al. (43) investigated *T. pyogenes* isolates for the genetic basis of tylosin resistance. In total, 10 of the 32 resistant isolates carried the *erm*(B) gene. Among the *erm*(B)-carrying isolates, no inducible resistance was detected, but five bovine strains already had MICs of $\geq2,048$ mg/liter without induction, and therefore a possible increase of the MICs might not be detectable (43). The constitutive expression of *erm*(B) in porcine strains with a MIC of 128 mg/liter is in accordance with the missing leader peptide being involved in inducible resistance (43). Differences of the MIC values of bovine and porcine isolates might be due to an additional resistance determinant present in the bovine strains, which could be confirmed by the preparation of *erm*(B) knockout mutants of one of the bovine strains, which showed an increase of the tylosin MICs from ≤0.06 to $\geq2,048$ mg/liter after tylosin induction (43). Jost et al. (42) found tylosin-resistant (MICs: ≥64 mg/liter) *T. pyogenes* harboring the resistance gene *erm*(X),

showing also elevated MICs for erythromycin, oleandomycin, spiramycin, clindamycin, and lincomycin. This finding indicates that the *erm*(X) gene confers a macrolide-lincosamide-streptogramin B phenotype (42). The *erm*(X) gene on plasmid pAP2 (AY255627) was colocated with the tetracycline resistance gene *tet*(33) (42). An inducible phenotype was detected for all but one of the *erm*(X)-carrying isolates, while for the remaining isolate the MIC was above the detection limit (42). Seven isolates with tylosin MICs of 128 to 1,024 mg/liter showed MICs of $\geq2,048$ mg/liter after induction, whereas the remaining two isolates with MICs of 2 mg/liter and 8 mg/liter showed MIC values of 128 mg/liter after induction (42). The finding of the different MIC values of the *erm*(X)-carrying isolates might be due to the presence of additional macrolide resistance determinants or differences in the plasmid copy numbers (42). Cloning of the *erm*(X) gene in the vector pEP2 in the *T. pyogenes* strain BBR1 revealed an increase of the tylosin MIC from ≤0.06 mg/liter for the empty vector to 64 mg/liter for the vector carrying *erm*(X) (42).

The *T. pyogenes erm*(X) gene had significant identity with the *erm*(X) genes of *C. diptheriae* (97.7%), *Corynebacterium striatum* (97.5%), *Corynebacterium jeikeium* (94.7%), and *Propionibacterium acnes* (97.5%) (42). Moreover, the *erm*(X) gene was also detected in 23 of the 32 *T. pyogenes* isolates in a subsequent study by Jost et al. (43). In another study, Jost et al. (70) found *T. pyogenes* isolates with high MICs for erythromycin (>64 mg/liter), oleandomycin (>64 mg/liter), and spiramycin (≥8 mg/liter) and differences in the resistance properties regarding tylosin and clindamycin. These isolates [negative for the *erm*(B) and *erm*(X) genes] were investigated for mutations in the 23S rRNA gene, which are known to mediate resistance to different macrolides (70). One strain had the 23S rRNA mutation A2058T; it was considered clindamycin-resistant because of its MIC of 8 mg/liter but had a tylosin MIC of only 0.5 mg/liter (70). Tylosin and clindamycin MICs of 8 mg/liter were seen in an isolate with the 23S rRNA mutations A2058T and G2137C (70). The 23S rRNA mutation A2058G was seen in an isolate with high-level clindamycin resistance (MIC: >64 mg/liter) and a tylosin MIC of 0.25 mg/liter, while the 23S rRNA mutation C2611G was found in an isolate with low MICs for tylosin (0.125 mg/liter) and clindamycin (1 mg/liter) (70). In the BfT-GermVet study the MIC values for erythromycin (≤0.016 to ≥64 mg/liter), tilmicosin (≤0.03 to ≥128 mg/liter), spiramycin (≤0.06 to ≥256 mg/liter), tulathromycin (0.06 to ≥128 mg/liter), and clindamycin (≤0.03 to ≥128 mg/liter) included a wide range of dilution steps (12), and identified erythromycin- and clindamycin-resistant isolates (10). In total, six isolates with erythromycin MICs of ≥64 mg/liter were positive for the *erm*(X) gene (12). The resistance genes *erm*(X) and *erm*(B) were also detected in *T. pyogenes* from bovine mastitis (47).

Resistance to Tetracyclines

Resistance to tetracyclines was observed in bovine isolates from uterine samples, including resistance to oxytetracycline (breakpoint ≥64 mg/liter), tetracycline (breakpoint ≥4 mg/liter), and doxycycline (breakpoint ≥8 mg/liter) (44). However, the CLSI breakpoints for tetracycline and doxycycline classify isolates with ≤4 mg/liter as susceptible and those with 8 mg/liter as intermediate (10). Tell et al. (46) classified isolates from white-tailed deer as resistant (MIC: ≥8 mg/liter) or intermediate (MIC: 4 mg/liter) to oxytetracycline and chlortetracycline. In a study by de Boer et al. (49), two bovine uterine *T. pyogenes* isolates revealed elevated oxytetracycline MICs of 16 mg/liter and 128 mg/liter, respectively. MIC ranges of 1 to ≥64 mg/liter for tetracycline and 0.125 to ≥64 mg/liter for oxytetracycline were detected in bovine uterine isolates, suggesting the presence of resistant isolates (10, 45). Tetracycline MICs of 16 mg/liter were seen in *T. pyogenes* from ewes with mastitis (14). Among the isolates from the BfT-GermVet study, tetracycline MIC_{90} values of 32 mg/liter and 16 mg/liter were observed for the bovine and porcine isolates, respectively (10, 12). Tetracycline resistance was detected in 70% of the bovine mastitis isolates from four farms in China when using a breakpoint of ≥16 mg/liter (10, 50).

Billington et al. (40) investigated tetracycline-resistant isolates from pigs, cattle, and a macaw for the genetic basis of the resistance and found the *tet*(W) gene in a bovine strain. This *tet*(W) gene had 92% sequence identity to *tet*(W) from *Butyrivibrio fibrisolvens* (40). Despite the detection of sequences similar to those involved in the regulation of *tet*(M) in transposon Tn*916*, an induction of *tet*(W) was not seen in the *T. pyogenes* isolates tested (40). The tetracycline-resistant isolates, as well as tetracycline-susceptible control isolates, were tested for the presence of the *tet*(W) gene via dot blot and a specific PCR assay, confirming the presence of this gene in all resistant isolates, while it was not seen in the susceptible ones (40). Trinh et al. (41) found *T. pyogenes* MIC_{90} values of 8 mg/liter for chlortetracycline and oxytetracycline, while the MIC_{90} for tetracycline was 16 mg/liter. Using 4 mg/liter as the breakpoint, a resistance rate of 41.7% was seen for all three substances, with the same 20 isolates being

classified as resistant and carrying the *tet*(W) gene (41). However, the resistance breakpoint in the most recent CLSI document is ≥16 mg/liter (10). Isolates with MICs in the range of 0.5 to 8 mg/liter were tested for an inducible phenotype, which was not present in any of the isolates (41). Jost et al. (42) detected the tetracycline resistance gene *tet*(33) colocated with the *erm*(X) gene on plasmid pAP2. The *tet*(33) gene was detected in 55.6% of the *erm*(X)-carrying isolates but in only 5.1% of the *erm*(X)-negative isolates (42). The *tet*(33) gene conferred tetracycline MICs of 1 mg/liter, compared to ≤0.06 mg/liter for susceptible strains (42). In contrast to the tetracycline resistance gene *tet*(W), which confers tetracycline MICs of up to 8 mg/liter, *tet*(33) apparently only confers low-level resistance, whereas the presence of both genes resulted in a MIC value of up to 16 mg/liter (42). Zastempowska and Lassa (47) found the *tet*(W) gene in all bovine *T. pyogenes* isolates that showed a tetracycline MIC of at least 4 mg/liter. In her study, Alešík (71) investigated the tetracycline susceptibility of *T. pyogenes* isolates and found 36 isolates with tetracycline MICs of ≥8 mg/liter. The resistance gene *tet*(W) was detected alone or in combination with *tet*(33) (71). Moreover, the *tet*(Z) gene, present in a single isolate, has been described for the first time in *T. pyogenes* (71) but was previously detected in *Corynebacterium glutamicum* (72).

Resistance to Aminoglycosides

Among the *T. pyogenes* isolates from ewes with mastitis, gentamicin MICs of 2 mg/liter were determined, while the kanamycin MICs ranged from 0.5 to 8 mg/liter (14). Gentamicin resistance in *T. pyogenes* isolates from bovine mastitis was detected when applying a breakpoint of ≥16 mg/liter (10, 50). Isolates from white-tailed deer with a MIC of 8 mg/liter were classified as intermediate to gentamicin (10, 46), while all isolates were susceptible to spectinomcin (MIC: ≤16 mg/liter) (46). The neomycin MIC distribution ranged from 4 to 32 mg/liter (46). Testing of *T. pyogenes* from the BfT-GermVet study for gentamicin, neomycin, and spectinomycin resulted in MIC_{90} values of 1 mg/liter, 4 mg/liter, and 4 mg/liter for the bovine and 0.5 mg/liter, 8 mg/liter, and 1 mg/liter for the porcine isolates, respectively (12). A single bovine isolate with a MIC of 32 mg/liter was classified as gentamicin-resistant (10, 12). The streptomycin susceptibility testing of bovine uterine isolates revealed a MIC_{90} of 16 mg/liter (45). For spectinomycin, a MIC_{90} value of ≥64 mg/liter was determined (45).

Zhao et al. (57) detected kanamycin and amikacin resistance in isolates from forest musk deer by agar dilution, using a breakpoint of 16 mg/liter for both substances. Gentamicin resistance based on a breakpoint of 2 mg/liter, which is below the resistance breakpoint from the CLSI ($\geq$16 mg/liter) (10). Aminoglycoside resistance was observed in 17 isolates (60.7%), while the total detection rate for the resistance genes *aacC*, *aadA1*, and *aadA2* was 57.1% (57). Liu et al. (44) found MICs of up to $\geq$64 mg/liter for streptomycin, 0.25 to $\geq$32 mg/liter for gentamicin, and 0.5 to $\geq$64 mg/liter for amikacin in isolates from bovine metritis and endometritis. Investigations of the genetic basis of aminoglycoside resistance identified gene cassettes with the resistance genes *aadA1*, *aadA5*, *aadA24*, and *aadB* (44).

Resistance to Phenicols

High MIC_{90} values of $\geq$64 mg/liter for chloramphenicol and 32 mg/liter for florfenicol were detected in *T. pyogenes* from bovine uterine samples (45). Resistant isolates were detected when using $\geq$8 mg/liter as the breakpoint (45). Among the isolates from the BfT-GermVet study, the MIC_{90} values for chloramphenicol and florfenicol were 2 mg/liter and 1 mg/liter for the bovine isolates and 1 mg/liter and 1 mg/liter for the porcine isolates, respectively (12). Fernández et al. (14) found chloramphenicol MICs of 4 mg/liter in ovine *T. pyogenes* isolates. Florfenicol resistance was detected in three bovine uterine isolates based on a breakpoint of 8 mg/liter, and the phenicol resistance gene *cmlA6* was detected (44).

Resistance to Sulfonamides and Diaminopyrimidines

In the BfT-GermVet study, bovine isolates were found to be resistant to sulfamethoxazole based on human breakpoints ($\geq$512 mg/liter), while all porcine isolates were classified as susceptible (12). In comparison, all bovine and porcine isolates had MICs of $\leq$0.12/2.38 to trimethoprim/sulfamethoxazole (12), which classifies them as susceptible by using the *T. pyogenes* breakpoint of $\leq$0.12/2.38 mg/liter (10). Liu et al. (44) classified all *T. pyogenes* isolates in their study as resistant to sulfadiazine and sulfamethoxydiazine, since the MIC_{50} and MIC_{90} values were $\geq$128 mg/liter for both substances. Zastempowska and Lassa (47) found that all bovine mastitis isolates in their collection also had sulfadimethoxine MICs of $\geq$128 mg/liter. Tell et al. (46) found all isolates with MICs of 2/38 mg/liter to trimethoprim/sulfamethoxazole and classified them as susceptible. Fernández et al. (14) tested trimethoprim and sulfisoxazole as separate compounds, resulting in MICs of 0.5 mg/liter and 64 mg/liter, respectively. Resistance to trimethoprim/sulfamethoxazole was seen

in 90% of the *T. pyogenes* isolates from four Chinese dairy farms, with MICs of $\geq$4/76 mg/liter (10, 50).

Trimethoprim resistance was detected by agar dilution in 46.4% of the *T. pyogenes* isolates from forest musk deer, using 16 mg/liter as breakpoint; the resistance gene *dfrB2a* was detected in only 28.6% of the isolates (57). This suggests the presence of another resistance determinant in these isolates.

Resistance to Fluoroquinolones

The enrofloxacin MICs obtained for *T. pyogenes* isolates from bovine uterine samples were 0.5 mg/liter or 1 mg/liter (49). Tell et al. (46) found all isolates from white-tailed deer to be resistant to danofloxacin (MICs: 0.5 mg/liter and 1 mg/liter) and resistant (MIC: 2 mg/liter) or intermediate (MICs: 0.5 mg/liter and 1 mg/liter) to enrofloxacin. Liu et al. (44) reported *T. pyogenes* from bovine metritis and endometritis exhibiting MIC_{90} values of 2 mg/liter, 2 mg/liter, 1 mg/liter, and 0.5 mg/liter to ciprofloxacin, ofloxacin, enrofloxacin, and gatifloxacin, respectively. For the first two substances, $\geq$16 mg/liter and for the latter two, $\geq$4 mg/liter were used as resistance breakpoints (44). Ciprofloxacin MICs of 2 mg/liter were seen in ovine mastitis isolates (14). The human-specific ciprofloxacin breakpoints available for coryneforms would classify isolates with MICs of 2 mg/liter as intermediate (9). A bovine mastitis isolate showed an enrofloxacin MIC of 0.25 mg/liter (36). Werckenthin et al. (12) described an enrofloxacin MIC_{90} of 1 mg/liter for both the bovine and the porcine *T. pyogenes* isolates from the BfT-GermVet study. Resistance to fluoroquinolones was detected among isolates with ciprofloxacin MICs of $\geq$4 mg/liter and enrofloxacin MICs of $\geq$1 mg/liter (50).

Resistance to Other Antimicrobial Agents

Rifampicin MICs of up to 2 mg/liter were seen in ovine *T. pyogenes* isolates (14). In the study conducted by Alkasir et al. (50), resistance to rifampicin has been detected in only two of the 50 bovine mastitis isolates. These isolates had MICs of $\geq$4 mg/liter, which is in accordance with the CLSI breakpoints for coryneform bacteria (10). Liu et al. (44) found all bovine *T. pyogenes* isolates from metritis and endometritis to be resistant to Zn-bacitracin, with MICs of $\geq$32 mg/liter. Fernández et al. (14) found vancomycin MICs of 0.5 mg/liter in isolates from ewes with mastitis, which would be classified as susceptible according to the CLSI breakpoint of $\leq$2 mg/liter for coryneform bacteria (10). Tell et al. (46) found all isolates from white-tailed deer to be susceptible to tiamulin (MIC: $\leq$2 mg/liter). A novobiocin MIC of 0.25 mg/liter was determined by Watts et al. (36).

Zastempowska and Lassa (47) reported that all 55 bovine mastitis isolates had MICs of 0.5 to 1 mg/liter for the combination of penicillin and novobiocin. The colistin MIC_{90} value of ≥ 64 mg/liter detected among all bovine and porcine *T. pyogenes* isolates (12) confirmed that colistin is not active against Gram-positive bacteria.

CONCLUDING REMARKS

This article has provided an overview of the antimicrobial susceptibility of *Corynebacterium* spp., *Arcanobacterium* spp., and *T. pyogenes*. However, the interpretation and comparability of the results is hampered by the use of different AST methods and test parameters. As described, agar disk diffusion, agar dilution, and broth microdilution using different media, supplements, incubation times, and incubation temperatures have been applied for these bacteria (Table 1). In recent years, the CLSI has provided major improvements with regard to the harmonization of AST of bacteria of the genera *Corynebacterium*, *Arcanobacterium*, and *Trueperella* by approving and publishing standard broth dilution methods accompanied by clinical breakpoints for *Corynebacterium* spp. and related coryneform genera/coryneforms (9, 10), as well as an additional method with differenttest conditions for *T. pyogenes* (10). For the *T. pyogenes* AST method, which requires a CO_2 atmosphere for incubation, only a few breakpoints are available, with the ones for penicillin, erythromycin, and trimethoprim/sulfamethoxazole differing from those for the coryneform bacteria (10). Moreover, there is a gap of knowledge with regard to the genetic basis of antimicrobial resistance in *Corynebacterium* spp., *Arcanobacterium* spp., and *T. pyogenes*. Expanded studies have been conducted on macrolide/lincosamide- and tetracycline resistance genes in *T. pyogenes*, while reports of genes and mutations accounting for other resistance properties are rare.

Acknowledgments. We thank PD Dr. Christiane Werckenthin for critical reading of the manuscript and many helpful comments.

Citation. Feßler AT, Schwarz S. 2017. Antimicrobial resistance in *Corynebacterium* spp., *Arcanobacterium* spp., and *Trueperella pyogenes*. Microbiol Spectrum 5(6):ARBA-0021-2017.

References

1. Skerman VBD, McGowan V, Sneath PHA. 1980. Approved lists of bacterial names. *Int J Syst Evol Microbiol* 30:225–420.

2. Markey B, Leonard F, Archambault M, Cullinane A, Maguire D. 2013. *Clinical Veterinary Microbiology*, 2nd ed. Mosby Elsevier, Edinburgh, United Kingdom.

3. Judson R, Songer JG. 1991. *Corynebacterium pseudotuberculosis*: *in vitro* susceptibility to 39 antimicrobial agents. *Vet Microbiol* 27:145–150.

4. Collins MD, Jones D, Schofield GM. 1982. Reclassification of 'Corynebacterium haemolyticum' (MacLean, Liebow & Rosenberg) in the genus *Arcanobacterium* gen. nov. as *Arcanobacterium haemolyticum* nom.rev., comb. nov. *J Gen Microbiol* 128:1279–1281.

5. Sammra O, Rau J, Wickhorst JP, Alssahen M, Hassan AA, Lämmler C, Kämpfer P, Glaeser SP, Busse HJ, Kleinhagauer T, Knauf-Witzens T, Prenger-Berninghoff E, Abdulmawjood A, Klein G. 2017. *Arcanobacterium wilhelmae* sp. nov., isolated from the genital tract of a rhinoceros (*Rhinoceros unicornis*). *Int J Syst Evol Microbiol* 67:2093–2097.

6. Yassin AF, Hupfer H, Siering C, Schumann P. 2011. Comparative chemotaxonomic and phylogenetic studies on the genus *Arcanobacterium* Collins et al. 1982 emend. Lehnen et al. 2006: proposal for *Trueperella* gen. nov. and emended description of the genus *Arcanobacterium*. *Int J Syst Evol Microbiol* 61:1265–1274.

7. Ribeiro MG, Risseti RM, Bolaños CA, Caffaro KA, de Morais AC, Lara GH, Zamprogna TO, Paes AC, Listoni FJ, Franco MM. 2015. *Trueperella pyogenes* multispecies infections in domestic animals: a retrospective study of 144 cases (2002 to 2012). *Vet Q* 35:82–87.

8. Watts JL, Sweeney MT, Lubbers BV. 2017. Antimicrobial susceptibility testing of bacteria of veterinary origin. *In* Aarestrup FM, Cavaco L, Schwarz S, Shen Y (ed), *Antimicrobial Resistance in Bacteria from Livestock and Companion Animals*. ASM Press, Washington, DC.

9. CLSI. 2016. Methods for antimicrobial dilution and disk susceptibility testing of infrequently isolated or fastidious bacteria, 3rd ed. CLSI guideline M45. Clinical and Laboratory Standards Institute, Wayne, PA.

10. CLSI. 2017. Methods for antimicrobial susceptibility testing of infrequently isolated or fastidious bacteria isolated from animals. CLSI supplement VET06. Clinical and Laboratory Standards Institute, Wayne, PA.

11. Schwarz S, Silley P, Simjee S, Woodford N, van Duijkeren E, Johnson AP, Gaastra W. 2010. Assessing the antimicrobial susceptibility of bacteria obtained from animals. *Vet Microbiol* 141:1–4.

12. Werckenthin C, Alesík E, Grobbel M, Lübke-Becker A, Schwarz S, Wieler LH, Wallmann J. 2007. Antimicrobial susceptibility of *Pseudomonas aeruginosa* from dogs and cats as well as *Arcanobacterium pyogenes* from cattle and swine as determined in the BfT-GermVet monitoring program 2004–2006. *Berl Munch Tierarztl Wochenschr* 120:412–422.

13. Watts JL, Rossbach S. 2000. Susceptibilities of *Corynebacterium bovis* and *Corynebacterium amylocolatum* isolates from bovine mammary glands to 15 antimicrobial agents. *Antimicrob Agents Chemother* 44:3476–3477.

14. Fernández EP, Vela AI, Las Heras A, Domínguez L, Fernández-Garayzábal JF, Moreno MA. 2001. Antimicrobial susceptibility of corynebacteria isolated from ewe's mastitis. *Int J Antimicrob Agents* 18:571–574.

15. Foley JE, Spier SJ, Mihalyi J, Drazenovich N, Leutenegger CM. 2004. Molecular epidemiologic features of *Corynebacterium pseudotuberculosis* isolated from horses. *Am J Vet Res* 65:1734–1737.

16. Bailiff NL, Westropp JL, Jang SS, Ling GV. 2005. *Corynebacterium urealyticum* urinary tract infection in dogs and cats: 7 cases (1996–2003). *J Am Vet Med Assoc* 226: 1676–1680.

17. Katsukawa C, Komiya T, Yamagishi H, Ishii A, Nishino S, Nagahama S, Iwaki M, Yamamoto A, Takahashi M. 2012. Prevalence of *Corynebacterium ulcerans* in dogs in Osaka, Japan. *J Med Microbiol* 61:266–273.

18. Rhodes DM, Magdesian KG, Byrne BA, Kass PH, Edman J, Spier SJ. 2015. Minimum inhibitory concentrations of equine *Corynebacterium pseudotuberculosis* isolates (1996–2012). *J Vet Intern Med* 29:327–332.

19. Adamson PJ, Wilson WD, Hirsh DC, Baggot JD, Martin LD. 1985. Susceptibility of equine bacterial isolates to antimicrobial agents. *Am J Vet Res* 46:447–450.

20. Prescott JF, Yielding KM. 1990. *In vitro* susceptibility of selected veterinary bacterial pathogens to ciprofloxacin, enrofloxacin and norfloxacin. *Can J Vet Res* 54: 195–197.

21. Olson ME, Ceri H, Morck DW, Buret AG, Read RR. 2002. Biofilm bacteria: formation and comparative susceptibility to antibiotics. *Can J Vet Res* 66:86–92.

22. Farrag H, Oof F. 1967. Sensitivity of organisms isolated from cases of bovine and goat mastitis to various antibiotics. *Indian Vet J* 44:640–646.

23. Wilkins RJ, Helland DR. 1973. Antibacterial sensitivities of bacteria isolated from dogs with tracheobronchitis. *J Am Vet Med Assoc* 162:47–50.

24. Swartz R, Jooste PJ, Novello JC. 1984. Antibiotic susceptibility patterns of mastitis pathogens isolated from Bloemfontein dairy herds. *J S Afr Vet Assoc* 55:187–193.

25. Gomez A, Nombela C, Zapardiel J, Soriano F. 1995. An encrusted cystitis caused by *Corynebacterium urealyticum* in a dog. *Aust Vet J* 72:72–73.

26. Guedeja-Marrón J, Blanco JL, Ruperez C, Garcia ME. 1998. Susceptibility of bacterial isolates from chronic canine otitis externa to twenty antibiotics. *Zentralbl Veterinarmed B* 45:507–512.

27. Lin CT, Petersen-Jones SM. 2007. Antibiotic susceptibility of bacterial isolates from corneal ulcers of dogs in Taiwan. *J Small Anim Pract* 48:271–274.

28. Aalbæk B, Bemis DA, Schjærff M, Kania SA, Frank LA, Guardabassi L. 2010. Coryneform bacteria associated with canine otitis externa. *Vet Microbiol* 145:292–298.

29. Kireçci E, Ozkanlar Y, Aktas MS, Uyanik MH, Yazgi H. 2010. Isolation of pathogenic aerobic bacteria from the blood of septicaemic neonatal calves and the susceptibility of isolates to various antibiotics. *J S Afr Vet Assoc* 81: 110–113.

30. Henneveld K, Rosychuk RA, Olea-Popelka FJ, Hyatt DR, Zabel S. 2012. *Corynebacterium* spp. in dogs and cats with otitis externa and/or media: a retrospective study. *J Am Anim Hosp Assoc* 48:320–326.

31. Oliveira M, Barroco C, Mottola C, Santos R, Lemsaddek A, Tavares L, Semedo-Lemsaddek T. 2014. First report

of *Corynebacterium pseudotuberculosis* from caseous lymphadenitis lesions in Black Alentejano pig (*Sus scrofa domesticus*). *BMC Vet Res* 10:218.

32. Johnson SP, Jang S, Gulland FM, Miller MA, Casper DR, Lawrence J, Herrera J. 2003. Characterization and clinical manifestations of *Arcanobacterium phocae* infections in marine mammals stranded along the central California coast. *J Wildl Dis* 39:136–144.

33. Tyrrell KL, Citron DM, Jenkins JR, Goldstein EJ. 2002. Periodontal bacteria in rabbit mandibular and maxillary abscesses. *J Clin Microbiol* 40:1044–1047.

34. Ülbegi-Mohyla H, Hassan AA, Alber J, Lämmler C, Prenger-Berninghoff E, Weiss R, Zschöck M. 2010. Identification of *Arcanobacterium pluranimalium* isolated from a dog by phenotypic properties and by PCR mediated characterization of various molecular targets. *Vet Microbiol* 142:458–460.

35. Hassan AA, Ülbegi-Mohyla H, Kanbar T, Alber J, Lämmler C, Abdulmawjood A, Zschöck M, Weiss R. 2009. Phenotypic and genotypic characterization of *Arcanobacterium haemolyticum* isolates from infections of horses. *J Clin Microbiol* 47:124–128.

36. Watts JL, Salmon SA, Yancey RJ Jr, Nickerson SC, Weaver LJ, Holmberg C, Pankey JW, Fox LK. 1995. Antimicrobial susceptibility of microorganisms isolated from the mammary glands of dairy heifers. *J Dairy Sci* 78:1637–1648.

37. Morck DW, Olson ME, Louie TJ, Koppe A, Quinn B. 1998. Comparison of ceftiofur sodium and oxytetracycline for treatment of acute interdigital phlegmon (foot rot) in feedlot cattle. *J Am Vet Med Assoc* 212:254–257.

38. Narayanan S, Nagaraja TG, Staats J, Chengappa MM, Oberst RD. 1998. Biochemical and biological characterizations and ribotyping of *Actinomyces pyogenes* and *Actinomyces pyogenes*-like organisms from liver abscesses in cattle. *Vet Microbiol* 61:289–303.

39. Nagaraja TG, Beharka AB, Chengappa MM, Carroll LH, Raun AP, Laudert SB, Parrott JC. 1999. Bacterial flora of liver abscesses in feedlot cattle fed tylosin or no tylosin. *J Anim Sci* 77:973–978.

40. Billington SJ, Songer JG, Jost BH. 2002. Widespread distribution of a *tet* W determinant among tetracycline-resistant isolates of the animal pathogen *Arcanobacterium pyogenes*. *Antimicrob Agents Chemother* 46:1281–1287.

41. Trinh HT, Billington SJ, Field AC, Songer JG, Jost BH. 2002. Susceptibility of *Arcanobacterium pyogenes* from different sources to tetracycline, macrolide and lincosamide antimicrobial agents. *Vet Microbiol* 85:353–359.

42. Jost BH, Field AC, Trinh HT, Songer JG, Billington SJ. 2003. Tylosin resistance in *Arcanobacterium pyogenes* is encoded by an *erm* X determinant. *Antimicrob Agents Chemother* 47:3519–3524.

43. Jost BH, Trinh HT, Songer JG, Billington SJ. 2004. A second tylosin resistance determinant, Erm B, in *Arcanobacterium pyogenes*. *Antimicrob Agents Chemother* 48: 721–727.

44. Liu MC, Wu CM, Liu YC, Zhao JC, Yang YL, Shen JZ. 2009. Identification, susceptibility, and detection of integron-gene cassettes of *Arcanobacterium pyogenes* in bovine endometritis. *J Dairy Sci* 92:3659–3666.

45. Santos TM, Caixeta LS, Machado VS, Rauf AK, Gilbert RO, Bicalho RC. 2010. Antimicrobial resistance and presence of virulence factor genes in *Arcanobacterium pyogenes* isolated from the uterus of postpartum dairy cows. *Vet Microbiol* **145**:84–89.

46. Tell LA, Brooks JW, Lintner V, Matthews T, Kariyawasam S. 2011. Antimicrobial susceptibility of *Arcanobacterium pyogenes* isolated from the lungs of white-tailed deer (*Odocoileus virginianus*) with pneumonia. *J Vet Diagn Invest* **23**:1009–1013.

47. Zastempowska E, Lassa H. 2012. Genotypic characterization and evaluation of an antibiotic resistance of *Trueperella pyogenes* (*Arcanobacterium pyogenes*) isolated from milk of dairy cows with clinical mastitis. *Vet Microbiol* **161**:153–158.

48. Zhang DX, Tian K, Han LM, Wang QX, Liu YC, Tian CL, Liu MC. 2014. Resistance to β-lactam antibiotic may influence *nanH* gene expression in *Trueperella pyogenes* isolated from bovine endometritis. *Microb Pathog* **71-72**:20–24.

49. de Boer M, Heuer C, Hussein H, McDougall S. 2015. Minimum inhibitory concentrations of selected antimicrobials against *Escherichia coli* and *Trueperella pyogenes* of bovine uterine origin. *J Dairy Sci* **98**:4427–4438.

50. Alkasir R, Wang J, Gao J, Ali T, Zhang L, Szenci O, Bajcsy ÁC, Han B. 2016. Properties and antimicrobial susceptibility of *Trueperella pyogenes* isolated from bovine mastitis in China. *Acta Vet Hung* **64**:1–12.

51. Guérin-Faublée V, Flandrois JP, Broye E, Tupin F, Richard Y. 1993. *Actinomyces pyogenes*: susceptibility of 103 clinical animal isolates to 22 antimicrobial agents. *Vet Res* **24**:251–259.

52. Cohen RO, Bernstein M, Ziv G. 1995. Isolation and anti-microbial susceptibility of *Actinomyces pyogenes* re-covered from the uterus of dairy cows with retained fetal membranes and post parturient endometritis. *Theriogenology* **43**:1389–1397.

53. Jousimies-Somer H, Pyörälä S, Kanervo A. 1996. Susceptibilities of bovine summer mastitis bacteria to antimicrobial agents. *Antimicrob Agents Chemother* **40**:157–160.

54. Chirino-Trejo M, Woodbury MR, Huang F. 2003. Antibiotic sensitivity and biochemical characterization of *Fusobacterium* spp. and *Arcanobacterium pyogenes* isolated from farmed white-tailed deer (*Odocoileus virginianus*) with necrobacillosis. *J Zoo Wildl Med* **34**:262–268.

55. Yoshimura H, Kojima A, Ishimaru M. 2000. Antimicrobial susceptibility of *Arcanobacterium pyogenes* isolated from cattle and pigs. *J Vet Med B Infect Dis Vet Public Health* **47**:139–143.

56. Sheldon IM, Bushnell M, Montgomery J, Rycroft AN. 2004. Minimum inhibitory concentrations of some antimicrobial drugs against bacteria causing uterine infections in cattle. *Vet Rec* **155**:383–387.

57. Zhao KL, Liu Y, Zhang XY, Palahati P, Wang HN, Yue BS. 2011. Detection and characterization of antibiotic-resistance genes in *Arcanobacterium pyogenes* strains from abscesses of forest musk deer. *J Med Microbiol* **60**:1820–1826.

58. Kunter E. 1963. Sensitivity of mastitis pathogens to antibiotics and sulfonamides and mastitis pathogens. *Mh Vet Med* **18**:88–92. (In German.)

59. Kunter E. 1975. Sensitivity of mastitis pathogens to antibiotics and chemotherapeutic agents. *Arch Exp Veterinarmed* **29**:1–32. (In German.)

60. Hariharan H, Barnum DA, Mitchell WR. 1974. Drug resistance among pathogenic bacteria from animals in Ontario. *Can J Comp Med* **38**:213–221.

61. Mohan K, Uzoukwu M. 1980. Certain characteristics of *Corynebacterium pyogenes* infection. *Vet Rec* **107**:252–253.

62. Lämmler C, Blobel H. 1988. Comparative studies on *Actinomyces pyogenes* and *Arcanobacterium haemolyticum*. *Med Microbiol Immunol (Berl)* **177**:109–114.

63. Vogel G, Nicolet J, Martig J, Tschudi P, Meylan M. 2001. Pneumonia in calves: characterization of the bacterial spectrum and the resistance patterns to antimicrobial drugs. *Schweiz Arch Tierheilkd* **143**:341–350. (In German.)

64. Martel A, Meulenaere V, Devriese LA, Decostere A, Haesebrouck F. 2003. Macrolide and lincosamide resistance in the Gram-positive nasal and tonsillar flora of pigs. *Microb Drug Resist* **9**:293–297.

65. Wettstein K, Frey J. 2004. Comparison of antimicrobial resistance pattern of selected respiratory tract pathogens isolated from different animal species. *Schweiz Arch Tierheilkd* **146**:417–422. (In German.)

66. Kidanemariam A, Gouws J, van Vuuren M, Gummow B. 2005. *In vitro* antimicrobial susceptibility of *Mycoplasma mycoides mycoides* large colony and *Arcanobacterium pyogenes* isolated from clinical cases of ulcerative balanitis and vulvitis in Dorper sheep in South Africa. *J S Afr Vet Assoc* **76**:204–208.

67. Schröder A, Hoedemaker M, Klein G. 2005. Resistance of mastitis pathogens in northern Germany. *Berl Munch Tierarztl Wochenschr* **118**:393–398. (In German.)

68. Markowska-Daniel I, Urbaniak K, Stepniewska K, Pejsak Z. 2010. Antibiotic susceptibility of bacteria isolated from respiratory tract of pigs in Poland between 2004 and 2008. *Pol J Vet Sci* **13**:29–36.

69. Brodzki P, Bochniarz M, Brodzki A, Wrona Z, Wawron W. 2014. *Trueperella pyogenes* and *Escherichia coli* as an etiological factor of endometritis in cows and the susceptibility of these bacteria to selected antibiotics. *Pol J Vet Sci* **17**:657–664.

70. Jost BH, Trinh HT, Songer JG, Billington SJ. 2004. Ribosomal mutations in *Arcanobacterium pyogenes* confer a unique spectrum of macrolide resistance. *Antimicrob Agents Chemother* **48**:1021–1023.

71. Alešík E. 2006. Antimicrobial susceptibility of *Arcanobacterium pyogenes*: Evaluation and application of a broth micro-dilution method for susceptibility testing and genotypic characterization of tetracycline resistant strains. (In German with English summary.) Thesis, Ludwig-Maximilians University, Munich, Germany.

72. Tauch A, Pühler A, Kalinowski J, Thierbach G. 2000. TetZ, a new tetracycline resistance determinant discovered in Gram-positive bacteria, shows high homology to Gram-negative regulated efflux systems. *Plasmid* **44**:285–291.

Antimicrobial Resistance in Bacteria from Livestock and Companion Animals
Edited by Frank Møller Aarestrup, Stefan Schwarz, Jianzhong Shen, and Lina Cavaco
© 2018 American Society for Microbiology, Washington, DC
doi:10.1128/microbiolspec.ARBA-0005-2017

Antimicrobial Resistance in *Stenotrophomonas* spp.

19

Yang Wang,[1] Tao He,[2] Zhangqi Shen,[1] and Congming Wu[1]

INTRODUCTION

The genus *Stenotrophomonas* comprises 16 characterized species (Table 1), and 13 validated species are included in the List of Prokaryotic names with Standing in Nomenclature (1). The first *Stenotrophomonas* species—*Stenotrophomonas maltophilia*—was isolated in 1943 from human pleural fluid. It was classified as *Bacterium bookeri* and subsequently renamed *Pseudomonas maltophilia/Xanthomonas maltophilia* (1, 2). Another 12 *Stenotrophomonas* species were first identified residing in soil, sewage, or plants. Of the remaining three species, *Stenotrophomonas* sp. D-1 and *Stenotrophomonas koreensis* were first isolated from deer fur and animal compost, respectively, and *Stenotrophomonas africana* was initially isolated from a sample of cerebrospinal fluid from a human immunodeficiency virus seropositive Rwandan refugee with primary meningoencephalitis (3). *S. maltophilia* is the most widely distributed bacterium of the *Stenotrophomonas* spp. in the environment and is isolated from soil, water, plants, animals, and humans. Moreover, the number of nosocomial infections caused by this opportunistic pathogen is increasing (4). Therefore, various studies of *Stenotrophomonas* in both animals and humans focus on the emergence, infections, treatment, and antimicrobial resistance of *S. maltophilia* as an opportunistic pathogen (4, 5). The main purpose of this article is to describe the antimicrobial resistance of *S. maltophilia* isolated from animals.

The earliest study of *S. maltophilia* reported its isolation from sources associated with rabbits, raw milk, and frozen fish in 1961 (6). It is the predominant bacterial species in swine and chicken feces (7), as well as in composted swine manure (8). *S. maltophilia* isolates have been found to coexist with influenza virus in the oral, nasal, and tracheal tissues of pigs and horses (9, 10). *S. maltophilia* is a predominant bacterial species in raw milk, milk processing plants, and milk products such as cheese (11–13) and is likely a constituent of the normal microflora of the mouth and cloacae of squirrels and captive healthy snakes (14, 15). In aquaculture, *Stenotrophomonas* spp. are predominant members of bacterial communities found in the internal organs of cultured snow crabs (*Chionoecetes*) (16) and are commonly isolated from cultured yellowtail (17), shrimp (18), and samples taken from salmon farms (19, 20).

Although *Stenotrophomonas* spp. are less frequently considered as primary pathogens, *S. maltophilia* is the major cause of the bacteriospermia in porcine or bovine semen in the United States and United Kingdom (21–23), as well as the infection of *Xenopus laevis* oocytes (24). It was also found to be associated with an outbreak of lymphadenitis in Omani goats (25) and causes fleece rot in sheep (26). Closely related *S. maltophilia* strains were isolated from an outbreak of bovine mastitis (27), which may be explained by the higher adhesion of these isolates to bovine mammary gland epithelial cells (28). *S. maltophilia* was identified as a cause of pyogranulomatous hepatitis in a female buffalo (*Bubalus bubalis*) in a herd in Serres, Greece (29), as well as the cause of necrosis and friability of the nictitating membrane of the giant panda (*Ailuropoda melanoleuca*) (30). It is also associated with chronic respiratory disease among horses, dogs, and cats (31, 32), as well as septicemia in pigs and crocodiles (33, 34). Moreover, the DNA of *S. maltophilia* is identified most frequently in the knee joints of dogs with inflammatory arthritis (35).

[1]Beijing Advanced Innovation Center for Food Nutrition and Human Health, College of Veterinary Medicine, China Agricultural University, Beijing, 100193, China; [2]Jiangsu Key Laboratory of Food Quality and Safety—State Key Laboratory Cultivation Base of MOST, Institute of Food Safety, Jiangsu Academy of Agricultural Sciences, Nanjing 210014, China.

Table 1 Characterization of *Stenotrophomonas* species

Species	Year of first identification/designation	Host when first identified	Characterization	Countries/continents	Ref.
S. maltophilia	1943	Human	*S. maltophilia*, a new bacterial genus for *X. maltophilia*, is first identified from a specimen of pleural fluid	England/Europe	99
S. africana	1997	Human	Opportunistic pathogen from cerebrospinal fluid	Rwanda/Africa	3
S. nitritireducens	2000	Ammonia-supplied biofilters	It reduced nitrite, but not nitrate, without production of nitrogen	Germany/Europe	100
S. sp. D-1	2002	Animal (deer fur)	A keratin-degrading bacterium isolated from soil containing deer fur; 16S rDNA revealed it has only 90.6% homology with *S. nitritireducens*	Japan/Asia	101
S. acidaminiphila	2002	Upflow anaerobic sludge blanket (UASB) reactor	A strictly aerobic, mesophilic bacterium isolated from UASB reactor treating a petrochemical wastewater	Burkina Faso/Africa	102
S. rhizophila	2002	Environment (plant)	Plant-associated bacterium with antifungal properties	Germany/Europe	103
S. dokdonensis	2006	Environment (soil)	The levels of 16S rDNA sequence similarity between *S. dokdonensis* and the type strains of *Stenotrophomonas* species ranged from 95.5 to 97.5%	Korea/Asia	104
S. koreensis	2006	Environment (animal compost)	A Gram-negative, rod-shaped, non-spore-forming bacterium was isolated from compost near Daejeon city	Korea/Asia	105
S. humi	2007	Environment (soil)	The nitrate-reducing bacterium was isolated from soil	Belgium/Europe	106
S. terrae	2007	Environment (soil)	The nitrate-reducing bacterium was isolated from soil	Belgium/Europe	106
S. chelatiphaga	2009	Environment (sewage)	An EDTA-utilizing gammaproteobacterial strain was isolated from municipal sewage sludge	Russia/Europe	107
S. ginsengisoli	2010	Environment (soil)	A Gram-negative, non-spore-forming, rod-shaped bacterium was isolated from soil from a ginseng field	Korea/Asia	108
S. daejeonensis	2011	Environment (sewage)	Comparative 16S rDNA analysis showed it was related most closely to *S. acidaminiphila* (97.9% similarity)	Korea/Asia	109
S. pavanii	2011	Environment (plant)	A Gram-negative, rod-shaped, non-spore-forming, and nitrogen-fixing bacterium was isolated from stems of a Brazilian sugar cane variety	Brazil/South America	110
S. tumulicola	2015	Environment (spot and gels)	A major contaminant of the stone chamber interior in blackish moldy spots and viscous gels (biofilms) collected from both tumuli	Japan/Asia	111

ANTIMICROBIAL SUSCEPTIBILITY

The susceptibility testing methods for *S. maltophilia* include disk diffusion, agar/broth dilution, commercially available microdilution strips, and microtiter panels (Table 2). Although the Clinical Laboratory Standards Institute (CLSI) has not defined breakpoints for *S. maltophilia* isolated from animals, the breakpoints for human isolates of *S. maltophilia* for sulfamethoxazole/trimethoprim (SXT), minocycline, levofloxacin, ticarcillin-clavulanic acid, ceftazidime, and chloramphenicol have been commonly adopted (36). The breakpoints for *Enterobacteriaceae* and *Pseudomonas* spp. are also frequently employed to interpret the susceptibility data for *S. maltophilia* (29, 32). Other breakpoints, such as those specified by the National Reference Laboratory for Antibiotics (National Institute of Public Health, Prague, Czech Republic) and the Antibiogram Committee of the French Microbiology Society, have also been used (13, 15).

Available data are limited for the antimicrobial susceptibility of *S. maltophilia*, because it is not considered as a major pathogen in animals. However, *S. maltophilia* isolates from animals are resistant to numerous antimicrobials that are commonly used in human and veterinary medicine, including β-lactams (penicillins and cephalosporins), aminoglycosides, macrolides, and tetracyclines (except minocyline) (Table 2). In contrast, they are often susceptible to fluoroquinolones, polymyxins (mainly including polymyxin B and polymyxin E [colistin]), and SXT. The antibiotic resistance of *S. maltophilia* varies among different animal species. For example, one isolate from swine in China showed high resistance to most antimicrobials, including fluoroquinolones, polymyxins, and SXT (33), whereas isolates from Omani goats were susceptible to all tested antimicrobials except β-lactams (25). Despite its intrinsic resistance to β-lactams, the resistance rates of *S. maltophilia* isolates from captive snakes to these antimicrobials range from 36.2 to 95.7% (15, 37). Moreover, antimicrobial resistance varies with the incubation temperature and time. For instance, the MICs at 37°C and 30°C (after 24 h or 48 h) of 24 antibiotics were determined (microdilution method) for *S. maltophilia* isolates from captive snakes, but resistance rates increased when the strains were incubated at 30°C or for 48 h (37). However, SXT and levofloxacin were the most effective drugs at both temperatures. In addition, the *S. maltophilia* isolates from animal products also exhibit a multidrug-resistant (MDR) phenotype. For example, *S. maltophilia* was the most frequently isolated species among a large collection of Gram-negative bacteria isolated from milk and cheese in France. These *S. maltophilia* isolates showed high resistance rates to β-lactams, chloramphenicol, and tetracycline (13), representing a potential risk to food safety and public health.

MOLECULAR MECHANISMS OF ANTIMICROBIAL RESISTANCE

S. maltophilia employs an array of mechanisms that singularly or collectively, intrinsic or acquired contribute to antimicrobial resistance (Table 3). The following subsections provide detailed descriptions of the major mechanisms.

Multidrug Efflux Pumps

The genome of *S. maltophilia* encodes multidrug efflux pumps, which contribute to intrinsic or acquired antibiotic resistance, as follows: ATP-binding cassette (ABC)-type (SmrA, FuaABC, and MacABCsm), major facilitator superfamily (MFS)-type (EmrCABsm, MsfA), and eight predicted resistance nodulation cell division (RND)-type efflux systems with SmeABC, SmeDEF, SmeVWX, SmeIJK, SmeYZ, and SmeOP-TolCSm characterized (38–47) and SmeMN and SmeGH uncharacterized (45). Most of the efflux pumps are superficially quiescent or expressed at low levels (39, 42, 44), and their overexpression is associated with reduced antibiotic susceptibility. Acquired resistance may be due to mutations in regulatory genes of these efflux systems (43, 46, 48).

SmrA, the first ABC-type efflux pump identified in *S. maltophilia*, confers acquired resistance to fluoroquinolones, tetracycline, doxorubicin, and multiple dyes (38). FuaABC, a fusaric acid (5-butylpicolinic acid, a mycotoxin) efflux pump, which is classified as a member of a subfamily of the ABC-type family, is induced by fusaric acid and contributes to fusaric acid resistance when overexpressed (41). The MacABCsm efflux pump confers intrinsic resistance to aminoglycosides, macrolides, and polymyxins and contributes to oxidative and envelope stress tolerance as well as biofilm formation (39). The MFS-type pump EmrCABsm is involved in the extrusion of hydrophobic compounds, including the antibiotics nalidixic acid and erythromycin, as well as the uncoupling agents carbonyl cyanide 3-chlorophenylhydrazone, and tetrachlorosalicylanilide (40). A novel MFS efflux pump (MfsA) with 14 transmembrane domains plays an important role in mediating resistance to paraquat (49), as well as to antibiotics such as aminoglycosides (kanamycin, streptomycin, and neomycin), cephalosporins (cefazolin and cefalexin), fluoroquinolones (ciprofloxacin, norfloxacin, levofloxacin,

Table 2 Antimicrobial resistance of *S. maltophilia* isolated from animals and animal products

Origin	Year of identification	Country	Strain no.	Standards and methods of susceptibility testing[a]	β-Lactams (penicillins, cephalosporins, carbapenems)	Macrolides
Swine semen	2000	USA	6	NCCLS M31-A, 1999; disk diffusion	AMP (100)	ERY (100) and TIL (100)
Omani goats	2003	Oman	15	NCCLS M2-A4, 1992; disk diffusion	PEN, AMP, AMC, and TIC (100) CAZ, CTX, and CEP (100)	ERY (0)
Salmon farm	2003	Chile	1	NCCLS M7-A5, 1998; agar dilution		
Yellowtail (*Seriola quinqueradiata*)	2005	Japan	6	Sensi-Disks (Showa, Tokyo, Japan); disk diffusion	AMP (100) CTX and CAZ (100)	
13-lined ground squirrel	2007	USA	1	*Clinical Microbiology Procedures Handbook*; broth microdilution	AMP and AMX (R)	
Captive snakes[c]	2007	Czech Republic	47	NCCLS M2-A8, 2003; breakpoints from National Reference Laboratory for Antibiotics (National Institute of Public Health, Prague, Czech Republic); broth microdilution	AMP (87.2), ATM (89.4), CAZ (68.1), CFP (63.8), CFZ (95.7), CPS (51.1), CTX (85.1), CXM (95.7), FEP (80.9), FOX (95.7), MEM (74.5), PIP (48.3), SAM (68.1), TZP (36.2)	
Horse, cat, dog, and python	2009	Germany	7	Automated susceptibility test strips ATB PSE 5 and ATB VET strips (BioMérieux); microdilution	TIC, PIP, IPM, and CAZ (100)	
Giant panda	2010	USA	1	Unknown	AMC, AMP, CAZ, CTX, CEF, and CEP (R)	AZI (R)
Captive snakes	2010	Czech Republic	45	CLSI M100-S19, 2009; broth microdilution	CAZ (44.4)	
Buffalo (*Bubalus bubalis*)	2010	Greece	1	CLSI M100-S15, 2005; breakpoints of *Pseudomonas* spp. used; broth microdilution	TIC and PIP (R)CAZ and IPM (R)	
Horse	2010	Denmark	7	CLSI M100-S13, 2003; broth microdilution	PEN, AMP, and AMC (100)CF, CPD, and IPM (100)	ERY (100)
Oocytes of *Xenopus laevis*	2011	USA	5	Unknown; disk diffusion	AMX, AMC, and TIC (100), CZ, CF, CTX, CPD, CEF, CXM, and CN (100) CRO (80), CAZ and IPM (0)	
Milk and Cheese	2012	France	3	Antibiogram Committee of the French Microbiology Society (CA-SFM), 2008/2009; disk diffusion	AM, PIP, AMX, AMC, TIM, CTX, and CAZ (100)IPM (66.7)	
Pig	2012	China	7	Unknown; disk diffusion	AMP, AMX, and novobiocin (100) CTX and CAZ (100)	
Bovine mastitis	2012	Japan	13	CLSI M31-A3 (2008) and M100-S21 (2011); commercially prepared microtiter panel (Opt Panel MP) and disk diffusion	MOX (0), CAZ (92.3)	
Pig	2015	China	1	CLSI VET01-A4 (2013) and M100-S24 (2014); broth microdilution	AMP, AMC, CEF, CAZ, and MEM (R)	ERY and AZI (R)

[a]For more than one strain, the resistance rate was calculated, and the susceptibility results were interpreted as resistant/intermediate/susceptible (R/I/S) for single strains. CLSI breakpoints were only available for *S. maltophilia* from humans for SXT, MIN, LEV, TIM, CAZ, SXT, and CHL determined using disk diffusion or dilution methods. For other antimicrobials, the breakpoints for *Enterobacteriaceae* or *Pseudomonas* spp. were used to interpret the susceptibility results for *S. maltophilia*.
[b]PEN, penicillin G; AMP, ampicillin; AMX, amoxicillin; PIP, piperacillin; TIC, ticarcillin; TIM, ticarcillin/clavulanic acid; AMC, amoxicillin/clavulanic acid; SAM, ampicillin/sulbactam; TZP, piperacillin/tazobactam; CAZ, ceftazidime; CTX, cefotaxime; CEF, ceftiofur; CEP, cephalothin; CFZ, cefazolin; CFP, cefoperazone; CN, cephalexin; CRO, ceftriaxone; CPS, cefoperazone/sulbactam; CF, cephalothin; CXM, cefuroxime; FEP, cefepime; FOX, cefoxitin; CPD, cefpodoxime; CZ, cefazolin; MOX, moxalactam; IPM, imipenem; MEM, meropenem; ERY, erythromycin; TIL, tilmicosin; AZI, azithromycin; CHL, chloramphenicol; FFC, florfenicol; GEN, gentamicin; KAN, kanamycin; AMK, amikacin; SPT, spectinomycin; STR, streptomycin; NEO, neomycin; TOB, tobramycin; TET, tetracycline; DOX, doxycycline; OTC, oxytetracycline; MIN, minocycline; CIP, ciprofloxacin; LVX, levofloxacin; OFX, ofloxacin; ENO, enrofloxacin; MAR, marbofloxacin; DIF, difloxacin; OFX, ofloxacin; OBX, orbifloxacin; CL, colistin; CLI, clindamycin; VAN, vancomycin; S3, sulfonamides; SMX, sulfamethoxazole; TMP, trimethoprim; SXT, trimethoprim-sulfamethoxazole.
[c]Resistance rates varied with incubation temperature (30°C or 37°C) and time (24 h or 48 h). Susceptibility data presented here were determined when isolates were incubated at 37°C for 24 h.

Antimicrobial agents used for susceptibility testing (resistance rates, %)[b]

Phenicols	Aminoglycosides	Tetracyclines	Fluoroquinolones	Polymyxins	Lincosamides/ glycopeptides	Sulfonamides	Ref.
	GEN and SPT (100)	OTC (100)		CL (0)		Triple sulfa (100)	21
CHL (0)	KAN, GEN, and AMK (0)	TET (0)	ENO (0)			SXT (0)	25
		OTC (R), DOX (R), MIN (S)					19
							17
CHL (R)	GEN and SPT (R)	TET (R)					14, 113
CHL (61.7)	AMK (31.9), GEN (25.5), TOB (57.4)	TET (89.4)	LVX (0), OFX (2.1), CIP (42.6)	CL (21.3)		SXT (2.1)	15
CHL (28.6)	AMK (42.9), GEN (71.4), TOB (57.1)	TET (100)	CIP and ENO (0)	CL (0)		SXT (14.3)	31
CHL (S)	GEN, NEO, and TOB (R)	DOX (S) OTC and TET (R)	CIP and ENO (S)	CL (R)	CLI and VAN (R)	SXT (I)	30
CHL (28.9)			LVX (0)			SMX (2.2)	37
CHL (S)	AMK, GEN, and TOB (R)	TET (R)	CIP and ENO (S)	CL (S)		SXT (S)	(29)
	GEN and AMK (100)	TET (0)	MAR and ENO (0)			SXT (0)	32
CHL (100)	GEN and TOB (100) AMK (0)	TET (100)	CIP (0)DIF, ENO, OFX, and OBX (100) MAR (80)				24
CHL (100)		TET (100)					13
	GEN and STR (100)					S3 and TMP (100)	10
CHL (7.7)			CIP (7.7) ENO (0)			SXT (15.4)	27
CHL and FFC (R)	GEN, STR, and SPT (R)	TET and DOX (R)	ENO (R), LVX (I), CIP (R)	CL (R)		SMX and SXT (R)	33

TABLE 3 Molecular mechanisms of antimicrobial resistance of *S. maltophilia*[a]

Resistance mechanisms and related genes	Products	Antibiotic resistance phenotype	Intrinsic/acquired resistance	Gene location	Ref.
Multidrug efflux pumps					
smrA	ABC-type efflux pump	Fluoroquinolones, tetracycline, doxorubicin	NK/yes	C	38
fuaABC	ABC-type efflux pump	Fusaric acid	Yes/no	C	41
macABCsm	ABC-type efflux pump	Macrolides, aminoglycosides, polymyxins	Yes/NK	C	39
emrCABsm	MFS-type efflux pump	Nalidixic acid, erythromycin	No/yes	C	40
mfsA	MFS-type efflux pump	Aminoglycosides, cephalosporins, fluorpquinolones, erythromycin, rifampicin, tetracycline, chloramphenicol	Yes/NK	C	50
smeABC	RND-type efflux pump	β-lactams, aminoglycosides and quinolones	No/yes	C	42
smeDEF	RND-type efflux pump	Quinolones, tetracyclines, macrolides, chloramphenicol, novobiocin, SXT	Yes/yes	C	43, 53
smeVWX	RND-type efflux pump	Chloramphenicol, quinolones, tetracyclines	No/yes	C	44
smeIJK	RND-type efflux pump	Aminoglycosides, tetracyclines, fluorpquinolones, leucomycin	Yes/yes	C	46, 55
smeYZ	RND-type efflux pump	Aminoglycosides, SXT	Yes/yes	C	45, 54
smeOP-TolC$_{Sm}$	RND-type efflux pump	Nalidixic acid, doxycycline, aminoglycosides, macrolides	Yes/no	C	47
β-lactamases					
bla$_{L1}$	Metallo-β-lactamase	β-Lactams except monobactams	Yes/yes	C or P	56, 97
bla$_{L2}$	Cephalosporinase	Penicillins and cephalosporins	Yes/yes	C	57, 97
bla$_{TEM-2}$, bla$_{TEM-116}$, bla$_{TEM-127}$, bla$_{CTX-M-1}$, bla$_{SHV-1}$ and bla$_{CTX-M-15}$	β-lactamase	Penicillins and/or cephalosporins	No/yes	P	62–65
bla$_{NDM-1}$	Metallo-β-lactamase	β-Lactams except monobactams	No/yes	C	66
Aminoglycoside-inactivating enzymes					
aac(6')-Iz	Aminoglycoside acetyltransferase	Amikacin, netilmicin, sisomicin, tobramycin	Yes/no	C	67
aph(3')-IIc	Aminoglycoside phosphotransferase	Kanamycin, neomycin, butirosin, paromomycin	Yes/no	C	68
aac(6')-Iak	Aminoglycoside acetyltransferase	Amikacin, arbekacin, dibekacin, isepamicin, kanamycin, neomycin, netilmicin, sisomicin, tobramycin	Yes/no	C	69
aac(6')-Iam	Aminoglycoside acetyltransferase	NK	NK	C	45
Qnr family					
Smqnr	Pentapeptide repeat proteins	Low-level quinolone resistance	Yes/no	C	76–78
SXT resistance					
sul1 and sul2	Folate reductase enzyme	Trimethoprim/sulfamethoxazole	No/yes	C or P	82–84
dfrA1, dfrA5, dfrA12, dfrA17, and dfrA27	Dihydrofolate reductase enzyme	Trimethoprim/sulfamethoxazole	No/yes	C or P	85
Phenicol exporters					
floR	MFS exporter protein	Chloramphenicol, florfenicol	No/yes	P	83
floRv	MFS exporter protein	Chloramphenicol, florfenicol	No/yes	GI in C	33
cmlA	MFS exporter protein	Chloramphenicol	No/yes	I-integron	90
Lipopolysaccharide					
spgM	Phosphoglucomutase	Polymyxin B/E, nalidixic acid, gentamicin	Yes/NK	C	92
phoPQ	Two-component regulatory system	Polymyxin B, chloramphenicol, ampicillin, aminoglycosides	Yes/yes	C	96

[a]NK, not known.

and ofloxacin), the macrolide erythromycin, rifampicin, tetracycline, and chloramphenicol (50).

SmeABC is involved in acquired, but not intrinsic, resistance to β-lactams, aminoglycosides, and quinolones. The deletion of *smeC* (encoding a porin) affects susceptibility to certain antibiotics, suggesting the relationship of porin to other unidentified efflux pumps (42). SmeDEF is involved in intrinsic and acquired (in the condition of overexpression) resistance to quinolones, tetracyclines, macrolides, chloramphenicol, novobiocin, and SXT, as well as acquired resistance to triclosan (51–53). SmeVWX mediates acquired resistance to chloramphenicol, quinolones, and tetracyclines and when overexpressed, increases susceptibility to aminoglycosides (44). SmeYZ mediates intrinsic resistance to aminoglycosides and SXT (45, 54), while SmeIJK is involved in intrinsic reduced susceptibility to gentamicin, amikacin, tetracycline, minocycline, ciprofloxacin, and leucomycin (45, 55). SmeIJK also mediated acquired resistance to levofloxacin, when overexpressed alone or in coordinate hyperproduction with SmeYZ (46). The activity of the SmeOP-TolCSm efflux pump is associated with the decreases in susceptibility to nalidixic acid, doxycycline, aminoglycosides (amikacin and gentamicin), and macrolides (erythromycin and leucomycin), as well as several nonantibiotic compounds including carbonyl cyanide 3-chlorophenylhydrazone, crystal violet, sodium dodecyl sulfate, and tetrachlorosalicylanilide (47).

Resistance to β-Lactam Antibiotics

The *S. maltophilia* genome encodes the inducible β-lactamases L1 and L2. L1 is a class B Zn^{2+}-dependent metallo-β-lactamase with substrate preference for penicillins, cephalosporins, and carbapenems, except for monobactams; and L2 is a class A clavulanic acid-sensitive cephalosporinase that hydrolyzes penicillins, cephalosporins, and monobactams (56, 57). The expression of L1 and L2 is simultaneously regulated by AmpR, a transcriptional regulator encoded by *ampR*, located upstream of bla_{L2}, which acts as a weak repressor or activator of the bla_{L2} in the presence or absence of β-lactam antibiotics, respectively (58). The induction of β-lactamases is inhibited by the deletion of the *ampN-ampG* operon, which encodes a permease transporter (59). The hyperproduction of L1/L2 β-lactamases occurs when the transcription of *mrcA* or $ampD_I$ (encoding penicillin-binding protein 1a [PBP1a] and a cytoplasmic N-acetyl-muramyl-L-alanine amidase [$AmpD_I$], respectively) is inhibited (60, 61). In addition, the β-lactamases TEM-2, TEM-116, TEM-127, CTX-M-1, SHV-1, and CTX-M-15 and the globally disseminated metallo-β-lactamase NDM-1 are present in human clinical and environmental isolates of *S. maltophilia* (62–66), suggesting that this pathogen may serve as a reservoir for mobile genes that encode β-lactamases.

Resistance to Aminoglycosides

The mechanisms employed by *S. maltophilia* that mediate resistance to aminoglycosides primarily involve aminoglycoside-modifying enzymes and multidrug efflux pumps. These enzymes include the aminoglycoside acetyltransferase AAC(6′)-Iz (67) and the aminoglycoside phosphotransferase APH(3′)-IIc (68), both of which confer low-level resistance to aminoglycosides, with the exception of gentamicin. The novel aminoglycoside acetyltransferase AAC(6′)-Iak, which exhibits 86.3% amino acid identity to AAC(6′)-Iz, is expressed by an MDR *S. maltophilia* strain isolated from Nepal and acetylates amikacin, arbekacin, dibekacin, isepamicin, kanamycin, neomycin, netilmicin, sisomicin, and tobramycin, but not apramycin, gentamicin, or lividomycin (69). Moreover, AAC(6′)-Iam [84.3% amino acid sequence identity to AAC(6′)-Iak], was detected in a clinical isolate of *S. maltophilia* (45). However, the resistance phenotype conferred by this enzyme is unknown. In addition, the efflux pumps SmeABC, SmeYZ, SmeOP-TolCsm, and MacABCsm are associated with aminoglycoside resistance (Table 3).

Resistance to Quinolones

Mutations in the quinolone-resistance-determining region of genes encoding topoisomerases (*gyrA*, *gyrB*, *parC*, and *parE*) are associated with the major mechanism of quinolone resistance employed by bacteria (70). So far, mutations have not been detected in the quinolone-resistance-determining region of *gyrA* of *S. maltophilia* (71, 72). Amino acid residue substitutions are present in the quinolone-resistance-determining region-encoding regions of *gyrB*, *parC*, and *parE* of clinical isolates of *S. maltophilia* that cause bacteremia; however, these alterations have not been directly associated with quinolone resistance (73). The specific mechanisms associated with the quinolone resistance of *S. maltophilia* are mediated by both the efflux pumps and the chromosomal *qnr* gene (Sm*qnr*) that protects gyrase and topoisomerase IV from quinolones (74). Sm*qnr* and its functional 12 variants belong to the *qnr* family (75) and contribute to low-level intrinsic quinolone resistance (76–78). Genes that encode efflux pumps that mediate quinolone resistance are as follows: *smeDEF*, *smeIJK*, *smeABC*, and *smeVWX* (Table 3). The most prevalent cause of quinolone resistance in

S. maltophilia is the overproduction of multidrug efflux pumps, among which the SmeDEF plays the most important role (79). Furthermore, overexpression of *smeVWX* in clinical isolates of *S. maltophilia* is associated with high-level resistance to quinolones (80).

Resistance to Trimethoprim-Sulfamethoxazole
The resistance of Gram-negative bacteria to sulfonamides is mainly conferred by the acquisition of either *sul1* or *sul2*, encoding dihydropteroate synthases (81). The *sul1* gene carried by class 1 integrons and *sul2*, which is linked to insertion sequence common region (ISCR) elements, was identified in SXT-resistant *S. maltophilia* isolates (82–84). The resistance of *S. maltophilia* to trimethoprim is mainly conferred by the dihydrofolate reductase *dfr* genes. For instance, the *dfrA* variant genes (*dfrA1*, *dfrA5*, *dfrA12*, *dfrA17*, and *dfrA27*), which are located within class 1 integrons as part of various resistance gene cassettes, are associated with high-level trimethoprim resistance in *S. maltophilia* isolates. Both types of *sul* and *dfr* genes can occur together in high-level SXT-resistant isolates (85, 86). Moreover, the efflux pumps SmeDEF, TolCsm, and SmeYZ are associated with SXT resistance (54, 87, 88).

Resistance to Phenicols
The main phenicol resistance determinant in *S. maltophilia* is *floR*, which encodes an exporter protein of the MFS family that mediates resistance to chloramphenicol and florfenicol (83). Florfenicol is extensively used in livestock to prevent or cure bacterial infections (89). In addition, the MFS exporter gene *cmlA1* and chloramphenicol acetyltransferase genes *catB2* and *catB8*, which separately reside in a gene cassette of class 1 integrons, confer resistance to chloramphenicol in *S. maltophilia* (82, 85, 90). Reports of the prevalence of *floR* in *S. maltophilia* are rare. One report that investigated an international collection of 55 clinical isolates of *S. maltophilia* found that four strains harbored *floR* (83). The novel variant *floRv* was detected in one porcine *S. maltophilia* isolate in China. The *floRv* gene encodes an exporter protein of 404 amino acids, which is 84.1 to 91.8% identical to FloR sequences deposited in GenBank. This FloR variant mediates resistance to chloramphenicol and florfenicol (33).

Alteration of Lipopolysaccharide and Two-Component Regulatory Systems
As in other Gram-negative bacteria, lipopolysaccharide (LPS) is an important structural component of the outer membrane of *S. maltophilia* and forms an effective barrier to exogenous compounds (91). The *spgM* gene

encodes a phosphoglucomutase that is associated with LPS biosynthesis in *S. maltophilia* (92). Mutants lacking *spgM*, which produce less LPS compared with the SpgM$^+$ strain, synthesize shorter O-polysaccharide chains and exhibit modest increases in susceptibility to polymyxin B, colistin, nalidixic acid, and gentamicin but increased resistance to vancomycin (92). The mobile colistin resistance gene *mcr-1*, which encodes a phosphoethanolamine transferase, couples phosphoethanolamine to the lipid A domain of the LPS component of the outer membrane of Gram-negative bacteria, and negates the efficacy of polymixins (93), has not been detected in *Stenotrophomonas* spp. The two-component regulatory system PhoPQ is involved in the resistance of numerous Gram-negative bacteria, including *S. maltophilia*, to cationic antimicrobial polypeptides, i.e., polymyxin B (94–96). Mutation of *S. maltophilia* PhoP increases susceptibility to polymyxin B, chloramphenicol, ampicillin, gentamicin, kanamycin, streptomycin, and spectinomycin (96). Moreover, downregulation of the SmeZ efflux transporter expressed by a PhoP mutant contributes to increased drug susceptibility, particularly to aminoglycosides (96).

DISSEMINATION, COSELECTION, AND PERSISTANCE OF RESISTANCE DETERMINANTS
As described above, the reduced susceptibility of *S. maltophilia* to most antibiotics can be attributed to intrinsic and acquired resistance. The proteins mediating intrinsic resistance of *S. maltophilia* include chromosomally encoded multidrug efflux pumps, antibiotic-inactivating enzymes (L1/L2 β-lactamases and aminoglycoside-inactivating enzymes), and the chromosomally encoded Qnr pentapeptide repeat proteins (74), which are present in most, if not all, strains of *S. maltophilia*, suggesting they did not arise during the recent evolution of resistance caused by antibiotic therapy. In addition, *S. maltophilia* can acquire mechanisms to increase its resistance through horizontal gene transfer via integrons, transposons, plasmids, and genomic islands (GIs). The *sul1* gene is always associated with the class 1 integron in *S. maltophilia*, indicating the role of the latter in the acquisition and dissemination of *sul1* within this species (82–86, 90). The *qacE1* gene, which encodes resistance to quaternary amines, coexists with *sul1* at the 3′-termini of class 1 integrons (83, 85, 90). The gene cassettes, which comprise the variable regions of integrons, integrate different combinations of drug-resistance genes donated by other Gram-negative bacteria, including those encoding resistance to

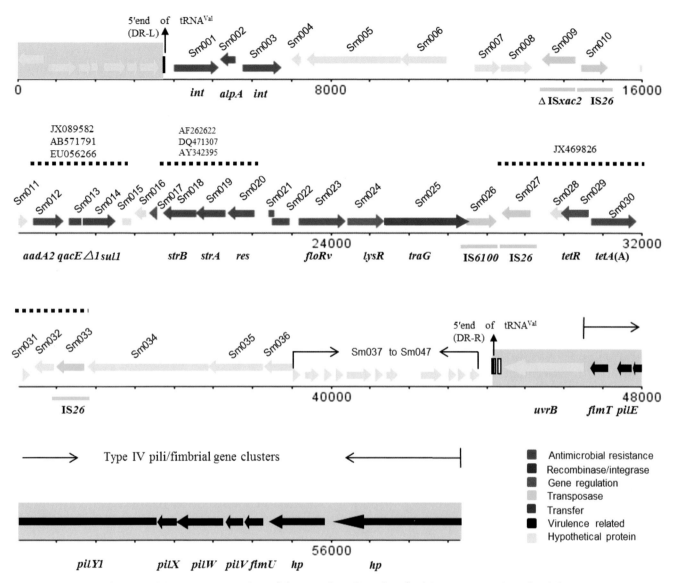

Figure 1 Linear representation of the complete GI and its flanking regions in *S. maltophilia* GZP-Sm1. The regions in gray represent the flanking regions of the GI when inserted into the bacterial chromosome. The arrows indicate the directions of gene transcription, and truncated genes are indicated by rectangles without arrowheads. Genes are depicted in different colors, and the regions of particular relevance (≥95% nucleotide sequence identity) are indicated by the dotted lines (33).

aminoglycosides [*aacA4*, *aacA7*, *aadA1*, *aadA2*, *aadA4*, *aadA5*, *aadB*, *aac(6′)-II*, *aac(6′)-Ib*, *aac(3′)-Ia*, and *ant (3″)-Ia*], trimethoprim (*dfrA1*, *dfrA5*, *dfrA12*, *dfrA17* and *dfrA27*), β-lactams (*bla*CARB-8), rifampicin (*arr-3*), and chloramphenicol (*catB2*, *catB8*, *cmlA1*) (82, 85, 90).

ISCR elements are frequently associated with antimicrobial resistance genes and are always linked to *sul2* in *S. maltophilia*. For example, seven *sul2*-positive *S. maltophilia* isolates harbor ISCR elements (five

ISCR2 and two ISCR3 elements) on a plasmid (83). Moreover, *sul2* and *floR* are linked to ISCR2 in all *sul2*-positive *S. maltophilia* isolates. Constitutively expressed *bla*TEM-2 resides within a novel Tn1/Tn3-type transposon in the genome of *S. maltophilia* isolate J675Ia (65). The transposon could mobilize *bla*TEM-2 onto the broad host-range conjugative plasmid R388, which is then transferred to *E. coli*.

The genes encoding β-lactamases L1 and L2 are invariably chromosomal and reside on an approximately

200-kb plasmid present in 10 clinical isolates of *S. maltophilia* (97). However, the sequences of the L1 and L2 genes diverge from that of the published strain IID 1275, indicating that the presence of β-lactamase genes on a plasmid may lead to their relatively quick evolution (97).

A literature search identified only a single report of an MDR GI in the *S. maltophilia* isolate GZP-Sm1 in China (33). GZP-Sm1 was isolated from swine with septicemia, and susceptibility testing revealed that the isolate was resistant to most antimicrobials employed in human and veterinary clinical practice (33). Whole-genome sequencing identified a GI of 40,226 bp, which contains an MDR region (19,364 bp) and is flanked by IS26 in opposite orientations (Fig. 1). Furthermore, six resistance genes exist in this region, including *floRv* (phenicol resistance), *tet*(A)-*tetR* (tetracycline resistance), *strA/strB* (streptomycin resistance), *sul1* (sulfonamide resistance), and *aadA2* (streptomycin/spectinomycin resistance). The MDR region comprises several segments with sequence similarity to plasmids or chromosomal sequences of other Gram-negative bacteria. For example, the *aadA2* cassette and the 3′-CS region (*qacE1-sul1-Δorf5*), which form part of an integron structure identified in this GI, occur in diverse bacterial species such as *Salmonella* spp., *Pseudomonas* spp., and *E. coli*. The 4,766-bp segment of Δ*sul-floRv-lysR-traG* is 86.3% identical to the corresponding region of plasmid pAB (accession no. HQ917128) detected in a clinical isolate of *Acinetobacter baumannii* from Chile. The composite transposon comprising IS26-*tet*(A)-*tetR*-IS26 flanked by a direct repeat of GC is 95.1% identical to the corresponding region of the plasmid pB12 from uncultivable bacteria (accession no. JX469826). Inverse PCR showed that the GI could be excised from the chromosome by recombination between the direct repeats to generate a circular extrachromosomal form (Fig. 1). The emerging resistance of *S. maltophilia* to numerous antimicrobials raises the concern that the presence of resistance genes in the novel MDR GI drastically limit therapeutic options and may enhance their coselection when antimicrobials are administered.

S. maltophilia could acquire antibiotic resistance from Gram-positive bacteria. For example, a gene cluster involved in resistance to antibiotics and heavy metals was detected in a clinical isolate of *S. maltophilia* (98). These genes encode a macrolide phosphotransferase (*mphBM*) and a cadmium efflux determinant (*cadA*), as well as its transcriptional regulator (*cadC*), encoding its cognate transcriptional regulator. The *cadC-cadA* region is flanked by a truncated IS257 sequence and a region coding for a *bin3* invertase. The sequences of these genetic elements are highly similar to those of *Staphylococcus aureus*, indicating their Gram-positive origin.

CONCLUSION

S. maltophilia is the most widely distributed environmental species among *Stenotrophomonas*, and it is also an opportunistic pathogen associated with the increased number of infections in both humans and animals. *S. maltophilia* isolates from animals are resistant to most antimicrobials used in both human and veterinary medicine, which compromise the design of optimal therapeutic strategies in clinical chemotherapy. The antimicrobial resistances in *S. maltophilia* are conferred not only by intrinsic mechanisms, but also by multiple acquired resistance mechanisms, which are commonly associated with mobile genetic elements such as integrons, transposons, and plasmids. Moreover, for the first time, the transmission mechanism conferred by MDRGI was identified in a porcine *S. maltophilia* isolate. Therefore, continued surveillance of MDR *S. maltophilia* from animals is warranted for not only optimizing treatment of infections caused by this bacterium, but also tackling the transmission of antimicrobial resistance from animals to humans by either food-chain or environmental routes.

Acknowledgments. This work was supported in part by the National Natural Science Foundation of China (grant no. 31422055) and the National Key Basic Research Program of China (grant no. 2013CB127200).

Citation. Wang Y, He T, Shen Z, Wu C. 2017. Antimicrobial resistance in *Stenotrophomonas* spp. Microbiol Spectrum 6(1): ARBA-0005-2017.

References

1. http://www.bacterio.net/stenotrophomonas.html.
2. Swings J, De Vos P, Van den Mooter M, De Ley J. 1983. Transfer of *Pseudomonas maltophilia* Hugh 1981 to the genus *Xanthomonas* as *Xanthomonas* maltophilia. *Int J Syst Bacteriol* 33:409–413.
3. Drancourt M, Bollet C, Raoult D. 1997. *Stenotrophomonas africana* sp. nov., an opportunistic human pathogen in Africa. *Int J Syst Bacteriol* 47:160–163.
4. Brooke JS. 2012. *Stenotrophomonas maltophilia*: an emerging global opportunistic pathogen. *Clin Microbiol Rev* 25:2–41.
5. Ryan RP, Monchy S, Cardinale M, Taghavi S, Crossman L, Avison MB, Berg G, van der Lelie D, Dow JM. 2009. The versatility and adaptation of bacteria from the genus *Stenotrophomonas*. *Nat Rev Microbiol* 7:514–525.
6. Hugh R, Ryschenkow E. 1961. *Pseudomonas maltophilia*, an alcaligenes-like species. *J Gen Microbiol* 26: 123–132.

7. Chien YC, Chen CJ, Lin TH, Chen SH, Chien YC. 2011. Characteristics of microbial aerosols released from chicken and swine feces. *J Air Waste Manag Assoc* 61:882–889.

8. Guo Y, Zhu N, Zhu S, Deng C. 2007. Molecular phylogenetic diversity of bacteria and its spatial distribution in composts. *J Appl Microbiol* 103:1344–1354.

9. Mancini DA, Mendonça RM, Dias AL, Mendonça RZ, Pinto JR. 2005. Co-infection between influenza virus and flagellated bacteria. *Rev Inst Med Trop São Paulo* 47:275–280.

10. Hou D, Bi Y, Sun H, Yang J, Fu G, Sun Y, Liu J, Pu J. 2012. Identification of swine influenza A virus and *Stenotrophomonas maltophilia* co-infection in Chinese pigs. *Virol J* 9:169.

11. Munsch-Alatossava P, Alatossava T. 2006. Phenotypic characterization of raw milk-associated psychrotrophic bacteria. *Microbiol Res* 161:334–346.

12. Cleto S, Matos S, Kluskens L, Vieira MJ. 2012. Characterization of contaminants from a sanitized milk processing plant. *PLoS One* 7:e40189.

13. Coton M, Delbés-Paus C, Irlinger F, Desmasures N, Le Fleche A, Stahl V, Montel MC, Coton E. 2012. Diversity and assessment of potential risk factors of Gram-negative isolates associated with French cheeses. *Food Microbiol* 29:88–98.

14. Cloud-Hansen KA, Villiard KM, Handelsman J, Carey HV. 2007. Thirteen-lined ground squirrels (*Spermophilus tridecemlineatus*) harbor multiantibiotic-resistant bacteria. *J Am Assoc Lab Anim Sci* 46:21–23.

15. Hejnar P, Bardon J, Sauer P, Kolár M. 2007. *Stenotrophomonas maltophilia* as a part of normal oral bacterial flora in captive snakes and its susceptibility to antibiotics. *Vet Microbiol* 121:357–362.

16. Kim M, Kwon TH, Jung SM, Cho SH, Jin SY, Park NH, Kim CG, Kim JS. 2013. Antibiotic resistance of bacteria isolated from the internal organs of edible snow crabs. *PLoS One* 8:e70887.

17. Furushita M, Okamoto A, Maeda T, Ohta M, Shiba T. 2005. Isolation of multidrug-resistant *Stenotrophomonas maltophilia* from cultured yellowtail (*Seriola quinqueradiata*) from a marine fish farm. *Appl Environ Microbiol* 71:5598–5600.

18. Matyar F, Kaya A, Dinçer S. 2008. Antibacterial agents and heavy metal resistance in Gram-negative bacteria isolated from seawater, shrimp and sediment in Iskenderun Bay, Turkey. *Sci Total Environ* 407:279–285.

19. Miranda CD, Kehrenberg C, Ulep C, Schwarz S, Roberts MC. 2003. Diversity of tetracycline resistance genes in bacteria from Chilean salmon farms. *Antimicrob Agents Chemother* 47:883–888.

20. Miranda CD, Zemelman R. 2002. Antimicrobial multiresistance in bacteria isolated from freshwater Chilean salmon farms. *Sci Total Environ* 293:207–218.

21. Althouse GC, Kuster CE, Clark SG, Weisiger RM. 2000. Field investigations of bacterial contaminants and their effects on extended porcine semen. *Theriogenology* 53:1167–1176.

22. Althouse GC, Lu KG. 2005. Bacteriospermia in extended porcine semen. *Theriogenology* 63:573–584.

23. Kilburn C, Rooks DJ, McCarthy AJ, Murray RD. 2013. Antimicrobial resistance in some Gram-negative bacteria isolated from the bovine ejaculate. *Reprod Domest Anim* 48:525–528.

24. O'Connell D, Mruk K, Rocheleau JM, Kobertz WR. 2011. *Xenopus laevis* oocytes infected with multi-drug-resistant bacteria: implications for electrical recordings. *J Gen Physiol* 138:271–277.

25. Johnson EH, Al-Busaidy R, Hameed MS. 2003. An outbreak of lymphadenitis associated with *Stenotrophomonas* (*Xanthomonas*) *maltophilia* in Omani goats. *J Vet Med B Infect Dis Vet Public Health* 50:102–104.

26. Macdiarmid JA, Burrell DH. 1986. Characterization of *Pseudomonas maltophilia* isolates from fleece rot. *Appl Environ Microbiol* 51:346–348.

27. Ohnishi M, Sawada T, Marumo K, Harada K, Hirose K, Shimizu A, Hayashimoto M, Sato R, Uchida N, Kato H. 2012. Antimicrobial susceptibility and genetic relatedness of bovine *Stenotrophomonas maltophilia* isolates from a mastitis outbreak. *Lett Appl Microbiol* 54:572–576.

28. Hagi T, Sasaki K, Aso H, Nomura M. 2013. Adhesive properties of predominant bacteria in raw cow's milk to bovine mammary gland epithelial cells. *Folia Microbiol (Praha)* 58:515–522.

29. Petridou E, Filioussis G, Karavanis E, Kritas SK. 2010. *Stenotrophomonas maltophilia* as a causal agent of pyogranulomatous hepatitis in a buffalo (*Bubalus bubalis*). *J Vet Diagn Invest* 22:772–774.

30. Boedeker NC, Walsh T, Murray S, Bromberg N. 2010. Medical and surgical management of severe inflammation of the nictitating membrane in a giant panda (*Ailuropoda melanoleuca*). *Vet Ophthalmol* 13(Suppl):109–115.

31. Albini S, Abril C, Franchini M, Hüssy D, Filioussis G. 2009. *Stenotrophomonas maltophilia* isolated from the airways of animals with chronic respiratory disease. *Schweiz Arch Tierheilkd* 151:323–328.

32. Winther L, Andersen RM, Baptiste KE, Aalbæk B, Guardabassi L. 2010. Association of *Stenotrophomonas maltophilia* infection with lower airway disease in the horse: a retrospective case series. *Vet J* 186:358–363.

33. He T, Shen J, Schwarz S, Wu C, Wang Y. 2015. Characterization of a genomic island in *Stenotrophomonas maltophilia* that carries a novel *floR* gene variant. *J Antimicrob Chemother* 70:1031–1036.

34. Harris NB, Rogers DG. 2001. Septicemia associated with *Stenotrophomonas maltophilia* in a West African dwarf crocodile (*Osteolaemus tetraspis* subsp. *tetraspis*). *J Vet Diagn Invest* 13:255–258.

35. Muir P, Oldenhoff WE, Hudson AP, Manley PA, Schaefer SL, Markel MD, Hao Z. 2007. Detection of DNA from a range of bacterial species in the knee joints of dogs with inflammatory knee arthritis and associated degenerative anterior cruciate ligament rupture. *Microb Pathog* 42:47–55.

36. Clinical and Laboratory Standards Institute. 2015. Performance Standards for Antimicrobial Susceptibility

Testing. Twenty-Fifth Informational Supplement M-S, CLSI, Wayne, PA.

37. Hejnar P, Kolár M, Sauer P. 2010. Antibiotic resistance of *Stenotrophomonas maltophilia* strains isolated from captive snakes. *Folia Microbiol (Praha)* **55**:83–87.

38. Al-Hamad A, Upton M, Burnie J. 2009. Molecular cloning and characterization of SmrA, a novel ABC multidrug efflux pump from *Stenotrophomonas maltophilia*. *J Antimicrob Chemother* **64**:731–734.

39. Lin YT, Huang YW, Liou RS, Chang YC, Yang TC. 2014. MacABCsm, an ABC-type tripartite efflux pump of *Stenotrophomonas maltophilia* involved in drug resistance, oxidative and envelope stress tolerances and biofilm formation. *J Antimicrob Chemother* **69**:3221–3226.

40. Huang YW, Hu RM, Chu FY, Lin HR, Yang TC. 2013. Characterization of a major facilitator superfamily (MFS) tripartite efflux pump EmrCABsm from *Stenotrophomonas maltophilia*. *J Antimicrob Chemother* **68**:2498–2505.

41. Hu RM, Liao ST, Huang CC, Huang YW, Yang TC. 2012. An inducible fusaric acid tripartite efflux pump contributes to the fusaric acid resistance in *Stenotrophomonas maltophilia*. *PLoS One* **7**:e51053.

42. Li XZ, Zhang L, Poole K. 2002. SmeC, an outer membrane multidrug efflux protein of *Stenotrophomonas maltophilia*. *Antimicrob Agents Chemother* **46**:333–343.

43. Alonso A, Martínez JL. 2000. Cloning and characterization of SmeDEF, a novel multidrug efflux pump from *Stenotrophomonas maltophilia*. *Antimicrob Agents Chemother* **44**:3079–3086.

44. Chen CH, Huang CC, Chung TC, Hu RM, Huang YW, Yang TC. 2011. Contribution of resistance-nodulation-division efflux pump operon smeU1-V-W-U2-X to multidrug resistance of *Stenotrophomonas maltophilia*. *Antimicrob Agents Chemother* **55**:5826–5833.

45. Crossman LC, Gould VC, Dow JM, Vernikos GS, Okazaki A, Sebaihia M, Saunders D, Arrowsmith C, Carver T, Peters N, Adlem E, Kerhornou A, Lord A, Murphy L, Seeger K, Squares R, Rutter S, Quail MA, Rajandream MA, Harris D, Churcher C, Bentley SD, Parkhill J, Thomson NR, Avison MB. 2008. The complete genome, comparative and functional analysis of *Stenotrophomonas maltophilia* reveals an organism heavily shielded by drug resistance determinants. *Genome Biol* **9**:R74.

46. Gould VC, Okazaki A, Avison MB. 2013. Coordinate hyperproduction of SmeZ and SmeJK efflux pumps extends drug resistance in *Stenotrophomonas maltophilia*. *Antimicrob Agents Chemother* **57**:655–657.

47. Lin CW, Huang YW, Hu RM, Yang TC. 2014. SmeOP-TolCSm efflux pump contributes to the multidrug resistance of *Stenotrophomonas maltophilia*. *Antimicrob Agents Chemother* **58**:2405–2408.

48. Cho HH, Sung JY, Kwon KC, Koo SH. 2012. Expression of Sme efflux pumps and multilocus sequence typing in clinical isolates of *Stenotrophomonas maltophilia*. *Ann Lab Med* **32**:38–43.

49. Srijaruskul K, Charoenlap N, Namchaiw P, Chattrakarn S, Giengkam S, Mongkolsuk S, Vattanaviboon P. 2015. Regulation by SoxR of *mfsA*, which encodes a major facilitator protein involved in paraquat resistance in *Stenotrophomonas maltophilia*. *PLoS One* **10**:e0123699.

50. Dulyayangkul P, Charoenlap N, Srijaruskul K, Mongkolsuk S, Vattanaviboon P. 2016. Major facilitator superfamily MfsA contributes to multidrug resistance in emerging nosocomial pathogen *Stenotrophomonas maltophilia*. *J Antimicrob Chemother* **71**:2990–2991.

51. Zhang L, Li XZ, Poole K. 2001. SmeDEF multidrug efflux pump contributes to intrinsic multidrug resistance in *Stenotrophomonas maltophilia*. *Antimicrob Agents Chemother* **45**:3497–3503.

52. Hernández A, Ruiz FM, Romero A, Martínez JL. 2011. The binding of triclosan to SmeT, the repressor of the multidrug efflux pump SmeDEF, induces antibiotic resistance in *Stenotrophomonas maltophilia*. *PLoS Pathog* **7**:e1002103.

53. Sánchez MB, Martínez JL. 2015. The efflux pump SmeDEF contributes to trimethoprim-sulfamethoxazole resistance in *Stenotrophomonas maltophilia*. *Antimicrob Agents Chemother* **59**:4347–4348.

54. Lin YT, Huang YW, Chen SJ, Chang CW, Yang TC. 2015. The SmeYZ efflux pump of *Stenotrophomonas maltophilia* contributes to drug resistance, virulence-related characteristics, and virulence in mice. *Antimicrob Agents Chemother* **59**:4067–4073.

55. Huang YW, Liou RS, Lin YT, Huang HH, Yang TC. 2014. A linkage between SmeIJK efflux pump, cell envelope integrity, and σ^E-mediated envelope stress response in *Stenotrophomonas maltophilia*. *PLoS One* **9**:e111784.

56. Crowder MW, Walsh TR, Banovic L, Pettit M, Spencer J. 1998. Overexpression, purification, and characterization of the cloned metallo-β-lactamase L1 from *Stenotrophomonas maltophilia*. *Antimicrob Agents Chemother* **42**:921–926.

57. Walsh TR, MacGowan AP, Bennett PM. 1997. Sequence analysis and enzyme kinetics of the L2 serine β-lactamase from *Stenotrophomonas maltophilia*. *Antimicrob Agents Chemother* **41**:1460–1464.

58. Okazaki A, Avison MB. 2008. Induction of L1 and L2 β-lactamase production in *Stenotrophomonas maltophilia* is dependent on an AmpR-type regulator. *Antimicrob Agents Chemother* **52**:1525–1528.

59. Huang YW, Lin CW, Hu RM, Lin YT, Chung TC, Yang TC. 2010. AmpN-AmpG operon is essential for expression of L1 and L2 β-lactamases in *Stenotrophomonas maltophilia*. *Antimicrob Agents Chemother* **54**:2583–2589.

60. Yang TC, Huang YW, Hu RM, Huang SC, Lin YT. 2009. AmpD$_I$ is involved in expression of the chromosomal L1 and L2 β-lactamases of *Stenotrophomonas maltophilia*. *Antimicrob Agents Chemother* **53**:2902–2907.

61. Lin CW, Lin HC, Huang YW, Chung TC, Yang TC. 2011. Inactivation of mrcA gene derepresses the basal-level expression of L1 and L2 β-lactamases in

Stenotrophomonas maltophilia. J Antimicrob Chemother 66:2033–2037.

62. al Naiemi N, Duim B, Bart A. 2006. CTX-M extended-spectrum β-lactamase in *Pseudomonas aeruginosa* and *Stenotrophomonas maltophilia. J Med Microbiol* 55:1607–1608.

63. Lavigne JP, Gaillard JB, Bourg G, Tichit C, Lecaillon E, Sotto A. 2008. Extended-spectrum β-lactamases-producing *Stenotrophomonas maltophilia* strains: CTX-M enzymes detection and virulence study. *Pathol Biol (Paris)* 56:447–453. (In French.)

64. Maravić A, Skočibušić M, Fredotović Z, Cvjetan S, Samanić I, Puizina J. 2014. Characterization of environmental CTX-M-15-producing *Stenotrophomonas maltophilia. Antimicrob Agents Chemother* 58:6333–6334.

65. Avison MB, von Heldreich CJ, Higgins CS, Bennett PM, Walsh TR. 2000. A TEM-2 β-lactamase encoded on an active Tn1-like transposon in the genome of a clinical isolate of *Stenotrophomonas maltophilia. J Antimicrob Chemother* 46:879–884.

66. Liu W, Zou D, Wang X, Li X, Zhu L, Yin Z, Yang Z, Wei X, Han L, Wang Y, Shao C, Wang S, He X, Liu D, Liu F, Wang J, Huang L, Yuan J. 2012. Proteomic analysis of clinical isolate of *Stenotrophomonas maltophilia* with bla_{NDM-1}, bla_{L1} and bla_{L2} β-lactamase genes under imipenem treatment. *J Proteome Res* 11:4024–4033.

67. Li XZ, Zhang L, McKay GA, Poole K. 2003. Role of the acetyltransferase AAC(6′)-Iz modifying enzyme in aminoglycoside resistance in *Stenotrophomonas maltophilia. J Antimicrob Chemother* 51:803–811.

68. Okazaki A, Avison MB. 2007. Aph(3′)-IIc, an aminoglycoside resistance determinant from *Stenotrophomonas maltophilia. Antimicrob Agents Chemother* 51:359–360.

69. Tada T, Miyoshi-Akiyama T, Dahal RK, Mishra SK, Shimada K, Ohara H, Kirikae T, Pokhrel BM. 2014. Identification of a novel 6′-N-aminoglycoside acetyltransferase, AAC(6′)-Iak, from a multidrug-resistant clinical isolate of *Stenotrophomonas maltophilia. Antimicrob Agents Chemother* 58:6324–6327.

70. Sánchez MB. 2015. Antibiotic resistance in the opportunistic pathogen *Stenotrophomonas maltophilia. Front Microbiol* 6:658.

71. Ribera A, Doménech-Sanchez A, Ruiz J, Benedi VJ, Jimenez de Anta MT, Vila J. 2002. Mutations in *gyrA* and *parC* QRDRs are not relevant for quinolone resistance in epidemiological unrelated *Stenotrophomonas maltophilia* clinical isolates. *Microb Drug Resist* 8:245–251.

72. Valdezate S, Vindel A, Echeita A, Baquero F, Cantó R. 2002. Topoisomerase II and IV quinolone resistance-determining regions in *Stenotrophomonas maltophilia* clinical isolates with different levels of quinolone susceptibility. *Antimicrob Agents Chemother* 46:665–671.

73. Cha MK, Kang CI, Kim SH, Cho SY, Ha YE, Chung DR, Peck KR, Song JH. 2016. Emergence of fluoroquinolone-resistant *Stenotrophomonas maltophilia* in blood isolates causing bacteremia: molecular epidemiology and

microbiologic characteristics. *Diagn Microbiol Infect Dis* 85:210–212.

74. Sanchez MB, Hernandez A, Martinez JL. 2009. *Stenotrophomonas maltophilia* drug resistance. *Future Microbiol* 4:655–660.

75. Gordon NC, Wareham DW. 2010. Novel variants of the Sm*qnr* family of quinolone resistance genes in clinical isolates of *Stenotrophomonas maltophilia. J Antimicrob Chemother* 65:483–489.

76. Sánchez MB, Hernández A, Rodríguez-Martínez JM, Martínez-Martínez L, Martínez JL. 2008. Predictive analysis of transmissible quinolone resistance indicates *Stenotrophomonas maltophilia* as a potential source of a novel family of Qnr determinants. *BMC Microbiol* 8:148.

77. Sánchez MB, Martínez JL. 2010. SmQnr contributes to intrinsic resistance to quinolones in *Stenotrophomonas maltophilia. Antimicrob Agents Chemother* 54:580–581.

78. Shimizu K, Kikuchi K, Sasaki T, Takahashi N, Ohtsuka M, Ono Y, Hiramatsu K. 2008. Sm*qnr*, a new chromosome-carried quinolone resistance gene in *Stenotrophomonas maltophilia. Antimicrob Agents Chemother* 52:3823–3825.

79. Garcia-Leon G, Salgado F, Oliveros JC, Sanchez MB, Martinez JL. 2014. Interplay between intrinsic and acquired resistance to quinolones in *Stenotrophomonas maltophilia. Environ Microbiol* 16:1282–1296.

80. García-León G, Ruiz de Alegría Puig C, García de la Fuente C, Martínez-Martínez L, Martínez JL, Sánchez MB. 2015. High-level quinolone resistance is associated with the overexpression of sme*VWX* in *Stenotrophomonas maltophilia* clinical isolates. *Clin Microbiol Infect* 21:464–467.

81. Rådström P, Swedberg G. 1988. RSF1010 and a conjugative plasmid contain *sulII*, one of two known genes for plasmid-borne sulfonamide resistance dihydropteroate synthase. *Antimicrob Agents Chemother* 32:1684–1692.

82. Barbolla R, Catalano M, Orman BE, Famiglietti A, Vay C, Smayevsky J, Centrón D, Piñeiro SA. 2004. Class 1 integrons increase trimethoprim-sulfamethoxazole MICs against epidemiologically unrelated *Stenotrophomonas maltophilia* isolates. *Antimicrob Agents Chemother* 48:666–669.

83. Toleman MA, Bennett PM, Bennett DM, Jones RN, Walsh TR. 2007. Global emergence of trimethoprim/sulfamethoxazole resistance in *Stenotrophomonas maltophilia* mediated by acquisition of *sul* genes. *Emerg Infect Dis* 13:559–565.

84. Chung HS, Kim K, Hong SS, Hong SG, Lee K, Chong Y. 2015. The *sul1* gene in *Stenotrophomonas maltophilia* with high-level resistance to trimethoprim/sulfamethoxazole. *Ann Lab Med* 35:246–249.

85. Hu LF, Chang X, Ye Y, Wang ZX, Shao YB, Shi W, Li X, Li JB. 2011. *Stenotrophomonas maltophilia* resistance to trimethoprim/sulfamethoxazole mediated by acquisition of *sul* and *dfrA* genes in a plasmid-mediated class 1 integron. *Int J Antimicrob Agents* 37:230–234.

86. Hu LF, Chen GS, Kong QX, Gao LP, Chen X, Ye Y, Li JB. 2016. Increase in the prevalence of resistance determinants to trimethoprim/sulfamethoxazole in clinical *Stenotrophomonas maltophilia* isolates in China. *PLoS One* 11:e0157693.

87. Huang YW, Hu RM, Yang TC. 2013. Role of the *pcmtolCsm* operon in the multidrug resistance of *Stenotrophomonas maltophilia*. *J Antimicrob Chemother* 68: 1987–1993.

88. Sánchez MB, Martínez JL. 2015. The efflux pump SmeDEF contributes to trimethoprim-sulfamethoxazole resistance in *Stenotrophomonas maltophilia*. *Antimicrob Agents Chemother* 59:4347–4348.

89. He T, Shen Y, Schwarz S, Cai J, Lv Y, Li J, Feßler AT, Zhang R, Wu C, Shen J, Wang Y. 2016. Genetic environment of the transferable oxazolidinone/phenicol resistance gene *optrA* in *Enterococcus faecalis* isolates of human and animal origin. *J Antimicrob Chemother* 71: 1466–1473.

90. Chang LL, Lin HH, Chang CY, Lu PL. 2007. Increased incidence of class 1 integrons in trimethoprim/ sulfamethoxazole-resistant clinical isolates of *Stenotrophomonas maltophilia*. *J Antimicrob Chemother* 59: 1038–1039.

91. Rahmati-Bahram A, Magee JT, Jackson SK. 1995. Growth temperature-dependent variation of cell envelope lipids and antibiotic susceptibility in *Stenotrophomonas (Xanthomonas) maltophilia*. *J Antimicrob Chemother* 36:317–326.

92. McKay GA, Woods DE, MacDonald KL, Poole K. 2003. Role of phosphoglucomutase of *Stenotrophomonas maltophilia* in lipopolysaccharide biosynthesis, virulence, and antibiotic resistance. *Infect Immun* 71: 3068–3075.

93. Liu YY, Wang Y, Walsh TR, Yi LX, Zhang R, Spencer J, Doi Y, Tian G, Dong B, Huang X, Yu LF, Gu D, Ren H, Chen X, Lv L, He D, Zhou H, Liang Z, Liu JH, Shen J. 2016. Emergence of plasmid-mediated colistin resistance mechanism MCR-1 in animals and human beings in China: a microbiological and molecular biological study. *Lancet Infect Dis* 16:161–168.

94. Gooderham WJ, Hancock RE. 2009. Regulation of virulence and antibiotic resistance by two-component regulatory systems in *Pseudomonas aeruginosa*. *FEMS Microbiol Rev* 33:279–294.

95. Bader MW, Sanowar S, Daley ME, Schneider AR, Cho U, Xu W, Klevit RE, Le Moual H, Miller SI. 2005. Recognition of antimicrobial peptides by a bacterial sensor kinase. *Cell* 122:461–472.

96. Liu MC, Tsai YL, Huang YW, Chen HY, Hsueh PR, Lai SY, Chen LC, Chou YH, Lin WY, Liaw SJ. 2016. *Stenotrophomonas maltophilia* PhoP, a two-component response regulator, involved in antimicrobial susceptibilities. *PLoS One* 11:e0153753.

97. Avison MB, Higgins CS, von Heldreich CJ, Bennett PM, Walsh TR. 2001. Plasmid location and molecular heterogeneity of the L1 and L2 β-lactamase genes of *Stenotrophomonas maltophilia*. *Antimicrob Agents Chemother* 45:413–419.

98. Alonso A, Sanchez P, Martínez JL. 2000. *Stenotrophomonas maltophilia* D457R contains a cluster of genes from Gram-positive bacteria involved in antibiotic and heavy metal resistance. *Antimicrob Agents Chemother* 44:1778–1782.

99. Palleroni NJ, Bradbury JF. 1993. Stenotrophomonas, a new bacterial genus for *Xanthomonas maltophilia* (Hugh 1980) Swings et al. 1983. *Int J Syst Bacteriol* 43: 606–609.

100. Finkmann W, Altendorf K, Stackebrandt E, Lipski A. 2000. Characterization of N_2O-producing *Xanthomonas*-like isolates from biofilters as *Stenotrophomonas nitritireducens* sp. nov., *Luteimonas mephitis* gen. nov., sp. nov. and *Pseudoxanthomonas broegbernensis* gen. nov., sp. nov. *Int J Syst Evol Microbiol* 50:273–282.

101. Yamamura S, Morita Y, Hasan Q, Rao SR, Murakami Y, Yokoyama K, Tamiya E. 2002. Characterization of a new keratin-degrading bacterium isolated from deer fur. *J Biosci Bioeng* 93:595–600.

102. Assih EA, Ouattara AS, Thierry S, Cayol JL, Labat M, Macarie H. 2002. *Stenotrophomonas acidaminiphila* sp. nov., a strictly aerobic bacterium isolated from an upflow anaerobic sludge blanket (UASB) reactor. *Int J Syst Evol Microbiol* 52:559–568.

103. Wolf A, Fritze A, Hagemann M, Berg G. 2002. *Stenotrophomonas rhizophila* sp. nov., a novel plant-associated bacterium with antifungal properties. *Int J Syst Evol Microbiol* 52:1937–1944.

104. Yoon JH, Kang SJ, Oh HW, Oh TK. 2006. *Stenotrophomonas dokdonensis* sp. nov., isolated from soil. *Int J Syst Evol Microbiol* 56:1363–1367.

105. Yang HC, Im WT, Kang MS, Shin DY, Lee ST. 2006. *Stenotrophomonas koreensis* sp. nov., isolated from compost in South Korea. *Int J Syst Evol Microbiol* 56: 81–84.

106. Heylen K, Vanparys B, Peirsegaele F, Lebbe L, De Vos P. 2007. *Stenotrophomonas terrae* sp. nov. and *Stenotrophomonas humi* sp. nov., two nitrate-reducing bacteria isolated from soil. *Int J Syst Evol Microbiol* 57:2056–2061.

107. Kaparullina E, Doronina N, Chistyakova T, Trotsenko Y. 2009. *Stenotrophomonas chelatiphaga* sp. nov., a new aerobic EDTA-degrading bacterium. *Syst Appl Microbiol* 32:157–162.

108. Kim HB, Srinivasan S, Sathiyaraj G, Quan LH, Kim SH, Bui TP, Liang ZQ, Kim YJ, Yang DC. 2010. *Stenotrophomonas ginsengisoli* sp. nov., isolated from a ginseng field. *Int J Syst Evol Microbiol* 60:1522–1526.

109. Lee M, Woo SG, Chae M, Shin MC, Jung HM, Ten LN. 2011. *Stenotrophomonas daejeonensis* sp. nov., isolated from sewage. *Int J Syst Evol Microbiol* 61:598–604.

110. Ramos PL, Van Trappen S, Thompson FL, Rocha RC, Barbosa HR, De Vos P, Moreira-Filho CA. 2011. Screening for endophytic nitrogen-fixing bacteria in Brazilian sugar cane varieties used in organic farming and description of *Stenotrophomonas pavanii* sp. nov. *Int J Syst Evol Microbiol* 61:926–931.

111. Handa Y, Tazato N, Nagatsuka Y, Koide T, Kigawa R, Sano C, Sugiyama J. 2016. *Stenotrophomonas tumulicola*

sp. nov., a major contaminant of the stone chamber interior in the Takamatsuzuka Tumulus. *Int J Syst Evol Microbiol* **66:**1119–1124.

112. **Pan X, Lin D, Zheng Y, Zhang Q, Yin Y, Cai L, Fang H, Yu Y.** 2016. Biodegradation of DDT by *Stenotrophomonas* sp. DDT-1: characterization and genome functional analysis. *Sci Rep* **6:**21332.

113. **Hindler JF, Tamashiro L.** 2004. Broth microdilution MIC test, p 5.2.1–5.2.17. *In* Clarke L, Della-Latta P, Denys GA, Douglas SD, Garcia LS, Hazen KC, Hindler JF, Jenkins SG, Mangels JI, Miller JM, Nachamkin I, Pfaller MA, Snyder JW, Weissfeld AS, York MK (ed), *Clinical Microbiology Procedures Handbook*, 2nd ed. ASM Press, Washington, DC.

Antimicrobial Resistance in Bacteria from Livestock and Companion Animals
Edited by Frank Møller Aarestrup, Stefan Schwarz, Jianzhong Shen, and Lina Cavaco
© 2018 American Society for Microbiology, Washington, DC
doi:10.1128/microbiolspec.ARBA-0030-2018

Antimicrobial Resistance in *Mycoplasma* spp.

20

Anne V. Gautier-Bouchardon[1]

INTRODUCTION

Mycoplasmas belong to the phylum *Firmicutes* (Gram-positive bacteria with low G+C content), to the class *Mollicutes* (from Latin: *mollis*, soft; *cutis*, skin), to the order *Mycoplasmatales*, and to the family *Mycoplasmataceae*. They presumably evolved by degenerative evolution from Gram-positive bacteria and are phylogenetically most closely related to some clostridia. Mycoplasmas are the smallest self-replicating prokaryotes (diameter of approximately 0.2 to 0.3 μm) with the smallest genomes (500 to 1,000 genes). They are characterized by the lack of a cell wall. The mycoplasma cell contains the minimum set of organelles essential for growth and replication: a plasma membrane, ribosomes, and a genome consisting of a double-stranded circular DNA molecule (1). The mycoplasma genome is characterized by a low G+C content and by the use of the universal stop codon UGA as a tryptophan codon. As a result of their limited genetic information, mycoplasmas express a small number of cell proteins and lack many enzymatic activities and metabolic pathways (1). Their nutritional requirements are therefore complex, and they are dependent on their host for many nutrients. This phenomenon explains the great difficulty of *in vitro* cultivation of mycoplasmas, with complex media containing serum (as a source of fatty acids and cholesterol) and a metabolizable carbohydrate (as a source of energy, for example, glucose, arginine, or urea).

All mycoplasmas cultivated and identified so far are parasites of humans or animals (2–5), with a high degree of host and tissue specificity. The primary habitats of mycoplasmas are epithelial surfaces of the respiratory and urogenital tracts, serous membranes, and mammary glands in some animal species. Many *Mycoplasma* species are pathogens, causing various diseases and significant economic losses in livestock productions. Mycoplasmas have developed mechanisms to resist their hosts' immune systems: modulatory effects on the host immune system, a highly plastic set of variable surface proteins responsible for rapid changes in major surface protein antigens (6, 7) and invasion of nonphagocytic host cells (8–11). These mechanisms contribute to the persistence of mycoplasmas in their hosts and to the establishment of chronic infections. The main pathogenic species in humans and animals are listed in Table 1.

Since *in vitro* culture of mycoplasmas is difficult to achieve (only performed by specialized laboratories) because of their specific requirements and slow growth, diagnosis of mycoplasmal infections is usually based on serologic tests (enzyme-linked immunosorbent assay, rapid plate agglutination) or specific PCR tests.

Vaccination, when available, can be an effective way of reducing clinical signs and improving herd performances. However, vaccination provides only partial protection and does not prevent infection (12–15). Eradication programs have also been implemented for several *Mycoplasma* species such as *Mycoplasma gallisepticum* and *Mycoplasma meleagridis* in poultry (16). However, the use of antimicrobials can be necessary in case of outbreaks and to control infections of *Mycoplasma* species for which vaccines and control programs are not available.

Without a cell wall, mycoplasmas are unaffected by many antibiotics such as β-lactams, glycopeptides, and fosfomycin that target cell-wall synthesis. Mycoplasmas are also naturally resistant to rifampicin, polymixins, sulfonamides, first-generation quinolones such as nalidixic acid, and trimethoprim (17, 18). Resistance to rifampicin was found to be due to a natural mutation in the *rpoB* gene of the RNA polymerase β subunit,

[1]Mycoplasmology, Bacteriology, and Antimicrobial Resistance Unit, Ploufragan-Plouzané Laboratory, French Agency for Food, Environmental, and Occupational Health and Safety (ANSES), Ploufragan, France.

Table 1 Main pathogenic *Mycoplasma* species in humans and livestock animals[a]

Host	*Mycoplasma* species	Clinical signs or syndrome
Humans	*M. genitalium*	Urethritis, often associated with bacterial vaginosis and cervicitis
	M. hominis	Urogenital tract infections
	M. pneumoniae	Upper respiratory disease, bronchopneumonia
Cattle	*M. bovis*	Infectious enzootic bronchopneumonia, mastitis, arthritis, otitis
Chickens, turkeys	*M. gallisepticum*	Chronic respiratory disease, infectious sinusitis
	M. synoviae	Subclinical respiratory tract infections, infectious synovitis, eggshell apex abnormality syndrome in laying-hen flocks
Swine	*M. hyopneumoniae*	Enzootic pneumonia
	M. hyorhinis	Polyserositis, arthritis
	M. hyosynoviae	Arthritis, polyarthritis

[a]From references 67, 69, 84, 95, 97, 145–147.

which prevents the antibiotic from binding to its target (19, 20). Resistance to polymyxins and sulfonamides/trimethoprim is due to the absence in mycoplasmas of lipopolysaccharides and folic acid synthesis, respectively, which are the initial targets of these antimicrobials (21, 22). The most active and widely used antimicrobial agents in animals against mycoplasmal infections are tetracyclines, macrolides, fluoroquinolones, and pleuromutilins (12, 23, 24).

Methods used for antibiotic susceptibility testing of pathogenic *Mycoplasma* species of major veterinary interest (Table 1) will be described in this article. Activities of antimicrobials and resistance mechanisms will also be reviewed.

IN VITRO DETERMINATION OF ANTIMICROBIAL ACTIVITY

The effectiveness on antimicrobials *in vivo* can be indirectly assessed by *in vitro* susceptibility testing to determine the MIC and minimum bactericidal concentration (MBC) of an antimicrobial agent toward *Mycoplasma* strains.

MIC Determination

Numerous studies of the MIC determination of different antimicrobial agents for animal mycoplasmas have been published (for review see 23–25). However, because of their slow growth, very small size of colonies, and complex growth medium requirements, standard procedures used to test the susceptibility of classic bacteria, such as the disk diffusion method, are not recommended for mycoplasmas. The lack of consensus procedures (several culture media and methods, different presentation of results; see Table 2 for examples) and quality control (QC) strains makes comparisons between studies difficult or impossible. Studies comparing several testing methods for the same strains under-

lined the importance of using standardized methods, especially for the titer of the strains tested and the time of reading (initial versus final MIC values) (25–29).

Recommendations for antimicrobial susceptibility testing of animal *Mycoplasma* species were proposed in 2000 by the International Research Programme on Comparative Mycoplasmology (IRPCM) (25). More recently, the Clinical and Laboratory Standards Institute (CLSI) established standardized antimicrobial susceptibility testing guidelines to determine MICs for human mycoplasma pathogens (30). However, these guidelines cannot be used for all mycoplasmas because nutritional requirements, metabolic capacities, and fitness vary among species, as evidenced by an international multilaboratory collaborative study performed with human mycoplasmas (31): sufficient consensus of results necessary to generate 3- to 4-dilution QC ranges for some antimicrobial agents were not obtained, evidencing the difficulties generated by the fastidious nature of mycoplasmas. Such a collaborative study has not been conducted yet with animal mycoplasmas, and no veterinary reference strains well characterized for MICs are available and shared by laboratories for QC purposes. Recent studies performed with animal mycoplasmas therefore often take the IRPCM recommendations (32–35) or CLSI guidelines for human mycoplasmas (36–38) as a basis for MIC determinations, but with different media and controls.

Titration of strains is important since the inoculum concentration can influence MIC values obtained in broth or on agar medium (25, 30, 31). Because of their small size, titration of mycoplasmas cannot be performed by optical density determination like for classical bacteria. Titrations are performed in different broth or agar media, depending on the *Mycoplasma* species studied (Table 2). For broth titrations, series of 1:10 dilutions of cultures are performed in broth medium with a metabolic indicator (for example, phenol-red to

Table 2 Examples of methods used (culture media, methods and measurement, expression of results) for the determination of antimicrobial activities toward animal mycoplasmas[a]

Mycoplasma species	Culture medium (agar or broth)	Methods and measurement	Expression of results[b]
M. agalactiae	Eaton's medium Hayflick's type medium Mycoplasma medium with pyruvate PH medium PPLO culture medium	Agar dilution: colonies on agar Broth dilution: color changes (sodium pyruvate fermentation), growth in wells after centrifugation (inverted mirror) Etest method: intersection of the inhibition zone with the MIC scale Flow cytometry: cell counts at different times	MIC per strain, MIC distribution (range), MIC_{50} and/or MIC_{90} Growth curves (flow cytometry)
M. bovis	Eaton's medium Friis medium Hayflick's type medium *Mycoplasma* medium *M. bovis* medium PPLO broth	Agar dilution: colonies on agar Agar diffusion: inhibition diameters Broth dilution (prepared or Sensititre plates): color changes (glucose fermentation, sodium pyruvate fermentation, AlamarBlue reagent, redox reagent resazurin), growth in wells after centrifugation (inverted mirror) Etest method: intersection of the inhibition zone with the MIC scale Flow cytometry: cell counts at different times	Initial and/or final MIC MIC per strain, MIC distribution (range), MIC_{50} and/or MIC_{90} Growth curves (flow cytometry)
M. gallisepticum	FM4 medium Frey's medium Frey's modified medium Friis medium Hayflick's modified medium	Agar dilution: colonies on agar Broth dilution (prepared or Sensititre plates): color changes (glucose fermentation) Etest method: intersection of the inhibition zone with the MIC scale	Initial and/or final MIC MIC per strain, MIC distribution (range), MIC_{50} and/or MIC_{90} Means
M. hyopneumoniae	Difco Turkey Serum (D-TS) medium Friis medium Friis modified medium Hank's-lactalbumin medium Hayflick's type medium	Agar dilution: colonies on agar Agar diffusion: inhibition diameters Broth dilution (prepared or Sensititre plates): color changes (glucose fermentation) Flow cytometry: cell counts at different times Microtiter biphasic agar-broth medium: colonies on agar	Initial and/or final MIC MIC per strain, MIC distribution (range), MIC_{50} and/or MIC_{90} Growth curves (flow cytometry)
M. hyorhinis	Friis medium Friis modified medium Hayflick's type medium M medium	Agar dilution: colonies on agar Agar diffusion: inhibition diameters Broth dilution (prepared or Sensititre plates): color changes (glucose fermentation)	Initial and/or final MIC MIC per strain, MIC distribution (range), MIC_{50} and/or MIC_{90}
M. hyosynoviae	Friis medium with mucin Hayflick's type medium Arginin/mucin-enriched Hayflick's medium Modified Difco medium with arginine	Agar dilution: colonies on agar Broth dilution (prepared or Sensititre plates): color changes (arginine hydrolysis)	Initial and/or final MIC MIC per strain, MIC distribution (range), MIC_{50} and/or MIC_{90}
M. synoviae	FM4 medium Frey's medium Frey's modified medium Friis medium with NAD	Agar dilution: colonies on agar Broth dilution (prepared or Sensititre plates): color changes (glucose fermentation) Etest method: intersection of the inhibition zone with the MIC scale	Initial and/or final MIC MIC per strain, MIC distribution (range), MIC_{50} and/or MIC_{90}

[a]These examples were compiled from references 18, 29, 34, 36, 38–43, 47, 49, 56–59, 62–66, 73–76, 81, 86, 87, 93, 94, 98–100, 102, 107–112, 148, 149.
[b]MIC_{50}, MIC which inhibits 50% of the tested isolates; MIC_{90}: MIC which inhibits 90% of the isolates tested.

detect pH changes due to glucose fermentation). Dilution of the last tube to show growth is taken as the number of color-changing units. For agar titrations, the number of colonies is determined by observation with a stereomicroscope. Titers are obtained after several days, depending on the growth of the *Mycoplasma* species being studied. According to IRPCM recommendations, strain dilutions should be performed to yield 10^3 to 10^5

color-changing units/ml in broth medium or 10^3 to 10^5 CFU/ml on agar medium, whereas CLSI recommends 10^4 to 10^5 CFU/ml for broth and agar assays. For broth dilution MIC testing, MIC is generally defined as the lowest antibiotic concentration that inhibits growth (usually detected by a color change of the medium) when growth is compared to the growth observed in the control without antibiotic (25, 30, 31). However, final MIC values (when strains are incubated for longer periods) are also reported in several studies performed in broth medium (29, 39, 40). For agar dilution MIC testing, strains are usually transferred onto agar via a replicator, and MIC is generally defined as the lowest antibiotic concentration that prevents colony formation (visualized under a stereomicroscope) when colonies are observed on the antibiotic-free control plate (30, 31). However, MIC is sometimes defined as the concentration resulting in strong reduction (50% or more, depending on the studies performed) in colony number (25, 39, 41) or size (39, 42, 43).

No QC reference strains are currently available for MIC assays with animal mycoplasmas, whereas Waites and collaborators (31) published values for QC reference strains of human mycoplasmas. It is therefore important to repeat MIC determination assays several times on separate occasions and to include, when available, one or several strains already tested, with known MIC values for the antibiotics studied, to validate the results obtained.

The absence of interpretation criteria (breakpoint concentrations) for mycoplasmas makes it difficult to evaluate the likely *in vivo* therapeutic efficacy from MIC data established *in vitro*. MIC values are often compared to breakpoints given for classical bacteria (44, 45) or to breakpoints suggested by Hannan and collaborators (25) or Ter Laak and collaborators (39).

Finally, it should be noted that, because of their fastidious nature, only a few laboratories are able to isolate animal mycoplasmas (especially slow-growing ones such as *Mycoplasma hyopneumoniae* and *Mycoplasma hyosynoviae* in pigs and *Mycoplasma synoviae* in poultry, for example), and susceptibility testing methods have to be carried out over several weeks (from titration to MIC determinations). Susceptibility testing of mycoplasmas is therefore not performed as routine monitoring like it is for classical bacteria, and studies are often performed with strains from one *Mycoplasma* species from one country.

MBC Determination

Antibiotics are commonly classified into bactericidal and bacteriostatic agents based on their antimicrobial action: bacteriostatic agents prevent the growth of bacteria, and bactericidal agents kill bacteria. Determination of MBC is performed to know if an antibiotic has more a bacteriostatic or a bactericidal activity toward bacteria. MBC is defined as the lowest antibiotic concentration that kills ≥99.9% of the cells. If the MBC value is close to the MIC value, the antimicrobial agent has a bactericidal effect, and if the MBC value is significantly higher than the MIC value, the antimicrobial agent has a bacteriostatic effect.

Very few studies determining minimum bactericidal (or mycoplasmacidal) concentrations against animal *Mycoplasma* species have been published, and no standardized method has been described for veterinary or human mycoplasmas. Guidelines for performing bactericidal tests with classical bacteria were published in 1999 (46) but cannot be applied strictly to mycoplasmas because of their slow growth and medium requirements.

Several methods have been used: killing curves with *M. hyopneumoniae* (41), subcultures on agar at the same time as recording of initial MIC with *M. synoviae* (47), or antibiotic dilution for *Mycoplasma bovis* (48, 49) or *M. hyopneumoniae* (50). Two methods (dilution or filtration) were also described by Taylor-Robinson to remove antibiotics from the surviving mycoplasmas (51). Subculture on agar medium is the most widely used method for the determination of MBC for human mycoplasmas (52–54), but dilutions in broth medium are also described (55). Flow cytometric assessment of *in vitro* antimicrobial activity toward strains of *M. agalactiae* (56, 57), *M. bovis* (58), and *M. hyopneumoniae* (59) also provided information on the bactericidal or bacteriostatic activity of antibiotics.

Among the antibiotics tested, fluoroquinolones were shown to be mycoplasmacidal *in vitro* (41, 49, 54), whereas antibiotics of the tetracycline group and tiamulin were mycoplasmastatic (41, 47). Macrolides, lincosamides, and spectinomycin are usually classified as mycoplasmastatic antibiotics but showed a better mycoplasmacidal activity for *M. synoviae* in the Kleven and Anderson study (47) than did tetracycline antibiotics.

Finally, it should be noted that, due to their instability under *in vitro* conditions, the antimicrobial activity of some antibiotics may be underestimated during *in vitro* susceptibility tests. Moreover, the stability of several antimicrobials is known to be affected *in vitro* by light, composition of the medium, temperature, and pH (60, 61). This degradation can be associated with an increase of the MIC and MBC values, which may be clinically significant for slow-growing bacteria such as mycoplasmas. Due to the very slow growth of mycoplasmas, the time required for the determination of

MICs can vary from 1 day to 1 week. These longer incubation times can lead to degradation or loss of activity of some antibiotics *in vitro* and thus lead to an underestimation of the actual activity of these antibiotics. Results of *in vitro* assays should therefore always be taken with precaution because they do not always reflect the *in vivo* action of antimicrobial agents. Host-linked factors also contribute to success or failure of a treatment on *in vitro* susceptible bacteria (pH values and cation concentrations in different body compartments, differences between intracellular and extracellular antibiotic concentrations, etc.).

IN VITRO ACTIVITIES OF ANTIBIOTICS AGAINST MYCOPLASMAS OF VETERINARY ORIGIN

Mycoplasmas are intrinsically resistant to all antimicrobials targeting the cell wall, such as fosfomycin, glycopeptides, or β-lactam antibiotics (23). Several studies evidenced high MICs for β-lactam antibiotics in several *Mycoplasma* species (18, 39, 42, 58, 62–65). Mycoplasmas are also intrinsically resistant to sulfonamides (18, 21, 22), first-generation quinolones such as nalidixic acid (41, 50), trimethoprim (18, 66), polymixins, and rifampicin (19–22).

The antibiotics most frequently used to control *Mycoplasma* infections in animals are macrolides and tetracyclines. Other antimicrobial agents—lincosamides, fluoroquinolones, pleuromutilins, phenicols, and aminoglycosides—can also be active against mycoplasmas.

Ribosomes are targets for most of these classes of antimicrobials. Macrolides, lincosamides, and pleuromutilins inhibit protein synthesis by binding to the peptidyl transferase component of the 50S subunit of ribosomes. Tetracyclines also inhibit protein synthesis in the ribosome by binding to the 30S ribosomal subunit. Florfenicol binds to the 50S ribosomal subunit, inhibiting the peptidation reaction and the translation of bacterial mRNA, whereas aminoglycosides disturb peptide elongation at the 30S ribosomal subunit level, giving rise to inaccurate mRNA translation. Fluoroquinolones have affinity for DNA gyrase and topoisomerase IV and prevent DNA replication of bacteria.

Susceptibility profiles (ranges of MIC) of the main *Mycoplasma* species of veterinary interest are presented in Table 3 (avian mycoplasmas), Table 4 (porcine mycoplasmas), and Table 5 (ruminant mycoplasmas).

Poultry

Avian mycoplasmoses can cause significant economic losses on poultry farms. *M. gallisepticum* is responsible for chronic respiratory disease of chickens and infectious sinusitis of turkeys (67). *M. synoviae* causes subclinical respiratory tract infections and infectious synovitis (68) and is also responsible for the eggshell apex abnormality syndrome (69). *M. meleagridis* and *Mycoplasma iowae* are mainly observed in turkeys and may cause growth retardations and embryonic mortality (70, 71).

Several studies report *in vitro* susceptibility levels of *M. gallisepticum* field isolates (26, 29, 33, 41, 62, 72–80) (Table 3). Tiamulin MICs are consistently lower than those for other antimicrobial agents tested *in vitro*, even if strains with reduced susceptibility were found in old (before 2000) and recent (after 2000) studies (33, 74). Most *M. gallisepticum* isolates are also susceptible to tetracycline antibiotics (Table 3), with lower MIC values for oxytetracycline and doxycycline than for chlortetracycline (77, 79). *M. gallisepticum* is not intrinsically resistant to 14-membered ring macrolides such as erythromycin, and most strains are susceptible to macrolides (Table 3). However, high MIC levels of erythromycin, tylosin, and tilmicosin were evidenced in strains isolated before and after 2000 in several countries (26, 33, 62, 72, 74, 75, 78, 79). For example, Gerchman and collaborators (78) reported that acquired resistance to tylosin and tilmicosin was present in 50% of *M. gallisepticum* strains isolated in Israel from 1997 to 2010. An increase in MIC levels was also reported for enrofloxacin, especially in studies comparing old and recent isolates (29, 79), even if most strains remained susceptible to this fluoroquinolone antimicrobial *in vitro*, with low MIC values (29, 74, 77, 79, 80). A marked decrease in susceptibility to fluoroquinolones was evidenced in field strains of *M. gallisepticum* in Israel (29), and 72% of the strains isolated since 2006 showed acquired resistance to enrofloxacin and macrolides (78). Only one study reported florfenicol MIC determination for *M. gallisepticum* isolates and showed good activity, with MICs ranging from 0.125 to 4 µg/ml (79).

Several studies report *in vitro* susceptibility levels of *M. synoviae* field isolates (29, 32, 41, 47, 74–76, 81, 82) (Table 3). *M. synoviae* was shown to be intrinsically resistant to 14-membered ring macrolides such as erythromycin (47, 82), and recent studies (published after 2000) evidenced strains with reduced susceptibility to other macrolides and lincosamides (82). In several studies, *M. synoviae* was found to be intrinsically less susceptible to fluoroquinolones than *M. gallisepticum* (29, 83) and resistant to flumequine (75). Recent *M. synoviae* strains (isolated between 2009 and 2012) with decreased susceptibility to enrofloxacin (MIC ranging

Table 3 MIC values (range in µg/ml) for various antimicrobials against avian *Mycoplasma* species (*M. gallisepticum* and *M. synoviae*)

Antimicrobials[b]	*M. gallisepticum*		*M. synoviae*	
	Old strains[a]	Recent strains[a]	Old strains[a]	Recent strains[a]
Tetracyclines:				
Tetracycline	0.08–0.64	ND	1–2	ND
Oxytetracycline	0.05–0.5	≤0.03–4	0.1–>100	0.39–3.12
Doxycycline	ND[d]	≤0.03–0.79	ND	ND
Chlortetracycline	ND	0.2–32	1–2	0.32–>12.5
Macrolides:				
Erythromycin	0.02–>80	≤0.03–>64	>40	32–>128
Tylosin	0.0025–10	≤0.03–5	0.025–10	≤0.006–2
Tilmicosin	ND	≤0.03–32	ND	0.03–>8
Josamycin	ND	0.2–>50	ND	ND
Spiramycin	0.5–>20	ND	ND	ND
Tylvalosin	ND	ND	ND	≤0.006–0.012
Lincosamides:				
Lincomycin	1.25–40	0.1–12.5	1–2	0.125–8
Pleuromutilins:				
Tiamulin	0.0005–1	≤0.03–2	0.1–1	0.012–0.12
Fluoroquinolones:				
Flumequine	2.5–10	ND	5–50	ND
Enrofloxacin	0.005–1[c]	≤0.03–10	0.1–10[c]	0.03–8
Danofloxacin	0.01–0.5	ND	0.1–0.5	ND
Amphenicols:				
Florfenicol	ND	0.125–4	ND	ND
Aminoglycosides:				
Spectinomycin	0.5–10	≤0.03–2	0.5–2	ND
Gentamicin	≥10–≥50	1–32	1	ND

[a]Data were compiled from studies performed on old strains (before 2000) (26, 41, 47, 62, 72–75) and more recent strains (2000 to 2016) (29, 32, 33, 76–82). Several methods were used to determine these MIC values.
[b]Antimicrobial family and antibiotics belonging to this family.
[c]For enrofloxacin, one study (29) compared isolates from 1997 to 2003 and from 2005 to 2006; results obtained for isolates from 1997 to 2003 are classified as old strains in this table.
[d]ND, no data found.

from 1 to 16 µg/ml) were found in Italy, Austria, and Israel (32), and several strains isolated between 1996 and 2008 in Israel already showed decreased susceptibility to this antibiotic (29). Tetracycline antimicrobials and tiamulin showed a relatively good *in vitro* activity against *M. synoviae* strains (Table 3), but strains with higher tetracycline MICs have been reported (75, 81).

Very few MIC determination studies have been performed with *M. meleagridis* and *M. iowae* strains. Two studies reported MIC values of enrofloxacin, tylosin, and tiamulin for very few strains (mainly reference strains of *M. iowae* and *M. meleagridis*) (41, 74), whereas a third study reported values of several antimicrobials for 19 strain of *M. iowae* (75). All the antibiotics tested showed a good activity against most strains. Danofloxacin, enrofloxacin, and tiamulin were the most effective antibiotics *in vitro*, whereas higher MIC values were observed for flumequine and tylosin (75).

Swine

Pathogenic swine mycoplasmas are considered to play an important role in pig production. *M. hyopneumoniae* is one of the primary pathogens associated with the porcine respiratory disease complex, one of the most common and economically important diseases for swine producers worldwide (84). *M. hyopneumoniae* is the etiological agent of enzootic pneumonia in swine, a chronic respiratory disease characterized by high morbidity and low mortality rates. Polyserositis and arthritis, induced by *Mycoplasma hyorhinis* and *M. hyosynoviae*, generally affect growing pigs (84). *Mycoplasma flocculare* is isolated in the swine respiratory tract and is genetically close to *M. hyopneumoniae*. Its role is still unclear, and it is often considered a commensal bacterium (85).

Several studies reported *in vitro* susceptibility levels of *M. hyopneumoniae* field isolates (39, 41, 50, 63, 75,

Table 4 MIC values (range in μg/ml) for various antimicrobials against swine *Mycoplasma* species (*M. hyopneumoniae*, *M. hyorhinis*, and *M. hyosynoviae*)

Antimicrobials[b]	M. hyopneumoniae		M. hyorhinis		M. hyosynoviae	
	Old strains[a]	Recent strains[a]	Old strains[a]	Recent strains[a]	Old strains[a]	Recent strains[a]
Tetracyclines:						
Tetracycline	0.025–1	ND[c]	≤0.03–0.5	≤0.5–2	0.01–10	ND
Oxytetracycline	0.025–2	0.03–12.5	0.025–10	0.1–6.3	0.1–10	0.5–>4
Doxycycline	≤0.03–1	0.03–6.25	≤0.03–0.5	ND	ND	ND
Chlortetracycline	0.12–50	3.12–100	0.12–8	0.2–12.5	ND	0.5–>4
Macrolides:						
Erythromycin	16–>16	6.25–>400	>16	>16	ND	ND
Tylosin	≤0.006–6.25	0.008–16	≤0.03–25	0.4–100	0.025–>10	≤0.25–1
Tilmicosin	ND	≤0.25–>16	ND	≤0.25–8	ND	≤2–32
Josamycin	≤0.006–0.2	0.1–>12.5	0.2–50	0.2–50	ND	ND
Spiramycin	0.06–0.5	0.03–25	≤0.03–4	ND	ND	ND
Tylvalosin	ND	0.016–0.06	ND	ND	ND	ND
Tulathromycin	≤0.004–0.125	ND	ND	ND	ND	1–≥32
Lincosamides:						
Lincomycin	0.025–1.56	≤0.025–>12.5	0.06–200	≤0.25–50	0.03–1	ND
Clindamycin	0.12–0.25	ND	0.06–1	ND	ND	≤0.12–0.25
Pleuromutilins:						
Tiamulin	≤0.006–0.3	≤0.01–0.125	0.025–0.78	0.2–1.56	0.0025–0.1	≤0.25
Valnemulin	0.00025–0.001	0.08	ND	ND	0.0001–0.00025	ND
Fluoroquinolones:						
Flumequine	0.25–1	0.25–>16	2.5–25	ND	5–50	ND
Enrofloxacin	0.0025–0.1	0.015–25	≤0.03–2	0.06–4	0.05–0.5	0.12–0.5
Danofloxacin	0.01–0.05	ND	0.25–1	ND	0.1–0.5	0.25–0.5
Amphenicols:						
Florfenicol	ND	ND	ND	ND	ND	0.25–4
Chloramphenicol	0.5–2	0.5–4	0.5–4	ND	ND	ND
Thiamphenicol	ND	ND	0.2–12.5	1.56–12.5	ND	ND
Aminoglycosides:						
Spectinomycin	0.5–6.5	0.06–2	0.12–4	≤1–8	ND	4
Gentamicin	0.1–2.5	≤0.125–1	ND	1–4	0.25–0.5	0.5

[a]Data were compiled from studies on old strains (isolated before 2000) (39–42, 63, 75, 86, 87, 89, 90, 93, 94) and more recent strains (2000 to 2016) (18, 43, 50, 66, 91–93). Several methods were used to determine these MIC values.
[b]Antimicrobial family and antibiotics belonging to this family.
[c]ND, no data found.

86–93) (Table 4). *M. hyopneumoniae* was shown to be intrinsically resistant to erythromycin (39, 50, 63, 93) but usually susceptible to 16-membered ring macrolides such as tylosin and tilmicosin (Table 4). However, strains with reduced susceptibility or resistance to macrolides and lincomycin were evidenced in studies performed in Belgium, Spain, and Thailand between 2004 and 2014 (50, 91, 93). Comparison between *M. hyopneumoniae* strains isolated from 1970 to 1981 and 1989 to 1990 in Japan and from 1997 to 1998 and 2006 to 2011 in Thailand suggested a decrease in chlortetracycline susceptibility (88, 93). As already seen for avian mycoplasmas, MIC values of chlortetracycline were higher than values for oxytetracycline and doxycycline, and most strains remained susceptible to

these antibiotics (Table 4). Pleuromutilins (tiamulin and valnemulin) were the most active antimicrobials *in vitro*, with MIC values not higher than 0.3 μg/ml. Most studied strains were also susceptible to fluoroquinolones, but strains with reduced susceptibility or resistance were isolated in Thailand and Belgium after 2000 (91, 93).

Like *M. hyopneumoniae*, *M. hyorhinis* is intrinsically resistant to erythromycin (39, 66). Even if macrolides and lincosamides still had good *in vitro* activity against most strains, several studies evidenced the selection of resistant strains (39, 42, 43, 66, 75). Strains of *M. hyorhinis* with resistance to 16-membered macrolides and lincomycin four times higher than 10 years before were isolated in Japan (43), and two strains

Table 5 MIC values (range in μg/ml) for various antimicrobials against ruminant *Mycoplasma* species (*M. bovis* and *M. agalactiae*)

Antimicrobials[b]	M. bovis		M. agalactiae	
	Old strains[a]	Recent strains[a]	Old strains[a]	Recent strains[a]
Tetracyclines:				
Tetracycline	0.05–1	0.05–>256	ND	0.125–32
Oxytetracycline	0.1–128	0.05–>256	0.1–4	0.06–16
Doxycycline	ND[c]	0.023–8	ND	0.008–1
Chlortetracycline	3.12–100	0.25–>32	ND	0.125–8
Macrolides:				
Erythromycin	50–>100	1–>512	ND	6–>256
Tylosin	0.025–>100	0.125–>256	0.1–1	0.03–12.8
Tilmicosin	1–>128	0.5–>1024	0.12–1	0.12–64
Spiramycin	0.39–>100	ND	ND	0.125–4
Gamithromycin	32–>128	128–>128	ND	4–32
Tulathromycin	1–64	0.25–>1024	ND	1–8
Azythromycin	ND	0.25–>256	ND	ND
Lincosamides:				
Lincomycin	0.39–3.12	0.06–>256	ND	0.125–4
Clindamycin	ND	≤0.03–>256	ND	≤0.12
Pleuromutilins:				
Tiamulin	0.05–1	ND	0.05–0.25	0.125–0.5
Valnemulin	ND	≤0.03	ND	ND
Fluoroquinolones:				
Flumequine	10–100	ND	ND	>128
Enrofloxacin	0.05–1	≤0.03–32	0.05–1	0.06–1.6
Danofloxacin	0.125–2.5	0.08–32	0.05–2.5	0.25–0.5
Marbofloxacin	0.25–1	0.25–>32	ND	0.1–12.8
Amphenicols:				
Chloramphenicol	6.25–25	0.25–32	ND	1–8
Florfenicol	1–64	0.06–32	1–8	2–8
Aminoglycosides:				
Spectinomycin	1–>128	0.38–>256	1–8	0.25–8
Gentamicin	ND	2.8	ND	0.5–16

[a]Data were compiled from studies performed on old strains (before 2000) (36, 38, 41, 49, 75, 87, 101) and more recent strains (2000 to 2016) (34, 36, 38, 58, 64, 65, 98–100, 102–105, 107–114). Several methods were used to determine these MIC values.
[b]Antimicrobial family and antibiotics belonging to this family.
[c]ND, No data found.

were resistant to all macrolides and lincomycin. However, this resistance reverted to susceptibility by serial *in vitro* subcultures without antibiotics. Fluoroquinolone MIC values were higher for *M. hyorhinis* than for *M. hyopneumoniae* (Table 4), and isolates with reduced susceptibility were evidenced in studies performed with strains isolated before and after 2000 (39, 42, 43, 66, 75). Tiamulin remained one of the most active antimicrobials *in vitro* against *M. hyorhinis*, but MIC values for recent strains (isolated after 2000) were 10 times higher than for old strains (isolated before 2000) (Table 4).

Several studies published before 2000 and one recent study (2012) report *in vitro* susceptibility levels of *M. hyosynoviae* field isolates (18, 40, 41, 75, 87, 89,

94) (Table 4). Resistance to macrolide antibiotics was evidenced in strains isolated before 2000: 2 of 54 old Japanese strains of *M. hyosynoviae* isolated between 1980 and 1995 showed resistance to all 14- and 16-membered macrolide antibiotics tested (94). Reduced susceptibility or resistance to tylosin was also evidenced for several Danish *M. hyosynoviae* strains isolated from 1995 to 1996 compared to older strains (1968 to 1971) (40). However, another study showed good *in vitro* activity of tylosin and clindamycin against U.S. strains isolated between 1997 and 2011 but higher MIC values for tilmicosin and tulathromycin (18). *M. hyosynoviae* strains isolated from 1994 to 1995 were less susceptible to tetracyclines than strains isolated from 1980 to 1984 (40). All strains of *M. hyosynoviae* were susceptible to

tiamulin, valnemulin, gentamicin, enrofloxacin, and danofloxacin (Table 4).

Only a very limited number of reports are available on MIC values for *M. flocculare*. Two studies, published in 1991 and 1994, reported good *in vitro* activity of tetracyclines, lincosamides, tiamulin, enrofloxacin, and spectinomycin (39, 87). *M. flocculare* strains were resistant to erythromycin but susceptible to tylosin and spiramycin (Table 4).

Cattle and Other Ruminants

In cattle, *M. bovis* causes respiratory disease, mastitis, arthritis, and otitis (95). This *Mycoplasma* species is frequently implicated in cases of bovine respiratory disease in calves raised in feedlots (96). *Mycoplasma agalactiae* is the causative agent of contagious agalactia, a serious disease of sheep and goats, affecting mammary glands, joints, and eyes and causing severe economic losses (97).

Several studies reported *in vitro* susceptibility levels of *M. bovis* field isolates to several antimicrobials (34, 36, 41, 49, 58, 64, 65, 75, 87, 98–105) (Table 5). All *M. bovis* strains were found to be resistant to erythromycin (64, 99, 106), suggesting an intrinsic resistance to the 14-membered ring macrolides. Resistance to tetracyclines and macrolides was already reported in strains isolated before 2000 (36, 49, 75), but resistant isolates were more frequently found in recent isolates (34, 36, 100, 102, 103) (Table 5). In France, an overall decrease in antimicrobial susceptibility was evidenced for *M. bovis* isolates by comparison between old (1978 to 1979) and recent (2010 to 2012) strains isolated from cattle (36): susceptibility of *M. bovis* decreased significantly for eight antimicrobials from the tetracycline, fluoroquinolone, aminoglycoside, and macrolide families. This led to a high prevalence of multiresistant strains of *M. bovis* in France (36): 100% of the *M. bovis* isolates tested harbored a reduced susceptibility or resistance to eight antimicrobials. However, no high-level resistance to fluoroquinolones was evidenced in recent French isolates of *M. bovis*: 2- to 4-fold increases of the MIC levels of fluoroquinolones were evidenced in most of these strains, suggesting an ongoing shift of French isolates toward a low-level resistance phenotype (36). Resistant strains were also found in other countries. Strains with acquired resistance to spectinomycin, clindamycin, tetracycline, and azithromycin were found in Canada between 2001 and 2003 (99), enrofloxacin being the most effective antibiotic, with MICs of ≤0.5 µg/ml. Recent Chinese isolates (2011 to 2013) were susceptible or had medium sensitivity to enrofloxacin and doxycycline but were

frequently resistant to macrolides (103). All recent Japanese strains of *M. bovis* isolated from milk samples were susceptible to fluoroquinolones, but several strains were resistant to kanamycin (aminoglycoside), oxytetracycline, and macrolides (102).

Fluoroquinolone-resistant strains were isolated in Europe (105), with marbofloxacin MICs ranging from 0.5 to 4 µg/ml. *M. bovis* strains isolated between 2008 and 2014 in the Netherlands also harbored high MIC values for several antimicrobial agents (34). In this study, fluoroquinolones appeared to be the most efficacious in inhibiting *M. bovis* growth *in vitro*, followed by tulathromycin and oxytetracycline. However, strains with reduced susceptibility or resistance were observed for these antibiotics. The highest MIC values were obtained for macrolides. For tulathromycin, MIC_{50} (MIC inhibiting 50% of the strains studied) for respiratory isolates was higher than for isolates from mastitis or arthritis (34), which can probably be explained by the frequent use of this antibiotic to treat respiratory infections and the absence of registration for mastitis or arthritis. Similarly, a significant difference in the susceptibility levels between quarter milk and lung isolates was found for spectinomycin (58), showing that the sample source can have an effect on antimicrobial activity profiles. Moreover, Gerchman and collaborators showed that local strains (isolated from cattle in Israel) were significantly more resistant to macrolides than strains from imported animals but were more susceptible to fluoroquinolones and spectinomycin (100). All these results also showed that the frequency of resistance in *M. bovis* isolates varies considerably from one country to another and that resistance can be observed for all the families of antimicrobials tested (tetracyclines, macrolides, fluoroquinolones, lincosamides, amphenicols, and aminoglycosides) except pleuromutilins (Table 5).

Old and recent studies reporting *in vitro* susceptibility levels of *M. agalactiae* field isolates showed that antimicrobial susceptibility profiles for this *Mycoplasma* species were different from antimicrobial susceptibility profiles of *M. bovis* field isolates (38, 75, 107–114) (Table 5). Even if resistance to macrolides and tetracyclines was evidenced in recent studies (38, 110), levels and frequencies of resistance were lower. Most strains remained susceptible or intermediate for fluoroquinolones and lincosamides (Table 5). One Spanish study found a wide MIC range for marbofloxacin (0.1 to 12.8 µg/ml) compared to other fluoroquinolones (114). Poumarat and collaborators, comparing old (1980 to 1990) and recent (2008 to 2012) strains from ovine or caprine origin, showed that a moderate shift toward higher MICs (two to four times higher) was observed for most of the antimicrobials tested, whereas the increase was more marked in ovine isolates but was restricted to macrolides (38): ovine isolates were shown to remain mainly susceptible over time. The authors hypothesized that this difference between caprine and ovine isolates could be due to different antimicrobial uses. Similarly, Paterna and collaborators found higher MIC values for several antimicrobials with *M. agalactiae* isolates from goat herds with clinical symptoms than from asymptomatic animals (114).

MYCOPLASMA RESISTANCE TO ANTIMICROBIALS

Several studies showed that resistance to antibiotics could be selected *in vitro* by several passages in subinhibitory concentrations of various antibiotics such as macrolides, fluoroquinolones, tetracyclines, or pleuromutilins (43, 115, 116). The rate of selection of resistant mutants appeared to be dependent on both the *Mycoplasma* species and the antibiotic (or family of antibiotics) used to select these mutants. Macrolide-resistant mutants were rapidly selected in *M. gallisepticum*, *M. synoviae*, *M. iowae*, and *M. bovis*, whereas more *in vitro* passages in the presence of subinhibitoty concentrations of antibiotics were necessary for fluoroquinolones, tetracyclines, and pleuromutilins (115–117). High MIC levels for tylosin were also reported in *M. hyopneumoniae* within five to seven *in vitro* passages whereas only a slight increase of MIC for oxytetracycline and no significant increase in MIC of valnemulin or tiamulin for two strains of *M. hyopneumoniae* were evidenced after 10 *in vitro* passages (89). This progressive increase in the level of resistance of strains to some antibiotics suggests a progressive selection of resistance mechanisms, such as point mutations, in different sites or target genes, whereas a rapid increase suggests the selection of a single mechanism conferring a high level of resistance.

Selection of mutants with reduced susceptibility or resistance to antimicrobials has also been reported after *in vivo* fluoroquinolone treatments of hens experimentally infected with *M. synoviae* (83) or *M. hyopneumoniae*-infected pigs (118). Links between field usage of antimicrobials and development of resistance were also evidenced: for example, according to Khalil and collaborators (119), the shift of *M. bovis* strains toward resistance to oxytetracycline happened earlier than for macrolides, which is in accordance with the earlier marketing authorization date for tetracycline and its earlier use in field conditions than macrolides.

Several recent studies described resistance mechanisms of animal *Mycoplasma* species in clinical isolates or in mutants obtained *in vitro*. Since mycoplasmas do not harbor plasmids, most resistance mechanisms described in mycoplasmas are point mutations in their chromosome, and few mechanisms are associated with a transposon.

Macrolides

Macrolide and lincosamide antibiotics are chemically distinct but share a similar mode of action. Bacteria become resistant to macrolide and lincosamide antibiotics (i) through target-site modification by methylation or mutation that prevents the binding of the antibiotic to its ribosomal target, (ii) through efflux of the antibiotic, and (iii) by drug inactivation. Modification of the ribosomal target confers broad-spectrum resistance to macrolides and lincosamides, whereas efflux and drug inactivation affect only some of these molecules (120).

Macrolides bind within the tunnel of the 50S ribosomal subunit and interact mainly with the A2058 nucleotide of the 23S rRNA (domain V), with an additional interaction with and around the G748 nucleotide (23S rRNA, domain II) and with the surface of proteins L4 and L22 (121, 122). Most of the point mutations described in *Mycoplasma* isolates harboring decreased susceptibility or resistance to macrolides are described at these positions or nearby (Table 6).

Several point mutations in domain V of the 23S rRNA gene were evidenced in macrolide-resistant *M. gallisepticum* isolates from Egypt (33), China (117), and Israel (78): the G2057A, A2058G, and A2059G substitutions were shown to be implicated in reduced susceptibility or resistance to macrolide antibiotics (Table 6).

Reduced susceptibility or resistance to macrolides or lincosamides in *M. synoviae* was also correlated with the presence of several amino acid substitutions in the 23S rRNA alleles (82) (Table 6). *M. synoviae* has an intrinsic resistance to 14-membered macrolides such as erythromycin, correlated with a G2057A substitution in the 23S rRNAs in all strains (82). The presence of point mutations A2058G and A2059G was correlated with a significant decrease in susceptibility to tylosin, tilmicosin, and lincomycin. A nucleotide substitution G748A in domain II was also evidenced: its presence in one or both 23S rRNA alleles may be responsible for a slight increase in MICs to macrolides, but no correlation between the presence of G748A and decreased susceptibility to lincomycin was found. Mutations G64E and Q90K/H were identified in the L4 and L22 proteins, respectively, but their impact on decreased

Table 6 Mutations in the 23S rRNA genes and in the ribosomal proteins L4 and L22 conferring resistance in animal *Mycoplasma* species

Mutations in[a]	*Mycoplasma* species (host species)	Impact on MIC values[b]	References
23S rRNA domain II			
G748A in one or both alleles (*rrl3* and *rrl4*)	*M. synoviae* (chicken, turkey)	Increase for Ty (up to 16-fold) and Tm (up to 67-fold)	82
G748A in both alleles (*rrl3* and *rrl4*)	*M. bovis* (cattle)	Increase for Ty (up to 64-fold) and Tm (up to 256-fold)	116, 119, 123
C752T in *rrl4*	*M. bovis* (cattle)	No clear impact	123
G954A in *rrl3*	*M. bovis* (cattle)	ND: no isolate with only this single mutation	119
23S rRNA domain V			
G2057A	*M. hyopneumoniae* (swine)	Intrinsic resistance to Ery	92
	M. synoviae (chicken, turkey)	Intrinsic resistance to Ery	82
	M. gallisepticum (chicken)	Increase for Ery (up to 128-fold)	33, 117
A2058G in one or both alleles (*rrl3* and *rrl4*)	*M. synoviae* (chicken, turkey)	Significant increase for Ty (up to 67-fold), Tm (up to 267-fold) and Ln (up to 64-fold)	82
	M. gallisepticum (chicken, turkey)	Significant increase for Ery (up to 8,533-fold), Ty (up to 125-fold), Tm (up to 1,000-fold) and Ln (up to 128-fold)	33, 78, 117
	M. bovis (cattle)	Significant increase for Ty (up to 32-fold) and Tm (up to 512-fold)	103, 119, 123
	M. agalactiae (sheep and goats)	Significant increase for Ty (8- to 64-fold)	111
A2059G in one or both alleles (*rrl3* and *rrl4*)	*M. synoviae* (chicken, turkey)	Significant increase for Ty (up to 67-fold), Tm (up to 267-fold), and Ln (up to 64-fold)	82
	M. gallisepticum (chicken, turkey)	Significant increase for Ery, Ty, Tm, and Ln	33, 78, 117
	M. bovis (cattle)	Significant increase for Ty, Tm, and Ln (up to 32-fold)	116, 123
	M. agalactiae (sheep and goats)	Significant increase for Ty (320-fold) and Ln (320-fold)	111
G2144A in *rrl3*	*M. bovis* (cattle)	No clear impact	119
C2152 in *rrl4*	*M. bovis* (cattle)	No clear impact	119
A2503U	*M. gallisepticum* (*in vitro*-selected mutants)	ND: mutation always described combined with A2058G or A2059G	117
G2526A	*M. bovis* (cattle)	No clear impact	119
C2611G	*M. gallisepticum* (chicken)	ND: no isolate with this single mutation	33
C2611T	*M. agalactiae* (sheep and goats)	Increase for Ty (3- to 10-fold) and Ln (2-fold) when associated with a A2059G substitution	111
L4 protein			
G64E	*M. synoviae* (chicken, turkey)	No clear impact	82
G185R/W	*M. bovis* (cattle)	No effect alone	119
G185A/L/R/V/W	*M. bovis* (cattle)	No clear impact alone	123
T186P	*M. bovis* (cattle)	No clear impact alone	123
L22 protein			
S89L	*M. agalactiae* (sheep and goats)	Slight increase for Ty (2- to 8-fold) and no impact for Ln	111
Q90K/H	*M. agalactiae* (sheep and goats)	Slight increase for Ty (2-fold) and Ln (2-fold)	111
	M. synoviae (chicken, turkey)	No clear impact	82
Q93K/H	*M. bovis* (cattle)	Increase for Ty (up to 8-fold) and Tm (up to 16-fold)	119
Q90H	*M. bovis* (cattle)	No clear impact	123

[a]*Escherichia coli* numbering.
[b]A quantitative impact is given into brackets when the MIC increase could be calculated (when the mutation was observed alone and/or when MIC values were available to compare isolates with or without this mutation). Ery, erythromycin; Ty, tylosin; Tm, tilmicosine; Ln, lincomycin; ND, not determined (or impact difficult to evaluate because several mutations were observed at the same time).

susceptibility to macrolides and lincomycin was not clear (82).

M. hyopneumoniae has an intrinsic resistance to 14-membered macrolides due to a G2057A transition in their 23S rRNA (92). An additional, acquired A2058G point mutation was found in the 23S rRNA of a field strain resistant to 16-membered macrolides such as tylosin and to lincosamides (Table 6).

M. hyorhinis has an intrinsic resistance to 14-membered macrolides such as erythromycin or oleandomycin, but most strains remained susceptible to tylosin and tilmicosin (42, 94). Mutants of *M. hyorhinis* that were resistant to macrolides/lincosamides were selected *in vitro* by serial passages in subinhibitory concentrations of tylosin or lincomycin (43). The same A2059G mutation was found in mutants selected in tylosin and in field strains. Other mutations were evidenced in domains II and V of 23S rRNA of the mutant selected in lincomycin: addition of an adenine at pentameric adenine sequence in domain II, G2597U, and C2611 in domain V. After 11 tylosin passages of this lincomycin-resistant mutant, another point mutation at position A2062G was detected (Table 6).

In *M. bovis*, the presence of any of the point mutations G748A or C752T (domain II), A2058G, or A2059G/C (domain V) in one or both alleles of the 23S rRNA was correlated with decreased susceptibility to tylosin and tilmicosin (123). The A2058G substitution was also evidenced in Chinese macrolide-resistant clinical isolates (103). However combination of mutations in the two domains seems to be necessary to achieve higher MICs (123). Point mutations in domain II may play a more critical role in acquired resistance to tilmicosin than tylosin, suggesting that there may be differences in the way these two macrolides interact within the binding site (122, 124). Sulyok and collaborators suggested that mutations in domain II (position 748 and insertion after nucleotide C752) were necessary to achieve tilmicosin and tylosin MICs of ≥128 and ≤32 µg/ml, respectively, whereas an additional mutation in domain V (positions 2059, 2060, 2063, and 2067) was needed to reach highly elevated tylosin (MIC, ≥128 µg/ml) and lincomycin (MIC, ≥64 µg/ml) MICs (116). Several mutations in L4 and L22 proteins were evidenced in *M. bovis* isolates (Table 6), but their contribution to increased MIC levels was difficult to establish since other point mutations were often present in the same isolates in domain II of both *rrl* alleles (123).

Two substitutions in protein L22 (Ser89-Leu and Gln90-Lys/His) were evidenced in clinical isolates of *M. agalactiae* with reduced susceptibility to macrolides,

whereas a mutation A2058G in domain V of the 23S rRNA gene was involved in a higher level of resistance (111) (Table 6). The substitutions Ser89-Leu and Gln90-Lys were also observed in protein L22 of *in vitro*-selected mutants. The A2058G substitution was not observed in mutants, but the mutation A2059G in both alleles led to a high level of resistance to macrolides (MIC, >128 µg/ml for tylosin and tilmicosin) and lincosamides (MIC, 6.4 µg/ml for lincomycin and clindamycin). Selection in lincomycin led to the selection of a C2611T substitution in both alleles of domain V, with an increase of MIC values for macrolides (3- to 10-fold) and lincosamides (2-fold) when associated with the A2059G substitution in one allele (Table 6).

Resistance to macrolides can also be the result of methylation of key nucleotides in domains II and/or V in bacteria (120). Methylation of DNA is an epigenetic modification (thus reversible) which concerns cytosines associated with guanine, by adding a methyl-CH3 group on carbon 5. This chemical modification, ensured by DNA-methyltransferases, may cause inhibition of the expression of certain genes without changing the sequence. Methylation has been reported in mycoplasmas (125), and methyltransferases responsible for methylation have been described in several *Mycoplasma* species (126–128), but no methylated G748 or A2058 has been identified until now.

No efflux mechanism involved in macrolide resistance has been described so far in *Mycoplasma* species, but an *erm*B methylase gene and three subtypes of active efflux *msr* gene have been reported in a macrolide- and lincosamide-resistant *Ureaplasma urealyticum* strain, which belongs to the *Mycoplasmataceae* family (129).

Tetracyclines

Tetracyclines bind to the 30S ribosomal subunit. Their binding pocket is formed by an irregular minor grove of helix 34 (residues 1196 to 1200:1053 to 1056) in combination with residues 964 to 967 from the helix 31 stem-loop (130).

Decreased susceptibilities to tetracycline in *M. bovis* strains (MICs, ≥2 µg/ml) were associated with mutations at two (A965T and A967T/C) or three (A965T, A967T/C, and G1058A/C) positions of the two 16S rRNA-encoding genes (*rrs3* and *rrs4* alleles) (116, 131). Another study showed that for *M. bovis* resistance to oxytetracycline, a single A967T point mutation in one *rrs* allele of 16S rRNA had a minor impact on MIC values (119). Homozygote mutations in positions 965 and 967 of the *rrs* genes are necessary and sufficient to increase oxytetracycline MICs and to categorize such isolates as resistant. Other point mutations evidenced in these *rrs* genes in positions 1058, 1192, and 1199 did not further modify MIC values (119). Cross-resistance between tetracycline and spectinomycin was reported in tetracycline-resistant mutants obtained *in vitro* (116).

Fluoroquinolones

Fluoroquinolones kill dividing bacteria by inhibiting the topoisomerases II and IV, which are required for DNA replication (132). Resistance to fluoroquinolones in several *Mycoplasma* species is due to alterations in the quinolone resistance-determining regions (QRDR) of the *gyr*A and *gyr*B genes encoding DNA-gyrase and the *par*C and *par*E genes encoding topoisomerase IV. The targeting of either DNA-gyrase or topoisomerase IV as the primary target by fluoroquinolones varies with the bacterial species and specific fluoroquinolone (132). Alteration of the primary target site can be followed by secondary mutations in lower-affinity binding sites, and highly resistant organisms typically carry a combination of mutations within DNA-gyrase and topoisomerase IV (133, 134).

In *M. gallisepticum*, substitutions Ser83-Arg in GyrA and Ser80-Leu/Trp in ParC QRDR were shown to have the greatest impact on resistance to fluoroquinolones (133–136). Even if DNA-gyrase seemed to be the primary target of enrofloxacin in *M. gallisepticum*, several mutations in both DNA-gyrase and topoisomerase IV were needed to reach high-level resistance to fluoroquinolones in mutant strains selected *in vitro* (134). The position and the nature of the amino acid also influenced the resistance level (134).

Reduced susceptibility or resistance to enrofloxacin in *M. synoviae* was correlated with the presence of several amino acid substitutions in the ParC QRDR (32) (Table 7): 26/43 strains with MICs between 1 and 16 µg/ml harbored the Thr80-Ile. A Ser81-Pro was also evidenced in the ParC QRDR of *M. synoviae* isolates after an *in vivo* treatment with marbofloxacin of a hen experimentally infected with *M. synoviae* (83).

Mutations in the QRDR of ParC (Ser80-Phe and Asp84-Asn) were detected in *M. hyopneumoniae* strains with reduced susceptibility to marbofloxacin isolated from infected pigs after an *in vivo* marbofloxacin treatment (118). A Ser80-Tyr substitution was also evidenced in the ParC QRDR of five field strains isolated from pig herds in Belgium and harboring reduced susceptibility to flumequine and enrofloxacin (137), and an extra mutation, Ala83-Val, leading to further increase of the enrofloxacin MIC, was also evidenced in GyrA for one of these strains (Table 7).

For *M. bovis*, point mutations detected in the GyrA and ParC QRDR could be different according to the strain origin (country of isolation, field strains versus selected mutants) (Table 7). Results from Lysnyansky and collaborators' study of strains isolated in Israel suggested that a Ser83-Phe point mutation in GyrA is sufficient to reach an intermediate level of susceptibility to enrofloxacin (MICs between 0.5 and 2 µg/ml) but that an Asp84-Asn substitution in ParC is required for resistance (MIC, >2 µg/ml) (138). Japanese field isolates with fluoroquinolone MICs of ≤2 µg/ml harbored no QRDR mutations and no Ser83-Leu point mutation in GyrA, whereas resistant isolates (MICs, ≥4 µg/ml) had a Ser83-Leu mutation in GyrA and a Ser81-Pro mutation in ParC, or a Ser83-Phe substitution in GyrA and a Ser80-Ile mutation in ParC (139). Laboratory-derived fluoroquinolone-resistant mutants selected from two isolates with a Ser83-Leu mutation in GyrA had an amino acid substitution in ParC at the same position (Ser80-Ile or Ser81-Tyr) as fluoroquinolone-resistant isolates, suggesting that a substitution in ParC at position Ser80 or Ser81 is important in fluoroquinolone resistance in *M. bovis* isolates (139). No mutations in the GyrA and ParC QRDR regions of recent French *M. bovis* strains (2009 to 2014) were evidenced to explain the slight loss of susceptibility to fluoroquinolones compared to old strains (1978 to 1983) (37). The only recurrent mutation that was present in all recent strains and absent from old ones was Asp362-Asn in the GyrB QRDR. However, alterations in GyrB have rarely been associated with a loss of susceptibility to fluoroquinolones, except in *M. gallisepticum*, where the Asp362-Asn substitution was detected in mutants selected *in vitro* (133) (Table 7). The most frequently observed substitutions in fluoroquinolone-resistant *M. bovis* clones selected *in vitro* from French clinical isolates were Ser83-Phe in GyrA and Asp84-Asn/Tyr in ParC, leading to 8- to 16-fold increases in the MICs. The Ser83-Phe in GyrA and Ser80-Ile in ParC combination of mutations was observed less frequently (only 3 of 72 selected clones) and was associated with 16- to 128-fold increases in the MICs (37). This combination of mutations was observed for Japanese and Chinese clinical isolates of *M. bovis* (139, 140).

In vitro resistance selection studies clearly confirmed the existence of hot spots for mutations conferring high resistance levels and the cumulative effects of mutations in GyrA and ParC on the MICs in several *Mycoplasma* species (37, 133, 139). Moreover, Khalil and collaborators showed that different clinical isolates, with different initial MICs and different genetic subtypes, were not equal in their ability to gain resistance to fluoroquinolones *in vitro*: some isolates were more likely to rapidly accumulate mutations in their QRDRs under selective pressure *in vitro* and hence to become resistant (37). Sulyok and collaborators showed that *in vitro*-selected fluoroquinolone-resistant mutants of *M. bovis* remained resistant after serial passages in antibiotic-free medium (116).

For *M. agalactiae*, point mutations were detected in the ParC QRDR of strains isolated between 2013 and 2015 (112): Asp83-Asn/Lys or Thr80-Ile point mutations resulted in 2- to 8-fold increases in MICs of fluoroquinolones (Table 7). Other mutations were evidenced in GyrB (position 424), ParC (positions 78, 79, 80, and 84), and ParE (positions 429 and 459) in mutants selected *in vitro* (112). The *parC* gene was the first gene harboring point mutations in isolates or mutants with reduced susceptibility to fluoroquinolones, suggesting that it could be the primary target of fluoroquinolones for *M. agalactiae*.

Target mutations are the main mechanisms conferring resistance to fluoroquinolones in *Mycoplasma* species. However, the active efflux mechanism is an alternative mechanism in mycoplasmas that could lead to acquired resistance to fluoroquinolones and explain a moderate shift in susceptibility. It has been described for *Mycoplasma hominis*, a human urogenital mycoplasma that belongs to the same phylogenetic group as *M. bovis*, and was linked to the overexpression of genes *md1* and *md2*, encoding multidrug resistance ATP-binding cassette transporters (141). In another ruminant mycoplasma, *Mycoplasma mycoides* subsp. *capri*, orthovanadate, an inhibitor of ATP-binding cassette efflux pumps, was able to induce a 2-fold decrease of the MICs of three fluoroquinolones in both clinical and *in vitro* mutants, suggesting the contribution of an efflux mechanism to the overall resistance patterns of isolates (142). Since the moderate increase of the MICs observed between the recent (2009 to 2012) and old (1978 to 1983) *M. bovis* populations could be a consequence of an efflux system, which usually confers low levels of resistance, this efflux hypothesis was explored in a set of isolates with reduced susceptibility to fluoroquinolones, without success (37).

Other Antibiotics

Pleuromutilin antibiotics inhibit protein synthesis by binding to the bacterial 50S ribosomal subunit at the peptidyl transferase center, therefore inhibiting the peptide bond formation (143). Point mutations in the 23S rRNA gene and L3 protein are associated with decreased susceptibility to pleuromutilins (tiamulin or valnemulin) in several bacterial species. No mutation

in protein L3 was evidenced in pleuromutilin-resistant mutants of *M. gallisepticum* selected *in vitro* (144). However, several point mutations were found in *rrn*A and/or *rrn*B alleles of domain V of the 23S rRNA gene at positions 2058, 2059, 2061, 2447, and 2503. Although a single mutation could cause an increase of tiamulin and valnemulin MICs, combinations of two or three mutations were necessary to produce high-level resistance (144). All pleuromutilin-resistant mutants exhibited cross-resistance to lincomycin, chloramphenicol, and florfenicol. Mutants with the A2058G or the A2059G mutation showed cross-resistance to macrolides (erythromycin, tilmicosin, and tylosin). In another study, all mutants selected *in vitro* for resistance to tiamulin showed cross-resistance to florfenicol and elevated lincomycin MICs (116). Substitutions C2035A, A2060G, G2062T, and C2500A were found in pleuromutilin-resistant mutants; these positions are closely associated with the pleuromutilin binding sites on the 23S rRNA genes.

Resistance to florfenicol was shown to be associated with a G2062T or a A2063T substitution in at least one allele of the 23S rRNA genes. In addition, a substitution G2506A showed cross-resistance with tiamulin (116).

Hungarian field strains of *M. bovis* with high spectinomycin MICs (≥256 µg/ml) and mutants selected *in vitro* in the presence of subinhibitory concentrations of spectinomycin harbored a single mutation: C1192A for field isolates and C1192T in mutants (116).

CONCLUSIONS

Several recent studies have shown a significant decrease in the susceptibility of animal mycoplasmas to several families of antibiotics. Some strains of *M. bovis* show currently high *in vitro* MIC levels for several antibiotics usually used to treat these infections *in vivo*. The highest resistances of the main veterinary *Mycoplasma* species are observed for macrolides, followed by tetracyclines. Although resistant strains have been described for fluoroquinolones, most strains remain susceptible to this family of antibiotics. Pleuromutilins are the most effective antibiotics *in vitro*. However, due to different usage practices of antimicrobials, frequencies of resistance can vary considerably from one country to another but also within a country between isolates from different origins (e.g., mastitis versus respiratory disease). It is therefore important to perform antimicrobial susceptibility testing periodically, on a regional basis, to monitor levels of susceptibility to several antibiotics for rational *in vivo* treatment strategies. The development of next-generation sequencing techniques

Table 7 Mutations in DNA-gyrase (GyrA and GyrB) and topoisomerase IV (ParC and ParE) associated with fluoroquinolone resistance in animal *Mycoplasma* species

Mutations in[a]	*Mycoplasma* species (host species for clinical isolates)	Origin of strains[b]	Impact on MIC values for enrofloxacin[c]	References
GyrA				
Thr58-Ile	*M. gallisepticum* (chicken, turkey)	CI	ND	136
His59-Tyr	*M. gallisepticum* (chicken, turkey)	CI	ND	136
Gly81-Ala	*M. gallisepticum*	M	4-fold increase	134
Asp82-Asn	*M. bovis*	M	ND	116
Ser83-Ile	*M. gallisepticum* (chicken, turkey)	M, CI	2-fold increase	80, 133–136
Ser83-Asn	*M. gallisepticum* (chicken, turkey)	M, CI	2-fold increase	80, 133, 134
Ser83-Arg	*M. gallisepticum*	M	32-fold increase	134
Ser83-Phe	*M. bovis* (cattle)	M, CI	32-fold increase	37, 116, 138
Ser83-Tyr	*M. bovis*	M	No impact	37, 116
Ala83-Val	*M. hyopneumoniae* (swine)	CI	>2-fold increase	137
Ala84-Pro	*M. gallisepticum*	M	2-fold increase	134
Glu87-Gly	*M. gallisepticum*	M	ND	134
Glu87-Gly/Lys/Val	*M. bovis*	M	No impact	37, 116
Glu87-Lys	*M. gallisepticum* (chicken, turkey)	M, CI	ND	80, 134, 136
Asn87-Ser/Lys	*M. synoviae* (chicken, turkey)	CI	4-fold increase	32
Asn87-Lys	*M. synoviae* (chicken, turkey)	CI	No impact	32
GyrB				
Val320-Ala	*M. bovis* (cattle)	CI	ND	116
Asp362-Asn	*M. bovis* (cattle)	M, CI	Slight increase (up to 2-fold)	37
Ser401-Tyr	*M. synoviae* (chicken, turkey)	CI	ND	32
Ser402-Asn	*M. synoviae* (chicken, turkey)	CI	ND	32
Ile423-Asn	*M. bovis*	M	ND	116
Asn424-Lys	*M. agalactiae*	M	8-fold increase	112
Asp426Asn	*M. gallisepticum* (chicken, turkey)	M, CI	2-fold increase	134, 136
Asp437-Asn	*M. gallisepticum* (chicken, turkey)	CI	ND	136
Asn464-Asp	*M. gallisepticum*	M	4-fold increase	134
Glu465-Lys	*M. gallisepticum*	M	No impact	134
Glu465-Gly	*M. gallisepticum*	M	2-fold increase	134
ParC				
Ala64-Ser	*M. gallisepticum*	M	4-fold increase	134
Gly78-Cys	*M. bovis*	M	ND	116
	M. agalactiae	M	2- to 8-fold increase	112
Asp79-Asn	*M. synoviae* (chicken, turkey)	CI	2-fold increase	32
	M. agalactiae	M	ND	112
Ser80-Leu	*M. gallisepticum* (chicken, turkey)	M, CI	8-fold increase	80, 101, 134–136
Ser80-Trp	*M. gallisepticum* (chicken)	M, CI	16-fold increase	134, 135
Ser80-Ile	*M. bovis* (cattle)	M, CI	2- to 8-fold increase	37, 116
Ser80-Phe	*M. hyopneumoniae* (swine)	EI	8-fold increase	118
Ser80-Tyr	*M. hyopneumoniae* (swine)	CI	8-fold increase	137
Thr80-Ile	*M. agalactiae*	M, CI	4- to 8-fold increase	112
Thr80-Ala/Ile	*M. synoviae* (chicken, turkey)	CI	2 to 8-fold increase	32
Ser81-Pro	*M. gallisepticum*	M	2 to 4-fold increase	134
	M. synoviae (chicken, turkey)	CI, EI	2 to 4-fold increase	32, 83
Glu84-Gly	*M. gallisepticum*	M	4-fold increase	134
Glu84-Gln	*M. gallisepticum*	M	2-fold increase	134
Glu84-Lys	*M. gallisepticum*	M	4-fold increase	134

(Continued)

Table 7 (Continued)

Mutations in[a]	Mycoplasma species (host species for clinical isolates)	Origin of strains[b]	Impact on MIC values for enrofloxacin[c]	References
Asp84-Asn	M. bovis (cattle)	M, CI	2-fold increase	37, 116, 138
	M. agalactiae (sheep and goats)	M, CI	2- to 8-fold increase	112
	M. synoviae (chicken, turkey)	CI	4-fold increase	32
	M. hyopneumoniae (swine)	EI	8-fold increase	118
Asp84-Tyr	M. agalactiae (sheep and goats)	M, CI	4- to 8-fold increase	112
Asp84-Tyr/Gly	M. bovis (cattle)	M, CI	ND	37
Thr98-Arg	M. bovis	M	ND	37
ParE				
Asp420-Asn	M. gallisepticum	M	2-fold increase	134
	M. synoviae (chicken, turkey)	CI	ND	32
Asp420-Lys	M. gallisepticum	M	ND	133
Gly429-Ser	M. agalactiae	M	ND	112
Glu459-Lys	M. agalactiae	M	8-fold increase	112
Ser463-Leu	M. gallisepticum	M	4-fold increase	134
Cys467-Phe	M. gallisepticum	M	ND	134

[a]Genes and amino acid substitutions (Escherichia coli numbering).
[b]M, mutants after in vitro selection, CI, clinical isolates, EI, experimental infection.
[c]A quantitative impact is given when the MIC increase could be calculated (when the mutation was observed alone and/or when MIC values were available to compare isolates or mutants with or without this mutation). ND, not determined (or impact difficult to evaluate because several mutations were observed at the same time).

in recent years has made it easier to study the resistance mechanisms of mycoplasmas to antibiotics and could rapidly detect mutations that have a significant impact on the resistance of mycoplasma species to antimicrobial agents, avoiding the long and tedious steps of in vitro culture. Further work should be carried out to determine breakpoints for veterinary mycoplasmas, based on molecular mutations, so that in vitro information can be used to provide advice for a prudent and targeted use of antimicrobials that are likely to be effective in vivo, to limit the development of antimicrobial resistance. However, the true measure of the effectiveness of an antimicrobial is its in vivo activity against mycoplasmas as well as other bacteria which are often associated with mycoplasmas and which often contribute to a more severe expression of the disease.

Citation. Gautier-Bouchardon AV. 2018. Antimicrobial Resistance in Mycoplasma spp., Microbiol Spectrum 6(4):ARBA-0030-2018.

References

1. Razin S. 1996. Mycoplasmas. In Baron S (ed), Medical Microbiology. University of Texas Medical Branch at Galveston, Galveston, TX.
2. Taylor-Robinson D. 1996. Infections due to species of Mycoplasma and Ureaplasma: an update. Clin Infect Dis 23:671–682, quiz 683–684.
3. Brown DR, Zacher LA, Wendland LD, Brown MB. 2005. Emerging mycoplasmoses in wildlife, p 383–414. In Blanchard A, Browning G (ed), Mycoplasmas:

Molecular Biology, Pathogenicity and Strategies for Control. Horizon Bioscience, Norfolk, UK.
4. Markham PF, Noormohammadi AH. 2005. Diagnosis of mycoplasmosis in animals, p 355–382. In Blanchard A, Browning G (ed), Mycoplasmas: Molecular Biology, Pathogenicity and Strategies for Control. Horizon Bioscience, Norfolk, UK.
5. Waites K, Talkington D. 2005. New developments in human diseases due to mycoplasmas, p 289–354. In Blanchard A, Browning G (ed), Mycoplasmas: Molecular Biology, Pathogenicity and Strategies for Control. Horizon Bioscience, Norfolk, UK.
6. Razin S, Yogev D, Naot Y. 1998. Molecular biology and pathogenicity of mycoplasmas. Microbiol Mol Biol Rev 62:1094–1156.
7. Chopra-Dewasthaly R, Baumgartner M, Gamper E, Innerebner C, Zimmermann M, Schilcher F, Tichy A, Winter P, Jechlinger W, Rosengarten R, Spergser J. 2012. Role of Vpma phase variation in Mycoplasma agalactiae pathogenesis. FEMS Immunol Med Microbiol 66:307–322.
8. Bürki S, Gaschen V, Stoffel MH, Stojiljkovic A, Frey J, Kuehni-Boghenbor K, Pilo P. 2015. Invasion and persistence of Mycoplasma bovis in embryonic calf turbinate cells. Vet Res (Faisalabad) 46:53.
9. Hegde S, Hegde S, Spergser J, Brunthaler R, Rosengarten R, Chopra-Dewasthaly R. 2014. In vitro and in vivo cell invasion and systemic spreading of Mycoplasma agalactiae in the sheep infection model. Int J Med Microbiol 304:1024–1031.
10. Buim MR, Buzinhani M, Yamaguti M, Oliveira RC, Mettifogo E, Ueno PM, Timenetsky J, Santelli GM, Ferreira AJ. 2011. Mycoplasma synoviae cell invasion:

elucidation of the *Mycoplasma* pathogenesis in chicken. *Comp Immunol Microbiol Infect Dis* **34**:41–47.

11. **Much P, Winner F, Stipkovits L, Rosengarten R, Citti C.** 2002. *Mycoplasma gallisepticum*: influence of cell invasiveness on the outcome of experimental infection in chickens. *FEMS Immunol Med Microbiol* **34**:181–186.

12. **Maes D, Segales J, Meyns T, Sibila M, Pieters M, Haesebrouck F.** 2008. Control of *Mycoplasma hyopneumoniae* infections in pigs. *Vet Microbiol* **126**:297–309.

13. **Pieters M, Fano E, Pijoan C, Dee S.** 2010. An experimental model to evaluate *Mycoplasma hyopneumoniae* transmission from asymptomatic carriers to unvaccinated and vaccinated sentinel pigs. *Can J Vet Res* **74**:157–160.

14. **Feberwee A, Landman WJ, von Banniseht-Wysmuller T, Klinkenberg D, Vernooij JC, Gielkens AL, Stegeman JA.** 2006. The effect of a live vaccine on the horizontal transmission of *Mycoplasma gallisepticum*. *Avian Pathol* **35**:359–366.

15. **Feberwee A, Dijkman R, Klinkenberg D, Landman WJM.** 2017. Quantification of the horizontal transmission of *Mycoplasma synoviae* in non-vaccinated and MS-H-vaccinated layers. *Avian Pathol* **46**:346–358.

16. **Kleven SH.** 2008. Control of avian mycoplasma infections in commercial poultry. *Avian Dis* **52**:367–374.

17. **Taylor-Robinson D, Bébéar C.** 1997. Antibiotic susceptibilities of mycoplasmas and treatment of mycoplasmal infections. *J Antimicrob Chemother* **40**:622–630.

18. **Schultz KK, Strait EL, Erickson BZ, Levy N.** 2012. Optimization of an antibiotic sensitivity assay for *Mycoplasma hyosynoviae* and susceptibility profiles of field isolates from 1997 to 2011. *Vet Microbiol* **158**:104–108.

19. **Bébéar CM, Bébéar C.** 2002. Antimicrobial agents, p 545–566. *In* Razin S, Herrmann R (ed), *Molecular Biology and Pathogenicity of Mycoplasmas*. Kluwer Academic/Plenum Publishers, New York, NY.

20. **Gaurivaud P, Laigret F, Bove JM.** 1996. Insusceptibility of members of the class *Mollicutes* to rifampin: studies of the *Spiroplasma citri* RNA polymerase beta-subunit gene. *Antimicrob Agents Chemother* **40**:858–862.

21. **Olaitan AO, Morand S, Rolain JM.** 2014. Mechanisms of polymyxin resistance: acquired and intrinsic resistance in bacteria. *Front Microbiol* **5**:643.

22. **McCormack WM.** 1993. Susceptibility of mycoplasmas to antimicrobial agents: clinical implications. *Clin Infect Dis* **17**(Suppl 1):S200–S201.

23. **Bébéar CM, Kempf I.** 2005. Antimicrobial therapy and antimicrobial resistance, p 535–568. *In* Blanchard A, Browning G (ed), *Mycoplasmas: Molecular Biology, Pathogenicity and Strategies for Control*. Horizon Bioscience, Norfolk, UK.

24. **Aarestrup FM, Kempf I.** 2006. Mycoplasma, p 239–248. *In* Aarestrup FM (ed), *Antimicrobial Resistance in Bacteria of Animal Origin*. ASM Press, Washington, DC.

25. **Hannan PC.** 2000. Guidelines and recommendations for antimicrobial minimum inhibitory concentration (MIC) testing against veterinary mycoplasma species. International Research Programme on Comparative Mycoplasmology. *Vet Res* **31**:373–395.

26. **Whithear KG, Bowtell DD, Ghiocas E, Hughes KL.** 1983. Evaluation and use of a micro-broth dilution procedure for testing sensitivity of fermentative avian mycoplasmas to antibiotics. *Avian Dis* **27**:937–949.

27. **Kenny GE.** 1996. Problems and opportunities in susceptibility testing of mollicutes, p 185–188. *In* Tully JG, Razin S (ed), Molecular and Diagnostic Procedures in Mycoplasmology, **vol II**, *Diagnostic Procedures*. Academic Press, London, UK.

28. **Bébéar C, Robertson JA.** 1996. Determination of minimal inhibitory concentrations, p 189–197. *In* Tully JG, Razin S (ed), Molecular and Diagnostic Procedures in Mycoplasmology, **vol II**, *Diagnostic Procedures*. Academic Press, London, UK.

29. **Gerchman I, Lysnyansky I, Perk S, Levisohn S.** 2008. *In vitro* susceptibilities to fluoroquinolones in current and archived *Mycoplasma gallisepticum* and *Mycoplasma synoviae* isolates from meat-type turkeys. *Vet Microbiol* **131**:266–276.

30. **CLSI.** 2011. M43A: Methods for antimicrobial susceptibility testing for human mycoplasmas. Approved guideline. Clinical and Laboratory Standards Institute, Wayne, PA.

31. **Waites KB, Duffy LB, Bébéar CM, Matlow A, Talkington DF, Kenny GE, Totten PA, Bade DJ, Zheng X, Davidson MK, Shortridge VD, Watts JL, Brown SD.** 2012. Standardized methods and quality control limits for agar and broth microdilution susceptibility testing of *Mycoplasma pneumoniae*, *Mycoplasma hominis*, and *Ureaplasma urealyticum*. *J Clin Microbiol* **50**:3542–3547.

32. **Lysnyansky I, Gerchman I, Mikula I, Gobbo F, Catania S, Levisohn S.** 2013. Molecular characterization of acquired enrofloxacin resistance in *Mycoplasma synoviae* field isolates. *Antimicrob Agents Chemother* **57**:3072–3077.

33. **Ammar AM, Abd El-Aziz NK, Gharib AA, Ahmed HK, Lameay AE.** 2016. Mutations of domain V in 23S ribosomal RNA of macrolide-resistant *Mycoplasma gallisepticum* isolates in Egypt. *J Infect Dev Ctries* **10**:807–813.

34. **Heuvelink A, Reugebrink C, Mars J.** 2016. Antimicrobial susceptibility of *Mycoplasma bovis* isolates from veal calves and dairy cattle in the Netherlands. *Vet Microbiol* **189**:1–7.

35. **Zhang N, Ye X, Wu Y, Huang Z, Gu X, Cai Q, Shen X, Jiang H, Ding H.** 2017. Determination of the mutant selection window and evaluation of the killing of *Mycoplasma gallisepticum* by danofloxacin, doxycycline, tilmicosin, tylvalosin and valnemulin. *PLoS One* **12**:e0169134.

36. **Gautier-Bouchardon AV, Ferré S, Le Grand D, Paoli A, Gay E, Poumarat F.** 2014. Overall decrease in the susceptibility of *Mycoplasma bovis* to antimicrobials over the past 30 years in France. *PLoS One* **9**:e87672.

37. **Khalil D, Becker CA, Tardy F.** 2015. Alterations in the quinolone resistance-determining regions and fluoroquinolone resistance in clinical isolates and laboratory-derived mutants of *Mycoplasma bovis*: not all genotypes may be equal. *Appl Environ Microbiol* **82**:1060–1068.

38. Poumarat F, Gautier-Bouchardon AV, Bergonier D, Gay E, Tardy F. 2016. Diversity and variation in antimicrobial susceptibility patterns over time in *Mycoplasma agalactiae* isolates collected from sheep and goats in France. *J Appl Microbiol* **120**:1208–1218.

39. Ter Laak EA, Pijpers A, Noordergraaf JH, Schoevers EC, Verheijden JH. 1991. Comparison of methods for *in vitro* testing of susceptibility of porcine *Mycoplasma* species to antimicrobial agents. *Antimicrob Agents Chemother* **35**:228–233.

40. Aarestrup FM, Friis NF. 1998. Antimicrobial susceptibility testing of *Mycoplasma hyosynoviae* isolated from pigs during 1968 to 1971 and during 1995 and 1996. *Vet Microbiol* **61**:33–39.

41. Hannan PC, O'Hanlon PJ, Rogers NH. 1989. *In vitro* evaluation of various quinolone antibacterial agents against veterinary mycoplasmas and porcine respiratory bacterial pathogens. *Res Vet Sci* **46**:202–211.

42. Kobayashi H, Morozumi T, Munthali G, Mitani K, Ito N, Yamamoto K. 1996. Macrolide susceptibility of *Mycoplasma hyorhinis* isolated from piglets. *Antimicrob Agents Chemother* **40**:1030–1032.

43. Kobayashi H, Nakajima H, Shimizu Y, Eguchi M, Hata E, Yamamoto K. 2005. Macrolides and lincomycin susceptibility of *Mycoplasma hyorhinis* and variable mutation of domain II and V in 23S ribosomal RNA. *J Vet Med Sci* **67**:795–800.

44. CLSI. 2013. VET01-A4: Performance standards for antimicrobial disk and dilution susceptibility tests for bacteria isolated from animals, 4th ed. Clinical and Laboratory Standards Institute, Wayne, PA.

45. CLSI. 2015. VET01S: Performance standards for antimicrobial disk and dilution susceptibility tests for bacteria isolated from animals, 3rd ed. Clinical and Laboratory Standards Institute, Wayne, PA.

46. CLSI. 1999. M26A: Methods for determining bactericidal activity of antibacterial agents. Approved guideline. Clinical and Laboratory Standards Institute, Wayne, PA.

47. Kleven SH, Anderson DP. 1971. *In vitro* activity of various antibiotics against *Mycoplasma synoviae*. *Avian Dis* **15**:551–557.

48. Ball HJ, Craig Reilly GA, Bryson DG. 1995. Antibiotic susceptibility in *Mycoplasma bovis* strains in Northern Ireland. *Ir Vet J* **48**:316–318.

49. Ayling RD, Baker SE, Peek ML, Simon AJ, Nicholas RA. 2000. Comparison of *in vitro* activity of danofloxacin, florfenicol, oxytetracycline, spectinomycin and tilmicosin against recent field isolates of *Mycoplasma bovis*. *Vet Rec* **146**:745–747.

50. Tavío MM, Poveda C, Assunção P, Ramírez AS, Poveda JB. 2014. *In vitro* activity of tylvalosin against Spanish field strains of *Mycoplasma hyopneumoniae*. *Vet Rec* **175**:539.

51. Taylor-Robinson D. 1996. Cidal activity testing, p 199–204. *In* Tully JG, Razin S (ed), Molecular and Diagnostic Procedures in Mycoplasmology, **vol II**, *Diagnostic Procedures*. Academic Press, London, UK.

52. Hayes MM, Foo HH, Timenetsky J, Lo SC. 1995. *In vitro* antibiotic susceptibility testing of clinical isolates of *Mycoplasma penetrans* from patients with AIDS. *Antimicrob Agents Chemother* **39**:1386–1387.

53. Ikejima H, Yamamoto H, Ishida K, Kaku M, Shimada J. 2000. Evaluation of *in-vitro* activity of new quinolones, macrolides, and minocycline against *Mycoplasma pneumoniae*. *J Infect Chemother* **6**:148–150.

54. Hamamoto K, Shimizu T, Fujimoto N, Zhang Y, Arai S. 2001. *In vitro* activities of moxifloxacin and other fluoroquinolones against *Mycoplasma pneumoniae*. *Antimicrob Agents Chemother* **45**:1908–1910.

55. Waites KB, Crabb DM, Bing X, Duffy LB. 2003. *In vitro* susceptibilities to and bactericidal activities of garenoxacin (BMS-284756) and other antimicrobial agents against human mycoplasmas and ureaplasmas. *Antimicrob Agents Chemother* **47**:161–165.

56. Assunção P, Antunes NT, Rosales RS, de la Fe C, Poveda C, Poveda JB, Davey HM. 2006. Flow cytometric method for the assessment of the minimal inhibitory concentrations of antibacterial agents to *Mycoplasma agalactiae*. *Cytometry A* **69**:1071–1076.

57. Assunção P, Antunes NT, Rosales RS, Poveda C, Poveda JB, Davey HM. 2006. Flow cytometric determination of the effects of antibacterial agents on *Mycoplasma agalactiae*, *Mycoplasma putrefaciens*, *Mycoplasma capricolum* subsp. *capricolum*, and *Mycoplasma mycoides* subsp. *mycoides* large colony type. *Antimicrob Agents Chemother* **50**:2845–2849.

58. Soehnlen MK, Kunze ME, Karunathilake KE, Henwood BM, Kariyawasam S, Wolfgang DR, Jayarao BM. 2011. *In vitro* antimicrobial inhibition of *Mycoplasma bovis* isolates submitted to the Pennsylvania Animal Diagnostic Laboratory using flow cytometry and a broth microdilution method. *J Vet Diagn Invest* **23**:547–551.

59. Assunção P, Antunes NT, Rosales RS, Poveda C, de la Fe C, Poveda JB, Davey HM. 2007. Application of flow cytometry for the determination of minimal inhibitory concentration of several antibacterial agents on *Mycoplasma hyopneumoniae*. *J Appl Microbiol* **102**:1132–1137.

60. Wick WE. 1964. Influence of antibiotic stability on the results of *in vitro* testing procedures. *J Bacteriol* **87**:1162–1170.

61. Lallemand EA, Lacroix MZ, Toutain PL, Boullier S, Ferran AA, Bousquet-Melou A. 2016. *In vitro* degradation of antimicrobials during use of broth microdilution method can increase the measured minimal inhibitory and minimal bactericidal concentrations. *Front Microbiol* **7**:2051.

62. Tanner AC, Wu CC. 1992. Adaptation of the Sensititre broth microdilution technique to antimicrobial susceptibility testing of *Mycoplasma gallisepticum*. *Avian Dis* **36**:714–717.

63. Tanner AC, Erickson BZ, Ross RF. 1993. Adaptation of the Sensititre broth microdilution technique to antimicrobial susceptibility testing of *Mycoplasma hyopneumoniae*. *Vet Microbiol* **36**:301–306.

64. Rosenbusch RF, Kinyon JM, Apley M, Funk ND, Smith S, Hoffman LJ. 2005. *In vitro* antimicrobial inhibition profiles of *Mycoplasma bovis* isolates recovered from

various regions of the United States from 2002 to 2003. *J Vet Diagn Invest* 17:436–441.

65. **Hendrick SH, Bateman KG, Rosengren LB.** 2013. The effect of antimicrobial treatment and preventive strategies on bovine respiratory disease and genetic relatedness and antimicrobial resistance of *Mycoplasma bovis* isolates in a western Canadian feedlot. *Can Vet J* 54:1146–1156.

66. **Wu CC, Shryock TR, Lin TL, Faderan M, Veenhuizen MF.** 2000. Antimicrobial susceptibility of *Mycoplasma hyorhinis*. *Vet Microbiol* 76:25–30.

67. **Kleven SH.** 2003. Mycoplasmosis, p 719–721. *In* Saif YM, Barnes HJ, Glisson JR, Fadly AM, McDougald LR, Swayne DE (ed), *Diseases of Poultry*, 11th ed. Iowa State Press, Ames, IA.

68. **Kleven SH.** 2003. *Mycoplasma synoviae* infection, p 756–766. *In* Saif YM, Barnes HJ, Glisson JR, Fadly AM, McDougald LR, Swayne DE (ed), *Diseases of Poultry*, 11th ed. Iowa State Press, Ames, IA.

69. **Feberwee A, de Wit JJ, Landman WJ.** 2009. Induction of eggshell apex abnormalities by *Mycoplasma synoviae*: field and experimental studies. *Avian Pathol* 38:77–85.

70. **Chin RP, Ghazikhanian GY, Kempf I.** 2003. *Mycoplasma meleagridis* infection, p 744–756. *In* Saif YM, Barnes HJ, Glisson JR, Fadly AM, McDougald LR, Swayne DE (ed), *Diseases of Poultry*, 11th ed. Iowa State Press, Ames, IA.

71. **Bradbury JM, Kleven SH.** 2003. *Mycoplasma iowae* infection, p 766–771. *In* Saif YM, Barnes HJ, Glisson JR, Fadly AM, McDougald LR, Swayne DE (ed), *Diseases of Poultry*, 11th ed. Iowa State Press, Ames, IA.

72. **Levisohn S.** 1981. Antibiotic sensitivity patterns in field isolates of *Mycoplasma gallisepticum* as a guide to chemotherapy. *Isr J Med Sci* 17:661–666.

73. **Jordan FT, Knight D.** 1984. The minimum inhibitory concentration of kitasamycin, tylosin and tiamulin for *Mycoplasma gallisepticum* and their protective effect on infected chicks. *Avian Pathol* 13:151–162.

74. **Jordan FT, Gilbert S, Knight DL, Yavari CA.** 1989. Effects of Baytril, tylosin and tiamulin on avian mycoplasmas. *Avian Pathol* 18:659–673.

75. **Hannan PC, Windsor GD, de Jong A, Schmeer N, Stegemann M.** 1997. Comparative susceptibilities of various animal-pathogenic mycoplasmas to fluoroquinolones. *Antimicrob Agents Chemother* 41:2037–2040.

76. **Wang C, Ewing M, Aarabi SY.** 2001. *In vitro* susceptibility of avian mycoplasmas to enrofloxacin, sarafloxacin, tylosin, and oxytetracycline. *Avian Dis* 45:456–460.

77. **Pakpinyo S, Sasipreeyajan J.** 2007. Molecular characterization and determination of antimicrobial resistance of *Mycoplasma gallisepticum* isolated from chickens. *Vet Microbiol* 125:59–65.

78. **Gerchman I, Levisohn S, Mikula I, Manso-Silván L, Lysnyansky I.** 2011. Characterization of *in vivo*-acquired resistance to macrolides of *Mycoplasma gallisepticum* strains isolated from poultry. *Vet Res (Faisalabad)* 42:90.

79. **Gharaibeh S, Al-Rashdan M.** 2011. Change in antimicrobial susceptibility of *Mycoplasma gallisepticum* field isolates. *Vet Microbiol* 150:379–383.

80. **Lysnyansky I, Gerchman I, Levisohn S, Mikula I, Feberwee A, Ferguson NM, Noormohammadi AH, Spergser J, Windsor HM.** 2012. Discrepancy between minimal inhibitory concentration to enrofloxacin and mutations present in the quinolone-resistance determining regions of *Mycoplasma gallisepticum* field strains. *Vet Microbiol* 160:222–226.

81. **Cerdá RO, Giacoboni GI, Xavier JA, Sansalone PL, Landoni MF.** 2002. *In vitro* antibiotic susceptibility of field isolates of *Mycoplasma synoviae* in Argentina. *Avian Dis* 46:215–218.

82. **Lysnyansky I, Gerchman I, Flaminio B, Catania S.** 2015. Decreased susceptibility to macrolide-lincosamide in *Mycoplasma synoviae* is associated with mutations in 23S ribosomal RNA. *Microb Drug Resist* 21:581–589.

83. **Le Carrou J, Reinhardt AK, Kempf I, Gautier-Bouchardon AV.** 2006. Persistence of *Mycoplasma synoviae* in hens after two enrofloxacin treatments and detection of mutations in the *parC* gene. *Vet Res* 37:145–154.

84. **Ross RF.** 1999. Mycoplasmal diseases, p 537–551. *In* Straw BE, D'allaire S, Mengeling WL, Taylor DJ (ed), *Diseases of Swine*, 8th ed. Iowa State University Press, Ames, IA.

85. **Paes JA, Lorenzatto KR, de Moraes SN, Moura H, Barr JR, Ferreira HB.** 2017. Secretomes of *Mycoplasma hyopneumoniae* and *Mycoplasma flocculare* reveal differences associated to pathogenesis. *J Proteomics* 154:69–77.

86. **Zimmermann BJ, Ross RF.** 1975. Determination of sensitivity of *Mycoplasma hyosynoviae* to tylosin and selected antibacterial drugs by a microtiter technique. *Can J Comp Med* 39:17–21.

87. **Friis NF, Szancer J.** 1994. Sensitivity of certain porcine and bovine mycoplasmas to antimicrobial agents in a liquid medium test compared to a disc assay. *Acta Vet Scand* 35:389–394.

88. **Inamoto T, Takahashi H, Yamamoto K, Nakai Y, Ogimoto K.** 1994. Antibiotic susceptibility of *Mycoplasma hyopneumoniae* isolated from swine. *J Vet Med Sci* 56:393–394.

89. **Hannan PC, Windsor HM, Ripley PH.** 1997. *In vitro* susceptibilities of recent field isolates of *Mycoplasma hyopneumoniae* and *Mycoplasma hyosynoviae* to valnemulin (Econor), tiamulin and enrofloxacin and the *in vitro* development of resistance to certain antimicrobial agents in *Mycoplasma hyopneumoniae*. *Res Vet Sci* 63:157–160.

90. **Bousquet E, Morvan H, Aitken I, Morgan JH.** 1997. Comparative *in vitro* activity of doxycycline and oxytetracycline against porcine respiratory pathogens. *Vet Rec* 141:37–40.

91. **Vicca J, Stakenborg T, Maes D, Butaye P, Peeters J, de Kruif A, Haesebrouck F.** 2004. *In vitro* susceptibilities of *Mycoplasma hyopneumoniae* field isolates. *Antimicrob Agents Chemother* 48:4470–4472.

92. **Stakenborg T, Vicca J, Butaye P, Maes D, Minion FC, Peeters J, De Kruif A, Haesebrouck F.** 2005. Characterization of *in vivo* acquired resistance of *Mycoplasma*

hyopneumoniae to macrolides and lincosamides. *Microb Drug Resist* 11:290–294.

93. Thongkamkoon P, Narongsak W, Kobayashi H, Pathanasophon P, Kishima M, Yamamoto K. 2013. *In vitro* susceptibility of *Mycoplasma hyopneumoniae* field isolates and occurrence of fluoroquinolone, macrolides and lincomycin resistance. *J Vet Med Sci* 75:1067–1070.

94. Kobayashi H, Sonmez N, Morozumi T, Mitani K, Ito N, Shiono H, Yamamoto K. 1996. *In vitro* susceptibility of *Mycoplasma hyosynoviae* and *M. hyorhinis* to antimicrobial agents. *J Vet Med Sci* 58:1107–1111.

95. Maunsell FP, Woolums AR, Francoz D, Rosenbusch RF, Step DL, Wilson DJ, Janzen ED. 2011. *Mycoplasma bovis* infections in cattle. *J Vet Intern Med* 25:772–783.

96. Nicholas RA. 2011. Bovine mycoplasmosis: silent and deadly. *Vet Rec* 168:459–462.

97. Bergonier D, Berthelot X, Poumarat F. 1997. Contagious agalactia of small ruminants: current knowledge concerning epidemiology, diagnosis and control. *Rev Sci Tech* 16:848–873.

98. Ayling RD, Rosales RS, Barden G, Gosney FL. 2014. Changes in antimicrobial susceptibility of *Mycoplasma bovis* isolates from Great Britain. *Vet Rec* 175:486.

99. Francoz D, Fortin M, Fecteau G, Messier S. 2005. Determination of *Mycoplasma bovis* susceptibilities against six antimicrobial agents using the E test method. *Vet Microbiol* 105:57–64.

100. Gerchman I, Levisohn S, Mikula I, Lysnyansky I. 2009. *In vitro* antimicrobial susceptibility of *Mycoplasma bovis* isolated in Israel from local and imported cattle. *Vet Microbiol* 137:268–275.

101. Hirose K, Kobayashi H, Ito N, Kawasaki Y, Zako M, Kotani K, Ogawa H, Sato H. 2003. Isolation of mycoplasmas from nasal swabs of calves affected with respiratory diseases and antimicrobial susceptibility of their isolates. *J Vet Med B Infect Dis Vet Public Health* 50:347–351.

102. Kawai K, Higuchi H, Iwano H, Iwakuma A, Onda K, Sato R, Hayashi T, Nagahata H, Oshida T. 2014. Antimicrobial susceptibilities of *Mycoplasma* isolated from bovine mastitis in Japan. *Anim Sci J* 85:96–99.

103. Kong LC, Gao D, Jia BY, Wang Z, Gao YH, Pei ZH, Liu SM, Xin JQ, Ma HX. 2016. Antimicrobial susceptibility and molecular characterization of macrolide resistance of *Mycoplasma bovis* isolates from multiple provinces in China. *J Vet Med Sci* 78:293–296.

104. Godinho KS. 2008. Susceptibility testing of tulathromycin: interpretive breakpoints and susceptibility of field isolates. *Vet Microbiol* 129:426–432.

105. Kroemer S, Galland D, Guérin-Faublée V, Giboin H, Woehrlé-Fontaine F. 2012. Survey of marbofloxacin susceptibility of bacteria isolated from cattle with respiratory disease and mastitis in Europe. *Vet Rec* 170:53.

106. Devriese LA, Haesebrouck F. 1991. Antibiotic susceptibility testing of *Mycoplasma bovis* using Tween 80 hydrolysis as an indicator of growth. *Zentralbl Veterinarmed B* 38:781–783.

107. Antunes NT, Tavío MM, Assunção P, Rosales RS, Poveda C, de la Fé C, Gil MC, Poveda JB. 2008.

108. de Garnica ML, Rosales RS, Gonzalo C, Santos JA, Nicholas RA. 2013. Isolation, molecular characterization and antimicrobial susceptibilities of isolates of *Mycoplasma agalactiae* from bulk tank milk in an endemic area of Spain. *J Appl Microbiol* 114:1575–1581.

In vitro susceptibilities of field isolates of *Mycoplasma agalactiae*. *Vet J* 177:436–438.

109. Loria GR, Sammartino C, Nicholas RA, Ayling RD. 2003. *In vitro* susceptibilities of field isolates of *Mycoplasma agalactiae* to oxytetracycline, tylosin, enrofloxacin, spiramycin and lincomycin-spectinomycin. *Res Vet Sci* 75:3–7.

110. Filioussis G, Petridou E, Giadinis ND, Kritas SK. 2014. *In vitro* susceptibilities of caprine *Mycoplasma agalaciae* field isolates to six antimicrobial agents using the E test methodology. *Vet J* 202:654–656.

111. Prats-van der Ham M, Tatay-Dualde J, de la Fe C, Paterna A, Sánchez A, Corrales JC, Contreras A, Gómez-Martín Á. 2017. Molecular resistance mechanisms of *Mycoplasma agalactiae* to macrolides and lincomycin. *Vet Microbiol* 211:135–140.

112. Tatay-Dualde J, Prats-van der Ham M, de la Fe C, Paterna A, Sánchez A, Corrales JC, Contreras A, Gómez-Martín Á. 2017. Mutations in the quinolone resistance determining region conferring resistance to fluoroquinolones in *Mycoplasma agalactiae*. *Vet Microbiol* 207:63–68.

113. Regnier A, Laroute V, Gautier-Bouchardon A, Gayrard V, Picard-Hagen N, Toutain PL. 2013. Florfenicol concentrations in ovine tear fluid following intramuscular and subcutaneous administration and comparison with the minimum inhibitory concentrations against mycoplasmal strains potentially involved in infectious keratoconjunctivitis. *Am J Vet Res* 74:268–274.

114. Paterna A, Sánchez A, Gómez-Martín A, Corrales JC, De la Fe C, Contreras A, Amores J. 2013. Short communication: *in vitro* antimicrobial susceptibility of *Mycoplasma agalactiae* strains isolated from dairy goats. *J Dairy Sci* 96:7073–7076.

115. Gautier-Bouchardon AV, Reinhardt AK, Kobisch M, Kempf I. 2002. *In vitro* development of resistance to enrofloxacin, erythromycin, tylosin, tiamulin and oxytetracycline in *Mycoplasma gallisepticum*, *Mycoplasma iowae* and *Mycoplasma synoviae*. *Vet Microbiol* 88:47–58.

116. Sulyok KM, Kreizinger Z, Wehmann E, Lysnyansky I, Bányai K, Marton S, Jerzsele Á, Rónai Z, Turcsányi I, Makrai L, Jánosi S, Nagy SA, Gyuranecz M. 2017. Mutations associated with decreased susceptibility to seven antimicrobial families in field and laboratory-derived *Mycoplasma bovis* strains. *Antimicrob Agents Chemother* 61:e01983-16.

117. Wu CM, Wu H, Ning Y, Wang J, Du X, Shen J. 2005. Induction of macrolide resistance in *Mycoplasma gallisepticum in vitro* and its resistance-related mutations within domain V of 23S rRNA. *FEMS Microbiol Lett* 247:199–205.

118. Le Carrou J, Laurentie M, Kobisch M, Gautier-Bouchardon AV. 2006. Persistence of *Mycoplasma hyopneumoniae* in experimentally infected pigs after

marbofloxacin treatment and detection of mutations in the *parC* gene. *Antimicrob Agents Chemother* 50: 1959–1966.

119. Khalil D, Becker CAM, Tardy F. 2017. Monitoring the decrease in susceptibility to ribosomal RNAs targeting antimicrobials and its molecular basis in clinical *Mycoplasma bovis* isolates over time. *Microb Drug Resist* 23: 799–811.

120. Leclercq R. 2002. Mechanisms of resistance to macrolides and lincosamides: nature of the resistance elements and their clinical implications. *Clin Infect Dis* 34:482–492.

121. Novotny GW, Jakobsen L, Andersen NM, Poehlsgaard J, Douthwaite S. 2004. Ketolide antimicrobial activity persists after disruption of interactions with domain II of 23S rRNA. *Antimicrob Agents Chemother* 48:3677–3683.

122. Poehlsgaard J, Andersen NM, Warrass R, Douthwaite S. 2012. Visualizing the 16-membered ring macrolides tildipirosin and tilmicosin bound to their ribosomal site. *ACS Chem Biol* 7:1351–1355.

123. Lerner U, Amram E, Ayling RD, Mikula I, Gerchman I, Harrus S, Teff D, Yogev D, Lysnyansky I. 2014. Acquired resistance to the 16-membered macrolides tylosin and tilmicosin by *Mycoplasma bovis*. *Vet Microbiol* 168: 365–371.

124. Andersen NM, Poehlsgaard J, Warrass R, Douthwaite S. 2012. Inhibition of protein synthesis on the ribosome by tildipirosin compared with other veterinary macrolides. *Antimicrob Agents Chemother* 56:6033–6036.

125. Razin A, Razin S. 1980. Methylated bases in mycoplasmal DNA. *Nucleic Acids Res* 8:1383–1390.

126. Luo W, Tu AH, Cao Z, Yu H, Dybvig K. 2009. Identification of an isoschizomer of the HhaI DNA methyltransferase in *Mycoplasma arthritidis*. *FEMS Microbiol Lett* 290:195–198.

127. Wojciechowski M, Czapinska H, Bochtler M. 2013. CpG underrepresentation and the bacterial CpG-specific DNA methyltransferase M.MpeI. *Proc Natl Acad Sci USA* 110:105–110.

128. Lluch-Senar M, Luong K, Lloréns-Rico V, Delgado J, Fang G, Spittle K, Clark TA, Schadt E, Turner SW, Korlach J, Serrano L. 2013. Comprehensive methylome characterization of *Mycoplasma genitalium* and *Mycoplasma pneumoniae* at single-base resolution. *PLoS Genet* 9:e1003191.

129. Lu C, Ye T, Zhu G, Feng P, Ma H, Lu R, Lai W. 2010. Phenotypic and genetic characteristics of macrolide and lincosamide resistant *Ureaplasma urealyticum* isolated in Guangzhou, China. *Curr Microbiol* 61:44–49.

130. Brodersen DE, Clemons WM Jr, Carter AP, Morgan-Warren RJ, Wimberly BT, Ramakrishnan V. 2000. The structural basis for the action of the antibiotics tetracycline, pactamycin, and hygromycin B on the 30S ribosomal subunit. *Cell* 103:1143–1154.

131. Amram E, Mikula I, Schnee C, Ayling RD, Nicholas RA, Rosales RS, Harrus S, Lysnyansky I. 2015. 16S rRNA gene mutations associated with decreased susceptibility to tetracycline in *Mycoplasma bovis*. *Antimicrob Agents Chemother* 59:796–802.

132. Redgrave LS, Sutton SB, Webber MA, Piddock LJ. 2014. Fluoroquinolone resistance: mechanisms, impact on bacteria, and role in evolutionary success. *Trends Microbiol* 22:438–445.

133. Reinhardt AK, Bébéar CM, Kobisch M, Kempf I, Gautier-Bouchardon AV. 2002. Characterization of mutations in DNA gyrase and topoisomerase IV involved in quinolone resistance of *Mycoplasma gallisepticum* mutants obtained *in vitro*. *Antimicrob Agents Chemother* 46:590–593.

134. Reinhardt AK, Kempf I, Kobisch M, Gautier-Bouchardon AV. 2002. Fluoroquinolone resistance in *Mycoplasma gallisepticum*: DNA gyrase as primary target of enrofloxacin and impact of mutations in topoisomerases on resistance level. *J Antimicrob Chemother* 50:589–592.

135. Reinhardt AK. 2002. Résistance aux fluoroquinolones liées à la cible chez *Mycoplasma gallisepticum*: sélection de mutants et analyse des mécanismes génétiques. Thesis, University of Rennes 1, Rennes, France.

136. Lysnyansky I, Gerchman I, Perk S, Levisohn S. 2008. Molecular characterization and typing of enrofloxacin-resistant clinical isolates of *Mycoplasma gallisepticum*. *Avian Dis* 52:685–689.

137. Vicca J, Maes D, Stakenborg T, Butaye P, Minion F, Peeters J, de Kruif A, Decostere A, Haesebrouck F. 2007. Resistance mechanism against fluoroquinolones in *Mycoplasma hyopneumoniae* field isolates. *Microb Drug Resist* 13:166–170.

138. Lysnyansky I, Mikula I, Gerchman I, Levisohn S. 2009. Rapid detection of a point mutation in the *parC* gene associated with decreased susceptibility to fluoroquinolones in *Mycoplasma bovis*. *Antimicrob Agents Chemother* 53:4911–4914.

139. Sato T, Okubo T, Usui M, Higuchi H, Tamura Y. 2013. Amino acid substitutions in GyrA and ParC are associated with fluoroquinolone resistance in *Mycoplasma bovis* isolates from Japanese dairy calves. *J Vet Med Sci* 75:1063–1065.

140. Mustafa R, Qi J, Ba X, Chen Y, Hu C, Liu X, Tu L, Peng Q, Chen H, Guo A. 2013. *In vitro* quinolones susceptibility analysis of Chinese *Mycoplasma bovis* isolates and their phylogenetic scenarios based upon QRDRs of DNA topoisomerases revealing a unique transition in ParC. *Pak Vet J* 33:364–369.

141. Raherison S, Gonzalez P, Renaudin H, Charron A, Bébéar C, Bébéar CM. 2005. Increased expression of two multidrug transporter-like genes is associated with ethidium bromide and ciprofloxacin resistance in *Mycoplasma hominis*. *Antimicrob Agents Chemother* 49:421–424.

142. Antunes NT, Assunção P, Poveda JB, Tavío MM. 2015. Mechanisms involved in quinolone resistance in *Mycoplasma mycoides* subsp. *capri*. *Vet J* 204:327–332.

143. Yan K, Madden L, Choudhry AE, Voigt CS, Copeland RA, Gontarek RR. 2006. Biochemical characterization of the interactions of the novel pleuromutilin derivative retapamulin with bacterial ribosomes. *Antimicrob Agents Chemother* 50:3875–3881.

144. Li BB, Shen JZ, Cao XY, Wang Y, Dai L, Huang SY, Wu CM. 2010. Mutations in 23S rRNA gene associated with decreased susceptibility to tiamulin and valnemulin

in *Mycoplasma gallisepticum*. *FEMS Microbiol Lett* 308:144–149.

145. Waites KB, Schelonka RL, Xiao L, Grigsby PL, Novy MJ. 2009. Congenital and opportunistic infections: ureaplasma species and *Mycoplasma hominis*. *Semin Fetal Neonatal Med* 14:190–199.

146. Nir-Paz R, Saraya T, Shimizu T, Van Rossum A, Bébéar C. 2017. Editorial: *Mycoplasma pneumoniae* clinical manifestations, microbiology, and immunology. *Front Microbiol* 8:1916.

147. Pereyre S, Laurier Nadalié C, Bébéar C, Arfeuille C, Beby-Defaux A, Berçot B, Boisset S, Bourgeois N, Carles M-J, Decré D, Garand A-L, Gibaud S-A, Grob A, Jeannot K, Kempf M, Moreau F, Petitjean-Lecherbonnier J, Prère M-F, Salord H, Verhoeven P, investigator group. 2017. *Mycoplasma genitalium* and *Trichomonas vaginalis* in France: a point prevalence study in people screened for sexually transmitted diseases. *Clin Microbiol Infect* 23:122.e1–122.e7.

148. Aarestrup FM, Friis NF, Szancer J. 1998. Antimicrobial susceptibility of *Mycoplasma hyorhinis* in a liquid medium compared to a disc assay. *Acta Vet Scand* 39:145–147.

149. Lysnyansky I, Ayling RD. 2016. *Mycoplasma bovis*: mechanisms of resistance and trends in antimicrobial susceptibility. *Front Microbiol* 7:595.

Antimicrobial Resistance in Bacteria from Livestock and Companion Animals
Edited by Frank Møller Aarestrup, Stefan Schwarz, Jianzhong Shen, and Lina Cavaco
© 2018 American Society for Microbiology, Washington, DC
doi:10.1128/microbiolspec.ARBA-0020-2017

Antimicrobial Resistance in *Clostridium* and *Brachyspira* spp. and Other Anaerobes

21

Marie Archambault[1] and Joseph E. Rubin[2]

INTRODUCTION

Anaerobic bacteria are unable to grow in the presence of oxygen. However, most clinical isolates grow very well under anaerobic conditions. Anaerobes can be divided into two groups: strict anaerobes, which are killed by exposure to oxygen, and aerotolerant anaerobes, which can tolerate some exposure to oxygen. They colonize many anatomical sites of animals, most notably the oral cavity, the rumen, and the lower intestinal tract, where they are part of the microbiota. They have also been associated with bacteria-rich mucosal surfaces of the respiratory tract, urinary and genital tracts, and even the skin (1). Only a small proportion of anaerobes can cause primary diseases, examples of which include *Clostridium* spp. such as *Clostridium perfringens* and *Clostridium difficile*, enterotoxigenic *Bacteroides fragilis*, *Dichelobacter nodosus*, and some *Brachyspira* spp. Other anaerobes, such as *Actinobaculum suis*, *Prevotella* spp., *Porphyromonas* spp., *Fusobacterium* spp., some *Clostridium* spp., *Peptococcus* spp., and *Streptopeptococcus* spp., are considered mostly opportunistic pathogens. Their disease onsets usually require predisposing factors such as inoculation into a normally sterile site through local trauma or any other conditions that permit bacterial entry and colonization. Anaerobes are often associated with clinical conditions involving necrotic and suppurative lesions such as abscesses and cellulitis. These opportunist infections are frequently multiple and commonly involve mixtures of aerobic and anaerobic bacteria, the former reducing the environment to allow the anaerobes to flourish. They are also considered a potential reservoir of antimicrobial resistance genes for other bacterial species (2).

The Clinical and Laboratory Standards Institute (CLSI) has established standardized methodologies for antimicrobial susceptibility testing for most anaerobes, which can be found in document M11 (3). This standard provides reference methods for the determination of MICs of anaerobic bacteria by agar dilution and broth microdilution. However, the document M11 standard was developed with human pathogens using human-specific methods and interpretative criteria. The documents VET01, 01S, and 02 provide the currently recommended techniques for antimicrobial agent disk and dilution susceptibility testing, criteria for quality control testing, and interpretive criteria for veterinary use, but refer to CLSI document M11 for guidance concerning anaerobes (4–6). As of 30 January 2017, document VET06 provides guidance for antimicrobial agent disk and dilution susceptibility testing, criteria for quality control testing, and breakpoints for fastidious and infrequently tested bacteria for veterinary use (7). Document VET06 includes a table on anaerobic bacteria and breakpoints for agar dilution and broth microdilution susceptibility testing. It includes a table on *Brachyspira hyodysenteriae* which provides information and breakpoints for agar dilution and broth microdilution susceptibility testing. In most cases in which veterinary-specific breakpoints have not yet been established, human breakpoints have been used when appropriate (see CLSI document M11). The veterinary-specific breakpoints have been established following CLSI document VET02, with particular attention given

¹Département de Pathologie et Microbiologie, Faculté de Médecine Vétérinaire, Université de Montréal, Saint-Hyacinthe, Québec J2S 2M2, Canada; ²Department of Veterinary Microbiology, Western College of Veterinary Medicine, University of Saskatchewan, Saskatchewan S7N 5B4, Canada.

447

to product label indications and directions as approved by regulatory authorities. Acceptable quality control ranges of MICs for anaerobic reference strains using agar dilution and broth microdilution are also provided in VET06. The methods described in this document are generic reference procedures that can be used routinely for susceptibility testing by clinical laboratories. They can also be used to evaluate commercial devices for possible routine use. Nevertheless, the data presented in this article have been mainly collected under the umbrella of human-specific methods and interpretative criteria of document M11 or other previously published breakpoints. Other organizations from different countries have been involved with antimicrobial susceptibility testing standardization for anaerobes, such as EUCAST (www.eucast.org) and the World Organization for Animal Health (www.oie.int).

Agar dilution is usually the reference method for most anaerobic bacteria, but other techniques may be used as long as equivalence to the reference methods is established (3). The disadvantages of the agar dilution approach are the laborious, time-consuming steps required to produce testing plates, mainly when the number of antimicrobials to be tested is high or when only a limited number of bacteria are to be tested. The Epsilometer test (Etest) is a rapid commercially available gradient diffusion system for quantitative antimicrobial susceptibility testing routinely used by laboratories for anaerobes such as C. difficile (8, 9). The use of disk diffusion tests is not recommended for anaerobic microorganisms because results are not reproducible, presumably due to the varied or insufficient growth rates of anaerobes. In addition, they do not correlate with those of the reference agar dilution method.

Anaerobic bacteria are usually naturally susceptible to most classes of antimicrobial agents, with the exception of aminoglycosides. The natural resistance to aminoglycosides can be explained by their requirement in oxygen for their transport into the bacterial cytoplasm (10). Anaerobes are also naturally resistant to polymyxins and the older fluoroquinolones. Trimethoprim-sulfonamides may not be effective *in vivo* against anaerobes due to the presence of thymidine in necrotic tissue (11). Penicillin, metronidazole, or clindamycin can be used for usual anaerobic coverage. Nitroimidazole antimicrobials such as metronidazole are usually effective because their intracellular reduction to active antimicrobial metabolites occurs under anaerobic conditions. However, due to their genotoxicities, they are not allowed for use in food-producing animals in many countries such as Canada, the United States,

and the European Union. The use of chloramphenicol, an active antimicrobial against anaerobes, in treating food-producing animals is also prohibited. Among antimicrobial resistance particularities, the *B. fragilis* group of bacteria of animal origin are frequently resistant to penicillins and some cephalosporins because they produce beta-lactamases (12, 13), although the use of clavulanic acid in combination with beta-lactam antimicrobials may restore susceptibility (14). *Clostridium* spp. are considered naturally resistant to trimethoprim because they have trimethoprim-insensitive dihydrofolate reductases and also have a permeability barrier to trimethoprim (15, 16).

In general, bacterial antimicrobial resistance is acquired on mobile genetic elements (MGEs) such as plasmids, transposons, and/or conjugative transposons. However, for fluoroquinolones and rifampin, resistance-mediating mutations are the main and most efficient resistance mechanisms. These mutations are also acquired, but not located, on MGEs. Although underinvestigated, this is also true for many antimicrobial-resistant anaerobic species described in the literature. A mini-review that summarizes what is known about tetracycline and macrolide-lincosamide-streptogramin B (MLS$_B$) resistance in genera with anaerobic species has been published (17). It discusses the MGEs associated with acquired tetracycline and/or MLS$_B$ resistance genes. Briefly, various tetracycline resistance efflux genes such as *tet*(B), *tet*(K), *tet*(L), and *tetA*(P) have been found in anaerobic species as well as tetracycline resistance genes coding for ribosomal protection proteins such as *tet*(M), *tet*(O), *tetB*(P), *tet*(Q), *tet*(W), and *tet* (32). Enzymes which inactivate tetracycline have been described, of which *tet*(X) has been identified in *Bacteroides*, though it is not functional under anaerobic growth conditions. This was also observed with the genes conferring MLS$_B$ resistance. The rRNA methylase MLS$_B$ resistance genes *erm*(B), *erm*(C), *erm*(F), *erm*(G), and *erm*(Q) have been identified in anaerobes. Since then, many more resistance genes and mechanisms have been unraveled.

This article describes the antimicrobial resistance known to date of the most frequently encountered anaerobic bacterial pathogens of animals. The following sections show that antimicrobial resistance can vary depending on the antimicrobial, the anaerobe, and the resistance mechanism. The variability in antimicrobial resistance patterns is also associated with factors such as geographic region and local antimicrobial usage. On occasion, the same resistance gene was observed in many anaerobes, whereas some were limited to certain anaerobes. This article focuses on antimicrobial resistance data of veterinary origin.

CLOSTRIDIUM

Clostridia are anaerobic Gram-positive rods with a low G + C content that form heat-resistant endospores. They are prokaryotic bacteria of the phylum *Firmicutes*. The genus *Clostridium* belongs to the *Clostridiaceae* family in the order *Clostridiales*. Most *Clostridium* spp. are intestinal commensals or inhabitants of soil or both. Only a few are pathogenic microorganisms (1). Clostridial diseases can be divided into three groups according to the types of infection they cause in animals: (i) enteric diseases are associated with enterotoxin-producing clostridia such as *C. perfringens*, *C. difficile*, and *C. spiroforme*. These species produce toxins that may act locally and/or systematically in the intestinal tract. They have also been involved with antibiotic-associated diarrhea. (ii) neurotoxic diseases are associated with species that produce potent neurotoxins, such as *C. botulinum* and *C. tetani*. These are rarely treated with antimicrobials. Thus, data on their antimicrobial susceptibility are not reviewed in this article. (iii) Histotoxic diseases involve species that produce histotoxins, such as *C. chauvoei*, *C. novyi*, *C. septicum*, *C. sordellii*, *C. haemolyticum*, *C. perfringens*, and *C. colinum* (1).

Enterotoxin-Producing Clostridia: *C. perfringens*

C. perfringens has been recently divided into seven types, A to G, based on the toxins they produce (18). Type A can cause gas gangrene (malignant edema) in several animal species and yellow lamb disease. Type B is responsible for lamb dysentery, while type C is associated with hemorrhagic and necrotizing enteritis mainly in neonatal animals. Type D is the agent of enterotoxemia mainly in small ruminants, and type E is responsible for bovine hemorrhagic gastroenteritis and enterotoxemia in rabbits. *C. perfringens* type F consists of strains responsible for *C. perfringens*-mediated human food poisoning and antibiotic associated diarrhea. *C. perfringens* type G comprises isolates that produce NetB toxin and thereby cause necrotic enteritis in chickens (18).

Susceptibility data in the literature mainly concern *C. perfringens* isolates from broilers because necrotic enteritis is a common and economically significant poultry disease that can be controlled by antimicrobials worldwide. Various antimicrobials such as bacitracin, avilamycin, virginiamycin, and lincomycin are currently used as in-feed medication for prophylactic or treatment purposes against necrotic enteritis in broilers, whereas diseases associated with *C. perfringens* in other animal species are only rarely treated with antimicrobials, with the exception of canine enteritis.

Occurrence of antimicrobial resistance in *C. perfringens*

The occurrence of tetracycline, bacitracin, and virginiamycin resistances has been described worldwide in *C. perfringens* from chicken broilers (19–23). Earlier studies of *C. perfringens* poultry isolates reported resistance to oxytetracycline (MIC, >1 mg/liter) as one of the most frequent resistances in samples from Sweden (76%), Denmark (10%), Norway (29%) (19), and Belgium (66%) (20). Resistance to bacitracin has also been reported in *C. perfringens* poultry isolates from the United States (88%) (21) and Denmark (18%) (19). Virginiamycin resistance has also been described in broiler isolates from Norway (18%) (19) and from the United States (31%) (21). It is believed that the use of these antimicrobials in broilers in many countries reflects the pattern of antimicrobial resistance observed. Earlier studies of poultry and pigs reported on susceptibilities to ampicillin, amoxicillin, penicillin, avilamycin, vancomycin, avoparcin, and ionophores such as narasin, salinomycin, lasalocid, and monensin (19–21, 24–26).

More recent studies of *C. perfringens* poultry isolates reported resistance to bacitracin and tetracycline as frequently encountered resistances in samples from Canada (22, 27) and Korea (28). Sulfonamides, macrolides, and lincosamide resistances were recently described in a few reports (28–31). In Belgium, resistances to tetracycline (66%) and lincomycin (61%) were the most frequent resistances observed, while bacitracin resistance was not noted (29). This was also reported in a Taiwanese study (31). Elevated MIC_{50} for virginiamycin has been described but rarely documented in chicken isolates (22). High levels of resistances to many antimicrobials have been observed in only one Egyptian report (30), where beta-lactam resistance was found to be a rare event. Globally, recent studies of poultry are still reporting on susceptibilities to beta-lactams, fluoroquinolones, and phenicols (28, 29).

There are only a few reports on antimicrobial susceptibility of *C. perfringens* from other species (25, 32–39). Earlier studies of *C. perfringens* of porcine origin reported resistance to tetracycline, erythromycin, clindamycin, and lincomycin, indicating multidrug resistance, whereas isolates were generally quite susceptible to penicillin and chloramphenicol (25, 33). More recently, reduced susceptibility to clindamycin (28%), erythromycin (31%), and tetracycline was observed in *C. perfringens* isolates of swine origin from Canada (22). In a German study, resistance to linezolid, with simultaneous resistance to florfenicol and erythromycin was reported (34). A Brazilian study of *C. perfringens* isolated from piglets (35) reported susceptibility to amoxicillin and ceftiofur, whereas resistance to tetracycline and lincomycin was quite common. A study in Thailand reported that most of the *C. perfringens* isolates from piglets were susceptible to ampicillin, bacitracin, chlortetracycline, doxycycline, and oxytetracycline, with MIC_{50} values ranging from 0.32 to 8 mg/liter (32). However, high resistance rates were observed for ceftiofur, enrofloxacin, erythromycin, lincomycin, and tylosin, and among resistant isolates, 82% were resistant to more than one type of antimicrobial. *C. perfringens* of bovine origin with reduced susceptibility to clindamycin, florfenicol, and tetracycline was reported in a Canadian study (22). *C. perfringens* isolates from cooked beef sold in the streets of Cote d'Ivoire, Africa, were shown to exhibit resistance rates to tetracycline, doxycycline, chloramphenicol, and erythromycin ranging from 20 to 50% (36). A survey of 50 Swedish *C. perfringens* isolates from individual dogs with acute diarrhea (37) reported that 18% of the isolates showed resistance to tetracycline and 54% showed decreased susceptibility to metronidazole, with an MIC of 4 mg/liter. In this study, all isolates were shown to be susceptible to all beta-lactams tested as well as to chloramphenicol and clindamycin (37). In a study in Costa Rica, multiresistance to clindamycin, chloramphenicol, penicillin, and metronidazole was observed in 5% of *C. perfringens* strains of animal origin (38).

The presence of *C. perfringens* in water is generally regarded as an indicator of fecal contamination, and exposure to waterborne spores is considered a possible source of infection for animals. In a Spanish study, the antimicrobial susceptibility of *C. perfringens* in water sources in a zoological park located in Madrid was investigated (40). Most isolates displayed intermediate susceptibility (57%; MIC, 16 mg/liter) or resistance (5.7%; MIC, ≥32 mg/liter) to metronidazole. In this study, no resistance to other antimicrobials was detected, although some isolates showed elevated MICs to erythromycin and/or linezolid.

Recently, antimicrobial tolerance was shown to be mediated by biofilms in *C. perfringens* (41–44). Bio-

films are structured communities of bacterial cells enclosed in a self-produced extracellular polysaccharide matrix which provides increased resistance to environmental stresses (45). Studies have demonstrated that the biofilm formed by *C. perfringens* could protect the cells from an exposure to atmospheric oxygen and to high concentrations of penicillin (41, 42). More recently, antimicrobial tolerance mediated by biofilms in *C. perfringens* was observed for bacitracin, penicillin, lincomycin, virginiamycin, tylosin, and the anticoccidial agents salinomycin, narasin, and monensin (44).

Another interesting area of research concerning *C. perfringens* is the impact of antimicrobial resistance on fitness and virulence (46–49). Recently, using comparative transcriptomic analysis, a study demonstrated that *C. perfringens* exposure to fluoroquinolones affected virulence (toxin production) in addition to drug resistance (46). In another study, it was observed that both the genetic background of the strain and the fluoroquinolone which induced resistance affected the fitness of *C. perfringens*-resistant mutants (47). Also, a ciprofloxacin-resistant mutant of *C. perfringens* with stable mutations in the topoisomerase genes was shown to accumulate less norfloxacin and ethidium bromide than the wild type via an ABC transporter protein (NP_562422) which was also associated with reduced susceptibility to norfloxacin and ciprofloxacin (49). It will be interesting to follow these new areas of research in regard to antimicrobial resistance.

Genetic basis of antimicrobial resistance in *C. perfringens*

The most common genetic antimicrobial resistance determinants described to date are associated with bacitracin, tetracyclines, MLS, and chloramphenicol antimicrobials (Table 1). Bacitracin resistance has been associated with genes encoding for an ABC transporter and an overproduced undecaprenol kinase in *C. perfringens* of poultry origin (23). These two mechanisms were both shown to be encoded by a *bcr*ABD operon under the control of a regulatory gene, *bcr*R (23). These genes were shown to be located on the chromosome and expressed under bacitracin stress (23). More recently, it was demonstrated that the *bcr*RABD locus was also localized to an 89.7-kb plasmid, pJIR4150, on a novel genetic element, ICECp1, which is related to the Tn*916* family of integrative conjugative elements (50). It was shown to be conjugative and associated with the pCW3 family of conjugative antimicrobial resistance and toxin plasmids from *C. perfringens* (50).

Previous studies that have reported on reduced susceptibility to tetracycline in poultry *C. perfringens* have

Table 1 Overview of the genes or the mutations in genes associated with acquired antimicrobial resistance so far identified in the different anaerobes of animal origin

Resistance mechanism	Resistance gene(s)	Gene product(s)	Resistance phenotype	Anaerobes involved	References
Chemical modification	Cat(P,Q)	Acetyltransferases	Chloramphenicol	C. perfringens	16, 67
	lnu(A, B, P)	Nucleotidyl transferases	Lincosamides	C. perfringens	29, 62
	tet(X)	Oxidoreductase	Tetracyclines	Bacteroides	17
Efflux: decreased intracellular drug accumulation	tet(B), tet(K), tet(L), or tetA(P)	Efflux system of the major facilitator superfamily	Tetracyclines	C. perfringens, C. difficile, C. septicum, C. sordellii	20, 29, 52, 54, 108
	bcrRABD	ABC transporter and an overproduced undecaprenol kinase	Bacitracin	C. perfringens	23, 50
	mef(A)	Efflux system of the major facilitator family	14-,15-Membered macrolides	C. perfringens	72
Hydrolytic degradation	bla$_{\mathrm{OXA\text{-}63}}$ group genes	Beta-lactamases	Beta-lactam antibiotics	B. pilosicoli	163, 164
	cep(A)	Beta-lactamases	Beta-lactam antibiotics	Bacteroides	12
Methylation of the target site	erm(B, C, F, G, or Q)	rRNA methylase	MLS$_B$	Bacteroides, C. perfringens, C. difficile	17, 97
Mutational modification		Mutation in the gene rplD, encoding protein L4 of the 50S ribosomal subunit	Linezolid, florfenicol and erythromycin	C. perfringens	34
		Mutation in the 23S rRNA gene	One or more of these drugs: macrolides, lincosamides, streptogramins, pleuromutilins, tetracyclines	Brachyspira	158–161
		Mutation in the genes coding for ribosomal proteins, L2, L3, L4, and L22	Tiamulin	Brachyspira	159, 161
Protection of the target site		Mutation in the 16S rRNA gene	Doxycycline	Brachyspira	162
	tet(M, O, Q, W, 32, or B(P))	Ribosomal protection proteins	Tetracyclines	Bacteroides, C. perfringens, C. difficile, C. septicum, C. sordellii	12, 20, 29, 52, 54, 97, 106

identified the *tetA*(P), *tetB*(P), and *tet*(M) genes as the most common genetic determinants (19, 51–53). The *tet*(P) gene was first identified in the conjugative *C. perfringens* R-plasmid pCW3, which demonstrated two functional overlapping tetracycline resistance genes, *tetA*(P) and *tetB*(P) (54). The *tetA*(P) gene encodes for a transmembrane protein which mediates active efflux of tetracycline from the cell, while *tetB*(P) encodes a protein which has significant similarity to Tet M-like tetracycline resistance proteins associated with ribosomal protection (54). While *tetA*(P) seems to be associated with all tetracycline-resistant strains, it was demonstrated that most of the isolates carried a second tetracycline resistance gene, *tetB*(P) or *tet*(M) (53). The *tetB*(P) gene was shown not to disturb the MIC of tetracycline in *C. perfringens* isolates already carrying *tetA*(P) (19) and was only associated with low-level tetracycline resistance (54). Other studies have also reported tetracycline resistance genes such as *tet*(Q), *tet*(K), *tet*(L), *tet*(O), and *tet*(W) (20, 29). The conjugative tetracycline resistance plasmids are relatively common in *C. perfringens* and are closely related to the originally isolated pCW3 (55–57). More recently, a conjugative 49-kb tetracycline resistance plasmid which is very similar to pCW3 was recently described in a *netB*-positive necrotic enteritis-derived *C. perfringens* strain (58). In a study from the United-States, susceptibility to tetracycline and minocycline in *C. perfringens* was most common in strains isolated from chickens, followed by those from soils, clinical samples, and foods (59). The most common resistance genes in this study were *tetA*(P) and *tetB*(P), with only one tetracycline-resistant food isolate with an intact *tet*(M) gene (59). Fragments with high degrees of identity to parts of the *tet*(M) sequences were also found in other strains, mainly of clinical origin, and often in isolates with *tetB*(P) (59). Interestingly, in this study, no correlation was observed between the level of susceptibility to tetracycline or minocycline and the presence of *tetA*(P), *tetB*(P), or part of *tet*(M) (59). More recently, all bacitracin-resistant *C. perfringens* poultry isolates in a Canadian study were found to carry both *tetA*(P) and *tetB*(P) (23). Plasmid curing experiments revealed the loss of the *tet* genes, indicating, as expected, plasmid localization of these genes (23).

Macrolide resistance is usually mediated by *erm*, erythromycin resistance methylase, genes (17). The proteins encoded by the *erm* genes confer N^6 dimethylation of a specific adenine residue (A2058) of the 23S rRNA molecule (17). This alteration of the macrolide target site is catalyzed by an rRNA methyltransferase. This resistance mechanism confers cross-resistance to macrolides, lincosamides, and streptogramin B (MLS$_B$ phenotype) (17). The *erm*(B), *erm*(F), and *erm*(Q) genes have been described in *C. perfringens* (17). This resistance has been shown to be plasmid-mediated (17, 60). In a recent Canadian study, only one bacitracin- and tetracycline-resistant *C. perfringens* poultry isolate was shown to harbor an MLS$_B$ resistance gene, *erm*(B) (23). A mutational analysis of the Erm(B) protein from *C. perfringens* indicated that nine mutants with single point mutations in the *erm*(B) gene produced stable but nonfunctional Erm(B) proteins (61). All of the mutants had amino acid changes within conserved methyltransferase motifs that were important for either substrate binding or catalysis, indicating that the point mutations all involved residues important for the structure and/or function of this rRNA methyltransferase (61). Lincomycin resistance in *C. perfringens* is also common and is usually encoded by *erm* genes that confer MLS$_B$ resistance (62). In a 2006 study of *C. perfringens* in dogs, a relatively high prevalence of tetracycline resistance was reported, where 96% (119/124) of the isolates were positive for the *tetA*(P) gene, and 41% (51/124) were positive for both the *tetA*(P) and *tetB*(P) genes (63). In this study, only one isolate was positive for the *erm*(B) gene, and another was positive for the *erm*(Q) gene (63). Of the 15 tested isolates, 2 (13%) demonstrated transfer of tetracycline resistance via bacterial conjugation (63).

In contrast to the MLS$_B$ phenotype, specific resistance to lincosamides is due to enzymatic inactivation of those antibiotics, usually via phosphorylation and nucleotidylation of the hydroxyl group at position 3 of lincosamides (64). Lincosamide nucleotidyltransferases encoded by the *lnu*(A) and *lnu*(B) genes (formerly *lin*) have been observed in *C. perfringens* from Belgium broilers (29). The O-nucleotidyltransferases encoded by these genes inactivate lincosamides by adenylation (65, 66). An Australian study, using a *C. perfringens* lincomycin-resistant but erythromycin-susceptible strain, demonstrated that the lincomycin resistance *lnu*(P) gene was plasmid borne (plasmid pJIR2774) and could be transferred to other *C. perfringens* isolates by conjugation (62). This plasmid did not harbor tetracycline resistance. The *lnu*(P) gene was shown to encode for a putative lincosamide nucleotidyltransferase and was located on tISCpe8, a functional transposable genetic element and member of the IS*1595* family of transposon-like insertion sequences (62). This element was reported to have significant similarities to the mobilizable lincomycin resistance element tISSag10 from *Streptococcus agalactiae* (62). Like tISSag10, tISCpe8 carries a functional origin of transfer-like region within the resistance gene, allowing the element to be mobilized by the conjugative transposon Tn916 (62). Recently, a new mutation was detected in a C. perfringens strain isolated from pig manure, which was shown to be resistant to linezolid, florfenicol, and erythromycin (34). This mutation was described in a highly conserved region of rplD, encoding protein L4 of the 50S ribosomal subunit (34).

Chloramphenicol resistance has been shown to be mediated by chloramphenicol acetyltransferase (CAT) enzymes encoded by cat(P) and cat(Q) (67). The cat(Q) gene was shown to be distinct from the C. perfringens cat(P) gene. The deduced CATQ monomer had considerable amino acid sequence conservation compared with CATP (53% similarity) and other known CAT proteins (39 to 53%). The amino acid sequence of CATP was significantly similar to CAT monomers from Vibrio anguillarum and Campylobacter coli, whereas phylogenetic analysis revealed that the CATQ monomer was as closely related to CAT proteins from Staphylococcus aureus and C. coli as it was to CAT monomers from the clostridia (67). Chloramphenicol resistance has been located on mobilizable transposons in C. perfringens (68). Mobilizable transposons are transposable genetic elements that also encode mobilization functions but are not in themselves conjugative (69). To conjugate, they rely on coresident conjugative elements to facilitate their transfer to recipient cells. C. perfringens mobilizable transposons include Tn4451 and Tn4452, which are closely related (68, 69). The Tn4451 group of elements encodes resistance to chloramphenicol with an unusual transposition which is dependent upon a large resolvase protein rather than a more conventional transposase or integrase (69). This group also encodes the mobilization protein TnpZ, which acts at the RS (A), an upstream palindromic sequence, or origin of transfer site located on the transposon (69). In the presence of a coresident conjugative element, this promotes the movement of the nonreplicating circular intermediate and of plasmids on which the transposon is located (69).

The mef(A) gene encodes an efflux pump associated with resistance to macrolides in the absence of resistance to lincosamides and streptogramin B and was first described in Streptococcus pneumoniae (70, 71). This gene has been observed in C. perfringens recovered from water, soil, and sewage from 14 U.S. states (72). In this study, the antimicrobial resistance genes tetA(P), tetB(P), tet(M), erm(B), and erm(Q) were also observed, indicating that environmental C. perfringens organisms are capable of acting as reservoirs for these antimicrobial resistance genes.

Enterotoxin-Producing Clostridia: C. difficile

C. difficile is the agent of necrotizing enterocolitis, often antibiotic-associated, in several mammalian species (9, 73–77). The disease is especially observed in animals with large or expanded bowels such as horses, swine, rabbits, and guinea-pigs (1). It has also been described in calves, foals, piglets, and dogs (1). In human medicine, C. difficile is a major nosocomial pathogen that also causes antibiotic-associated diarrhea, often referred to as a pseudomembranous colitis (9, 73, 77). Healthy carriers have been described in humans and animals (78). Oral treatment with broad-spectrum antibiotics is reported as a risk factor for the disease to occur (9, 73). Erythromycin has been reported as an antimicrobial associated with C. difficile colitis in horses (79, 80). Other antimicrobials often associated with this disease in horses are trimethoprim-sulfonamides, beta-lactams, clindamycin, rifampicin, and gentamicin (74, 76). Other factors such as hospitalization and changes in diet may also contribute to the development of C. difficile infection (81).

The virulence of C. difficile is essentially mediated by two toxins of the large clostridial cytotoxin family named toxin A (TcdA), an enterotoxin, and toxin B (TcdB), a cytotoxin (1). The genes tcdA and tcdB are located on a large pathogenicity locus in the chromosome (1). An important increase in incidence of human C. difficile infection has been observed across the United States, Canada, and Europe over the past decade due to the emergence of highly virulent (or hypervirulent) strains of C. difficile (9). The most prominent hypervirulent type is categorized as PCR ribotype 027 (RT027), North American pulsed field gel electrophoresis type I, and restriction endonuclease analysis group B1 (9). Strain RT027 is characterized by severe infection, a high rate of recurrence, mortality, and resistance to traditional therapy (9). In addition to RT027, a number of emergent highly virulent ribotypes, correlated with RT027 or not, have recently been identified (82). The hypervirulent RT078 has been recognized as a cause of infections in humans in hospitals (83) and in the community (84) and in animals (85–89). The epidemic of RT027 infections marked an antimicrobial resistance turning point for C. difficile with the arrival of fluoroquinolone resistance, most likely due to overuse of this antimicrobial in human medicine (9). Since then, many reports have been published on the antimicrobial susceptibilities and resistance genes of C. difficile of human origin. Far less documentation is readily available in veterinary medicine. A recent review on the phenotypic and genotypic traits of antimicrobial resistance in C. difficile taking into consideration the most recent data has been published (9).

Occurrence of antimicrobial resistance in *C. difficile*

Acquired resistance in *C. difficile* isolates of animal origin to a diverse range of antimicrobials including chloramphenicol (80), rifampin (90, 91), metronidazole (91), tetracyclines (75, 80, 92), erythromycin (75, 80, 92), and vancomycin have been described (91). Earlier studies of *C. difficile* isolates reported on susceptibility to penicillin (80, 90, 92), but acquired resistance was described to be between 10 and 25% in a prospective study on equine diarrhea (92). In a Western Australian investigation over a 24-month period (2007 to 2009), *C. difficile* was isolated from 14 (23%) of 62 diarrheal horses (including 10 foals), and all isolates were reported as susceptible to metronidazole and vancomycin (93). A survey of 777 horses of different breeds, age, and sex and their environment revealed that all 52 strains of *C. difficile* recovered were susceptible to metronidazole (MIC, ≤4 mg/liter) and vancomycin (MIC, ≤2 mg/liter) (90). A cross-sectional observational study of *C. difficile* recovered from diarrheic and non-diarrheic foals (*n* = 153) resulted in 7 (4.6%) positive samples for *C. difficile* A/B toxin, all from diarrheic foals. All of the *C. difficile* isolates were susceptible to metronidazole and vancomycin (94). Resistance to metronidazole was reported in some strains of *C. difficile* from a prospective study of horses admitted to an intensive care unit for acute gastrointestinal tract disease with loose feces (*n* = 130) (95). Horses infected with these strains were 10 times more likely to have been treated with metronidazole prior to the onset of diarrhea than horses infected with other strains. The duration from onset of diarrhea to discharge was longer, systemic inflammatory response syndromes were more pronounced, and the mortality rate was higher in horses infected with these strains, indicating that metronidazole-resistant strains may be associated with severe disease (95). Also, in a retrospective study of 28 foals with *C. difficile*-associated diarrhea, 10 of 23 (43%) *C. difficile* isolates were resistant to metronidazole (96). In this study, molecular fingerprinting revealed marked heterogeneity among isolates, except for the metronidazole-resistant isolates (96). A Canadian study of *C. difficile* from horses admitted to a veterinary teaching hospital over a 7-month period recovered 10 isolates with high-level resistance to clindamycin and ceftiofur (81). Among these isolates, seven PCR ribotypes were identified, including RT014 (81). In a *C. difficile* study of horses with colitis in Sweden, all 36 clinical and 14

environmental isolates were shown to be susceptible to vancomycin and avilamycin, but 50% had bimodal MIC distributions of erythromycin, virginiamycin, spiramycin, and oxytetracycline (80). All isolates in this study were resistant to rifampin (80).

An earlier study of *C. difficile* isolated from diarrheic neonatal piglets from the United States reported a high occurrence of resistance to bacitracin and ceftiofur (MICs_{90}, ≥256 mg/liter) (75). In this study, the MIC_{90} (64 or ≥256 mg/liter) for erythromycin, tilmicosin, and tylosin suggested resistance of a proportion of *C. difficile* isolates, while susceptibility to tetracycline varied widely among isolates with MIC_{50} and MIC_{90} of 8 and 32 mg/liter, respectively. In this study, The MICs_{90} for tiamulin (8 mg/liter) and virginiamycin (16 mg/liter) suggested moderate susceptibility in those isolates. More recently, an investigation of antimicrobial resistance determinants of *C. difficile* isolated from swine raised in Ohio and North Carolina revealed that 19% (119/609) of *C. difficile* isolates were resistant to tetracycline, and 7% (44/609) were resistant to both erythromycin and tetracycline (97). In this study, the majority of *C. difficile* isolates (80.5%) were shown to have a MIC of >32 mg/liter for ciprofloxacin (98). An investigation of *C. difficile* among different age and production groups of swine in a vertically integrated swine operation in Texas revealed that all isolates (*n* = 131) were resistant to cefoxitin, ciprofloxacin, and imipenem, whereas all were susceptible to metronidazole, piperacillin/tazobactam, amoxicillin/clavulanic acid, and vancomycin (99). The majority of isolates were resistant to clindamycin, resistant or intermediate to ampicillin, and susceptible to tetracycline and chloramphenicol (99). In a study comparing the antimicrobial resistance patterns of *C. difficile* isolated from a closed, integrated population of humans and swine, antimicrobial susceptibility testing was performed on 523 *C. difficile* strains (100). Swine isolates originated from a vertically flowing swine population consisting of farrowing, nursery, breeding, and grower/finisher production groups, while human wastewater isolates were collected from swine worker and nonworker occupational group cohorts. All of the swine and human strains were susceptible to amoxicillin/clavulanic acid, piperacillin/tazobactam, and vancomycin (100). In addition, all of the human strains were susceptible to chloramphenicol (100). The majority of the human and swine strains were resistant to cefoxitin and ciprofloxacin (100). Statistically significant differences in antimicrobial susceptibility were found among the swine production groups for ciprofloxacin, tetracycline, amoxicillin/clavulanic acid, and clindamycin (100). No significant differences in antimicrobial susceptibility were found across the human occupational group cohorts. This study reported metronidazole resistance in 8.3% of the swine strains and in 13.3% of the human strains (100). The authors concluded that the finding of differences in susceptibility patterns between human and swine strains of *C. difficile* provides evidence that transmission between host species in this integrated population is unlikely (100).

In a survey of antimicrobial susceptibility of 144 Spanish *C. difficile* swine isolates, a high prevalence of the toxigenic RT078 (94.4%) was observed along with multidrug resistance (49.3%) among isolates tested (101). In this study, resistance to clindamycin, ertapenem, erythromycin, and moxifloxacin was common (≥27.8% in all cases). Also, all isolates were resistant to ciprofloxacin but susceptible to daptomycin, linezolid, meropenem, rifampicin, teicoplanin, tigecycline, metronidazole, and vancomycin. It was found that erythromycin and moxifloxacin resistance was associated with the geographic origin of the isolates and that metronidazole heteroresistance was observed. A study of commercial pigs at the preharvest food-safety level (68 sows and 251 young pigs from 5 farms) in North Carolina and Ohio (3 farms) revealed ciprofloxacin resistance as predominant in young pigs (91.3% of isolates) and sows (94%) (102). In this study, the ciprofloxacin-erythromycin-tetracycline resistance profile was detected in 21.4% and 11.7% of isolates from young pigs and sows, respectively. Also, erythromycin and tetracycline resistances were both significantly associated with toxin gene profiles (102). In a Japanese study, *C. difficile* from neonatal piglets less than 20 days of age recovered during June to August 2012 were shown to be susceptible to vancomycin and metronidazole (103). In this study, resistance against clindamycin, ceftriaxone, erythromycin, and ciprofloxacin were found in 59, 6, 46, and 75% of the isolates, respectively. Also, of the 61 toxigenic *C. difficile* isolates (toxin A⁺B⁺), the incidence of resistance to clindamycin, ceftriaxone, erythromycin, and ciprofloxacin was 71%, 10%, 43%, and 74%, respectively. It was also observed that the percentage of resistant isolates derived from piglets against all antimicrobials, particularly ceftriaxone, was lower than that clinically isolated from humans (8, 103). In a North Carolina study of free-ranging feral swine in areas with extensive commercial swine production, antimicrobial resistance was detected in *C. difficile* isolates for six of the eight antimicrobials tested (104). Briefly, isolates exhibited a high frequency of resistance to tetracycline (57%) and levofloxacin (30%), whereas none of the isolates exhibited resistance to metronidazole and vancomycin.

Characterization of *C. difficile* isolates from Italian swine and dogs revealed 10 PCR ribotypes in porcine strains and 6 in canine strains (105). The predominant type found in porcine strains was RT078 (50%), whereas canine strains carried the nontoxinogenic RT010 (64%). Among swine, resistance to erythromycine (60%), moxifloxacin (35%), clindamycin (15%), and rifampin (5%) was observed, whereas all isolates were susceptible to metronidazole or vancomycin. Among dogs, 51% of strains were resistant to clindamycin, 46% to erythromycin, 21% to metronidazole, and 5% to moxifloxacin or rifampin, but all isolates were susceptible to vancomycin. In this study, five porcine strains (10%) and nine canine isolates (41%) were multidrug resistant, and some multidrug-resistant canine strains (*n* = 8) were highly resistant to metronidazole, with MICs of ≥32 mg/liter. Also in this study, using the EUCAST cutoff for metronidazole (MIC, >2 mg/liter), 13 canine isolates and 1 porcine strain were found to have reduced susceptibility to metronidazole (MICs ranging from 3 to ≥256 mg/liter). Those strains belonged to RT010 and RT078, which have also been associated with reduced susceptibility to metronidazole in humans (105). A Cote d'Ivoire study in Abidjan looked at the antimicrobial susceptibilities of *C. difficile* in cooked beef sold in the streets, with a total of 395 kidney and meat samples from vendors (36). A prevalence of 12.4% for *C. difficile* (11.04% in kidney and 13.45% in meat) was determined, with resistance rates to tetracycline, doxycycline, chloramphenicol, and erythromycin against *C. difficile* isolates ranging from 2.05% to 8.16% (36). In this study, metronidazole and vancomycin were the most potent antimicrobial agents against *C. difficile*.

Genetic basis of antimicrobial resistance in *C. difficile*

Studies looking into the genetic basis of *C. difficile* antimicrobial resistance are available in the human medicine literature, but there is a paucity of comparable data from the veterinary discipline (Table 1). Multiple mechanisms for the acquisition of antimicrobial resistance have been described in *C. difficile*, mostly of human origin, such as mobilizable and conjugative transposons, other MGEs, and various mutations (9). To our knowledge, plasmids encoding antimicrobial resistance seem to not have been described in *C. difficile*.

Tetracycline resistance is commonly due to protection of the ribosomes, and the most widespread *tet* class in *C. difficile* is *tet*(M), usually found on conjugative Tn916-like elements such as Tn5397 (9, 106, 107). Other *tet* genes have been identified such as *tet*(P), *tet*

(K), and *tet*(L) (108). The presence of both *tet*(M) and *tet*(W) has been described in *C. difficile* isolates from humans and animals (97, 109). Indeed, a study of *C. difficile* isolated from swine raised in Ohio and North Carolina revealed that tetracycline resistance was mainly associated with *tet*(M) (97%), followed by *tet*(W) (32%) genes, with a subset of 31% (37/119) of these isolates carrying both *tet*(M) and *tet*(W) genes (97). In this study, isolates that carried both genes had a wide range of MICs within the category "resistance," indicating no benefit in carrying both genes. Also in this study, the majority (97%; 66/68) of isolates with an erythromycin MIC of >256 mg/liter were found to carry the *erm*(B) gene (91%, 68/75), and the majority of isolates that were resistant to both erythromycin and tetracycline tested positive for both the *erm*(B) and *tet*(M) genes. Both genes have been previously associated with a Tn*916*-like element in *C. difficile* of human origin (107), and this could also be the case in animal isolates. Ribosomal methylation is reported as the most widespread mechanism of resistance of the MLS$_B$ family in *C. difficile* and is mediated by the *erm*(B) gene (109). Characteristics of *C. difficile* strains with reduced susceptibility to metronidazole from 16 studies published between 2012 and 2015 have recently been reviewed (9). Generally, the percentage of *C. difficile* strains resistant to metronidazole is low. However, a number of *C. difficile* strains with MICs of >2 mg/liter, the EUCAST epidemiological cut-off, have been reported in both humans and animals (9). Genes conferring resistance to metronidazole have not yet been described in *C. difficile* (9).

The following reports on antimicrobial resistance genes are of human origin, and these genes have not yet been identified, to our knowledge, from animal sources (110–126). Briefly, the Tn*6164* containing the *tet*(44) and *ant*(6)-Ib genes, predicted to confer resistance to tetracycline and streptomycin, respectively, was described in a *C. difficile* human isolate (110). Resistance to fluoroquinolones in *C. difficile* has been reported to be due to alterations in the quinolone-resistance-determining region of either GyrA or GyrB; the DNA gyrase subunits and several amino acid substitutions have been identified in both GyrA and/or GyrB (9). The majority of *C. difficile* fluoroquinolone-resistant strains have shown the substitution Thr82Ile in GyrA (115–117). For rifampin and rifaximin resistance, mutations in the beta-subunit of the RNA polymerase, *rpoB*, have been described (9). Among the amino acid substitutions identified, Arg505Lys is the most common, particularly in *C. difficile* strain RT027 (118). Fusidic acid resistance has been associated with mutations in the *fusA*

gene, encoding for a protein elongation factor (119). Chloramphenicol resistance in *C. difficile* has been identified as mediated by the *cat*D gene, which encodes a CAT enzyme (120). This gene was found on mobilizable transposons Tn*4453a* and Tn*4453b* on the chromosome, and these are structurally and functionally related to the *C. perfringens* mobilizable element Tn*4451* (121). In humans, resistance to linezolid in *C. difficile* has been associated with a *cfr*-like gene, *cfr*(B), that encodes a Cfr RNA methyltransferase causing multiple resistances to peptidyl transferase inhibitors by methylation of A2503 in the 23S rRNA (122, 123). In addition to phenicol and linezolid, the *cfr*(B) gene has been shown to encode resistance to lincosamides, pleuromutilins, and streptogramin A (122). The vancomycin, metronidazole, and cephalosporins resistance mechanisms in *C. difficile* are still unclear (9, 124–126).

Histotoxic Clostridia: *C. chauvoei*, *C. novyi*, *C. septicum*, and *C. sordellii*

C. chauvoei is the causative agent of blackleg, a highly fatal disease characterized by a myonecrosis in cattle and more rarely in sheep. The infection has also been described in other animal species (1). It was suggested that *C. chauvoei* susceptibilities to antimicrobials reflects the fact that blackleg is not treated with antimicrobials due to its virulent appearance leading to rapid death of the animal (127). The MICs for *C. chauvoei* strain JF4335 using the microdilution method according to the CLSI guidelines (3) have been described as low, suggesting susceptibility to these antimicrobials.

Gas gangrene, otherwise known as malignant edema, is a necrotizing soft tissue infection. It is usually an acute, often fatal, toxemia affecting all species and ages of animals, with a higher incidence in ruminants and horses (1). This disease can be caused by *C. septicum*, *C. chauvoei*, *C. novyi* type A, *C. perfringens* type A, and *C. sordellii* (1). A study in 2001 reported low penicillin and ampicillin MICs in Japanese isolates of *C. septicum* and *C. sordellii* from cattle with gas gangrene (52). In this study, all *C. sordellii* isolates were reported as resistant to oxytetracycline, whereas 22% of *C. septicum* isolates were identified as resistant to this antimicrobial. Also, low MICs were reported for enrofloxacin, erythromycin, vancomycin, and chloramphenicol in these Japanese cattle isolates. In humans, resistance to sulfamethoxazole and trimethoprim but susceptibility to imipenem and cefoxitin have been reported in *C. sordellii* (128–130).

In sheep and cattle, *C. septicum* also causes a disease known as braxy, a necrotizing abomasitis, where affected animals are generally found dead (1). This highly fatal infection is characterized by toxemia and inflammation of the abomasal wall. A study in the 1980s in California that looked at *C. septicum* isolates from humans and animals demonstrated relatively good susceptibilities to many antimicrobials (131, 132), such as beta-lactams, macrolides, lincosamides, phenicols, nitro-imidazoles, rifamycins, bacitracin, and tetracyclines.

C. novyi type B causes acute hepatic necrosis, commonly known as black disease, in animals grazing in fluke-infested pastures (133). No information is available on antimicrobial resistance in this bacterium from animals, but data is available from humans (134).

Genetic basis of antimicrobial resistance in *C. chauvoei*, *C. septicum*, and *C. sordellii*

An earlier study on the antimicrobial resistance determinants of *C. septicum* and *C. sordellii* from cattle affected with gas gangrene in Japan identified the *tetA*(P), *tetB*(P), and *tet*(M) genes in tetracycline-resistant isolates (52) (Table 1). This study also reported on the sequences of the tetracycline resistance genes of some *C. septicum* strains which were completely or almost completely identical to those of strains belonging to other clostridial species. More recently, the draft genome of *C. chauvoei* JF4335 was revealed to contain 2,630 predicted open reading frames, of which 1,935 protein sequences could be assigned, along with 632 open reading frames representing hypothetical proteins that could not be assigned (127). Of the assigned proteins, 44 genes were shown to be involved in antibiotic and metal resistance. It was shown that *C. chauvoei* strain JF4335 harbors a genetic potential for penicillin resistance, a beta-lactamase (EC 3.5.2.6), as well as an elongator factor EF G type tetracycline resistance gene potentially involved in protection of ribosomes from tetracycline and catalysis and release of tetracycline [*tet*(M) and *tet*(O) analogue] and a vancomycin B-type resistance protein gene, *van*(W), with no further genes potentially involved in vancomycin resistance.

BRACHYSPIRA

Brachyspira are Gram-negative, fastidious, microaerophilic anaerobic spirochetes which inhabit the colon and cecum (135). There are currently seven species of *Brachyspira* with standing in nomenclature: *B. aalborgi*, *B. alvinipulli*, *B. hyodysenteriae*, *B. innocens*, *B. intermedia*, *B. murdochii*, and *B. pilosicoli* (136). A number of other taxa without standing in the nomenclature, including *B. hampsonii*, *B. canis*, *B. suanatina*, and *B. pulli*, have been described in the literature (137, 138).

Brachyspira-Associated Disease in Pigs

Swine dysentery, characterized by muco-hemorrhagic diarrhea, is the most economically significant disease caused by *Brachyspira* in domestic animals. Swine dysentery was first described in 1921 and has historically been caused by *B. hyodysenteriae*; since the late 2000s a clinically indistinguishable syndrome associated with a novel taxon proposed to be called "*B. hampsonii*" has been described in North America and Europe (139, 140). Spirochetal colitis is a milder syndrome caused by *B. pilosicoli* and is associated with nonhemorrhagic, loose stools and production losses (141, 142).

Brachyspira-Associated Disease in Avian Species

Avian intestinal spirochetosis in domestic poultry species, characterized by diarrhea and mucosal thickening, is most often associated with *B. pilosicoli*, although *B. intermedia* and *B. alvinipulli* have also been implicated (143). Necrotizing typhlitis in juvenile rheas has been reported in association with *B. hyodysenteriae*. Colonization of wild birds with *Brachyspira* spp. is well recognized; phylogenetically diverse microorganisms including recognized pathogens and species of unknown clinical significance have been described in wild birds, including ducks and geese (138, 144).

Brachyspira-Associated Disease in Other Species

Brachyspira spp. have been reported from other domestic animal species, although their significance in disease has not been clearly defined. In people, intestinal spirochetosis associated with *B. aalborgi* and *B. pilosicoli* is an infrequently encountered chronic syndrome most often associated with immunosuppression (135, 145).

Antimicrobial Susceptibility Testing Methods and Challenges

Brachyspira-associated diseases in animals are primarily treated with the pleuromutilins, macrolides/lincosamides, and in the United States, carbadox (146). Treatment is generally empiric, since antimicrobial susceptibility testing of *Brachyspira* is not routinely conducted by most diagnostic laboratories. Although descriptions of the susceptibility of these organisms have been reported in the literature, the lack of standardized testing methods is a critical limitation to the interpretation of these studies. The methods used for antimicrobial susceptibility of other bacteria are described in exquisite detail in highly prescriptive standards published by the CLSI and EUCAST (4, 147). These standards dictate test factors including incubation temperature and time, bacterial concentration, atmosphere, and test media composition. The application of these methods to *Brachyspira* is hindered by the "nonstandard" growth conditions required by *Brachyspira* spp. Furthermore, because *Brachyspira* spp. do not reliably produce surface growth (colonies) on solid media and grow unreliably in liquid media, defining reproducible test endpoints to allow MICs to be determined is challenging. Laboratories performing these assays therefore rely heavily on in-house-developed methods, which while consistent within the facility, may differ substantially between laboratories. Studies reporting the use of agar dilution-based testing describe methods utilizing highly variable inoculum sizes (10^4 to 5×10^5 CFU/spot), incubation temperatures (37 to 42°C), and incubation time (48 to 120 hours) and utilize 5% blood-containing media with variable bases (trypticase soy agar, Wilkins-Charlgren, or Mueller-Hinton) (148–151). The effects of the variability of test methods on diagnostic outcomes was highlighted by a 2005 multicenter ring trial which described inconsistent results between participating laboratories (152). The introduction of the commercially prepared VetMIC *Brachyspira* microdilution panel in the early 2000s was an important step toward standardization of test methods. This panel has helped to improve the uniformity of the test media used by laboratories (153). The VetMIC panel includes tiamulin, valnemulin, doxycycline, tylvalosin, lincomycin, and tylosin.

The paucity of validated interpretive criteria for categorizing *Brachyspira* susceptibility test results is another critical limitation to the application of laboratory data to clinical practice. While breakpoints based on the pharmacokinetic properties of various drugs have been proposed by researchers (Table 2), the CLSI has just started to publish some interpretive criteria for classifying isolates as susceptible or resistant (7) (Table 2). CLSI document VET06 provides guidance for antimicrobial agent disk and dilution susceptibility testing, criteria for quality control testing, and breakpoints for fastidious and infrequently tested bacteria for veterinary use (7). Document VET06 includes a table on anaerobic bacteria and breakpoints for agar dilution and broth microdilution susceptibility testing. It includes data on *B. hyodysenteriae* which provides information and breakpoints for agar dilution and broth microdilution susceptibility testing. Acceptable quality control ranges of MICs for anaerobic reference strains using agar dilution and broth microdilution are also provided in VET06. The methods described in this document are generic reference procedures that can be used routinely for susceptibility testing by clinical laboratories (7).

Emergence of Antimicrobial Resistance

The treatment of *Brachyspira*-associated diseases relies heavily on mechanistically similar drugs (primarily lincosamide- and pleuromutilin-type compounds) which inhibit protein synthesis by binding to the 50S ribosomal subunit. It therefore stands to reason that there is a high selection pressure for the development of resistance to these drugs. A number of research groups have reported longitudinal studies of diagnostic isolates from their regions, and it is clear that resistance to drugs critical for treating *Brachyspira*-associated disease is emerging. Decreases in the susceptibility (increasing MICs) of *B. hyodysenteriae* to tiamulin and valnemulin have been reported when isolates from as early as the late 1980s are compared to isolates from the mid- to late-2000s. These trends have been described in multiple European countries (Italy, Germany, the Czech Republic, and Sweden) and in Japan (149, 154–157). Fewer longitudinal studies including *B. pilosicoli* have been published, although a Swedish investigation found that in contrast to decreasing pleuromutilin susceptibility among *B. hyodysenteriae*, the susceptibility of *B. pilosicoli* appeared to be stable (156).

Mechanisms of Resistance

Genetic associations with elevated antimicrobial MICs have been identified for a number of species-drug combinations (Table 1). Most of the published studies have focused on either *B. hyodysenteriae* or *B. pilosicoli*.

Table 2 Proposed breakpoints for the interpretation of *Brachyspira* MICs

| Author | Proposed resistance breakpoint[a] or wildtype cutoff[a] (mg/liter) | | | | | | | | Reference |
	Valnemulin	Tiamulin	Lincomycin	Tylosin	Tylvalosin	Doxycycline	Genatmicin	Carbadox	
Burch	>0.125–0.25	>0.5–1	>50–100	>1632	>16–32				219
Pringle	>0.12	>0.25	>1	>16	>1	>0.5			156, 220
Duhamel		≥2	≥75				≥10	≥1	221

[a]Resistance breakpoint, Burch and Duhamel; wildtype cutoff, Pringle.

Single nucleotide polymorphisms (SNPs) in rRNA gene sequences have been found to be associated with elevated macrolide, lincosamide, streptogramin, pleuromutilin, and tetracycline MICs. The first SNP found to be associated with decreased drug susceptibility was an A → G substitution at position 2058 of the 23S rRNA gene (158). Subsequently, additional SNPs, including at positions 2032, 2055, 2057, 2447, 2504, 2535, 2572, and 2611, have also been related to decreased susceptibility to one or more of these drugs (159–160). Decreased susceptibility to tiamulin has also been associated with mutations in ribosomal proteins L2, L3, L4, and L22 (159, 161). Ribosomal RNA SNPs have also been associated with decreasing susceptibility to doxycycline in B. hyodysenteriae and B. intermedia. Specifically, a polymorphism at location 1058 of the 16S rRNA gene has been identified in B. hyodysenteriae with decreased susceptibility to doxycycline (162).

A number of narrow-spectrum oxacillinases (Ambler class D beta-lactamases which hydrolyze penicillin, ampicillin, and oxacillin) have been identified in B. pilosicoli (163). To date, 14 closely related enzymes (OXA-63, 136, 137, 192, and 470 to 479) have been identified (164). The impact of these beta-lactamases on the treatment of Brachyspira-associated disease is questionable, although a deeper understanding of their epidemiology may be helpful for developing a more holistic model of resistance in animal pathogens. To date, there are no publications describing the presence of these enzymes in species other than B. pilosicoli, although whether this is reflective of the relative propensity of this species to carry these genes or of researcher/publication bias is unknown.

There is a great paucity of data describing the role of horizontal gene transmission in the epidemiology of resistance among Brachyspira. Phage-mediated transfer of resistance to chloramphenicol and tylosin between B. hyodysenteriae has been reported following exposure to metronidazole and carbadox (165). Plasmids have not been demonstrated to facilitate the dissemination of resistance, and one of the few studies addressing conjugative elements did not identify an association between the phenotype and the presence or absence of plasmids (166). Further work on understanding the extent and basis of resistance is needed in view of the extensive use of antibiotics to control brachyspiral infection in swine and poultry.

BACTEROIDES

Bacteroides are anaerobic Gram-negative rods and are one of the major groups colonizing the large intestines of animals and humans (167, 168). The B. fragilis group species are commonly associated with intra-abdominal abscesses, bacteremia, and soft tissue infections in both animals and humans. Some strains of B. fragilis can produce enterotoxins and are involved in diarrhea in lambs, calves, piglets, foals, young rabbits, and children. Antimicrobial resistance data on Bacteroides of animal origin is limited, whereas information is far more documented for human strains.

Earlier studies of clinical Bacteroides isolates from various animal species have indicated that penicillin, ampicillin, and cephalothin resistance varied between 18 and 24%, whereas tetracycline resistance was found to be between 9 and 20%, depending on the study (169, 170). In these studies, Bacteroides strains were usually susceptible to clindamycin and metronidazole. In a study of abscesses in pigs, Bacteroides isolates were susceptible to clindamycin, penicillin, ampicillin, minocycline, chloramphenicol, and cefoxitin, with clindamycin being the most active antimicrobial tested, with a median MIC of 0.8 mg/liter (171). Among Bacteroides isolates recovered from the uteri of dairy cows with retained fetal membranes and postparturient endometritis, all isolates were found to be susceptible to clindamycin (MIC$_{90}$ of 0.064 mg/liter), and all but two were susceptible to metronidazole (172). In this study, the MIC$_{90}$ of tetracycline was >256 mg/liter, and susceptibility to ciprofloxacin was variable, with a bimodal distribution of MIC values. Earlier studies also reported on Bacteroides clinical isolates from dogs and cats, with 29% of isolates being resistant to ampicillin and 16% to clindamycin (173). In this study, all isolates were susceptible to amoxicillin-clavulanic acid and chloramphenicol, while most were susceptible to metronidazole. Beta-lactamase activity was also observed in all ampicillin-resistant isolates.

More recently, in a study of Bacteroides isolates (n = 10) recovered from clinical cases of caprine and ovine foot rot, a necrotic pododermatitis, strains were found to be generally resistant to penicillins, first-generation cephalosporins, tetracycline, and erythromycin and expressed a low level of beta-lactamase activity (12). The genes cep(A) and tet(Q) were the dominant resistance determinants conferring resistance to beta-lactams and tetracycline, respectively (12) (Table 1). In a study that analyzed 161 B. fragilis group bacteria isolated from calves with and without diarrhea, MIC values for cefoxitin ranged from 32 to >512 mg/liter, with 47 (29.2%) of them being resistant to cefoxitin using the breakpoint of 16 mg/liter (13). In this study, seven isolates were found to harbor plasmids varying from 6.0 to 5.0 kb, with a 5.5-kb plasmid B. fragilis

Bc5j which might be associated with cefoxitin resistance. Also, using the nitrocefin method, beta-lactamase was detected in 33 (70.2%) isolates. The *cep* (A) gene was observed in total DNA as well as in the 5.5-kb plasmid (13). In a study of enterotoxigenic and nonenterotoxigenic *B. fragilis* in fecal samples from calves with or without acute diarrhea, 124 and 92 members of the *B. fragilis* group were recovered from 54 diarrheal and 54 nondiarrheal samples, respectively (174). In this study, two enterotoxigenic strains were isolated from two diarrhea samples. All strains were found to be susceptible to chloramphenicol, imipenem, moxifloxacin, piperacillin/tazobactam, metronidazole, and tigecycline.

Bacteroides spp. recovered from human clinical specimens frequently exhibit resistance to several antimicrobials, particularly to beta-lactams, tetracycline, ciprofloxacin, and clindamycin (175–178). It has been reported that resistance to multiple antimicrobials has been increasing in *Bacteroides* spp. for decades in human medicine, primarily due to horizontal gene transfer of a plethora of mobile elements (179). A review that summarizes the mechanisms of action and resistance to antimicrobials used to treat *Bacteroides* spp. infections in humans and that highlights current information on conjugation-based DNA exchange has been published (179). Briefly, in humans, resistance to tetracycline has been associated with the *tet*(Q) gene, which encodes for ribosomal protection (175, 181). Resistance to beta-lactams has been associated with the production of beta-lactamases encoded by the *cep*(A) (175, 180, 181) and *cfi*A (181) genes. Clindamycin resistance has been linked with ribosomal modification (181) via the *erm*(B), *erm*(F), and *erm*(G) (183, 184) genes. The *lin*(A) gene has been associated with MLS$_B$ resistance (184). The *nim* genes of *Bacteroides* have been associated with metronidazole resistance via reduced uptake and altered reduction of the nitro group (183, 185–186). A study demonstrated that constitutive BmeB, a component of the RND (Resistance-Nodulation-Division) family efflux transport systems (BmeABC1-16), expression is prevalent in *B. fragilis* (187), and this involves the transport of antimicrobials such as beta-lactams, fluoroquinolones, and tetracycline (187). Mutations in *gyrA* have been documented in fluoroquinolone resistance (188). *BexA*, which codes for the fluoroquinolone efflux pump, was represented only in a minor proportion of moxifloxacin-resistant strains (184). Combinations of *cfx*A, *cep*A, *cfi*A, *nim*A, *nim*D, *nim*E, *nim*J, *tet*(Q), *erm*(B), *erm*(F), *bex*B, and possibly, *lin* and *mef* genes were recently identified in multidrug-resistant *B. fragilis* using whole-genome shotgun sequencing (183).

FUSOBACTERIUM

Fusobacterium are non-spore-forming Gram-negative rods that are usually found as normal flora in the mouth, the intestines, and the urogenital tract (189). *F. necrophorum* is considered the most virulent species, followed by other species such as *F. nucleatum*, *F. canifelinum*, and *F. varium* (189–191). *Fusobacterium* can cause a plethora of necrotic infections in animals, such as necrotic stomatitis, foot rot (interdigital necrobacillosis), gangrenous dermatitis, and pulmonary, hepatic, and jaw abscesses (189). These infections are often polymicrobial, and some of them (hepatic necrobacillosis, necrotic laryngitis, and foot rot) have important economic impacts in cattle (189). Antimicrobials can be used to reduce the risk of *Fusobacterium*-associated liver abscesses in cattle (192). The antimicrobials most commonly reported for usage in prophylaxis against this disease are bacitracin, chlortetracycline, oxytetracycline, tylosin, and virginiamycin. In humans, *Fusobacterium* is associated with clinically distinctive, severe septicemic infections variously known as necrobacillosis, postanginal sepsis, or Lemierre's syndrome (193). It may also occur after accidental trauma such as animal bites (194, 195). In earlier studies of *Fusobacterium* isolates from human bite wounds, susceptibility was reported to a range of beta-lactam antimicrobials as well as metronidazole; resistance to penicillin, clindamycin, and ciprofloxacin was seldom seen (194, 195). In contrast, a study in Taiwan reported a higher level of resistance (196). In humans, resistance to penicillin associated with beta-lactamase production has been described, and there is widespread resistance to erythromycin and other macrolides (193, 197).

Earlier studies of *Fusobacterium* from various animal species revealed susceptibility to penicillin, ampicillin, cephalothin, chloramphenicol, clindamycin, tetracycline, and metronidazole (169, 173). A Spanish study in the 1990s that investigated *F. necrophorum* isolates from hepatic abscesses in cattle and sheep described broad susceptibility to spiramycin, lincomycin, tylosin, oxytetracycline, chlortetracycline, metronidazole, cotrimoxazole, sulfadimethoxine, virginiamycin, and fosfomycin but resistance to clindamycin (42%) (198). In this study, out of the 13 beta-lactam antimicrobials tested, only 1, cefotetan, was not active against all isolates. In a U.S. study of *F. necrophorum* from bovine hepatic abscesses, isolates were generally found to be susceptible to penicillins, tetracyclines (chlortetracycline and oxytetracycline), lincosamides (clindamycin and lincomycin), and macrolides (tylosin and erythromycin) (199). In this study, bacitracin and virginiamycin were also active against *F. necrophorum*.

A Spanish and Portuguese study of *Fusobacterium* (n = 108) from 90 cases of foot rot in sheep described that most isolates were susceptible to beta-lactams (benzyl penicillin, ampicillin, cloxacillin, cefadroxil, cefuroxime, and cephalexine), chloramphenicol, clindamycin, and metronidazole, but resistance to erythromycin and spiramycin was observed in 77% and 60% of isolates, respectively (200). In this study, doxycycline was also quite active against *Fusobacterium*.

More recently, a survey of *Fusobacterium* strains isolated from caprine and ovine foot rot revealed that most isolates were generally susceptible to beta-lactams, whereas resistance to tetracycline and/or erythromycin was observed (12). In a study of subgingival plaque from dogs with and without periodontitis, *F. nucleatum* and *F. canifelinum* were susceptible to most of the antimicrobials tested; however, different resistance rates to clarithromycin, erythromycin, and metronidazole were observed (191). Intrinsic resistance (MIC, >4 mg/liter) to levofloxacin and other fluoroquinolones has been observed in *F. canifelinum* originating from cats or dogs (201). In this study, it was found that Ser79 was replaced with leucine, and Gly83 was replaced with arginine when compared to the quinolone resistance-determining region within *gyr*A of susceptible strains of *F. nucleatum*. A survey of clinical isolates of *Fusobacterium* (n = 23) recovered at necropsy over a 2-year period from the respiratory tracts of white-tailed deer indicated that susceptibility to antimicrobials was markedly different for *F. varium* compared to *F. necrophorum* and *F. funduliforme* (202). In this study, all isolates were susceptible to ampicillin, florfenicol, and trimethoprim-sulfamethoxazole, whereas fewer *F. varium* isolates were susceptible to chlortetracycline, clindamycin, oxytetracycline, tiamulin, tilmicosin, tulathromycin, and tylosin compared with *F. necrophorum*. Also, intermediate or variable susceptibilities were observed to ceftiofur, danofloxacin, penicillin, and sulfadimethoxine. Almost all isolates were resistant to enrofloxacin, indicating intrinsic resistance. In summary, despite observed resistance to macrolides and tetracyclines, *Fusobacterium* spp. of animal origin remain quite susceptible to antimicrobials, including those of the beta-lactam class. To date, to our knowledge, there has been no analysis of the genetic basis of acquired antimicrobial resistance.

DICHELOBACTER NODOSUS

D. nodosus, a Gram-negative non-spore-forming bacterium, is the principal etiologic agent of foot rot. It is a transmissible disease that involves the epiderma of the feet and results in lameness. It is an economically important and worldwide endemic disease affecting the sheep industry in terms of production losses and costs for treatment and prevention (203). Other animal species may also develop foot rot but in a milder form. Foot rot is a contagious infection involving the invasion of the epidermal tissues of the interdigital space of the foot and of the soft horn of the hoof (203). Eventually, the hoof and its underlying dermal tissues become separated. This hoof underrunning process can range from mild to severe, but the latter only occurs when virulent strains of *D. nodosus* are involved. Host and environmental factors can influence the disease (203–205). Virulent and benign variants of *D. nodosus* have recently been demonstrated by whole-genome sequencing, and they have been shown to correlate with the presence of *aprV2* and *aprB2*, respectively (206–208). These genes encode for distinct extracellular proteases with only a single amino acid substitution (206). The infection can also be polymicrobial and may involve *F. necrophorum* as well as other anaerobes, but the presence of *D. nodosus* seems to be mandatory for true foot rot to occur. When treatment is attempted, a footbath with bactericidal agents such as copper sulfate or zinc sulfate can be used after removal of necrotic debris and horn (209). Antimicrobials have been successfully used to control foot rot in particular settings, and penicillin-streptomycin (210), erythromycin (211), oxytetracycline (212), and lincomycin-spectinomycin (213) have been shown to be efficient.

A U.S. study performed in the 1980s of the antimicrobial resistance of *D. nodosus* reported penicillin as the most effective antimicrobial along with susceptibility to cefamandole, clindamycin, tetracycline, chloramphenicol, erythromycin, cefoxitin, tylosin, and nitrofurazone (214). Two Spanish studies of goats and sheep in the 1990s revealed more penicillin and tetracycline resistances in *D. nodosus* (215, 216). Their results also indicated that chloramphenicol, metronidazole, and rifampin were effective *in vitro*, but chloramphenicol and metronidazole are both restricted worldwide in food-producing animals. More recently, in a survey in Portugal and Spain of 90 clinical cases of ovine foot rot, 69 strains of *D. nodosus* were recovered, and 90% were susceptible to penicillin, ampicillin, erythromycin, spiramycin, tylosin, chloramphenicol, and enrofloxacin (200). In this study, resistance to metronidazole, oxytetracycline, doxycycline, and trimethoprim was observed in 17.5%, 42%, 14%, and 10% of the strains, respectively (200). In another survey, where *D. nodosus* was isolated from 48% of the sampled animals (n = 25) with foot rot, the susceptibility of 99 isolates to

5 antimicrobials (penicillin G, amoxicillin, spiramycin, erythromycin, and oxytetracycline) indicated that resistance was in all cases higher than 30% (217). In this study, the efficacy of erythromycin and oxytetracycline in the treatment of ovine foot rot using an intramuscular injection at the beginning of the treatment demonstrated that 75% of animals were cured within 15 days with one or the other antimicrobials used (217). More recently, in a Spanish survey of *Dichelobacter* and other anaerobes obtained from clinical cases of foot rot, beta-lactams, tetracyclines, and metronidazole were shown to have the highest *in vitro* efficacy (218). In this study, *D. nodosus* showed no resistance either to penicillins (penicillin G) or to cephalosporins (cefadroxil, cefuroxime, and cephalexin). To date, to our knowledge, there has been no analysis of the genetic basis of acquired antimicrobial resistance.

CONCLUSION

Antimicrobial resistance has been described in the most frequently encountered anaerobic bacterial pathogens of animals. However, because animal data are too limited in certain cases, this article focused not only on antimicrobial resistance data of veterinary origin, but also included antimicrobial resistance identified in anaerobes from humans. Many studies describe point prevalence but give little data about trends in the development of resistance over time. Overall, antimicrobial resistance can vary depending on the antimicrobial, the anaerobe, and the resistance mechanism. On occasion, the same resistance gene was observed in many anaerobes, whereas some genes were limited to certain anaerobes. Surprisingly, in some anaerobes, mechanisms of antimicrobial resistance have not been studied, and further attention should be given to the investigation of molecular mechanisms of resistance. This may be facilitated by the increasing use of routine genome sequencing as well as a shift of CLSI approaches to gene-based analysis of resistance. Additional work is indeed required to increase our knowledge about antimicrobial resistance in anaerobes.

Citation. Archambault M, Rubin JE. 2018. Antimicrobial resistance in *Clostridium* and *Brachyspira* spp. and other anaerobes. Microbiol Spectrum 6(3):ARBA-0020-2017.

References

1. Uzal FA, Songer G, Prescott JF, Popoff MR. 2016. *Clostridial Diseases of Animals*. John Wiley & Sons, Hoboken, NJ.

2. Salyers AA, Gupta A, Wang Y. 2004. Human intestinal bacteria as reservoirs for antibiotic resistance genes. *Trends Microbiol* 12:412–416.

3. Clinical and Laboratory Standards Institute. 2012. Standard on methods for antimicrobial susceptibility testing of anaerobic bacteria (M11-A8). Approved standard, 7th ed. CLSI, Wayne, PA.

4. Clinical and Laboratory Standards Institute. 2015. Performance standards for antimicrobial disk and dilution susceptibility tests for bacteria isolated from animals, 3rd ed. CLSI supplement VET01S. CLSI, Wayne, PA.

5. Clinical and Laboratory Standards Institute. 2008. *In vitro* susceptibility testing criteria and quality control parameters for veterinary antimicrobial agents, 3rd ed. CLSI VET02-A3. CLSI, Wayne, PA.

6. Clinical and Laboratory Standards Institute. 2013. Performance standards for antimicrobial disk and dilution susceptibility tests for bacteria isolated from animals, 4th ed. CLSI VET01-A4. CLSI, Wayne, PA.

7. Clinical and Laboratory Standards Institute. 2017. Methods for antimicrobial susceptibility testing of infrequently isolated or fastidious bacteria isolated from animals, 1st ed. CLSI VET06. CLSI, Wayne, PA.

8. Oka K, Osaki T, Hanawa T, Kurata S, Okazaki M, Manzoku T, Takahashi M, Tanaka M, Taguchi H, Watanabe T, Inamatsu T, Kamiya S. 2012. Molecular and microbiological characterization of *Clostridium difficile* isolates from single, relapse, and reinfection cases. *J Clin Microbiol* 50:915–921.

9. Spigaglia P. 2016. Recent advances in the understanding of antibiotic resistance in *Clostridium difficile* infection. *Ther Adv Infect Dis* 3:23–42.

10. Bryan LE, Kwan S. 1981. Mechanisms of aminoglycoside resistance of anaerobic bacteria and facultative bacteria grown anaerobically. *J Antimicrob Chemother* 8(Suppl D):1–8.

11. Indiveri MC, Hirsh DC. 1992. Tissues and exudates contain sufficient thymidine for growth of anaerobic bacteria in the presence of inhibitory levels of trimethoprim-sulfamethoxazole. *Vet Microbiol* 31:235–242.

12. Lorenzo M, García N, Ayala JA, Vadillo S, Píriz S, Quesada A. 2012. Antimicrobial resistance determinants among anaerobic bacteria isolated from footrot. *Vet Microbiol* 157:112–118.

13. dos Santos Almeida F, Avila-Campos MJ. 2006. Plasmid-related resistance to cefoxitin in species of the *Bacteroides fragilis* group isolated from intestinal tracts of calves. *Curr Microbiol* 53:440–443.

14. Appelbaum PC, Spangler SK, Jacobs MR. 1990. Beta-lactamase production and susceptibilities to amoxicillin, amoxicillin-clavulanate, ticarcillin, ticarcillin-clavulanate, cefoxitin, imipenem, and metronidazole of 320 non-*Bacteroides fragilis Bacteroides* isolates and 129 fusobacteria from 28 U.S. centers. *Antimicrob Agents Chemother* 34:1546–1550.

15. Then RL, Angehrn P. 1979. Low trimethoprim susceptibility of anaerobic bacteria due to insensitive dihydrofolate reductases. *Antimicrob Agents Chemother* 15:1–6.

16. Then RL. 1982. Mechanisms of resistance to trimethoprim, the sulfonamides, and trimethoprim-sulfamethoxazole. *Rev Infect Dis* 4:261–269.

17. Roberts MC. 2003. Acquired tetracycline and/or macrolide-lincosamides-streptogramin resistance in anaerobes. *Anaerobe* 9:63–69.

18. Rood JI, Adams V, Lacey J, Lyras D, McClane BA, Melville SB, Moore RJ, Popoff MR, Sarker MR, Songer GJ, Uzal FA, Van Immerseel F. 2018. Expansion of the *Clostridium perfringens* toxin-based typing scheme. *Anaerobe*.

19. Johansson A, Greko C, Engström BE, Karlsson M. 2004. Antimicrobial susceptibility of Swedish, Norwegian and Danish isolates of *Clostridium perfringens* from poultry, and distribution of tetracycline resistance genes. *Vet Microbiol* 99:251–257.

20. Martel A, Devriese LA, Cauwerts K, De Gussem K, Decostere A, Haesebrouck F. 2004. Susceptibility of *Clostridium perfringens* strains from broiler chickens to antibiotics and anticoccidials. *Avian Pathol* 33:3–7.

21. Watkins KL, Shryock TR, Dearth RN, Saif YM. 1997. *In-vitro* antimicrobial susceptibility of *Clostridium perfringens* from commercial turkey and broiler chicken origin. *Vet Microbiol* 54:195–200.

22. Slavić D, Boerlin P, Fabri M, Klotins KC, Zoethout JK, Weir PE, Bateman D. 2011. Antimicrobial susceptibility of *Clostridium perfringens* isolates of bovine, chicken, porcine, and turkey origin from Ontario. *Can J Vet Res* 75:89–97.

23. Charlebois A, Jalbert LA, Harel J, Masson L, Archambault M. 2012. Characterization of genes encoding for acquired bacitracin resistance in *Clostridium perfringens*. *PLoS One* 7:e44449.

24. Devriese LA, Daube G, Hommez J, Haesebrouck F. 1993. *In vitro* susceptibility of *Clostridium perfringens* isolated from farm animals to growth-enhancing antibiotics. *J Appl Bacteriol* 75:55–57.

25. Rood JI, Maher EA, Somers EB, Campos E, Duncan CL. 1978. Isolation and characterization of multiply antibiotic-resistant *Clostridum perfringens* strains from porcine feces. *Antimicrob Agents Chemother* 13:871–880.

26. Tansuphasiri U, Matra W, Sangsuk L. 2005. Antimicrobial resistance among *Clostridium perfringens* isolated from various sources in Thailand. *Southeast Asian J Trop Med Public Health* 36:954–961.

27. Chalmers G, Martin SW, Hunter DB, Prescott JF, Weber LJ, Boerlin P. 2008. Genetic diversity of *Clostridium perfringens* isolated from healthy broiler chickens at a commercial farm. *Vet Microbiol* 127:116–127.

28. Park JY, Kim S, Oh JY, Kim HR, Jang I, Lee HS, Kwon YK. 2015. Characterization of *Clostridium perfringens* isolates obtained from 2010 to 2012 from chickens with necrotic enteritis in Korea. *Poult Sci* 94:1158–1164.

29. Gholamiandehkordi A, Eeckhaut V, Lanckriet A, Timbermont L, Bjerrum L, Ducatelle R, Haesebrouck F, Van Immerseel F. 2009. Antimicrobial resistance in *Clostridium perfringens isolates* from broilers in Belgium. *Vet Res Commun* 33:1031–1037.

30. Osman KM, Elhariri M. 2013. Antibiotic resistance of *Clostridium perfringens* isolates from broiler chickens in Egypt. *Rev Sci Tech* 32:841–850.

31. Fan YC, Wang CL, Wang C, Chen TC, Chou CH, Tsai HJ. 2016. Incidence and antimicrobial susceptibility to *Clostridium perfringens* in premarket broilers in Taiwan. *Avian Dis* 60:444–449.

32. Ngamwongsatit B, Tanomsridachchai W, Suthienkul O, Urairong S, Navasakuljinda W, Janvilisri T. 2016. Multidrug resistance in *Clostridium perfringens* isolated from diarrheal neonatal piglets in Thailand. *Anaerobe* 38:88–93.

33. Rood JI, Buddle JR, Wales AJ, Sidhu R. 1985. The occurrence of antibiotic resistance in *Clostridium perfringens* from pigs. *Aust Vet J* 62:276–279.

34. Hölzel CS, Harms KS, Schwaiger K, Bauer J. 2010. Resistance to linezolid in a porcine *Clostridium perfringens* strain carrying a mutation in the *rpl*D gene encoding the ribosomal protein L4. *Antimicrob Agents Chemother* 54:1351–1353.

35. Salvarani FM, Silveira Silva RO, Pires PS, da Costa Cruz Júnior EC, Albefaro IS, de Carvalho Guedes RM, Faria Lobato FC. 2012. Antimicrobial susceptibility of *Clostridium perfringens* isolated from piglets with or without diarrhea in Brazil. *Braz J Microbiol* 43:1030–1033.

36. Kouassi KA, Dadie AT, N'Guessan KF, Dje KM, Loukou YG. 2014. *Clostridium perfringens* and *Clostridium difficile* in cooked beef sold in Côte d'Ivoire and their antimicrobial susceptibility. *Anaerobe* 28:90–94.

37. Gobeli S, Berset C, Burgener I, Perreten V. 2012. Antimicrobial susceptibility of canine *Clostridium perfringens* strains from Switzerland. *Schweiz Arch Tierheilkd* 154:247–250.

38. Gamboa-Coronado MM, Mau-Inchaustegui S, Rodríguez-Cavallini E. 2011. Molecular characterization and antimicrobial resistance of *Clostridium perfringens* isolates of different origins from Costa Rica. *Rev Biol Trop* 59:1479–1485. (In Spanish.)

39. Catalán A, Espoz MC, Cortés W, Sagua H, González J, Araya JE. 2010. Tetracycline and penicillin resistant *Clostridium perfringens* isolated from the fangs and venom glands of *Loxosceles laeta*: its implications in loxoscelism treatment. *Toxicon* 56:890–896.

40. Álvarez-Pérez S, Blanco JL, Peláez T, Martínez-Nevado E, García ME. 2016. Water sources in a zoological park harbor genetically diverse strains of *Clostridium perfringens* type A with decreased susceptibility to metronidazole. *Microb Ecol* 72:783–790.

41. Varga JJ, Therit B, Melville SB. 2008. Type IV pili and the CcpA protein are needed for maximal biofilm formation by the Gram-positive anaerobic pathogen *Clostridium perfringens*. *Infect Immun* 76:4944–4951.

42. Charlebois A, Jacques M, Archambault M. 2014. Biofilm formation of *Clostridium perfringens* and its exposure to low-dose antimicrobials. *Front Microbiol* 5:183.

43. Charlebois A, Jacques M, Archambault M. 2016. Comparative transcriptomic analysis of *Clostridium perfringens* biofilms and planktonic cells. *Avian Pathol* 45:593–601.

44. Charlebois A, Jacques M, Boulianne M, Archambault M. 2017. Tolerance of *Clostridium perfringens* biofilms to disinfectants commonly used in the food industry. *Food Microbiol* 62:32–38.

45. Costerton JW. 1999. Introduction to biofilm. *Int J Antimicrob Agents* 11:217–221; discussion 237–219.

46. Park S, Park M, Rafii F. 2013. Comparative transcription analysis and toxin production of two fluoroquinolone-resistant mutants of *Clostridium perfringens*. *BMC Microbiol* 13:50.

47. Park M, Sutherland JB, Kim JN, Rafii F. 2013. Effect of fluoroquinolone resistance selection on the fitness of three strains of *Clostridium perfringens*. *Microb Drug Resist* 19:421–427.

48. Rafii F, Park M, Gamboa da Costa G, Camacho L. 2009. Comparison of the metabolic activities of four wild-type *Clostridium perfringens* strains with their gatifloxacin-selected resistant mutants. *Arch Microbiol* 191:895–902.

49. Rafii F, Park M, Carman RJ. 2009. Characterization of an ATP-binding cassette from *Clostridium perfringens* with homology to an ABC transporter from *Clostridium hathewayi*. *Anaerobe* 15:116–121.

50. Han X, Du XD, Southey L, Bulach DM, Seemann T, Yan XX, Bannam TL, Rood JI. 2015. Functional analysis of a bacitracin resistance determinant located on ICECp1, a novel Tn916-like element from a conjugative plasmid in *Clostridium perfringens*. *Antimicrob Agents Chemother* 59:6855–6865.

51. Chopra I, Roberts M. 2001. Tetracycline antibiotics: mode of action, applications, molecular biology, and epidemiology of bacterial resistance. *Microbiol Mol Biol Rev* 65:232–260.

52. Sasaki Y, Yamamoto K, Tamura Y, Takahashi T. 2001. Tetracycline-resistance genes of *Clostridium perfringens*, *Clostridium septicum* and *Clostridium sordellii* isolated from cattle affected with malignant edema. *Vet Microbiol* 83:61–69.

53. Lyras D, Rood JI. 1996. Genetic organization and distribution of tetracycline resistance determinants in *Clostridium perfringens*. *Antimicrob Agents Chemother* 40:2500–2504.

54. Sloan J, McMurry LM, Lyras D, Levy SB, Rood JI. 1994. The *Clostridium perfringens* Tet P determinant comprises two overlapping genes: *tetA*(P), which mediates active tetracycline efflux, and *tetB*(P), which is related to the ribosomal protection family of tetracycline-resistance determinants. *Mol Microbiol* 11:403–415.

55. Abraham LJ, Wales AJ, Rood JI. 1985. Worldwide distribution of the conjugative *Clostridium perfringens* tetracycline resistance plasmid, pCW3. *Plasmid* 14:37–46.

56. Abraham LJ, Rood JI. 1985. Cloning and analysis of the *Clostridium perfringens* tetracycline resistance plasmid, pCW3. *Plasmid* 13:155–162.

57. Abraham LJ, Rood JI. 1985. Molecular analysis of transferable tetracycline resistance plasmids from *Clostridium perfringens*. *J Bacteriol* 161:636–640.

58. Bannam TL, Yan XX, Harrison PF, Seemann T, Keyburn AL, Stubenrauch C, Weeramantri LH, Cheung JK, McClane BA, Boyce JD, Moore RJ, Rood JI. 2011. Necrotic enteritis-derived *Clostridium perfringens* strain with three closely related independently conjugative toxin and antibiotic resistance plasmids. *MBio* 2:2.

59. Park M, Rooney AP, Hecht DW, Li J, McClane BA, Nayak R, Paine DD, Rafii F. 2010. Phenotypic and genotypic characterization of tetracycline and minocycline resistance in *Clostridium perfringens*. *Arch Microbiol* 192:803–810.

60. Brefort G, Magot M, Ionesco H, Sebald M. 1977. Characterization and transferability of *Clostridium perfringens* plasmids. *Plasmid* 1:52–66.

61. Farrow KA, Lyras D, Polekhina G, Koutsis K, Parker MW, Rood JI. 2002. Identification of essential residues in the Erm(B) rRNA methyltransferase of *Clostridium perfringens*. *Antimicrob Agents Chemother* 46:1253–1261.

62. Lyras D, Adams V, Ballard SA, Teng WL, Howarth PM, Crellin PK, Bannam TL, Songer JG, Rood JI. 2009. tISCpe8, an IS1595-family lincomycin resistance element located on a conjugative plasmid in *Clostridium perfringens*. *J Bacteriol* 191:6345–6351.

63. Kather EJ, Marks SL, Foley JE. 2006. Determination of the prevalence of antimicrobial resistance genes in canine *Clostridium perfringens* isolates. *Vet Microbiol* 113:97–101.

64. Marshall VP, Liggett WF, Cialdella JI. 1989. Enzymic inactivation of lincosaminide and macrolide antibiotics: divalent metal cation and coenzyme specificities. *J Antibiot (Tokyo)* 42:826–830.

65. Bozdogan B, Berrezouga L, Kuo MS, Yurek DA, Farley KA, Stockman BJ, Leclercq R. 1999. A new resistance gene, linB, conferring resistance to lincosamides by nucleotidylation in *Enterococcus faecium* HM1025. *Antimicrob Agents Chemother* 43:925–929.

66. Brisson-Noël A, Delrieu P, Samain D, Courvalin P. 1988. Inactivation of lincosaminide antibiotics in *Staphylococcus*. Identification of lincosaminide O-nucleotidyltransferases and comparison of the corresponding resistance genes. *J Biol Chem* 263:15880–15887.

67. Bannam TL, Rood JI. 1991. Relationship between the *Clostridium perfringens* catQ gene product and chloramphenicol acetyltransferases from other bacteria. *Antimicrob Agents Chemother* 35:471–476.

68. Abraham LJ, Rood JI. 1987. Identification of Tn4451 and Tn4452, chloramphenicol resistance transposons from *Clostridium perfringens*. *J Bacteriol* 169:1579–1584.

69. Adams V, Lyras D, Farrow KA, Rood JI. 2002. The clostridial mobilisable transposons. *Cell Mol Life Sci* 59:2033–2043.

70. Shortridge VD, Flamm RK, Ramer N, Beyer J, Tanaka SK. 1996. Novel mechanism of macrolide resistance in *Streptococcus pneumoniae*. *Diagn Microbiol Infect Dis* 26:73–78.

71. Sutcliffe J, Tait-Kamradt A, Wondrack L. 1996. *Streptococcus pneumoniae* and *Streptococcus pyogenes* resistant to macrolides but sensitive to clindamycin: a common resistance pattern mediated by an efflux system. *Antimicrob Agents Chemother* 40:1817–1824.

72. Soge OO, Tivoli LD, Meschke JS, Roberts MC. 2009. A conjugative macrolide resistance gene, *mef*(A), in environmental *Clostridium perfringens* carrying multiple

macrolide and/or tetracycline resistance genes. *J Appl Microbiol* **106**:34–40.

73. Thomas C, Stevenson M, Riley TV. 2003. Antibiotics and hospital-acquired *Clostridium difficile*-associated diarrhoea: a systematic review. *J Antimicrob Chemother* **51**:1339–1350.

74. Båverud V, Gustafsson A, Franklin A, Lindholm A, Gunnarsson A. 1997. *Clostridium difficile* associated with acute colitis in mature horses treated with antibiotics. *Equine Vet J* **29**:279–284.

75. Post KW, Songer JG. 2004. Antimicrobial susceptibility of *Clostridium difficile* isolated from neonatal pigs with enteritis. *Anaerobe* **10**:47–50.

76. Diab SS, Songer G, Uzal FA. 2013. *Clostridium difficile* infection in horses: a review. *Vet Microbiol* **167**:42–49.

77. Squire MM, Riley TV. 2013. *Clostridium difficile* infection in humans and piglets: a 'One Health' opportunity. *Curr Top Microbiol Immunol* **365**:299–314.

78. Schoster A, Arroyo LG, Staempfli HR, Shewen PE, Weese JS. 2012. Presence and molecular characterization of *Clostridium difficile* and *Clostridium perfringens* in intestinal compartments of healthy horses. *BMC Vet Res* **8**:94.

79. Gustafsson A, Båverud V, Gunnarsson A, Rantzien MH, Lindholm A, Franklin A. 1997. The association of erythromycin ethylsuccinate with acute colitis in horses in Sweden. *Equine Vet J* **29**:314–318.

80. Båverud V, Gunnarsson A, Karlsson M, Franklin A. 2004. Antimicrobial susceptibility of equine and environmental isolates of *Clostridium difficile*. *Microb Drug Resist* **10**:57–63.

81. Rodriguez C, Taminiau B, Brévers B, Avesani V, Van Broeck J, Leroux AA, Amory H, Delmée M, Daube G. 2014. Carriage and acquisition rates of *Clostridium difficile* in hospitalized horses, including molecular characterization, multilocus sequence typing and antimicrobial susceptibility of bacterial isolates. *Vet Microbiol* **172**: 309–317.

82. Valiente E, Dawson LF, Cairns MD, Stabler RA, Wren BW. 2012. Emergence of new PCR ribotypes from the hypervirulent *Clostridium difficile* 027 lineage. *J Med Microbiol* **61**:49–56.

83. Bauer MP, Notermans DW, van Benthem BH, Brazier JS, Wilcox MH, Rupnik M, Monnet DL, van Dissel JT, Kuijper EJ, ECDIS Study Group. 2011. *Clostridium difficile* infection in Europe: a hospital-based survey. *Lancet* **377**:63–73.

84. Limbago BM, Long CM, Thompson AD, Killgore GE, Hannett GE, Havill NL, Mickelson S, Lathrop S, Jones TF, Park MM, Harriman KH, Gould LH, McDonald LC, Angulo FJ. 2009. *Clostridium difficile* strains from community-associated infections. *J Clin Microbiol* **47**: 3004–3007.

85. Keel K, Brazier JS, Post KW, Weese S, Songer JG. 2007. Prevalence of PCR ribotypes among *Clostridium difficile* isolates from pigs, calves, and other species. *J Clin Microbiol* **45**:1963–1964.

86. Hammitt MC, Bueschel DM, Keel MK, Glock RD, Cuneo P, DeYoung DW, Reggiardo C, Trinh HT, Songer JG. 2008. A possible role for *Clostridium difficile* in the etiology of calf enteritis. *Vet Microbiol* **127**:343–352.

87. Goorhuis A, Debast SB, van Leengoed LA, Harmanus C, Notermans DW, Bergwerff AA, Kuijper EJ, Songer JG. 2008. *Clostridium difficile* PCR ribotype 078: an emerging strain in humans and in pigs? *J Clin Microbiol* **46**:1157–1158, author reply 1158.

88. Goorhuis A, Bakker D, Corver J, Debast SB, Harmanus C, Notermans DW, Bergwerff AA, Dekker FW, Kuijper EJ. 2008. Emergence of *Clostridium difficile* infection due to a new hypervirulent strain, polymerase chain reaction ribotype 078. *Clin Infect Dis* **47**:1162–1170.

89. Rupnik M, Widmer A, Zimmermann O, Eckert C, Barbut F. 2008. *Clostridium difficile* toxinotype V, ribotype 078, in animals and humans. *J Clin Microbiol* **46**:2146.

90. Båverud V, Gustafsson A, Franklin A, Aspán A, Gunnarsson A. 2003. *Clostridium difficile*: prevalence in horses and environment, and antimicrobial susceptibility. *Equine Vet J* **35**:465–471.

91. Jang SS, Hansen LM, Breher JE, Riley DA, Magdesian KG, Madigan JE, Tang YJ, Silva J Jr, Hirsh DC. 1997. Antimicrobial susceptibilities of equine isolates of *Clostridium difficile* and molecular characterization of metronidazole-resistant strains. *Clin Infect Dis* **25**(Suppl 2):S266–S267.

92. Weese JS, Staempfli HR, Prescott JF. 2001. A prospective study of the roles of *Clostridium difficile* and enterotoxigenic *Clostridium perfringens* in equine diarrhoea. *Equine Vet J* **33**:403–409.

93. Thean S, Elliott B, Riley TV. 2011. *Clostridium difficile* in horses in Australia: a preliminary study. *J Med Microbiol* **60**:1188–1192.

94. Silva RO, Ribeiro MG, Palhares MS, Borges AS, Maranhão RP, Silva MX, Lucas TM, Olivo G, Lobato FC. 2013. Detection of A/B toxin and isolation of *Clostridium difficile* and *Clostridium perfringens* from foals. *Equine Vet J* **45**:671–675.

95. Magdesian KG, Dujowich M, Madigan JE, Hansen LM, Hirsh DC, Jang SS. 2006. Molecular characterization of *Clostridium difficile* isolates from horses in an intensive care unit and association of disease severity with strain type. *J Am Vet Med Assoc* **228**:751–755.

96. Magdesian KG, Hirsh DC, Jang SS, Hansen LM, Madigan JE. 2002. Characterization of *Clostridium difficile* isolates from foals with diarrhea: 28 cases (1993–1997). *J Am Vet Med Assoc* **220**:67–73.

97. Fry PR, Thakur S, Abley M, Gebreyes WA. 2012. Antimicrobial resistance, toxinotype, and genotypic profiling of *Clostridium difficile* isolates of swine origin. *J Clin Microbiol* **50**:2366–2372.

98. Huang H, Weintraub A, Fang H, Nord CE. 2009. Antimicrobial resistance in *Clostridium difficile*. *Int J Antimicrob Agents* **34**:516–522.

99. Norman KN, Harvey RB, Scott HM, Hume ME, Andrews K, Brawley AD. 2009. Varied prevalence of *Clostridium difficile* in an integrated swine operation. *Anaerobe* **15**:256–260.

100. Norman KN, Scott HM, Harvey RB, Norby B, Hume ME. 2014. Comparison of antimicrobial susceptibility

among *Clostridium difficile* isolated from an integrated human and swine population in Texas. *Foodborne Pathog Dis* 11:257–264.

101. Peláez T, Alcalá L, Blanco JL, Álvarez-Pérez S, Marín M, Martín-López A, Catalán P, Reigadas E, García ME, Bouza E. 2013. Characterization of swine isolates of *Clostridium difficile* in Spain: a potential source of epidemic multidrug resistant strains? *Anaerobe* 22:45–49.

102. Thakur S, Putnam M, Fry PR, Abley M, Gebreyes WA. 2010. Prevalence of antimicrobial resistance and association with toxin genes in *Clostridium difficile* in commercial swine. *Am J Vet Res* 71:1189–1194.

103. Usui M, Nanbu Y, Oka K, Takahashi M, Inamatsu T, Asai T, Kamiya S, Tamura Y. 2014. Genetic relatedness between Japanese and European isolates of *Clostridium difficile* originating from piglets and their risk associated with human health. *Front Microbiol* 5:513.

104. Thakur S, Sandfoss M, Kennedy-Stoskopf S, DePerno CS. 2011. Detection of *Clostridium difficile* and *Salmonella* in feral swine population in North Carolina. *J Wildl Dis* 47:774–776.

105. Spigaglia P, Drigo I, Barbanti F, Mastrantonio P, Bano L, Bacchin C, Puiatti C, Tonon E, Berto G, Agnoletti F. 2015. Antibiotic resistance patterns and PCR-ribotyping of *Clostridium difficile* strains isolated from swine and dogs in Italy. *Anaerobe* 31:42–46.

106. Dong D, Chen X, Jiang C, Zhang L, Cai G, Han L, Wang X, Mao E, Peng Y. 2014. Genetic analysis of Tn*916*-like elements conferring tetracycline resistance in clinical isolates of *Clostridium difficile*. *Int J Antimicrob Agents* 43:73–77.

107. Spigaglia P, Barbanti F, Mastrantonio P. 2007. Detection of a genetic linkage between genes coding for resistance to tetracycline and erythromycin in *Clostridium difficile*. *Microb Drug Resist* 13:90–95.

108. Roberts MC, McFarland LV, Mullany P, Mulligan ME. 1994. Characterization of the genetic basis of antibiotic resistance in *Clostridium difficile*. *J Antimicrob Chemother* 33:419–429.

109. Spigaglia P, Barbanti F, Mastrantonio P. 2008. Tetracycline resistance gene *tet*(W) in the pathogenic bacterium *Clostridium difficile*. *Antimicrob Agents Chemother* 52:770–773.

110. Corver J, Bakker D, Brouwer MS, Harmanus C, Hensgens MP, Roberts AP, Lipman LJ, Kuijper EJ, van Leeuwen HC. 2012. Analysis of a *Clostridium difficile* PCR ribotype 078 100 kilobase island reveals the presence of a novel transposon, Tn*6164*. *BMC Microbiol* 12:130.

111. Farrow KA, Lyras D, Rood JI. 2001. Genomic analysis of the erythromycin resistance element Tn*5398* from *Clostridium difficile*. *Microbiology* 147:2717–2728.

112. Spigaglia P, Carucci V, Barbanti F, Mastrantonio P. 2005. ErmB determinants and Tn*916*-like elements in clinical isolates of *Clostridium difficile*. *Antimicrob Agents Chemother* 49:2550–2553.

113. Wasels F, Spigaglia P, Barbanti F, Mastrantonio P. 2013. *Clostridium difficile erm*(B)-containing elements and the burden on the *in vitro* fitness. *J Med Microbiol* 62:1461–1467.

114. Goh S, Hussain H, Chang BJ, Emmett W, Riley TV, Mullany P. 2013. Phage C2 mediates transduction of Tn*6215*, encoding erythromycin resistance, between *Clostridium difficile* strains. *MBio* 4:e00840-13.

115. Ackermann G, Tang YJ, Kueper R, Heisig P, Rodloff AC, Silva J Jr, Cohen SH. 2001. Resistance to moxifloxacin in toxigenic *Clostridium difficile* isolates is associated with mutations in *gyrA*. *Antimicrob Agents Chemother* 45:2348–2353.

116. Dridi L, Tankovic J, Burghoffer B, Barbut F, Petit JC. 2002. *gyrA* and *gyrB* mutations are implicated in cross-resistance to ciprofloxacin and moxifloxacin in *Clostridium difficile*. *Antimicrob Agents Chemother* 46:3418–3421.

117. Kuwata Y, Tanimoto S, Sawabe E, Shima M, Takahashi Y, Ushizawa H, Fujie T, Koike R, Tojo N, Kubota T, Saito R. 2015. Molecular epidemiology and antimicrobial susceptibility of *Clostridium difficile* isolated from a university teaching hospital in Japan. *Eur J Clin Microbiol Infect Dis* 34:763–772.

118. Pecavar V, Blaschitz M, Hufnagl P, Zeinzinger J, Fiedler A, Allerberger F, Maass M, Indra A. 2012. High-resolution melting analysis of the single nucleotide polymorphism hot-spot region in the *rpoB* gene as an indicator of reduced susceptibility to rifaximin in *Clostridium difficile*. *J Med Microbiol* 61:780–785.

119. Norén T, Akerlund T, Wullt M, Burman LG, Unemo M. 2007. Mutations in *fusA* associated with post-therapy fusidic acid resistance in *Clostridium difficile*. *Antimicrob Agents Chemother* 51:1840–1843.

120. Wren BW, Mullany P, Clayton C, Tabaqchali S. 1988. Molecular cloning and genetic analysis of a chloramphenicol acetyltransferase determinant from *Clostridium difficile*. *Antimicrob Agents Chemother* 32:1213–1217.

121. Lyras D, Storie C, Huggins AS, Crellin PK, Bannam TL, Rood JI. 1998. Chloramphenicol resistance in *Clostridium difficile* is encoded on Tn*4453* transposons that are closely related to Tn*4451* from *Clostridium perfringens*. *Antimicrob Agents Chemother* 42:1563–1567.

122. Hansen LH, Vester B. 2015. A *cfr*-like gene from *Clostridium difficile* confers multiple antibiotic resistance by the same mechanism as the *cfr* gene. *Antimicrob Agents Chemother* 59:5841–5843.

123. Marín M, Martín A, Alcalá L, Cercenado E, Iglesias C, Reigadas E, Bouza E. 2015. *Clostridium difficile* isolates with high linezolid MICs harbor the multiresistance gene *cfr*. *Antimicrob Agents Chemother* 59:586–589.

124. Chong PM, Lynch T, McCorrister S, Kibsey P, Miller M, Gravel D, Westmacott GR, Mulvey MR, Canadian Nosocomial Infection Surveillance Program (CNISP). 2014. Proteomic analysis of a NAP1 *Clostridium difficile* clinical isolate resistant to metronidazole. *PLoS One* 9:e82622.

125. Moura I, Monot M, Tani C, Spigaglia P, Barbanti F, Norais N, Dupuy B, Bouza E, Mastrantonio P. 2014. Multidisciplinary analysis of a nontoxigenic *Clostridium difficile* strain with stable resistance to metronidazole. *Antimicrob Agents Chemother* 58:4957–4960.

126. Vuotto C, Moura I, Barbanti F, Donelli G, Spigaglia P. 2016. Subinhibitory concentrations of metronidazole increase biofilm formation in *Clostridium difficile* strains. *Pathog Dis* 74:74.

127. Frey J, Falquet L. 2015. Patho-genetics of *Clostridium chauvoei*. *Res Microbiol* 166:384–392.

128. Stevens DL, Bisno AL, Chambers HF, Dellinger EP, Goldstein EJ, Gorbach SL, Hirschmann JV, Kaplan SL, Montoya JG, Wade JC. 2014. Practice guidelines for the diagnosis and management of skin and soft tissue infections: 2014 update by the infectious diseases society of America. *Clin Infect Dis* 59:147–159.

129. Butra ND, Vichivanives P. 1991. *Clostridium sordellii* in diarrhoeal stools, its medical significance. *J Med Assoc Thai* 74:264–270.

130. Nakamura S, Yamakawa K, Nishida S. 1986. Antibacterial susceptibility of *Clostridium sordellii* strains. *Zentralbl Bakteriol Mikrobiol Hyg A* 261:345–349.

131. Gabay EL, Rolfe RD, Finegold SM. 1981. Susceptibility of *Clostridium septicum* to 23 antimicrobial agents. *Antimicrob Agents Chemother* 20:852–853.

132. Leal J, Gregson DB, Ross T, Church DL, Laupland KB. 2008. Epidemiology of *Clostridium* species bacteremia in Calgary, Canada, 2000–2006. *J Infect* 57:198–203.

133. Aleman M, Watson JL, Jang SS. 2003. *Clostridium novyi* type A intra-abdominal abscess in a horse. *J Vet Intern Med* 17:934–936.

134. McGuigan CC, Penrice GM, Gruer L, Ahmed S, Goldberg D, Black M, Salmon JE, Hood J. 2002. Lethal outbreak of infection with *Clostridium novyi* type A and other spore-forming organisms in Scottish injecting drug users. *J Med Microbiol* 51:971–977.

135. Hovind-Hougen K, Birch-Andersen A, Henrik-Nielsen R, Orholm M, Pedersen JO, Teglbjaerg PS, Thaysen EH. 1982. Intestinal spirochetosis: morphological characterization and cultivation of the spirochete *Brachyspira aalborgi* gen. nov., sp. nov. *J Clin Microbiol* 16:1127–1136.

136. Euzéby JP. 1997. List of Bacterial Names with Standing in Nomenclature: a folder available on the Internet. *Int J Syst Bacteriol* 47:590–592.

137. Chander Y, Primus A, Oliveira S, Gebhart CJ. 2012. Phenotypic and molecular characterization of a novel strongly hemolytic *Brachyspira* species, provisionally designated "*Brachyspira hampsonii*". *J Vet Diagn Invest* 24:903–910.

138. Råsbäck T, Jansson DS, Johansson KE, Fellström C. 2007. A novel enteropathogenic, strongly haemolytic spirochaete isolated from pig and mallard, provisionally designated 'Brachyspira suanatina' sp. nov. *Environ Microbiol* 9:983–991.

139. Rubin JE, Costa MO, Hill JE, Kittrell HE, Fernando C, Huang Y, O'Connor B, Harding JC. 2013. Reproduction of mucohaemorrhagic diarrhea and colitis indistinguishable from swine dysentery following experimental inoculation with "*Brachyspira hampsonii*" strain 30446. *PLoS One* 8:e57146.

140. Whiting RA, Doyle LP, Spray RS. 1921. Swine dysentery. *Purdue Univ Agr Exp Sta Bull* 257:1–15.

141. Trott DJ, Stanton TB, Jensen NS, Duhamel GE, Johnson JL, Hampson DJ. 1996. *Serpulina pilosicoli* sp. nov., the agent of porcine intestinal spirochetosis. *Int J Syst Bacteriol* 46:206–215.

142. Hampson DJ, Duhamel GE. 2006. Porcine colonic spirochetosis/intestinal spirochetosis, p 755–767. In Straw BE, Zimmerman JJ, D'Allaire S, Taylor DJ (ed), *Diseases of Swine*, 9th ed. Blackwell Publishing, Ames, IA.

143. Mappley LJ, La Ragione RM, Woodward MJ. 2014. *Brachyspira* and its role in avian intestinal spirochaetosis. *Vet Microbiol* 168:245–260.

144. Rubin JE, Harms NJ, Fernando C, Soos C, Detmer SE, Harding JC, Hill JE. 2013. Isolation and characterization of *Brachyspira* spp. including "*Brachyspira hampsonii*" from lesser snow geese (*Chen caerulescens caerulescens*) in the Canadian Arctic. *Microb Ecol* 66:813–822.

145. Tateishi Y, Takahashi M, Horiguchi S, Funata N, Koizumi K, Okudela K, Hishima T, Ohashi K. 2015. Clinicopathologic study of intestinal spirochetosis in Japan with special reference to human immunodeficiency virus infection status and species types: analysis of 5265 consecutive colorectal biopsies. *BMC Infect Dis* 15:13.

146. Hampson DJ. 2012. Brachyspiral colitis, p 680–696. In Zimmerman JJ, Karriker LA, Ramirez A, Schwartz KJ, Stevenson GW (ed), *Diseases of Swine*, 10th ed. John Wiley & Sons, Hoboken, NJ.

147. EUCAST. 2017. The European Committee on Antimicrobial Susceptibility Testing - EUCAST. http://www.eucast.org/. Accessed 12 January 2017.

148. Kajiwara K, Kozawa M, Kanazawa T, Uetsuka K, Nakajima H, Adachi Y. 2015. Drug-susceptibility of isolates of *Brachyspira hyodysenteriae* isolated from colonic mucosal specimens of pigs collected from slaughter houses in Japan in 2009. *J Vet Med Sci* 78:517–519.

149. Prasek J, Sperling D, Lobova D, Smola J, Cizek A. 2014. Antibiotic susceptibility of *Brachyspira hyodysenteriae* isolates from Czech swine farms: a 10-year study. *Acta Vet Brno* 83:3–7.

150. Clothier KA, Kinyon JM, Frana TS, Naberhaus N, Bower L, Strait EL, Schwartz K. 2011. Species characterization and minimum inhibitory concentration patterns of *Brachyspira* species isolates from swine with clinical disease. *J Vet Diagn Invest* 23:1140–1145.

151. Lim S, Lee H, Nam H, Cho YS, Jung S, Joo Y. 2012. Prevalence and antimicrobial susceptibility of *Brachyspira* species in pigs in Korea. *Korean J Vet Res* 52:253–257.

152. Råsbäck T, Fellström C, Bergsjø B, Cizek A, Collin K, Gunnarsson A, Jensen SM, Mars A, Thomson J, Vyt P, Pringle M. 2005. Assessment of diagnostics and antimicrobial susceptibility testing of *Brachyspira* species using a ring test. *Vet Microbiol* 109:229–243.

153. SVA. 2011. VetMIC Brachy for antimicrobial susceptibility testing of *Brachyspira* spp. http://www.sva.se/globalassets/redesign2011/pdf/analyser_produkter/vetmic/vetmic_brachy.pdf. Accessed 5 May 2016.

154. Rugna G, Bonilauri P, Carra E, Bergamini F, Luppi A, Gherpelli Y, Magistrali CF, Nigrelli A, Alborali GL, Martelli P, La T, Hampson DJ, Merialdi G. 2015.

Sequence types and pleuromutilin susceptibility of *Brachyspira hyodysenteriae* isolates from Italian pigs with swine dysentery: 2003–2012. *Vet J* 203:115–119.

155. Herbst W, Schlez K, Heuser J, Baljer G. 2014. Antimicrobial susceptibility of *Brachyspira hyodysenteriae* determined by a broth microdilution method. *Vet Rec* 174:382.

156. Pringle M, Landén A, Unnerstad HE, Molander B, Bengtsson B. 2012. Antimicrobial susceptibility of porcine *Brachyspira hyodysenteriae* and *Brachyspira pilosicoli* isolated in Sweden between 1990 and 2010. *Acta Vet Scand* 54:54.

157. Ohya T, Sueyoshi M. 2010. *In vitro* antimicrobial susceptibility of *Brachyspira hyodysenteriae* strains isolated in Japan from 1985 to 2009. *J Vet Med Sci* 72:1651–1653.

158. Karlsson M, Fellström C, Heldtander MU, Johansson KE, Franklin A. 1999. Genetic basis of macrolide and lincosamide resistance in *Brachyspira (Serpulina) hyodysenteriae*. *FEMS Microbiol Lett* 172:255–260.

159. Hillen S, Willems H, Herbst W, Rohde J, Reiner G. 2014. Mutations in the 50S ribosomal subunit of *Brachyspira hyodysenteriae* associated with altered minimum inhibitory concentrations of pleuromutilins. *Vet Microbiol* 172:223–229.

160. Hidalgo Á, Carvajal A, Vester B, Pringle M, Naharro G, Rubio P. 2011. Trends towards lower antimicrobial susceptibility and characterization of acquired resistance among clinical isolates of *Brachyspira hyodysenteriae* in Spain. *Antimicrob Agents Chemother* 55:3330–3337.

161. Pringle M, Poehlsgaard J, Vester B, Long KS. 2004. Mutations in ribosomal protein L3 and 23S ribosomal RNA at the peptidyl transferase centre are associated with reduced susceptibility to tiamulin in *Brachyspira* spp. isolates. *Mol Microbiol* 54:1295–1306.

162. Pringle M, Fellström C, Johansson KE. 2007. Decreased susceptibility to doxycycline associated with a 16S rRNA gene mutation in *Brachyspira hyodysenteriae*. *Vet Microbiol* 123:245–248.

163. Meziane-Cherif D, Lambert T, Dupêchez M, Courvalin P, Galimand M. 2008. Genetic and biochemical characterization of OXA-63, a new class D beta-lactamase from *Brachyspira pilosicoli* BM4442. *Antimicrob Agents Chemother* 52:1264–1268.

164. La T, Neo E, Phillips ND, Hampson DJ. 2015. Genes encoding ten newly designated OXA-63 group class D β-lactamases identified in strains of the pathogenic intestinal spirochaete *Brachyspira pilosicoli*. *J Med Microbiol* 64:1425–1435.

165. Stanton TB, Humphrey SB, Sharma VK, Zuerner RL. 2008. Collateral effects of antibiotics: carbadox and metronidazole induce VSH-1 and facilitate gene transfer among *Brachyspira hyodysenteriae* strains. *Appl Environ Microbiol* 74:2950–2956.

166. Buller NB, Hampson DJ. 1994. Antimicrobial susceptibility testing of *Serpulina hyodysenteriae*. *Aust Vet J* 71:211–214.

167. Leser TD, Amenuvor JZ, Jensen TK, Lindecrona RH, Boye M, Møller K. 2002. Culture-independent analysis of gut bacteria: the pig gastrointestinal tract microbiota revisited. *Appl Environ Microbiol* 68:673–690.

168. Suau A, Bonnet R, Sutren M, Godon JJ, Gibson GR, Collins MD, Doré J. 1999. Direct analysis of genes encoding 16S rRNA from complex communities reveals many novel molecular species within the human gut. *Appl Environ Microbiol* 65:4799–4807.

169. Hirsh DC, Indiveri MC, Jang SS, Biberstein EL. 1985. Changes in prevalence and susceptibility of obligate anaerobes in clinical veterinary practice. *J Am Vet Med Assoc* 186:1086–1089.

170. Even H, Rohde J, Verspohl J, Ryll M, Amtsberg G. 1998. Investigations into the occurrence and the antibiotic susceptibility of Gram negative anaerobes of the genera *Bacteroides*, *Prevotella*, *Porphyromonas* and *Fusobacterium* in specimens obtained from diseased animals. *Berl Munch Tierarztl Wochenschr* 111:379–386. (In German.)

171. Benno Y, Mitsuoka T. 1984. Susceptibility of *Bacteroides* from swine abscesses to 13 antibiotics. *Am J Vet Res* 45:2631–2633.

172. Cohen RO, Colodner R, Ziv G, Keness J. 1996. Isolation and antimicrobial susceptibility of obligate anaerobic bacteria recovered from the uteri of dairy cows with retained fetal membranes and postparturient endometritis. *Zentralbl Veterinarmed B* 43:193–199.

173. Jang SS, Breher JE, Dabaco LA, Hirsh DC. 1997. Organisms isolated from dogs and cats with anaerobic infections and susceptibility to selected antimicrobial agents. *J Am Vet Med Assoc* 210:1610–1614.

174. Almeida FS, Nakano V, Avila-Campos MJ. 2007. Occurrence of enterotoxigenic and nonenterotoxigenic *Bacteroides fragilis* in calves and evaluation of their antimicrobial susceptibility. *FEMS Microbiol Lett* 272:15–21.

175. Sarkar A, Pazhani GP, Dharanidharan R, Ghosh A, Ramamurthy T. 2015. Detection of integron-associated gene cassettes and other antimicrobial resistance genes in enterotoxigenic *Bacteroides fragilis*. *Anaerobe* 33:18–24.

176. Karlowsky JA, Walkty AJ, Adam HJ, Baxter MR, Hoban DJ, Zhanel GG. 2012. Prevalence of antimicrobial resistance among clinical isolates of *Bacteroides fragilis* group in Canada in 2010-2011: CANWARD surveillance study. *Antimicrob Agents Chemother* 56:1247–1252.

177. Toprak NU, Yağci A, Celik C, Cakici O, Söyletir G. 2005. Comparison of antimicrobial resistance patterns of enterotoxin gene positive and negative *Bacteroides fragilis* isolates. *Mikrobiyol Bul* 39:145–152. (In Turkish.)

178. Paula GR, Falcão LS, Antunes EN, Avelar KE, Reis FN, Maluhy MA, Ferreira MC, Domingues RM. 2004. Determinants of resistance in *Bacteroides fragilis* strains according to recent Brazilian profiles of antimicrobial susceptibility. *Int J Antimicrob Agents* 24:53–58.

179. Vedantam G. 2009. Antimicrobial resistance in *Bacteroides* spp.: occurrence and dissemination. *Future Microbiol* 4:413–423.

180. Liu CY, Huang YT, Liao CH, Yen LC, Lin HY, Hsueh PR. 2008. Increasing trends in antimicrobial resistance

among clinically important anaerobes and *Bacteroides fragilis* isolates causing nosocomial infections: emerging resistance to carbapenems. *Antimicrob Agents Chemother* 52:3161–3168.

181. **Rasmussen BA, Bush K, Tally FP.** 1993. Antimicrobial resistance in *Bacteroides*. *Clin Infect Dis* 16(Suppl 4): S390–S400.

182. **das Graças Silva E Souza W, Avelar KE, Antunes LC, Lobo LA, Domingues RM, de Souza Ferreira MC.** 2000. Resistance profile of *Bacteroides fragilis* isolated in Brazil. Do they shelter the *cfiA* gene? *J Antimicrob Chemother* 45:475–481.

183. **Sydenham TV, Sóki J, Hasman H, Wang M, Justesen US, ESGAI (ESCMID Study Group on Anaerobic Infections).** 2015. Identification of antimicrobial resistance genes in multidrug-resistant clinical *Bacteroides fragilis* isolates by whole genome shotgun sequencing. *Anaerobe* 31:59–64.

184. **Eitel Z, Sóki J, Urbán E, Nagy E, ESCMID Study Group on Anaerobic Infection.** 2013. The prevalence of antibiotic resistance genes in *Bacteroides fragilis* group strains isolated in different European countries. *Anaerobe* 21:43–49.

185. **Gal M, Brazier JS.** 2004. Metronidazole resistance in *Bacteroides* spp. carrying *nim* genes and the selection of slow-growing metronidazole-resistant mutants. *J Antimicrob Chemother* 54:109–116.

186. **Snydman DR, Jacobus NV, McDermott LA, Goldstein EJ, Harrell L, Jenkins SG, Newton D, Patel R, Hecht DW.** 2017. Trends in antimicrobial resistance among *Bacteroides* species and *Parabacteroides* species in the United States from 2010–2012 with comparison to 2008–2009. *Anaerobe* 43:21–26.

187. **Pumbwe L, Ueda O, Yoshimura F, Chang A, Smith RL, Wexler HM.** 2006. *Bacteroides fragilis* BmeABC efflux systems additively confer intrinsic antimicrobial resistance. *J Antimicrob Chemother* 58:37–46.

188. **Oh H, El Amin N, Davies T, Appelbaum PC, Edlund C.** 2001. *gyrA* mutations associated with quinolone resistance in *Bacteroides fragilis* group strains. *Antimicrob Agents Chemother* 45:1977–1981.

189. **Tan ZL, Nagaraja TG, Chengappa MM.** 1996. *Fusobacterium necrophorum* infections: virulence factors, pathogenic mechanism and control measures. *Vet Res Commun* 20:113–140.

190. **Jang SS, Hirsh DC.** 1994. Characterization, distribution, and microbiological associations of *Fusobacterium* spp. in clinical specimens of animal origin. *J Clin Microbiol* 32:384–387.

191. **Senhorinho GN, Nakano V, Liu C, Song Y, Finegold SM, Avila-Campos MJ.** 2012. Occurrence and antimicrobial susceptibility of *Porphyromonas* spp. and *Fusobacterium* spp. in dogs with and without periodontitis. *Anaerobe* 18:381–385.

192. **Nagaraja TG, Chengappa MM.** 1998. Liver abscesses in feedlot cattle: a review. *J Anim Sci* 76:287–298.

193. **Riordan T.** 2007. Human infection with *Fusobacterium necrophorum* (necrobacillosis), with a focus on Lemierre's syndrome. *Clin Microbiol Rev* 20:622–659.

194. **Goldstein EJ, Citron DM, Merriam CV, Warren YA, Tyrrell K, Fernandez H.** 2001. Comparative *in vitro* activity of ertapenem and 11 other antimicrobial agents against aerobic and anaerobic pathogens isolated from skin and soft tissue animal and human bite wound infections. *J Antimicrob Chemother* 48:641–651.

195. **Aldridge KE, Ashcraft D, Cambre K, Pierson CL, Jenkins SG, Rosenblatt JE.** 2001. Multicenter survey of the changing *in vitro* antimicrobial susceptibilities of clinical isolates of *Bacteroides fragilis* group, *Prevotella*, *Fusobacterium*, *Porphyromonas*, and *Peptostreptococcus* species. *Antimicrob Agents Chemother* 45:1238–1243.

196. **Teng LJ, Hsueh PR, Tsai JC, Liaw SJ, Ho SW, Luh KT.** 2002. High incidence of cefoxitin and clindamycin resistance among anaerobes in Taiwan. *Antimicrob Agents Chemother* 46:2908–2913.

197. **Nyfors S, Könönen E, Syrjänen R, Komulainen E, Jousimies-Somer H.** 2003. Emergence of penicillin resistance among *Fusobacterium nucleatum* populations of commensal oral flora during early childhood. *J Antimicrob Chemother* 51:107–112.

198. **Mateos E, Piriz S, Valle J, Hurtado M, Vadillo S.** 1997. Minimum inhibitory concentrations for selected antimicrobial agents against *Fusobacterium necrophorum* isolated from hepatic abscesses in cattle and sheep. *J Vet Pharmacol Ther* 20:21–23.

199. **Lechtenberg KF, Nagaraja TG, Chengappa MM.** 1998. Antimicrobial susceptibility of *Fusobacterium necrophorum* isolated from bovine hepatic abscesses. *Am J Vet Res* 59:44–47.

200. **Jiménez R, Píriz S, Mateos E, Vadillo S.** 2004. Minimum inhibitory concentrations for 25 selected antimicrobial agents against *Dichelobacter nodosus* and *Fusobacterium* strains isolated from footrot in sheep of Portugal and Spain. *J Vet Med B Infect Dis Vet Public Health* 51:245–248.

201. **Conrads G, Citron DM, Goldstein EJ.** 2005. Genetic determinant of intrinsic quinolone resistance in *Fusobacterium canifelinum*. *Antimicrob Agents Chemother* 49:434–437.

202. **Brooks JW, Kumar A, Narayanan S, Myers S, Brown K, Nagaraja TG, Jayarao BM.** 2014. Characterization of *Fusobacterium* isolates from the respiratory tract of white-tailed deer (Odocoileus virginianus). *J Vet Diagn Invest* 26:213–220.

203. **Green LE, George TR.** 2008. Assessment of current knowledge of footrot in sheep with particular reference to *Dichelobacter nodosus* and implications for elimination or control strategies for sheep in Great Britain. *Vet J* 175:173–180.

204. **Escayg AP, Hickford JG, Bullock DW.** 1997. Association between alleles of the ovine major histocompatibility complex and resistance to footrot. *Res Vet Sci* 63: 283–287.

205. **Depiazzi LJ, Roberts WD, Hawkins CD, Palmer MA, Pitman DR, Mcquade NC, Jelinek PD, Devereaux DJ, Rippon RJ.** 1998. Severity and persistence of footrot in merino sheep experimentally infected with a protease

thermostable strain of *Dichelobacter nodosus* at five sites. *Aust Vet J* 76:32–38.

206. **Kennan RM, Gilhuus M, Frosth S, Seemann T, Dhungyel OP, Whittington RJ, Boyce JD, Powell DR, Aspán A, Jørgensen HJ, Bulach DM, Rood JI.** 2014. Genomic evidence for a globally distributed, bimodal population in the ovine footrot pathogen *Dichelobacter nodosus*. *MBio* 5:e01821-14.

207. **McPherson AS, Dhungyel OP, Whittington RJ.** 2017. Evaluation of genotypic and phenotypic protease virulence tests for *Dichelobacter nodosus* infection in sheep. *J Clin Microbiol* 55:1313–1326.

208. **Frosth S, König U, Nyman AK, Aspán A.** 2017. Sample pooling for real-time PCR detection and virulence determination of the footrot pathogen *Dichelobacter nodosus*. *Vet Res Commun* 41:189–193.

209. **Malecki JC, Coffey L.** 1987. Treatment of ovine virulent footrot with zinc sulphate/sodium lauryl sulphate footbathing. *Aust Vet J* 64:301–304.

210. **Egerton JR, Parsonson IM, Graham NP.** 1968. Parenteral chemotherapy of ovine foot-rot. *Aust Vet J* 44:275–283.

211. **Rendell DK, Callinan AP.** 1997. Comparison of erythromycin and oxytetracycline for the treatment of virulent footrot in grazing sheep. *Aust Vet J* 75:354.

212. **Jordan D, Plant JW, Nicol HI, Jessep TM, Scrivener CJ.** 1996. Factors associated with the effectiveness of antibiotic treatment for ovine virulent footrot. *Aust Vet J* 73:211–215.

213. **Venning CM, Curtis MA, Egerton JR.** 1990. Treatment of virulent footrot with lincomycin and spectinomycin. *Aust Vet J* 67:258–260.

214. **Gradin JL, Schmitz JA.** 1983. Susceptibility of *Bacteroides nodosus* to various antimicrobial agents. *J Am Vet Med Assoc* 183:434–437.

215. **Píriz Durán S, Cuenca Valera R, Valle Manzano J, Vadillo Machota S.** 1991. Comparative *in vitro* susceptibility of *Bacteroides* and *Fusobacterium* isolated from footrot in sheep to 28 antimicrobial agents. *J Vet Pharmacol Ther* 14:185–192.

216. **Piriz Duran S, Valle Manzano J, Cuenca Valera R, Vadillo Machota S.** 1990. *In-vitro* antimicrobial susceptibility of *Bacteroides* and *Fusobacterium* isolated from footrot in goats. *Br Vet J* 146:437–442.

217. **Píriz S, Pobel T, Jiménez R, Mateos EM, Martín-Palomino P, Vila P, Vadillo S.** 2001. Comparison of erythromycin and oxytetracycline for the treatment of ovine footrot. *Acta Vet Hung* 49:131–139.

218. **Lacombe-Antoneli A, Píriz S, Vadillo S.** 2007. *In vitro* antimicrobial susceptibility of anaerobic bacteria isolated from caprine footrot. *Acta Vet Hung* 55:11–20.

219. **Burch DGS.** 2005. Pharmacokinetic, pharmacodynamic and clinical correlations relating to the therapy of colonic infections in the pig and breakpoint determinations. *Pig J* 56:8–24.

220. **Hellman J, Aspevall O, Bengtsson B, Pringle M.** 2014. Consumption of antibiotics and occurrence of antibiotic resistance in Sweden. Public Health Agency of Sweden and National Veterinary Institute, Uppsala, Sweden.

221. **Duhamel GE, Kinyon JM, Mathiesen MR, Murphy DP, Walter D.** 1998. *In vitro* activity of four antimicrobial agents against North American isolates of porcine *Serpulina pilosicoli*. *J Vet Diagn Invest* 10:350–356.

Antimicrobial Resistance in Bacteria from Livestock and Companion Animals
Edited by Frank Møller Aarestrup, Stefan Schwarz, Jianzhong Shen, and Lina Cavaco
© 2018 American Society for Microbiology, Washington, DC
doi:10.1128/microbiolspec.ARBA-0029-2017

Antimicrobial Resistance in *Leptospira*, *Brucella*, and Other Rarely Investigated Veterinary and Zoonotic Pathogens

22

Darren J. Trott[1], Sam Abraham[2], and Ben Adler[3]

ANTIMICROBIAL RESISTANCE IN THE GENUS *LEPTOSPIRA*

Members of the genus *Leptospira* are classified into more than 20 species based on DNA relatedness and comprise over 350 serovars, based on surface agglutinating lipopolysaccharide antigens. However, they are best viewed as three groupings. Saprophytic species, e.g., *Leptospira biflexa*, are never associated with disease. Members of the pathogen group, e.g., *Leptospira interrogans* and *Leptospira borgpetersenii*, cause leptospirosis in humans and animals worldwide, with infection resulting in a range of syndromes from mild or asymptomatic infection to severe forms involving multiple organ failure and death. An intermediate group containing, e.g., *Leptospira fainei* and *Leptospira licerasiae*, may be associated with infection and mild disease (1, 2).

Leptospira spp. are intrinsically resistant to a range of antimicrobial agents, but the precise mechanisms responsible for this remain unknown. However, resistance to sulfonamides, neomycin, actidione, polymyxin, nalidixic acid, vancomycin, and rifampicin has allowed the development of selective media containing various combinations of these antimicrobial agents for isolation of leptospires (3–5).

In terms of resistance to antimicrobial agents used in human and veterinary medicine, the picture is not as clear-cut. Often, the studies involved only a single species or a small number of isolates which were tested for susceptibility *in vitro*. There are few data available on any

development of resistance *in vivo*; accordingly, this section concentrates on current knowledge about *in vitro* antimicrobial agent susceptibility of *Leptospira* spp. A caveat that must be borne in mind is that results for one or more species and from one geographical region may not necessarily be extrapolatable elsewhere. Moreover, comparisons using different testing methods may not be valid. Not surprisingly, the MICs against penicillin and tetracycline of leptospires growing in biofilm were 6-fold higher than those of planktonic cells (6). The significance, if any, of this finding for treatment is unknown.

There is no consensus on a method for susceptibility testing in *Leptospira*. The most commonly used method for determining MICs is broth dilution, although a disk sensitivity method using a modified agar medium has been developed (Table 1). The main findings of *in vitro* susceptibility testing are shown in Table 1. In general, there is little evidence of a significant emergence of antimicrobial resistance in *Leptospira*. One recent study (7) detected resistance against a range of antimicrobial agents in a small proportion of strains, although importantly, universal susceptibility to β-lactams remained. Nevertheless, the overall conclusion must be drawn that antimicrobial agent resistance has not emerged as a major problem in leptospirosis. However, it should be noted that there is no clear evidence of what constitutes a resistance breakpoint for *Leptospira* against most antimicrobial agents.

A similar picture emerges from the smaller number of studies that investigated the efficacy of antimicrobial

[1]Australian Centre for Antimicrobial Resistance Ecology, School of Animal and Veterinary Sciences, University of Adelaide, Roseworthy Campus, Roseworthy, South Australia, 5371, Australia; [2]School of Veterinary and Life Sciences, Murdoch University, Murdoch, Western Australia, 6150, Australia; [3]School of Biomedical Sciences, Monash University, Clayton, Victoria 3800, Australia.

Table 1 Reported *in vitro* antimicrobial susceptibilities of *Leptospira* spp.

Leptospiral species	Year	Region	No. of strains tested	Main source	Method	Susceptible	Resistant (no. of strains)	Ref
L. interrogans, *L. borgpetersenii*[a]	1977	New Zealand	14	Human	MIC broth dilution	Penicillin, tetracycline, minocycline		112
L. borgpetersenii[a]	1988	Canada	18	Cattle	MIC broth dilution	Penicillin, tetracycline, ampicillin, erythromycin, streptomycin	Sulfamethazine (18)	113
L. interrogans, *L. borgpetersenii*, *L. kirschneri*, *L. noguchii*, *L. santarosai*, *L. weilii*	2004	USA	24	Lab reference strains	MIC broth dilution	Penicillin and other β-lactams, macrolides, chloramphenicol, tetracycline, doxycycline, fluroquinolones, telithromycin	Aztreonam (24)	114
L. interrogans, *L. kirschneri*	2006	USA	4	Lab reference strains	MIC broth dilution	Amoxycillin, tilmicosin, enrofloxacin		15
L. interrogans, *L. borgpetersenii*	2010	Philippines	46	Rat	MIC broth dilution	Ampicillin, cefotaxime, fluroquinolones, doxycycline, erythromycin, streptomycin	Neomycin (46)[b], fosfomycin (46), sulfamethoxazole (46), trimethoprim (46), vancomycin (46)[c]	115
L. interrogans, *L. borgpetersenii*, *L. kirschneri*, *L. noguchii*, *L. weilii*	2011	USA	13	Human, lab reference strains, not stated	MIC broth dilution, hamster infection	Cephalexin, cefazolin		11
L. interrogans, *L. borgpetersenii*, *L. kirschneri*	2013	Mainly South East Asia	109	Mainly human	Etest	Penicillin, doxycycline, cefotaxime, ceftriaxone, chloramphenicol		116
L. interrogans	2013	Brazil	20	human, rat, dog, cattle	MIC broth dilution	Penicillin and other β-lactams, fluoroquinolones[d], tetracyclines gentamicin	Sulfamethoxazole-trimethoprim (20), neomycin (15)	117
L. interrogans	2015	Trinidad	67	Rodent, dog	MIC broth dilution	Amoxicillin, ceftriaxone, ciprofloxacin, clindamycin, doxycycline, erythromycin, imipenem, penicillin, polymyxin B[e]	Polymyxin B[e], gentamicin[f], sulfamethoxazole-trimethoprim[f]	118
L. interrogans, *L. borgpetersenii*, *L. kirschneri*, *L. weilii*	2015	Thailand	10	Not stated	Disk susceptibility	Amoxicillin, azithromycin, cefoxitin, ceftazidime, ceftriaxone, chloramphenicol, ciprofloxacin, clindamycin, doripenem, doxycycline, gentamicin, linezolid, nitrofurantoin, penicillin, piperacillin/tazobactam, tetracycline	Sulfamethoxazole-trimethoprim (10), fosfomycin (10), nalidixic acid (10), Rifampicin (10)	119
L. interrogans, *L. borgpetersenii*, *L. meyeri*, *L. santarosai*	2016	Brazil	47	Human, dog, rat, cattle, swine	MIC broth dilution	Penicillin, ampicillin[e]	Sulfamethoxazole-trimethoprim[g]	7
L. interrogans, *L. borgpetersenii*	2017	Malaysia	65	Dog, rat, human, swine, water	MIC broth dilution	Penicillin, ampicillin, doxycycline	Sulfamethoxazole-trimethoprim (65), chloramphenicol[f]	120

[a]Based on the probability that the isolates were serovar Hardjo-bovis.
[b]Assuming a breakpoint of 6.25 μg/ml.
[c]Assuming a breakpoint of 16μg/ml.
[d]Variable MICs among different isolates.
[e]Variable MICs with other antibiotics. See text.
[f]Intermediate level of susceptibility.
[g]Data for individual strains not shown.

agents *in vivo*. As early as 1955, erythromycin was shown to be effective in experimental hamster infection (8), as were other macrolides subsequently (9). Not surprisingly, fluoroquinolones and cephalosporins were likewise efficacious (10, 11). A study of gerbils showed that low-dose oral chlortetracycline was 100% successful in preventing renal colonization by leptospires (G. Andres-Fontaine, personal communication). In cattle infected with *Leptospira borgpetersenii*, oxytetracycline, tilmicosin, penicillin combined with dihydrostreptomycin, and ceftiofur were all effective in eliminating urinary shedding (12).

Accordingly, the current recommendations for treatment of human leptospirosis remain penicillin, ampicillin, ceftriaxone, or cefotaxime. Alternatives in cases of allergy or in nonhospital settings include oral doxycycline or azithromycin (13). In the veterinary setting a penicillin-streptomycin combination has been the antimicrobial agent therapy of choice for the treatment of acute leptospirosis, but ampicillin, amoxycillin, tetracyclines, tulathromycin, and third-generation cephalosporins have also been used (14). Tilmicosin offers an additional alternative (12, 15).

The apparent lack of any significant emergence of antimicrobial agent resistance in *Leptospira* raises an interesting question. Why has this not occurred? Any suggestions are, of course, purely speculative. In the environment, leptospires cohabit with many other bacterial species, but in the general absence of any therapeutically useful antimicrobial agents, there is no selective pressure. Leptospiral infections are usually monomicrobial, with leptospires present in internal organs, such as blood, liver, spleen, lungs, and renal proximal tubules. The opportunity for horizontal resistance gene acquisition from other bacterial species is therefore minimal. In addition, there is no experimental evidence to date of uptake of foreign DNA by *Leptospira* spp., although genomic analyses support this notion. Finally, in humans leptospirosis is a dead-end infection; human-to-human transmission is so rare as to be considered insignificant. The spread of any antimicrobial-resistant leptospires from infected people would thus be negligible.

ANTIMICROBIAL RESISTANCE IN THE GENUS *BRUCELLA*

Introduction

The genus *Brucella* comprises 10 recognized species (the three main zoonotic species *Brucella abortus*, *Brucella melitensis*, *Brucella suis*, and an additional seven species of limited or no zoonotic potential: *Brucella canis*, *Brucella ceti*, *Brucella inopinata*, *Brucella microti*, *Brucella neotomae*, *Brucella ovis*, and *Brucella pinnipedialis*) (16). Brucellosis caused by *B. abortus*, *B. melitensis*, or *B. suis* is a notifiable disease in humans and animals in many countries, particularly those that have undertaken vaccination, test, and slaughter eradication campaigns directed at eliminating *B. abortus* from cattle. Clinical signs in humans are highly variable and may be chronic in nature following dissemination and sequestration of the organism in bone, joints, brain, or the genitourinary system without prompt effective treatment. *Brucella* spp. are listed as category B bioterrorism agents by the U.S. Centers for Disease Control and Prevention (17).

B. abortus eradication has remained difficult in countries with significant sylvatic ruminant populations, which may act as reservoirs of infection that occasionally spill over into domestic cattle. *B. melitensis* infection remains endemic in ruminants in many countries in the Middle East, Africa, the Mediterranean basin, Asia, and Central and South America, with much higher rates of infection in humans compared to *B. abortus*, mainly due to ingestion of unpasteurized milk (18). *B. suis*, also a much more serious zoonotic pathogen than *B. abortus*, is endemic to countries with significant wild boar populations, with infections largely restricted to pig hunters and their dogs (19, 20). For example, since eradication of *B. abortus* in cattle and buffalo in Australia in the 1970s, very few human brucellosis cases have been reported in that country. *B. suis* is endemic in the feral pig populations of Queensland, northern New South Wales, and parts of Western Australia and the Northern Territory, and approximately 10 to 50 cases of *B. suis* infection in humans are diagnosed annually, with most cases occurring in pig hunters (21–24).

A number of recent cases of *B. suis* infection have been reported in pig-hunting dog breeds in Georgia, United States (20), as well as northern New South Wales and Queensland, with the main presenting signs being fever, malaise, back pain, and shifting lameness from associated discospondylitis in neutered animals or orchitis/epididymitis/abortion in entire animals (25). Humans and dogs may acquire *B. suis* infection during hunting and carcass dressing from either contamination of cuts and abrasions or from exposure to aerosols. Consumption of undercooked pig meat is also an important risk factor, especially for dogs (25). Veterinary laboratory staff may also be at risk of infection as the organism aerosolizes off the plate, requiring work to be undertaken in a biocontainment level 3 biosafety cabinet at all times.

Antimicrobial Susceptibility Testing for the Genus *Brucella*

Routine susceptibility testing of *Brucella* spp. is not generally recommended due to the risk to laboratory personnel, the fastidious nature of the organisms, and their overall susceptibility to the majority of antimicrobial agents used in combination for treatment (26). MIC testing using broth microdilution of *Brucella* isolates is hazardous for laboratory personnel due to the potential for creating aerosols and must be undertaken in a biocontainment level 3 biosafety cabinet (27). In early MIC studies, although a lack of standardization was apparent, most *Brucella* isolates were identified as susceptible to the antimicrobial agents tested, which was also demonstrated in one of the first MIC studies (undertaken in Spain in 1986) involving a large collection of isolates (28). Also, many early studies were flawed in the respect that quality control ranges for the media adopted did not exist, and therefore, quality control strains were rarely tested alongside clinical *Brucella* isolates (29). In a second Spanish study, also undertaken in 1986, *Brucella* spp. showed *in vitro* susceptibility to all seven antimicrobial agents tested, and the MICs of the isolates had no bearing on relapse rates (see "Antimicrobial Resistance Emergence and Spread in the Genus *Brucella*" below for a more complete description of relapse in relation to MIC) (30). *Brucella* MIC testing has utilized methods including broth macrodilution, broth microdilution, agar dilution (using Iso-Sensitest agar with the MIC determined to be the lowest concentration of antimicrobial agent that eliminates bacterial growth), and most recently, Etest strips (27, 28, 31, 32). Few studies have directly compared these methods, and the large disparities in frequencies of resistance reported in some countries compared to others (see "Antimicrobial Resistance Emergence and Spread in the Genus *Brucella*" below) bring into question the rigor of some of these studies and the techniques utilized. Lonsway et al. (26) noted in a multicenter study that for broth microdilution testing in *Brucella* broth, incubation in CO_2 decreased the doxycycline MIC by one $\log_2$ dilution, whereas for aminoglycosides, it increased by one dilution. The CLSI has produced guidelines and some clinical breakpoints (Table 2) for *Brucella* MIC testing within the methods for antimicrobial dilution and disk susceptibility testing of infrequently isolated or fastidious bacteria for potential bacterial agents of bioterrorism (33). The medium of choice for broth microdilution is pH-adjusted *Brucella* broth without additional supplementation. The three quality control strains and their ranges as recommended by the CLSI are shown in Table 3 below (29).

Antimicrobial Treatment Regimes for Brucellosis in Humans and Animals

The treatment of brucellosis in humans is challenging, particularly if the disease is not diagnosed in the early stages of infection. Treatment regimes recommended by the World Health Organization include the combination of high doses of doxycycline (200 mg/day) and rifampicin (900 mg/day) orally for 45 days or doxycycline (200 mg/day) or tetracycline orally for 45 days and streptomycin (1 g/day) intramuscularly for 21 days. Trimethoprim-sulfamethoxazole (320 to 1,600 mg/day) in combination with rifampicin (900 mg/day) (34, 35) or doxycycline (200 mg/day) orally for 45 days are cost-effective alternatives for some patient groups (36). Although streptomycin is known to be one of the most active agents against brucellosis, its potential adverse effects on the patient, such as ototoxicity, nephrotoxicity, and the requirement for intramuscular parenteral administration, preclude its wider use (27). However, a combination of rifampicin, doxycycline, and streptomycin is recommended for patients with spondylitis (37).

A similar combination regime of rifampicin (5 mg/kg *per os* once daily) and doxycycline (6 mg/kg *per os* twice daily) has been administered to dogs for *B. suis* infection (21, 25), although euthanasia is a recommended option for *B. suis* infection in dogs to prevent the risk of zoonotic exposure (21). However, evidence of dog-to-human transmission is scarce, with only a single case report implicating exposure to aborted dog fetuses (38). In one case of *B. suis* discospondylitis in a large-breed dog (the bull Arab, which are specifically bred for hunting wild boar), rifampicin-doxycycline treatment was continued for 25 months and successfully eliminated *Brucella* infection, with the rifampicin

Table 2 CLSI human-specific clinical breakpoints for MIC testing of *Brucella* spp.

Antimicrobial agent	CLSI breakpoint for *Brucella* (mg/liter)[a]		
	S	I	R
Doxycycline	≤4	8	≥16
Rifampin[b]	≤1	2	≥4
Streptomycin	≤8		
Gentamicin	≤4		
Trimethoprim-sulfamethoxazole	≤0.5	1–2	≥4
Ciprofloxacin[b]	≤1		
Moxifloxacin[b]	≤1		

[a]S, susceptible; I, intermediate; R, resistant.
[b]Extrapolated from CLSI breakpoints for slow-growing bacteria (*Haemophilus* spp.) (42).

Table 3 MIC_{50}, MIC_{90}, and MIC range values for 6 antimicrobial agents tested against 10 North American and European isolates of *L. intracellularis*[a,b]

Antimicrobial	MIC_{50} (µg/ml)		MIC_{90} (µg/ml)		MIC range (µg/ml)	
	IC	EC	IC	EC	IC	EC
Carbadox	0.125	4	0.25	16	0.125–0.25	1–32
Chlortetracycline	8–16	32	16–32	64	0.125–64	16–64
Lincomycin	16–32	>128	128	>128	1–>128	32–>128
Tiamulin	0.125	4–8	0.125	8–16	0.125–0.5	1–32
Tylosin	1	16	2-8	128	0.25–32	1–>128
Valnemulin	0.125	0.25	0.125	0.25–2	0.125	0.125–4

[a]Adapted from reference 110.
[b]IC, Intracellular; EC, Extracellular.

dose lowered after 2 weeks of treatment to prevent liver damage (21). In a case of *B. suis* orchitis, combination treatment was commenced for 2 weeks, the infected, enlarged testis was removed under general anesthesia, with all attending personnel wearing appropriate protective equipment, and combination antimicrobial therapy was then continued for another 4 weeks (21).

Antimicrobial dual therapy is also recommended for cases of *B. canis* infection in dogs, but high relapse rates have been noted, particularly in male dogs (39). In production animals, treatment of brucellosis with antimicrobial agents is usually not attempted; affected animals are slaughtered, and the carcass is disposed of appropriately to prevent zoonotic exposure. However, administration of oxytetracycline and streptomycin to cows with brucellosis infection did not influence the MIC of the causal agents (40).

Other antimicrobial agents reported to have been administered to humans or animals for the treatment of brucellosis with variable success rates include streptomycin (41), ampicillin (42), sulfamethoxazole-trimethoprim alone (43) or in combination with rifampin or doxycycline (35), fluoroquinolones (44), chloramphenicol, erythromycin and cephalosporins (36), doxycycline and netilmycin (45), tetracycline and streptomycin, and various combinations of gentamicin, doxycycline, fluoroquinolones, and rifampicin (46). It has been noted that critically important antimicrobial agents such as ciprofloxacin and ceftriaxone have been tested as monotherapy for brucellosis, but clinical outcomes are generally poor even though the isolates show *in vitro* susceptibility, though the MICs are often at the high end of the susceptibility range (35, 47). Newer-generation fluoroquinolones have lower MICs (48). Although there is future potential for dual therapy approaches with other antimicrobial agents, the high cost of fluoroquinolones and their critical importance

for acute Gram-negative infection such as urosepsis has led to recommendations precluding their use in chronic conditions such as brucellosis (35).

Antimicrobial Resistance Emergence and Spread in the Genus *Brucella*

Given the chronic nature of brucellosis, the intracellular location of the invading bacteria in reticuloendothelial cells, and their predilection to sequester within infected sites (e.g., bone) that are poorly penetrated by many antimicrobial classes, it is not surprising that there are numerous reports of relapses following therapy (estimated to range from 5 to 15% of uncomplicated cases) (35). Whether this is due to the development of resistance or the failure to eliminate residual bacteria within infection sites due to inappropriate choice, dose, and/or duration of therapy is somewhat equivocal. However, in the majority of MIC studies undertaken in countries where brucellosis is endemic, *Brucella* spp. have maintained their susceptibility to doxycycline and rifampicin (18, 49–51). An additional issue to consider in developing countries with higher rates of both brucellosis and tuberculosis is that the use of certain agents such as rifampicin for the treatment of one disease (brucellosis) may lead to the development of resistance to this drug in the other disease (i.e., tuberculosis) (35).

Hall and Spink (41) first reported the development of resistance during monotherapy with streptomycin. Subsequently, Lal et al. (43) reported that one of four patients with *B. abortus* infection treated with sulfamethoxazole-trimethoprim did not respond to therapy, presumably due to a 7-day time period during convalescence when only trimethoprim monotherapy was administered due to a perceived reaction to the sulfonamide. Recommencement of dual therapy did not eliminate the infection. In a prospective randomized trial, doxycycline-rifampicin was inferior to tetracycline-streptomycin in preventing relapses of *B. melitensis* infection, though it was noted that the patients in this treatment group only received antimicrobial therapy for 30 days rather than the recommended 45 days (52). The longer duration of rifampicin-doxycycline therapy was subsequently shown in a randomized double-blind trial to be as effective as tetracycline-streptomycin for the treatment of all cases of brucellosis infection except spondylitis (53). In a study of 75 prospective cases, Ariza et al. (28) showed no difference in the MIC of the *Brucella* spp. isolated from primary compared to relapsed infections.

Proof of development of rifampicin resistance during dual therapy with doxycycline was first reported in 1986 in a case of *B. melitensis* infection (45). An isolate obtained from a blood culture was susceptible to all six antimicrobial agents tested (rifampicin MIC of 1.0 µg/ml), and the patient initially responded to dual therapy for 6 weeks. Three months after the last dose, the patient re-presented with joint pain. Blood and joint fluid cultures were positive for *B. melitensis*, but this time, the isolate's rifampicin MIC had risen to 64 µg/ml. The patient was then treated successfully with doxycycline and netilmicin in combination. Other reports of very low numbers of *Brucella* isolates (mainly *B. melitensis*) exhibiting rifampicin resistance have been described in Turkey (54) and Kuwait (55). However, until the study of Abdel-Maksoud (described in the text below), the majority of *Brucella* isolates investigated exhibited susceptibility to rifampicin and doxycycline (56). In addition to this report, a high rate of reduced susceptibility to rifampicin, but interestingly, no resistant strains, has been reported among *B. melitensis* isolates from Iran (57, 58) and Turkey (59). No resistance to the main antimicrobial agents used to treat brucellosis in humans was identified in *B. abortus* isolates from the United Kingdom between 2011 and 2014 (17 isolates in total).

Resistance of *B. melitensis* to ciprofloxacin was noted by al-Sibai and Qadri (60), who documented an increase in MIC between initial (0.08 µg/ml) and follow-up isolates (5.0 µg/ml) obtained 3 weeks after commencement of ciprofloxacin therapy. In a study of 160 patients with brucellosis in Saudi Arabia, Memish et al. (61) noted that 29% of the isolates were resistant to sulfamethoxazole-trimethoprim, while only a handful of isolates were resistant to rifampicin (3.5%), doxycycline (0.6%), or streptomycin (0.6%). Bannatyne et al. (62) and Almuneef et al. (63) also noted the very high rate of sulfamethoxazole-trimethoprim resistance among *Brucella* isolates from Saudi Arabia; however, the resistance phenotype of the isolate had no bearing on relapse rates, presumably due to the use of sulfamethoxazole-trimethoprim in combination with rifampicin with or without streptomycin (64).

Few studies have examined the antimicrobial susceptibility of veterinary *Brucella* isolates. However, very low levels of resistance to the main agents used in the treatment of brucellosis were identified in a study of 147 *B. abortus* isolates from cattle in Brazil (1977 to 2009) (32). Three strains (2.0%) exhibited resistance to rifampicin, but 54 strains (36.7%) showed reduced susceptibility. In a similar study undertaken on 86 *B. abortus* isolates from Korea (1998 to 2006), antimicrobial susceptibilities to 13 antimicrobial agents were assayed using broth microdilution (65). A total of four isolates exhibited resistance to rifampicin, and again, a large number of isolates (63/86; 73.3%) exhibited nonsusceptibility. None of these isolates have been subjected to molecular testing, so it is impossible to determine if they possess *rpoB* gene mutations, or other possible resistance mechanisms, or whether they represent wild-type isolates at the upper range of rifampicin MICs.

Few molecular-based studies have been undertaken to confirm the genetic basis of resistance or reduced susceptibility to antimicrobial agents used in the treatment of brucellosis. Key mutations in the *rpoB* gene of laboratory-induced rifampicin-resistant *B. melitensis* mutants have been identified in at least two studies (66, 67). Similarly, overexpression of efflux pumps and mutations in *gyrA* associated with fluoroquinolone resistance have been induced *in vitro* in *Brucella* spp. strains (68–71). However, none of these mutations were identified in a collection of 67 clinical *Brucella* isolates from Spain (72). On the basis of CLSI broth microdilution and rifampicin breakpoints (MICs of ≥4.0 µg/ml), probable rifampicin resistance was noted in a large collection of *B. melitensis* isolates from Egypt between 1999 and 2007 (MIC_{50}, 2.0 µg/ml; MIC_{90}, 4.0 µg/ml; MIC range, 0.25 to 6.0 µg/ml; 19% of isolates with an MIC of ≥4.0 µg/ml) (56). However, none of the isolates were investigated further to confirm the basis of resistance/reduced susceptibility.

ANTIMICROBIAL RESISTANCE IN *BORRELIA BURGDORFERI*

The spirochete *B. burgdorferi sensu lato* is the agent of Lyme disease in humans and animals, a vector-borne disease resulting from an infected tick bite. Lyme disease typically manifests as a site-specific infection following primary multiplication at the cutaneous site of infection (often associated with a pathognomonic bull's-eye lesion around the tick bite, the erythema migrans) and secondary bacteremia. In animals, arthritis is the most common syndrome, but clinical signs can be vague and nonspecific, including fever, malaise, and potentially, cardiac, renal, or neurological disturbance. In humans, a subset of individuals experience persistent chronic symptoms of fatigue, neurocognitive difficulties, or musculoskeletal pains despite antimicrobial therapy, which has been considered a noninfectious syndrome; however, recent identification of antimicrobial-tolerant persister cells and biofilms have challenged this paradigm (73).

B. burgdorferi has a complicated pathogenesis and epidemiological cycle of infection involving ticks, tick maintenance (predominantly deer, sheep, and other large mammals), and tick reservoir hosts (small mammals including rodents and hedgehogs, lizards, and birds). In animals, Lyme disease is most commonly reported in dogs, but cases have also occurred in horses, cattle, and sheep (74–76). Acute Lyme disease in animals can be treated with amoxicillin or doxycycline, but the recommended treatment for dogs is doxycycline at 10 mg/kg every 24 h for at least 4 weeks (77). Prompt removal of ticks and frequent treatments with an acaricide are recommended in endemic regions where Lyme disease is common.

Early antimicrobial susceptibility testing of *B. burgdorferi* resulted in variation in MICs due to a lack of a standardized method and differences in endpoint determination. Isolates were reported to be highly susceptible *in vitro* to macrolides and third-generation cephalosporins and moderately susceptible to tetracyclines and penicillins. Newer agents such as fluoroquinolones, tigecycline, and ketolides have also demonstrated *in vitro* activity (78, 79). Dever et al. (80) developed a standardized, reproducible, and reliable susceptibility test based on broth microdilution in Barbour-Stoenner-Kelly II media, with an initial inoculum size of 10^6 bacterial cells per ml and an incubation time of 72 h. Wells were assessed visually for growth. A number of additional susceptibility tests have been developed (81), with some incorporating a calorimetric endpoint determination using phenol red, with the color change being indicative of the accumulation of nonvolatile acid produced by actively metabolizing spirochetes (78).

B. burgdorferi does not usually possess resistance mechanisms and is generally susceptible to antimicrobial agents *in vitro* (82, 83). However, a small number of studies have demonstrated acquired resistance in both laboratory and clinical settings. Development of resistance to erythromycin (100 to 500 mg/liter) has been reported in clinical isolates of *B. burgdorferi* (84). A low-passage clinical isolate with an unusually high level of resistance to macrolides and lincosamides was phenotypically shown to have a modified ribosome structure using radiolabeled erythromycin, but the genes encoding this resistance could not be identified. The resistance determinant appeared to be encoded by mobile genetic elements, because the phenotype was transferable to other bacterial species (85). The elements were hypothesized based on conjugation frequency to be constins or integrating conjugative elements. Resistance to coumermycin due to mutation in *gyrA*, to aminoglycosides due to homologous mutations in the small ribosomal RNA subunit, and to fluoroquinolones due to mutation in *parC* have been demonstrated following laboratory selection (86–88).

A novel, TolC-like efflux system, with the outer membrane porin BesC forming an integral role, has been identified in *B. burgdorferi* and demonstrated to have a dual role in both virulence and antimicrobial resistance. A *B. burgdorferi besC* knockout mutant became more susceptible to a wide range of antimicrobial classes compared to the wild-type, but it is important to note that the wild type strain was already highly susceptible to antimicrobial agents (89).

Bacterial persistence in the presence of antimicrobial, with no apparent increase in the MIC of the organism, appears to be a more common mechanism of antimicrobial resistance in *Borrelia* and may be associated with post-treatment Lyme disease syndrome (73, 90). The formation of drug-tolerant persister cells, which has been demonstrated *in vitro*, may be one explanation for chronic Lyme disease symptomology and lack of responsiveness to antimicrobial therapy (91). *B. burgdorferi* can form both round body cells and biofilm-like structures which are more resistant to antimicrobial agents (92, 93). In a primate model of Lyme disease, in which antimicrobial agents were administered 4 to 6 months after infection, antimicrobial-tolerant persister cells could be demonstrated/isolated following treatment, demonstrating that *B. burgdorferi* can withstand antimicrobial agent treatment administered post-dissemination. Eradication of persister cells *in vitro* has been achieved by pulse dosing with third-generation cephalosporins or daptomycin combinations with doxycycline and/or cephalosporins (73, 91).

ANTIMICROBIAL RESISTANCE IN *LAWSONIA INTRACELLULARIS*

L. intracellularis is the agent of porcine proliferative enteropathy (PPE) in pigs, which comprises porcine intestinal adenomatosis, regional ileitis, and necrotic enteritis in young growing pigs, as well as porcine hemorrhagic enteropathy in older immunologically naive animals (94). *L. intracellularis* or related organisms are also associated with a similar clinical syndrome and pathognomonic, PPE-like lesions in horses, in which it is considered to be an emerging pathogen, and acute necrotizing enteritis in recently weaned foals has been reported (95, 96). Other animal species in which clinical and/or pathological lesions associated with *L. intracellularis* infection have been found include hamsters, rabbits, ferrets, foxes, dogs, rats, sheep, deer, emus, ostriches, non-human primates, and guinea pigs (97).

L. intracellularis is an obligate, intracellular bacterium that can only be grown *in vitro* in cell culture systems (98). *In vitro* studies of the antimicrobial susceptibility of this obligate intracellular bacterium necessitate complicated cell culture systems (because *Lawsonia* cell division only occurs within the host cell), and only a few laboratories in the world have performed antimicrobial susceptibility testing, because few *L. intracellularis* strains have been successfully isolated and maintained in cell culture (99–101). Typically, these are monolayers of murine fibroblast-like McCoy cells incubated in a microaerophilic atmosphere containing both hydrogen and carbon dioxide (102). Hence, antimicrobial susceptibility testing needs to account for intracellular as well as extracellular drug concentrations attained during coculture.

Antimicrobial susceptibility of *L. intracellularis* was first reported by McOrist and colleagues (103) and McOrist and Gebhart (104). However, only three isolates were tested. The most comprehensive antimicrobial susceptibility study to date assessed the antimicrobial susceptibility of 10 North American ($n = 6$) and European ($n = 4$) *L. intracellularis* isolates (enough isolates to calculate MIC_{50} and MIC_{90} values) against carbadox, chlortetracycline, lincomycin, tiamulin, tylosin, and valnemulin (101). When tested for intracellular activity, carbadox, tiamulin, and valnemulin were most active (MICs of ≤ 0.5 mg/liter), tylosin MICs ranged from 0.25 to 32 mg/liter, and chlortetracycline (MICs of 0.125 to 64 mg/liter) and lincomycin (MICs of 8 to >128 mg/liter) were the least active (Table 3). Similar results were obtained when the isolates were tested for extracellular activity; however, MICs were often several $\log_2$ dilutions higher compared to their intracellular MICs, with only valnemulin showing high extracellular activity (MIC range, 0.125 to 4 mg/liter). Importantly, these results showed that *Lawsonia* isolates differ significantly in their susceptibility to common antimicrobial agents used in pig production. There was also a general trend for carbadox, chlortetracycline, lincomy-

cin, and tylosin MICs to be several $\log_2$ dilutions higher for North American isolates compared to European isolates, but the numbers of isolates are too low to confirm this trend with confidence. While there are no antimicrobial MIC breakpoints for intracellular organisms using a tissue culture system, making interpretation of the susceptibility data difficult, the results do suggest that *L. intracellularis* strains may develop resistance to some antimicrobial agents. The disparity between intracellular and extracellular MICs could be a true reflection of activity or may be due to variations in the protocol such as exposure time, or the accumulation of antimicrobial inside the cell, which may explain the higher activity of macrolides compared to other drug classes.

Yeh et al. (99) followed up this study by assessing two Asian strains of *L. intracellularis* for susceptibility against a total of 16 antimicrobial agents (lincomycin, carbadox, ampicillin, penicillin, tiamulin, chlortetracycline, bacitracin, colistin, tylosin, gentamicin, kanamycin, neomycin, spectinomycin, streptomycin, enrofloxacin, and tilmicosin). Interestingly, they found both tylosin (intracellular activity, 0.25 to 0.5 mg/liter; extracellular activity 1 mg/liter) and tilmicosin (intracellular activity, 0.25 to 2 mg/liter; extracellular activity 4 to 32 mg/liter) to be the most active antimicrobial agents against the two strains *in vitro*. Enrofloxacin MICs ranged from 2 to 4 mg/liter for intracellular activity and 8 to 16 mg/liter for extracellular activity, confirming that fluoroquinolones have relatively poor activity against *L. intracellularis*.

Antimicrobial agents shown to be efficacious in the field against *L. intracellularis* infection in pigs include tylosin, tiamulin, and tetracyclines. Following the European ban on use of antimicrobial agents with a growth-promotion claim, *L. intracellularis* (together with *E. coli*) was one of the pathogens that increased in prevalence, requiring a slight increase in therapeutic antimicrobial use (105). In young horses, antimicrobial agents recommended for therapy include macrolides (e.g., erythromycin), alone or in combination with rifampicin, chloramphenicol, oxytetracycline, doxycycline, or minocycline (106). The availability of an effective live *L. intracellularis* vaccine has resulted in reduced use of antimicrobial agents for the prevention and treatment of PPE (107).

In a randomized clinical trial conducted with nursery pigs, batch treatment with oxytetracycline for 5 days was superior in preventing high-level *Lawsonia* shedding and diarrhea compared to treatment of diarrheic pens or individual diarrheic pigs (108). Furthermore, no significant difference in the proportion of tetracycline-resistant coliforms was observed between treatment types (109). Additionally, orally administered oxytetracycline at a high dose was more effective at preventing high-level shedding and symptoms of diarrhea compared to a low dose (110). However, in some circumstances, complete elimination of the organism by antimicrobial agents can leave herds immunologically naive and thus prone to porcine hemorrhagic enteropathy at an older age (111). For example, low-level inclusion in the diet of olaquindox in countries where it is still registered for use in livestock provides a bacteriostatic effect, protecting against disease but allowing pigs to seroconvert at a younger age (P. McKenzie, personal communication).

Despite the limited number of *in vitro* studies showing some variation in the MICs of several antimicrobial agents that have been used in the treatment/prevention of PPE, There are few reports in the literature of antimicrobial resistance in *Lawsonia* isolates, and the genetic basis of resistance in strains with elevated MICs has not been determined.

Acknowledgments. The authors acknowledge the editorial assistance of Terence Lee.

Citation. Trott DJ, Abraham S, and Ben Adler B. 2018. Antimicrobial resistance in *Leptospira*, *Brucella*, and other rarely investigated veterinary and zoonotic pathogens. Microbiol Spectrum 6(3):ARBA-0029-2017.

References

1. Adler B, de la Peña Moctezuma A. 2010. *Leptospira* and leptospirosis. *Vet Microbiol* 140:287–296.

2. Fouts DE, Matthias MA, Adhikarla H, Adler B, Amorim-Santos L, Berg DE, Bulach D, Buschiazzo A, Chang Y-F, Galloway RL, Haake DA, Haft DH, Hartskeerl R, Ko AI, Levett PN, Matsunaga J, Mechaly AE, Monk JM, Nascimento ALT, Nelson KE, Palsson B, Peacock SJ, Picardeau M, Ricaldi JN, Thaipandungpanit J, Wunder EA Jr, Yang XF, Zhang J-J, Vinetz JM. 2016. What makes a bacterial species pathogenic? Comparative genomic analysis of the genus *Leptospira*. *PLoS Negl Trop Dis* 10:e0004403.

3. Adler B, Faine S, Christopher WL, Chappel RJ. 1986. Development of an improved selective medium for isolation of leptospires from clinical material. *Vet Microbiol* 12:377–381.

4. Cousineau JG, McKiel JA. 1961. *In vitro* sensitivity of *Leptospira* to varioqs antimicrobial agents. *Can J Microbiol* 7:751–758.

5. Schönberg A. 1981. Studies on the effect of antibiotic substances on leptospires and their cultivation from material with a high bacterial count. *Zentralbl Bakteriol A* 249:400–406.

6. Vinod Kumar K, Lall C, Raj RV, Vedhagiri K, Sunish IP, Vijayachari P. 2016. *In vitro* antimicrobial susceptibility

of pathogenic *Leptospira* biofilm. *Microb Drug Resist* 22:511–514.

7. Moreno LZ, Miraglia F, Lilenbaum W, Neto JSF, Freitas JC, Morais ZM, Hartskeerl RA, da Costa BLP, Vasconcellos SA, Moreno AM. 2016. Profiling of *Leptospira interrogans*, *L. santarosai*, *L. meyeri* and *L. borgpetersenii* by SE-AFLP, PFGE and susceptibility testing: a continuous attempt at species and serovar differentiation. *Emerg Microbes Infect* 5:e17.

8. Faine S, Kaipainen WJ. 1955. Erythromycin in experimental leptospirosis. *J Infect Dis* 97:146–151.

9. Moon JE, Ellis MW, Griffith ME, Hawley JS, Rivard RG, McCall S, Hospenthal DR, Murray CK. 2006. Efficacy of macrolides and telithromycin against leptospirosis in a hamster model. *Antimicrob Agents Chemother* 50:1989–1992.

10. Griffith ME, Moon JE, Johnson EN, Clark KP, Hawley JS, Hospenthal DR, Murray CK. 2007. Efficacy of fluoroquinolones against *Leptospira interrogans* in a hamster model. *Antimicrob Agents Chemother* 51:2615–2617.

11. Harris BM, Blatz PJ, Hinkle MK, McCall S, Beckius ML, Mende K, Robertson JL, Griffith ME, Murray CK, Hospenthal DR. 2011. *In vitro* and *in vivo* activity of first generation cephalosporins against *Leptospira*. *Am J Trop Med Hyg* 85:905–908.

12. Alt DP, Zuerner RL, Bolin CA. 2001. Evaluation of antibiotics for treatment of cattle infected with *Leptospira borgpetersenii* serovar Hardjo. *J Am Vet Med Assoc* 219:636–639.

13. Haake DA, Levett PN. 2015. Leptospirosis in humans, p 65–97. *In* Adler B (ed), *Leptospira and Leptospirosis*. Springer, Berlin, Germany.

14. Ellis WA. 2015. Animal leptospirosis, p 99–137. *In* Adler B (ed), *Leptospira and Leptospirosis*. Springer, Berlin, Germany.

15. Kim D, Kordick D, Divers T, Chang Y-F. 2006. *In vitro* susceptibilities of *Leptospira* spp. and *Borrelia burgdorferi* isolates to amoxicillin, tilmicosin, and enrofloxacin. *J Vet Sci* 7:355–359.

16. Olsen SC, Palmer MV. 2014. Advancement of knowledge of *Brucella* over the past 50 years. *Vet Pathol* 51:1076–1089.

17. Centers for Disease Control and Prevention. 2017. *Bioterrorism agents/diseases*. https://emergency.cdc.gov/agent/agentlist-category.asp.

18. Marianelli C, Graziani C, Santangelo C, Xibilia MT, Imbriani A, Amato R, Neri D, Cuccia M, Rinnone S, Di Marco V, Ciuchini F. 2007. Molecular epidemiological and antibiotic susceptibility characterization of *Brucella* isolates from humans in Sicily, Italy. *J Clin Microbiol* 45:2923–2928.

19. Leiser OP, Corn JL, Schmit BS, Keim PS, Foster JT. 2013. Feral swine brucellosis in the United States and prospective genomic techniques for disease epidemiology. *Vet Microbiol* 166:1–10.

20. Ramamoorthy S, Woldemeskel M, Ligett A, Snider R, Cobb R, Rajeev S. 2011. *Brucella suis* infection in dogs, Georgia, USA. *Emerg Infect Dis* 17:2386–2387.

21. James DR, Golovsky G, Thornton JM, Goodchild L, Havlicek M, Martin P, Krockenberger MB, Marriott D, Ahuja V, Malik R, Mor SM. 2017. Clinical management of *Brucella suis* infection in dogs and implications for public health. *Aust Vet J* 95:19–25.

22. Norton TH, Thomas AD. 1976. Letter: *Brucella suis* in feral pigs. *Aust Vet J* 52:293–294.

23. Eales KM, Norton RE, Ketheesan N. 2010. Brucellosis in northern Australia. *Am J Trop Med Hyg* 83:876–878.

24. Irwin MJ, Massey PD, Walker B, Durrheim DN. 2009. Feral pig hunting: a risk factor for human brucellosis in north-west NSW? *N S W Public Health Bull* 20:192–194.

25. Mor SM, Wiethoelter AK, Lee A, Moloney B, James DR, Malik R. 2016. Emergence of *Brucella suis* in dogs in New South Wales, Australia: clinical findings and implications for zoonotic transmission. *BMC Vet Res* 12:199.

26. Lonsway DR, Jevitt LA, Uhl JR, Cockerill FR III, Anderson ME, Sullivan MM, De BK, Edwards JR, Patel JB. 2010. Effect of carbon dioxide on broth microdilution susceptibility testing of *Brucella* spp. *J Clin Microbiol* 48:952–956.

27. Bayram Y, Korkoca H, Aypak C, Parlak M, Cikman A, Kilic S, Berktas M. 2011. Antimicrobial susceptibilities of *Brucella* isolates from various clinical specimens. *Int J Med Sci* 8:198–202.

28. Ariza J, Bosch J, Gudiol F, Liñares J, Viladrich PF, Martín R. 1986. Relevance of *in vitro* antimicrobial susceptibility of *Brucella melitensis* to relapse rate in human brucellosis. *Antimicrob Agents Chemother* 30:958–960.

29. Brown SD, Traczewski MM, the Brucella QC Working Group. 2005. Broth microdilution susceptibility testing of *Brucella* species: quality control limits for ten antimicrobial agents against three standard quality control strains. *J Clin Microbiol* 43:5804–5807.

30. Bosch J, Liñares J, López de Goicoechea MJ, Ariza J, Cisnal MC, Martin R. 1986. *In-vitro* activity of ciprofloxacin, ceftriaxone and five other antimicrobial agents against 95 strains of *Brucella melitensis*. *J Antimicrob Chemother* 17:459–461.

31. Clinical and Laboratory Standards Institute. 2010. *Performance standards for antimicrobial susceptibility testing*. CLSI, Wayne, PA.

32. Barbosa Pauletti R, Reinato Stynen AP, Pinto da Silva Mol J, Seles Dorneles EM, Alves TM, de Sousa Moura Souto M, Minharro S, Heinemann MB, Lage AP. 2015. Reduced susceptibility to rifampicin and resistance to multiple antimicrobial agents among *Brucella abortus* isolates from cattle in Brazil. *PLoS One* 10:e0132532.

33. Clinical and Laboratory Standards Institute. 2015. *Methods for antimicrobial dilution and disk susceptibility testing of infrequently isolates or fastidious bacteria, 3rd ed.* CLSI guidline M45. CLSI, Wayne PA.

34. Solís García del Pozo J, Solera J. 2012. Systematic review and meta-analysis of randomized clinical trials in the treatment of human brucellosis. *PLoS One* 7:e32090.

35. Ariza J, Bosilkovski M, Cascio A, Colmenero JD, Corbel MJ, Falagas ME, Memish ZA, Roushan MRH, Rubinstein E, Sipsas NV, Solera J, Young EJ, Pappas G, International Society of Chemotherapy, Institute of Continuing Medical Education of Ioannina. 2007. Perspectives for the treatment of brucellosis in the 21st century: the Ioannina recommendations. *PLoS Med* 4:e317.

36. Bertrand A. 1994. Antibiotic treatment of brucellosis. *Presse Med* 23:1128–1131. (In French).

37. Bayindir Y, Sonmez E, Aladag A, Buyukberber N. 2003. Comparison of five antimicrobial regimens for the treatment of brucellar spondylitis: a prospective, randomized study. *J Chemother* 15:466–471.

38. Nicoletti PL, Quinn BR, Minor PW. 1967. Canine to human transmission of brucellosis. *N Y State J Med* 67:2886–2887.

39. Mateu-de-Antonio EM, Martín M. 1995. *In vitro* efficacy of several antimicrobial combinations against *Brucella canis* and *Brucella melitensis* strains isolated from dogs. *Vet Microbiol* 45:1–10.

40. Guerra MA, Nicoletti P. 1986. Comparison of the susceptibility of *Brucella abortus* isolates obtained before and after cows were treated with oxytetracycline and streptomycin. *Am J Vet Res* 47:2612–2613.

41. Hall WH, Spink WW. 1947. *In vitro* sensitivity of *Brucella* to streptomycin; development of resistance during streptomycin treatment. *Proc Soc Exp Biol Med* 64:403–406.

42. Balandin GA. 1967. Ampicillin and brucellas. *Antibiotiki* 12:828–830. (In Russian.)

43. Lal S, Modawal KK, Fowle AS, Peach B, Popham RD. 1970. Acute brucellosis treated with trimethoprim and sulphamethoxazole. *BMJ* 3:256–257.

44. Qadri SM, Akhtar M, Ueno Y, al-Sibai MB. 1989. Susceptibility of *Brucella melitensis* to fluoroquinolones. *Drugs Exp Clin Res* 15:483–485.

45. De Rautlin de la Roy YM, Grignon B, Grollier G, Coindreau MF, Becq-Giraudon B. 1986. Rifampicin resistance in a strain of *Brucella melitensis* after treatment with doxycycline and rifampicin. *J Antimicrob Chemother* 18:648–649.

46. Reynes E, López G, Ayala SM, Hunter GC, Lucero NE. 2012. Monitoring infected dogs after a canine brucellosis outbreak. *Comp Immunol Microbiol Infect Dis* 35:533–537.

47. Falagas ME, Bliziotis IA. 2006. Quinolones for treatment of human brucellosis: critical review of the evidence from microbiological and clinical studies. *Antimicrob Agents Chemother* 50:22–33.

48. Kocagöz S, Akova M, Altun B, Gür D, Hasçelik G. 2002. *In vitro* activities of new quinolones against *Brucella melitensis* isolated in a tertiary-care hospital in Turkey. *Clin Microbiol Infect* 8:240–242.

49. Sayan M, Kılıc S, Uyanık MH. 2012. Epidemiological survey of rifampicin resistance in clinic isolates of *Brucella melitensis* obtained from all regions of Turkey. *J Infect Chemother* 18:41–46.

50. Maves RC, Castillo R, Guillen A, Espinosa B, Meza R, Espinoza N, Núñez G, Sánchez L, Chacaltana J, Cepeda D, González S, Hall ER. 2011. Antimicrobial

susceptibility of *Brucella melitensis* isolates in Peru. *Antimicrob Agents Chemother* 55:1279–1281.

51. Jiang H, Mao L, Zhao H-y, Li LY, Piao D, Yao WQ, Cui BY. 2010. MLVA typing and antibioticantimicrobial agent susceptibility of *Brucella* human isolates from Liaoning, China. *Trans R Soc Trop Med Hyg* 104:796–800.

52. Ariza J, Gudiol F, Pallarés R, Rufí G, Fernández-Viladrich P. 1985. Comparative trial of rifampin-doxycycline versus tetracycline-streptomycin in the therapy of human brucellosis. *Antimicrob Agents Chemother* 28:548–551.

53. Ariza J, Gudiol F, Pallares R, Viladrich PF, Rufi G, Corredoira J, Miravitlles MR. 1992. Treatment of human brucellosis with doxycycline plus rifampin or doxycycline plus streptomycin. A randomized, double-blind study. *Ann Intern Med* 117:25–30.

54. Baykam N, Esener H, Ergönül O, Eren S, Çelikbas AK, Dokuzoğuz B. 2004. *In vitro* antimicrobial susceptibility of *Brucella* species. *Int J Antimicrob Agents* 23:405–407.

55. Dimitrov TS, Panigrahi D, Emara M, Al-Nakkas A, Awni F, Passadilla R. 2005. Incidence of bloodstream infections in a speciality hospital in Kuwait: 8-year experience. *Med Princ Pract* 14:417–421.

56. Abdel-Maksoud M, House B, Wasfy M, Abdel-Rahman B, Pimentel G, Roushdy G, Dueger E. 2012. In vitro antibiotic susceptibility testing of *Brucella* isolates from Egypt between 1999 and 2007 and evidence of probable rifampin resistance. *Ann Clin Microbiol Antimicrob* 11:24.

57. Torkaman Asadi F, Hashemi SH, Alikhani MY, Moghimbeigi A, Naseri Z. 2017. Clinical and diagnostic aspects of brucellosis and antimicrobial susceptibility of *Brucella* isolates in Hamedan, Iran. *Jpn J Infect Dis* 70:235–238.

58. Razzaghi R, Rastegar R, Momen-Heravi M, Erami M, Nazeri M. 2016. Antimicrobial susceptibility testing of *Brucella melitensis* isolated from patients with acute brucellosis in a centre of Iran. *Indian J Med Microbiol* 34:342–345.

59. Sayan M, Yumuk Z, Dündar D, Bilenoğlu O, Erdenliğ S, Yaşar E, Willke A. 2008. Rifampicin resistance phenotyping of *Brucella melitensis* by rpoB gene analysis in clinical isolates. *J Chemother* 20:431–435.

60. al-Sibai MB, Qadri SM. 1990. Development of ciprofloxacin resistance in *Brucella melitensis*. *J Antimicrob Chemother* 25:302–303.

61. Memish Z, Mah MW, Al Mahmoud S, Al Shaalan M, Khan MY. 2000. *Brucella* bacteraemia: clinical and laboratory observations in 160 patients. *J Infect* 40:59–63.

62. Bannatyne RM, Rich M, Memish ZA. 2001. Cotrimoxazole resistant *Brucella*. *J Trop Pediatr* 47:60.

63. Almuneef M, Memish ZA, Al Shaalan M, Al Banyan E, Al-Alola S, Balkhy HH. 2003. *Brucella melitensis* bacteremia in children: review of 62 cases. *J Chemother* 15:76–80.

64. Shaalan MA, Memish ZA, Mahmoud SA, Alomari A, Khan MY, Almuneef M, Alalola S. 2002. Brucellosis in children: clinical observations in 115 cases. *Int J Infect Dis* 6:182–186.

65. Heo E-J, Kang S-I, Kim J-W, Her M, Cho D, Cho Y-S, Hwang I-Y, Moon J-S, Wee S-H, Jung S-C, Nam HM. 2012. *In vitro* activities of antimicrobials against *Brucella abortus* isolates from cattle in Korea during 1998-2006. *J Microbiol Biotechnol* 22:567–570.

66. Marianelli C, Ciuchini F, Tarantino M, Pasquali P, Adone R. 2004. Genetic bases of the rifampin resistance phenotype in *Brucella* spp. *J Clin Microbiol* 42:5439–5443.

67. Sandalakis V, Psaroulaki A, De Bock P-J, Christidou A, Gevaert K, Tsiotis G, Tselentis Y. 2012. Investigation of rifampicin resistance mechanisms in *Brucella abortus* using MS-driven comparative proteomics. *J Proteome Res* 11:2374–2385.

68. Turkmani A, Psaroulaki A, Christidou A, Samoilis G, Mourad TA, Tabaa D, Tselentis Y. 2007. Uptake of ciprofloxacin and ofloxacin by 2 *Brucella* strains and their fluoroquinolone-resistant variants under different conditions. An *in vitro* study. *Diagn Microbiol Infect Dis* 59:447–451.

69. Turkmani A, Psaroulaki A, Christidou A, Chochlakis D, Tabaa D, Tselentis Y. 2008. *In vitro*-selected resistance to fluoroquinolones in two *Brucella* strains associated with mutational changes in *gyrA*. *Int J Antimicrob Agents* 32:227–232.

70. Ravanel N, Gestin B, Maurin M. 2009. *In vitro* selection of fluoroquinolone resistance in *Brucella melitensis*. *Int J Antimicrob Agents* 34:76–81.

71. Lázaro FG, Rodríguez-Tarazona RE, García-Rodríguez JÁ, Muñoz-Bellido JL. 2009. Fluoroquinolone-resistant *Brucella melitensis* mutants obtained *in vitro*. *Int J Antimicrob Agents* 34:252–254.

72. Valdezate S, Navarro A, Medina-Pascual MJ, Carrasco G, Saéz-Nieto JA. 2010. Molecular screening for rifampicin and fluoroquinolone resistance in a clinical population of *Brucella melitensis*. *J Antimicrob Chemother* 65:51–53.

73. Feng J, Auwaerter PG, Zhang Y. 2015. Drug combinations against *Borrelia burgdorferi* persisters *in vitro*: eradication achieved by using daptomycin, cefoperazone and doxycycline. *PLoS One* 10:e0117207.

74. Stefancikóva A, Adaszek Ł, Pet'ko B, Winiarczyk S, Dudinák V. 2008. Serological evidence of *Borrelia burgdorferi sensu lato* in horses and cattle from Poland and diagnostic problems of Lyme borreliosis. *Ann Agric Environ Med* 15:37–43.

75. Stefancíkóva A, Stěpánová G, Derdákóva M, Pet'ko B, Kysel'ová J, Cigánek J, Strojný L, Cislákóva L, Trávnicek M. 2002. Serological evidence for *Borrelia burgdorferi* infection associated with clinical signs in dairy cattle in Slovakia. *Vet Res Commun* 26:601–611.

76. Ogden NH, Nuttall PA, Randolph SE. 1997. Natural Lyme disease cycles maintained via sheep by co-feeding ticks. *Parasitology* 115:591–599.

77. Littman MP, Goldstein RE, Labato MA, Lappin MR, Moore GE. 2006. ACVIM small animal consensus statement on Lyme disease in dogs: diagnosis, treatment, and prevention. *J Vet Intern Med* 20:422–434.

78. Hunfeld K-P, Kraiczy P, Kekoukh E, Schäfer V, Brade V. 2002. Standardised *in vitro* susceptibility testing of *Borrelia burgdorferi* against well-known and newly developed antimicrobial agents: possible implications for new therapeutic approaches to Lyme disease. *Int J Med Microbiol* 291(Suppl 33):125–137.

79. Ates L, Hanssen-Hübner C, Norris DE, Richter D, Kraiczy P, Hunfeld K-P. 2010. Comparison of *in vitro* activities of tigecycline, doxycycline, and tetracycline against the spirochete *Borrelia burgdorferi*. *Ticks Tick Borne Dis* 1:30–34.

80. Dever LL, Jorgensen JH, Barbour AG. 1992. *In vitro* antimicrobial susceptibility testing of *Borrelia burgdorferi*: a microdilution MIC method and time-kill studies. *J Clin Microbiol* 30:2692–2697.

81. Hunfeld K-P, Kraiczy P, Wichelhaus TA, Schäfer V, Brade V. 2000. New colorimetric microdilution method for *in vitro* susceptibility testing of *Borrelia burgdorferi* against antimicrobial substances. *Eur J Clin Microbiol Infect Dis* 19:27–32.

82. Embers ME, Barthold SW, Borda JT, Bowers L, Doyle L, Hodzic E, Jacobs MB, Hasenkampf NR, Martin DS, Narasimhan S, Phillippi-Falkenstein KM, Purcell JE, Ratterree MS, Philipp MT. 2012. Persistence of *Borrelia burgdorferi* in rhesus macaques following antibiotic treatment of disseminated infection. *PLoS One* 7:e29914.

83. Hunfeld K-P, Brade V. 2006. Antimicrobial susceptibility of *Borrelia burgdorferi sensu lato*: what we know, what we don't know, and what we need to know. *Wien Klin Wochenschr* 118:659–668.

84. Terekhova D, Sartakova ML, Wormser GP, Schwartz I, Cabello FC. 2002. Erythromycin resistance in *Borrelia burgdorferi*. *Antimicrob Agents Chemother* 46:3637–3640.

85. Jackson CR, Boylan JA, Frye JG, Gherardini FC. 2007. Evidence of a conjugal erythromycin resistance element in the Lyme disease spirochete *Borrelia burgdorferi*. *Int J Antimicrob Agents* 30:496–504.

86. Samuels DS, Marconi RT, Huang WM, Garon CF. 1994. *gyrB* mutations in coumermycin A1-resistant *Borrelia burgdorferi*. *J Bacteriol* 176:3072–3075.

87. Criswell D, Tobiason VL, Lodmell JS, Samuels DS. 2006. Mutations conferring aminoglycoside and spectinomycin resistance in *Borrelia burgdorferi*. *Antimicrob Agents Chemother* 50:445–452.

88. Galbraith KM, Ng AC, Eggers BJ, Kuchel CR, Eggers CH, Samuels DS. 2005. *parC* mutations in fluoroquinolone-resistant *Borrelia burgdorferi*. *Antimicrob Agents Chemother* 49:4354–4357.

89. Bunikis I, Denker K, Östberg Y, Andersen C, Benz R, Bergström S. 2008. An RND-type efflux system in *Borrelia burgdorferi* is involved in virulence and resistance to antimicrobial compounds. *PLoS Pathog* 4:e1000009.

90. Hunfeld K-P, Ruzic-Sabljic E, Norris DE, Kraiczy P, Strle F. 2005. *In vitro* susceptibility testing of *Borrelia burgdorferi sensu lato* isolates cultured from patients with erythema migrans before and after antimicrobial chemotherapy. *Antimicrob Agents Chemother* 49: 1294–1301.

91. Sharma B, Brown AV, Matluck NE, Hu LT, Lewis K. 2015. *Borrelia burgdorferi*, the causative agent of Lyme disease, forms drug-tolerant persister cells. *Antimicrob Agents Chemother* 59:4616–4624.

92. Sapi E, Kaur N, Anyanwu S, Luecke DF, Datar A, Patel S, Rossi M, Stricker RB. 2011. Evaluation of *in-vitro* antibiotic susceptibility of different morphological forms of *Borrelia burgdorferi*. *Infect Drug Resist* 4:97–113.

93. Sapi E, Theophilus PA, Pham TV, Burugu D, Luecke DF. 2016. Effect of RpoN, RpoS and LuxS pathways on the biofilm formation and antibiotic sensitivity of *Borrelia burgdorferi*. *Eur J Microbiol Immunol (Bp)* 6: 272–286.

94. Zimmerman JJ, Karriker LA, Ramirez A, Schwartz KJ, Stevenson GW. 2012. *Diseases of Swine*, 10 ed. Wiley-Blackwell, Chichester, UK.

95. Page AE, Slovis NM, Horohov DW. 2014. *Lawsonia intracellularis* and equine proliferative enteropathy. *Vet Clin North Am Equine Pract* 30:641–658.

96. Page AE, Fallon LH, Bryant UK, Horohov DW, Luna TW, Marsh PS, Slovis NM, Sprayberry KA, Loynachan AT. 2012. Acute deterioration and death with necrotizing enteritis associated with *Lawsonia intracellularis* in 4 weanling horses. *J Vet Intern Med* 26:1476–1480.

97. Vannucci FA, Gebhart CJ. 2014. Recent advances in understanding the pathogenesis of *Lawsonia intracellularis* infections. *Vet Pathol* 51:465–477.

98. McOrist S, Gebhart CJ, Boid R, Barns SM. 1995. Characterization of *Lawsonia intracellularis* gen. nov., sp. nov., the obligately intracellular bacterium of porcine proliferative enteropathy. *Int J Syst Bacteriol* 45:820–825.

99. Yeh J-Y, Lee J-H, Yeh H-R, Kim A, Lee JY, Hwang J-M, Kang B-K, Kim J-M, Choi I-S, Lee J-B. 2011. Antimicrobial susceptibility testing of two *Lawsonia intracellularis* isolates associated with proliferative hemorrhagic enteropathy and porcine intestinal adenomatosis in South Korea. *Antimicrob Agents Chemother* 55:4451–4453.

100. McOrist S, Smith SH, Shearn MF, Carr MM, Miller DJ. 1996. Treatment and prevention of porcine proliferative enteropathy with oral tiamulin. *Vet Rec* 139:615–618.

101. Wattanaphansak S, Singer RS, Gebhart CJ. 2009. *In vitro* antimicrobial activity against 10 North American and European *Lawsonia intracellularis* isolates. *Vet Microbiol* 134:305–310.

102. Vannucci FA, Wattanaphansak S, Gebhart CJ. 2012. An alternative method for cultivation of *Lawsonia intracellularis*. *J Clin Microbiol* 50:1070–1072.

103. McOrist S, Mackie RA, Lawson GH. 1995. Antimicrobial susceptibility of ileal symbiont intracellularis isolated from pigs with proliferative enteropathy. *J Clin Microbiol* 33:1314–1317.

104. McOrist S, Gebhart J. 1995. *In vitro* testing of antimicrobial agents for proliferative enteropathy (ileitis). *Swine Health Prod* 3:146–149.

105. Casewell M, Friis C, Marco E, McMullin P, Phillips I. 2003. The European ban on growth-promoting antibiotics and emerging consequences for human and animal health. *J Antimicrob Chemother* 52:159–161.

106. Pusterla N, Gebhart C. 2013. *Lawsonia intracellularis* infection and proliferative enteropathy in foals. *Vet Microbiol* 167:34–41.

107. Bak H, Rathkjen PH. 2009. Reduced use of antimicrobials after vaccination of pigs against porcine proliferative enteropathy in a Danish SPF herd. *Acta Vet Scand* 51:1.

108. Larsen I, Nielsen SS, Olsen JE, Nielsen JP. 2016. The efficacy of oxytetracycline treatment at batch, pen and individual level on *Lawsonia intracellularis* infection in nursery pigs in a randomised clinical trial. *Prev Vet Med* 124:25–33.

109. Græsbøll K, Damborg P, Mellerup A, Herrero-Fresno A, Larsen I, Holm A, Nielsen JP, Christiansen LE, Angen Ø, Ahmed S, Folkesson A, Olsen JE. 2017. Effect of tetracycline dose and treatment mode on selection of resistant coliform bacteria in nursery pigs. *Appl Environ Microbiol* 83:e00538-17.

110. Larsen I, Hjulsager CK, Holm A, Olsen JE, Nielsen SS, Nielsen JP. 2016. A randomised clinical trial on the efficacy of oxytetracycline dose through water medication of nursery pigs on diarrhoea, faecal shedding of *Lawsonia intracellularis* and average daily weight gain. *Prev Vet Med* 123:52–59.

111. Riber U, Cordes H, Boutrup TS, Jensen TK, Heegaard PM, Jungersen G. 2011. Primary infection protects pigs against re-infection with *Lawsonia intracellularis* in experimental challenge studies. *Vet Microbiol* 149:406–414.

112. Cameron GL. 1977. The susceptibility of New Zealand isolates of *Leptospira* to three antibiotics. *N Z Med J* 86:93–94.

113. Prescott JF, Nicholson VM. 1988. Antimicrobial drug susceptibility of *Leptospira interrogans* serovar Hardjo isolated from cattle. *Can J Vet Res* 52:286–287.

114. Murray CK, Hospenthal DR. 2004. Determination of susceptibilities of 26 *Leptospira* sp. serovars to 24 antimicrobial agents by a broth microdilution technique. *Antimicrob Agents Chemother* 48:4002–4005.

115. Chakraborty A, Miyahara S, Villanueva SYAM, Gloriani NG, Yoshida S. 2010. *In vitro* sensitivity and resistance of 46 *Leptospira* strains isolated from rats in the Philippines to 14 antimicrobial agents. *Antimicrob Agents Chemother* 54:5403–5405.

116. Wuthiekanun V, Amornchai P, Paris DH, Langla S, Thaipadunpanit J, Chierakul W, Smythe LD, White NJ, Day NPJ, Limmathurotsakul D, Peacock SJ. 2013. Rapid isolation and susceptibility testing of *Leptospira* spp. using a new solid medium, LVW agar. *Antimicrob Agents Chemother* 57:297–302.

117. Miraglia F, Matsuo M, Morais ZM, Dellagostin OA, Seixas FK, Freitas JC, Hartskeerl R, Moreno LZ, Costa BL, Souza GO, Vasconcellos SA, Moreno AM. 2013. Molecular characterization, serotyping, and antibiotic susceptibility profile of *Leptospira interrogans* serovar Copenhageni isolates from Brazil. *Diagn Microbiol Infect Dis* 77:195–199.

118. Suepaul SM, Carrington C, Campbell M, Borde G, Adesiyun AA. 2015. Antimicrobial susceptibility of *Leptospira* isolates from dogs and rats to 12 antimicrobial agents. *Trop Biomed* 32:1–10.

119. Wuthiekanun V, Amornchai P, Langla S, White NJ, Day NPJ, Limmathurotsakul D, Peacock SJ. 2015. Antimicrobial disk susceptibility testing of *Leptospira* spp. using *Leptospira* Vanaporn Wuthiekanun (LVW) agar. *Am J Trop Med Hyg* 93:241–243.

120. Benacer D, Zain SNM, Ooi PT, Thong KL. 2017. Antimicrobial susceptibility of *Leptospira* spp. isolated from environmental, human and animal sources in Malaysia. *Indian J Med Microbiol* 35:124–128.

Antimicrobial Resistance in Bacteria from Livestock and Companion Animals
Edited by Frank Møller Aarestrup, Stefan Schwarz, Jianzhong Shen, and Lina Cavaco
© 2018 American Society for Microbiology, Washington, DC
doi:10.1128/microbiolspec.ARBA-0003-2017

Antimicrobial Resistance in *Chlamydiales*, *Rickettsia*, *Coxiella*, and Other Intracellular Pathogens

23

Daisy Vanrompay,[1] Thi Loan Anh Nguyen,[1] Sally J. Cutler,[2] and Patrick Butaye[3]

BACKGROUND

The three groups of microbes considered in this article share some general lifestyle features. First, they are all multihost pathogens with the ability to infect diverse species ranging from arthropods, reptiles, and birds to mammalian species including companion animals, livestock, and humans and are thus considered as zoonoses. Second, they are all highly adapted to survival within their intracellular niche and, as such, have undergone significant genomic reduction that is largely responsible for their obligate requirement for intracellular growth (1, 2). This has been partially overcome in the case of *Coxiella*, whereby genomic sequencing provided insights into the nutritional requirements for propagation of this microbe and an axenic medium was subsequently produced (see section below). Both the *Chlamydiales* and *Coxiella* share the ability to produce small cell variants and larger replicative forms. These small cell variants facilitate environmental persistence that is key to long-term survival under adverse conditions.

Challenges for the manipulation of these microbes not only reside in their intracellular nature and thus infrequent *in vitro* investigative studies such as antimicrobial susceptibility testing, but also result from their classification as biosafety level 3 agents, necessitating their handling within suitable containment facilities. Consequently, data on both susceptibility testing and acquisition of resistance mechanisms are sparse. Initially, detection of infection was largely restricted to

serological methods, but more recently, molecular diagnostic approaches are favored and offer the potential to explore well-characterized resistance genes. Furthermore, these groups comprise variants that are considered to be endosymbionts within a range of arthropod species. This potentially offers targets for future development for control of arthropod vectors and their associated pathogens (3).

Chlamydia

In 1879, Jacob Ritter linked multiple pneumonia cases to the import of infected psittacine birds in Switzerland (4), and following a new outbreak in Paris 3 years later, the disease was called psittacosis, after the Greek word for parrot (*psittakos*, "ψιττακος"), the source of the disease (5). In 1907, Halberstaedter and Von Prowazek were the first to describe intracytoplasmatic inclusions containing large numbers of microorganisms in human conjunctival epithelial cells, as well as in orangutans experimentally infected with material from trachoma cases (6). Considered to be protozoa, these organisms were originally called chlamydozoa, after the Greek word *chlamys* ("χλαμῦς") for mantle, because a mantle seemed to surround the particles in Giemsa staining. Because these were not withheld by bacterial filters and because of the inability to grow them on artificial media, they were considered to be of viral origin. During pandemic outbreaks of human psittacosis in 1929–1930, small basophile particles were described in blood and tissues of infected birds and

[1]Department of Animal Production, Faculty of Bioscience Engineering, Ghent University, 9000 Ghent, Belgium; [2]School of Health, Sport, and Bioscience, University of East London, London, United Kingdom; [3]Department of BioSciences, Ross University, School of Veterinary Medicine, Basseterre, Saint Kitts and Nevis, West Indies and Department of Pathology, Bacteriology, and Poultry Diseases, Faculty of Veterinary Medicine, Ghent University, 9820 Merelbeke, Belgium.

humans (7–9), which were isolated shortly thereafter (10). The same year, the pathogenic agent causing lymphogranuloma venereum (a serious genital infection) was isolated from human tissue. Both particles were classified as viruses of the psittacosis-lymphogranuloma venereum group. Only 2 years later, the unique developmental cycle, characteristic of all *Chlamydiales*, was described (11). Although the agent was referred to as an "obligate intracellular parasite with bacterial affinities" (12), it was found to be more closely related to *Rickettsiae* than to bacteria because of its multiplication through binary fission. With the development of electron microscopy and cell culture in 1965, its bacterial nature could no longer be denied. The *Chlamydiaceae* were classified as Gram-negative bacteria because of the structure of their cell wall, the presence of DNA and RNA, a unique replicative cycle, and prokaryotic ribosomes susceptible to antibiotics (13).

Coxiella

Following its original recognition by Edward Derrick in 1937 (14) as a cause of zoonotic infection among abattoir workers with an outbreak of febrile infection in Brisbane, Australia, our understanding of this organism has expanded. Initial analysis of the agent of what became known as "Q fever," for query fever, and its subsequent isolation by Frank Burnet using experimental guinea pig infection coupled with its notable resemblance to *Rickettsia* resulted in the agent initially being called *Rickettsia burnetii*. Later, analogy was drawn between this agent and that recovered by Harold Cox (15) from *Dermacentor andersoni* ticks collected from Nine Mile Valley in Montana, resulting in a name change to *Coxiella burnetii* in recognition, but it was retained within the family *Rickettsiaceae*. With the advent of 16S rRNA phylogeny, and later corroborated by whole-genome sequencing, it was found that this microbe clustered with the gamma subdivision of *Proteobacteria*—hence its reclassification into the family *Francisellaceae* (16).

For many years *C. burnetii* was believed to be monophyletic, but not only have accumulating data shown significant sequence divergence within this species, with an excess of 35 genotypes (17), but additionally, new species have been proposed within the genus *Coxiella*, which has been divided into four clades, with *C. burnetii* being derived from clade A, closest to genotypes found residing among soft *Ornithodoros* tick species (16). Many of these appear to be endosymbionts of ticks, but their pathogenic potential is yet to be determined.

Rickettsia

Members of this genus have been described since 1906, with the initial description by Howard Ricketts of the causative agent of Rocky Mountain spotted fever (18). These early investigations demonstrated the association with tick vectors responsible for transmission of infection to humans. This microbe became known as *Rickettsia rickettsii* in honor of Ricketts' work. This was soon followed by the discovery of the agent of epidemic typhus, *Rickettsia prowazekii*, which unlike the aforementioned, was transmitted by the human clothing louse *Pediculus humanus* (19). Since these early descriptions, a plethora of other rickettsial species have been described, vectored mostly by ticks but also by other arthropod species. This group resides within the alpha-proteobacteria and are obligate intracellular pathogens with a Gram-negative cell wall structure. As a group, they are generally considered to fall into two clusters: the typhus group and spotted fever groups. However, this has been challenged over recent years with the description of transitional and ancestral lineages that disrupt this model (20). These organisms, unlike the examples above, rapidly escape from the phagocytic vacuole, typically multiplying within the cytoplasm of endothelial cells of their vertebrate host (21–23).

Application of molecular techniques has resulted in the description of many new species, mostly within the spotted fever group, but several remain with *Candidatus* status through their lack of cultivable strains. Indeed, this difficulty in obtaining isolates of this biosafety level 3 pathogen has hampered the assessment of its susceptibility testing to antimicrobial agents (24–26).

VETERINARY IMPORTANCE

Chlamydia

Members of the family *Chlamydiaceae* are obligate, intracellular, Gram-negative bacteria that cause a variety of diseases in humans, other mammals, and birds. They have a serious impact on both human and animal health and are therefore of major economic importance worldwide. The primary sites of replication are mucosal epithelial cells of the respiratory, urogenital, and gastrointestinal tracts; the conjunctival epithelium; and monocytes and macrophages (27). Currently, 11 *Chlamydia* species are identified, and some of the animal pathogens are well-known zoonotic agents (*Chlamydia psittaci* and *Chlamydia abortus*). Other species were occasionally found to be transmitted from animals to humans (*Chlamydia avium*, *Chlamydia caviae*, *Chlamydia felis*,

Chlamydia gallinacea) (28, 29). Recently, *Chlamydia suis* has been emerging in industrial swine production. The agent is mainly associated with conjunctivitis and reproductive failure and was also found in the human eye (30–32).

Currently, infections are treated with antibiotics. Generally, tetracyclines (chlortetracycline, oxytetracycline, and doxycycline) are the drugs of choice to control the disease because they are highly effective and they have (i) a low cost, (ii) a broad spectrum of activity, (iii) low toxicity, and (iv) excellent tissue distribution. Quinolones (enrofloxacin) or macrolides (erythromycin) can be administered in case of an infection with a tetracycline-resistant *C. suis* strain (33). The rest of this section on *Chlamydia* focuses on the major zoonotic pathogens *C. psittaci* and *C. abortus* and on *C. suis* as an emerging *Chlamydia* species in pigs that is transmitted to humans.

C. psittaci

C. psittaci infections have been reported in over 500 species of birds, where infection is either latent or can become systemic and clinically overt in the respiratory tract (34). The symptoms include conjunctivitis, anorexia, nasal discharge, rhinitis, diarrhea, polyuria, dyspnea, and dullness (35). *C. psittaci* is an important zoonotic pathogen. In humans, *C. psittaci* infections can vary from mild flu-like symptoms to a life-threatening pneumonia (36–38). Symptoms commonly reported are high fever, difficulty breathing and a nonproductive cough, low pulse, chills, headache, and myalgia. Transmission of *C. psittaci* occurs horizontally via inhalation of infected aerosols of pharyngeal or nasal excretions or dry feces and vertically via the eggshell (39). Sequencing of the *C. psittaci* major outer membrane protein (*ompA*) gene identified nine genotypes (A to F, E/B, M56, and WC) (40). The genotypes cluster with host species (41). Genotypes A and B are associated with psittacine birds (cockatoos, parrots, parakeets, and lories) and pigeons, respectively. Genotype C has been isolated from ducks and geese, whereas genotype D was found mainly in turkeys. The host range of genotype E is more diverse, since it has been isolated from pigeons, ratites, ducks, turkeys, and occasionally humans. Genotype F was isolated from psittacine birds and turkeys. Genotype E/B has been isolated mainly from ducks (40, 41). Genotypes WC and M56 represent isolates from epizootics in cattle and muskrats, respectively (42, 43). In contrast to *C. felis* and *C. abortus*, for which live attenuated and inactivated whole-organism vaccines are commercially available, there are no registered vaccines against *C. psittaci* to date.

C. abortus

C. abortus is phylogenetically closely related to *C. psittaci* (44). The species mainly infects small ruminants, but it can also be found in pigs and wild boars (45, 46). Chlamydial strains from ruminant abortion were formerly classified as serotype 1, biotype 1, immunotype 1, or outer membrane protein A (*ompA*) gene type B577 of ruminant *Chlamydiae* (47–50). *C. abortus* is recognized as a major cause of stillbirth and abortion in sheep, goats, and cattle in Europe, North America, and Africa (51). It is the etiological cause of ovine enzootic abortion. *C. abortus* has also been associated with abortion in pigs and horses (52). In addition, pregnant women working with animals infected with *C. abortus* are at risk because the agent can cause abortion, stillbirth, or premature delivery in humans (53–60).

C. suis

C. suis seems to be common and widespread in pigs (45). Recently, chlamydial species-specific nucleic acid amplification tests such as real-time PCR and microarray have been developed, which make it possible to examine the prevalence of *C. suis* in pigs (61–64). *C. suis* has been associated with arthritis, pericarditis, and polyserositis in piglets (65) and diarrhea (66), conjunctivitis (67), and the periparturient dysgalactiae syndrome in sows (68). In sows, *C. suis* was also the cause of vaginal discharge, endometritis, and poor reproductive performance such as return to estrus, abortion, mummification, delivery of weak piglets, and increased perinatal and neonatal mortality (45, 68–71). *C. suis* infections in boars have been correlated with orchitis, epididymitis, urethritis, and inferior semen quality (45, 72).

C. suis is phylogenetically closely related to the human pathogen *Chlamydia trachomatis* (42) and hence might be a potential zoonotic pathogen (45). Recently, *C. suis* was found in conjunctival samples from a few trachoma patients in Nepal (30). Furthermore, De Puysseleyr et al. (31, 63) detected *C. suis* in the eyes of two Belgian slaughterhouse employees without disease symptoms. These recent studies demonstrate the zoonotic potential of *C. suis*. *C. suis* infections are generally treated with tetracycline or its derivatives, since they are most effective and rather cheap (73).

Coxiella

Coxiella causes Q fever in humans, but veterinary infection is generally referred to as coxiellosis. Veterinary infection is the source of the majority of human Q fever cases, so control of infection in reservoir species holds the key to reducing human infection. *C. burnetii* has resulted in veterinary infections of goats, sheep, cattle, horses, and companion animal species including dogs and cats. Furthermore, it has been associated with numerous wildlife species. Infection of animals can range from asymptomatic carriage through to febrile, respiratory infections and abortion outbreaks, particularly among small ruminant species (74, 75). Episodes of abortion are associated with liberation of vast numbers of infective particles (reaching 109 infective guinea-pig doses per gram of placental tissue) and thus represent a major infective source. Significant dispersal from a contaminated source has been further facilitated by wind to susceptible hosts over a range of several miles (76, 77). Veterinary transmission has also been described through sexual transmission via seminal fluid (natural or artificial insemination) (78) and can be shed for significant periods of time in vaginal fluid and milk postpartum (74, 79). Detection of shedding through milk provides a useful cost-effective means of veterinary surveillance for infection (80). Alternatively, serological or molecular surveillance can be undertaken, though on a cautionary note, infection is best interpreted on a herd basis rather than from the individual animal because shedding can be intermittent and animals that are infected, but serologically negative, can still shed *C. burnetii* (79). Although ticks have often been suggested as a potential source of infection, it appears that their role might not be of major significance, but they may play more of a role in maintenance of *C. burnetii* in the environment (81).

Application of molecular typing to *C. burnetii* has revealed significant interspecies diversity that appears to correlate with host species infectivity. Indeed, from such studies we have learned that genotypes predominating among small ruminant species show the greatest zoonotic potential for human infection. Furthermore, genetic variants have been described to have hyper-virulence for humans associated with deletion of a type 1 secretion system (82, 83). These unusual variants cluster within a particular genotype (multispacer type 17) and appear to have a wildlife reservoir in the three-toed sloth (84).

Until recently, the *Coxiella* genus was thought to be composed of *C. burnetii* as the sole species, but new members showing homology with *C. burnetii* are now being recognized, namely, *Coxiella cheraxi* and a novel *Coxiella*-like organism identified in birds and nonvertebrate species. *C. cheraxi* was first isolated in 2000 from hepato-pancreatic tissues from crayfish with inclusion bodies with *Rickettsia*-like Gram-negative bacteria that displayed remarkable homology with

C. burnetii (85, 86). More recently, newer members of the genus have been described with potential significance for avian species with the *Coxiella*-like organism, "*Candidatus* Coxiella avium," causing inflammation of the liver, lung, and spleen, often with systemic infection leading to death of the host (86, 87).

Another report has described *Coxiella*-like organisms as endosymbionts of several ticks species (88), with remarkably high incidence (close to 100%). It proposed that these might represent an ancestral species of *C. burnetii* (89). Several molecular diagnostics fail to differentiate between these species and *C. burnetii*. Whether these species have veterinary significance other than complicating the diagnostic interpretation for coxiellosis remains to be established.

Veterinary vaccines are available and can reduce shedding and associated clinical signs but have had mixed success in preventing infection. As such, veterinary control is generally achieved through good husbandry practice to reduce contamination of the environment and subsequent spread, combined with isolation of cases and appropriate destruction of infective material. Control of a recent and particularly large outbreak in The Netherlands was achieved through a massive culling campaign of pregnant goats (90).

Rickettsia

The rickettsiae are established pathogens for humans, but their veterinary impact is less well known. Because most have ticks serve as both their reservoir and vector, with successful transovarial transmission, but are also transmitted via small rodent species consequently they are generally considered zoonotic. However, *R. prowazekii* could be considered the exception, being transmitted via the human clothing louse from human to human. Surprisingly, though, *R. prowazekii* has also been reported from American flying squirrels and their lice and fleas, suggesting a possible zoonotic origin (91). Rickettsial infections such as endemic or murine typhus caused by *Rickettsia typhi* cycle through rats and their fleas. Similarly, *Rickettsia felis* is flea-borne and thus likely to transmit to multiple vertebrate species. Infection is well documented in humans, but this species has also been detected in tissues collected from opossums (92). Although the veterinary impact of rickettsial infection remains poorly documented, these organisms are important human pathogens causing fever, rash, myalgia, meningitis, endocarditis, lymphadenopathy, and lymphangitis with cardiopulmonary, neurological, or hepatic disease complications (26, 93).

Veterinary rickettsiosis has been documented in dogs, in which its differential diagnosis is that of anaplasmosis or ehrlichiosis. The clinical course of *R. rickettsia* infection is generally more severe than that seen in ehrlichiosis (94, 95). Experimental canine infection has confirmed the susceptibility of dogs for rickettsiosis (96, 97). In Europe serological surveillance of dogs has suggested significant exposure to Rickettsia species, and others have correlated acute febrile infection with positive rickettsial serology (98). Clinical presentation is rarely characterized by petechial hemorrhages; instead, it usually presents as fever, depression, and lymphadenopathy accompanied by neurological signs. Mite-borne rickettsiosis caused by *Rickettsia akari* has also been reported in a dog (99). Surprisingly, given their extensive exposure to the arthropod-borne vectors of *Rickettsia*, remarkably few clinical cases of rickettsiosis in cats have been presented, despite positive PCR detection of *Rickettsia* in their blood (100). Studies of livestock have reported detection of *Rickettsia* in ticks removed from cattle, but without associated signs of infection (101), while others have suggested possible correlation with *R. helvetica* detected in *Amblyomma maculatum* ticks in animals presenting with "gotch ear," but further evaluations appear to correlate the presence of gotch ear more with ticks than with the *Rickettsia* carried by them (102–104).

ANTIMICROBIAL SUSCEPTIBILITY TESTING

Assessment of antimicrobial susceptibility of intracellular bacteria is rarely undertaken. In the case of human zoonotic infection, an assessment might be considered. On a cautionary note, it must be remembered that such assessment involves manipulation of fastidious and highly infectious agents under the constraints of working under level 3 biosafety containment and thus is not a light undertaking. Furthermore, these microbes have a longer mean generation time compared to many cultivable bacteria, so evaluation is not always timely for providing information for selecting appropriate therapeutic options. As a consequence, it is more appropriate to be familiar with trends in susceptibility to guide appropriate and timely therapeutic interventions.

In Vitro Antimicrobial Susceptibility Testing of Intracellular Bacteria

Intracellular bacteria are a specific subgroup of bacteria that need a living cell for their multiplication and survival as a species. This lifestyle has major implications for their treatment because the antimicrobials have to pass an extra barrier, the eukaryotic cell wall. It also has major implications for susceptibility testing since this has to be done within tissue cultures.

Because growth of these bacteria tends to be tedious, difficult, and for some even impossible, little phenotypic antimicrobial susceptibility testing has been done, and those evaluations undertaken to date have not benefitted from standardized methods for susceptibility testing. Moreover, the systems of susceptibility testing need to be adapted to the bacterial species investigated, since they have different growth requirements and reside within different subcellular locations. In this article we will present the possibilities for susceptibility testing for intracellular bacteria and discuss the influence the differences may have on the outcome.

Several methods have been developed to assess the susceptibility of intracellular microbes, and most of them include the use of tissue cultures. The only alternative method available is the molecular detection of resistance genes, though this is only possible when the genes have been previously described. For the detection of new genes without phenotypic detection, whole-genome sequencing may be a solution, but there should be enough homology with existing genes, and phenotypic confirmation should follow.

Phenotypic Detection of Antimicrobial Resistance: Tissue Culture Methods

Essentially, this method is the same as the MIC determination of other bacterial species, with the difference being the way these bacteria grow. The necessity of growing intracellular bacteria within cells means that only MIC values can be determined. The MIC data cannot be interpreted readily, but one has to use the microbiological or epidemiological criterion to assess for acquired resistance (105, 106). Hereby, one looks for a bimodal distribution of the population when based on the phenotypic analysis of the MICs. The link to the clinical efficacy of the tests remains to be explored, and considering the limited data on acquired resistance, it may prove difficult to determine a clinical breakpoint for now. However, clinical experience has demonstrated the efficacy of several antibiotics, though some clinical failures have also been described.

The main variables in the methods used to test the susceptibility of intracellular bacteria are discussed below. First, the cell lines used may vary, and second, frequently as a consequence, the tissue culture used, the detection of the intracellular bacteria, and finally, the inoculum. Their influence has not been assessed, but it is known from the susceptibility testing of bacteria growing extracellularly that differences in media, even slight, may have an influence on the MIC (107, 108).

The cell lines may influence the MIC in two ways. First, they may influence the growth of bacteria and inclusion bodies, and intracellular bacteria may be more clear when bacterial cells grow better and, as such, be easier to detect, even if slight growth has remained. The cell culture used should support the best possible growth of a bacterium. Moreover, antimicrobials are only effective on growing bacterial cells. A second reason why MICs may differ between cell lines is the differences in uptake of the antibiotic by the cells (109, 110). In *Chlamydia* susceptibility testing, the use of different cell lines has been shown to be of minor importance (111), but it has been shown for macrolide antibiotics and *Chlamydia* susceptibility testing that different cell lines may produce different MICs (112). In addition, some antibiotics may not be assessed, because they are unable to enter prokaryotic cells. A clear example of this is the use of the aminoglycosides such as gentamicin. It is used in studies assessing intracellular growth of facultative intracellular bacteria, by which it is necessary to eliminate the remaining extracellular bacteria (113). However, none of these possible variables have been studied to a great extent for the intracellular bacteria, so their influence is not well quantified. This leads to complications in comparing different studies of resistance in intracellular bacteria.

The composition of the media used may also influence the activity of the antimicrobial. Even a slight difference in protein composition may influence the activity of an antibiotic. This has been assessed for some antibiotics, and a clear example is the antibiotic flavomycin, for which differences in concentrations as low as 0.001% may have an influence on susceptibility testing (108). Another clear example is the influence of acidification of the media on the macrolide antibiotics. This has only been assessed for susceptibility testing in regular media, and it is known that, for example, incubating in CO_2, which creates an acidification of the culture media, influences the MICs (107). During the culture of prokaryotic cells, CO_2 is routinely added to the atmospheric conditions and which combined with the cellular metabolism of the cells, causes acidification of the media, and thus potentially causing difficulties in determination of an accurate MIC. Finally, cell culture systems are rarely conducted under oxygen-depleted conditions and thus do not mimic the local intracellular environment particularly well.

A third potential variable in susceptibility testing is the sensitivity of the detection method of the microorganisms. Several staining methods can be used for different microorganisms, but for a single microorganism, different staining methods can be used. Classical chemical staining methods and immunofluorescence differ in their ability to detect microorganisms. Moreover, the

microorganisms can also be detected using reverse transcriptase PCR as an indication of metabolic activity of the bacterial cells. This technique is less labor-intensive and time-consuming, but MICs are higher compared to classical immunofluorescence (114, 115). In the determination of the susceptibility of *Rickettsia*, one may also use the plaque assay (detecting cytopathogenic effect), though that does not work with those *Rickettsia* that do not show a cytopathogenic effect. In this case the dye uptake system may be used (116). However, the differences caused by the different detection methods have by and large not been quantified.

Finally, there is the inoculum. The inoculum can have an effect in two ways: the inoculum dose and the time between inoculation and application of the antibiotic. The inoculum dose, however, is only important if a dose is used that causes immediate cytopathogenic effect. Inoculum doses that are too low may pose difficulties in the detection of the bacteria. Optimal inoculum dosing should be installed, but this will need international agreement for each of the tested intracellular bacteria. A lot of work has yet to be done in that field. The time between inoculation and application of the antibiotic becomes significant only after 8 hours of incubation with an increase in MIC (112).

Non-Culture-Based Methods

Non-culture-based methods are promoted more and more, but they have some disadvantages. The current nonculture methods are based on the detection of resistance genes, which implies that you have to know the gene or have analytical methods that can detect genes that are related to genes involved in the resistance. This definitely reduces the sensitivity of the assay because it fails to embrace unknown resistance genes that would remain invisible by the current analytical pipelines for the analysis of sequence data. Nonculture methods are based on PCR, real-time PCR, hybridization techniques (colony hybridization, DNA hybridization, or micro array hybridization), and whole-genome sequencing.

For PCR and real time PCR, the exact sequences should be known, and only the known genes (or variant genes if the variation is between conserved primer sites) may be detected. When hybridization techniques are being used, the presence of a weak signal may be an indication that a gene similar to the known gene is present, but this needs to be confirmed by sequencing. Finally, whole-genome sequencing allows the detection of similar sequences potentially encoding a resistance gene.

The disadvantage of these nonculture methods is the low sensitivity. A clear and recent example of this is colistin resistance in *Enterobacteriaceae*. While the sequences were in the database and the strains had been investigated for antimicrobial resistance genes using available pipelines, they were not found until their first full description (117).

ANTIMICROBIAL RESISTANCE IN INTRACELLULAR MICROBES

Given these difficulties in susceptibility testing, coupled with the difficulties in isolating obligate intracellular bacteria, it is clear that little data is available on susceptibility and resistance in these bacterial species. Below, we summarize the available data for the intracellular bacteria that have been studied, detailing the strengths and limitations of these approaches.

Susceptibility and Resistance of *Chlamydia*

C. psittaci and susceptibility

C. psittaci infections in birds and humans are primarily treated with tetracycline and its derivatives (chlortetracycline, oxytetracycline, doxycycline) (73, 118). Tetracyclines interfere with the binding of aminoacyl tRNAs on the ribosome and thus impede bacterial protein synthesis. Butaye et al. (119) evaluated the antibiotic susceptibility of 14 European *C. psittaci* isolates from turkeys. For doxycycline, the MIC values ranged from 0.05 to 0.2 mg/ml, with an average of 0.1 mg/ml. For enrofloxacin, the MIC value was 0.25 mg/ml. Acquired resistance was not detected. Two other studies tested the MICs of 8 and 12 antimicrobials (quinolones, tetracyclines, macrolides), respectively, for *C. psittaci* strain Cal10 and Bud (120, 121). All antimicrobials were effective. Both chlamydial strains showed almost identical drug susceptibility. Results of both studies were thus comparable. Clarithromycin and minocycline showed the lowest MICs (range for each, 0.016 to 0.031 mg/ml), and the MIC at which 90% of the clinical isolates were inhibited (MIC$_{90}$) was 0.031 mg/ml for each of these agents (121).

Suchland et al. (112) tested the antibiotic susceptibility of the *C. psittaci* reference strain 6BC and found the following MIC values: 0.064 g/ml (doxycycline), 0.125 g/ml (azithromycin), and 0.5 g/ml (ofloxacin). The MCC (minimal chlamydicidal concentration following one passage in cell culture) values for strain 6BC were 0.250 g/ml (doxycycline), 0.50 g/ml (azithromycin), and 2.0 g/ml (ofloxacin). Acquired resistance was not detected.

C. abortus and susceptibility

Ovine enzootic abortion remains a common cause of infectious abortion in many sheep-rearing countries despite the existence of commercially available vaccines that protect against the disease (122). If ovine enzootic abortion is suspected to be present in a flock/herd, the administration of a long-acting oxytetracycline preparation (20 mg/kg body weight intramuscularly) will reduce the severity of infection and losses resulting from abortion. It is important that treatment is given soon after the 95th to 100th day of gestation, the point at which pathologic changes start to occur. Additional doses can be given at 2-week intervals until the time of lambing. Although such treatment reduces losses and limits the shedding of infectious organisms, it does not eliminate the infection or reverse any pathologic damage already done to the placenta, so abortions or the delivery of stillborn or weak lambs can still occur, and the shed organisms are a source of infection for other naive animals (123). Moreover, this practice generally selects for resistance and should thus be avoided. As far as we know, acquired resistance has not been reported.

C. suis and susceptibility

C. suis is generally highly sensitive to tetracycline antibiotics. However, tetracycline-resistant *C. suis* strains seem to be emerging. The first stably tetracycline-resistant *C. suis* strains were isolated from diseased and normal pigs during the 1990s in the United States, and some of these also exhibited a stable resistance to sulfadiazine (124). Di Francesco et al. (125) identified 14 additional tetracycline-resistant *C. suis* strains in Italy. Borel et al. (126) demonstrated rapid selection for tetracycline-resistant *C. suis* after antibiotic treatment in a pig farm with an outbreak of conjunctivitis and diarrhea. In addition, tetracycline-resistant *C. suis* strains have been found in the United States, Belgium, Cyprus, Germany, Israel, Italy, Switzerland, and The Netherlands (33, 125–127; D. Vanrompay, personal communication, 2016).

Lenart et al. (127) studied the intracellular development of two tetracycline-resistant *C. suis* strains: R19 and R27 (isolated in the United States). The strains grow in concentrations of up to 4 mg of tetracycline/ml, while a tetracycline-sensitive swine strain (S45) grows in up to 0.1 mg of tetracycline/ml. Inclusions formed in the presence of tetracycline may, however, contain large aberrant reticulate bodies (RBs) that do not differentiate into infectious elementary bodies. The percentage of inclusions containing typical developmental forms decreases with increasing tetracycline concentrations, and at 3 mg of tetracycline/ml, 100% of inclusions contain aberrant RBs. However, upon removal of tetracycline, the aberrant RBs revert to typical RBs, and a productive developmental cycle ensues.

The tetracycline-resistant phenotype is attributed to the presence of an acquired genomic island (ranging from 6 to 13.5 kb) in the chlamydial chromosome. Four genomic islands have been identified to date, all carrying genes encoding a tetracycline efflux pump, tet (C), a regulatory repressor, tetR(C), and additional genes involved in replication and mobilization of the genomic island (128). The membrane-associated tetracycline efflux pump prevents the tetracycline-mediated inhibition of protein synthesis through export of tetracycline entering the bacterial cell. The regulatory repressor encoded by the tetR(C) gene suppresses production of the tetracycline efflux pump, and its function is neutralized through binding of the antibiotic (73). Three of four tet(C)-containing islands also carry a unique insertion sequence (IScs605). It was demonstrated that a transposase within the IScs605 sequence is likely responsible for integration of the genomic islands into the C. suis chromosome (129). In all examined strains, the C. suis tet(C) is integrated in the inv-like gene, a gene of unknown function. The tet(C) islands represent the first identification of antibiotic resistance acquired through horizontal gene transfer in any obligate intracellular bacteria, but the exact nature of acquisition is still subject to scientific speculation.

Consequently, the emergence of tetracycline-resistant C. suis strains requires treatment with other, more expensive antibiotics and may become economically devastating to pig production. Besides the economic consequences, tetracycline-resistant C. suis strains pose an additional risk for human health. C. suis is phylogenetically closely related to the human pathogenic species C. trachomatis (42). If zoonotic transmission of C. suis occurs, human patients may become coinfected with tetracycline-resistant C. suis and tetracycline-sensitive C. trachomatis bacteria, providing the ideal environment for transfer of the resistance gene. Tetracycline treatment of these patients will even further enhance the emergence and spread of tetracycline-resistant C. trachomatis strains, endangering the treatment of millions of people worldwide (130, 131). Monitoring of the spread of tetracycline-resistant C. suis to commercial pigs and the zoonotic transmission to humans is therefore needed to assess the associated risk and to decide on the appropriate measures.

So far, no stable antibiotic resistance has been reported in C. trachomatis isolates from human patients. A few cases of treatment failure displayed "heterotypic resistance," a form of phenotypic resistance in which a small portion of an infecting microbial species survives after exposure to antibiotics. However, the isolates could not survive long-term passage or lost their resistance

upon passage (132, 133). Several alternative antibiotics are applied in clinical settings in case of treatment failure when using tetracycline. Although clinical genetically based resistance to these alternatives in Chlamydia has not been documented so far, in vitro studies demonstrate the rapid emergence of C. suis strains resistant to rifamycins and fluoroquinolones (134). Moreover, naturally occurring tetracycline and sulfadiazine doubly resistant C. suis strains have been already isolated from pigs in the United States (124). Horizontal gene transfer of tetracycline resistance genes was shown among the different chlamydial species in vitro (134), hence, sowing the potential emergence of multiresistant human chlamydial pathogens and representing a potential public health impact.

Suchland et al. (112) tested the antibiotic susceptibility of the tetracycline-resistant C. suis strain R19 (isolated in the United States) (124) and found the following MIC values: 1.0 g/ml (doxycycline), 0.125 g/ml (azithromycin), and 0.5 g/ml (ofloxacin). The MCC (minimal chlamydicidal concentration following one passage in cell culture) values for strain R19 were 2.0 g/ml (doxycycline), 0.25 g/ml (azithromycin), and 1.0 g/ml (ofloxacin).

The in vitro susceptibility to tetracycline of C. suis conjunctival isolates obtained in Italy showed MIC values ranging from 0.5 to 4 µg/ml (67). Tet(C) and tetR(C) transcripts were found in all the isolates, cultured in both the absence and presence of tetracycline. This contrasts with other Gram-negative bacteria in which both genes are repressed in the absence of the drug. Further investigation into tet gene regulation in C. suis is needed. Reproductive failure on Belgian, Cypriote, and Israeli pig farrowing to slaughter farms has been shown to be mediated by tetracycline-resistant C. suis strains (33). The MIC of doxycycline for these strains varied from 1.6 g/ml to 3.2 g/ml, compared to 0.05 g/ml for a susceptible C. suis control strain.

Susceptibility and Resistance of Coxiella

C. burnetii has the ability to undergo phase variation, which complicates susceptibility testing. Phase II is predominate upon in vitro cultivation, while phase I correlates with in vivo growth. Within its intracellular niche, a parasitophorous vacuole akin to a phagolysosomal compartment, the local conditions are extreme, with poor nutrient availability, a pH of 4.5, and the presence of numerous cationic peptides and hydrolases (135). This environment is challenging to reproduce and might mitigate in vitro-derived susceptibility data.

Therapeutic approaches have largely focused on human infection where doxycycline is the drug of choice

(136) and have been verified by assessment of the large cohort of human cases resulting from the recent large outbreak in The Netherlands (137). However, this treatment is used in conjunction with hydrochloroquine to reduce the *in vivo* acidity and thus preserve the efficacy of doxycycline (138–140). Alternative options such as azithromycin and co-trimoxazole are sometimes used in the case of pregnancy (141, 142). Studies of the use of antimicrobials in livestock are scarce, but a study of dairy cattle suggested that there was reduced *Coxiella* shedding when tetracycline was combined with vaccination (143).

Susceptibility testing is rarely undertaken, because it was believed that *C. burnetii* was predictably susceptible to recommended regimes; this view has recently been challenged by the detection of doxycycline-resistant isolates (144) coupled with the finding of a human endocarditis case resistant to doxycycline, with a fatal outcome (145). Where susceptibility testing has been undertaken, various approaches have been used such as evaluation using shell-vial tissue cultures (146–148) and, more recently, real-time PCR methods (149, 150), nuclear magnetic resonance spectroscopy (151), and flow cytometry (152). Indeed, flow cytometry was used to assess the emergent infections in French Guiana belonging to a unique MST 17 genotype with the detection of macrolide resistance to erythromycin, azithromycin, and one isolate additionally resistant to telithromycin (152).

Advances have been made through the development of axenic medium supplementing *C. burnetii* with the essential nutrients that it conventionally derives from its host cell. The medium has evolved through several iterations, from acidified citrate cysteine medium to a modified formulation and subsequent complex *Coxiella* medium, which when incubated under microaerophilic conditions enables *in vitro* passage of *C. burnetii* over several generations (153–156). Though not all isolates are amenable to propagation through this medium, this offers a momentous advance in our ability to test this microbe *in vitro* and could be used to assess antimicrobial susceptibility (157).

Novel therapeutic approaches are also being considered, with various drugs not previously considered as conventional antibiotics now being explored, including those that target cellular processes such as intracellular calcium signals, G protein-coupled receptors, and membrane cholesterol distribution, and showing promise *in vitro* (149). Similarly, the activity of antimicrobial peptides has been assessed (158).

The phylogeny of newly described members of the *Coxiella* genus (see section above) has disclosed common patterns of codivergence in tick species (tick species-specific clades) and evidence of horizontal gene transfer events complicating their phylogenetic separation (89). The genome is reduced compared to *C. burnetii* (159), and traditional cultivation methods have been unsuccessful (89). The evidence of lateral gene transfer is important in that it might facilitate dispersal of antibiotic resistance genes.

Susceptibility and Resistance of the *Rickettsiae*

Initial attempts to evaluate rickettsial susceptibility were conducted using embryonated eggs or animal models. These approaches are now superseded by alternative, less hazardous strategies for determining the susceptibility of isolates. Plaque assays have proven useful to determine susceptibility using cell cultures visualized by crystal violet staining formaldehyde-fixed monolayers after incubation, but cytopathic effects and plaque formation are not uniformly produced by all rickettsiae, particularly when using primary cell cultures. Rickettsial susceptibility (for *R. akari*, *Rickettsia conorii*, *R. prowazekii*, and *R. rickettsii*) has been evaluated for clarithromycin and its 14-hydroxy derivative together with tetracycline using tissue culture combined with immunofluorescence to assess the impact on intracellular multiplication (160) and later for fluoroquinolones (161). This method overcomes the shortcomings of working with strains that do not form demonstrable plaques. Although they provide useful insights into the susceptibility of isolates, such approaches have limitations in their requirement for containment level 3 facilities. Other groups have undertaken extensive assessment of a range of rickettsial species to selected therapeutically useful agents using molecular PCR-based methods. For this, replicate infected cells with varying dilutions of test antimicrobial are harvested each day over a 7-day period. Samples are frozen until the end of the test period, at which time they are washed and DNA is extracted. The harvested DNA is then subjected to real-time PCR, and the transcript copy number is calculated by comparison to a standard curve. This approach has been found to be both specific and reproducible for the evaluation of susceptibility to test antimicrobials.

The above protocols have revealed susceptibility differences among the rickettsiae tested, with doxycycline showing the greatest efficacy against the strains tested (MICs 0.06 to 0.25 g/ml). Poor MIC results were found for amoxicillin (128 to 256 g/ml) and gentamicin (4 to 16 g/ml), while chloramphenicol (0.5 to 4.0 g/ml) and fluoroquinolone (0.25 to 2 g/ml) were effective.

Erythromycin proved to be variable (MICs ranging from 0.125 to 0.5 for the typhus group but only 2 to 8 g/ml for the spotted fever group). Similarly, rifampicin was variable with the typhus group and some spotted fever rickettsiae, giving MICs of 0.03 to 1 g/ml; however, *Rickettsia massiliae*, *Rickettsia montanensis*, *Rickettsia rhipicephali*, *Rickettsia aeschlimannii*, and *R. felis* were more resistant, with MICs ranging from 2 to 4 g/ml (24).

The basis for the differential susceptibility for erythromycin between typhus and spotted fever rickettsiae likely resides in a three-amino acid difference revealed in the L22 ribosomal protein. The rifampicin resistance observed among members of the *R. massiliae* subgroup is likely to be associated with mutation of *rboB* (24).

Novel agents that are currently not considered to be antimicrobial, as mentioned above for *C. burnetii*, have also been assessed for their ability to inhibit *R. conorii*, with some promising results using a cell culture test system and statins assessed with rickettsiae using a plaque assay (162, 163). Intriguingly, known resistance mechanisms have been identified in *R. felis*, potentially accounting for observed resistance, namely, a class C and class D B-lactamase, penicillin acylase homologue, and ABC-multidrug transporter system (24). By analogy with other resistance mechanisms described for different microbial groups, resistance to sulfamethoxazole and trimethoprim is likely to correlate with the absence of *folA* and/or *folP* from the typhus groups, while members of the spotted fever group only have *folA* (24).

The therapeutic response of dogs with rickettsiosis has been assessed *in vivo* comparing the efficacy of long-acting tetracycline and doxycycline, both showing successful recovery (164).

Though antimicrobial testing is rarely undertaken and, thus, emerging resistance to antimicrobials is not often considered, on a cautionary note it must be remembered that *Orienta tsutsugamushi*, formerly *Rickettsia tsutsugamushi*, has been reported using flow cytometry to have resistance to doxycycline, though it has remained susceptible to azithromycin (165). Furthermore, strains of *O. tsutsugamushi* have been recorded with quinolone resistance mediated through *gyrA* mutation (166, 167). Indeed, poorer clinical response has been noted in patients with *R. conorii* infection that have been treated with fluoroquinolones in contrast to doxycycline, though these observations were not corroborated by *in vitro* laboratory evaluation (168). Furthermore, genetic manipulation of *R. prowazekii* using electroporation has been successfully achieved incorporating a resistance-selective marker on a plasmid that was stably expressed (169).

This demonstrates the ability of rickettsiae to harbor selective resistance markers.

CONCLUDING REMARKS

Because of the cost and workload required to determine the susceptibility of intracellular bacteria, few data are available, and it is not expected that a lot of data will be generated in the future. Meanwhile, we see antimicrobial resistance increasing, including in intracellular bacteria, though definitely not as dramatically as in many other bacterial species. However, we should remain vigilant and have good methods to follow up the further evolution of resistance. Because the mechanism of resistance for intracellular bacteria may be different than that of other bacteria, the use of molecular techniques such as whole-genome sequencing may be difficult and may be prone to missing emerging resistance.

Citation. Vanrompay D, Nguyen TLA, Cutler SJ, Butaye P. 2017. Antimicrobial resistance in *Chlamydiales*, *Rickettsia*, *Coxiella*, and other intracellular pathogens. Microbiol Spectrum 6(2):ARBA-0003-2017.

References

1. Seshadri R, Samuel J. 2005. Genome analysis of *Coxiella burnetii* species: insights into pathogenesis and evolution and implications for biodefense. *Ann N Y Acad Sci* 1063:442–450.
2. Merhej V, Raoult D. 2011. Rickettsial evolution in the light of comparative genomics. *Biol Rev Camb Philos Soc* 86:379–405.
3. Zhong J, Jasinskas A, Barbour AG. 2007. Antibiotic treatment of the tick vector *Amblyomma americanum* reduced reproductive fitness. *PLoS One* 2:e405.
4. Ritter J. 1880. Beitrag zur Frage des Pneumotyphus [Eine Hausepidem ie in Uster (Schweiz) betreffendd]. *Dtsch A rchiv für Klin Medizin* 25:5, 53–59.
5. Morange A. 1895. *De la psittacose, ou Infection Speciale Determinee par les Peruches*. Academie de Paris, Paris, France.
6. Longbottom D, Coulter LJ. 2003. Animal chlamydioses and zoonotic implications. *J Comp Pathol* 128:217–244.
7. Coles AC. 1930. Micro-organisms in psittacosis. *Lancet* 218:1011–1012.
8. Levinthal W. 1930. Die aetiologe der psittakosis. *Klin Wchnsch* 9:654.
9. Lillie RD. 1930. Psittacosis-rickettsia-like inclusions in man and in experimental animals. *Publ Hlth Rep Wash* 45:773–778.
10. Bedson SP, Western GT, Simpson SL. 1930. Observations on the aetiology of psittacosis. *Lancet* 1:235–236.
11. Bedson SP, Bland JW. 1932. A morphological study of psittacosis virus, with the description of a developmental cycle. *Br J Exp Pathol* 13:461–466.

12. Bedson SP, Gostling JV. 1954. A study of the mode of multiplication of psittacosis virus. *Br J Exp Pathol* **35:** 299–308.

13. Moulder JW. 1966. The relation of the psittacosis group (Chlamydiae) to bacteria and viruses. *Annu Rev Microbiol* **20:**107–130.

14. Derrick EH. 1937. "Q" fever, a new fever entity: clinical features, diagnosis and laboratory investigation. *Med J Aust* **2:**281–299.

15. Davis GE, Cox HR. 1938. Weekly reports for December 30, 1938. *Public Health Rep* **53:**2259–2309.

16. Eldin C, Mélenotte C, Mediannikov O, Ghigo E, Million M, Edouard S, Mege J-L, Maurin M, Raoult D. 2017. From Q fever to *Coxiella burnetii* infection: a paradigm change. *Clin Microbiol Rev* **30:**115–190.

17. Hornstra HM, Priestley RA, Georgia SM, Kachur S, Birdsell DN, Hilsabeck R, Gates LT, Samuel JE, Heinzen RA, Kersh GJ, Keim P, Massung RF, Pearson T. 2011. Rapid typing of *Coxiella burnetii*. *PLoS One* **6:**e26201.

18. Ricketts HT. 1911. A Summary of Investigations of the Nature and Means of Transmission of Rocky Mountain Spotted Fever. Contributions to Medical Science by Howard Taylor Ricketts, 1870–1910. University of Chicago Press, Chicago, IL.

19. Bechah Y, Capo C, Mege JL, Raoult D. 2008. Epidemic typhus. *Lancet Infect Dis* **8:**417–426.

20. Gillespie JJ, Williams K, Shukla M, Snyder EE, Nordberg EK, Ceraul SM, Dharmanolla C, Rainey D, Soneja J, Shallom JM, Vishnubhat ND, Wattam R, Purkayastha A, Czar M, Crasta O, Setubal JC, Azad AF, Sobral BS. 2008. Rickettsia phylogenomics: unwinding the intricacies of obligate intracellular life. *PLoS One* **3:**e2018.

21. Rahman MS, Ammerman NC, Sears KT, Ceraul SM, Azad AF. 2010. Functional characterization of a phospholipase A(2) homolog from *Rickettsia typhi*. *J Bacteriol* **192:**3294–3303.

22. Elfving K, Lukinius A, Nilsson K. 2012. Life cycle, growth characteristics and host cell response of *Rickettsia helvetica* in a Vero cell line. *Exp Appl Acarol* **56:** 179–187.

23. Walker DH. 2007. Rickettsiae and rickettsial infections: the current state of knowledge. *Clin Infect Dis* **45**(Suppl 1):S39–S44.

24. Rolain JM. 2007. Antimicrobial susceptibility of rickettsial agents, p 361–369. *In* Raoult D, Parola P (ed), *Rickettsial Diseases*. Informa Healthcare, New York, NY.

25. Tahir D, Socolovschi C, Marié J-L, Ganay G, Berenger J-M, Bompar J-M, Blanchet D, Cheuret M, Mediannikov O, Raoult D, Davoust B, Parola P. 2016. New *Rickettsia* species in soft ticks *Ornithodoros hasei* collected from bats in French Guiana. *Ticks Tick Borne Dis* **7:**1089–1096.

26. Oteo JA, Portillo A. 2012. Tick-borne rickettsioses in Europe. *Ticks Tick Borne Dis* **3:**271–278.

27. Pospischil A, Borel N, Andersen AA. 2010. Chlamydia, p 575–588. *In* Gyles C, Prescott J, Songer J, Thoen C (ed), *Pathogenesis of Bacterial Infections in Animals*. Wiley-Blackwell, Oxford, United Kingdom.

28. Longbottom D, Livingstone M. 2006. Vaccination against chlamydial infections of man and animals. *Vet J* **171:**263–275.

29. Sachse K, Bavoil PM, Kaltenboeck B, Stephens RS, Kuo C-C, Rosselló-Móra R, Horn M. 2015. Emendation of the family *Chlamydiaceae*: proposal of a single genus, *Chlamydia*, to include all currently recognized species. *Syst Appl Microbiol* **38:**99–103.

30. Dean D, Rothschild J, Ruettger A, Kandel RP, Sachse K. 2013. Zoonotic *Chlamydiaceae* species associated with trachoma, Nepal. *Emerg Infect Dis* **19:**1948–1955.

31. De Puysseleyr K, De Puysseleyr L, Dhondt H, Geens T, Braeckman L, Morré SA, Cox E, Vanrompay D. 2014. Evaluation of the presence and zoonotic transmission of *Chlamydia suis* in a pig slaughterhouse. *BMC Infect Dis* **14:**560.

32. De Puysseleyr L, De Puysseleyr K, Braeckman L, Morré SA, Cox E, Vanrompay D. 2015. Assessment of *Chlamydia suis* infection in pig farmers. *Transbound Emerg Dis* **64:**826–833.

33. Schautteet K, De Clercq E, Miry C, Van Groenweghe F, Delava P, Kalmar I, Vanrompay D. 2013. Tetracycline-resistant *Chlamydia suis* in cases of reproductive failure on Belgian, Cypriote and Israeli pig production farms. *J Med Microbiol* **62:**331–334.

34. Stewardson AJ, Grayson ML. 2010. Psittacosis. *Infect Dis Clin North Am* **24:**7–25.

35. Vanrompay D, Ducatelle R, Haesebrouck F. 1995. *Chlamydia psittaci* infections: a review with emphasis on avian chlamydiosis. *Vet Microbiol* **45:**93–119.

36. Smith KA, Campbell CT, Murphy J, Stobierski MG, Tengelsen LA. 2011. Compendium of measures to control *Chlamydophila psittaci* infection among humans (psittacosis) and pet birds (avian chlamydiosis), 2010 National Association of State Public Health Veterinarians (NASPHV). *J Exot Pet Med* **20:**32–45.

37. Beeckman DS, Vanrompay DCG. 2009. Zoonotic *Chlamydophila psittaci* infections from a clinical perspective. *Clin Microbiol Infect* **15:**11–17.

38. NASPHV, Centers for Disease Control and Prevention, Council of State and Territorial Epidemiologists, American Veterinary Medical Association. 2011. Compendium of measures to prevent disease associated with animals in public settings, 2009: National Association of State Public Health Veterinarians, Inc. (NASPHV). *MMWR Recomm Rep* **58**(RR-5):1–21.

39. Ahmed B, De Boeck C, Dumont A, Cox E, De Reu K, Vanrompay D. 2015. First experimental evidence for the transmission of *Chlamydia psittaci* in poultry through eggshell penetration. *Transbound Emerg Dis* **64:**167–170.

40. Geens T, Desplanques A, Van Loock M, Bönner BM, Kaleta EF, Magnino S, Andersen AA, Everett KDE, Vanrompay D. 2005. Sequencing of the *Chlamydophila psittaci* ompA gene reveals a new genotype, E/B, and the need for a rapid discriminatory genotyping method. *J Clin Microbiol* **43:**2456–2461.

41. Pannekoek Y, Dickx V, Beeckman DSA, Jolley KA, Keijzers WC, Vretou E, Maiden MCJ, Vanrompay D,

van der Ende A. 2010. Multi locus sequence typing of *Chlamydia* reveals an association between *Chlamydia psittaci* genotypes and host species. *PLoS One* 5: e14179.

42. Everett KD, Bush RM, Andersen AA. 1999. Emended description of the order *Chlamydiales*, proposal of *Parachlamydiaceae* fam. nov. and *Simkaniaceae* fam. nov., each containing one monotypic genus, revised taxonomy of the family *Chlamydiaceae*, including a new genus and five new species, and standards for the identification of organisms. *Int J Syst Bacteriol* 49:415–440.

43. Spalatin J, Fraser CE, Connell R, Hanson RP, Berman DT. 1966. Agents of psittacosis-lymphogranuloma venereum group isolated from muskrats and snowshoe hares in Saskatchewan. *Can J Comp Med Vet Sci* 30: 260–264.

44. Stephens RS, Myers G, Eppinger M, Bavoil PM. 2009. Divergence without difference: phylogenetics and taxonomy of *Chlamydia* resolved. *FEMS Immunol Med Microbiol* 55:115–119.

45. Schautteet K, Vanrompay D. 2011. *Chlamydiaceae* infections in pig. *Vet Res (Faisalabad)* 42:29.

46. Di Francesco A, Baldelli R, Donati M, Cotti C, Bassi P, Delogu M. 2013. Evidence for *Chlamydiaceae* and *Parachlamydiaceae* in a wild boar (*Sus scrofa*) population in Italy. *Vet Ital* 49:119–122.

47. Schachter J, Banks J, Sugg N, Sung M, Storz J, Meyer KF. 1975. Serotyping of *Chlamydia*: isolates of bovine origin. *Infect Immun* 11:904–907.

48. Storz J, Spears P. 1979. Pathogenesis of chlamydial polyarthritis in domestic animals: characteristics of causative agent. *Ann Rheum Dis* 38(Suppl 1):111–115.

49. Perez-Martinez JA, Storz J. 1985. Antigenic diversity of *Chlamydia psittaci* of mammalian origin determined by microimmunofluorescence. *Infect Immun* 50:905–910.

50. Kaltenboeck B, Kousoulas KG, Storz J. 1993. Structures of and allelic diversity and relationships among the major outer membrane protein (ompA) genes of the four chlamydial species. *J Bacteriol* 175:487–502.

51. Aitken ID. 2000. Chlamydial abortion, p 81–86. *In* Martin WB, Aitken ID (ed), *Diseases of Sheep*. Blackwell Scientific, Oxford, United Kingdom.

52. Everett KDE. 2000. *Chlamydia* and *Chlamydiales*: more than meets the eye. *Vet Microbiol* 75:109–126.

53. Rodolakis A, Laroucau K. 2015. *Chlamydiaceae* and chlamydial infections in sheep or goats. *Vet Microbiol* 181:107–118.

54. Omori T, Morimoto T, Harada K, Inaba Y, Ishii S, Matumoto M. 1957. Miyagawanella: psittacosis-lymphogranuloma group of viruses. I. Excretion of goat pneumonia virus in feces. *Jpn J Exp Med* 27:131–143.

55. Kawakami Y, Kaji T, Sugimura K, Omori T, Matumoto M. 1958. Miyagawanella: psittacosis-lymphogranuloma group of viruses. V. Isolation of a virus from feces of naturally infected sheep. *Jpn J Exp Med* 28:51–58.

56. Storz J. 1963. Superinfection of pregnant ewes latently infected with a psittacosis-lymphogranuloma agent. *Cornell Vet* 53:469–480.

57. Pospischil A, Thoma R, Hilbe M, Grest P, Gebbers J-O. 2002. Abortion in woman caused by caprine *Chlamydophila abortus* (*Chlamydia psittaci* serovar 1). *Swiss Med Wkly* 132:64–66.

58. Walder G, Hotzel H, Brezinka C, Gritsch W, Tauber R, Würzner R, Ploner F. 2005. An unusual cause of sepsis during pregnancy: recognizing infection with *Chlamydophila abortus*. *Obstet Gynecol* 106:1215–1217.

59. Kampinga GA, Schröder FP, Visser IJ, Anderson JM, Buxton D, Möller AV. 2000. [Lambing ewes as a source of severe psittacosis in a pregnant woman]. *Ned Tijdschr Geneeskd* 144:2500–2504. (In Dutch.)

60. Wong SY, Gray ES, Buxton D, Finlayson J, Johnson FW. 1985. Acute placentitis and spontaneous abortion caused by *Chlamydia psittaci* of sheep origin: a histological and ultrastructural study. *J Clin Pathol* 38: 707–711.

61. Sachse K, Hotzel H, Slickers P, Ellinger T, Ehricht R. 2005. DNA microarray-based detection and identification of *Chlamydia* and *Chlamydophila* spp. *Mol Cell Probes* 19:41–50.

62. Pantchev A, Sting R, Bauerfeind R, Tyczka J, Sachse K. 2010. Detection of all *Chlamydophila* and *Chlamydia* spp. of veterinary interest using species-specific real-time PCR assays. *Comp Immunol Microbiol Infect Dis* 33:473–484.

63. De Puysseleyr K, De Puysseleyr L, Geldhof J, Cox E, Vanrompay D. 2014. Development and validation of a real-time PCR for *Chlamydia suis* diagnosis in swine and humans. *PLoS One* 9:e96704.

64. Lis P, Kumala A, Spalinski M, Rypula K. 2014. Novel locked nucleic acid (LNA)-based probe for the rapid identification of *Chlamydia suis* using real-time PCR. *BMC Vet Res* 10:225.

65. Willigan DA, Beamer PD. 1955. Isolation of a transmissible agent from pericarditis of swine. *J Am Vet Med Assoc* 126:118–122.

66. Hoffmann K, Schott F, Donati M, Di Francesco A, Hässig M, Wanninger S, Sidler X, Borel N. 2015. Prevalence of chlamydial infections in fattening pigs and their influencing factors. *PLoS One* 10:e0143576.

67. Donati M, Balboni A, Laroucau K, Aaziz R, Vorimore F, Borel N, Morandi F, Vecchio Nepita E, Di Francesco A. 2016. Tetracycline susceptibility in *Chlamydia suis* pig isolates. *PLoS One* 11:e0149914.

68. Eggemann G, Wendt M, Hoelzle LE, Jäger C, Weiss R, Failing K. 2000. Prevalence of Chlamydia infections in breeding sows and their importance in reproductive failure. *Dtsch Tierarztl Wochenschr* 107:3–10. (In German.)

69. Woollen N, Daniels EK, Yeary T, Leipold HW, Phillips RM. 1990. Chlamydial infection and perinatal mortality in a swine herd. *J Am Vet Med Assoc* 197:600–601.

70. Schiller I, Koesters R, Weilenmann R, Thoma R, Kaltenboeck B, Heitz P, Pospischil A. 1997. Mixed infections with porcine *Chlamydia trachomatis/pecorum* and infections with ruminant *Chlamydia psittaci* serovar 1 associated with abortions in swine. *Vet Microbiol* 58:251–260.

71. Kauffold J, Melzer F, Berndt A, Hoffmann G, Hotzel H, Sachse K. 2006. *Chlamydiae* in oviducts and uteri of repeat breeder pigs. *Theriogenology* 66:1816–1823.

72. Sarma DK, Tamuli MK, Rahman T, Boro BR, Deka BC, Rajkonwar CK. 1983. Isolation of *Chlamydia* from a pig with lesions in the urethra and prostate gland. *Vet Rec* 112:525.

73. Chopra I, Roberts M. 2001. Tetracycline antibiotics: mode of action, applications, molecular biology, and epidemiology of bacterial resistance. *Microbiol Mol Biol Rev* 65:232–260.

74. Berri M, Rousset E, Champion JL, Russo P, Rodolakis A. 2007. Goats may experience reproductive failures and shed *Coxiella burnetii* at two successive parturitions after a Q fever infection. *Res Vet Sci* 83:47–52.

75. Rousset E, Berri M, Durand B, Dufour P, Prigent M, Delcroix T, Touratier A, Rodolakis A. 2009. *Coxiella burnetii* shedding routes and antibody response after outbreaks of Q fever-induced abortion in dairy goat herds. *Appl Environ Microbiol* 75:428–433.

76. Hawker JI, Ayres JG, Blair I, Evans MR, Smith DL, Smith EG, Burge PS, Carpenter MJ, Caul EO, Coupland B, Desselberger U, Farrell ID, Saunders PJ, Wood MJ. 1998. A large outbreak of Q fever in the West Midlands: windborne spread into a metropolitan area? *Commun Dis Public Health* 1:180–187.

77. Boden K, Brasche S, Straube E, Bischof W. 2014. Specific risk factors for contracting Q fever: lessons from the outbreak Jena. *Int J Hyg Environ Health* 217:110–115.

78. Schimmer B, Luttikholt S, Hautvast JLA, Graat EAM, Vellema P, Duynhoven YT. 2011. Seroprevalence and risk factors of Q fever in goats on commercial dairy goat farms in the Netherlands, 2009–2010. *BMC Vet Res* 7:81.

79. de Cremoux R, Rousset E, Touratier A, Audusseau G, Nicollet P, Ribaud D, David V, Le Pape M. 2012. *Coxiella burnetii* vaginal shedding and antibody responses in dairy goat herds in a context of clinical Q fever outbreaks. *FEMS Immunol Med Microbiol* 64:120–122.

80. Astobiza I, Ruiz-Fons F, Piñero A, Barandika JF, Hurtado A, García-Pérez AL. 2012. Estimation of *Coxiella burnetii* prevalence in dairy cattle in intensive systems by serological and molecular analyses of bulk-tank milk samples. *J Dairy Sci* 95:1632–1638.

81. Duron O, Sidi-Boumedine K, Rousset E, Moutailler S, Jourdain E. 2015. The importance of ticks in Q fever transmission: what has (and has not) been demonstrated? *Trends Parasitol* 31:536–552.

82. Mahamat A, Edouard S, Demar M, Abboud P, Patrice JY, La Scola B, Okandze A, Djossou F, Raoult D. 2013. Unique clone of *Coxiella burnetii* causing severe Q fever, French Guiana. *Emerg Infect Dis* 19:1102–1104.

83. D'Amato F, Eldin C, Georgiades K, Edouard S, Delerce J, Labas N, Raoult D. 2015. Loss of TSS1 in hypervirulent *Coxiella burnetii* 175, the caus ative agent of Q fever in French Guiana. *Comp Immunol Microbiol Infect Dis* 41:35–41.

84. Davoust B, Marié JL, Pommier de Santi V, Berenger JM, Edouard S, Raoult D. 2014. Three-toed sloth as putative reservoir of *Coxiella burnetii*, Cayenne, French Guiana. *Emerg Infect Dis* 20:1760–1761.

85. Tan CK, Owens L. 2000. Infectivity, transmission and 16S rRNA sequencing of a rickettsia, *Coxiella cheraxi* sp. nov., from the freshwater crayfish *Cherax quadricarinatus*. *Dis Aquat Organ* 41:115–122.

86. Cooper A, Layton R, Owens L, Ketheesan N, Govan B. 2007. Evidence for the classification of a crayfish pathogen as a member of the genus *Coxiella*. *Lett Appl Microbiol* 45:558–563.

87. Vapniarsky N, Barr BC, Murphy B. 2012. Systemic *Coxiella*-like infection with myocarditis and hepatitis in an eclectus parrot (*Eclectus roratus*). *Vet Pathol* 49:717–722.

88. Duron O. 2015. The IS1111 insertion sequence used for detection of *Coxiella burnetii* is widespread in *Coxiella*-like endosymbionts of ticks. *FEMS Microbiol Lett* 362:fnv132.

89. Duron O, Noël V, McCoy KD, Bonazzi M, Sidi-Boumedine K, Morel O, Vavre F, Zenner L, Jourdain E, Durand P, Arnathau C, Renaud F, Trape JF, Biguezoton AS, Cremaschi J, Dietrich M, Léger E, Appelgren A, Dupraz M, Gómez-Díaz E, Diatta G, Dayo GK, Adakal H, Zoungrana S, Vial L, Chevillon C. 2015. The recent evolution of a maternally-inherited endosymbiont of ticks led to the emergence of the Q fever pathogen, *Coxiella burnetii*. *PLoS Pathog* 11:e1004892.

90. Roest HIJ, Tilburg JJHC, van der Hoek W, Vellema P, van Zijderveld FG, Klaassen CHW, Raoult D. 2011. The Q fever epidemic in The Netherlands: history, onset, response and reflection. *Epidemiol Infect* 139:1–12.

91. Bozeman FM, Masiello SA, Williams MS, Elisberg BL. 1975. Epidemic typhus *Rickettsiae* isolated from flying squirrels. *Nature* 255:545–547.

92. Abramowicz KF, Wekesa JW, Nwadike CN, Zambrano ML, Karpathy SE, Cecil D, Burns J, Hu R, Eremeeva ME. 2012. *Rickettsia felis* in cat fleas, *Ctenocephalides felis* parasitizing opossums, San Bernardino County, California. *Med Vet Entomol* 26:458–462.

93. Walker DH, Ismail N, Olano JP, Valbuena G, McBride J. 2007. Pathogenesis, immunity, pathology, and pathophysiology in rickettsial diseases, p 15–26. *In* Raoult D, Parola P (ed), *Rickettsial Diseases*. Informa Healthcare, New York, NY.

94. López Del PJ, Abarca VK, Azócar AT. 2007. Clinical and serological evidence of canine rickettsiosis in Chile. *Rev Chilena Infectol* 24:189–193. (In Spanish.)

95. Fortes FS, Biondo AW, Molento MB. 2011. Brazilian spotted fever in dogs. *Semina Cienc Agrar Londrina* 32:339–354.

96. Inokuma H, Matsuda H, Sakamoto L, Tagawa M, Matsumoto K. 2011. Evaluation of *Rickettsia japonica* pathogenesis and reservoir potential in dogs by experimental inoculation and epidemiologic survey. *Clin Vaccine Immunol* 18:161–166.

97. Levin ML, Killmaster LF, Zemtsova GE, Ritter JM, Langham G. 2014. Clinical presentation, convalescence, and relapse of rocky mountain spotted fever in dogs

experimentally infected via tick bite. *PLoS One* **9:** e115105.

98. Solano-Gallego L, Kidd L, Trotta M, Di Marco M, Caldin M, Furlanello T, Breitschwerdt E. 2006. Febrile illness associated with *Rickettsia conorii* infection in dogs from Sicily. *Emerg Infect Dis* **12:**1985–1988.

99. Zavala-Castro JE, Zavala-Velázquez JE, del Rosario García M, León JJA, Dzul-Rosado KR. 2009. A dog naturally infected with *Rickettsia akari* in Yucatan, México. *Vector Borne Zoonotic Dis* **9:**345–347.

100. Bayliss DB, Morris AK, Horta MC, Labruna MB, Radecki SV, Hawley JR, Brewer MM, Lappin MR. 2009. Prevalence of *Rickettsia* species antibodies and *Rickettsia* species DNA in the blood of cats with and without fever. *J Feline Med Surg* **11:**266–270.

101. Mediannikov O, Diatta G, Zolia Y, Balde MC, Kohar H, Trape JF, Raoult D. 2012. Tick-borne *Rickettsiae* in Guinea and Liberia. *Ticks Tick Borne Dis* **3:**43–48.

102. Edwards KT. 2011. Gotch ear: a poorly described, local, pathologic condition of livestock associated primarily with the Gulf Coast tick, *Amblyomma maculatum*. *Vet Parasitol* **183:**1–7.

103. Edwards KT, Goddard J, Jones TL, Paddock CD, Varela-Stokes AS. 2011. Cattle and the natural history of *Rickettsia parkeri* in Mississippi. *Vector Borne Zoonotic Dis* **11:**485–491.

104. Edwards KT, Varela-Stokes AS, Paddock CD, Goddard J. 2011. Gotch ear in a goat: a case report. *Vector Borne Zoonotic Dis* **11:**1217–1219.

105. Butaye P, Devriese LA, Haesebrouck F. 2003. Antimicrobial growth promoters used in animal feed: effects of less well known antibiotics on Gram-positive bacteria. *Clin Microbiol Rev* **16:**175–188.

106. Butaye P, Devriese LA, Haesebrouck F. 1999. Phenotypic distinction in *Enterococcus faecium* and *Enterococcus faecalis* strains between susceptibility and resistance to growth-enhancing antibiotics. *Antimicrob Agents Chemother* **43:**2569–2570.

107. Butaye P, Devriese LA, Haesebrouck F. 1998. Effects of different test conditions on the minimal inhibitory concentration of growth promoting antibacterial agents with enterococci. *J Clin Microbiol* **36:**1907–1911.

108. Butaye P, Devriese LA, Haesebrouck F. 2000. Influence of different medium components on the *in vitro* activity of the growth-promoting antibiotic flavomycin against enterococci. *J Antimicrob Chemother* **46:**713–716.

109. Van Bambeke F, Glupczynski Y, Plésiat P, Pechère JC, Tulkens PM. 2003. Antibiotic efflux pumps in prokaryotic cells: occurrence, impact on resistance and strategies for the future of antimicrobial therapy. *J Antimicrob Chemother* **51:**1055–1065.

110. Van Bambeke F, Michot JM, Tulkens PM. 2003. Antibiotic efflux pumps in eukaryotic cells: occurrence and impact on antibiotic cellular pharmacokinetics, pharmacodynamics and toxicodynamics. *J Antimicrob Chemother* **51:**1067–1077.

111. Henning K, Krauss H. 1986. Zur methodik der bestimmung der antobiotikumempfindlichkeit von Chlamydien *in vitro*. *J Vet Med Ser B* **33:**447–461.

112. Suchland RJ, Geisler WM, Stamm WE. 2003. Methodologies and cell lines used for antimicrobial susceptibility testing of *Chlamydia* spp. *Antimicrob Agents Chemother* **47:**636–642.

113. Bonventre PF, Hayes R, Imhoff J. 1967. Autoradiographic evidence for the impermeability of mouse peritoneal macrophages to tritiated streptomycin. *J Bacteriol* **93:** 445–450.

114. Khan MA, Potter CW, Sharrard RM. 1996. A reverse transcriptase-PCR based assay for *in-vitro* antibiotic susceptibility testing of *Chlamydia pneumoniae*. *J Antimicrob Chemother* **37:**677–685.

115. Cross NA, Kellock DJ, Kinghorn GR, Taraktchoglou M, Bataki E, Oxley KM, Hawkey PM, Eley A. 1999. Antimicrobial susceptibility testing of *Chlamydia trachomatis* using a reverse transcriptase PCR-based method. *Antimicrob Agents Chemother* **43:**2311–2313.

116. Rolain JM, Maurin M, Vestris G, Raoult D. 1998. *In vitro* susceptibilities of 27 rickettsiae to 13 antimicrobials. *Antimicrob Agents Chemother* **42:**1537–1541.

117. Hasman H, Hammerum AM, Hansen F, Hendriksen RS, Olesen B, Agersø Y, Zankari E, Leekitcharoenphon P, Stegger M, Kaas RS, Cavaco LM, Hansen DS, Aarestrup FM, Skov RL. 2015. Detection of mcr-1 encoding plasmid-mediated colistin-resistant *Escherichia coli* isolates from human bloodstream infection and imported chicken meat, Denmark 2015. *Euro Surveill* **20:**49.

118. Michalova E, Novotna P, Schlegelova J. 2004. Tetracyclines in veterinary medicine and bacterial resistance to them. *Vet Med Czech* **49:**79–100.

119. Butaye P, Ducatelle R, De Backer P, Vermeersch H, Remon JP, Haesebrouck F. 1997. *In vitro* activities of doxycycline and enrofloxacin against European *Chlamydia psittaci* strains from turkeys. *Antimicrob Agents Chemother* **41:**2800–2801.

120. Niki Y, Kimura M, Miyashita N, Soejima R. 1994. *In vitro* and *in vivo* activities of azithromycin, a new azalide antibiotic, against chlamydia. *Antimicrob Agents Chemother* **38:**2296–2299.

121. Miyashita N, Niki Y, Kishimoto T, Nakajima M, Matsushima T. 1997. *In vitro* and *in vivo* activities of AM-1155, a new fluoroquinolone, against *Chlamydia* spp. *Antimicrob Agents Chemother* **41:**1331–1334.

122. Entrican G, Wheelhouse N, Wattegedera SR, Longbottom D. 2012. New challenges for vaccination to prevent chlamydial abortion in sheep. *Comp Immunol Microbiol Infect Dis* **35:**271–276.

123. Stuen S, Longbottom D. 2011. Treatment and control of chlamydial and rickettsial infections in sheep and goats. *Vet Clin North Am Food Anim Pract* **27:**213–233.

124. Andersen A, Rogers D. 1998. Resistance to tetracycline and sulfadiazine in swine *C. trachomatis* isolates, 313–316. *In* Stephens RS (ed), *Chlamydial infections*. Proceedings of the Ninth International Symposium on Human Chlamydial Infection. International Chlamydia Symposium, San Francisco, CA.

125. Di Francesco A, Donati M, Rossi M, Pignanelli S, Shurdhi A, Baldelli R, Cevenini R. 2008. Tetracycline-resistant *Chlamydia suis* isolates in Italy. *Vet Rec* 163: 251–252.

126. Borel N, Regenscheit N, Di Francesco A, Donati M, Markov J, Masserey Y, Pospischil A. 2012. Selection for tetracycline-resistant *Chlamydia suis* in treated pigs. *Vet Microbiol* 156:143–146.

127. Lenart J, Andersen AA, Rockey DD. 2001. Growth and development of tetracycline-resistant *Chlamydia suis*. *Antimicrob Agents Chemother* 45:2198–2203.

128. Dugan J, Rockey DD, Jones L, Andersen AA. 2004. Tetracycline resistance in *Chlamydia suis* mediated by genomic islands inserted into the chlamydial *inv*-like gene. *Antimicrob Agents Chemother* 48:3989–3995.

129. Dugan J, Andersen AA, Rockey DD. 2007. Functional characterization of *IScs605*, an insertion element carried by tetracycline-resistant *Chlamydia suis*. *Microbiology* 153:71–79.

130. Mabey D. 2008. Trachoma: recent developments. *Adv Exp Med Biol* 609:98–107.

131. WHO. 2008. *Global Incidence and Prevalence of Selected Curable Sexually Transmitted Infections-2008*. WHO, Geneva, Switzerland.

132. Wang SA, Papp JR, Stamm WE, Peeling RW, Martin DH, Holmes KK. 2005. Evaluation of antimicrobial resistance and treatment failures for *Chlamydia trachomatis*: a meeting report. *J Infect Dis* 191:917–923.

133. Jones RB, Van der Pol B, Martin DH, Shepard MK. 1990. Partial characterization of *Chlamydia trachomatis* isolates resistant to multiple antibiotics. *J Infect Dis* 162:1309–1315.

134. Suchland RJ, Sandoz KM, Jeffrey BM, Stamm WE, Rockey DD. 2009. Horizontal transfer of tetracycline resistance among *Chlamydia* spp. *in vitro*. *Antimicrob Agents Chemother* 53:4604–4611.

135. Hicks LD, Raghavan R, Battisti JM, Minnick MF. 2010. A DNA-binding peroxiredoxin of *Coxiella burnetii* is involved in countering oxidative stress during exponential-phase growth. *J Bacteriol* 192:2077–2084.

136. Anderson A, Bijlmer H, Fournier PE, Graves S, Hartzell J, Kersh GJ, Limonard G, Marrie TJ, Massung RF, McQuiston JH, Nicholson WL, Paddock CD, Sexton DJ. 2013. Diagnosis and management of Q fever–United States, 2013: recommendations from CDC and the Q Fever Working Group. *MMWR Morb Mortal Wkly Rep* 62:1–30.

137. Dijkstra F, Riphagen-Dalhuisen J, Wijers N, Hak E, Van der Sande MAB, Morroy G, Schneeberger PM, Schimmer B, Notermans DW, Van der Hoek W. 2011. Antibiotic therapy for acute Q fever in The Netherlands in 2007 and 2008 and its relation to hospitalization. *Epidemiol Infect* 139:1332–1341.

138. Raoult D, Houpikian P, Tissot Dupont H, Riss JM, Arditi-Djiane J, Brouqui P. 1999. Treatment of Q fever endocarditis: comparison of 2 regimens containing doxycycline and ofloxacin or hydroxychloroquine. *Arch Intern Med* 159:167–173.

139. Darmon A, Million M, Audoly G, Lepidi H, Brouqui P, Raoult D. 2014. Q fever: still a diagnostic and therapeutic challenge in 2014. *Rev Francoph Lab* 2014: 51–59.

140. Raoult D, Drancourt M, Vestris G. 1990. Bactericidal effect of doxycycline associated with lysosomotropic agents on *Coxiella burnetii* in P388D1 cells. *Antimicrob Agents Chemother* 34:1512–1514.

141. Carcopino X, Raoult D, Bretelle F, Boubli L, Stein A. 2007. Managing Q fever during pregnancy: the benefits of long-term cotrimoxazole therapy. *Clin Infect Dis* 45: 548–555.

142. Cerar D, Karner P, Avsic-Zupanc T, Strle F. 2009. Azithromycin for acute Q fever in pregnancy. *Wien Klin Wochenschr* 121:469–472.

143. Taurel AF, Guatteo R, Joly A, Beaudeau F. 2012. Effectiveness of vaccination and antibiotics to control *Coxiella burnetii* shedding around calving in dairy cows. *Vet Microbiol* 159:432–437.

144. Rolain JM, Lambert F, Raoult D. 2005. Activity of telithromycin against thirteen new isolates of *C. burnetii* including three resistant to doxycycline. *Ann N Y Acad Sci* 1063:252–256.

145. Rouli L, Rolain JM, El Filali A, Robert C, Raoult D. 2012. Genome sequence of *Coxiella burnetii* 109, a doxycycline-resistant clinical isolate. *J Bacteriol* 194: 6939–6939.

146. Gikas A, Spyridaki I, Psaroulaki A, Kofterithis D, Tselentis Y. 1998. *In vitro* susceptibility of *Coxiella burnetii* to trovafloxacin in comparison with susceptibilities to pefloxacin, ciprofloxacin, ofloxacin, doxycycline, and clarithromycin. *Antimicrob Agents Chemother* 42:2747–2748.

147. Gikas A, Spyridaki I, Scoulica E, Psaroulaki A, Tselentis Y. 2001. *In vitro* susceptibility of *Coxiella burnetii* to linezolid in comparison with its susceptibilities to quinolones, doxycycline, and clarithromycin. *Antimicrob Agents Chemother* 45:3276–3278.

148. Spyridaki I, Psaroulaki A, Vranakis I, Tselentis Y, Gikas A. 2009. Bacteriostatic and bactericidal activities of tigecycline against *Coxiella burnetii* and comparison with those of six other antibiotics. *Antimicrob Agents Chemother* 53:2690–2692.

149. Boulos A, Rolain J-M, Maurin M, Raoult D. 2004. Measurement of the antibiotic susceptibility of *Coxiella burnetii* using real time PCR. *Int J Antimicrob Agents* 23:169–174.

150. Brennan RE, Samuel JE. 2003. Evaluation of *Coxiella burnetii* antibiotic susceptibilities by real-time PCR assay. *J Clin Microbiol* 41:1869–1874.

151. García-Álvarez L, Busto JH, Peregrina JM, Fernández Recio MA, Avenoza A, Oteo JA. 2013. Nuclear magnetic resonance applied to antimicrobial drug susceptibility. *Future Microbiol* 8:537–547.

152. Eldin C, Perreal C, Mahamat A, Djossou F, Edouard S, Raoult D. 2015. Antibiotic susceptibility determination for six strains of *Coxiella burnetii* MST 17 from Cayenne, French Guiana. *Int J Antimicrob Agents* 46: 600–602.

153. Omsland A. 2012. Axenic growth of *Coxiella burnetii*. *Adv Exp Med Biol* 984:215–229.

154. Omsland A, Beare PA, Hill J, Cockrell DC, Howe D, Hansen B, Samuel JE, Heinzen RA. 2011. Isolation from animal tissue and genetic transformation of *Coxiella burnetii* are facilitated by an improved axenic growth medium. *Appl Environ Microbiol* 77:3720–3725.

155. Omsland A, Cockrell DC, Fischer ER, Heinzen RA. 2008. Sustained axenic metabolic activity by the obligate intracellular bacterium *Coxiella burnetii*. *J Bacteriol* 190:3203–3212.

156. Omsland A, Cockrell DC, Howe D, Fischer ER, Virtaneva K, Sturdevant DE, Porcella SF, Heinzen RA. 2009. Host cell-free growth of the Q fever bacterium *Coxiella burnetii*. *Proc Natl Acad Sci USA* 106:4430–4434.

157. Singh S, Eldin C, Kowalczewska M, Raoult D. 2013. Axenic culture of fastidious and intracellular bacteria. *Trends Microbiol* 21:92–99.

158. Unsworth NB, Dawson RM, Wade JD, Liu CQ. 2014. Susceptibility of intracellular *Coxiella burnetii* to antimicrobial peptides in mouse fibroblast cells. *Protein Pept Lett* 21:115–123.

159. Smith TA, Driscoll T, Gillespie JJ, Raghavan R. 2015. A *Coxiella*-like endosymbiont is a potential vitamin source for the Lone Star tick. *Genome Biol Evol* 7:831–838.

160. Ives TJ, Marston EL, Regnery RL, Butts JD, Majerus TC. 2000. *In vitro* susceptibilities of *Rickettsia* and *Bartonella* spp. to 14-hydroxy-clarithromycin as determined by immunofluorescent antibody analysis of infected vero cell monolayers. *J Antimicrob Chemother* 45:305–310.

161. Ives TJ, Marston EL, Regnery RL, Butts JD. 2001. *In vitro* susceptibilities of *Bartonella* and *Rickettsia* spp. to fluoroquinolone antibiotics as determined by immunofluorescent antibody analysis of infected Vero cell monolayers. *Int J Antimicrob Agents* 18:217–222.

162. Czyż DM, Potluri LP, Jain-Gupta N, Riley SP, Martinez JJ, Steck TL, Crosson S, Shuman HA, Gabay JE. 2014. Host-directed antimicrobial drugs with broad-spectrum efficacy against intracellular bacterial pathogens. *MBio* 5:e01534-14.

163. Edouard S, Raoult D. 2013. Use of the plaque assay for testing the antibiotic susceptibility of intracellular bacteria. *Future Microbiol* 8:1301–1316.

164. de Almeida AJ, Rodrigues HF, Rodrigues ABF, Di Filippo PA, Pinto ABT. 2014. Comparative study of therapeutic protocols used in the treatment of infections caused by *Rickettsiales* in dogs. *Comp Clin Pathol* 24:555–560.

165. Strickman D, Sheer T, Salata K, Hershey J, Dasch G, Kelly D, Kuschner R. 1995. *In vitro* effectiveness of azithromycin against doxycycline-resistant and -susceptible strains of *Rickettsia tsutsugamushi*, etiologic agent of scrub typhus. *Antimicrob Agents Chemother* 39:2406–2410.

166. Jang HC, Choi SM, Jang MO, Ahn JH, Kim UJ, Kang SJ, Shin JH, Choy HE, Jung SI, Park KH. 2013. Inappropriateness of quinolone in scrub typhus treatment due to *gyrA* mutation in *Orientia tsutsugamushi* Boryong strain. *J Korean Med Sci* 28:667–671.

167. Tantibhedhyangkul W, Angelakis E, Tongyoo N, Newton PN, Moore CE, Phetsouvanh R, Raoult D, Rolain J-M. 2010. Intrinsic fluoroquinolone resistance in *Orientia tsutsugamushi*. *Int J Antimicrob Agents* 35:338–341.

168. Botelho-Nevers E, Rovery C, Richet H, Raoult D. 2011. Analysis of risk factors for malignant Mediterranean spotted fever indicates that fluoroquinolone treatment has a deleterious effect. *J Antimicrob Chemother* 66:1821–1830.

169. Wood DO, Hines A, Tucker AM, Woodard A, Driskell LO, Burkhardt NY, Kurtti TJ, Baldridge GD, Munderloh UG. 2012. Establishment of a replicating plasmid in *Rickettsia prowazekii*. *PLoS One* 7:e34715.

Antimicrobial Resistance in Bacteria from Livestock and Companion Animals
Edited by Frank Møller Aarestrup, Stefan Schwarz, Jianzhong Shen, and Lina Cavaco
© 2018 American Society for Microbiology, Washington, DC
doi:10.1128/microbiolspec.ARBA-0017-2017

Antimicrobial Drug Resistance in Fish Pathogens

Ron A. Miller[1] and Heather Harbottle[1]

24

INTRODUCTION TO ANTIMICROBIAL AGENT USE IN AQUACULTURE

With an increasing global population, aquaculture can provide a source for inexpensive protein. However, many of these sources are and will continue to be located in developing countries where medicated feeds are inexpensive and widely available for broad application on farms. These feeds can contain antimicrobial agents from classes generally considered unsafe for use in food-producing animals due to their critical importance to human medicine (e.g., fluoroquinolones).

The availability of antimicrobial agents over the counter in many developing countries with little to no veterinarian oversight can contribute directly to the emergence of antimicrobial resistance in bacterial pathogens of fish (Table 1) and of humans. Some environmental or commensal bacteria may also pass their resistance determinants to veterinary and zoonotic pathogens.

In any given farm situation, many factors can contribute to the perceived need for chemotherapeutic intervention. The reality is, in some countries where medicated feeds can be obtained inexpensively, there is widespread and unrestricted use of antimicrobial agents to prevent bacterial infections. The use of a wide variety of antimicrobial agent classes, including nonbiodegradable antimicrobial agents useful in human medicine, ensures that they remain in the aquatic environment, exerting their selective pressure for long periods of time. This process has resulted in the emergence of antimicrobial resistant bacteria in aquaculture environments, the increase of antimicrobial resistance in fish pathogens, and the increasing potential for transfer of these resistance determinants to bacterial pathogens of terrestrial animals and humans.

Conversely, when a disease outbreak is believed to be imminent, improved water quality and/or metaphylactic treatment can be used efficiently to reduce animal suffering and economic losses. The timeliness of such interventions is absolutely critical, particularly in aquatic animal medicine, where declines in water quality and/or increases in pathogen shedding can quickly result in catastrophic losses and facility closures.

FACTORS CONTRIBUTING TO ANTIMICROBIAL RESISTANCE IN AQUACULTURE

Therapeutic Use on the Farm

Antimicrobial agents are most commonly administered in aquaculture settings using broadcasted medicated feeds. Often, the largest and strongest fish on farms consume the majority of the medicated feed, likely affording them a positive clinical outcome, whereas the smaller and/or sick fish are likely to be underdosed and considerably more prone to disease and ultimately death (1, 2). Alternative dosing strategies (i.e., pulse, increased dose) can circumvent some of these issues, but optimization of medicated feed dosages and durations in fish can be extremely challenging. Logistical difficulties confronted in pharmacokinetic investigations of fish include determination of both the amount of ingested antimicrobial agent in each animal studied and serum drug concentrations during the dosing regimen without introducing significant handling stress. Miller et al. used a gastric lavage technique and preweighed, homogenized oxytetracycline-medicated feed to standardize the amount of antimicrobial agent ingested per gram of body weight (3). Destructive sampling was used to reduce experimental bias and ensure sufficient blood volumes. Low standards of deviation were noted at all sampling time points. Environmental factors can also complicate therapy because

[1]U.S. Food and Drug Administration, Center for Veterinary Medicine, Division of Human Food Safety, Rockville, MD 20855.

Table 1 Frequently isolated bacterial pathogens of fish

Organism	Disease
Aeromonas caviae	Motile aeromonad septicemia
Aeromonas hydrophila	
Aeromonas sobria	
Aeromonas salmonicida	Furunculosis, ulcer disease, carp erythrodermatitis
Edwardsiella ictaluri	Enteric septicemia of catfish
Edwardsiella tarda-like organisms	Motile Edwardsiella septicemia (Edwardsiella piscicida), nonmotile Edwardsiella septicemia (Edwardsiella anguillarum)
Flavobacterium branchiophilum	Bacterial gill disease
Flavobacterium columnare	Columnaris disease
Flavobacterium psychrophilum	Cold-water disease, rainbow trout fry syndrome
Francisella spp.	Francisellosis
Lactococcus garvieae	Lactococcosis, Lactococcus septicemia
Moritella viscosa	Winter ulcer disease
Mycobacterium spp.	Mycobacteriosis
Photobacterium damselae subsp. damselae	Vibriosis
P. damselae subsp. piscicida	Photobacteriosis, fish pasteurellosis, pseudotuberculosis
Piscirickettsia salmonis	Piscirickettsiosis, salmonid piscirickettsial septicemia
Plesiomonas shigelloides	Winter disease
Pseudomonas spp.	Pseudomoniasis
Pseudomonas anguilliseptica	Red spot disease
Renibacterium salmoninarum	Bacterial kidney disease
Streptococcus agalactiae	Group B streptococcosis
Streptococcus dysgalactiae	Group C streptococcosis
Streptococcus iniae	Streptococcosis
Streptococcus phocae	Warm-water streptococcosis
Tenacibaculum maritimum	Salt-water columnaris, marine flexibacteriosis
Vagococcus salmoninarum	Cold-water streptococcosis
Vibrio salmonicida	Cold-water vibriosis, Hitra disease
Vibrio spp.	Vibriosis
Yersinia ruckeri	Enteric redmouth disease

temperature, water salinity, and the presence of inactivating divalent cations (e.g., Mg^{+2} and Ca^{+2}) can affect drug absorption and ultimately the amount of bioavailable free drug.

Agricultural Runoff and Human Pollution
Release of antimicrobial-resistant pathogens from an aquaculture facility or from agricultural runoff into surrounding areas can have an impact on the overall movement of resistance through microbial communities. Petersen et al. showed that integrated farming strongly favored antimicrobial-resistant bacteria in a pond environment (4). As the source, they attributed the selective pressure of the antimicrobial agents used or the direct introduction of antimicrobial-resistant bacteria from animal manure. Leaching of antimicrobial agents from fish farming operations into surrounding waterways may also contribute to the spread of antimicrobial-resistant animal and zoonotic pathogens. Additional research in this area is needed to fully characterize the extent of the issue at the national level, and then a determination can be made as to the breadth of the animal and human health risk. Due to the vast disparity between countries and regions in availability of antimicrobial agent classes and types of aquaculture farming practices, inherent risk profiles will be different.

ANTIMICROBIAL RESISTANCE GENES FOUND IN FISH PATHOGENS
The widespread use of antimicrobial agents to treat and control fish diseases has led to the emergence of antimicrobial resistance to single and multiple classes of antimicrobial agents in important fish pathogens. In one of the first reports of resistance, in fish pathogens, Aoki et al. investigated mobile R plasmids in three Aeromonas salmonicida strains (5), one of which was isolated in 1959 by S. F. Snieszko in the United States and has been considered the standard A. salmonicida strain of reference for many later genetic investigations. The R plasmids were transmissible to Escherichia coli, transferring two resistant phenotypes. The standard U.S. strain transmitted resistance to sulfathiazole and tetracycline, and the two Japanese strains transmitted resistance to chloramphenicol and dihydrostreptomycin. Aoki and collaborators, over a series of natural transformation and DNA-DNA hybridization studies in the 1970s and 1980s, were the first to fully characterize a number of fish-pathogenic bacterial species (Edwardsiella tarda, Vibrio anguillarum, A. hydrophila, and Pasteurella piscicida [since reclassified as Photobacterium damselae subsp. piscicida]) containing R plasmids and their associated antimicrobial resistance genes (6–9).

The rising concern regarding the development of antimicrobial resistance and the reporting of the discovery of antimicrobial resistance genes in fish pathogens and commensals in and around aquaculture systems has increased due to the occasional close proximity of human populations, recreational fisheries, and other animal production systems. These relationships have prompted a number of notable investigations, review articles, and opinion articles (10–13).

A. salmonicida

Considerable antimicrobial resistance and corresponding resistance genes in *A. salmonicida* have been identified from clinical infections of fish, with one of the first reports of resistance being described in 1971 (5). Transmissible resistance was found conferring resistance to sulfathiazole and tetracycline on one R plasmid and a second R plasmid conferring phenotypic resistance to chloramphenicol and dihydrostreptomycin. In addition to this early report of resistance to four classes of antimicrobial agents (tetracyclines, sulfonamides, phenicols, and aminoglycosides), quinolone resistance has also been observed in *A. salmonicida*. Tetracyclines are commonly used to treat furunculosis caused by *A. salmonicida*. Genes conferring resistance to tetracycline are commonly associated with transfer *via* mobile genetic elements, and quinolones are of particular concern because they are used to treat *Aeromonas* infections in humans and are widely used in some parts of the world in aquaculture. Oxytetracycline-resistant strains (MIC ≥ 8 µg/ml) and oxolinic acid-resistant strains (MIC ≥ 1 µg/ml) from Korea were screened for multidrug resistance (MDR) phenotypes (i.e., resistant to more than two classes) and antimicrobial resistance determinants, revealing that a majority of the strains were considered MDR (14). One strain was found to be resistant to ampicillin, gentamicin, oxytetracycline, enrofloxacin, and oxolinic acid. The tetracycline resistance gene *tet*(A) was identified in most tetracycline-resistant isolates, and one isolate was positive for *tet*(E). Screening for mobile genetic elements was not conducted in this study; however, the sequenced *tet*(A) and *tet*(E) genes showed 100% homology to *tet*(A) in pRAS1 (GenBank accession no. AJ517790.2) and *tet*(E) in pAsa4 (GenBank accession no. CP000645.1). These plasmids have been associated with carriage in *A. salmonicida*. The quinolone-resistance-determining regions (QRDRs) consisting of the *gyrA* and *parC* genes were sequenced and, among the quinolone-resistant *A. salmonicida* strains, all harbored point mutations in the *gyrA* codon-83 which are responsible for the corresponding amino acid substitutions of Ser83→Arg83 or Ser83→Asn83. The authors detected no point mutations in other QRDRs, such as *gyrA* codons-87 and -92, and *parC* codons-80 and -84; the mobile *qnr* genes were not detected. Genetic similarity was assessed *via* pulsed-field gel electrophoresis, and the results indicated high clonality among the Korean antimicrobial-resistant strains of *A. salmonicida* (14). In agreement

with this study, another investigation of the mechanism of quinolone resistance in seven oxolinic acid-resistant *A. salmonicida* isolates from Atlantic salmon was conducted by PCR amplification and sequencing of the *gyrA* gene. All strains with MICs ≥ 1 µg/ml (defined as resistant) were positive for a serine to isoleucine mutation at the 83 position in the *gyrA*- encoded amino acid. These mutations conferring quinolone resistance were identified solely at the 83 position in the *gyrA*-encoded protein and were nontransmissible (15).

Integrons carrying antimicrobial resistance genes have been widely identified in *A. salmonicida* and associated with multiple antimicrobial resistance phenotypes. In an effort to screen for class 1 integrons in *A. salmonicida* over a wide geographic range, PCR amplification of the class 1 integron structural component *sul1* gene was utilized as a marker for integron carriage (16). Twenty-one sulfonamide-resistant *A. salmonicida* strains from France, Japan, Switzerland, Norway, Scotland, and the United States were determined to carry class 1 integrons. Of the strains positive for class 1 integrons, 19 possessed a single gene cassette and one possessed two resistance genes within the cassette. A variety of resistance genes were identified in the gene cassettes: *aadA1* (three strains), *aadA2* (eight strains), *dfrA16* (five strains), *dfrB2c* (three strains), and *qacG* and *orfD* (one strain). Twenty strains were tetracycline-resistant and positive for either *tet*(A) (*n* = 16) or *tet*(E) (*n* = 4), with *tet*(A) being frequently associated with a Tn*1721* transposon. Seven integron-negative sulfonamide-resistant strains possessed the *sul2* gene. Geographic associations were reported, with aminoglycoside resistance being associated with the *aadA2* gene in Scotland and with the *aadA1* gene in Switzerland and France. The *dfrA16* gene cassette was found only in Norwegian strains, whereas *dfrB2c* was identified as causing trimethoprim resistance in Scotland.

Mobile genetic elements associated with MDR phenotypes have been identified in *A. salmonicida* since the earliest reports of resistance by Aoki et al. (5). Early plasmids associated with drug resistance to sulfonamides, phenicols, and streptomycins were associated with the pAr-32 plasmid isolated in Japan in 1970 from an *A. salmonicida* isolate carrying a class 1 integron. Molecular characterization of a similar pRA3 plasmid from *A. hydrophila* in Japan revealed that these plasmids were nearly identical, suggesting transmission between *A. hydrophila* and *A. salmonicida* for some time (17). The plasmid pRA3 is the reference plasmid for the incompatibility group U (IncU). Atypical and typical *A. salmonicida* strains were resistant to tetracycline and potentiated sulfonamides and were found to carry the

IncU pRAS1 plasmid, which is responsible for the resistance phenotypes. Molecular mapping of the pRAS1 plasmid from *A. salmonicida* showed that a 12-kb antimicrobial resistance-determining region was encoded, including a class 1 integron carrying the *dfrA16*, *sul1*, *qac*, and *tet*(A) genes conferring resistance to trimethoprim, sulfonamides, quaternary ammonium compounds, and tetracyclines. Molecular analysis of pAr-32 and pRAS1 showed that the backbone of pRAS1 is similar to that of pAr-32, indicating that pRAS1 may have evolved from pAr-32, with the addition of and rearrangement of antimicrobial resistance genes. Conjugation experiments showed the potential for the effective spread of the IncU pRAS1 plasmid to other aquatic pathogens such as *Vibrio cholerae*, *Vibrio parahaemolyticus*, and *Yersinia ruckeri* (17).

Since their identification in the United States in 1959, MDR *A. salmonicida* strains have been extensively studied for their rich and diverse plasmid repertoire. *A. salmonicida* was reported to carry three cryptic plasmids not conferring antimicrobial resistance genes [pAsa1 (pAsal2), pAsa2 (pAsal3), pAsa3], and four plasmids not conferring antimicrobial resistance genes (pAsal1, pAsal1B, pAsa5, pAsa6) (18). The cryptic plasmids [pAsa1 (pAsal2), pAsa2 (pAsal3), pAsa3] are ColE1- and ColE2-type plasmids and have been reported to encode genes responsible for replication, stability, and mobilization (19). Further investigation is ongoing with regard to the functions of the pAsal-type plasmids; however, pAsa5, pAsal1, pAsal1B, and pAsa6 are known to bear genes encoding type III secretion systems and effectors. Plasmids in *A. salmonicida* which carry antimicrobial resistance genes have been reported to include pRAS1 and pAr-32 (described above); pASOT, pASOT2, and pASOT3 [*aadA2*, *tet*(A)]; pSN254b [*tet*(A), *floR*, *sul1*, *sul2*, *bla*CMY, *aadA*, *strA*, *strB*, *sugE2*, *qacE1*]; pAB5S9b [*tet*(H), *floR*, *sul2*, *strA*, *strB*]; pAsa7 (*cat*); and pAasa4 [*tet*(E), *sul1*, *aadA*, *cat*] (18, 19). A new pAsa8 plasmid was characterized in Canada from *A. salmonicida* carrying a large number of antimicrobial resistance genes [*tet*(A), *tet*(G), *floR*, *sul1*, *bla*PSE-1, and *aadA2*] and a complex class 1 integron with similarity to the *Salmonella* genomic island 1 (SGI132) found in *Salmonella enterica* (20). Plasmid exchange between terrestrial pathogens such as *S. enterica* serotypes has been shown previously (21), as exemplified by the IncA/C pSN254b plasmid, a variant of pSN254 found in *S. enterica*. The plasmids of the IncA/C group are known to be conjugative and found, in addition to *A. salmonicida* and *S. enterica*, in a broad range of bacteria such as *Yersinia pestis*, *Klebsiella pneumonia*, *Aeromonas hydrophila*, *Photobacte-*

rium damselae subsp. *piscicida*, and *E. coli*. The IncA/C plasmids are also known to regulate the excision of SGI132 and to serve as helpers for its mobilization in trans (20).

While it is beyond the scope of this chapter to go into intimate detail of all known plasmids identified in *A. salmonicida* strains, it is obvious that the rich and varied plasmid profiles of this important fish pathogen have allowed strains to persist after antimicrobial agent therapy, and they may serve as a considerable reservoir for transmissible antimicrobial resistance elements.

Edwardsiella ictaluri and *E. tarda*

Despite the U.S. Food and Drug Administration approval of oxytetracycline, ormetoprim-sulfadimethoxine, and florfenicol in channel catfish, reports of antimicrobial resistance of the enteric septicemia of the catfish pathogen *E. ictaluri* are scarce. In 1993, ormetoprim-sulfadimethoxine-resistant *E. ictaluri* was isolated from treated catfish in Virginia and Mississippi (22). A 55-kb conjugative plasmid was found to be responsible for the resistance to ormetoprim-sulfadimethoxine. It also conferred resistance to tetracycline, oxytetracycline, streptomycin, trimethoprim, and trimethoprim-sulfamethoxazole.

In 2009, florfenicol resistance in *E. ictaluri* was found to be conferred *via* an MDR IncA/C plasmid, pM07-1 (23). The plasmid was self-transmissible and conferred resistance to florfenicol, chloramphenicol, tetracycline, streptomycin, ampicillin, amoxicillin-clavulanic acid, ceftiofur, and cefoxitin and reduced susceptibility to trimethoprim-sulfamethoxazole and ceftriaxone. The *floR* and *bla*CMY-2 genes were detected on the plasmid *via* PCR and subsequently sequenced, revealing 100% nucleotide identity of the *bla*CMY-2 gene from plasmids in the human pathogens *S. enterica*, *E. coli*, and *K. pneumoniae*. Discovery of IncA/C plasmids carrying *floR* and *bla*CMY-2 resistance determinants in *S. enterica* serotype Newport and *A. salmonicida* highlight the mobility and potential promiscuity of these plasmids in aquatic and terrestrial environments (21, 24).

E. tarda has a broad host range and can be pathogenic to fish including economically important species such as catfish, turbot, flounder, and salmon (25) and to humans. Transferable, plasmid-mediated antimicrobial resistance has been identified in *E. tarda* going back to the 1970s (6) when naturally occurring R plasmids were found to confer resistance to up to five classes of antimicrobial agents (sulfonamides, tetracyclines, streptogramins, phenicols, and aminoglycosides). In China, a pathogenic *E. tarda* strain, TX01, from an outbreak at a fish farm was found to be resistant to kanamycin, tetracycline, and chloramphenicol and possessed associated antimicrobial resistance genes (25). The strain was positive for known kanamycin resistance determinants, *catA3*, and *tet*(A) genes which were cloned, sequenced, and compared to human and animal strains. These genes were 99 to 100% identical to genes on plasmids and transposons in human and terrestrial animal strains. Further, the carrier plasmid of the *tet* and *catA3* genes, pETX, demonstrated its transferability among different genera of bacteria. Due to its transmissibility among a wide variety of genera and the high level of resistance gene identity between human, environmental, and fish strains, this plasmid has likely played a persistent role in the dissemination of antimicrobial resistance within and possibly between environments (25).

Plasmid typing, in addition to other molecular subtyping methods, can expand on our knowledge surrounding the potential for transmission between environments and geographic locations. Ninety-four *E. tarda* isolates from diseased eels were tested for their susceptibility to eight commonly used antimicrobial agents in Taiwan (26). The isolates were highly susceptible to ampicillin, amoxicillin, florfenicol, oxolinic acid, and flumequine. However, 21.3% were oxytetracycline resistant and positive for *tet*(A), and 90% also carried *tet*(M). Interestingly, the efflux pump inhibitor omeprazole reduced oxytetracycline MICs 2- to 8-fold, suggesting that an intact efflux pump, presumably encoded by *tet*(A), is required for high-level tetracycline resistance. Real-time PCR experiments showed that increased expression levels of *tetA* and *tetR* contribute to oxytetracycline resistance. Southern blot hybridization revealed that all oxytetracycline-resistant isolates carried the *tet*(A) gene on a 50- to 70-kb plasmid. Plasmid typing and restriction fragment length polymorphism analysis identified similarities across different farms in the same region, indicating that horizontal spread and local transmission of the plasmid in the oxytetracycline-resistant *E. tarda* population has occurred.

In addition to antimicrobial resistance determinants, plasmids and other mobile genetic elements can simultaneously carry virulence genes, giving pathogens even greater potential to cause disease and persist during and after antimicrobial agent exposure. A genetic analysis of a South Korean *E. tarda* strain (*E. tarda* CK41) with reduced susceptibility to kanamycin, ampicillin, tetracycline, and streptomycin revealed a 70-kb plasmid responsible for transferring kanamycin and tetracycline resistance genes (27). These authors hypothesized that virulence genes were concomitantly housed on plasmids in *E. tarda* and conducted survival experiments

with a plasmid-cured strain, *E. tarda* CK108, and its parent strain, CK41. Of the fish infected with *E. tarda*, 80% survived infection with *E. tarda* CK108, while only 20% survived infection with the parent strain, CK41, which contained the antimicrobial resistance and virulence genes. Due to the difference in survival rate, it is clear that additional virulence genes can be transmitted with antimicrobial resistance genes on plasmids in *Edwardsiella* spp.

Y. ruckeri

Y. ruckeri causes the economically devastating enteric redmouth disease in several fish species, including rainbow trout (*Onchorynchus mykiss*) (28). Because of the economic impact, antimicrobial agents such as quinolones and potentiated sulfonamides are often used to combat infections, prompting investigations into the development of antimicrobial resistance to these and other antimicrobial agents.

MDR *Y. ruckeri* has been reported worldwide. *Y. ruckeri* isolates (*n* = 116) from geographically separated areas of Turkey were tested for their susceptibility to oxytetracycline, streptomycin, florfenicol, ampicillin, trimethoprim-sulfamethoxazine, and oxolinic acid (29). Of the isolates tested, 16.3% were MDR. Although the authors tested for class 1 and 2 integrons, none were identified, and the presence of plasmids was not determined. Oxytetracycline resistance was mediated by *tet*(A) (36.3%) and *tet*(B) (4.5%). Other variants of the *tet* genes were not screened. Ampicillin resistance was identified in 29% of isolates, but all were negative for bla_{TEM} and bla_{SHV}. Other beta-lactamases were not tested, and the authors proposed that a low-level AmpC-type enzyme may have been expressed in some *Y. ruckeri* isolates, as was reported by Schiefer et al. (30).

To characterize antimicrobial-resistant outbreak strains, 10 representative *Y. ruckeri* isolates with reduced enrofloxacin and nalidixic acid susceptibility were screened for resistance determinants (28). The authors sequenced the QRDR of the isolates and tested for plasmid-borne resistance in one isolate which displayed reduced susceptibility to the potentiated sulfonamides. Isolates with low-level resistance to enrofloxacin (MICs of 0.06 to 0.25 µg/ml) and nalidixic acid (MICs from 8 to 32 µg/ml) possessed a single *gyrA* mutation in the QRDR. These changes represented an 8- to 32-fold increase in the enrofloxacin MIC and a 32- to 128-fold increase in the nalidixic acid MIC. This finding is in agreement with other studies in which a single *gyrA* mutation conferred resistance to quinolones but only a slight increase for fluoroquinolones, which require more than one mutation to achieve clinical resistance

(31). In one isolate with elevated MICs to potentiated sulfonamides, the *sul2*, *strB*, and *dfrA14* gene cassette was identified to be housed on an 8.9-kb transmissible plasmid. This study confirmed that *Y. ruckeri* is able to develop mutations resulting in reduced fluoroquinolone susceptibility and can also acquire plasmid-borne resistance genes (28).

Plasmid acquisition and genomic content plasticity are significant in antimicrobial resistance development for *Y. ruckeri*, *Aeromonas* spp., and other important fish pathogens. Welch et al. investigated the genomic similarities of three MDR IncA/C plasmids identified in the human pathogen *Y. pestis* (pIP1202), the foodborne pathogen *S.* Newport (pSN254), and the fish pathogen *Y. ruckeri* (pYR1) (24). Sequencing analysis showed that the three plasmid backbones shared an IncA/C backbone with an overall backbone sequence identity of 99 to 100%. Similar codon usage was observed in the plasmid backbones encoding functions such as type IV secretion systems and plasmid maintenance/replication, further strengthening the assertion that these plasmids evolved from a common ancestor. These plasmids contained antimicrobial gene cassettes within Tn*21* or Tn*10* transposons, with the *Y. ruckeri* plasmid containing only the Tn*10* transposon. The Tn*10* transposon encoded the *strA/B* and *tet*(A) genes in this plasmid, conferring streptomycin and tetracycline resistance, respectively. The *Y. ruckeri* plasmid also encoded *dfrA1* conferring trimethoprim resistance and a *sul2* gene conferring sulfonamide resistance, which is common to all three plasmids and is believed to be the selective factor in the evolution of these plasmids. The *Y. ruckeri* plasmid was the smallest of the three, and the *S.* Newport plasmid was the largest and encoded the most numerous antimicrobial resistance genes including three cephalosporin resistance genes (bla_{SHV-1}, and two copies of bla_{CMY-2}), tetracycline resistance genes [*tet*(A)], aminoglycoside resistance genes (two copies of *aadA*), streptomycin resistance genes (*strA/B*), chloramphenicol resistance genes (*cat*), florfenicol resistance genes (*floR*), and mercury resistance genes (*merRTPABDE*), to name a few. Salmonellae carrying similar MDR IncA/C plasmids were also identified in retail meats between 2002 and 2005 (24). This highlights the dissemination ability of isolates harboring these MDR plasmids in aquaculture and food animals and in human health.

More-recent studies have included comparisons of these IncA/C plasmids with plasmids from *Y. ruckeri*, *P. damselae*, and terrestrial pathogens. Call et al. investigated the relatedness of IncA/C plasmids in *S.* Newport (pAM04528 from a human) and *E. coli* (peH4H and pAR060302 from cattle) against the published plasmid sequences of pSN254 from *S.* Newport, the fish pathogen *Y. ruckeri* (pYR1) (24), and the fish pathogen *P. damselae* (pP91278 and pP99-108) (32). While all of the plasmids shared a similar IncA/C backbone, the plasmids originating from fish pathogens were evolutionarily the most dissimilar. The *Y. ruckeri* plasmid pYR1 was the most dissimilar with the smallest number of antimicrobial resistance genes. Based on bootstrap analysis of all of the plasmids, those from *E. coli* and *S.* Newport clustered together, the *P. damselae* plasmids clustered together, and the *Y. ruckeri* plasmid clustered separately from the others, indicating evolutionary distance. The authors proposed that although the plasmids evolved from a common ancestor, those sourced from terrestrial animals and humans diverged a considerable time ago compared to those sourced from fish.

In a similar study, Fricke et al. compared the sequences of historical and contemporary MDR IncA/C plasmids from aquatic and terrestrial environments to investigate the evolution of these plasmids *via* gene cassette insertions and single nucleotide polymorphisms (SNPs) in the core plasmid backbones (33). Sequences of pRAx (the cryptic plasmid), pRA1 (*A. hydrophila*), pYR1 (*Y. ruckeri*), pIP1202 (*Y. pestis*), pP91278 and pP99-018 (*P. damselae* subsp. *piscicida*), and pSN245 (*S.* Newport) were compared. The authors found that the oldest plasmid in the study, pRA1, and the more contemporary plasmids shared a highly conserved plasmid backbone, with 80% identity. In addition, the core plasmid is largely identical between pRA1 and pYR1 (*Y. ruckeri*), pIP1202 (*Y. pestis*), and pSN245 (*S.* Newport). The pRAx plasmid was identified after conjugative experiments transferring pRA1 from *A. hydrophila* to *E. coli*, and despite the significantly reduced plasmid size and reduced antimicrobial resistance gene carriage compared to pRA1, no SNP difference was identified between the two plasmids. Data indicated that these plasmids evolved primarily by gene cassette rearrangement rather than mutational change. This assertion is supported by the observation that pIP1202, isolated from *Y. pestis* in 1995 from Madagascar, and pP99-018, isolated in 1999 in Japan from *P. damselae* subsp. *piscicida*, do not vary by SNPs in the 100-kb plasmid backbone. Further, pP91278 which was isolated from *P. damselae* subsp. *piscicida* in 1991 in the United States differs by one SNP. Even though these plasmids have almost identical plasmid backbones, they carry very different resistance islands, varying from as few as two resistance genes in the most evolutionarily primary plasmids in *A. hydrophila* [*tet*(A) and *sul2* in pRAx and pRA1] to nine resistance genes in the

S. enterica plasmid pSN254 [*bla*_{CMY-2}, *strA/B*, *aacA/C*, *tet*(A), *floR*, *sul1/2*]. IncA/C plasmids have evolved through gene cassette rearrangement from a common ancestor, which likely originated from an aquatic environment and subsequently spread to terrestrial environments.

Motile Aeromonads

Mobile genetic elements have played a role in the dissemination of antimicrobial resistance in *Aeromonas* spp. In 2012, 50 Taiwanese *A. hydrophila* isolates from tilapia were screened for class 1, 2, and 3 integrons; resistance gene cassettes; mutations in the QRDR; and their susceptibility to 15 antimicrobial agents (34). Nineteen isolates were resistant to enrofloxacin and/or ciprofloxacin (MIC of 4 to 16 µg/ml) and had mutations in their *gyrA* and *parC* genes in the QRDR. All 50 isolates were resistant to at least one antimicrobial agent, and 94% were MDR. Forty-six percent were positive for class 1 integrons, with six resistance gene profiles identified. The most common resistance gene cassette identified in 26% of the class 1-positive isolates contained *dfrA12* and *aad2*. This was one of the first studies to report both a class 1 integron and more than one resistance gene cassette carried on a class 1 integron in an *Aeromonas* sp. in finfish (16, 35). High percentages of resistance were found to streptomycin (92%), trimethoprim (88%), and sulfamethoxazole (62%). The identification of multiple gene cassettes on integrons underscores the risk of resistance coselection following repeated use of a single antimicrobial agent class.

Another investigation of class 1 integrons was performed in 112 *Aeromonas* spp. isolates from aquacultured food fish, ornamental fish, shrimp, turtles, and amphibians in China (36). Isolates positive for the *int1* gene, indicating the presence of a class 1 integron, were subsequently screened for resistance gene cassettes and other resistance genes. Of the strains tested, 19.6% were positive for *int1*, and all of these carried the *sul1* and *qacE1* genes, indicating that these were structurally complete integrons. Many of the class 1 integron-positive strains were *A. hydrophila* and *Aeromonas veronii* isolated from aquacultured fish. Similar to other studies, common class 1 integron gene cassettes were found to contain the *dfrA17* gene alone (20%) or *dfrA12-orfF-aadA2* gene cassettes (80%). All of the class 1 integron-positive strains from aquacultured food fish had mutations in the QRDR genes *gyrA* and *parC*, and two were positive for *tet*(A). Phenotypic resistance profiles varied for the class 1 integron-positive strains; however, every strain was MDR and showed reduced susceptibility to at least ampicillin, sulfon-amides, trimethoprim-sulfamethoxazole, nalidixic acid, tetracycline, or streptomycin.

Class 1 integrons have also been identified in *Aeromonas* spp. from ornamental carp, with 100% of isolates from one study containing the *sul1* gene (37). Gene cassettes were identified on the class 1 integrons containing either the *aadA2* gene or *dfrA12-aadA2* genes, in agreement with other reports (34, 36).

As discussed earlier in this article for *A. salmonicida* and *Yersinia* spp., *Aeromonas* spp. have long been identified to have conjugative plasmids carrying varied antimicrobial resistance gene cassettes (33, 38). The first *floR*-containing plasmid in an *Aeromonas* sp. (pAB5S9) was discovered in *Aeromonas bestarium* (39). Researchers identified and performed conjugation experiments with pAB5S9, showing the presence of genes that conferred resistance to phenicols, streptomycin, tetracycline, and sulfonamides. Sequencing revealed that pAB5S9 carried the *floR*, *sul2*, *strA-strB*, and a *tetR-tet*(Y) resistance determinant. This was the first description of the combination *tetR-tet*(Y) determinant. Further, in the region of the plasmid containing the *floR* gene, an ISCR2 insertion element, the *sul2* and *strA-strB* genes matched with 100% identity to the SXT region, an integrating and conjugative element which has been reported *via* a BLAST search to carry resistance genes for potentiated sulfonamides and streptomycins in *Vibrio cholerae*.

P. damselae subsp. *piscicida*

Historically, *P. damselae* subsp. *piscicida*, the causative agent of photobacteriosis, has commonly been reported to carry R plasmids. One of the first reports in 1988 analyzed 168 MDR plasmids taken from *P. damselae* subsp. *piscicida* isolates from Japanese yellowtail farms (38). Plasmids conferred resistance to chloramphenicol, tetracycline, ampicillin, and sulfonamides; however, the resistance determinants housed on these plasmids were not identified. Later, investigators screened MDR isolates for R plasmids and used DNA probes to characterize and compare the DNA structure of detected R plasmids (40). These R plasmids included an *amp* gene for ampicillin; *tet*(A), *cat1*, and *cat2* for chloramphenicol; a kanamycin resistance gene postulated to be *aphA7*; *floR*; and *sul*. Resistance to kanamycin, sulfonamides, and tetracyclines was most often transferred by the R plasmids, and DNA probe hybridization revealed that there was significant homology between nine plasmids, indicating persistence of plasmids in *P. damselae* subsp. *piscicida* in these environments. A complex transposon-like structure consisting of insertion element 26 (IS26), *tet*(A), and *kan* was identified in *P. damselae* subsp.

piscicida, which conferred resistance to tetracycline and kanamycin. This study showed that the ease of genetic rearrangement due to flanking IS26 elements on the transposon-like structure in the plasmid was likely the cause of the carriage of a kanamycin resistance gene postulated to be *aphA7* on this plasmid (41). Full sequencing has been conducted on two MDR plasmids from *P. damselae* subsp. *piscicida*, pP99-018 (Japan) and pP91278 (United States). Both plasmids were categorized as belonging to a novel incompatibility group closely related to incompatibility group IncJ. Multiple mobilizable elements, including IS26, were identified on pP99-018 as well as *catA1*, *aphA7*, *tet*(A), *tet*(R), and *sul2*. The plasmid from the United States, pP91278, was 99% identical to pP99-018, from Japan, except that it carried fewer resistance elements including *tet*(A), *sul2*, and *dfrA8* (42).

A novel MDR IncP-1 plasmid, pP9014, was identified in *P. damselae* subsp. *piscicida* isolates from cultured yellowtail (*Seriola quinqueradiata*) in Japan (43). This MDR plasmid carried *tet*, *bla*, and *catA2* and is the first IncP-1 group plasmid identified from a fish pathogen. The authors performed comparative sequencing analysis of the pP9014 plasmid with other plasmid sequences in fish pathogens and in the National Center for Biotechnology Information database and identified no other IncP-1 plasmids in fish pathogens. This plasmid, however, is closely related to IncP-1 plasmids isolated from genera from wastewater treatment plants, marine biofilms, soil, and humans. The authors postulated that IncP-1 plasmids in aquaculture pathogens could be a vehicle for transmission of resistance genes within and between these environments.

Other Halophiles

Infections in fish caused by resistant *V. anguillarum* have been reported in the literature since the 1970s, including resistance to quinolones. In a study of 25 *V. anguillarum* strains obtained from cultured Japanese ayu (*Plecoglossus altivelis*), characterization of the *gyrA*, *gyrB*, *parC*, and *parE* gene mutations compared to reduced susceptibility to oxolinic acid was investigated (44). Of the 25 strains, 10 were oxolinic acid-susceptible, and for those with reduced susceptibility, MICs ranged from 0.006 µg/ml to 25 µg/ml. No *gyrB* or *parE* mutations were detected in any of the strains showing reduced susceptibility. In strains with MICs > 12.5 µg/ml, point mutations were identified in both *gyrA* (conferring a change in amino acid composition at position 83 from serine to isoleucine) and *parC* (conferring a change in amino acid composition at position 85 from serine to leucine). An intermediate interpretive category was defined by an MIC of 6.25 µg/ml and correlated only with a mutation in *gyrA* (conferring a change in amino acid composition at position 83 from serine to isoleucine).

In addition to chromosomal resistance determinant carriage, *V. anguillarum* strains were found to carry transmissible R plasmids containing tetracycline resistance genes. DNA-DNA hybridization analyses have differentiated the tetracycline resistance genes into four classes: A, B, C, and D. Aoki et al. analyzed tetracycline resistance determinants in R plasmids belonging to incompatibility types IncA/C and IncE in representative *V. anguillarum* isolates collected from 1973 to 1987 (8). The authors found that many strains of *V. anguillarum* obtained from 1973 to 1977 carried class B tetracycline resistance genes. However, a novel tetracycline resistance determinant, *tet*(G), which emerged in 1981, was identified on pJA8122 from *V. anguillarum* (8, 45). Interestingly, the authors also found that the DNA structure of the R plasmid changed in 1981 to a structure similar to that of pJA8122 and was different from R plasmids known at the time in other fish pathogens. Therefore, the origin of this new structure of plasmid similar to pJA8122 likely emerged in *V. anguillarum* with greater fitness over previous plasmids from sources not associated with other common fish pathogens (8).

Gliding Pathogens (Flavobacteria)

Flavobacterium psychrophilum causes bacterial cold water disease and rainbow trout fry syndrome in salmonids, ayu, and other species of finfish, resulting in major economic losses. Quinolone resistance has been reported in strains recovered from diseased fish. Izumi et al. characterized 244 isolates of *F. psychrophilum* from diseased fish using a genotyping method utilizing PCR restriction fragment length polymorphism and analyzing the *gyrA* gene to identify mutations in the QRDR (46). They amplified the *gyrA* gene and digested the product with restriction enzyme *Mph*1103I, resulting in the identification of quinolone-resistant isolates possessing an alanine residue at the GyrA 83 position. Overall, 62.7% of *F. psychrophilum* isolates were quinolone resistant and possessed the GyrA 83 mutation. Ayu isolates were found to have the same mutation at a rate of 82.5%.

Tetracycline resistance in *F. psychrophilum* has been noted as a result of six nucleotide polymorphisms in the 16s rRNA *via* 16s rDNA microarray experiments. Soule et al. reported that two genetic lineages of *F. psychrophilum* have been identified in diseased rainbow trout as defined by restriction fragment length polymorphism and microarray analysis, and tetracycline resistance is associated with one lineage (47).

A study to assess the variability in resistance genotypes of 25 *F. psychrophilum* isolates from Spain was conducted *via* plasmid profiling (48). Twenty isolates possessed 3.5-kb (*n* = 13) or 5.5-kb (*n* = 7) plasmids, but plasmid-mediated resistance was not found to be correlated with resistance to oxytetracycline or florfenicol, suggesting a chromosomal location for the source of the resistance genotype. Reduced susceptibility to oxytetracycline was identified in 80% of isolates, with MICs ranging from 2.4 to 9.7 µg/ml, and all isolates were susceptible to florfenicol.

Streptococcaceae

Streptococcus iniae, *Streptococcus parauberis*, and *Lactococcus garvieae* cause streptococcosis in a number of fish species, including olive flounder. Farmed olive flounder are common in Korea and can suffer heavy losses due to streptococcosis. This disease is usually treated with tetracycline and erythromycin. Park et al. investigated tetracycline and erythromycin susceptibility and corresponding resistance genes in *S. iniae* and *S. parauberis* isolates from Korean fish farms (49). The authors reported pan-susceptibility in *S. iniae*; however, a large number of the *S. parauberis* isolates were resistant to tetracycline (63%) and erythromycin (58%). PCR screening for resistance genes was conducted, and *tet*(M), *tet*(O), and *tet*(S) genes were found in most tetracycline-resistant isolates. Fourteen erythromycin-resistant isolates were positive for the *erm*B gene. The presence of both *tet*(S) and *erm*B genes was responsible for high-level resistance to both erythromycin and tetracycline in *S. parauberis* in olive flounder.

S. agalactiae (group B) is associated with high mortality of cultured tilapia worldwide. Dangwetngam et al. reported the antimicrobial susceptibilities of 144 *S. agalactiae* strains isolated from infected tilapia cultured in Thailand and screened oxytetracycline-resistant isolates for tetracycline resistance genes (50). Phenotypic resistance was observed against oxolinic acid, gentamicin, sulfamethoxazole, trimethoprim, and oxytetracycline. As determined by PCR and sequencing, 17 isolates were resistant to oxytetracycline and were positive for the *tet*(M) gene. All of these isolates were also resistant to trimethoprim, oxolinic acid, gentamicin, sulfamethoxazole, and oxytetracycline; however, investigation of any associations with mobile elements was not conducted.

Other Important Pathogens of Fish

Piscirickettsia salmonis causes piscirickettsiosis in a variety of species of salmonids, causing notable economic losses in Chile. Although oxytetracycline and/or florfenicol have been used to control *P. salmonis* for many years, few reports have characterized the antimicrobial resistance profiles of this key Chilean aquaculture pathogen. Cartes et al. conducted whole-genome sequencing of three Chilean *P. salmonis* strains to correlate oxytetracycline and florfenicol resistance genes with reduced susceptibility (51). After bioinformatic comparative genomic analysis, the authors identified resistance genes encoding transmembrane domains belonging to transporters and efflux pumps such as the major facilitator superfamily, which contributed to tetracycline resistance and concurrent tetracycline and florfenicol resistance. All antimicrobial resistance genes found were observed in the two field strains. One putative tetracycline resistance gene was found on a pathogenicity island, while another was postulated to be located on a transposon, due to the proximity of transposases detected. These genes have been identified in other fish pathogens (*Photobacterium*, *Vibrio*, *Pseudomonas* spp., and others). Membrane permeability, as studied by accumulated intracellular ethidium bromide after exposure to subinhibitory florfenicol concentrations, revealed that most of the accumulation occurred in the more susceptible strain. This demonstrated that the membrane transporters and pumps identified are capable of pumping out multiple classes of compounds and may be responsible for the MDR phenotype (51). This comprehensive study investigated the mechanism for oxytetracycline and florfenicol resistance, which may be transmissible or cohoused with virulence genes on pathogenicity islands.

Aliivibrio salmonicida, formerly known as *Vibrio salmonicida*, causes a bacterial septicemia called cold water vibriosis in farmed salmon and cod. Due to the long-term use of antimicrobial agents to combat this disease, resistance to multiple antimicrobial agents has been reported, in many cases mediated by transmissible mobile elements. Resistance plasmids in *A. salmonicida* have been reported to be associated with three separate transposon gene cassettes and resistance to trimethoprim, sulfonamides, and tetracyclines. Trimethoprim resistance has been associated with the *dfrA1* gene cassette contained in a class II transposon, which does not contain other drug resistance genes. Tetracycline resistance was associated with the *tet*(E) gene and sulfonamide resistance with the *sul2* gene. Both genes were located between two identical insertion elements (11).

While antimicrobial resistance has been identified for many of these key fish pathogens, at the writing of this arcticle, reports characterizing genetic determinants conferring resistance have not been identified for

Tenacibaculum maritimum, *Flavobacterium columnare*, or *Francisella noatunensis* subsp. *orientalis*. One study described the complete genome sequencing of *F. noatunensis* subsp. *orientalis*, in which a putative resistance island was identified; however, further characterization of the underlying antimicrobial resistance genes and their correlation with phenotypes were not reported (52).

Rhodes et al. (53) investigated macrolide susceptibility and mechanisms of resistance in the bacterial kidney disease pathogen *Renibacterium salmoninarum* Due to the practice of using erythromycin or azithromycin in female brood stock to prevent vertical transmission of *R. salmoninarum*, antimicrobial resistance has been postulated to be a risk. The authors screened isolates from fish treated multiple times for their susceptibility to erythromycin and azithromycin. Four isolates displayed higher MICs than the *R. salmoninarum* control strain, ATCC 33209, with MICs for erythromycin ranging between 0.125 and 0.25 µg/ml and MICs for azithromycin ranging between 0.016 and 0.03 µg/ml. Sequence analyses of both the 23S rDNA gene and the open reading frames of ribosomal proteins L4 and L22 revealed identical sequences among all isolates. This finding indicates that the phenotype was not a result of mutations in the drug-binding site of 23S rRNA, and the mechanism of resistance was not identified. This study represents the first report of *R. salmoninarum* isolates from fish that have received multiple macrolide treatments and exhibit reduced susceptibility.

ANTIMICROBIAL SUSCEPTIBILITY TESTING OF FISH PATHOGENS

Historical Perspective

When adjustments to aquatic animal husbandry approaches fail, are economically impractical, or are unlikely to resolve a disease outbreak, veterinarians and farmers typically turn to chemotherapy. Selection of an appropriate treatment, in general, should be made by a veterinarian after considering the anticipated pharmacokinetics of the antimicrobial agent in the target population under the given conditions (i.e., water temperature, salinity, hardness), as well as which antimicrobial agent has shown prior success against the etiological agent. When such information is unavailable or when additional reassurance is desired, performance of a well-controlled, standardized antimicrobial susceptibility test (AST) (i.e., disk diffusion, broth microdilution) can be used as a surrogate. When AST data are used correctly in combination with validated clinical breakpoints (susceptible, intermediate, resistant), these

data have a high likelihood of accurately predicting clinical outcome, especially if the normal dosage regimen recommended for the indicated disease is used (54). To date, the only fish pathogen with attributable and internationally accepted clinical breakpoints is *A. salmonicida* (55). In the absence of clinical breakpoints, AST data can be interpreted using epidemiological cutoff values (ECOFFs or ECVs; wild type, non-wild type) to determine if an isolate harbors antimicrobial resistance genes or resistance-mediating mutations. In *Salmonella*, the presence of resistance genes has been shown to be highly correlated (99%) with an increase in MIC (56). Although ECOFFs are most useful for the phenotypic detection of resistance mechanisms, veterinarians may be forced to select a therapy using available ECOFFs and/or susceptibility distributions from the published literature. However, effort should be made to select a therapy based on susceptibility results in conjunction with empirical evidence of effectiveness and knowledge of the pharmacokinetics and pharmacodynamics of the antimicrobial agent(s). At present, only *A. salmonicida* has published ECOFFs (55, 57), but data analyses are forthcoming for other key fish pathogens. In January 2017, the CLSI's Subcommittee on Veterinary Antimicrobial Susceptibility Testing approved MIC ECOFFs for the key fish pathogen *F. psychrophilum*. These will be published in the next edition of the CLSI's VET03/VET04-S2 (55).

Importance of Understanding the Scope of an AST Testing Program

When conducting investigations of the AST of fish pathogens, it is important for workers to understand the scope and goals of their work. If a project intends to monitor for clinically relevant resistance, then clinical breakpoints should be used when available. If the surveillance and detection of emerging low-level resistance is the goal, then ECOFFs should be used. If one of the program's goals is to provide meaningful susceptibility comparisons across borders and even worldwide, then serious consideration should be given to whether clinical breakpoints should be used. This is because clinical breakpoints are established based partly on pharmacokinetics and pharmacodynamics using the normal dosage regimen (58), which may differ greatly by country, thus altering the practical definitions of susceptible, intermediate, and resistant, and ultimately the clinical usefulness of the clinical breakpoints. Also, in most cases use of clinical breakpoints as the sole interpretive criteria in an antimicrobial resistance surveillance program of bacterial pathogens of fish or any other animal species may not be as sensitive in the detection of emerging resistance. This is because clinical breakpoints are often one to three 2-fold dilutions higher than the corresponding ECOFFs (Fig. 1).

Standard AST Methods

Prior to 2001, aquatic animal disease researchers commonly used AST methods and clinical breakpoints developed in their own laboratories. The use of different methods and breakpoint values limited accurate interlaboratory comparisons and correlation to clinical cases. The magnitude of the issue was brought to light by Smith (59) when he surveyed 32 fish health laboratories in 18 countries and found that 25 laboratories used predominantly disk diffusion testing procedures and only 4 used the standard CLSI procedure found in the original M42-A guideline published in 2003 and again in 2006 as VET03-A (60). Alarmingly, 22 of the 25 laboratories reported that for any given antimicrobial agent they employed the same clinical breakpoints for all nonfas-

tidious pathogens. Due to outreach efforts over the past decade by Smith and other members, advisors, and observers of the CLSI's Subcommittee on Veterinary Antimicrobial Susceptibility Testing, the authors have confidence that the percentage accordance with standardized CLSI methods has risen significantly. However, it is clear that additional educational opportunities are warranted on what constitutes use of a standardized AST method and quality control, data interpretation, clinical breakpoints, and ECOFFs.

Currently, there are two fish pathogen-specific CLSI guidelines: one for disk diffusion AST (60) and an updated guideline for broth microdilution AST (61). These guidelines provide standardized methods and quality control procedures that allow internationally harmonized testing of nonfastidious aquaculture pathogens (group 1 organisms) on unsupplemented Mueller-Hinton media, and *F. columnare* and *F. psychrophilum* in diluted cation-adjusted Mueller-Hinton broth (Table 2). For other

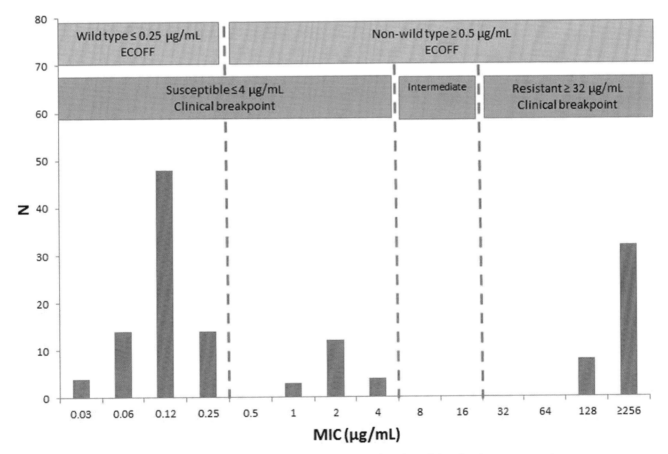

Figure 1 Distribution of MICs and categorization by clinical breakpoints contrasted to ECOFFs.

Table 2 Antimicrobial susceptibility testing methods of aquatic bacterial pathogens[a]

Organism	Medium[c]	Incubation
Group 1: nonfastidious bacteria		
Enterobacteriaceae	**MHA**	22°C (24–28 h and/or 44–48 h or 28°C (24–28 h) or 35°C (16–18 h)
Aeromonas salmonicida (nonpsychrophilic strains)	**CAMHB**	22°C (24–28 h and/or 44–48 h or 28°C (24–28 h) or 35°C (16–20 h)
Aeromonas hydrophila and other mesophilic aeromonads		
Pseudomonas spp.		
Plesiomonas shigelloides		
Shewanella spp.		
Group 3: gliding bacteria[b]		
Flavobacterium columnare	**Diluted CAMHB (4 g/liter)**	28°C (44–48 h)
Flavobacterium psychrophilum	**Diluted CAMHB (4 g/liter)**	18°C (92–96 h)
Group 2: strictly halophilic *Vibrionaceae*		
Vibrio vulnificus, V. parahaemolyticus, V. alginolyticus, V. anguillarum, V. fischeri, V. metschnikovii, V. ichthyoenteri	CAMHB + NaCl (1%)	22°C (24–28 h and/or 44–48 h) or 28°C (24–28 h and/or 44–48 h)
	MHA + NaCl (1%)	22°C (24–28 h and/or 44–48 h) or 28°C (24–28 h and/or 44–48 h)
Group 4: Streptococci		
Lactococcus spp., *Vagococcus salmoninarum*	MHA + 5% sheep blood	22°C (44–48 hours) + CO_2
	CAMHB + LHB (2.5–5% vol/vol)	22°C (44–48 h) + CO_2
Streptococcus spp., *Carnobacterium maltaromaticum*, and other streptococci	MHA + 5% sheep blood	28°C (24–28 h and/or 44–48 h) + CO_2
	CAMHB + LHB (2.5% to 5% v/v)	28°C (24–28 h and/or 44–48 h) + CO_2
Group 5: other fastidious bacteria		
Atypical *Aeromonas salmonicida*	CAMHB	15°C (44–48 h)
	MHA	15°C (44–48 h)
Aliivibrio salmonicida (formerly *V. salmonicida*) and *Moritella viscosa*	MHA + NaCl (1.5%)	4°C (*A. salmonicida*) or 15°C (*M. viscosa*) (6 days)
Tenacibaculum maritimum	FMM or diluted MHB (1:7) + inorganic ion supplementation	25°C (44–48 h)
	FMM or diluted MHA (1:7) + inorganic ion supplementation	25°C (44–48 h)
Francisella spp.	CAMHB + IsoValitex (2%) + 0.1% glucose	28°C (44–48 h)
Renibacterium salmoninarum	KDM	15°C (with agitation for 96 h)
Piscirickettsia salmonis	AUSTRAL-SRS	18°C (92–96 h and/or 116–120 h)

[a]Bold text indicates that the method has been standardized and quality control guidelines are available (60, 61).
[b]Disk diffusion testing has proven difficult. Some modification may be necessary for testing *F. branchiophilum*, which may include cations, horse or fetal calf serum, or NaCl.
[c]CAMHB, cation-adjusted Mueller-Hinton broth; FMM, *Flexibacter maritimum* medium; KDM, kidney disease medium; LHB, lysed horse blood; MHA, Mueller-Hinton agar.

fastidious species pathogenic for fish, recommendations are provided to develop laboratory-specific methods until a method can be standardized.

Non-fastidious bacterial pathogens

Nonfastidious bacterial pathogens of fish (termed group 1 by the CLSI) are those that grow adequately in unsupplemented Mueller-Hinton media at 22°C for 24 to 28 hours and/or 44 to 48 hours, 28°C for 24 to 28 hours, or 35°C for 16 to 20 hours (16 to 18 hours for disk diffusion). These organisms typically include

members of the *Enterobacteriaceae*, some members of the *Vibrionaceae*, *A. salmonicida*, *A. hydrophila* and other mesophilic aeromonads, *Pseudomonas* spp., and *Plesiomonas shigelloides*. These organisms should be tested using CLSI guidelines (60–62) with quality control.

Investigations of *A. salmonicida* using standardized AST methods far outnumber those of any other fish pathogen. Miller and Reimschuessel published oxytetracycline, ormetoprim-sulfadimethoxine, oxolinic acid, and florfenicol MIC and zone diameter distributions for 217 *A. salmonicida* isolates (57). They used the

Table 3 CLSI-approved MIC and zone diameter CBP and ECOFFs for *A. salmonicida* (55)[a]

Antimicrobial agent	MIC CBP			MIC ECOFF	Zone diameter CBP			Zone diameter ECOFF
	S	I	R	WT	S	I	R	WT
Gentamicin								≥18
Florfenicol				≤4				≥27
Oxytetracycline	≤1	2-4	≥8	≤1	≥28	22–27	≤21	≥28
Oxolinic acid	≤0.12	0.25-0.5	≥1	≤0.12	≥30	25–29	≤24	≥30
Erythromycin								≥14
Ormetoprim-sulfadimethoxine				≤0.5/9.5				≥20
Trimethoprim-sulfamethoxazole				[b]				≥20

[a]S, susceptible; I, intermediate; R, resistant; WT, wild type.
[b]MIC ECOFF for ormetoprim-sulfadimethoxine can be used for interpretations of this antimicrobial.

data to establish the first consensus-approved, CLSI-endorsed ECOFFs for a fish pathogen (Table 3). Later, the distributions were used in conjunction with available pharmacokinetics, pharmacodynamics, and clinical effectiveness data to establish MIC and zone diameter clinical breakpoints for oxytetracycline and oxolinic acid (55). Douglas et al. determined trimethoprim-sulfamethoxazole, trimethoprim, and sulfamethoxazole zone diameters for 106 *A. salmonicida* isolates (63). Their analysis showed that testing trimethoprim-sulfamethoxazole together was unreliable for predicting a susceptibility phenotype for trimethoprim and sulfamethoxazole if tested alone. In a similar study by the same group of investigators, Ruane et al. determined oxolinic acid, flumequine, and enrofloxacin zone diameters for 106 *A. salmonicida* isolates (64). They proposed laboratory-specific ECOFFs for each species and argued that oxolinic acid is the best quinolone representative to monitor for the presence of resistance mechanisms. Other *A. salmonicida* susceptibility testing studies employed similar testing methods but lacked available quality control parameters at the time, thus making direct comparisons with current data more difficult (65, 66).

Čížek et al. evaluated the antimicrobial susceptibility of *Aeromonas* spp. from ornamental (koi) carp and common carp in the Czech Republic to investigate differences in resistance patterns resulting from different on-farm usage practices (37). While it is permitted in the Czech Republic to treat common carp with oxytetracycline, the regulation of antimicrobial use is not enforced on ornamental carp production, resulting in more widespread use. Significant differences in reduced susceptibility were identified in isolates from ornamental carp versus common carp, and 60% of isolates were resistant to one or more antimicrobial agents. Ornamental carp isolates were significantly more resistant to more than one antimicrobial agent and more resis-

tant to ciprofloxacin than those from common carp. Resistance to oxytetracycline was detected in 50% of aeromonads from ornamental carp and slightly less (41%) in common carp.

Despite *E. ictaluri* being a major pathogen of catfish, few susceptibility investigations using standard or nonstandard methods are available. Hawke et al. used standard broth microdilution testing methods for eight *E. ictaluri* isolates from laboratory-held zebrafish and reported all as lacking resistance mechanisms to florfenicol, enrofloxacin, and trimethoprim-sulfamethoxazole (67). Dung et al. used nonstandard testing conditions to measure the MICs of 15 antimicrobial agents for 64 *E. ictaluri* isolates from Vietnam (68). Study-specific ECOFFs for streptomycin, oxolinic acid, flumequine, oxytetracycline, and trimethoprim were calculated using the current "gold-standard" statistical method published by Turnidge and Paterson (69). All isolates were highly susceptible to florfenicol, with MICs ≤ 0.25 µg/ml. McGinnis et al. (70) noted similar findings for florfenicol, using nonstandard conditions. Dung et al. were the first to report widespread resistance emergence to streptomycin, with 82.8% of isolates identified as non-wild type (68).

E. tarda is primarily isolated from diseased eels and flounder. In a Taiwanese study, 94 isolates were tested at 25°C for 18 hours in broth microdilution panels (26). Susceptibility to five classes of antimicrobial agents was determined, with decreased susceptibility to potentiated sulfonamides and tetracyclines reported. It is important to note that these investigators stated that the methods used were in accordance with CLSI guidelines; however, they used a nonstandard incubation temperature of 25°C, and the use of human-specific interpretive categories are only reliable for data generated at 35°C and when the data are generated for human medical application.

Enteric redmouth disease, caused by *Y. ruckeri*, is an important disease in rainbow trout aquaculture. Huang et al. used standardized broth microdilution testing to obtain MICs of 24 antimicrobial agents for 82 clinical isolates from Germany (28). Using wide test concentration ranges and quality control parameters when possible, this study accurately captured the current antibiogram for *Y. ruckeri*. Researchers noted that measurements after 24 hours and 48 hours often revealed an increase in calculated MIC_{50} and MIC_{90} values with time. Due to the adequate growth of *Y. ruckeri* at 22°C after 24 to 28 hours, investigators recommended this incubation time for future research. For most of the antimicrobial agents tested, a unimodal distribution of MICs was observed. All isolates that showed low enrofloxacin MICs also showed low nalidixic acid MICs. Seventy-two isolates had elevated nalidixic acid and enrofloxacin MICs of 0.06 to 0.25 µg/ml and 8 to 64 µg/ml, respectively. Only one isolate had elevated MICs for sulfamethoxazole (≥1,024 µg/ml) and for trimethoprim-sulfamethoxazole (≥32/608 µg/ml). Three isolates had colistin MICs of ≥32 µg/ml. It is envisaged that these data will be combined with others derived from the same standardized methodology to establish ECOFFs that can be useful to detect emerging resistance concerns in this economically important fish pathogen. Balta et al. obtained zone diameters for 116 *Y. ruckeri* isolates from infected rainbow trout in commercial farms in Turkey (29). The authors stated that CLSI methods, quality control, and clinical breakpoints were used, but it is unclear if this is, in fact, the case since detailed methods were not provided and no clinical breakpoints are available for *Y. ruckeri* at this time. The authors did find the presence of resistance genes for oxytetracycline in 35.3% of isolates, ampicillin in 29%, oxolinic acid in 11.1%, streptomycin in 10.2%, sulfamethoxazole in 9.4%, trimethoprim-sulfamethoxazole in 9.4%, florfenicol in 4.2%, and enrofloxacin in 2.3% of the isolates.

At least one member of the family *Vibrionaceae* (*V. cholerae*) does not require NaCl supplementation for *in vitro* susceptibility testing, but others such as *V. parahaemolyticus*, *V. alginolyticus*, *V. vulnificus*, *V. anguillarum*, *V. fischeri*, *V. metschnikovii*, and *V. ichthyoenteri* have been shown to need NaCl at least in agar media (71, 72). The methods, quality control parameters, and interpretive categories described in the CLSI's M45-A3 guideline (62) should be used for tests of *V. cholerae*, but additional investigation is clearly warranted for tests of other vibrios to ensure accurate phenotypic characterization.

Motile aeromonad septicemia caused by mesophilic motile *Aeromonas* species is probably the most common bacterial disease in freshwater aquarium fish (73). *A. hydrophila* has often been the primary implicated

pathogen, but others including *A. veronii* and *Aeromonas caviae* have been shown to play important roles. Jagoda et al. used disk diffusion methods described in CLSI M31-A3 (74) to test 53 motile aeromonads at 35°C and found resistance to tetracycline (58.5%), erythromycin (54.7%), trimethoprim-sulfamethoxazole (26.4%), nitrofurantoin (22.6%), neomycin (9.4%), chloramphenicol (7.5%), and enrofloxacin (7.5%) (75). A total of 49% of the isolates were found to be resistant to more than one antimicrobial agent class. Deng et al. tested 112 motile *Aeromonas* spp. by disk diffusion against 14 antimicrobial agents (36). Tests were conducted under standard conditions at 35°C. Although not all antimicrobial agents had interpretive criteria available, the authors noted that 49.1% of isolates were MDR. Most isolates (≥90%) were susceptible to cefotaxime, amikacin, ciprofloxacin, norfloxacin, and doxycycline. Interestingly, *A. hydrophila* and *A. veronii* displayed greater levels of resistance compared to *A. caviae*, *Aeromonas sobria*, *Aeromonas dhakensis*, *Aeromonas jandaei*, *Aeromonas trota*, and *Aeromonas media*. Čížek et al. conducted nonstandardized agar dilution testing at 28°C with 72 motile *Aeromonas* spp. isolated from common carp and koi carp (37). The authors noted that they cautiously used clinical breakpoints appropriate for tests conducted at 35°C (62). Resistance rates of 50% to oxytetracycline, 15% to ciprofloxacin, and 7% to chloramphenicol were noted. A significantly higher incidence of class 1 integrons and ciprofloxacin resistance in motile aeromonads from koi carp was ascribed to a distinct Czech policy on antimicrobial use in ornamental fish farms (koi) versus in traditional aquaculture (common carp). Antimicrobial resistance linked to class 1 integrons has also been shown by other researchers (34).

Gliding pathogens (group 3)

Fish health specialists have a standard broth microdilution method for the nutritionally fastidious aquatic gliding bacteria family, *Flavobacteriaceae* (61, 76). Recently, ECOFFs have been proposed for *F. columnare* (77) (Table 4) and *F. psychrophilum* (78, 79) (Table 5). Gieseker et al. proposed provisional ECOFFs for ampicillin, enrofloxacin, erythromycin, florfenicol, flumequine, oxolinic acid, and oxytetracycline using MIC distributions of 120 geographically diverse *F. columnare* isolates (77). ECOFFs were calculated using the ECOFFinder method (69). These ECOFFs combined with existing pharmacokinetic and clinical data may be used in the future to establish clinical breakpoints. Van Vliet et al. recently published 10 MIC distributions for 50 Michigan *F. psychrophilum* isolates (79). Their

Table 4 Provisional MIC ECOFFs for *F. columnare* (77)

Antimicrobial agent	MIC ECOFF (ECOFFinder) Wild type
Ampicillin	≤0.25
Florfenicol	≤4
Oxytetracycline	≤0.12
Oxolinic acid	≤0.25
Flumequine	≤0.12
Enrofloxacin	≤0.03
Erythromycin	≤4

data revealed a unimodal, wild-type distribution for all antimicrobial agents tested except oxytetracycline, for which there were some non-wild-type isolates. Using normalized resistance interpretation and the ECOFFinder method to calculate an ECOFF, these researchers proposed provisional ECOFFs that largely agree with those presented by Smith (78) in 2017 and were approved by the CLSI Subcommittee on Veterinary Antimicrobial Susceptibility Testing (Table 5). Earlier, using nonstandard agar dilution and disk diffusion methods to generate MIC and zone diameter data distributions, Miranda et al. calculated ECOFFs using normalized resistance interpretation for amoxicillin, florfenicol, oxytetracycline, and three quinolones (80). These data from 125 *F. psychrophilum* isolates from farm-raised salmonids in Chile revealed that agar dilution testing was more precise than disk diffusion at determining a non-wild-type phenotype for all antimicrobial agents tested. The authors concluded that the disk diffusion testing method is not suitable for investigating the susceptibility of *F. psychrophilum* isolates. Henríquez-Núñez et al. came to a similar conclusion when they used nonstandard broth microdilution and disk diffusion methods on 40

F. psychrophilum isolates from Chilean salmonid farms (81). They determined susceptibility to oxytetracycline, florfenicol, and oxolinic acid and noted very high levels of resistance to all three antimicrobial agents, and again found that the disk diffusion testing method was difficult with this species.

Nonstandard, Recommended AST Methods

Strictly halophilic *Vibrionaceae* (group 2)

As mentioned earlier, some noncholera vibrios should be tested *in vitro* with NaCl present. Israil et al. used agar dilution testing to show that resistant phenotypes were observed when tests were conducted in Mueller-Hinton agar supplemented with 1%, 2%, and 3% NaCl, but not in unsupplemented media (71). Until a standardized susceptibility testing method can be developed for noncholera vibrios, the methods and quality control parameters described in the CLSI's M45-A3 guideline (62) should be employed, but with caution. Tang et al. tested fluoroquinolone activity against 46 human clinical *V. vulnificus* isolates by agar dilution in unsupplemented Mueller-Hinton agar (82). They found a lack of decreased susceptibility in all isolates to all fluoroquinolones. Similarly, Hsueh et al. investigated 19 *V. vulnificus* isolates from Taiwanese patients and found them to be pan-susceptible to 17 antimicrobial agents tested and resistant only to clindamycin (83). All isolates were tested on unsupplemented media. A recent Iranian investigation of two *P. damselae* subsp. *damselae* isolates tested on unsupplemented Mueller-Hinton agar showed zone diameters indicative of susceptibility to ciprofloxacin, chloramphenicol, and nalidixic acid (84). Zones suggesting a clinically resistant phenotype were noted for ampicillin, amoxicillin, gentamicin, streptomycin, erythromycin, clindamycin,

Table 5 MIC ECOFFs and zone diameter ECOFFs for *F. psychrophilum* (78–80)

Antimicrobial agent	MIC ECOFF (ECOFFinder + NRI)[a] Wild type	MIC ECOFF (ECOFFinder) Wild type	MIC ECOFF (NRI) Wild type	Zone diameter ECOFF Wild type
Amoxicillin				≥44
Florfenicol	≤2	≤2	≤2	≥46
Oxytetracycline	≤0.12	≤0.06	≤0.12	≥47
Oxolinic acid	≤0.25	≤0.25	≤0.25	≥29
Flumequine	≤0.12	≤0.12	≤0.12	≥47
Enrofloxacin	≤0.03	≤0.015	≤0.03	≥49
Erythromycin	≤8	≤8	≤8	
Ormetoprim-sulfadimethoxine		≤0.5/9.5	≤1/19	
Trimethoprim-sulfamethoxazole		≤0.12/2.38	≤0.5/9.5	

[a]Accepted by the CLSI Subcommittee for Veterinary Antimicrobial Susceptibility Testing in January 2017.

and novobiocin. Clearly, additional research is needed to determine not only whether NaCl is required for testing all halophilic vibrios, but also if an incubation temperature lower than 35°C may be required for some fish-pathogenic vibrios.

Streptococcaceae (group 4)

Most streptococcal fish pathogens can likely be grown and tested under standard testing conditions as described in the CLSI's VET01 standard (58). The recommended agar medium for testing streptococci is Mueller-Hinton agar supplemented with 5% defibrinated sheep blood. Incubation conditions are at 35°C ± 2°C in an atmosphere of 5% ± 2% CO_2 for 20 to 24 hours. For fish pathogens that cannot grow satisfactorily under these conditions, adjustments may be necessary, including longer incubation times and probably lower incubation temperatures. Broth microdilution testing should be performed using cation-adjusted Mueller-Hinton broth supplemented with 2.5 to 5% lysed horse blood. Incubation conditions are 35°C for 20 to 24 hours without CO_2. Some streptococcal fish pathogens likely require lower incubation temperatures (22°C for *Lactococcus* spp. and *Vagococcus salmoninarum*; 28°C for some *Streptococcus* spp. and *Carnobacterium maltaromaticum*) and CO_2 supplementation (55).

Other fastidious bacterial pathogens (group 5)

Those organisms that do not grow in standardized Mueller-Hinton media or under standardized conditions have been classified by the CLSI as group 5 organisms (55). These included atypical *A. salmonicida*, psychrophilic members of *Vibrionaceae*, *T. maritimum*, *Francisella* spp., *R. salmoninarum*, and *P. salmonis*.

Atypical *A. salmonicida* isolates have optimal temperatures *in vitro* of <22°C but can be tested in cation-adjusted Mueller-Hinton broth. Disk diffusion results of these isolates should be read with caution because extended incubation times may be required and drug stability can be an issue.

Some psychrophilic vibrios including *Moritella viscosa* and *A. salmonicida* (formerly *V. salmonicida*) may have optimal temperatures *in vitro* of between 4 and 15°C. At these temperatures extended incubation times will almost certainly be required, and drug stability can be an issue. Coyne et al. conducted agar dilution and disk diffusion susceptibility testing on clinical *M. viscosa* isolates in Mueller-Hinton media at 15°C and used a 6-day incubation period (85).

Similar to the group 3 organisms, *T. maritimum* is a gliding bacterium and a member of the class *Flavobacteriaceae*. However, this species has been shown to require a specialized *Flexibacter maritimum* medium prepared with seawater (86) and an *in vitro* growth temperature of 24°C (87). Zone diameter and MIC determinations on this media for seven antimicrobial agents appeared to provide reproducible results when conducted in duplicate. However, the lack of a source of commercial grade seawater has precluded the standardization of a method for this organism.

F. noatunensis subsp. *orientalis* is an emerging warm-water fish pathogen and the causative agent of francisellosis in tilapia. Soto and colleagues are close to standardizing a broth microdilution testing method for this important species (88). Testing at 28°C for 48 hours in cation-adjusted Mueller-Hinton broth supplemented with 2% IsoVitalex and 0.1% glucose tested at a pH of 6.4 ±1 provided optimal growth and reproducible results. The authors noted that the lower pH did affect the inhibitory properties of the potentiated sulfonamides.

The Gram-positive fish pathogen *R. salmoninarum* is the causative agent of bacterial kidney disease. *R. salmoninarum* can be transmitted horizontally as well as vertically, and fish can be susceptible to disease throughout their life cycle. For veterinarians, the windows of opportunity for chemotherapy can be limited, and macrolides are typically the most common choice. Rhodes et al. used a specialized medium (kidney disease medium) to conduct broth micro- and macro-dilution tests at 15°C with 150 rpm agitation for 4 days (measurements every 24 hours) (53). The authors found that broth microdilution did not provide optimal growth conditions due to a generation time twice that calculated in the broth macrodilution tests. Reduced susceptibility to erythromycin and azithromycin was noted in isolates obtained from fish that received multiple macrolide treatments.

Piscirickettsiosis caused by *P. salmonis* is by far the most damaging infectious disease in the Chilean salmon industry. The recommended AST conditions for this pathogen can be found in CLSI VET03/VET04-S2 (55) and are based on the research of Yañez et al. (89). AUSTRAL-SRS medium was found to perform well when inoculated and incubated at 18°C for 92 to 96 hours and/or 116 to 120 hours. More recently, Henríquez et al. conducted a large-scale field study and obtained susceptibility profiles of 292 *P. salmonis* isolates (90). They used a new medium called ADL-PSB to conduct broth microdilution tests at 19°C ± 2°C for 5 to 7 days. The authors analyzed the MIC data using a method similar to the ECOFFinder method (69) to establish laboratory-specific epidemiological cutoff values for oxolinic acid, flumequine, and oxytetracycline.

FUTURE RESEARCH

Whether it is routine culture and susceptibility testing in a diagnostic laboratory or epidemiological surveillance of antimicrobial resistance, incorporation of a standard AST method when available should always be the priority. In the absence of a standard method, researchers can optimize their testing methods and eventually lead a multilaboratory method standardization trial (74). Alternatively, laboratory-specific methods, quality control, and interpretive criteria can be developed. Although this route precludes a lab's data from being internationally harmonized, it may be appropriate in some situations.

Aquatic animal disease diagnosticians need additional standard testing methods, as well as internationally harmonized criteria for interpreting zones of inhibition and MICs. Clinical breakpoints are notoriously difficult to establish for fish for a multitude of reasons. Pharmacokinetic and pharmacodynamic data are very difficult to ascertain because antimicrobial exposure data during the dosing interval can be extremely challenging. Clinical effectiveness data are difficult to interpret due to on-farm predation and cannibalism. Lastly, available susceptibility data in large numbers is traditionally hard to locate because of the lack of a centralized database and the general lack of standardized methods until recently and because there are not standardized, reproducible methods for all fish pathogens. To compensate for the lack of clinical breakpoints, laboratories should instead use ECOFFs to determine whether their isolate harbors resistance genes that may confer clinically relevant resistance.

Citation. Miller RA, Harbottle H. 2017. Antimicrobial drug resistance in fish pathogens. Microbiol Spectrum 6(1):ARBA-0017-2017.

References

1. Coyne R, Bergh Ø, Samuelsen O, Andersen K, Lunestad BT, Nilsen H, Dalsgaard I, Smith P. 2004. Attempt to validate breakpoint MIC values estimated from pharmacokinetic data obtained during oxolinic acid therapy of winter ulcer disease in Atlantic salmon (*Salmo salar*). *Aquaculture* 238:51–66.
2. Austin B, Austin DA. 1993. *Bacterial Fish Pathogens: Diseases in Farmed and Wild Fish*. Ellis Horwood, Chichester, United Kingdom.
3. Miller RA, Pelsor FR, Qiu J, Kane AS, Reimschuessel R. 2016. Determination of oxytetracycline absorption and effectiveness against *Aeromonas salmonicida* in rainbow trout (*Oncorhynchus mykiss*). *J Vet Sci Anim Welf* 1:1–9.
4. Petersen A, Andersen JS, Kaewmak T, Somsiri T, Dalsgaard A. 2002. Impact of integrated fish farming on antimicrobial resistance in a pond environment. *Appl Environ Microbiol* 68:6036–6042.
5. Aoki T, Egusa S, Kimura T, Watanabe T. 1971. Detection of R-factors in naturally occurring *Aeromonas salmonicida* strains. *Appl Microbiol* 22:716–717.
6. Aoki T, Arai T, Egusa S. 1977. Detection of R plasmids in naturally occurring fish-pathogenic bacteria, *Edwardsiella tarda*. *Microbiol Immunol* 21:77–83.
7. Aoki T, Kitao T. 1981. Drug resistance and transferrable R plasmids in *Edwardsiella tarda* from fish culture ponds. *Fish Pathol* 15:277–281.
8. Aoki T, Satoh T, Kitao T. 1987. New tetracycline resistance determinant on R plasmids from *Vibrio anguillarum*. *Antimicrob Agents Chemother* 31:1446–1449.
9. Aoki T, Takahashi A. 1987. Class D tetracycline resistance determinants of R plasmids from the fish pathogens *Aeromonas hydrophila*, *Edwardsiella tarda*, and *Pasteurella piscicida*. *Antimicrob Agents Chemother* 31: 1278–1280.
10. Miranda CD, Tello A, Keen PL. 2013. Mechanisms of antimicrobial resistance in finfish aquaculture environments. *Front Microbiol* 4:233.
11. Sørum H. 1998. Mobile drug resistance genes among fish bacteria. *APMIS Suppl* 106:74–76.
12. Cabello FC, Godfrey HP, Buschmann AH, Dölz HJ. 2016. Aquaculture as yet another environmental gateway to the development and globalisation of antimicrobial resistance. *Lancet Infect Dis* 16:e127–e133.
13. Cabello FC, Godfrey HP, Tomova A, Ivanova L, Dölz H, Millanao A, Buschmann AH. 2013. Antimicrobial use in aquaculture re-examined: its relevance to antimicrobial resistance and to animal and human health. *Environ Microbiol* 15:1917–1942.
14. Kim JH, Hwang SY, Son JS, Han JE, Jun JW, Shin SP, Choresca C Jr, Choi YJ, Park YH, Park SC. 2011. Molecular characterization of tetracycline- and quinolone-resistant *Aeromonas salmonicida* isolated in Korea. *J Vet Sci* 12:41–48.
15. Oppegaard H, Sørum H. 1994. *gyrA* mutations in quinolone-resistant isolates of the fish pathogen *Aeromonas salmonicida*. *Antimicrob Agents Chemother* 38: 2460–2464.
16. L'Abée-Lund TM, Sørum H. 2001. Class 1 integrons mediate antibiotic resistance in the fish pathogen *Aeromonas salmonicida* worldwide. *Microb Drug Resist* 7: 263–272.
17. Sørum H, L'Abée-Lund TM, Solberg A, Wold A. 2003. Integron-containing IncU R plasmids pRAS1 and pAr-32 from the fish pathogen *Aeromonas salmonicida*. *Antimicrob Agents Chemother* 47:1285–1290.
18. Dallaire-Dufresne S, Tanaka KH, Trudel MV, Lafaille A, Charette SJ. 2014. Virulence, genomic features, and plasticity of *Aeromonas salmonicida* subsp. *salmonicida*, the causative agent of fish furunculosis. *Vet Microbiol* 169: 1–7.
19. Vincent AT, Emond-Rheault JG, Barbeau X, Attéré SA, Frenette M, Lagüe P, Charette SJ. 2016. Antibiotic resistance due to an unusual ColE1-type replicon plasmid in *Aeromonas salmonicida*. *Microbio* 162:942–953.
20. Trudel MV, Vincent AT, Attéré SA, Labbé M, Derome N, Culley AI, Charette SJ. 2016. Diversity of antibiotic-

resistance genes in Canadian isolates of *Aeromonas salmonicida* subsp. *salmonicida*: dominance of pSN254b and discovery of pAsa8. *Sci Rep* **6**:35617.

21. McIntosh D, Cunningham M, Ji B, Fekete FA, Parry EM, Clark SE, Zalinger ZB, Gilg IC, Danner GR, Johnson KA, Beattie M, Ritchie R. 2008. Transferable, multiple antibiotic and mercury resistance in Atlantic Canadian isolates of *Aeromonas salmonicida* subsp. *salmonicida* is associated with carriage of an IncA/C plasmid similar to the *Salmonella enterica* plasmid pSN254. *J Antimicrob Chemother* **61**:1221–1228.

22. Starliper CE, Cooper RK, Shotts EB, Taylor PW. 1993. Plasmid-mediated Romet resistance of *Edwardsiella ictaluri*. *J Aquat Anim Health* **5**:1–8.

23. Welch TJ, Evenhuis J, White DG, McDermott PF, Harbottle H, Miller RA, Griffin M, Wise D. 2009. IncA/C plasmid-mediated florfenicol resistance in the catfish pathogen *Edwardsiella ictaluri*. *Antimicrob Agents Chemother* **53**:845–846.

24. Welch TJ, Fricke WF, McDermott PF, White DG, Rosso ML, Rasko DA, Mammel MK, Eppinger M, Rosovitz MJ, Wagner D, Rahalison L, Leclerc JE, Hinshaw JM, Lindler LE, Cebula TA, Carniel E, Ravel J. 2007. Multiple antimicrobial resistance in plague: an emerging public health risk. *PLoS One* **2**:e309.

25. Sun K, Wang H, Zhang M, Ziao Z, Sun L. 2009. Genetic mechanisms of multi-antimicrobial resistance in a pathogenic *Edwardsiella tarda* strain. *Aquaculture* **289**:134–139.

26. Lo DY, Lee YJ, Wang JH, Kuo HC. 2014. Antimicrobial susceptibility and genetic characterisation of oxytetracycline-resistant *Edwardsiella tarda* isolated from diseased eels. *Vet Rec* **175**:203.

27. Yu JE, Cho MY, Kim JW, Kang HY. 2012. Large antibiotic-resistance plasmid of *Edwardsiella tarda* contributes to virulence in fish. *Microb Pathog* **52**:259–266.

28. Huang Y, Michael GB, Becker R, Kaspar H, Mankertz J, Schwarz S, Runge M, Steinhagen D. 2014. Pheno- and genotypic analysis of antimicrobial resistance properties of *Yersinia ruckeri* from fish. *Vet Microbiol* **171**:406–412.

29. Balta F, Sandalli C, Kayis S, Ozgumus OB. 2010. Molecular analysis of antimicrobial resistance in *Yersinia ruckeri* strains isolated from rainbow trout (*Oncorhynchus mykiss*) grown in commercial farms in Turkey. *Bull Eur Assoc Fish Pathol* **30**:211–219.

30. Schiefer AM, Wiegand I, Sherwood KJ, Wiedemann B, Stock I. 2005. Biochemical and genetic characterization of the beta-lactamases of *Y. aldovae*, *Y. bercovieri*, *Y. frederiksenii* and "*Y. ruckeri*" strains. *Int J Antimicrob Agents* **25**:496–500.

31. Vanni M, Meucci V, Tognetti R, Cagnardi P, Montesissa C, Piccirillo A, Rossi AM, Di Bello D, Intorre L. 2014. Fluoroquinolone resistance and molecular characterization of *gyrA* and *parC* quinolone resistance-determining regions in *Escherichia coli* isolated from poultry. *Poult Sci* **93**:856–863.

32. Call DR, Singer RS, Meng D, Broschat SL, Orfe LH, Anderson JM, Herndon DR, Kappmeyer LS, Daniels JB, Besser TE. 2010. bla$_{CMY-2}$-positive IncA/C plasmids from *Escherichia coli* and *Salmonella enterica* are a distinct component of a larger lineage of plasmids. *Antimicrob Agents Chemother* **54**:590–596.

33. Fricke WF, Welch TJ, McDermott PF, Mammel MK, LeClerc JE, White DG, Cebula TA, Ravel J. 2009. Comparative genomics of the IncA/C multidrug resistance plasmid family. *J Bacteriol* **191**:4750–4757.

34. Lukkana M, Wongtavatchai J, Chuanchuen R. 2012. Class 1 integrons in *Aeromonas hydrophila* isolates from farmed Nile tilapia (*Oreochromis nilotica*). *J Vet Med Sci* **74**:435–440.

35. Ndi OL, Barton MD. 2011. Incidence of class 1 integron and other antibiotic resistance determinants in *Aeromonas* spp. from rainbow trout farms in Australia. *J Fish Dis* **34**:589–599.

36. Deng Y, Wu Y, Jiang L, Tan A, Zhang R, Luo L. 2016. Multidrug resistance mediated by class 1 integrons in *Aeromonas* isolated from farmed freshwater animals. *Front Microbiol* **7**:935.

37. Čížek A, Dolejská M, Sochorová R, Strachotová K, Piacková V, Veselý T. 2010. Antimicrobial resistance and its genetic determinants in aeromonads isolated in ornamental (koi) carp (*Cyprinus carpio koi*) and common carp (*Cyprinus carpio*). *Vet Microbiol* **142**:435–439.

38. Aoki T. 1988. Drug-resistant plasmids from fish pathogens. *Microbiol Sci* **5**:219–223.

39. Gordon L, Cloeckaert A, Doublet B, Schwarz S, Bouju-Albert A, Ganière JP, Le Bris H, Le Flèche-Matéos A, Giraud E. 2008. Complete sequence of the *floR*-carrying multiresistance plasmid pAB5S9 from freshwater *Aeromonas bestiarum*. *J Antimicrob Chemother* **62**:65–71.

40. Kim EH, Aoki T. 1993. Drug resistance and broad geographical distribution of identical R plasmids of *Pasteurella piscicida* isolated from cultured yellowtail in Japan. *Microbiol Immunol* **37**:103–109.

41. Kim EH, Aoki T. 1994. The transposon-like structure of IS26-tetracycline, and kanamycin resistance determinant derived from transferable R plasmid of fish pathogen, *Pasteurella piscicida*. *Microbiol Immunol* **38**:31–38.

42. Kim MJ, Hirono I, Kurokawa K, Maki T, Hawke J, Kondo H, Santos MD, Aoki T. 2008. Complete DNA sequence and analysis of the transferable multiple-drug resistance plasmids (R plasmids) from *Photobacterium damselae* subsp. *piscicida* isolates collected in Japan and the United States. *Antimicrob Agents Chemother* **52**:606–611.

43. del Castillo CS, Jang HB, Hikima J, Jung TS, Morii H, Hirono I, Kondo H, Kurosaka C, Aoki T. 2013. Comparative analysis and distribution of pP9014, a novel drug resistance IncP-1 plasmid from *Photobacterium damselae* subsp. *piscicida*. *Int J Antimicrob Agents* **42**:10–18.

44. Rodkhum C, Maki T, Hirono I, Aoki T. 2008. gyrA and parC associated with quinolone resistance in *Vibrio anguillarum*. *J Fish Dis* **31**:395–399.

45. Zhao J, Aoki T. 1992. Nucleotide sequence analysis of the class G tetracycline resistance determinant from *Vibrio anguillarum*. *Microbiol Immunol* **36**:1051–1060.

46. Izumi S, Ouchi S, Kuge T, Arai H, Mito T, Fujii H, Aranishi F, Shimizu A. 2007. PCR-RFLP genotypes associated with quinolone resistance in isolates of *Flavobacterium psychrophilum*. *J Fish Dis* 30:141–147.

47. Soule M, LaFrentz S, Cain K, LaPatra S, Call DR. 2005. Polymorphisms in 16S rRNA genes of *Flavobacterium psychrophilum* correlate with elastin hydrolysis and tetracycline resistance. *Dis Aquat Organ* 65:209–216.

48. Del Cerro A, Márquez I, Prieto JM. 2010. Genetic diversity and antimicrobial resistance of *Flavobacterium psychrophilum* isolated from cultured rainbow trout, *Onchorynchus mykiss* (Walbaum), in Spain. *J Fish Dis* 33:285–291.

49. Park YK, Nho SW, Shin GW, Park SB, Jang HB, Cha IS, Ha MA, Kim YR, Dalvi RS, Kang BJ, Jung TS. 2009. Antibiotic susceptibility and resistance of *Streptococcus iniae* and *Streptococcus parauberis* isolated from olive flounder (*Paralichthys olivaceus*). *Vet Microbiol* 136:76–81.

50. Dangwetngam M, Suanyuk N, Kong F, Phromkunthong W. 2016. Serotype distribution and antimicrobial susceptibilities of *Streptococcus agalactiae* isolated from infected cultured tilapia (*Oreochromis niloticus*) in Thailand: nine-year perspective. *J Med Microbiol* 65:247–254.

51. Cartes C, Isla A, Lagos F, Castro D, Muñoz M, Yañez A, Haussmann D, Figueroa J. 2016. Search and analysis of genes involved in antibiotic resistance in Chilean strains of *Piscirickettsia salmonis*. *J Fish Dis* 40:1025–1039.

52. Gonçalves LA, de Castro Soares S, Pereira FL, Dorella FA, de Carvalho AF, de Freitas Almeida GM, Leal CA, Azevedo V, Figueiredo HC. 2016. Complete genome sequences of *Francisella noatunensis* subsp. *orientalis* strains FNO12, FNO24 and FNO190: a fish pathogen with genomic clonal behavior. *Stand Genomic Sci* 11:30.

53. Rhodes LD, Nguyen OT, Deinhard RK, White TM, Harrell LW, Roberts MC. 2008. Characterization of *Renibacterium salmoninarum* with reduced susceptibility to macrolide antibiotics by a standardized antibiotic susceptibility test. *Dis Aquat Organ* 80:173–180.

54. CLSI. 2011. Generation, presentation, and application of antimicrobial susceptibility test data for bacteria of animal origin. Report VET05. Clinical and Laboratory Standards Institute, Wayne, PA.

55. CLSI. 2014. Performance standards for antimicrobial susceptibility testing of bacteria isolated from aquatic animals. Informational supplement VET03/VET04. Clinical and Laboratory Standards Institute, Wayne, PA.

56. McDermott PF, Tyson GH, Kabera C, Chen Y, Li C, Folster JP, Ayers SL, Lam C, Tate HP, Zhao S. 2016. Whole-genome sequencing for detecting antimicrobial resistance in nontyphoidal *Salmonella*. *Antimicrob Agents Chemother* 60:5515–5520.

57. Miller RA, Reimschuessel R. 2006. Epidemiologic cutoff values for antimicrobial agents against *Aeromonas salmonicida* isolates determined by frequency distributions of minimal inhibitory concentration and diameter of zone of inhibition data. *Am J Vet Res* 67:1837–1843.

58. CLSI. 2013. Performance standards for antimicrobial disk and dilution susceptibility tests for bacteria isolated from animals. Approved standard VET01. Clinical and Laboratory Standards Institute, Wayne, PA.

59. Smith P. 2006. Breakpoints for disc diffusion susceptibility testing of bacteria associated with fish diseases: a review of current practice. *Aquaculture* 261:1113–1121.

60. CLSI. 2006. Methods for antimicrobial disk susceptibility testing of bacteria isolated from aquatic animals. Approved guideline VET03. Clinical and Laboratory Standards Institute, Wayne, PA.

61. CLSI. 2014. Methods for broth dilution susceptibility testing of bacteria isolated from aquatic animals. Approved guideline VET04. Clinical and Laboratory Standards Institute, Wayne, PA.

62. CLSI. 2016. Methods for antimicrobial dilution and disk susceptibility testing of infrequently isolated or fastidious bacteria. Approved guideline M45. Clinical and Laboratory Standards Institute, Wayne, PA.

63. Douglas I, Ruane NM, Geary M, Carroll C, Fleming GTA, McMurray J, Smith P. 2007. The advantages of the use of discs containing single agents in disc diffusion testing of the susceptibility of *Aeromonas salmonicida* to potentiated sulfonamides. *Aquaculture* 272:118–125.

64. Ruane NM, Douglas I, Geary M, Carroll C, Fleming GTA, Smith P. 2007. Application of normalised resistance interpretation to disc diffusion data on the susceptibility of *Aeromonas salmonicida* to three quinolone agents. *Aquaculture* 272:156–167.

65. Inglis V, Richards RH. 1991. The *in vitro* susceptibility of *Aeromonas salmonicida* and other fish-pathogenic bacteria to 29 antimicrobial agents. *J Fish Dis* 14:641–650.

66. Giraud E, Blanc G, Bouju-Albert A, Weill FX, Donnay-Moreno C. 2004. Mechanisms of quinolone resistance and clonal relationship among *Aeromonas salmonicida* strains isolated from reared fish with furunculosis. *J Med Microbiol* 53:895–901.

67. Hawke JP, Kent M, Rogge M, Baumgartner W, Wiles J, Shelley J, Savolainen LC, Wagner R, Murray K, Peterson TS. 2013. Edwardsiellosis caused by *Edwardsiella ictaluri* in laboratory populations of zebrafish *Danio rerio*. *J Aquat Anim Health* 25:171–183.

68. Dung TT, Haesebrouck F, Nguyen AT, Sorgeloos P, Baele M, Decostere A. 2008. Antimicrobial susceptibility pattern of *Edwardsiella ictaluri* isolates from natural outbreaks of bacillary necrosis of *Pangasianodon hypophthalmus* in Vietnam. *Microb Drug Resist* 14:311–316.

69. Turnidge J, Paterson DL. 2007. Setting and revising antibacterial susceptibility breakpoints. *Clin Microbiol Rev* 20:391–408.

70. McGinnis A, Gaunt P, Santucci T, Simmons R, Endris R. 2003. *In vitro* evaluation of the susceptibility of *Edwardsiella ictaluri*, etiological agent of enteric septicemia in channel catfish, *Ictalurus punctatus* (Rafinesque), to florfenicol. *J Vet Diagn Invest* 15:576–579.

71. Israil AM, Balotescu-Chifiriuc MC, Delcaru C, Aramă M. 2012. Influence of salinity upon the phenotypic expression of antibiotic resistance in nonhalophilic and halophilic vibrios. *Roum Arch Microbiol Immunol* 71:5–10.

72. **Lee DC, Han HJ, Choi SY, Kronvall G, Park CI, Kim DH.** 2012. Antibiograms and the estimation of epidemiological cutoff values for *Vibrio ichthyoenteri* isolated from larval olive flounder, *Paralichthys olivaceus*. *Aquaculture* **342**:31–35.

73. **Lewbart G.** 2001. Bacteria and ornamental fish. *Semin Avian Exotic Pet Med* **10**:48–56.

74. **CLSI.** 2008. Performance standards for antimicrobial disk and dilution susceptibility tests for bacteria isolated from animals. Approved standard M31. Clinical and Laboratory Standards Institute, Wayne, PA.

75. **Jagoda SS, Wijewardana TG, Arulkanthan A, Igarashi Y, Tan E, Kinoshita S, Watabe S, Asakawa S.** 2014. Characterization and antimicrobial susceptibility of motile aeromonads isolated from freshwater ornamental fish showing signs of septicaemia. *Dis Aquat Organ* **109**: 127–137.

76. **Gieseker CM, Mayer TD, Crosby TC, Carson J, Dalsgaard I, Darwish AM, Gaunt PS, Gao DX, Hsu HM, Lin TL, Oaks JL, Pyecroft M, Teitzel C, Somsiri T, Wu CC.** 2012. Quality control ranges for testing broth microdilution susceptibility of *Flavobacterium columnare* and *F. psychrophilum* to nine antimicrobials. *Dis Aquat Organ* **101**:207–215.

77. **Gieseker CM, Crosby TC, Woods LC III.** 2016. Provisional epidemiological cutoff values for standard broth microdilution susceptibility testing of *Flavobacterium columnare*. *J Fish Dis* (Sep):1–8.

78. **Smith P.** 2017. MIC for *Flavobacterium psychrophilum*: analysis of the data from 5 laboratories. Presentation to the Clinical and Laboratory Standards Institute – Subcommittee on Veterinary Antimicrobial Susceptibility Testing. January 2017. Tempe, AZ.

79. **Van Vliet D, Loch TP, Smith P, Faisal M.** 2017. Antimicrobial susceptibilities of *Flavobacterium psychrophilum* isolates from the Great Lakes Basin, Michigan. *Microb Drug Resist* **23**:791–798.

80. **Miranda CD, Smith P, Rojas R, Contreras-Lynch S, Vega JM.** 2016. Antimicrobial susceptibility of *Flavobacterium psychrophilum* from Chilean salmon farms and their epidemiological cut-off values using agar dilution and disk diffusion methods. *Front Microbiol* **7**:1880.

81. **Henríquez-Núñez H, Evrard O, Kronvall G, Avendaño-Herrera R.** 2012. Antimicrobial susceptibility and plasmid profiles of *Flavobacterium psychrophilum* strains isolated in Chile. *Aquaculture* **354**:38–44.

82. **Tang HJ, Chang MC, Ko WC, Huang KY, Lee CL, Chuang YC.** 2002. *In vitro* and *in vivo* activities of newer fluoroquinolones against *Vibrio vulnificus*. *Antimicrob Agents Chemother* **46**:3580–3584.

83. **Hsueh PR, Chang JC, Chang SC, Ho SW, Hsieh WC.** 1995. *In vitro* antimicrobial susceptibility of *Vibrio vulnificus* isolated in Taiwan. *Eur J Clin Microbiol Infect Dis* **14**:151–153.

84. **Hassanzadeh Y, Bahador N, Baseri-Salehi M.** 2015. First time isolation of *Photobacterium damselae* subsp. *damselae* from *Caranx sexfasciatus* in Persian Gulf, Iran. *Iran J Microbiol* **7**:178–184.

85. **Coyne R, Smith P, Dalsgaard I, Nilsen H, Kongshaug H, Bergh Ø, Samuelsen O.** 2006. Winter ulcer disease of post-smolt Atlantic salmon: an unsuitable case for treatment? *Aquaculture* **253**:171–178.

86. **Pazos F, Santos Y, Macias AR, Nuñez S, Toranzo AE.** 1996. Evaluation of media for the successful culture of *Flexibacter maritimus*. *J Fish Dis* **19**:193–197.

87. **Avendaño-Herrera R, Nuñez S, Barja JL, Toranzo AE.** 2008. Evolution of drug resistance and minimum inhibitory concentration to enrofloxacin in *Tenacibaculum maritimum* strains isolates in fish farms. *Aquacult Int* **16**: 1–11.

88. **Soto E, Halliday-Simmonds I, Francis S, Fraites T, Martínez-López B, Wiles J, Hawke JP, Endris RD.** 2016. Improved broth microdilution method for antimicrobial susceptibility testing of *Francisella noatunensis orientalis*. *J Aquat Anim Health* **28**:199–207.

89. **Yañez AJ, Valenzuela K, Silva H, Retamales J, Romero A, Enriquez R, Figueroa J, Claude A, Gonzalez J, Avendaño-Herrera R, Carcamo JG.** 2012. Broth medium for the successful culture of the fish pathogen *Piscirickettsia salmonis*. *Dis Aquat Organ* **97**:197–205.

90. **Henríquez P, Kaiser M, Bohle H, Bustos P, Mancilla M.** 2016. Comprehensive antibiotic susceptibility profiling of Chilean *Piscirickettsia salmonis* field isolates. *J Fish Dis* **39**:441–448.

Antimicrobial Resistance in Bacteria from Livestock and Companion Animals
Edited by Frank Møller Aarestrup, Stefan Schwarz, Jianzhong Shen, and Lina Cavaco
© 2018 American Society for Microbiology, Washington, DC
doi:10.1128/microbiolspec.ARBA-0009-2017

Antimicrobial Resistance: a One Health Perspective

25

Scott A. McEwen[1] and Peter J. Collignon[2]

INTRODUCTION

Antimicrobial resistance is a global public health crisis that threatens our ability to successfully treat bacterial infections (1, 2). Microbiologists and infectious disease specialists have long recognized the problem—the discoverer of penicillin Sir Alexander Fleming himself drew attention to the threat of resistance from underdosing (3)—but realization of the vast scale of the resistant threat is only now reaching wider audiences. Many infectious agents that could once be successfully treated with any one of several drug classes have acquired resistance to most, and in some cases, virtually all of these drugs (4, 5). The threat is most acute for antibiotics and synthetic antibacterial antimicrobial agents, the focus of this paper, but also threatened are antifungals, antiparasitics, and antivirals (6). How did we get from the point where antimicrobials were truly "wonder drugs" that could be relied upon to cure a wide range of life-threatening infections to the point today, where resistance to most antimicrobials is widely prevalent and the supply of new classes of drugs has dwindled to a trickle? The complete answer is not simple, nor unfortunately, is the solution. One thing seems certain: that overuse of these precious drugs in multiple sectors (human, animal, agriculture) is the main problem and one that must be addressed (4, 7).

Through the process of Darwinian selection, microorganisms faced with antimicrobial selection pressure enhance their fitness by acquiring and expressing resistance genes and then share those genes with other bacteria. Thus, antimicrobial use and overuse are important drivers of the resistance phenomenon; the other main drivers are factors that promote the spread of resistant bacteria and their genes locally and globally (8). These include poor infection control, environmental contamination, and geographical movement of infected

humans and animals (9, 10). Wherever antimicrobials are used, there are reservoirs of resistance, including within humans and the local environments of hospitals and the community, as well as in animals and the farm and aquaculture environments, but also in water, soil, wildlife, and many other ecological niches, due to pollution by sewage, pharmaceutical industry waste, and manure runoff from farms (Fig. 1) (10, 11). Bacteria and their genes move relatively easily within and between humans, animals, and the environment. Microbial adaptations to antimicrobial use and other selection pressures within any one sector are reflected in any other sector (8, 12). Similarly, actions taken (or not taken) to contain antimicrobial resistance in one sector affect other sectors (13, 14). Antimicrobial resistance is an ecological problem that is characterized by complex interactions involving diverse microbial populations affecting the health of humans, animals, and the environment. It makes sense to address the resistance problem by taking this complexity and ecological nature into account using a coordinated, multisectoral approach, such as One Health (6, 15–19).

One Health is defined as "the collaborative effort of multiple health science professions, together with their related disciplines and institutions—working locally, nationally, and globally—to attain optimal health for people, domestic animals, wildlife, plants, and our environment" (20). The origins of One Health are centuries old and are based on the mutual dependency of humans and animals and the recognition that they share not only the same environment, but also many infectious diseases (19). It has been estimated that as many as 75% of human infectious diseases that have emerged or re-emerged in recent decades are zoonotic; that is, they originated in animals (21). Rudolf Virchow

[1]Department of Population Medicine, University of Guelph, Guelph, Canada N1G 2W1; [2]Infectious Diseases and Microbiology, Canberra Hospital, Canberra, Australia and Medical School, Australian National University, Acton, Australia.

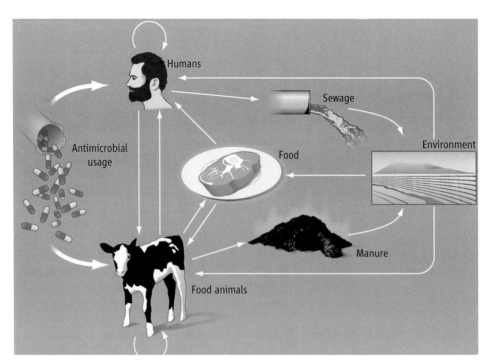

Figure 1 Diagrammatic representation of the routes of transmission of antimicrobial resistance between farm animals, the wider environment, and humans. Reprinted from *Science* (12) with permission of the publisher.

and William Osler were medical pioneers that recognized the importance of a comparative approach to medical investigation, and veterinarian Calvin Schwabe coined the term "One Medicine" to denote the many commonalities in human and animal medicine and in recognition that most veterinary activities benefit human health, either directly or indirectly (19, 22). One Health goes further, embracing the health of the environment as well as human and animal health, and promotes the view that with the ever-increasing human population growth that is accompanied by climate change, increasing pollution, and depletion of the earth's resources, health disciplines and others must work together to provide for the future health and well-being of humans, animals, and the environment (19, 20).

In this chapter, we take a One Health perspective on the problem of antimicrobial resistance by showing its multisectoral and interrelated nature, highlighting important risks to the health of humans and animals, and describing One Health approaches to the containment of antimicrobial resistance, particularly at the international level. We then offer some reflections on challenges facing the One Health approach in reconciling the sometimes-conflicting interests that deter some measures to addressing antimicrobial resistance. At the outset, we state our belief that human health and well-

being are the most important considerations for preserving the continued effectiveness of antimicrobials, even within a One Health perspective, but that it is also in the greater, long-term interest of humankind to adequately care for animals and the environment.

USE OF ANTIMICROBIALS IN HUMANS, ANIMALS, AND PLANTS

A few antimicrobial classes are reserved more or less exclusively for humans, in particular those used to treat tuberculosis (e.g., isoniazid) or other infections for which animals are typically not treated (e.g., cattle with bovine tuberculosis are usually destroyed rather than treated). A few others are limited to veterinary use (e.g., flavophospholipols, ionophores), mainly because of toxicity to humans. However, the great majority of antimicrobial classes are used in both humans and animals, including domestic mammals, birds, farmed fish and shellfish, honey bees, and others (23–27). In horticulture, tetracyclines, streptomycin, and some other antimicrobials are sometimes used for the treatment and prophylaxis of bacterial infections of fruit, such as apples and pears (e.g., "fire blight" caused by *Erwinia amylovora*) (28). In people, antimicrobials are mostly used for the treatment of clinical infections in individual patients, but there is also limited prophylactic use in individuals (e.g., postsurgery) or in groups (e.g., prevention of meningococcal disease). In veterinary medicine there are notable differences in the ways that antimicrobials are used in companion animals (e.g., dogs, cats, pet birds, horses) compared to food-producing animals. Antimicrobial use practices in companion animals are broadly similar to those in humans; that is, the drugs are mostly administered on an individual animal basis for the treatment of clinical infection, with some use for prophylaxis in individual animals, such as postsurgery (29, 30). In the case of food animals, however, when some animals in a group are clinically infected and in need of antimicrobial therapy, for reasons of practicality and efficiency, the drugs are frequently administered through feed or water to the entire group (e.g., pens of pigs, flocks of broilers), even when the majority of the animals are not displaying signs of infection (in effect, prophylaxis). This is, however, now defined inappropriately by many in the animal health sector as "therapeutic" use. In addition, there is use in food animals similar to what happens in people, when antimicrobials are used to treat individual clinically sick animals (e.g., dairy cows with mastitis) (23). "Metaphylaxis" is a term used variously to describe therapeutic and/or prophylactic treatment at the group level, usually in the context of mass administration of therapeutic doses of an antimicrobial to a group of animals at high risk of infection, e.g., administration of an injectable antimicrobial to groups of calves upon arrival at a feedlot because of a high risk of bovine respiratory disease (23, 31). Antimicrobial prophylaxis in groups of people is uncommon and is usually limited to the management of serious, highly communicable infections such as meningococcal disease. Even in those cases, for example, meningococcal disease in a child at school, antimicrobials are recommended to be limited to those with prolonged and close contact (usually those in the same household) and not to be given to all pupils in same school or classroom (32).

Many in industry justify group-level treatments as therapeutic when clinical infections are observed in at least some of the animals in the pen or flock, or prophylactic when there are no sick animals present, but they are at high risk of clinical bacterial infection due to exposure to infectious agents (e.g., mixing of animals from different sources), unsanitary or crowded conditions, or other factors (e.g., age, stress of transport) (31).

The most controversial type of group treatment in food animals is long-term, low-dose mass medication for purposes of growth promotion. The controversy is rooted partially in the propensity of this practice to select for antimicrobial resistance and partially in its justification on economic grounds, rather than for treatment of clinical infection. Antimicrobial growth promoters are important contributors to antimicrobial resistance because they are administered to entire groups of animals, usually for prolonged periods of time and often at subtherapeutic doses—conditions which favor the selection and spread of resistant bacteria within and between groups of animals, as well as to humans through food or other environmental pathways (33). The period of exposure is usually greater than 2 weeks and often is for almost the entire life of an animal, e.g., in chickens for 36 days. It is imprudent to extensively use antimicrobials for economic reasons alone when it is clear that such use selects for resistance to antimicrobials of importance to human and animal health (6, 27, 34, 35) and also may have relatively little or no economic benefits (35, 36). Based on experimental studies, mostly conducted decades ago, the purported production benefits of antimicrobial growth promoters range widely (1 to 10%), but surveillance and animal production data from Europe suggest that benefits in animals reared in good conditions are probably quite small and may now be nonexistent. In the past, benefits were derived mainly from the disease prophylaxis properties of the antimicrobials used, rather than enhancement of feed efficiency or other production effect (35). Some large poultry corporations are now marketing chicken raised without antimicrobials administered at the hatchery or farm levels (36).

Concerns are expressed that antimicrobial growth promoters are used to compensate for poor hygiene and housing and as a replacement for proper animal health management (14, 34, 35). For these reasons, the World Health Organization (WHO) advocates for the termination of the use of antimicrobials for growth promotion (6, 34, 37), and the practice has been banned in Europe and elsewhere and phased out in some other countries, such as the United States and Canada (38–40). Recently, the World Organization for Animal Health (OIE) reported that 41% of 146 countries reporting on antimicrobial use in animals allow the use of antimicrobial growth promoters. This represents a reduction from 51% of 151 reporting countries in 2012 (41). Among the drugs allowed are several categorized by WHO as critically important to humans, for example, colistin, fluoroquinolones, and macrolides (42).

ONE HEALTH ANTIMICROBIAL RESISTANCE CASE STUDIES

The following two case studies illustrate some of the antimicrobial resistance problems that arise from the use of the same classes of antimicrobials in humans and animals, as well as the challenges that arise from competing interests and imbalances of risk and benefit in various sectors. The first case, which focuses on the third-generation cephalosporins, illustrates One Health issues concerning an antimicrobial intended mainly for therapeutic purposes in animals, but in some important situations it is also used prophylactically. The second case features colistin, which illustrates One Health considerations arising from an older class of antimicrobial that has long been used in animals for therapeutic, prophylactic, and in some countries, growth promotion purposes, but quite recently has gained importance to human health.

Third-Generation Cephalosporins

Third-generation cephalosporins are broad-spectrum beta-lactam antimicrobials that are widely used in humans and animals. Cefotaxime, ceftriaxone, and several other members of the class are used for a wide variety of frequently serious infections of humans, particularly in hospital settings, e.g., urinary tract, abdominal, lung, and bloodstream infections due to *Escherichia coli*, *Klebsiella pneumoniae*, and other bacteria, but also in community settings, e.g., *Neisseria gonorrhoeae* (42). Because of their important role in the therapy of many bacterial infections where resistance has become a major problem, third-generation cephalosporins have been classified as "critically important" for human health (42).

Ceftiofur is the principal third-generation cephalosporin for veterinary use; others include cefpodoxime, cefoperazone, and cefovecin. Ceftiofur is approved in many countries for the treatment of several bacterial infections, predominantly in food-producing animals. It is limited to parenteral administration, so treatment usually is administered to individual animals, either singly or in groups (43). Depending on the species, it is used to treat pneumonia, arthritis, polyserositis, septicemia, metritis, meningitis, and infections of other body systems (44). However, it is also sometimes used in mass therapy (metaphylaxis or prophylaxis). This can be either under an approved label claim (e.g., injection of feedlot cattle for control of bovine respiratory disease) or off-label (e.g., injection of hatching eggs or day-old chicks for prevention of *E. coli* infections). Factors that favor the use of ceftiofur include its broad-spectrum activity, clinical efficacy, zero withdrawal time of milk from treated lactating dairy animals (due to its high maximum residual level [MRL]), and availability of a long-acting preparation (43, 44).

In Europe, where high-quality data on antimicrobial consumption in animals are available, approximately 14 tonnes of third- and fourth-generation cephalosporins were used in 2014, mainly in food animals (25). This represented about 0.16% of total antimicrobial consumption in animals in Europe. In the United States, total consumption of all cephalosporins (not just third-generation) in animals was approximately 32.3 tonnes in 2015 (45).

In many countries, cephalosporins are commonly used in humans. For example, in Europe, as a percentage of total defined daily dose per 1,000 inhabitants per day for systemic use, cephalosporins accounted for a range of 0.2% (Denmark) to 23.5% (Malta) in 2012; a total of 101 tonnes of third-generation cephalosporins for use in Europe were consumed overall in humans (26). In the United States, approximately 82 tonnes of third-generation cephalosporins for use in humans were consumed in 2011 (46). Among countries that report antimicrobial consumption data, quantities of third-generation cephalosporins used in humans are greater than in animals.

Resistance to the third-generation cephalosporins is mediated by extended-spectrum beta-lactamases (ESBLs) and AmpC beta-lactamases (43). ESBL genes are highly mobile and are transmitted on plasmids, transposons, and other genetic elements. AmpC beta-lactamases were originally reported to be chromosomal but have also been identified on plasmids and shown to have spread horizontally among *Enterobacteriaceae* (43). Unfortunately, in many countries resistance to third-generation cephalosporins is common among *E. coli* and *K. pneumoniae* from severe human infections (47, 48), placing greater reliance on the few remaining classes of available antimicrobials, such as carbapenems. Resistance to these drugs is accompanied by serious public health consequences; a systematic review conducted by the WHO reported that patients with third-generation cephalosporin-resistant *E. coli* infections had a 2-fold increase in all-cause mortality, bacterium-attributable mortality, and 30-day mortality compared with susceptible infections (1). Resistance has also been reported in *Salmonella*, particularly mediated by CMY-2 AmpC beta-lactamase genes, and these are frequently colocated with genes encoding resistance to other classes of antimicrobials, including tetracyclines, aminoglycosides, and sulfonamides. As a consequence, coselection of beta-lactam resistance in *Enterobacteriaceae* (including cephalosporin resistance) by use of other antimicrobials in animals, including tetracyclines administered in feed, has been reported (49).

Much of the spread of *E. coli* with ESBL and other beta-lactamases is thought to be clonal, but there is also horizontal dissemination of the responsible genes in a variety of bacterial species from humans, animals, and the environment (43, 50). Several studies conducted in Europe and the United States have attempted to determine the relatedness of ESBL-bearing *E. coli* from humans, animals (particularly poultry), and food (50–52). In some studies, there was only limited relatedness of ESBL-containing *E. coli* isolates (53), but other studies comparing isolates from animals, food, and human infections have found higher similarity in ESBL genes in plasmids as well as some similar clones (53–55). This includes studies using whole-genome sequencing. One group failed to demonstrate evidence for recent clonal transmission of cephalosporin-resistant *E. coli* strains from poultry to humans but instead found evidence that cephalosporin resistance genes are mainly disseminated in animals and humans via distinct plasmids (50). If one considers the large numbers of different *E. coli* clones likely to be present in food animals, plus the wide distribution of foods and their ingestion by people, it is not surprising that "clonal" transmission is only rarely detected compared to plasmid distribution and exchange. However, it is still unclear to what extent beta-lactamase-bearing *E. coli* strains from animals are directly responsible for human infections. Given the high human disease burden from these organisms, however, even if this was only a small fraction, it is still very important.

The critical importance of third-generation cephalosporins to human health and serious concerns about the ease with which resistance emerges and spreads, both clonally and horizontally, have focused considerable attention on their use in animals, particularly with regard to mass medication of ceftiofur to groups of animals (26, 33, 43). As mentioned above, the requirement for parenteral administration places practical limits on mass medication to certain situations, such as injection of steers on arrival at the feedlot or routine injection of pigs. However, one such mass exposure application that is now severely restricted in many countries has been convincingly shown to provide powerful selection pressure for resistance in *E. coli* and *Salmonella*. It involves administration of ceftiofur to eggs or day-old chicks at the hatchery using highly automated equipment that injects small quantities of the drug to the many thousands of hatching eggs or chicks intended for treated flocks (56, 57). The main reason for this treatment is prophylaxis against *E. coli* infections and/or yolk sac infections. This practice has been shown to select for cephalosporin resistance in *Salmonella enterica* serovar Heidelberg, an important cause of human illness in many countries that is typically associated with consumption of contaminated poultry

products (58). Surveillance conducted by the Canadian Integrated Program for Antimicrobial Resistance Surveillance detected a high degree of temporal correlation in trends of resistance to ceftiofur (and ceftriaxone, a drug of choice for the treatment of severe cases of salmonellosis in children and pregnant women) among *Salmonella* Heidelberg from clinical infections in humans, from poultry samples collected at retail stores, and in *E. coli* from poultry samples collected at retail stores (56) (Fig. 2). Voluntary termination of this use of ceftiofur in hatcheries in the province of Quebec was followed by a precipitous drop in the prevalence of resistance to ceftiofur; subsequent reintroduction of its use, apparently in a more limited way, was followed by a return to higher levels of resistance (57).

In recognition of the resultant human health risks, in 2014, the Canadian poultry industry placed a voluntary ban on the use of ceftiofur and other critically important antimicrobials for disease prophylaxis (Chicken Farmers of Canada, http://www.chickenfarmers.ca/what-we-do/antibiotics/faq/). In Japan, voluntary withdrawal of the off-label use of ceftiofur in hatcheries in 2012 was also followed by a significant decrease in broad-spectrum cephalosporin resistance in *E. coli* from broilers (59). Some other countries (e.g., Denmark) have also placed voluntary restrictions on its use (60). The label claim for day-old injection of poultry flocks was withdrawn in Europe, while some countries banned off-label use of third-generation cephalosporins (e.g., the United States) (43, 61), and in other countries there is a requirement that use be restricted to situations where no other effective approved drugs are available for treatment (62).

From the One Health antimicrobial resistance perspective, the third-generation cephalosporins are good examples of antimicrobials that are considered critically important for both human and animal health (Table 1) and for which the main concerns for selection and spread of resistance from animals to humans derive from their use as mass medications in large numbers of animals, for either therapy or prophylaxis. In this regard, there are parallels with fluoroquinolones, another class of critically important antimicrobials, to which resistance among *Campylobacter jejuni* isolates emerged following mass medication of poultry flocks (63–65). In Australia, where fluoroquinolones were never approved in food animals, fluoroquinolone-resistant strains in food animals remain very rare (66).

Given the critical importance of these two classes of antimicrobials to human medicine and the clear evidence that treatment of entire groups of animals selects for resistance in important pathogens that

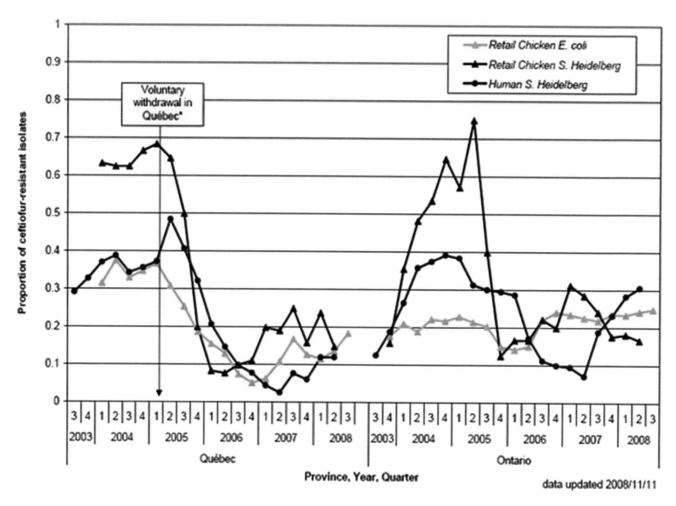

Figure 2 Ceftiofur resistance in chicken and human *Salmonella* Heidelberg and chicken
E. coli. Reprinted from the Public Health Agency of Canada (56) with permission of the
publisher.

spread from animals to humans (57, 65), third- and
fourth-generation cephalosporins and fluoroquinolones
should be used rarely, if at all, in animals, and only
when supporting laboratory data demonstrate that no
suitable alternatives of less human health importance
are available (37). Their use as mass medications should
be restricted.

Colistin

Colistin is a member of the polymixin class of antimicrobials, which have been used in both human and
veterinary medicine for over 50 years (67). Polymixins,
which cause nephrotoxicity and neurotoxicity in people
(68), were until recently mainly limited to topical use in
humans and treatment of infections in cystic fibrosis
patients (by inhalation as colistimethate sodium). Colistin is gaining importance as a drug of last resort for

parenteral use in the treatment of multiresistant Gram-
negative infections including carbapenem-resistant
Pseudomonas aeruginosa, *Acinetobacter baumannii*,
K. pneumoniae, and *E. coli*, mainly in intensive care
units in certain countries (69–71). Where approved
for use in food animals (e.g., Brazil, Europe, China),
most colistin is administered orally to entire groups of
pigs, poultry, and in some cases calves, for treatment
and prophylaxis of diarrhea due to Gram-negative infections (67, 71, 72). In some countries colistin is also
used for growth promotion (41). Other claims for
polymixins exist, including mastitis in cows, systemic
endotoxemia in horses, and skin and eye infections in
companion animals, but the quantities used for these
purposes are small (67). In countries where colistin is
approved for use in food animals and for which antimicrobial consumption data are available, the quantities

Table 1 Classification of importance of antimicrobial classes for human health and animal health

Category	Human health (WHO) (42)	Animal health (OIE) (162)
Critically important	Aminoglycosides Ansamycins Carbapenems and other penems Cephalosporins (3rd and 4th generation) Phosphonic acid derivatives Glycopeptides Glycylcyclines Lipopeptides Macrolides and ketolides Monobactams Oxazolidinones Penicillins (natural, aminopenicillins, and antipseudomonal) Polymyxins Quinolones Drugs used solely to treat tuberculosis or other mycobacterial diseases	Aminoglycosides Amphenicols Cephalosporins (3rd and 4th generation) Macrolides Penicillins (natural, aminopenicillins, aminopenicillins with beta-lactamase inhibitor, antistaphylococcal) Fluoroquinolones Sulfonamides Diaminopyrimidines Tetracyclines
Highly important	Amidinopenicillins Amphenicols Cephalosporins (1st and 2nd generation) and cephamycins Lincosamides Penicillins (antistaphylococcal) Pleuromutilins Pseudomonic acids Riminofenazines Steroid antibacterials Streptogramins Sulfonamides, dihydrofolate reductase inhibitors, and combinations Tetracyclines	Ansamycin—rifamycins Cephalosporins (1st and 2nd generation) Ionophores Lincosamides Phosphonic acid Pleuromutilins Polymyxins (including bacitracin and other polypeptides) 1st-generation quinolones (flumequin, miloxacin, nalidixic acid, oxolinic acid)
Important	Aminocyclitols Cyclic polypeptides Nitrofurantoins Nitroimidazoles	Aminocoumarin Arsenical Bicyclomycin Fusidic acid Orthosomycins Quinoxalines Streptogramins Thiostrepton

consumed for animal production vastly exceed those used in humans. In Europe, for example, colistin use in humans is quite low overall, at 0.012 defined daily doses per 1,000 inhabitants per day in 2014, although there is considerable between-country variation, and there has been an increase in recent years (73). Animal use of colistin in Europe also varies widely, for example, from 0 mg/population correction unit (PCU) (Finland, Iceland, and Norway) to 34 mg/PCU (Spain) in 2013 (67). In 2013, total consumption in animals in Europe was 495 tonnes—99.7% in oral form (e.g., for oral solution, medicated feed premix, and oral powder)

(67). Liu et al. reported that in China, with the world's largest production of pigs and poultry, an estimated 12,000 tonnes of colistin was used in food animal production (72).

Until recently, limited data on colistin resistance were available, partly because of technical difficulties in phenotypic susceptibility testing (67, 74), and it was not included in panels for routine resistance surveillance in Gram-negative bacteria from animals, food, the environment, and humans. Mandatory monitoring for colistin resistance in *Salmonella* and *E. coli* from animals and some foods was initiated in Europe in

2014 (75), when it was reported that 0.9% of 4,037 *E. coli* isolates from broilers and 7.4% of 1,663 *E. coli* isolates from fattening turkeys demonstrated phenotypic colistin resistance (>2 mg/liter.) (67). Resistance was also found in 8.3% of isolates from broilers, 4.4% from broiler meat, 2% from turkeys, and 27.7% from turkey meat; a large proportion of resistant isolates were *S. enterica* serovar Enteritidis (but this may represent a type of intrinsic resistance rather than resistance by an acquired chromosomal or plasmid-mediated mechanism [75]). Multidrug resistance was common; among 162 colistin-resistant *E. coli* isolates from poultry or poultry meat, 91.4% were resistant to three or more other antimicrobials; 120 (74.1%) of the isolates were also resistant (using epidemiological cutoff values) to either ciprofloxacin or ceftriaxone. Multidrug resistance was less common among *Salmonella* isolates with phenotypic colistin resistance (67).

Until very recently it was thought that acquired colistin resistance was limited to chromosomal mutation and was essentially nontransferable (67). In November 2015, however, Liu et al. (72) reported a transferable plasmid-mediated colistin resistance gene, *mcr-1*, in *E. coli* isolates obtained from animals, food, and human bloodstream infections from China. Spread of the gene by conjugation has been shown in *K. pneumoniae*, *Enterobacter aerogenes*, other *Enterobacter* spp., and *P. aeruginosa* (72). Aided by the rapid application of whole-genome sequencing techniques to strain collections around the world, retrospective analyses have revealed the *mcr-1* gene in several bacterial species isolated from human, animal, and environmental samples in numerous countries (76–79), and the gene was found in about 5% of healthy travelers (80). The earliest identification of the gene thus far was in *E. coli* from poultry collected in the 1980s in China (81). In Europe, the *mcr-1* gene is still relatively uncommon; for example, Doumith et al. reported that within large United Kingdom databases, *mcr-1* was detected in 15 of 24,000 (0.0625%) isolates of *Salmonella* spp., *E. coli*, *Klebsiella* spp., *Enterobacter* spp., and *Campylobacter* spp., from human and food samples collected between 2012 and 2015 (82). The *mcr-1* gene has also been detected in isolates obtained from wildlife and surface water samples, demonstrating environmental contamination (83). Now even more plasmid-mediated colistin resistance genes have been reported. This started with a novel *mcr-2* gene in *E. coli* from pigs in Belgium (84), and *mcr-3*, *mcr-4*, and *mcr-5* genes have been reported in many other bacterial species and in many countries (85).

Colistin illustrates some important One Health dimensions of antimicrobial resistance that differ from those of the third-generation cephalosporins. These relate, in particular, to the history and patterns of colistin use in humans and animals and to the subsequent emergence of resistance to the polymyxin class of antimicrobials, probably driven by large volumes of colistin used in animals rather than by use in humans. As mentioned above, for many years the toxicity and availability of other safer and more effective antimicrobials limited colistin to mainly topical uses in people. However, with the emergence of multidrug resistance in many Gram-negative bacteria, there has been increasing need for this drug to treat severe, life-threatening infections in humans in some countries. The colistin case demonstrates (once again) that using large quantities of antimicrobials for group treatments or growth promotion in animals can lead to significant antimicrobial resistance problems for human health, even if the drug class is initially believed to be less important, because the relative importance of antimicrobials to human health changes. The European Medicines Agency (EMA) has recommended an overall reduction of the use of polymixins in animals, with national targets of 5 mg/PCU and 1 or below 1 mg/PCU for countries with previous high and moderate use, respectively (67).

This closely parallels the experience of the 1990s with avoparcin, a glycopeptide antimicrobial growth promoter used widely in pig and poultry production that was initially thought not to be of public health importance. However, another glycopeptide, vancomycin, was critically important in the treatment of life-threatening methicillin resistant *Staphylococcus aureus* (MRSA) and for enterococcal infections of humans (the latter especially in penicillin-allergic patients) (86). Surveillance and research eventually were able to show that avoparcin use in animals contributed to the selection and widespread dissemination of vancomycin-resistant enterococci and glycopeptide resistance genes in enterococci from animals, food, humans, and the environment (87). There should be no need to repeat this lesson; antimicrobials, even if at some times regarded as only of minor importance to human health (e.g., colistin), should not be administered to groups of animals for routine disease prophylaxis or growth promotion.

HISTORY OF ONE HEALTH DIMENSIONS OF ANTIMICROBIAL RESISTANCE

The history of efforts to address the One Health dimensions of antimicrobial use in food animals is in some ways a study of country-by-country variation in the application of the available scientific evidence to antimicrobial policy (for more detail see reference 88). Public health concerns about antimicrobial use in animals have since the 1950s focused on both microbiological and toxicological effects (89, 90). While the latter are largely beyond the scope of this article, it can be argued that the generally successful approaches that quickly evolved to assess and manage the toxicological risks have made it more difficult to address the more challenging microbiological risks from antimicrobial resistance. It is fairly straightforward, using pharmaco-kinetics and pharmacodynamics, to predict rates of depletion of antimicrobial residues in edible products (meat, milk, eggs) from treated animals and, along with toxicological dose-response data from animal studies, to determine the concentrations of antimicrobial residue in foods (so-called maximum residue levels, or MRLs) that are compatible with acceptable levels of risk in exposed humans (91). This enables the establishment of a "withdrawal time," the time from administration of a drug until residues in foods from animals are reliably below the MRL for that drug. Regulations requiring avoidance of above-MRL (i.e., unsafe) and potentially chemically toxic concentrations of antimicrobial residues were widely established many years ago and are enforced with testing programs and penalties (31). For decades, veterinarians and farmers administering therapeutic antimicrobials to animals have been well aware of the need to adhere to withdrawal times to maintain product quality. This is a simple concept that was straightforward in application, easily communicated and enforced, and did not really interfere with the veterinarian's access to antimicrobials, so long as the withdrawal times and other label requirements were followed. On the other hand, this does not take into account antimicrobial resistance. The dynamics of antimicrobial resistance are not nearly as predictable, and microbiological risks cannot so easily be assessed, managed, and communicated in such a simple, straightforward manner as drug toxicity (33, 92, 93), and this has plagued the timely development and implementation of One Health approaches to address antimicrobial resistance in animals.

Concerns about the human health antimicrobial resistance risks from antimicrobial use in animals initially focused on administration of antimicrobials in animal feeds, particularly those administered without veterinary prescription for growth promotion (88). In 1968, the Swann Committee recommended separate regulation of "feed antibiotics" and "therapeutic antibiotics," such that the latter should be available for use in animals only under veterinary prescription (94). These recommendations were soon adopted in the United Kingdom and elsewhere in Europe, and as a consequence, the use

of penicillins, tetracyclines, sulfonamides, and other antimicrobials with therapeutic applications in humans and animals became no longer available over-the-counter in Europe for use as growth promoters (95). However, the United States, Canada, and many other countries did not follow the European example of distinctly separating antimicrobials for food animals into those for veterinary use and those for feed additives.

Concerns about antimicrobial feed additives were not limited to Europe; since 1969, several U.S. organizations (e.g. National Academy of Sciences, Food and Drug Administration ([FDA], Office of Technology Assessment) have deliberated on the use of antimicrobial drugs in animals, particularly in feeds (96–100), but early attempts to withdraw approval for "subtherapeutic" (growth-promotion) administration of antimicrobials from animal feeds were met with arguments that there was inadequate epidemiological evidence that the resultant antimicrobial-resistant bacteria are commonly transmitted to humans and cause serious illness (98). In 1987, the FDA asked the National Academy of Sciences Institute of Medicine to review the human health consequences and risk associated with including subtherapeutic levels of penicillin and tetracyclines in animal feed (101). The Institute of Medicine committee concluded that there was insufficient direct evidence to establish conclusively the presence of a human health hazard from such use, but the committee found a substantial body of indirect evidence, particularly for *Salmonella*. They developed a quantitative risk assessment model, the first in this field, using data from epidemiological surveillance and published literature, and concluded that the estimated annual number of fatal antimicrobial-resistant salmonellosis cases in the United States due to subtherapeutic use of penicillin and tetracycline was most likely about 40 but ranged from 1 to 400. They went on to use the risk assessment model to identify the fraction of these cases attributable to antimicrobial uses in livestock feed and estimated that these "excess deaths" were in the range of 6 per year in the United States (101). Unfortunately, the assembled indirect evidence and formal quantitative risk assessment findings were apparently insufficient for U.S. regulatory purposes, since the FDA proposal to withdraw "subtherapeutic" (low-dose, long-term administration) use of penicillin and tetracycline from animal feeds was not implemented (98). It is remarkable that the finding of excess deaths could be considered acceptable from a regulatory perspective. After another 3 decades of evidence gathering, and with greater societal and stakeholder acceptance that something must be done about growth promoters, the FDA recently introduced guidance for the voluntary removal of claims for growth promotion and other "production uses" of medically important antimicrobials in the United States (40). The choice of a voluntary approach may at least in part reflect the previous difficulties with forced withdrawals where the burden of proof is placed on the regulator.

The 1990s saw a resurgence in concerns about antimicrobial resistance in the human, agricultural, and veterinary sectors. In particular, growth promoter use of avoparcin and therapeutic use of fluoroquinolones featured prominently in these concerns, along with the emergence and spread of multiple-resistant *S. enterica* serovar Typhimurium DT104 (34, 102). As mentioned previously, avoparcin was a glycopeptide antimicrobial that was used as a feed additive in Europe, Australia, and many other countries and that selected for resistance to vancomycin, another glycopeptide (34, 103). At the same time, increasing concerns about resistance to the fluoroquinolone class among important human pathogens focused attention on the use of these drugs in animals, particularly in poultry, where they were typically administered in water at the flock level (102). Endtz and coworkers demonstrated convincingly that fluoroquinolone resistance among *C. jejuni* isolated from poultry and clinical infections of humans emerged soon after veterinary use of the drugs was introduced (63). In the United States, an application to approve fluoroquinolone use in poultry was met with concern that it would compromise the effectiveness of the drug class for the treatment of human infections. The FDA eventually approved the application, but to address resistance concerns restricted off-label use of the drug in food animals and established the U.S. National Antimicrobial Resistance Monitoring program in 1996 to improve food chain surveillance of antimicrobial resistance of human health concern. Within a short time, surveillance and research confirmed that fluoroquinolone use in poultry did indeed adversely affect human health by selecting for resistance to this class of drugs in *C. jejuni*, and the FDA withdrew its approval of its use in poultry, but this required a prolonged legal process (65).

In 1986, Sweden was the first European country to ban antimicrobial growth promoters in food animals (34). Denmark, through a combination of voluntary industry initiatives and regulatory action, terminated the use of avoparcin in 1995 and then other antimicrobial growth promoters by 1999 (35). Subsequently, the European Union terminated the use of all antimicrobial growth promoters as of January 1, 2006. The European Union has continued to permit therapeutic use of approved antimicrobials in animals, including fluoroquinolones and some other critically important antimicrobials for humans, with some restrictions, for example, that third-generation cephalosporins should not be used in poultry (104).

The history of some of these major attempts to address One Health antimicrobial resistance issues reveals remarkable differences between countries in the speed and efficiency with which they made major regulatory changes to the availability of antimicrobials for use in animals on the basis of concerns about human health. This is especially the case for drugs that had been on the market for years. Globally, Europe and the United States have been the dominant centers of regulatory activity, with some other countries more or less following suit, particularly with U.S. approaches. Broadly speaking, European countries have been more nimble in moving forward with major regulatory changes to antimicrobial availability (e.g., implementation of the Swann recommendations and, later, the outright ban on antimicrobial growth promoters), and this may reflect a greater willingness in Europe to exercise precaution in favor of public health when making antimicrobial policy. The United States, while quite ready to exercise precaution in some stages of the drug licensing process (e.g., preapproval human safety evaluation), has been hampered by demands for higher levels of proof of adverse effects on human health (by legislatures and industry groups) to justify revoking specific drug authorizations for animals (e.g., subtherapeutic uses of penicillin and tetracycline in livestock feed and fluoroquinolone for the treatment of poultry).

RISKS TO PUBLIC HEALTH AND ANIMAL HEALTH

Antimicrobial resistance is harmful to health because it reduces the effectiveness of antimicrobial therapy and tends to increase the severity, incidence, and cost of infection (4, 105). Antimicrobial use in humans has been associated with resistance in numerous important human pathogens affecting various body systems (2), and there is now considerable evidence that antimicrobial use in animals is an important contributor to antimicrobial resistance among pathogens of humans, in particular, common enteric pathogens such as *Salmonella* spp., *Campylobacter* spp., *Enterococcus* spp., and *E. coli* and in some cases other bacteria that can also be zoonotic, e.g., *S. aureus* (7, 14, 23, 33, 34). There is also increasing concern that exposure of bacteria to heavy metals and biocides (e.g., disinfectants, antiseptics) in animals and environmental niches may coselect for resistance to antimicrobials (106).

Nontyphoidal *Salmonella* is among the most common bacteria isolated from foodborne infections of humans. It has been estimated that globally, there are around 94 million cases, including 155,000 deaths, of nontyphoidal *Salmonella* gastroenteritis each year (1). Animals are the most important reservoirs of nontyphoidal *Salmonella* for humans, and resistance has been associated with antimicrobial use in animals, along with other management factors such as mixing of animals from different sources and transport (33, 94, 101, 107). Fecal shedding by carrier animals is an important source of antimicrobial-resistant *Salmonella* contamination of meat and poultry products (33) and may also be responsible for fruit and vegetable contamination through fecal contamination of the environment (108). *Salmonella* resistance to any medically important antimicrobial is a public health concern, but particularly to those critically important to human health, such as cephalosporins and fluoroquinolones (33, 34, 57), for which therapeutic options can be limited. Therapy in some groups (e.g., children and pregnant women) can be very restricted because of issues of toxicity with many antibiotics. Beta-lactams such as third-generation cephalosporins often may be the only therapy available to treat serious infections.

Concerns have been expressed that fluoroquinolone use in food animals is linked to quinolone resistance in *Salmonella* (34, 102, 109, 110). Surveillance data compiled by WHO indicate that rates of fluoroquinolone resistance in nontyphoidal *Salmonella* vary widely by geographical region. For example, rates are relatively low in Europe (2 to 3%), higher in the Eastern Mediterranean region (up to 40 to 50%), and wide-ranging in the Americas (0 to 96%) (1). Many *Salmonella* strains are also resistant to antimicrobials that have long been used as growth promoters in many countries (e.g., Canada, the United States), including tetracyclines, penicillins, and sulfonamides (34, 107). Antimicrobial resistance in some of the more virulent *Salmonella* serovars (e.g., Heidelberg, Newport, Typhimurium) has been associated with more severe infections in humans (33, 101, 105, 111). Resistance to other critically important antimicrobials continues to emerge in *Salmonella*; for example, a carbapenem-resistant strain of *Salmonella* was identified on a pig farm that routinely administered prophylactic cephalosporin (ceftiofur) to piglets (112).

C. jejuni infections are among the most common food- and waterborne infections in many countries, and while antimicrobial treatment is typically not indicated in uncomplicated cases, because they are usually self-limiting, resistance to some antimicrobials, e.g.,

fluoroquinolones, has been associated with greater severity, including longer duration of infection (105, 113). As mentioned above, fluoroquinolone resistance is associated with the use of this drug in animals, especially in poultry, where it is typically administered as a mass medication in drinking water (63, 64). In Australia, where fluoroquinolones have never been licensed for use in poultry but are widely used in humans, quinolone resistance among *C. jejuni* isolates from human infections remains very low (66). Macrolides are widely used in animals, and in many countries they are administered in feed to groups of animals and in some cases as growth promoters, and such uses have been associated with macrolide resistance in *Campylobacter* (33, 40).

E. coli is an important pathogen of both humans and animals. In humans, *E. coli* is a common cause of serious bacterial infections, including enteritis, urinary tract infection, and sepsis. For example, reported rates of bloodstream *E. coli* infections in developed countries ranged between 30 and 50 episodes per 100,000 population annually in the past (114, 115). Currently in England, the rate is about 64 cases per 100,000 per year and rising. A large and increasing proportion is antimicrobial resistant (116). These higher rates are also being seen in countries with good surveillance systems in place, e.g., Denmark (60).

In animals, *E. coli* is responsible for enteritis, various extra-intestinal infections such as mastitis in lactating animals, and septicemia. In poultry, *E. coli* causes cellulitis, salpingitis, synovitis, and omphalitis (yolk sac infections) (117). Some *E. coli* strains appear to be species-specific pathogens, while others are capable of infecting multiple species, including humans. Many *E. coli* strains appear to behave as commensals of the gut of animals and humans but may be opportunistic pathogens as well as donors of resistance genetic elements for pathogenic *E. coli* or other species of bacteria (51, 118). Although antimicrobial resistance is a rapidly increasing problem in *E. coli* infections of both animals and humans, the problem is better documented for isolates from human infections, where resistance is extensive, particularly in developing countries (1, 119). Humans are regularly exposed to antimicrobial-resistant *E. coli* through foods and inadequately treated drinking water (120, 121). Resistance to third-generation cephalosporins, fluoroquinolones, and/or carbapenems is increasing in many regions, particularly in developing countries (1, 119). Travelers from developed countries are at risk of acquiring multiresistant *E. coli* from other people or contaminated food and/or water (114, 121, 122). There are now serious problems with ESBL *E. coli* in both developing and developed countries, and foods from animals, poultry in particular, have been implicated as sources for humans (50, 53, 55), although the magnitude of the contribution from food animals is uncertain. WHO is attempting to improve this situation by the establishment and expansion of integrated surveillance of antimicrobial resistance in foodborne bacteria using the application of a One Health approach, which will help establish links and calculate risks including by using newer methodologies such as whole-genome sequencing (123). WHO has also reported wide-ranging rates of *E. coli* resistance to third-generation cephalosporins, for example, up to 48% in the Americas and 70% in Africa and South-East Asia (1). A systematic review of the health burden from third-generation cephalosporin resistance (including ESBL) in *E. coli* infections relative to susceptible infections revealed a significant 2-fold increase in all-cause mortality, bacterium-attributable mortality, and 30-day mortality. Patients with fluoroquinolone-resistant *E. coli* infections experienced a significant 2-fold increase in all-cause mortality and 30-day mortality (1).

MRSA is an important pathogen of humans in both community and hospital settings, causing skin, wound, bloodstream, and other types of infection (1, 124, 125). Serious staphylococcal infections in people are common: about 10 to 30 per 100,000 inhabitants per year (126). WHO reports that beta-lactam resistance (i.e., MRSA) is a global problem, with rates of resistance of up to 80 to 100% in Africa, up to 90% in the Americas, and up to 60% in Europe (1). Systematic review of the health burden of MRSA relative to methicillin-susceptible *S. aureus* showed that patients with predominantly healthcare-associated MRSA infections experienced a significant increase in all-cause mortality, bacterium-attributable mortality, and intensive care unit mortality and septic shock (1). Community acquired MRSA bacteremia has increased with time, and the disease is associated with more necrotizing pneumonia and cutaneous abscesses, although with less endovascular infection compared to more sensitive strains of *S. aureus*. Unlike healthcare-associated infections, patients with community-acquired MRSA bacteremia did not have higher mortality than did patients with more sensitive strains of *S. aureus* (127).

S. aureus and other staphylococci are also recognized pathogens of animals; for example, they are responsible for cases of mastitis in cattle and skin infections in pigs and companion animals (128, 129). MRSA was until recently relatively rare in animals, but strains pathogenic to humans have emerged in several animal species (129–132). Transmission to humans is currently thought to be mainly through contact with carrier animals (132).

The predominant strain isolated from animals, sequence type 398, while pathogenic to humans, is not considered a major epidemic strain (128, 129). Antimicrobial use in livestock, as well as lapses in biosecurity within and between farms and international trade in animals, food, or other products are factors contributing to the spread of this pathogen in animals (129, 133).

ONE HEALTH CONSIDERATIONS FROM THE ENVIRONMENT

Antimicrobial resistance in other pathogens as well as gut commensals and bacteria in other ecological niches can also be driven by antimicrobial use in animals and humans. One Health includes consideration of the environment as well as human and animal health (19, 134). The ecological nature of antimicrobial resistance is a reflection and consequence of the interconnectedness and incredible diversity of life on the planet (18). Many pathogenic bacteria, the antimicrobials that we use to treat them, and genes that confer resistance have environmental origins (e.g., soil) (8, 16, 135). Some important resistance genes, such as beta-lactamases, are millions of years old (135, 136). Soil and other environmental matrices are rich sources of highly diverse populations of bacteria and their genes (135, 137). Antimicrobial resistance to a wide variety of drugs has been demonstrated in environmental bacteria isolated from the preantibiotic era, as well as from various sites (e.g., caves) free of other sources of exposure to modern antimicrobials (8, 134, 136, 138). Despite having ancient origins, there is abundant evidence that human activity has an impact on the resistome, which is the totality of resistance genes in the wider environment (135, 137, 138). Hundreds of thousands of tonnes of antimicrobials are produced annually and find their way into the environment (14, 24). Waste from treatment plants and the pharmaceutical industry, particularly if inadequately treated, has been shown to release high concentrations of antimicrobials into surface water (14, 15, 139, 140). Residues and metabolites of antimicrobials are constituents of human sewage, livestock manure, and aquaculture, along with fecal bacteria and resistance genes (137, 141–143). Sewage treatment and composting of manure reduce concentrations of some but not all antimicrobials and microorganisms, which are introduced to soil upon land application of human and animal biosolids (144).

Various environmental pathways are important routes of human exposure to resistant bacteria and their genes from animal and plant reservoirs (14, 112) and provide opportunities for better regulations to control antimicrobial resistance (Fig. 3). In developed countries with good-quality sewage and drinking water treatment, and where most people have little to no direct contact with food-producing animals, transmission of bacteria and resistance genes from agricultural sources is largely foodborne, either from direct contamination of meat and poultry during slaughter and processing, or indirectly from fruit and vegetables contaminated by manure or irrigation water (33, 65, 108). In countries with poor sewage and water treatment, drinking water is likely to be very important in the transmission of resistant bacteria and/or genes from animals (114, 134, 139). Poor sanitation also facilitates indirect person-person water-

borne transmission of enteric bacteria among residents as well as international travelers who return home colonized with resistant bacteria acquired locally (119, 145). Through these and other means, including globalized trade in animals and food and long-distance migratory patterns of wildlife, antimicrobial-resistant bacteria are globally disseminated.

General measures to address antimicrobial resistance in the wider environment include improved controls on pollution from industrial, residential, and agricultural sources. Improved research as well as environmental monitoring and risk assessment are required to better understand the role of the environment in the selection

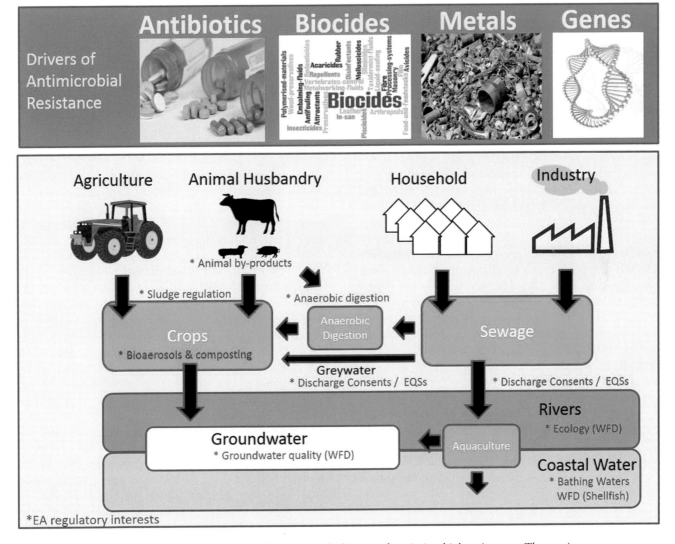

Figure 3 Schematics of the hotspots and drivers of antimicrobial resistance. The environmental compartments that are currently monitored or regulated by the Environmental Agency (EA; England) are denoted by an asterisk in red. WDF, Water Framework Directive. Reprinted from *Frontiers in Microbiology* (140) with permission of the publisher.

and spread of antimicrobial resistance and to identify more specific measures to address resistance in this sector (11, 14, 116, 119, 135, 146).

ONE HEALTH STRATEGIES TO ADDRESS ANTIMICROBIAL RESISTANCE

WHO and other international agencies (e.g., Food and Agriculture Organization [FAO], OIE), along with many individual countries, have developed comprehensive action plans to address the antimicrobial resistance crisis (6, 147–153). The WHO Global Action Plan seeks to address five major objectives, discussed in the following subsections. The WHO Global Action Plan embraces a One Health approach to address antimicrobial resistance, and it calls on member countries to do the same when developing their own action plans (6).

Improve Awareness and Understanding of Antimicrobial Resistance through Effective Communication, Education, and Training

Antimicrobial resistance is a rapidly evolving, highly complex topic, not least its One Health dimensions, which feature various forms of antimicrobial use within human, animal, and environmental sectors, accompanied by selection of antimicrobial resistance among bacteria in a wide variety of niches and with serious consequences to the health of humans and animals. At the most basic level, everyone should understand the principles of basic hygiene to prevent the spread of infections, understand the need to follow the antimicrobial prescriber's instructions for treatment, and have a basic appreciation of the risks to themselves and others associated with antimicrobial use, in addition to the benefits (4, 6). This applies to antimicrobial use in humans as well as animals. While all can benefit from a more in-depth understanding of the One Health dimensions of antimicrobial resistance, those with particular need include companion animal owners, farmers, veterinarians, and others involved in food production and the wider food industry. The depth of understanding that these groups require varies. Animal owners should understand that some bacterial infections are shared by animals and humans and that they should follow veterinary advice on antimicrobial use and prevention of disease transmission. Farmers should understand how to raise animals, fruits, and vegetables with no or minimal use of antimicrobials and ideally use them only for the treatment of clinically ill individual animals. They also need to know how to reduce the need for antimicrobial treatment by improving overall levels of husbandry and minimizing overcrowded, unsanitary, and

stressful conditions that promote the spread of disease in populations of animals and plants (154, 155). Veterinarians who prescribe antimicrobials and advise farmers on disease prevention obviously require a deeper understanding of the One Health dimensions of antimicrobial resistance. Veterinarians should possess the knowledge, attitudes, and behaviors that characterize good antimicrobial stewardship, thereby protecting the health and welfare of their patients, the economic interests of their clients, as well as the health of the wider community (147, 153–155). Human health professionals would also benefit from a good understanding of the One Health aspects of antimicrobial resistance and a better understanding and implementation of the mechanisms that help control the spread of pathogens, including resistant bacteria, e.g., by infection control, improved hygiene, improved sanitation, etc. All health professionals should have a good understanding of the modifiable drivers of antimicrobial resistance (Fig. 4) and be motivated to reduce their impact on antimicrobial resistance selection and spread.

Opportunities to enhance awareness and understanding of One Health dimensions of antimicrobial resistance include the health promotion and health protection programs offered by pubic health and animal health organizations, consumer information campaigns (public, animal owners), farmer outreach activities, veterinary consultations, farm industry publications (farmers), veterinary curricula, and professional development programs (veterinarians, physicians).

Strengthen the Knowledge and Evidence Base through Surveillance and Research

Surveillance and research are essential because they identify antimicrobial resistance problems and how to prevent them (1, 6). There are many gaps in our understanding of the complex biology that characterizes the One Health dimensions of resistance, but many advances have been made in recent years that support evidence-based interventions to address antimicrobial resistance (4, 7, 136).

Surveillance of antimicrobial resistance and antimicrobial use in both human and nonhuman sectors is necessary to estimate the extent, patterns, and health burden of resistance at the national, regional, and international levels (123, 156). Such surveillance should be able to detect emerging trends in antimicrobial resistance of clinical significance to humans and animals (1, 26, 56). Surveillance should inform educational efforts to minimize antimicrobial resistance, as well as antimicrobial use policies and antimicrobial stewardship programs (4, 6, 7). Surveillance is also needed to mea-

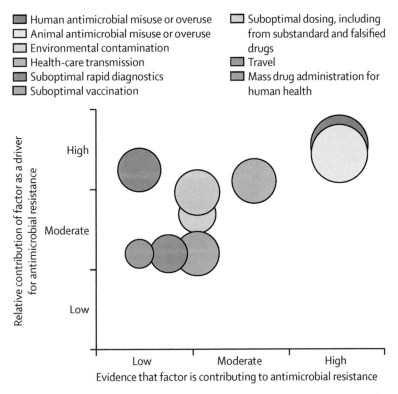

■ Human antimicrobial misuse or overuse
□ Animal antimicrobial misuse or overuse
□ Environmental contamination
■ Health-care transmission
■ Suboptimal rapid diagnostics
□ Suboptimal vaccination

□ Suboptimal dosing, including
from substandard and falsified
drugs
■ Travel
■ Mass drug administration for
human health

Relative contribution of factor as a driver
for antimicrobial resistance

High

Moderate

Low

Low   Moderate   High
Evidence that factor is contributing to antimicrobial resistance

Figure 4 Role of modifiable drivers for antimicrobial resistance: a conceptual framework.
Reprinted from Lancet (8) with permission of the publisher.

sure the effectiveness of interventions and other measures that are taken to control antimicrobial resistance
(17, 157). One Health surveillance of antimicrobial
resistance should include sampling of appropriate bacteria from specimens collected in various human, animal, and environmental settings including hospitals,
extended-care and community settings, veterinary clinics, farms, food, and the environment (e.g., wildlife,
soil, water) (17, 123, 155). Surveillance of antimicrobial use should also be conducted in human, veterinary,
and agricultural settings and should provide estimates
of antimicrobial consumption in humans and animal
species at the national level along with suitable de-
nominators (e.g., population size, numbers of animals,
PCUs) to enable comparisons among countries (17, 60,
123). To provide information that is useful for assessing and guiding prescribing practices and antimicrobial
use behaviors, antimicrobial use monitoring should
also take place at the level of prescribing (e.g., hospitals, community, veterinary clinic, farm) (60, 123, 158).
Surveillance data should be analyzed, interpreted, and
presented in an integrated fashion across sectors, and
reports should be timely in order to be useful to relevant stakeholders (60). WHO has provided guidance
on harmonized, integrated surveillance of antimicrobial

resistance and antimicrobial use to assist developed
and developing countries in implementing their own
national surveillance programs and to contribute to improved global surveillance activities which are essential
for better coordination of international efforts to contain antimicrobial use (123).

Targeted research is essential to demonstrate how
resistance develops and spreads within and between
ecological niches and species of bacteria, including
pathogens as well as enteric commensals and environmental bacteria (4, 11, 33). To reduce antimicrobial use
in animals, additional research is needed for suitable
cost-effective alternatives to antimicrobials for disease
prevention and enhancement of growth and production
efficiency (7, 14, 15). Additional research is also needed
to support antimicrobial stewardship such as improved
diagnostic tools, ways to improve antimicrobial prescribing and utilization behaviors, and better vaccines (4–6).

Reduce the Incidence of Infection
through Effective Sanitation, Hygiene,
and Infection Prevention Measures

Infection control in healthcare settings, particularly
hospitals, is a well-recognized and important means to
limit the spread of antimicrobial resistance in humans

(16, 118). In veterinary clinics, however, formal infection control programs are underutilized (159, 160). At the farm level, infection control in the form of biosecurity and other disease control programs is important in most food animal industries, particularly for intensive production in the poultry and swine sectors (7, 23). Some animal disease control programs are applied at the national level, particularly to prevent the introduction of exotic animal pathogens to the national herd, while others are applied at the farm level (147, 154, 155). These programs usually target production-limiting animal pathogens or specific zoonoses, and the extent to which they are effective in limiting the spread of antimicrobial resistance, particularly in nonpathogenic bacteria, is rarely if ever evaluated. Nevertheless, to reduce the need for antimicrobial use in animals, whether for treatment or prophylaxis, it is important to adopt health management measures to prevent disease in animals, particularly those responsible for the largest quantities of medically important antimicrobials (e.g., *Streptococcus suis* infections and diarrhea in pigs, pneumonia in calves, *E. coli* infections in broilers, mastitis in dairy cows) (31, 155).

To reduce human exposure to the spread of antimicrobial resistance from environmental sources and pathways, it is also important to implement measures to improve the safety of food and drinking water, particularly in underdeveloped countries, and to control environmental pollution from the pharmaceutical industry (118, 135, 140). Foodborne pathogen reduction programs at the farm, slaughter, and further processing levels are important for controlling the spread of enteric bacteria such as *Salmonella* and *Campylobacter* to humans (154). Likewise, measures to improve the microbiological quality of drinking water (from source water protection through to disinfection) as well as proper sewage treatment are important to reduce exposure to bacteria from environmental sources, as well as to reduce indirect human-human transmission of enteric bacteria (both susceptible and resistant) (16, 114).

Optimize the Use of Antimicrobial Medicines in Human and Animal Health

A One Health approach to improved antimicrobial stewardship involves a range of regulatory, voluntary, and other means to preserve the effectiveness of antimicrobials in human, animal, and agricultural settings (4). This approach should include interventions to promote judicious use of antimicrobials, as well as monitoring of antimicrobial utilization and mechanisms for continued improvement of prescribing and utilization (7, 147, 160). A One Health approach to stewardship

requires some alignment of activities in the various sectors (human, veterinary, agriculture) to achieve the overall goal of preserving antimicrobial effectiveness for both humans and animals (6, 160). This involves finding a way of balancing the sometimes-competing interests that exist in the different sectors, and this can be contentious. Typically, human health interests predominate, but animal health and welfare are also important considerations (37). In our view, economic interests are subordinate to health considerations. From the One Health perspective, antimicrobial stewardship programs should seek to ensure that antimicrobials are reserved for the treatment of clinical infections in humans and animals that occur despite the existence of good infection control and other programs designed to minimize the need for treatment (147, 155, 160). Overall, there is greater emphasis on national regulatory interventions to control antimicrobial resistance in the veterinary/agricultural sectors than in human medicine (160). This is a reflection of the importance that society places on the health of humans relative to other interests, and with it, a more frequent need in the veterinary/agricultural sectors for mandatory controls and restrictions that are best applied at a systems level, rather than relying on voluntary measures at the prescriber or user level. Regulatory approval of antimicrobials for use in animals normally depends on the demonstration that such use is safe for humans (through exposure to residues in food and selection of antimicrobial resistance) as well as being safe for animals and efficacious (31, 40, 62). Examples of regulatory interventions taken to address antimicrobial resistance include the ban on the use of antimicrobial growth promoters in food-producing animals in the European Union, restriction of the extra-label use of fluoroquinolones and third-generation cephalosporin in animals in the United States, and the prescription-only availability of antimicrobials for veterinary use in many countries (7, 35, 61).

Drug classification is an important tool for addressing antimicrobial resistance. From the One Health perspective, the most important classification schemes are those that categorize antimicrobials with respect to their importance to human and animal health (Table 1). Beginning in 2005 and then updated at regular intervals, WHO has developed a scheme to classify antimicrobials used in humans into three categories: critically important, highly important, and important (42, 161). The purpose of the classification is to guide risk management strategies to prevent and control antimicrobial resistance from food animal production. Two criteria are used for classification, and additional criteria are used to prioritize those antimicrobial classes in the critically important category. Examples of the highest-priority classes are quinolones and third- and fourth-generation cephalosporins (42, 161).

The OIE has developed a system of classification of antimicrobials of importance to animal health (162). The list was first adopted by the OIE in 2007 and then updated in 2013 and 2015. It was based on information obtained from a survey of OIE member countries. There is considerable overlap of the WHO and OIE lists; for example, third- and fourth-generation cephalosporins, fluoroquinolones, and macrolides are found in the critically important category of antimicrobials on both lists (Table 1). Some individual countries (e.g., Canada, United States) and the European Union have developed their own approaches to categorizing antimicrobial classes with respect to importance to human health (62). It would be useful to harmonize the criteria used in these different classifications of antimicrobials with respect to human health and to make progress in reconciling the overlap in the human and animal lists (163).

There are several ways to incorporate this antimicrobial classification into antimicrobial risk management strategies. One example is to eliminate the growth promotion uses of medically important antimicrobials (i.e., classes within the critically important, highly important, and important categories of the WHO list) (34, 37, 155). This strategy has been used in the European Union and Korea and is being implemented in other countries (e.g., Canada, United States) (38, 39). Another way is to completely restrict the use in animals of certain microbials that are critically important in humans. For example, in the European Union carbapenems, glycopeptides, monobactams, and some other classes are not licensed for use in food animal species, nor may they be used off-label in these species, and in companion animals they may be used only in exceptional circumstances (38, 62). It is also possible to utilize categorization in schemes involving treatment cascades or formularies (e.g., first-line, second-line, etc. choices). For example, the European Union stipulates that in consideration of their importance to human health, third- and fourth-generation cephalosporins and fluoroquinolones should be used only when there are no alternative antimicrobials authorized for the target species and indications (38, 62). Another application of antimicrobial classification is the promotion of antimicrobial stewardship by industry. For example, the McDonald's corporation, Perdue, Tyson Foods, and other major food companies have adopted antimicrobial use policies that require suppliers to restrict food animal use of antimicrobials classified by WHO as critically important for human medicine (36, 164, 165).

Develop the Economic Case for Sustainable Investment that Takes Account of the Needs of All Countries and Increase Investment in New Medicines, Diagnostic Tools, Vaccines, and Other Interventions

While this particular objective of the WHO Global Action Plan is aimed largely at the human health sector, there is also a need for investments in the animal health sector that reduce the need for antimicrobials, such as additional vaccines and other nonantimicrobial disease control strategies.

CURRENT ROLES OF INTERNATIONAL ORGANIZATIONS IN ONE HEALTH ASPECTS OF ANTIMICROBIAL RESISTANCE

Several international organizations have made important One Health contributions to the containment of antimicrobial resistance. Since the early 1990s, WHO has undertaken several expert, multidisciplinary, multisectoral consultations and advisory groups, compiled considerable objective evidence of and scientific opinion about the human health impacts of antimicrobial use in animals, and formulated wide-ranging recommendations applicable to all stakeholders (e.g., regulatory authorities, pharmaceutical industry, animal production industry, veterinarians, farmers, public health, consumers) (155). The first was the 1997 report Medical Impact of the Use of Antimicrobials in Food Animals (34), which was quickly followed by numerous others (6, 35, 102, 155). The need to consider the human health importance of antimicrobials when managing antimicrobial resistance in animals led to the previously mentioned work by WHO to categorize antimicrobial classes according to their relative importance in human medicine (42, 161). Furthermore, since 2008, the WHO Advisory Group on Integrated Surveillance of Antimicrobial Resistance has issued six reports that include scientific information, guidelines for integrated surveillance of antimicrobial resistance and antimicrobial use, and recommendations in support of global efforts to contain antimicrobial resistance, particularly in the developing world (37, 123, 166). WHO recently launched new guidelines on the use of medically important antimicrobials in food-producing animals, recommending that farmers and the food industry stop using antimicrobials routinely to promote growth and prevent disease in healthy animals. The purpose of the guidelines is to preserve the effectiveness of antimicrobials that are important for human health by reducing their excessive use in animals (37).

The OIE has contributed technical guidance on antimicrobial resistance and antimicrobial use monitoring, antimicrobial resistance risk analysis, and the prudent use of antimicrobials in veterinary medicine and aquaculture (167, 168). As mentioned previously, the OIE also developed a list of critically important antimicrobials for animal health (162).

Codex Alimentarius is a set of international food standards administered under the auspices of the FAO and WHO. In 2001, in recognition of the importance of antimicrobials to human health as well as animal health, Codex recommended that the FAO, OIE, and WHO jointly address antimicrobial resistance issues. One outcome was a series of joint FAO/WHO/OIE expert workshops on nonhuman antimicrobial usage and antimicrobial resistance that implicitly took a One Health perspective (33, 154, 163, 169).

The 29th session of the Codex Alimentarius Commission established the Ad Hoc Intergovernmental Task Force on Antimicrobial Resistance with a mandate to propose guidelines for risk analysis of foodborne antimicrobial resistance (170). These guidelines are most applicable to national public health agencies that regulate the nonhuman use of antimicrobials (92). There is a focus on foodborne antimicrobial resistance (to the exclusion of nonhuman sectors, such as companion animals and the environment) because Codex is a food standards organization. This undertaking built on previous work on risk assessment and management of foodborne chemical and microbiological hazards conducted by Codex, as well as the OIE and VICH (International Cooperation on Harmonization of Technical Requirements for Registration of Veterinary Medicinal Products). The resulting Guidelines for Risk Analysis of Foodborne Antimicrobial Resistance (CAC/GL 77-2011) provide a methodology for evidence-based decision-making and policy formation on One Health dimensions of antimicrobial resistance and will be particularly important if antimicrobial resistance control becomes an international trade issue (170).

On the international front, the European Union has been very active in One Health antimicrobial resistance activities, particularly with regard to the regulation of antimicrobials for veterinary use and in the integrated surveillance of antimicrobial resistance and antimicrobial use (17, 25, 26, 38, 43, 67, 104, 110, 124, 171–173). The European action plan to address antimicrobial resistance declared the need for a One Health approach to address antimicrobial resistance, in view of the interconnection between animal health, human health, and ecosystems (147). In many ways, the European approach is a model for other regions/

countries to follow because it is relatively proactive, thorough, consistent with international standards, policy oriented, and well communicated through abundant publicly available information on antimicrobial use policies and the scientific information on which they are based. European agencies with important responsibilities in this One Health approach include the EMA, the European Center for Disease Control (ECDC), and the European Food Standards Agency (EFSA). The Committee for Medicinal Products for Veterinary Use of the EMA regulates veterinary drugs across the European Union and has articulated a strategy to address antimicrobial resistance concerns that includes periodic re-evaluation of marketing authorizations, public release of decisions, promotion of alternatives to antimicrobials, advice, and reflection papers (172). An example of the latter is the recent review of colistin use in human and veterinary medicine in Europe that addresses resistance mechanisms, evidence of the selection and spread of colistin resistance, a profiling of the risks to public health from the use of colistin in animals, and risk management options, including those rejected and those recommended with full discussion of the rationale (67).

Monitoring of veterinary antimicrobial use from countries within the European Union and European Economic Area (EEA) has been conducted since 2009 under the ESVAC (European Surveillance of Veterinary Antimicrobial Consumption) project (17, 25). ESVAC has been instrumental in developing national-level antimicrobial use data collection methodologies for the veterinary sector, technical units of measurement, and approaches for the collection of antimicrobial consumption data by animal species. ESVAC publishes annual reports on sales of veterinary antimicrobial agents in European Union/European Economic Area countries (25). Monitoring of antimicrobial use in the human health sector, conducted by the ECDC through ESAC-Net, has been in place since 2001 and focuses on consumption in the community and hospital sectors. Certain ESAC projects studied antimicrobial consumption in the community and hospital sectors. The ESAC has also conducted point-prevalence surveys of antimicrobial prescribing in hospitals and in long-term care facilities and developed indicators of appropriate antimicrobial prescribing in primary care. The ESAC data were used to explain the variation of antibiotic resistance in Europe and to assess the impact of interventions in the community (72).

Surveillance of antimicrobial resistance in Europe is conducted by the ECDC (bacteria from human infections) and EFSA (bacteria from animals and food). The ECDC and EFSA publish annual summaries of antimicrobial resistance (as well as zoonotic infections and food-borne outbreaks) for individual member states within the European Union (75). The ECDC, EFSA, and EMA have also published Joint Interagency Antimicrobial Consumption and Resistance Analysis integrated reports and analyses of antimicrobial resistance and antimicrobial use data from Europe, including analyses of statistical associations between antimicrobial resistance and antimicrobial use data across sectors (26, 171). While recognizing the limitations in the data, the analyses demonstrated positive ecologic (national level) associations between consumption of antimicrobials and resistance in bacteria to corresponding antimicrobials in both humans and animals. There were also some positive associations between antimicrobial consumption in animals and resistance in bacteria from humans. These findings reinforce the need for many countries to reduce the overall consumption of antimicrobials in both the human and animal sectors (26).

ONGOING ONE HEALTH CHALLENGES IN ADDRESSING ANTIMICROBIAL RESISTANCE

The need for a One Health approach to address antimicrobial resistance is now firmly established at the international level and is included in the action plans of many countries around the world (6, 147–153). This is fostering communication among sectors that for too long operated in isolation and offers the potential for greater coordination and understanding across sectors. Other positive developments include the establishment of integrated antimicrobial resistance and antimicrobial use surveillance systems in many countries, explicit consideration of antimicrobial resistance issues in the regulation of veterinary use of antimicrobials, a trend toward more countries terminating the use of medically important antimicrobials as growth promoters, and actions by some major food industries to use their buying power to limit the use of medically important antimicrobials in food animals. However, despite these positive signs, the available data indicate that globally, antimicrobial use is still far too excessive in both the human and animal sectors and antimicrobial resistance among important pathogens continues to increase at alarming rates (2, 4, 16, 24). Much more progress is needed in addressing these issues in the human and animal sectors on a global basis, in both developed and developing countries.

There are many challenges to improving antimicrobial stewardship in humans and animals (155, 160). These include a lack of adequate motivation for change and awareness of the need for all prescribers and users to be good antimicrobial stewards, a lack of oversight and controls on antimicrobial availability in many countries, and pressures on prescribers from patients and animal owners to use antimicrobials even when they are unnecessary (4, 7, 154). Reflection on the history of antimicrobial use shows, not surprisingly, that we have been very quick to adopt uses for these drugs but exceedingly slow to cut back on use when it is harmful to the wider community. In the veterinary/agricultural sectors, most antimicrobials were authorized for use before there was any systematic evaluation of the potential adverse effects on antimicrobial resistance. Like pesticides, improved genetics of animals and crops, and advances in animal nutrition, large-scale use of antimicrobials was widely adopted during the post-WWII intensification and scaling-up of agriculture and is still considered in many circles as necessary for efficient food production. In some countries, agricultural interests and veterinary medical organizations have been too slow to accept the scientific evidence of harm to public health from excessive antimicrobial use in animal production and to make the changes needed to raise animals humanely with reduced use of antimicrobials. Notwithstanding the tremendous new insights provided by antimicrobial resistance research and surveillance, and major improvements in antimicrobial resistance risk analysis methodologies, there will always be uncertainties and data gaps in a subject as complex as antimicrobial resistance. Improvements in our ability to analyze bacteria and their genes using whole-genome sequencing and metagenomics in animals, people, and the environment, along with metadata analysis and phylogenetic studies should allow us to make better links and understand with more precision the ways they multiply and spread. More importantly, it will help us better track how antimicrobial resistance genes that have long been in existence spread and recirculate in plants, insects, animals, people, soil, and water. This will help us better understand what is driving the development and the spread of antimicrobial resistance and better manage it.

Nevertheless, given the highly unpredictable nature of antimicrobial resistance, and the propensity of resistance to spread between ecological niches in the human, animal, and environmental sectors, we need to be much more cautious. Antimicrobial stewardship programs should be aggressive in setting their targets to reduce antimicrobial use, and not simply focus on those practices that are most obviously linked to resistance selection, such as growth promotion. All mass medication should be aggressively addressed.

Other antimicrobial stewardship barriers to overcome include the lack of controls on the over-the-counter availability of antimicrobials for use in humans and animals in many countries, particularly in the developing world, the lack of data from most countries on the quantities and types of antimicrobials that are used, and the relatively limited uptake of animal treatment guidelines and formularies in most countries (147, 155, 123, 174). To address antimicrobial resistance on a global scale, it is important that all countries have the basic regulatory, infrastructure, oversight, and enforcement capabilities to control antimicrobial availability and use as laid out by international guidelines, such as those from WHO and OIE (147, 155, 123). Related to this is the need for good antimicrobial consumption data from all countries. Antimicrobial consumption is an essential indicator of resistance selection pressure and, when adjusted for population size, allows for comparison between countries, regions, hospitals, veterinary clinics, farms, etc. This can be a powerful tool for improving antimicrobial stewardship, as has been shown in countries that are using it (60, 158). When collected regularly at the level of prescriber or use (e.g., farm), these data can be used to evaluate and improve stewardship and to set benchmarks and reduction targets.

CONCLUSION

History has shown that it is not feasible to neatly separate antimicrobial classes into those exclusively for use in humans or animals, with the exception of new antimicrobial classes. These should probably be reserved for use in humans as long as few or no alternatives are available. The majority of classes, however, will be available for use in both sectors, and the challenge for One Health is to ensure that the use of these drugs is optimal overall. This is likely to be achieved when antimicrobials used in both sectors are used for therapy, only rarely for prophylaxis, and never for growth promotion and when we better control the types and amounts of antimicrobials plus the numbers of resistant bacteria that we allow to be placed into the environment.

Citation. McEwen SA, Collignon PJ. 2017. Antimicrobial resistance: a one health perspective. Microbiol Spectrum 6(2): ARBA-0009-2017.

References

1. World Health Organization (WHO). 2014. *Antimicrobial Resistance: Global Report on Surveillance.* WHO, Geneva, Switzerland.

2. Centers for Disease Control (CDC). 2013. *Antibiotic Resistance Threats in the United States.* Centers for Disease Control and Prevention, Atlanta, GA.

3. Fleming A. 1945. Penicillin. Nobel lecture.

4. O'Neill J. 2016. Tackling drug-resistant infections globally: final report and recommendations. The review on antimicrobial resistance. https://amr-review.org/.

5. Laxminarayan R, Duse A, Wattal C, Zaidi AKM, Wertheim HFL, Sumpradit N, Vlieghe E, Hara GL, Gould IM, Goossens H, Greko C, So AD, Bigdeli M, Tomson G, Woodhouse W, Ombaka E, Peralta AQ, Qamar FN, Mir F, Kariuki S, Bhutta ZA, Coates A, Bergstrom R, Wright GD, Brown ED, Cars O. 2013. Antibiotic resistance: the need for global solutions. *Lancet Infect Dis* 13:1057–1098.

6. World Health Organization (WHO). 2015. *Global Action Plan on Antimicrobial Resistance.* WHO, Geneva, Switzerland.

7. Aarestrup FM, Wegener HC, Collignon P. 2008. Resistance in bacteria of the food chain: epidemiology and control strategies. *Expert Rev Anti Infect Ther* 6:733–750.

8. Holmes AH, Moore LSP, Sundsfjord A, Steinbakk M, Regmi S, Karkey A, Guerin PJ, Piddock LJ. 2016. Understanding the mechanisms and drivers of antimicrobial resistance. *Lancet* 387:176–187.

9. Burow E, Käsbohrer A. 2017. Risk factors for antimicrobial resistance in *Escherichia coli* in pigs receiving oral antimicrobial treatment: a systematic review. *Microb Drug Resist* 23:194–205.

10. Marti E, Variatza E, Balcazar JL. 2014. The role of aquatic ecosystems as reservoirs of antibiotic resistance. *Trends Microbiol* 22:36–41.

11. Huijbers PMC, Blaak H, de Jong MCM, Graat EAM, Vandenbroucke-Grauls CMJE, de Roda Husman AM. 2015. Role of the environment in the transmission of antimicrobial resistance to humans: a review. *Environ Sci Technol* 49:11993–12004.

12. Woolhouse MEJ, Ward MJ. 2013. Sources of antimicrobial resistance. *Science* 341:1460–1461.

13. Heuer OE, Kruse H, Grave K, Collignon P, Karunasagar I, Angulo FJ. 2009. Human health consequences of use of antimicrobial agents in aquaculture. *Clin Infect Dis* 49:1248–1253.

14. O'Neill J. 2015. Antimicrobials in agriculture and the environment: reducing unnecessary use and waste. The review on antimicrobial resistance. https://amr-review.org/. Accessed January 3, 2018.

15. So AD, Shah TA, Roach S, Ling Chee Y, Nachman KE. 2015. An integrated systems approach is needed to ensure the sustainability of antibiotic effectiveness for both humans and animals. *J Law Med Ethics* 43(Suppl 3):38–45.

16. Collignon P. 2013. The importance of a One Health approach to preventing the development and spread of antibiotic resistance, p 19–36. *In* Mackenzie JS, Jeggo M, Daszak P, Richt JA (ed), *One Health: the Human-Animal-Environment Interfaces in Emerging Infectious Diseases.* Springer, Berlin, Germany.

17. Torren-Edo J, Grave K, Mackay D. 2015. "One Health": the regulation and consumption of antimicrobials for animal use in the EU. *IHAJ* 2:14–16.

18. Robinson TP, Bu DP, Carrique-Mas J, Fèvre EM, Gilbert M, Grace D, Hay SI, Jiwakanon J, Kakkar M, Kariuki S, Laxminarayan R, Lubroth J, Magnusson U, Thi Ngoc P, Van Boeckel TP, Woolhouse MEJ. 2016. Antibiotic resistance is the quintessential One Health issue. *Trans R Soc Trop Med Hyg* 110:377–380.

19. Zinsstag J, Meisser A, Schelling E, Bonfoh B, Tanner M. 2012. From 'two medicines' to 'One Health' and beyond. *Onderstepoort J Vet Res* 79:492.

20. One Health Commission. 2018. What is One Health? https://www.onehealthcommission.org/en/why_one_health/what_is_one_health/. Accessed January 3, 2017.

21. Woolhouse MEJ, Gowtage-Sequeria S. 2005. Host range and emerging and reemerging pathogens. *Emerg Infect Dis* 11:1842–1847.

22. Schwabe CW. 1984. *Veterinary Medicine and Human Health*, 3rd ed. Williams & Wilkins, Baltimore, MD.

23. McEwen SA, Fedorka-Cray PJ. 2002. Antimicrobial use and resistance in animals. *Clin Infect Dis* 34(Suppl 3):S93–S106.

24. Van Boeckel TP, Brower C, Gilbert M, Grenfell BT, Levin SA, Robinson TP, Teillant A, Laxminarayan R. 2015. Global trends in antimicrobial use in food animals. *Proc Natl Acad Sci USA* 112:5649–5654.

25. European Medicines Agency, European Surveillance of Veterinary Antimicrobial Consumption. 2016. Sales of veterinary antimicrobial agents in 29 European countries in 2014. (EMA/61769/2016).

26. ECDC (European Centre for Disease Prevention and Control), EFSA (European Food Safety Authority), EMA (European Medicines Agency). 2015. ECDC/EFSA/EMA first joint report on the integrated analysis of the consumption of antimicrobial agents and occurrence of antimicrobial resistance in bacteria from humans and food-producing animals. *EFSA J* 13:4006.

27. Food and Agriculture Organization (FAO). 2016. *Drivers, Dynamics and Epidemiology of Antimicrobial Resistance in Animal Production*. FAO, Rome, Italy. http://www.fao.org/publications/card/en/c/d5f6d40d-ef08-4fcc-866b-5e5a92a12dbf/.

28. Vidaver AK. 2002. Uses of antimicrobials in plant agriculture. *Clin Infect Dis* 34(Suppl 3):S107–S110.

29. Sykes JE. 2013. Antimicrobial drug use in dogs and cats, p 473–494. *In* Giguère S, Prescott JF, Dowling PM (ed), *Antimicrobial Therapy in Veterinary Medicine*, 5th ed. John Wiley & Sons, Hoboken, NJ.

30. Giguère S, Abrams-Ogg ACG, Kruth SA. 2013. Prophylactic use of antimicrobial agents, and antimicrobial chemotherapy for the neutropenic patient, p 357–378. *In* Giguère S, Prescott JF, Dowling PM (ed), *Antimicrobial Therapy in Veterinary Medicine*, 5th ed. John Wiley & Sons, Hoboken, NJ.

31. National Research Council. 1999. *The Use of Drugs in Food Animals: Benefits and Risks*. The National Academies Press, Washington, DC.

32. Health Protection Agency. 2012. Guidance for public health management of meningococcal disease in the UK. Health Protection Agency. Meningococcus and Haemophilus Forum. Updated March 2012. https://www.gov.uk/government/publications/meningococcal-disease-guidance-on-public-health-management. Accessed 20 December 2017.

33. FAO/OIE/WHO. 2003. Joint FAO/OIE/WHO expert workshop on non-human antimicrobial usage and antimicrobial resistance: scientific assessment. FAO/OIE/WHO, Geneva, Switzerland.

34. World Health Organization (WHO). 1997. *The Medical Impact of the Use of Antimicrobials in Food Animals*. WHO, Berlin, Germany.

35. World Health Organization (WHO). 2003. Impacts of antimicrobial growth promoter termination in Denmark. The WHO international review panel's evaluation of the termination of the use of antimicrobial growth promoters in Denmark. WHO, Geneva, Switzerland.

36. Zuraw L. 2014. Perdue announces dramatic reduction in antibiotic use in its chickens. *Food Safety News*. 4 September 2014. http://www.foodsafetynews.com/2014/09/perdue-dramatically-reduces-antibiotic-use-in-chickens/#.VQZbbtKUd8E.

37. World Health Organization (WHO). 2017. *WHO Guidelines on Use of Medically Important Antimicrobials in Food-Producing Animals*. WHO, Geneva, Switzerland.

38. European Union (EU). 2015. Guidelines for the prudent use of antimicrobials in veterinary medicine (2015/C 299/04). *Official Journal of the European Union* 11.9.2015. C 299/7-26.

39. Health Canada. 2014. Notice to stakeholders: collaborative efforts to promote the judicious use of medically-important antimicrobial drugs in food animal production. http://www.hc-sc.gc.ca/dhp-mps/vet/antimicrob/amr-notice-ram-avis-20140410-eng.php. Accessed 3 January 2017.

40. Food and Drug Administration (FDA). 2013. New animal drugs and new animal drug combination products administered in or on medicated feed or drinking water of food-producing animals: recommendations for drug sponsors for voluntarily aligning product use conditions with GFI #209. U.S. Department of Health and Human Services, Washington, DC.

41. World Organisation for Animal Health (OIE). 2018. OIE annual report on the use of antimicrobial agents in animals. Second report. http://www.oie.int/fileadmin/Home/eng/Our_scientific_expertise/docs/pdf/AMR/Annual_Report_AMR_2.pdf.

42. WHO Advisory Group on Integrated Surveillance of Antimicrobial Resistance (AGISAR). 2016. *Critically Important Antimicrobials for Human Medicine*, 4th revision. WHO, Geneva, Switzerland.

43. European Medicines Agency (EMA). 2009. Revised reflection paper on the use of 3rd and 4th generation cephalosporins in food producing animals in the European Union: development of resistance and impact on human and animal health. EMA, London, United Kingdom. EMEA/CVMP/SAGAM/81730/2006-Rev.1.

44. Prescott JF. 2013. Beta-lactam antibiotics, p 153–173. *In* Giguère S, Prescott JF, Dowling PM (ed), *Antimicrobial Therapy in Veterinary Medicine*, 5th ed. John Wiley & Sons, Hoboken, NJ.

45. Food and Drug Administration (FDA). 2016. Summary report on antimicrobials sold or distributed for use in food-producing animals. FDA, Department of Health and Human Services. Washington, DC. http://www.fda.gov/downloads/ForIndustry/UserFees/AnimalDrugUserFeeActADUFA/UCM534243.pdf.

46. Food and Drug Administration (FDA). 2012. Drug use review. FDA, Department of Health and Human Services. Washington, DC. http://www.fda.gov/downloads/Drugs/DrugSafety/InformationbyDrugClass/UCM319435.pdf.

47. de Kraker MEA, Wolkewitz M, Davey PG, Koller W, Berger J, Nagler J, Icket C, Kalenic S, Horvatic J, Seifert H, Kaasch A, Paniara O, Argyropoulou A, Bompola M, Smyth E, Skally M, Raglio A, Dumpis U, Melbarde Kelmere A, Borg M, Xuereb D, Ghita MC, Noble M, Kolman J, Grabljevec S, Turner D, Lansbury L, Grundmann H. 2011. Burden of antimicrobial resistance in European hospitals: excess mortality and length of hospital stay associated with bloodstream infections due to *Escherichia coli* resistant to third-generation cephalosporins. *J Antimicrob Chemother* 66:398–407.

48. Park SH. 2014. Third-generation cephalosporin resistance in Gram-negative bacteria in the community: a growing public health concern. *Korean J Intern Med* 29:27–30.

49. Kanwar N, Scott HM, Norby B, Loneragan GH, Vinasco J, McGowan M, Cottell JL, Chengappa MM, Bai J, Boerlin P. 2013. Effects of ceftiofur and chlortetracycline treatment strategies on antimicrobial susceptibility and on *tet*(A), *tet*(B), and *bla* CMY-2 resistance genes among *E. coli* isolated from the feces of feedlot cattle. *PLoS One* 8:e80575.

50. de Been M, Lanza VF, de Toro M, Scharringa J, Dohmen W, Du Y, Hu J, Lei Y, Li N, Tooming-Klunderud A, Heederik DJJ, Fluit AC, Bonten MJM, Willems RJL, de la Cruz F, van Schaik W. 2014. Dissemination of cephalosporin resistance genes between *Escherichia coli* strains from farm animals and humans by specific plasmid lineages. *PLoS Genet* 10:e1004776.

51. Hammerum AM, Larsen J, Andersen VD, Lester CH, Skovgaard Skytte TS, Hansen F, Olsen SS, Mordhorst H, Skov RL, Aarcstrup FM, Agcrsø Y. 2014. Characterization of extended-spectrum β-lactamase (ESBL)-producing *Escherichia coli* obtained from Danish pigs, pig farmers and their families from farms with high or no consumption of third- or fourth-generation cephalosporins. *J Antimicrob Chemother* 69:2650–2657.

52. Willemsen I, Oome S, Verhulst C, Pettersson A, Verduin K, Kluytmans J. 2015. Trends in extended spectrum beta-lactamase (ESBL) producing *Enterobacteriaceae* and ESBL genes in a Dutch teaching hospital, measured in 5 yearly point prevalence surveys (2010–2014). *PLoS One* 10:e0141765.

53. Lazarus B, Paterson DL, Mollinger JL, Rogers BA. 2015. Do human extraintestinal *Escherichia coli* infections resistant to expanded-spectrum cephalosporins originate from food-producing animals? A systematic review. *Clin Infect Dis* 60:439–452.

54. Johnson JR, Sannes MR, Croy C, Johnston B, Clabots C, Kuskowski MA, Bender J, Smith KE, Winokur PL, Belongia EA. 2007. Antimicrobial drug-resistant *Escherichia coli* from humans and poultry products, Minnesota and Wisconsin, 2002–2004. *Emerg Infect Dis* 13:838–846.

55. Jakobsen L, Kurbasic A, Skjøt-Rasmussen L, Ejrnaes K, Porsbo LJ, Pedersen K, Jensen LB, Emborg H-D, Agersø Y, Olsen KEP, Aarestrup FM, Frimodt-Møller N, Hammerum AM. 2010. *Escherichia coli* isolates from broiler chicken meat, broiler chickens, pork, and pigs share phylogroups and antimicrobial resistance with community-dwelling humans and patients with urinary tract infection. *Foodborne Pathog Dis* 7:537–547.

56. Canadian Integrated Program for Antimicrobial Resistance (CIPARS). 2009. Update: *Salmonella* Heidelberg ceftiofur-related resistance in human and retail chicken isolates—2006 to 2008. Public Health Agency of Canada. http://www.phac-aspc.gc.ca/cipars-picra/heidelberg/heidelberg_090326-eng.php.

57. Dutil L, Irwin R, Finley R, Ng LK, Avery B, Boerlin P, Bourgault AM, Cole L, Daignault D, Desruisseau A, Demczuk W, Hoang L, Horsman GB, Ismail J, Jamieson F, Maki A, Pacagnella A, Pillai DR. 2010. Ceftiofur resistance in *Salmonella enterica* serovar Heidelberg from chicken meat and humans, Canada. *Emerg Infect Dis* 16:48–54.

58. Smith KE, Medus C, Meyer SD, Boxrud DJ, Leano F, Hedberg CW, Elfering K, Braymen C, Bender JB, Danila RN. 2008. Outbreaks of salmonellosis in Minnesota (1998 through 2006) associated with frozen, microwaveable, breaded, stuffed chicken products. *J Food Prot* 71:2153–2160.

59. Hiki M, Kawanishi M, Abo H, Kojima A, Koike R, Hamamoto S, Asai T. 2015. Decreased resistance to broad-spectrum cephalosporin in *Escherichia coli* from healthy broilers at farms in Japan after voluntary withdrawal of ceftiofur. *Foodborne Pathog Dis* 12:639–643.

60. DANMAP. 2014. 2015. *Use of Antimicrobial Agents and Occurrence of Antimicrobial Resistance in Bacteria from Food Animals, Food and Humans in Denmark*. DANMAP, Denmark.

61. Food and Drug Administration. New animal drugs; cephalosporin drugs; extralabel animal drug use; order of prohibition. *Fed Reg* 77:735–745.

62. European Medicines Agency (EMA). 2014. Answers to the requests for scientific advice on the impact on public health and animal health of the use of antibiotics in animals. http://www.ema.europa.eu/docs/en_GB/document_library/Other/2014/07/WC500170253.pdf.

63. Endtz HP, Ruijs GJ, van Klingeren B, Jansen WH, van der Reyden T, Mouton RP. 1991. Quinolone resistance in *Campylobacter* isolated from man and poultry following the introduction of fluoroquinolones in veterinary medicine. *J Antimicrob Chemother* 27:199–208.

64. McDermott PF, Bodeis SM, English LL, White DG, Walker RD, Zhao S, Simjee S, Wagner DD. 2002.

Ciprofloxacin resistance in *Campylobacter jejuni* evolves rapidly in chickens treated with fluoroquinolones. *J Infect Dis* 185:837–840.

65. Nelson JM, Chiller TM, Powers JH, Angulo FJ. 2007. Fluoroquinolone-resistant *Campylobacter* species and the withdrawal of fluoroquinolones from use in poultry: a public health success story. *Clin Infect Dis* 44:977–980.

66. Cheng AC, Turnidge J, Collignon P, Looke D, Barton M, Gottlieb T. 2012. Control of fluoroquinolone resistance through successful regulation, Australia. *Emerg Infect Dis* 18:1453–1460.

67. European Medicines Agency (EMA). 2016. Updated advice on the use of colistin products in animals within the European Union: development of resistance and possible impact on human and animal health. EMA, London, United Kingdom.

68. Falagas ME, Kasiakou SK. 2006. Toxicity of polymyxins: a systematic review of the evidence from old and recent studies. *Crit Care* 10:R27.

69. Falagas ME, Kasiakou SK, Saravolatz LD. 2005. Colistin: the revival of polymyxins for the management of multidrug-resistant Gram-negative bacterial infections. *Clin Infect Dis* 40:1333–1341.

70. Linden PK, Kusne S, Coley K, Fontes P, Kramer DJ, Paterson D. 2003. Use of parenteral colistin for the treatment of serious infection due to antimicrobial-resistant *Pseudomonas aeruginosa*. *Clin Infect Dis* 37:e154–e160.

71. Fernandes MR, Moura Q, Sartori L, Silva KC, Cunha MPV, Esposito F, Lopes R, Otutumi LK, Gonçalves DD, Dropa M, Matté MH, Monte DFM, Landgraf M, Francisco GR, Bueno MFC, de Oliveira Garcia D, Knöbl T, Moreno AM, Lincopan N. 2016. Silent dissemination of colistin-resistant *Escherichia coli* in South America could contribute to the global spread of the *mcr-1* gene. *Euro Surveill* 21:30214. http://www.eurosurveillance.org/content/10.2807/1560-7917.ES.2016.21.17.30214.

72. Liu Y-Y, Wang Y, Walsh TR, Yi L-X, Zhang R, Spencer J, Doi Y, Tian G, Dong B, Huang X, Yu L-F, Gu D, Ren H, Chen X, Lv L, He D, Zhou H, Liang Z, Liu J-H, Shen J. 2016. Emergence of plasmid-mediated colistin resistance mechanism MCR-1 in animals and human beings inChina: a microbiological and molecular biological study. *Lancet Infect Dis* 16:161–168.

73. European Center for Disease Prevention and Control (ECDC). 2015. Summary of the latest data on antibiotic consumption in the European Union. https://ecdc.europa.eu/en/publications-data/summary-latest-data-antibiotic-consumption-eu-2015.

74. Landman D, Georgescu C, Martin DA, Quale J. 2008. Polymyxins revisited. *Clin Microbiol Rev* 21:449–465.

75. European Food Safety Authority (EFSA), European Centre for Disease Prevention and Control (ECDC). 2016. The European Union summary report on antimicrobial resistance in zoonotic and indicator bacteria from humans, animals and food in 2014. *EFSA J* 14:4380.

76. Catry B, Cavaleri M, Baptiste K, Grave K, Grein K, Holm A, Jukes H, Liebana E, Lopez Navas A, Mackay D, Magiorakos A-P, Moreno Romo MA, Moulin G, Muñoz Madero C, Matias Ferreira Pomba MC, Powell M, Pyörälä S, Rantala M, Ružauskas M, Sanders P, Teale C, Threlfall EJ, Törneke K, van Duijkeren E, Torren Edo J. 2015. Use of colistin-containing products within the European Union and European Economic Area (EU/EEA): development of resistance in animals and possible impact on human and animal health. *Int J Antimicrob Agents* 46:297–306.

77. Prim N, Rivera A, Rodríguez-Navarro J, Español M, Turbau M, Coll P, Mirelis B. 2016. Detection of mcr-1 colistin resistance gene in polyclonal *Escherichia coli* isolates in Barcelona, Spain, 2012 to 2015. *Euro Surveill* 21:30183. http://www.eurosurveillance.org/content/10.2807/1560-7917.ES.2016.21.13.30183.

78. Irrgang A, Roschanski N, Tenhagen B-A, Grobbel M, Skladnikiewicz-Ziemer T, Thomas K, Roesler U, Käsbohrer A. 2016. Prevalence of *mcr-1* in *E. coli* from livestock and food in Germany, 2010–2015. *PLoS One* 11:e0159863.

79. Hasman H, Hammerum AM, Hansen F, Hendriksen RS, Olesen B, Agersø Y, Zankari E, Leekitcharoenphon P, Stegger M, Kaas RS, Cavaco LM, Hansen DS, Aarestrup FM, Skov RL. 2015. Detection of *mcr-1* encoding plasmid-mediated colistin-resistant *Escherichia coli* isolates from human bloodstream infection and imported chicken meat, Denmark 2015. *Euro Surveill* 20:30085. http://www.eurosurveillance.org/content/10.2807/1560-7917.ES.2015.20.49.30085.

80. von Wintersdorff CJH, Wolffs PFG, van Niekerk JM, Beuken E, van Alphen LB, Stobberingh EE, Oude Lashof AML, Hoebe CJPA, Savelkoul PHM, Penders J. 2016. Detection of the plasmid-mediated colistin-resistance gene *mcr-1* in faecal metagenomes of Dutch travellers. *J Antimicrob Chemother* 71:3416–3419.

81. Shen Z, Wang Y, Shen Y, Shen J, Wu C. 2016. Early emergence of *mcr-1* in *Escherichia coli* from food-producing animals. *Lancet Infect Dis* 16:293.

82. Doumith M, Godbole G, Ashton P, Larkin L, Dallman T, Day M, Day M, Muller-Pebody B, Ellington MJ, de Pinna E, Johnson AP, Hopkins KL, Woodford N. 2016. Detection of the plasmid-mediated *mcr-1* gene conferring colistin resistance in human and food isolates of *Salmonella enterica* and *Escherichia coli* in England and Wales. *J Antimicrob Chemother* 71:2300–2305.

83. Zurfuh K, Poirel L, Nordmann P, Nüesch-Inderbinen M, Hächler H, Stephan R. 2016. Occurrence of the plasmid-borne *mcr-1* colistin resistance gene in extended-spectrum-β-lactamase-producing *Enterobacteriaceae* in river water and imported vegetable samples in Switzerland. *Antimicrob Agents Chemother* 60:2594–2595.

84. Xavier BB, Lammens C, Ruhal R, Kumar-Singh S, Butaye P, Goossens H, Malhotra-Kumar S. 2016. Identification of a novel plasmid-mediated colistin-resistance gene, *mcr-2*, in *Escherichia coli*, Belgium, June 2016. *Eurosurveillance* 21(27). http://www.eurosurveillance.org/content/10.2807/1560-7917.ES.2016.21.27.30280.

85. Borowiak M, Fischer J, Hammerl JA, Hendriksen RS, Szabo I, Malorny B. 2017. Identification of a novel transposon-associated phosphoethanolamine transferase

gene, *mcr-5*, conferring colistin resistance in d-tartrate fermenting *Salmonella enterica* subsp. *enterica* serovar Paratyphi B. *J Antimicrob Chemother* **72:**3317–3324.

86. **Levine DP.** 2006. Vancomycin: a history. *Clin Infect Dis* **42**(Suppl 1):S5–S12.

87. **Bager F, Madsen M, Christensen J, Aarestrup FM.** 1997. Avoparcin used as a growth promoter is associated with the occurrence of vancomycin-resistant *Enterococcus faecium* on Danish poultry and pig farms. *Prev Vet Med* **31:**95–112.

88. **Prescott JF.** 2017. History and current use of antimicrobial drugs in veterinary medicine. *Microbiol Spectr* **5**(6).

89. **National Academy of Sciences – National Research Council (NAS-NRC).** 1956. *Proceedings, First International Conference on the Use of Antibiotics in Agriculture.* National Academies Press, Washington, DC.

90. *Food and Drug Administration (FDA).* Guidance for Industry no. 209. 2012. The judicious use of medically important antimicrobial drugs in food-producing animals. FDA, Washington, DC.

91. **Food and Drug Administration (FDA).** 2016. Guidance for Industry no. 3. General principles for evaluating the human food safety of new animal drugs used in food-producing animals. FDA Center for Veterinary Medicine, Washington, DC. http://www.fda.gov/downloads/AnimalVeterinary/GuidanceComplianceEnforcement/GuidanceforIndustry/ucm052180.pdf. Accessed 3 January 2017.

92. **Codex Alimentarius.** 2011. Guidelines for risk analysis of foodborne antimicrobial resistance. Codex Alimentarius. CAC/GL 77- 2011.

93. **Food and Drug Administration (FDA).** 2003. Guidance for Industry no. 152. Evaluating the safety of antimicrobial new animal drugs with regard to their microbiological effects on bacteria of human health concern. FDA, Washington, DC. http://www.fda.gov/AnimalVeterinary/GuidanceComplianceEnforcement/GuidanceforIndustry/ucm123614.htm. Accessed 3 January 2017.

94. **Swann MM.** 1969. *The Use of Antibiotics in Animal Husbandry and Veterinary Medicine.* Her Majesty's Stationery Office, London, United Kingdom.

95. **Kirchhelle C.** 2016. Toxic confusion: the dilemma of antibiotic regulation in West German food production (1951–1990). *Endeavour* **40:**114–127.

96. **Harrison P, Lederberg J** (eds). 1998. "Antimicrobial Resistance: Issues and Options." Workshop Report, Forum on Emerging Infections, Division of Health and Sciences Policy, Institute of Medicine. National Academy Press: Washington, D.C.

97. **National Academy of Sciences (NAS).** 1980. *The Effects on Human Health of Subtherapeutic Use of Antimicrobials in Animal Feeds.* National Academy Press, Washington, DC.

98. **O'Brien B.** 1996. Animal welfare reform and the magic bullet: the use and abuse of subtherapeutic doses of antibiotics in livestock. *Univ Colo Law Rev* **67:**407.

99. **National Academy of Sciences (NAS).** 1969. *The Use of Drugs in Animal Feeds: Proceedings of a Symposium.* National Academy Press, Washington, DC.

100. **U.S. Congress Office of Technology Assessment.** 1995. Impacts of antibiotic-resistant bacteria, OTA-H-629. U.S. Government Printing Office, Washington, DC.

101. **Institute of Medicine.** 1989. *Human Health Risks with the Subtherapeutic Use of Penicillin or Tetracyclines in Animal Feed.* National Academy Press, Washington, DC.

102. **World Health Organization (WHO).** 1998. *Use of Quinolones in Food Animals and Potential Impact on Human Health.* WHO, Geneva, Switzerland.

103. **Joint Expert Advisory Committee on Antibiotic Resistance (JETACAR).** 1999. The use of antibiotic in food producing animals: antibiotic-resistant bacteria in animals and humans. Commonwealth of Australia.

104. **European Medicines Agency (EMA).** 2012. Referral procedure on veterinary medicinal products containing 3rd and 4th generation cephalosporins under Article 35 of Directive 2001/82/EC, as amended. EMA/253066/2012.

105. **Barza M.** 2002. Potential mechanisms of increased disease in humans from antimicrobial resistance in food animals. *Clin Infect Dis* **34**(Suppl 3):S123–S125.

106. **Wales AD, Davies RH.** 2015. Co-selection of resistance to antibiotics, biocides and heavy metals, and its relevance to foodborne pathogens. *Antibiotics (Basel)* **4:** 567–604.

107. **Anderson ES.** 1968. Drug resistance in *Salmonella typhimurium* and its implications. *BMJ* **3:**333–339.

108. **Hanning IB, Nutt JD, Ricke SC.** 2009. Salmonellosis outbreaks in the United States due to fresh produce: sources and potential intervention measures. *Foodborne Pathog Dis* **6:**635–648.

109. **Chiu CH, Wu TL, Su LH, Chu C, Chia JH, Kuo AJ, Chien MS, Lin TY.** 2002. The emergence in Taiwan of fluoroquinolone resistance in *Salmonella enterica* serotype Choleraesuis. *N Engl J Med* **346:**413–419.

110. **European Medicines Agency (EMA).** 2006. Reflection paper on the use of fluoroquinolones in food-producing animals in the European Union: development of resistance and impact on human and animal health. EMA, London, United Kingdom. EMEA/CVMP/SAGAM/184651/2005.

111. **Helms M, Simonsen J, Mølbak K.** 2004. Quinolone resistance is associated with increased risk of invasive illness or death during infection with *Salmonella* serotype Typhimurium. *J Infect Dis* **190:**1652–1654.

112. **Mollenkopf DF, Stull JW, Mathys DA, Bowman AS, Feicht SM, Grooters SV, Daniels JB, Wittum TE.** 2017. Carbapenemase-producing *Enterobacteriaceae* recovered from the environment of a swine farrow-to-finish operation in the United States. *Antimicrob Agents Chemother* **61:**e02348-16.

113. **Helms M, Simonsen J, Olsen KEP, Mølbak K.** 2005. Adverse health events associated with antimicrobial drug resistance in *Campylobacter* species: a registry-based cohort study. *J Infect Dis* **191:**1050–1055.

114. **Kennedy K, Collignon P.** 2010. Colonisation with *Escherichia coli* resistant to "critically important" antibiotics: a high risk for international travellers. *Eur J Clin Microbiol Infect Dis* **29:**1501–1506.

115. Laupland KB, Church DL. 2014. Population-based epidemiology and microbiology of community-onset bloodstream infections. *Clin Microbiol Rev* 27:647–664.

116. Bou-Antoun S, Davies J, Guy R, Johnson AP, Sheridan EA, Hope RJ. 2016. Descriptive epidemiology of *Escherichia coli* bacteraemia in England, April 2012 to March 2014. *Euro Surveill* 21:30329. http://www.eurosurveillance.org/content/10.2807/1560-7917.ES.2016.21.35.30329.

117. Mellata M. 2013. Human and avian extraintestinal pathogenic *Escherichia coli*: infections, zoonotic risks, and antibiotic resistance trends. *Foodborne Pathog Dis* 10:916–932.

118. Collignon P. 2015. Antibiotic resistance: are we all doomed? *Intern Med J* 45:1109–1115.

119. Walsh TR, Weeks J, Livermore DM, Toleman MA. 2011. Dissemination of NDM-1 positive bacteria in the New Delhi environment and its implications for human health: an environmental point prevalence study. *Lancet Infect Dis* 11:355–362.

120. Graham DW, Collignon P, Davies J, Larsson DG, Snape J. 2014. Underappreciated role of regionally poor water quality on globally increasing antibiotic resistance. *Environ Sci Technol* 48:11746–11747.

121. Tängdén T, Cars O, Melhus A, Löwdin E. 2010. Foreign travel is a major risk factor for colonization with *Escherichia coli* producing CTX-M-type extended-spectrum beta-lactamases: a prospective study with Swedish volunteers. *Antimicrob Agents Chemother* 54:3564–3568.

122. Vieira AR, Collignon P, Aarestrup FM, McEwen SA, Hendriksen RS, Hald T, Wegener HC. 2011. Association between antimicrobial resistance in *Escherichia coli* isolates from food animals and blood stream isolates from humans in Europe: an ecological study. *Foodborne Pathog Dis* 8:1295–1301.

123. World Health Organization (WHO). 2017. *Integrated Surveillance of Antimicrobial Resistance in Foodborne Bacteria. Application of a One Health Approach.* WHO, Geneva, Switzerland. http://www.who.int/foodsafety/publications/agisar_guidance2017/en/.

124. ECDC (European Centre for Disease Prevention and Control), EFSA (European Food Safety Authority) and EMA (European Medicines Agency). 2009. Joint scientific report of ECDC, EFSA and EMEA on meticillin resistant *Staphylococcus aureus* (MRSA) in livestock, companion animals and foods. EFSA-Q-2009-00612 (EFSA Scientific Report (2009) 301, 1–10) and EMEA/CVMP/SAGAM/62464/2009.

125. European Centre for Disease Prevention and Control (ECDC). 2015. *Antimicrobial Resistance Surveillance in Europe 2014. Annual Report of the European Antimicrobial Resistance Surveillance Network.* EARS-Net, Stockholm, Sweden.

126. Tong SY, Davis JS, Eichenberger E, Holland TL, Fowler VG Jr. 2015. *Staphylococcus aureus* infections: epidemiology, pathophysiology, clinical manifestations, and management. *Clin Microbiol Rev* 28:603–661.

127. Wang JL, Chen SY, Wang JT, Wu GH, Chiang WC, Hsueh PR, Chen YC, Chang SC. 2008. Comparison of both clinical features and mortality risk associated with bacteremia due to community-acquired methicillin-resistant *Staphylococcus aureus* and methicillin-susceptible *S. aureus*. *Clin Infect Dis* 46:799–806.

128. Price LB, Stegger M, Hasman H, Aziz M, Larsen J, Andersen PS, Pearson T, Waters AE, Foster JT, Schupp J, Gillece J, Driebe E, Liu CM, Springer B, Zdovc I, Battisti A, Franco A, Żmudzki J, Schwarz S, Butaye P, Jouy E, Pomba C, Porrero MC, Ruimy R, Smith TC, Robinson DA, Weese JS, Arriola CS, Yu F, Laurent F, Keim P, Skov R, Aarestrup FM. 2012. *Staphylococcus aureus* CC398: host adaptation and emergence of methicillin resistance in livestock. *MBio* 3:e00305-11.

129. Weese JS, van Duijkeren E. 2010. Methicillin-resistant *Staphylococcus aureus* and *Staphylococcus pseudintermedius* in veterinary medicine. *Vet Microbiol* 140:418–429.

130. Boost MV, O'Donoghue MM, Siu KHG. 2007. Characterisation of methicillin-resistant *Staphylococcus aureus* isolates from dogs and their owners. *Clin Microbiol Infect* 13:731–733.

131. Lewis HC, Mølbak K, Reese C, Aarestrup FM, Selchau M, Sørum M, Skov RL. 2008. Pigs as source of methicillin-resistant *Staphylococcus aureus* CC398 infections in humans, Denmark. *Emerg Infect Dis* 14:1383–1389.

132. Voss A, Loeffen F, Bakker J, Klaassen C, Wulf M. 2005. Methicillin-resistant *Staphylococcus aureus* in pig farming. *Emerg Infect Dis* 11:1965–1966.

133. Dorado-García A, Dohmen W, Bos ME, Verstappen KM, Houben M, Wagenaar JA, Heederik DJ. 2015. Dose-response relationship between antimicrobial drugs and livestock-associated MRSA in pig farming. *Emerg Infect Dis* 21:950–959.

134. Finley RL, Collignon P, Larsson DGJ, McEwen SA, Li X-Z, Gaze WH, Reid-Smith R, Timinouni M, Graham DW, Topp E. 2013. The scourge of antibiotic resistance: the important role of the environment. *Clin Infect Dis* 57:704–710.

135. Gaze WH, Krone SM, Larsson DG, Li XZ, Robinson JA, Simonet P, Smalla K, Timinouni M, Topp E, Wellington EM, Wright GD, Zhu YG. 2013. Influence of humans on evolution and mobilization of environmental antibiotic resistome. *Emerg Infect Dis* 19:e120871.

136. Perry JA, Wright GD. 2014. Forces shaping the antibiotic resistome. *BioEssays* 36:1179–1184.

137. Ruuskanen M, Muurinen J, Meierjohan A, Pärnänen K, Tamminen M, Lyra C, Kronberg L, Virta M. 2016. Fertilizing with animal manure disseminates antibiotic resistance genes to the farm environment. *J Environ Qual* 45:488–493.

138. Wellington EMH, Boxall AB, Cross P, Feil EJ, Gaze WH, Hawkey PM, Johnson-Rollings AS, Jones DL, Lee NM, Otten W, Thomas CM, Williams AP. 2013. The role of the natural environment in the emergence of antibiotic resistance in Gram-negative bacteria. *Lancet Infect Dis* 13:155–165.

139. Aubertheau E, Stalder T, Mondamert L, Ploy M-C, Dagot C, Labanowski J. 2017. Impact of wastewater treatment plant discharge on the contamination of river

biofilms by pharmaceuticals and antibiotic resistance. *Sci Total Environ* **579:**1387–1398.

140. **Singer AC, Shaw H, Rhodes V, Hart A.** 2016. Review of antimicrobial resistance in the environment and its relevance to environmental regulators. *Front Microbiol* **7:**1728.

141. **Rizzo L, Manaia C, Merlin C, Schwartz T, Dagot C, Ploy MC, Michael I, Fatta-Kassinos D.** 2013. Urban wastewater treatment plants as hotspots for antibiotic resistant bacteria and genes spread into the environment: a review. *Sci Total Environ* **447:**345–360.

142. **Zhang QQ, Ying GG, Pan CG, Liu YS, Zhao JL.** 2015. Comprehensive evaluation of antibiotics emission and fate in the river basins of China: source analysis, multimedia modeling, and linkage to bacterial resistance. *Environ Sci Technol* **49:**6772–6782.

143. **Cabello FC, Godfrey HP, Buschmann AH, Dölz HJ.** 2016. Aquaculture as yet another environmental gateway to the development and globalisation of antimicrobial resistance. *Lancet Infect Dis* **16:**e127–e133.

144. **Rahube TO, Marti R, Scott A, Tien Y-C, Murray R, Sabourin L, Duenk P, Lapen DR, Topp E.** 2016. Persistence of antibiotic resistance and plasmid-associated genes in soil following application of sewage sludge and abundance on vegetables at harvest. *Can J Microbiol* **62:**600–607.

145. **Collignon P, Kennedy KJ.** 2015. Long-term persistence of multidrug-resistant *Enterobacteriaceae* after travel. *Clin Infect Dis* **61:**1766–1767.

146. **Ashbolt NJ, Amézquita A, Backhaus T, Borriello P, Brandt KK, Collignon P, Coors A, Finley R, Gaze WH, Heberer T, Lawrence JR, Larsson DGJ, McEwen SA, Ryan JJ, Schönfeld J, Silley P, Snape JR, Van den Eede C, Topp E.** 2013. Human Health Risk Assessment (HHRA) for environmental development and transfer of antibiotic resistance. *Environ Health Perspect* **121:**993–1001.

147. **World Organisation for Animal Health (OIE).** 2016. *The OIE Strategy on Antimicrobial Resistance and the Prudent Use of Antimicrobials.* Paris, France.

148. **Department of Health and Department for Environment Food & Rural Affairs.** 2013. *UK Five Year Antimicrobial Resistance Strategy 2013 to 2018.* Department of Health. London, United Kingdom.

149. **Public Health Agency of Canada.** 2015. Federal action plan on antimicrobial resistance and use in Canada. http://healthycanadians.gc.ca/alt/pdf/publications/drugs-products-medicaments-produits/antibiotic-resistance-a-ntibiotique/action-plan-daction-eng.pdf.

150. **Commonwealth of Australia.** 2016. Responding to the threat of antimicrobial resistance. Australia's First National Antimicrobial Resistance Strategy 2015–2019. https://www.health.gov.au/internet/main/publishing.nsf/Content/1803C433C71415CACA257C8400121B1F/$-File/amr-strategy-2015-2019.pdf

151. **European Commission, Directorate-General for Health and Consumers.** 2011. *Communication from the Commission to the European Parliament and the Council. Action plan against the rising threats from Antimicrobial Resistance.* COM (2011) 748, November 2011.

152. **The White House.** 2015. National action plan for combating antibiotic-resistant bacteria. The White House, Washington, DC.

153. **Food and Agriculture Organization (FAO).** 2016. *The FAO Action Plan on Antimicrobial Resistance 2016–2020.* Food and Agriculture Organization of the United Nations, Rome, Italy.

154. **FAO/OIE/WHO.** 2004. Second Joint FAO/OIE/WHO expert workshop on non-human antimicrobial usage and antimicrobial resistance: management options, Oslo, Norway. WHO, Geneva, Switzerland.

155. **World Health Organization (WHO).** 2000. Global principles for the containment of antimicrobial resistance in animals for food. Report of a WHO consultation with the participation of the Food and Agriculture Organization of the United Nations and the Office International des Epizooties. WHO, Geneva, Switzerland.

156. **Collignon P, Voss A.** 2015. China: what antibiotics and what volumes are used in food production animals? *Antimicrob Resist Infect Control* **4:**16.

157. **Dorado-García A, Mevius DJ, Jacobs JJH, Van Geijlswijk IM, Mouton JW, Wagenaar JA, Heederik DJ.** 2016. Quantitative assessment of antimicrobial resistance in livestock during the course of a nationwide antimicrobial use reduction in the Netherlands. *J Antimicrob Chemother* **71:**3607–3619.

158. **Speksnijder DC, Mevius DJ, Bruschke CJM, Wagenaar JA.** 2015. Reduction of veterinary antimicrobial use in the Netherlands. The Dutch success model. *Zoonoses Public Health* **62**(Suppl 1):79–87.

159. **Murphy CP, Reid-Smith RJ, Weese JS, McEwen SA.** 2010. Evaluation of specific infection control practices used by companion animal veterinarians in community veterinary practices in southern Ontario. *Zoonoses Public Health* **57:**429–438.

160. **Weese JS, Page SW, Prescott JF.** 2013. Antimicrobial stewardship in animals, p 117–132. *In* Giguère S, Prescott JF, Dowling PM (ed), *Antimicrobial Therapy in Veterinary Medicine*, 5th ed. John Wiley & Sons, Hoboken, NJ.

161. **Collignon PC, Conly JM, Andremont A, McEwen SA, Aidara-Kane A, Agerso Y, Andremont A, Collignon P, Conly J, Dang Ninh T, Donado-Godoy P, Fedorka-Cray P, Fernandez H, Galas M, Irwin R, Karp B, Matar G, McDermott P, McEwen S, Mitema E, Reid-Smith R, Scott HM, Singh R, DeWaal CS, Stelling J, Toleman M, Watanabe H, Woo GJ, World Health Organization Advisory Group, Bogotá Meeting on Integrated Surveillance of Antimicrobial Resistance (WHO-AGISAR).** 2016. World Health Organization ranking of antimicrobials according to their importance in human medicine: a critical step for developing risk management strategies to control antimicrobial resistance from food animal production. *Clin Infect Dis* **63:**1087–1093.

162. **World Organisation for Animal Health (OIE).** 2015. *OIE list of antimicrobial agents of veterinary importance.* OIE, Paris, France.

163. **FAO/OIE/WHO.** 2007. *Joint FAO/OIE /WHO Expert Meeting on Critically Important Antimicrobials.* FAO, Rome, Italy.

164. **McDonald's Corporation.** McDonald's global vision for antimicrobial stewardship in food animals. 2017. http://corporate.mcdonalds.com/content/mcd/sustainability/sourcing/animal-health-and-welfare/issues-we-re-focusing--on/vision-for-antimicrobial-stewardship-for-food-animals.html. Accessed 3 January 2018.

165. **Tysons Foods.** Antibiotic use. https://www.tysonfoods.com/news/viewpoints/antibiotic-use. Accessed 3 January 2018.

166. **WHO Advisory Group on Integrated Surveillance of Antimicrobial Resistance.** 2015. *Report of the 6th Meeting of the WHO Advisory Group on Integrated Surveillance of Antimicrobial Resistance with AGISAR 5-Year Strategic Framework to Support Implementation of the Global Action Plan on Antimicrobial Resistance (2015–2019), Seoul.* WHO, Geneva, Switzerland.

167. **World Organisation for Animal Health (OIE).** 2016. Terrestrial animal health code, 25th ed. http://www.oie.int/en/international-standard-setting/terrestrial-code/access-online/. Accessed 3 January 2017.

168. **World Organisation for Animal Health (OIE).** 2016. Aquatic animal health code, 19th ed, 2016. http://www.oie.int/en/international-standard-setting/aquatic-code/access-online/. Accessed 3 January 2017.

169. **FAO/OIE/WHO.** 2006. *Antimicrobial Use in Aquaculture and Antimicrobial Resistance. Report of a Joint FAO/OIE/WHO Expert Consultation on Antimicrobial Use in Aquaculture and Antimicrobial Resistance, Seoul.* WHO, Geneva, Switzerland.

170. **Codex Alimentarius Commission.** 2009. Report of the 3rd session of the Codex ad hoc intergovernmental task force on antimicrobial resistance, Jeju, Republic of Korea. http://www.who.int/foodsafety/publications/thirdsession-codex/en/.

171. **ECDC (European Centre for Disease Prevention and Control), EFSA (European Food Safety Authority), EMA (European Medicines Agency).** 2017. ECDC/EFSA/EMA second joint report on the integrated analysis of the consumption of antimicrobial agents and occurrence of antimicrobial resistance in bacteria from humans and food-producing animals – Joint Interagency Antimicrobial Consumption and Resistance Analysis (JIACRA) Report. *EFSA J* 15:4872.

172. **European Medicines Agency (EMA).** 2015. *CVMP strategy on antimicrobials 2016–2020. EMA/CVMP/209189/2015. Draft.* http://www.ema.europa.eu/docs/en_GB/document_library/Scientific_guideline/2015/11/WC500196645.pdf.

173. **European Medicines Agency (EMA).** 2015. Guideline on the assessment of the risk to public health from antimicrobial resistance due to the use of an antimicrobial veterinary medicinal product in food-producing animals. EMA/CVMP/AWP/706442/2013. Draft. http://www.ema.europa.eu/docs/en_GB/document_library/Scientific_guideline/2015/03/WC500183774.pdf.

174. **Grace D.** 2015. Review of evidence on antimicrobial resistance and animal agriculture in developing countries. International Livestock Research Institute (ILRI). http://www.evidenceondemand.info/review-of-evidence-on-antimicrobial-resistance-and-animal-agriculture-in-developing-countries.

Antimicrobial Resistance in Bacteria from Livestock and Companion Animals
Edited by Frank Møller Aarestrup, Stefan Schwarz, Jianzhong Shen, and Lina Cavaco
© 2018 American Society for Microbiology, Washington, DC
doi:10.1128/microbiolspec.ARBA-0016-2017

Licensing and Approval of Antimicrobial Agents for Use in Animals

Constança Pomba,[1] Boudewijn Catry,[2] Jordi Torren Edo,[3] and Helen Jukes[4]

26

INTRODUCTION

Veterinary medicines and vaccines are indispensable for the treatment and prevention of farm animal and pet diseases around the world. To ensure that these medications are high quality and appropriately produced, countries require that animal health medicines are manufactured to specific standards of quality, with proven safety and efficacy. The responsible authority in a given country must authorize that a veterinary medicine can be manufactured, sold, and used. The marketing authorization, also known as "registration" or "license," implies that the responsible authority has approved not only the product to be marketed, but also the conditions that will characterize the use of the product. These conditions become part of the labelling, packaging, and information leaflets of the product and include (i) the characteristics of the active substance, its purity and concentration, and the complete composition of the medicinal product; (ii) the pharmaceutical form in which the medicine will be delivered (e.g., tablet, powder, cream, solution for injection), and the way it will be administered to the animal (e.g., injection, by mouth, in feed or water, or by topical application); (iii) the animals for which it is intended to be used, including specific ages and weights where relevant; (iv) what diseases or conditions it can be used to prevent, treat, or control, also known as the "indications"; (v) the dosages for each indication, the duration of treatment, and the withdrawal period, which means the number of days the medication must be withheld from farm animals prior to their produce entering the food system; and (vi) other circumstances regarding its use, including storage, shelf life, safety warnings, disposal instructions, and possible contra-indications. The sponsor develops this data package (or "application" or "dossier") according to the testing requirements and standards of the authorizing legislation in place in the jurisdiction. Authorised veterinary medicines have a clear positive benefit associated with their use while considering the risk to public health, animal health, and the environment. The authorization and production of veterinary medicinal products also require manufacturing controls for the active substance(s) and the final product and sampling and testing of products. Regular manufacturing site inspections and pharmacovigilance ensure continued monitoring once the medicine has been authorised and is being marketed. Additionally, many countries have monitoring systems in place to ensure compliance with maximum residue limits (MRLs). This means that any residues of the medicine in food from its use in food-producing animals must remain below the established safe levels for the consumer.

International food standards are developed by the Codex Alimentarius, which was established in 1962 by the Food and Agriculture Organization of the United Nations and the World Health Organization (WHO) (1). The Codex international food standards, guidelines, and codes of practice are voluntary for countries to reference or implement as part of their national regulations. While the Codex Alimentarius Commission is responsible for food safety from primary processing through to consumption, the World Organisation for Animal Health (OIE) is responsible for

[1]Faculty of Veterinary Medicine, University of Lisbon and Antimicrobial and Biocide Resistance Laboratory, Centre for Interdisciplinary Research in Animal Health (CIISA), Lisbon, Portugal; [2]Sciensano, Brussels, Belgium; [3]European Medicines Agency, London, UK and Facultat de Veterinària, UAB, Cerdanyola del Vallès, Spain; [4]Veterinary Medicines Directorate, Addlestone, UK.

setting standards in the domains of animal health and veterinary public health, including animal production food safety, to manage risks arising from the farm through to primary processing. The OIE and Codex collaborate closely in the development of standards relevant to the whole food production continuum. As a consequence of world trade globalization, a trend toward harmonization of the data requirements for authorization of veterinary medicines has occurred because approved veterinary medicines must satisfy the concerns about public health, animal health, and the environment. VICH—the International Cooperation on Harmonisation of Technical Requirements for Registration of Veterinary Medicinal Products—is the trilateral (European Union-Japan-United States) program that aims at harmonizing technical requirements for veterinary product registration (http://www.vichsec.org). VICH was officially launched in April 1996 by the animal health industry and regulators from the European Union, Japan, and the United States, with Australia, New Zealand and Canada joining as observers. It has the support and network of the OIE, and countries that are not part of VICH are invited to provide comments on the guidelines. It was based on a comparable international effort to harmonize technical requirements for human medicines called the International Conference on Harmonisation of Technical Requirements for Registration of Pharmaceuticals for Human Use. The main objectives of VICH are (i) to harmonize regulatory requirements in the VICH regions to ensure high quality, safety, and efficacy standards; (ii) to provide a basis for broader international harmonization of registration requirements; (iii) to monitor and maintain existing VICH guidelines, and (iv) to encourage constructive technical dialogue between regulators and industry (http://www.vichsec.org). VICH does not usually address issues regarding the assessment of data. That important task is kept for the regulatory authorities in each of the VICH countries.

The approval of veterinary antimicrobials is based on the principles of risk analysis. The risks considered in the approval of veterinary antimicrobials are (i) the consequences of the uncontrolled quality of the antimicrobial product, (ii) the direct exposure of people to the antimicrobial product (human occupational safety and consumer safety), (iii) the inadvertent exposure of organisms to the antimicrobial product (environmental safety), (iv) the antimicrobial product causing harm in the treated animals (target animal safety), and (v) failure to achieve claims (efficacy). Antimicrobial resistance constitutes another hazard emerging from the use of antimicrobial veterinary products. Adequate preapproval risk assessment must include the potential increase in the number of resistant bacteria in the gastrointestinal tract of exposed animals due to the use of the antimicrobial product and the probability that humans will be exposed to the resistant bacteria or resistant determinants and that this exposure will result in adverse human health consequences.

This article will focus on the licensing and approval of antimicrobial agents for use in animals including current initiatives on antimicrobial resistance.

PREAPPROVAL INFORMATION FOR REGISTERING NEW VETERINARY ANTIMICROBIAL AGENTS FOR FOOD-PRODUCING ANIMALS WITH RESPECT TO ANTIMICROBIAL RESISTANCE

In 2003, harmonized technical guidance was agreed upon in the European Union, Japan, and the United States for registration of antimicrobial veterinary medicinal products intended for use in food-producing animals with regard to characterization of the potential for a given antimicrobial agent to select for resistant bacteria of human health concern (2). This guidance outlines the types of studies and data recommended to characterize the potential resistance development in the food-producing animal that may arise from the use of an antimicrobial agent. The necessary information includes the attributes of the drug substance, the drug product, the nature of the resistance, and the potential exposure of the gut microbiota (flora) in the target animal species. The VICH GL27 guideline recommends that sponsors provide basic information regarding (i) antimicrobial class (common name, chemical name, chemical abstract services registry number, chemical structure, and manufacturer's code number and/or synonyms), (ii) mechanism and type of antimicrobial action, (iii) antimicrobial spectrum of activity, (iv) antimicrobial resistance (AMR) mechanisms and genetics, (v) occurrence and rate of transfer of AMR genes, (vi) occurrence of cross-resistance and coresistance, and (vii) pharmacokinetic data (2). The sponsor must provide information on the antimicrobial spectrum of activity, including data from MIC susceptibility testing against a wide variety of microorganisms or studies from the literature regarding (i) the target animal pathogens (as per product label claim) and (ii) foodborne pathogens (*Salmonella enterica* and *Campylobacter* spp.) and commensal organisms (*Escherichia coli* and *Enterococcus* spp.) (2).

The sponsor may present additional information regarding *in vitro* mutation frequency studies, antimicrobial agent activity in the intestinal tract, and other animal studies aiming to characterize the rate and extent (coselection due to linked resistance genes) of resistance development associated with the proposed use of the antimicrobial product (2). The overall submitted information should characterize the potential for the use of the veterinary medicinal product to select for antimicrobial-resistant bacteria of human health concern in terms of the exposure of foodborne pathogens and commensal organisms to the microbiologically active substance in the target animal after administration of the veterinary medicinal product under the proposed conditions of use (2).

SAFETY REQUIREMENTS FOR VETERINARY MEDICINAL PRODUCTS CONTAINING ANTIMICROBIAL SUBSTANCES

Target Animal Safety
International standards for studies for the demonstration of target animal safety for pharmaceutical veterinary medicines (for terrestrial animals) have been agreed on by VICH in their guideline 43 (3). The aim of the studies is to provide information on the margin of safety of the medicine and to identify adverse effects associated with an overdose or treatment beyond the recommended duration. The designs of the studies are based on the known pharmacological and toxicological properties of the active pharmaceutical ingredient, based on data from preliminary studies in target and nontarget laboratory animals, and the proposed conditions of use of the medicine (formulation, dosing regimen, target species, and production type) (3). Target animal safety studies are conducted on relatively small numbers of experimental animals in observance of the 3Rs principle of animals in research (replacement: replace with nonanimal system or with phylogenetically lower species; refinement: lessen or eliminate pain or distress in animals; reduction: lower the number of test animals needed) (3). Specific reproductive safety studies are required for medicines intended for use in breeding animals and for products to be administered locally into the mammary gland (3–5).

In addition to laboratory safety studies, safety data are also collected from field studies intended to evaluate the effectiveness of the medicine under conditions of field use—that is, in a typical population with or at risk of the disease of interest and under normal conditions of care. These studies collect data from a much larger number of animals and may therefore detect adverse events occurring at lower frequency than could be observed in the target animal safety study or that are related to particular animal characteristics (3).

Similar principles apply for demonstration of safety in aquatic species, although with flexibility in study design and interpretation considering differences in practicality of clinical sampling and the possible need to extrapolate between different species and varying environmental conditions (6).

Environmental Safety
International harmonized guidance for conducting environmental impact assessments (EIAs) for veterinary drugs consists of a two-phase procedure stated in Ecotoxicity Phase I VICH Harmonized Tripartide Guideline GL6 and Ecotoxicity Phase II VICH Harmonized Tripartite Guideline GL38 (7, 8). In phase I, the intended use of the drug determines the potential for environmental exposure. It is anticipated that drugs with limited use and limited environmental exposure will have limited environmental effects. Consequently, they stop at phase I (7). Phase I also recognizes veterinary drugs that require a more extensive EIA under phase II. The phase I EIA for a veterinary drug uses a decision tree via which an applicant determines that their veterinary drug needs or does not need an EIA (7). High potential exposure is defined by the initial route by which the veterinary drug enters the environment. Two main ecosystems are targeted: veterinary drugs intended for treatment of species reared in the aquatic environment and for treatment of species reared in the terrestrial environment. Veterinary drugs introduced directly into the aquatic environment or used in animals raised on pasture have a greater potential to contaminate aquatic habitats and the terrestrial environment, respectively. If the veterinary drug is an ecto- and/or endoparasiticide, its ecotoxicological potential needs to be assessed by conducting aquatic and terrestrial effects tests, respectively, in phase II. The exposure level of both ecosystems are also addressed in the guidelines (7, 8). A veterinary drug released from aquaculture facilities with an environmental introduction concentration of less than 1 µg/liter (the level shown to have adverse effects in aquatic ecotoxicity studies with human drugs) may stop at phase I (9). If the predicted environmental concentration of the veterinary drug in soil is less than 100 µg/kg, then the EIA for the veterinary drug may stop in phase I (9, 10). For a veterinary drug that has no possible mitigation measures aimed at reducing its aquatic environmental introduction concentration or predicted environmental concentration in soil, phase II guidance provides recommendations for standard datasets and conditions for determining whether more

information should be generated (8). The phase II guidance contains sections for each of the major branches: (i) aquaculture, (ii) intensively reared terrestrial animals, and (iii) pasture animals, each containing decision trees. Figure 1 shows the decision tree/flow diagram for veterinary drugs used for aquaculture according to ecotoxicity phase II VICH Harmonized Tripartide Guideline GL38 (8).

The presence of antimicrobials in the environment exerts a selective pressure for resistance genes in bacteria, and thus the importance of the environment as a reservoir for AMR genes is now widely recognized (11). The cycling of resistance genes between the different ecosystems deserves great attention; in particular, further consideration should be given to the contribution of veterinary antimicrobial use to the environmental resistome. Assessing the risk of AMR transmission from the environment to humans is also difficult, given that a nondirect proportionality between abundance and risk may exist (11). There are currently no legal requirements to monitor or prevent possible effects of antibiotic residues on the development or spread of AMR in the environment. Yet worldwide concern is growing about the role of polluted soil and water environments in the spread of AMR, and frameworks that regulate environmental risk assessment are considering the feasibility of including a risk assessment of AMR in the environment in their assessment schemes and thus of establishing the role of the contaminant resistome due to food-producing animal antimicrobial treatment.

Human Food Safety

The safety of food containing residues of veterinary drugs is generally assessed in laboratory animals (12). The requirements for toxicological testing of veterinary drugs are based on the toxicological tests for human medicines, food additives, and pesticides. International guidelines indicate the tests particularly relevant to the identification of a no-observed-adverse-effect level for veterinary drugs. These are (i) basic tests required for all new drugs used in food-producing animals to assess the safety of drug residues in human food (repeat-dose toxicity testing, reproduction toxicity testing, developmental toxicity testing, and genotoxicity testing), (ii) additional tests that may be required depending on specific toxicological concerns such as those associated with the structure, class, and mode of action of the drug (testing for effects on the human intestinal microbiota, pharmacological effects testing, immunotoxicity testing, neurotoxicity testing, and carcinogenicity

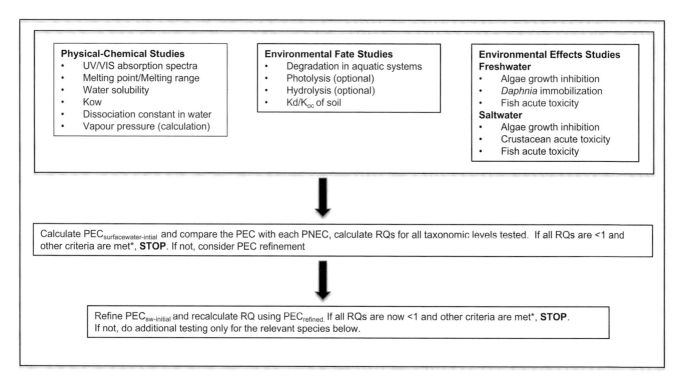

Figure 1 Partial decision tree/flow diagram for veterinary medicinal products used for aquaculture according to the Ecotoxicity Phase II VICH Harmonized Tripartide Guideline GL38 (8).

testing), and (iii) special tests which might assist in the interpretation of data obtained in the basic or additional tests (12).

Repeat-dose (90-day) toxicity testing is performed in a rodent and a nonrodent species to assess the toxic effects on target organs based on repeated and/or cumulative exposures to the compound and/or its metabolites, the incidence and severity of the effect in relation to dose and/or duration of exposure, the doses associated with toxic and biological responses, and the no-observed-adverse-effect level (13, 14). Additionally, reproduction toxicity testing is performed to detect any effect on mammalian reproduction (male and female fertility, mating, conception, implantation, ability to maintain pregnancy to term, parturition, lactation, survival, growth and development of the offspring from birth through to weaning, sexual maturity and the subsequent reproductive function of the offspring as adults) (15). Further basic testing involves developmental toxicity and genotoxicity testing (16, 17).

Among additional testing for specific toxicological properties of a veterinary drug, testing for effects on the human intestinal microbiota of antimicrobial compounds involves the determination of the effects of residues of the drug on the human intestinal microbiota (17). The ecology of the intestinal microbiota may be potentially altered by the ingestion of an antimicrobial drug. A drug may reach the colon either due to incomplete absorption or by the enterohepatic cycle. VICH guideline 36 outlines the steps for determining the need for establishing a microbiological acceptable daily intake (ADI) and how to derive those recommends test systems and methods for determining no-observable-adverse-effect concentrations (NOAECs) and (no-observed-adverse-effect levels) for the endpoints of health concern (18).

A harmonized approach to determine the threshold dose that might adversely disturb the human intestinal microbiota has not been established. International regulatory bodies have used a formula-based approach that takes into consideration relevant data including MIC data against human intestinal bacteria for determining microbiological ADIs for antimicrobial drugs (18). If the endpoint of concern is the disruption of the colonization barrier, the ADI may be derived from MIC data, fecal slurries, and semicontinuous, continuous, and fed-batch culture test systems as shown in Table 1. If the endpoint of concern is an increase in the population(s) of resistant bacteria to establish a microbiological ADI, NOAECs derived from semicontinuous, continuous, and fed-batch culture test systems may be used as in the previous case (18).

Residues of veterinary drugs, namely antimicrobial agents, in food are routinely evaluated for effects following chronic exposures, and a corresponding ADI is established, as described previously. Yet sometimes there is a potential for veterinary drug residues to cause adverse effects in humans following only a single meal. The ADI in such cases may not be the most appropriate value for quantifying the level above which a single exposure (after a single meal or during 1 day) can produce adverse effects (19). The acute reference dose is the appropriate approach. The acute reference dose is the estimate of the amount of a substance in food or drinking water, expressed in milligrams of the chemical per kilogram of body weight, which can be ingested in a period of 24 h or less without appreciable health risk to the consumer (19, 20). Regarding acute effects of antimicrobial agents on the human intestinal microbiota, the most relevant microbiological endpoint for acute exposure would be disruption of the colonization barrier. It is considered that a single exposure is unlikely to provide the selective pressure necessary to change the susceptibility of the bacterial population within the microbiome (20).

Maximum Residue Limits

The various toxicological tests previously described provide data for the establishment of a toxicological and microbiological ADI. The overall ADI (pharmacological, toxicological, and microbiological), generally expressed as microgram (μg) or milligram (mg)/kg body

Table 1 Derivation of ADI from *in vitro* data[a]

ADI derived from MIC data	ADI derived from other *in vitro* test systems
ADI = MICcalc[b] × mass of colon content (220 g/day)[d]/ (fraction of oral dose available to microorganisms)[e] × (60 kg person)	ADI = NOAEC[c] × mass of colon content (220 g/day)[d]/ (fraction of oral dose available to microorganisms)[e] × (60 kg person)

[a]Source: reference 18.
[b]The MICcalc is derived from the lower 90% confidence limit for the mean MIC_{50} of the relevant genera for which the drug is active.
[c]The NOAEC derived from the lower 90% confidence limit for the mean NOAEC from *in vitro* systems should be used to account for the variability of the data. Therefore, in this formula uncertainty factors are not generally needed to determine the microbiological ADI.
[d]The 220-g value is based on the colon content measured from accident victims.
[e]The fraction of an oral dose available for colonic microorganisms should be based on *in vivo* measurements for the drug administered orally.

weight per day, is the amount of antimicrobial residues that can be consumed by an adult daily for a lifetime without appreciable risk to human health (21). The overall ADI provides the basis for determining the MRL of an antimicrobiological agent in a treated animal intended for human consumption. The MRL is the maximum concentration of residue accepted in a food product obtained from an animal that has received a veterinary medicine or that has been exposed to a biocidal product for use in animal husbandry (21). In the European Union/European Economic Area, the assessment of the safety of residues is carried out by the European Medicines Agency (EMA) Committee for Medicinal Products for Veterinary Use (CVMP) and in the United States by the Food and Drug Administration (FDA). The European Union requires by law that foodstuffs, such as meat, milk, and eggs obtained from animals treated with veterinary medicines or exposed to biocidal products used in animal husbandry must not contain any residue that might represent a hazard to the health of the consumer. Once the substances have been assessed and following the adoption of a commission regulation confirming the classification of the substances, the substances that may be used are listed in Table 1 of the annex to Commission Regulation (European Union) no. 37/2010. An external database (https://www.globalmrl.com/home) contains maximum acceptable levels of pesticides and veterinary drugs in food and agricultural products in the United States, as well as 70 other countries, the European Union, and the Codex Alimentarius Commission (https://www.fas.usda.gov/maximum-residue-limits-mrl-database).

EFFICACY REQUIREMENTS FOR VETERINARY MEDICINAL PRODUCTS CONTAINING ANTIMICROBIAL SUBSTANCES

Among the larger jurisdictions, only the European Union provides a specific guidance for industry on the design of pharmacological and clinical studies to support demonstration of the efficacy of antimicrobial veterinary medicines (22). An applicant for a marketing authorization for such a product must provide these data to support a specified "claim"/"indication." The indication concerns a clinical disease associated with named bacterial pathogens in a particular animal species. In the European Union, indications are usually related to "treatment" alone or in association with "metaphylaxis" (22). Treatment relates to administration of a product to animals that are showing clinical

signs of disease, whereas metaphylaxis is administration to animals in close contact and presumably infected but not yet showing signs of disease (22). Prevention claims (administration to healthy animals to prevent infection) are nowadays rare and only considered when the risk for infection is high and consequences are severe. The definitions and terminology differ between different areas of the world.

In accordance with European Union guidance, preclinical studies are required. Pharmacodynamic and pharmacokinetic data that are used to support the indications and dosing regimen for the product (22). The pharmacodynamics data should include information on the mechanism of action of the antimicrobial and MIC data determined using an accepted standardized methodology. The derived MIC distribution should include a sufficient number of isolates of target pathogen(s) obtained from recent European Union clinical cases, and ideally the epidemiological cut-off value should be available (22). Pharmacokinetics studies should provide data on the bioavailability of the product according to its route of administration and the concentration of the antimicrobial in the plasma and, if feasible, at the site of infection over time. These data can be used to explore a pharmacokinetics/pharmacodynamics relationship, which can be used to support the dosing regimen (22).

Dose determination studies investigate the dose level, dosing interval, and number of administrations of the product required. They are usually conducted in a small number of experimental animals that have been challenged with a strain of the target pathogen known to elicit a predictable level of disease. The efficacy of the selected dosing regimen is then corroborated in dose-confirmation studies, preferably using naturally infected animals, but conducted under well-controlled conditions.

Finally, the effectiveness and safety of the proposed antimicrobial medicine are investigated in clinical field trials. These involve a much larger number of animals, representative of the target population, under conditions of a natural disease outbreak. Clinical field trials should be multicentric randomized controlled studies. In the European Union they may use a negative or placebo control group, but more often, for animal welfare reasons, the control product is an authorized medicine with the same indication. The presence of the target pathogens and their antimicrobial susceptibility should be determined prior to treatment in diagnostic samples from a representative number of animals. The response to treatment is determined based primarily on the clinical response rate, which is evaluated on clinically relevant endpoints for the disease (e.g., pyrexia, respiratory and depression scores for swine respiratory disease). The microbiological cure rate is also an important (or often coprimary) endpoint. The outcomes of field trials must be statistically robust, and therefore it is important that studies are suitably designed and powered. Guidance is further provided on the statistical design and evaluation (23).

In addition to the above-mentioned guidance for antimicrobials, in the European Union and other VICH regions, clinical studies of all types of products should be conducted in accordance with VICH Harmonized Tripartite Guideline GL9 on good clinical practice (24). The purpose of the guideline is to establish guidance for the conduct of clinical studies that ensures the accuracy, integrity, and correctness of data, ensuring the welfare of the study animals and the effects on the environment and on residues in the edible products derived from food-producing study animals. Public access to information on clinical trial databases could be generalized; see as an example the European Union Clinical Trials Register (https://www.clinicaltrialsregister.eu/), which does not, however, include veterinary medicinal products.

Several jurisdictions (4, 5, 25) provide more detailed guidance on the data requirements for the demonstration of effectiveness of antimicrobial medicines intended for treatment and prevention of mastitis in cattle. In general, for subclinical mastitis, effectiveness is based on elimination of the udder pathogen and normalization of quarter somatic cell counts. Additionally,

for clinical mastitis, resolution of local clinical signs of the udder and the quality of milk should be demonstrated. Prevention claims relating to protection from the establishment of new intramammary infections during the dry period can also be considered for products intended for dry cows.

RISK ANALYSIS FRAMEWORK IN THE APPROVAL OF VETERINARY MEDICINAL PRODUCTS CONTAINING ANTIMICROBIAL SUBSTANCES

The risk to public health from the development, emergence, and spread of resistance consequent to the use of antimicrobials in veterinary medicine is dependent on multiple risk factors (26, 27). Figure 2 summarises the chain of events that may lead from use of antimicrobials in animals to a compromised antimicrobial treatment in humans. The OIE and the Codex Alimentarius Commission have developed risk analysis guidance. VICH has developed guidance the data required to assess the potential for the use of new antimicrobial products to select for resistant bacteria of human health concern, as stated regarding the preapproval requirements (2).

The OIE indicates that authorities regulating antimicrobials should have in place a policy framework for monitoring, measuring, assessing, and managing risk involved with the use of antimicrobials in food-producing animals. To assist risk assessors and risk managers, the

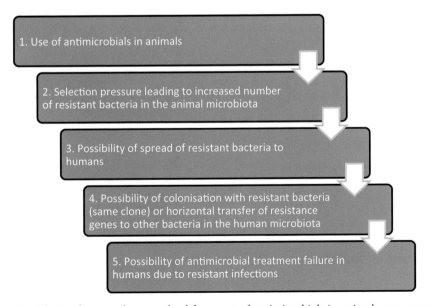

Figure 2 Chain of events that may lead from use of antimicrobials in animals to a compromised antimicrobial treatment in humans.

OIE has provided guidance on the principles for conducting a transparent and objective risk analysis (28, 29). The OIE risk analysis process is divided into four components: hazard identification, risk assessment, risk management, and risk communication, based on the terminology of the Covello-Merkhofer system. The hazard is defined as "the resistant microorganism or resistance determinant that emerges as a result of the use of a specific antimicrobial in animals." The resistant organism may itself be pathogenic or pass its resistance determinant to other organisms that are pathogenic. The risk assessment is based on scientific data, and the process is divided into four steps (Table 2). The OIE recommends that a qualitative risk assessment is always conducted as a preliminary evaluation. This will help to identify risk pathways which are feasible and those that can be discounted. The model should only be as complex as necessary to evaluate the risk management options available. It is acknowledged that a lack of appropriate data often prevents a complete quantitative risk assessment; alternatively, a semiquantitative approach can be adopted in which estimates of the probability and size of potential consequences are assigned to well-defined categories which can be combined into a severity score for the risk. This allows risks to be compared systematically and a threshold to be set for unacceptable risks.

Although there should be communication between risk assessors and risk managers, the responsibilities should be kept separate to ensure independence of the evaluation of the risk and decision-making. Risk managers should have a policy framework that explains the risk management options that are available under the legislative and regulatory framework of the country and the level of risk deemed acceptable. The final step of the risk analysis is risk communication, defined as "the interactive transmission and exchange of information and opinion throughout the risk analysis process concerning risk, risk-related factors and risk perceptions among risk assessors, risk managers, risk communicators, the general public and interested parties." It is noted that communication is essential to avoid failure of the risk analysis process (28, 29).

As previously mentioned, the Codex Alimentarius Commission develops international standards and guidelines to protect the health of consumers and to ensure fair practices in the food trade. In 2005, the Codex Alimentarius Commission produced its code of practice to minimize and contain AMR, which provides guidance for the responsible and prudent use of antimicrobials in food-producing animals (30). The code aims to minimize the potential adverse impact on public health resulting from the use of antimicrobial agents in food-producing animals. The code addresses in a summary manner the assessment of the efficacy of antimicrobials, the potential of veterinary antimicrobial drugs to select for resistant microorganisms, the establishment of ADIs and MRLs, and withdrawal periods for those products. The code of practice will be revised to address risk mitigation measures and other factors such as strategies that prevent or reduce the need to use antimicrobial agents, the use of lists of critically important antimicrobials, and the use of antimicrobials as growth promoters. Furthermore, the Codex Alimentarius Commission has developed a guideline providing a risk analysis framework to address the risks to human health associated specifically with foodborne AMR linked to nonhuman use of antimicrobial agents (30). The guideline address the risks associated with veterinary applications, plant protection, and food processing. The initial step of the framework is a scoping exercise in which an AMR food safety issue is identified by the risk manager followed by the development of an AMR risk profile to consider the context of the problem. This includes consideration of the food production chain, information on adverse public health effects, and available risk management options and leads to the establishment of a risk assessment policy.

The foodborne AMR risk assessment uses a science-based approach to identify the frequency and amount of AMR microorganisms to which humans are exposed through the consumption of food and the resulting magnitude and severity of the adverse health effects. To achieve this, the risk assessment is performed in four steps (Table 2). Risk management options should be evaluated with regard to their capacity to achieve an "appropriate level of protection" (WTO Agreement on the Application of Sanitary and Phytosanitary Measures) or other public health criterion (Table 2) (31). In keeping with the OIE guidance, the need for early communication between risk managers and risk assessors, and with consumer and industry representatives (producers, food processors, pharma), is recommended.

The Codex guidelines additionally highlight the importance of surveillance programs for the use of antimicrobials and prevalence of foodborne AMR in providing data for use throughout the risk analysis process.

Regional risk analysis frameworks for veterinary medicinal products also exist in the United States (32), the European Union (33), Canada (34), Australia (35), and Japan. (In Japan, the risk assessment for AMR arising from the use of antimicrobials in animals is performed by the Food Safety Commission of Japan at http://fsc.go.jp/english/index.html.)

Table 2 Risk analysis frameworks in the approval of veterinary medicinal products containing antimicrobial substances[a]

OIE hazard identification and risk assessment process	Codex Alimentarius Commission foodborne AMR risk assessment	OIE risk management process	Codex Alimentarius Commission foodborne AMR risk management process
Hazard identification: Resistant microorganism or resistance determinant that emerges as a result of the use of a specific antimicrobial in animals.	Hazard identification: Identification of the foodborne antimicrobial-resistant microorganisms or determinants of concern in the food commodity.	NA	NA
Release assessment: Biological pathways that may lead to release of resistant microorganisms or resistance determinants into a particular environment due to the use of a specific antimicrobial agent in animals. Exposure assessment: Biological pathways necessary for exposure of animals and/or humans to the hazards released from a given source and the probability of the exposure occurring.	Exposure assessment: Detailing of the exposure pathways both preharvest, in the environment, and postharvest. The objective is to provide an estimate of the probability and level of contamination of the food product with AMR microorganisms at the time of food consumption.	Risk evaluation: The process of comparing the risk estimated in the risk assessment with the reduction in the risk expected from the proposed risk management measures. Option evaluation: The evaluation of a range of risk management measures, which may include regulatory and non regulatory measures, such as development of codes of practice and disease control measures.	RMOs, pre- and postharvest risk factors, and approaches already adopted under good agricultural practice, good veterinary practices, good hygiene practices, and hazard analysis and critical control point Regulatory controls on the use of veterinary antimicrobial medicines (limiting marketing authorizations), non regulatory controls (e.g., development of treatment and responsible use guidelines), and checking compliance of food products with microbiological criteria.
Consequence assessment: Describes the potential adverse health consequences, which may in turn lead to socioeconomic consequences, due to the specified exposures of humans or animals to resistant microorganisms. The probability of the potential consequences should also be estimated.	Hazard characterization: Considers the characteristics of the hazard, food commodity, and host to determine the probability of disease in humans and to estimate the additional frequency and severity of disease due to resistant pathogens, including the risk of treatment failure.	Development of an implementation plan.	Development of an implementation plan.
Risk estimation: Integrates the results from the release assessment, exposure assessment, and consequence assessment to provide an overall measure of the risks associated with the identified hazard(s).	Risk characterization: Considers the key findings from the first three steps to estimate the risk according to the risk manager's needs, e.g., increased rates of hospitalization and mortality due to resistant infections, risks to sensitive subgroups, existence of alternative treatments.	Monitoring and review of the effectiveness of risk management measures.	Monitoring and review of the effectiveness of risk management measures, including evaluation against specific food safety metrics such as those used for national surveillance programs.

[a]NA, not applicable; RMO, risk management option.

The FDA's methodology includes a qualitative approach to the risk assessment and provides guidance on the ranking of certain risk factors as high, medium, or low. A matrix is used to integrate the qualitative outcomes of the release, exposure, and consequence assessments into an overall risk estimation for the antimicrobial as having either low, medium, or high risk potential for human health due to selection of resistant foodborne bacteria associated with the use of the drug in food-producing animals (32). Whether a new antimicrobial animal drug is considered approvable is dependent on whether the FDA can conclude that "there is a reasonable certainty of no harm to human health when the drug is approved under specific use restrictions."

The legislative framework for veterinary medicinal products in the European Union is currently under review. Key among the objectives of the review is to address the public health risk of AMR and to strengthen the benefit-risk assessment for antimicrobial veterinary medicinal products. In this respect, the CVMP, in collaboration with its Antimicrobials Working Party, have prepared draft guidance on the assessment of the risk to public health from AMR due to the use of antimicrobial veterinary medicinal products in food-producing animals (36). The guidance predominantly relates to the foodborne route of exposure, although transmission of AMR through direct contact by handling animals or animal produce should also be considered. The EMA's risk assessment methodology is adapted closely from the OIE framework but also takes account of that provided by Codex and other regulatory jurisdictions. The CVMP Antimicrobials Working Party has also provided over the past decade a series of reflection papers addressing the use of certain antimicrobial classes in food-producing animals in the European Union and the development of resistance and its impact on human and animal health (37–39). Based on these papers, the CVMP has made recommendations which have been followed up, according to priority, by "class referral" procedures aimed at amending the summary of product characteristics (SPCs) of groups of related veterinary medicinal products to ensure that they are in line with the CVMP's risk profiling and responsible use principles (40, 41). Following a referral procedure, a decision is issued by the European Commission (EC), requiring member states to implement the CVMP's recommendations. In 2015 the EMA/CVMP published a reflection paper on the risk of AMR transfer from companion animals (42, 43). Although it was recognized that the use in companion animals of antimicrobials that are critically important for human health and the close contact between humans and pets

increases the risks for transfer of important resistances, owing to the extensive knowledge gaps at the time, it was concluded that currently only an abbreviated risk assessment would be possible when approving veterinary antimicrobials for companion animals.

COMBATING ANTIMICROBIAL RESISTANCE
In addition to the risk analysis framework for veterinary medicinal products, many authorities provide general guidance on how to use antimicrobials to minimize the risks related to AMR. Novel main areas of awareness include the categorization of antimicrobials, responsible use guidance, and monitoring and surveillance strategies.

Critically Important Antimicrobial Categorization and Restrictions on Use
Lists categorizing antimicrobials have become popular, because they allow for targeting of risk management measures and provide overall recommendations on the prudent use of antimicrobials. Those recommendations take the lists as one of the factors, or the basis, for the recommendations on antimicrobial use and adapt them to the local situation. Lists of critically important antimicrobials (CIAs) provide a ranking of the antimicrobials currently used in medicine for humans or animals. For most risk assessors and regulators the most important criteria for the preparation of such lists is the impact of the use of those antimicrobials on public health, followed by animal health. Different institutions, such as the WHO, OIE, EMA, and FDA, have considered the impact of some of those factors and created lists ranking antimicrobials for use in animals; those lists might vary depending on the above-listed objectives and other factors such as the availability of medicinal products, including the pharmaceutical form in which they are available, or the area/region for which the lists are produced. In most cases the lists are based on the WHO list of CIAs for human medicine, highlighting the importance of the WHO list.

WHO list of CIAs
The WHO follows a One Health approach, so the list of Critically Important Antimicrobials is of use for public and animal health. According to the WHO, the list is intended to be used by "authorities, practicing physicians and veterinarians, and other interested stakeholders involved in managing antimicrobial resistance." Most of the lists that have been produced, including the WHO list, aim to help prioritize risk assessment and risk management. Importantly, the WHO indicates that the list should not be "considered as the

sole source of information to guide a risk management approach" (44).

Criteria for the ranking

According to the WHO list, the criteria for the ranking of antimicrobials are the following:

- **Criterion 1:** The antimicrobial class is the sole or one of limited available therapies to treat serious bacterial infections in people.
- **Criterion 2:** The antimicrobial class is used to treat infections in people caused by either (i) bacteria that may be transmitted to humans from nonhuman sources or (ii) bacteria that may acquire resistance genes from nonhuman sources.

In addition, the criteria for prioritizing the antimicrobials of the critically important category are as follows:

- **Prioritization criterion 1:** A high absolute number of people are affected by diseases for which the antimicrobial class is the sole or one of few alternatives to treat serious infections in humans.
- **Prioritization criterion 2:** There is a high frequency of use of the antimicrobial class for any indication in human medicine, since use may favor selection of resistance.
- **Prioritization criterion 3:** The antimicrobial class is used to treat infections in people for which there is evidence of transmission of resistant bacteria (e.g., nontyphoidal *Salmonella* and *Campylobacter* spp.) or resistance genes (high for *E. coli* and *Enterococcus* spp.) from nonhuman sources.

Categories of antimicrobials

The WHO divides antimicrobials into three categories: (i) critically important—antimicrobial classes which meet the first and second criteria, (ii) highly important— antimicrobials that meet one of the two criteria, and (iii) important—antimicrobials that do not meet either of the two criteria.

The WHO also includes a group of substances categorized as being highest-priority CIAs. These are those CIAs that meet all three prioritization criteria listed above.

As a summary, the classes of antimicrobials include:

- **Critically important antimicrobials:** Aminoglycosides, ansamycins, carbapenems (and other penems), cephalosporins (third and fourth generation), phosphonic acid derivatives, glycopeptides, glycylcyclines, lipopeptides, macrolides and ketolides, monobactams, oxazolidinones, penicillins (natural, aminopenicillins,

and antipseudomonal), polymyxins, quinolones, and drugs used solely to treat tuberculosis or other mycobacterial diseases
- **Highly important antimicrobials:** Amidinopenicillins, amphenicols, cephalosporins (first and second generation) and cephamycins, lincosamides, penicillins (antistaphylococcal), pleuromutilins, pseudomonic acids, riminofenazines, steroid antibacterials, streptogramins, sulfonamides, dihydrofolate reductase inhibitors and combinations, sulfones, and tetracyclines
- **Important antimicrobials:** Aminocyclitols, cyclic polypeptides, nitrofurantoins and nitroimidazoles
- **Highest-priority CIAs:** Quinolones; third-, fourth-, and fifth-generation cephalosporins; polymyxins; glycopeptides; macrolides; and ketolides

WHO guidelines on use of medically important antimicrobials in food-producing animals

The WHO has recently published guidelines on the use of medically important antimicrobials in food-producing animals (45). According to the WHO, the guidelines are "evidence-based recommendations and best practice statements on use of medically important antimicrobials in food-producing animals, based on the WHO CIA List."

The WHO recommendations are based on different themes and ranked according to their type of recommendation (e.g., strong) and the quality of the evidence. A summary of WHO recommendations is presented in Table 3.

WHO best practices statements

In addition to the above recommendations, the WHO has produced two best practice statements. Of relevance for this article is the second one, "Medically important antimicrobials that are not currently used in food production should not be used in the future in food production including in food-producing animals or plants" (45).

OIE list of antimicrobials of veterinary importance

The OIE has produced a list of antimicrobials of veterinary importance (46). The list is the result of a questionnaire that was sent to the OIE member states and other institutions. The main difference between the WHO list and the OIE list is that the OIE list aims to establish the degree of importance for classes of veterinary antimicrobials.

Criteria for the ranking

The first criterion for the OIE list is the response rate to the questionnaire that was sent. The second criterion

Table 3 Summary of WHO recommendations on use of medically important antimicrobials in food-producing animals[a]

Theme (subject)	Recommendation	Type and quality of evidence
Overall antimicrobial use	We recommend an overall reduction in the use of all classes of medically important antimicrobials in food-producing animals.	Strong recommendation, low-quality evidence
Growth promotion use	We recommend complete restriction of use of all classes of medically important antimicrobials in food-producing animals for growth promotion.	Strong recommendation, low-quality evidence
Preventive use (in the absence of disease)	We recommend complete restriction of use of all classes of medically important antimicrobials in food-producing animals for prevention of infectious diseases that have not yet been clinically diagnosed.	Strong recommendation, low-quality evidence
Control and treatment use (in the presence of disease)[b]	We suggest that antimicrobials classified as critically important for human medicine should not be used for control of the dissemination of a clinically diagnosed infectious disease identified within a group of food-producing animals.	Conditional recommendation, very low-quality evidence
Control and treatment use (in the presence of disease)[b]	We suggest that antimicrobials classified as highest priority critically important for human medicine should not be used for treatment of food- producing animals with a clinically diagnosed infectious disease.	Conditional recommendation, very low-quality evidence

[a]Source: reference 45.
[b]To prevent harm to animal health and welfare, exceptions can be made when veterinary professionals judge that culture and sensitivity tests demonstrate that the selected drug is the only treatment option.

refers to the treatment of serious animal disease and the availability of alternative antimicrobials.

In line with the WHO list, the OIE list is divided between veterinary CIAs, veterinary highly important antimicrobials, and veterinary important antimicrobials. Taking into account the two above-listed criteria, the following categories were established:

- **Veterinary CIAs:** Those that meet both criteria 1 and 2
- **Veterinary highly important antimicrobials:** Those that meet criteria 1 or 2
- **Veterinary important antimicrobials:** Those that meet neither criteria 1 nor 2

The three categories of antimicrobials include the following classes of antimicrobials:

- **Veterinary CIAs:** Aminoglycosides, cephalosporins (all generations), macrolides, penicillins, phenicols, quinolones, sulfonamides (including trimethoprim), and tetracyclines
- **Veterinary highly important antimicrobials:** Ansamycin/rifamycins, fosfomycin, ionophores, lincosamides, pleuromutilins, and polypeptides
- **Veterinary important antimicrobials:** Bicyclomycin, fusidic acid, novobiocin, orthosomycins, quinoxalines, and streptogramins

The EMA categorization of antimicrobials

The EMA, following a request from the EC, has produced a categorization of antimicrobials for use in food-producing animals (47). The categorization was

part of the answer to a request from the EC concerning the impact of the use of antibiotics in animals on public and animal health and measures to manage the possible risk to humans. For the categorization, the EMA assembled a group of experts, including experts on the use of antibiotics and resistance in humans. The group was named the Antimicrobial Advice ad hoc Expert Group. The group's opinions, including the categorization, were adopted by the CVMP and the Committee for Medicinal Products for Human Use. Specifically, the answer to the question of categorization was adopted in December 2014. Two main factors were taken into account for the categorization: the need for antimicrobials in human medicine and the risk for spread of resistance from animals to humans. One of the main intentions of the ranking was to take into account the use of veterinary medicinal antimicrobials in the European Union and to adapt the recommendations to the specific conditions of the European Union.

Criteria for the ranking

As indicated above, the two main factors for the ranking were (i) the need for a specific class of antimicrobials in human medicine and (ii) the risk for spread of resistance from animals to humans. These two criteria were addressed as follows: hazard of zoonotic relevance (e.g., *Campylobacter* spp., *Salmonella* spp.), probability of resistance transfer (e.g., low or high), use in veterinary medicine (indicating if the substance is approved for use in the European Union and if it is authorized for group treatment), and information from member states' marketing authorizations. For each antimicrobial class it was considered which are the bacterial targets in human medicine in the European Union for which the availability of a class/substance is critically important because there are few alternatives. For the classification of antimicrobial classes according to their probability of transfer of resistance genes and resistant bacteria, the following parameters were considered: vertical transmission of resistance genes, mobile genetic element-mediated transfer of resistance, coselection of resistance, potential for transmission of resistance through zoonotic and commensal foodborne bacteria, and evidence of similarity of resistance (genes, mobile genetic elements, and resistant bacteria). In addition, the recommendations were product independent and apply across the whole of the European Union independently of the animal health situation and of the availability of antimicrobial products for animals in individual member states.

Categories of antimicrobials

The EMA/Antimicrobial Advice ad hoc Expert Group categorization was divided into three categories:

- **Category 1:** Antimicrobials used in veterinary medicine where the risk for public health is currently estimated as low or limited
- **Category 2:** Antimicrobials used in veterinary medicine where the risk for public health is currently estimated as higher
- **Category 3:** Antimicrobials currently not approved for use in veterinary medicine

Category 1 includes substances which are considered the first choice in treatment guidelines and for which no specific associated hazards were identified to which people could be exposed from use in animals in the European Union. Category 2 includes substances that should be reserved for the treatment of clinical conditions which have responded poorly, or are expected to respond poorly, to other antimicrobials. The recommendations also indicate that "these reserved antimicrobials should be included in treatment guidelines only when there are no alternatives that could be used." The recommendations also indicate that all efforts should be made to reduce the need for the use of category substances and to convince companies to seek marketing authorizations for alternative substances presenting less risk for public health. Category 3 includes antimicrobials currently not approved for use in veterinary medicine (but used for human medicine in the European Union). According to their legal status these substances may only be used by way of exception and only in companion animals (non-food producing species).

Lists of antimicrobials by category

Category 1 includes some classes of antimicrobial that have widespread use in veterinary medicine (48) and substances which are regarded as the first choice in animal treatments. These are certain penicillins, tetracyclines, and macrolides (polymyxins were initially included but later were moved to category 2). In addition, there is some limited use of rifampicin (a rifamycin) in veterinary medicine. Penicillins with a narrow spectrum of activity (e.g., penicillin G and penicillin V) belong with tetracyclines in a category in which the risk to public health is estimated as low.

In human medicine, certain macrolides (e.g., azithromycin) are being increasingly used in developing countries to treat invasive *Salmonella* spp. and *Shigella* spp. infections in humans, such as those caused by typhoidal salmonellae (e.g., *Salmonella enterica* serovar Typhi) or by *Shigella dysenteriae* type 1 (Shiga's bacillus), when patients fail to respond to treatment with more conventional antimicrobials such as the fluoroquinolones. So far, use of these antimicrobials is limited in the European Union, and *S.* Typhi, *S. enterica* serovar Paratyphi, and *S. dysenteriae* 1 are not zoonotic hazards, but there is a need for awareness because in the future, macrolide-resistant *Salmonella* spp. other than typhoidal serovars may become a concern. For more information on the most extensively used polymyxin in veterinary medicine, i.e., colistin, see the response to the first request from the EC (49, 50). Currently, there are no recommendations to avoid the use of category 1 substances beyond what is stated by general responsible use principles. Nevertheless, these antimicrobials are not devoid of negative impact on resistance development and spread, and even if extensive use in veterinary medicine is to be expected, it is also important to ensure that any use is responsible. Category 1 substances might be of concern, e.g., if they facilitate spread of multidrug-resistant strains due to coresistance. This is a known problem for, e.g., livestock-associated methicillin-resistant *Staphylococcus aureus* where many antimicrobials, and in particular tetracyclines, (51), might collaborate to resistance selection. Likewise, resistance by coselection through the use of macrolides has also been involved in the persistence of vancomycin-resistant enterococci in livestock (39).

Category 2 includes antimicrobials used in veterinary medicine where the risk for public health is currently estimated as higher than the risk for category 1. Fluoroquinolones and third- and fourth-generation cephalosporins are of special concern. These antimicrobials have been used in some countries as the first-line treatment for a variety of infections in veterinary medicine. The EMA/CVMP Scientific Advisory Group on Antimicrobials (SAGAM) has provided risk profiles for fluoroquinolones and third- and fourth-generation cephalosporins (37, 38), and the CVMP concluded, among other recommendations, that an appropriate level of risk mitigation would be to reserve these agents for the treatment of clinical conditions which have responded poorly, or are expected to respond poorly, to other antimicrobials. These reserved antimicrobials should be included in treatment guidelines only when there are no alternatives that could be used. In some member states these category 2 substances are the only available choices approved for certain species and infections. In such cases, all efforts should be made to reduce the need for their use and to convince companies to seek marketing authorizations for alternative substances (including nonantimicrobial agents) presenting less risk for public health. The recommendations for these category 2 substances as reserved antimicrobials have been implemented in all summaries of product characteristics for veterinary medicinal products for food-producing species. For fluoroquinolones, regulatory actions have been taken (by the EMA), as they have for systemically active (parenteral and oral) third- and fourth-generation cephalosporins (40, 41). These actions have resulted in partial harmonization of relevant parts of the scientific literature concerning those medicinal products.

Aminoglycosides and some penicillins are classes of antimicrobials for which no risk profiling has yet been done by the EMA/CVMP. These classes have been added to category 2 based on the information available on criticality of use in human medicine and probability of spread of resistance. The EMA/CVMP/Committee for Medicinal Products for Human Use/Antimicrobial Advice ad hoc Expert Group recommends profiling the risk to public health related to the use of these classes in veterinary medicine. Future assessments could result in a change of the categorization.

Aminoglycosides are used extensively in veterinary medicine and are also given as oral group/flock medication; no use restrictions apply for this class. Because they may be effective against multidrug-resistant *Enterobacteriaceae* in humans and because the risk for spread of resistance from animals to humans is ranked as high, there might be a concern with the use of this class which is currently not addressed. To further elaborate on possible risks from aminoglycoside use in animals, a more detailed risk profile would be needed.

Penicillins are a diverse class that includes substances such as penicillin G and V, which have no activity against *Enterobacteriacea*, and substances that have an extended spectrum. Those with an extended spectrum could be a concern if their ability to facilitate spread of extended-spectrum beta-lactamases is similar to that of third- and fourth-generation cephalosporins. Therefore, a more detailed risk profile on penicillins with activity against *Enterobacteriaceae* is recommended. It is recommended to consider the diversity of the penicillin class when discussing the risk to public health from a veterinary treatment guideline perspective.

A number of the classes/substances listed are not currently approved for use in veterinary medicine, and these are classified as category 3. The extent of use of these classes would be low provided the restrictions detailed in articles 10 and 11 of Directive 2001/82/EC. According to these restrictions, they may only be used by way of exception and only in companion animals (non-food producing species), as MRLs have not been established to allow their use in food-producing animals.

Categorization may be considered one element when deciding on when/whether to use a certain class/substance in veterinary medicine, but it may not be used as the sole basis when creating treatment guidelines or when deciding on risk mitigation activities. It should not be interpreted as a recommendation for treatment guidelines. The categorization could also be taken into account when considering hazard characterization for the risk assessment in applications for marketing authorizations for veterinary medicinal products. Development and implementation of evidence-based national and regional treatment guidelines is encouraged.

FDA list of medically important antimicrobials

In 2003, the FDA published the Guidance for Industry number 152, "Evaluating the Safety of Antimicrobial New Animal Drugs with Regard to their Microbiological Effects on Bacteria of Human Health Concern," for the evaluation of antimicrobial substances for food-producing species (33). Annex A of the this guidance provides the categorization of antimicrobials according to their importance for antimicrobial use.

Criteria for the ranking

The annex of the criteria for the ranking defines the criteria as follows:

- **Antimicrobial drugs used to treat enteric pathogens that cause foodborne disease:** The Infectious Disease

Society of America guidelines on the treatment of diarrhea and other sources such as the Sanford Guide provide the drugs typically used in the treatment of foodborne diseases.

- **Sole therapy or one of few alternatives to treat serious human disease or the drug is an essential component among many antimicrobials in treatment of human disease:**
- Includes antimicrobials such as vancomycin and linezolid for methicillin-resistant *S. aureus* infections. Although they are not the "sole" therapy, they are one of only a few alternatives.
- This would also include a drug like polymyxin, which is one of few alternatives for multidrug-resistant *Pseudomonas aeruginosa* infections.
- Rifampin is not only a drug used to treat tuberculosis, but is also an essential part of the treatment regimen, because the cure rate is lower without it.
- Serious diseases are defined as those with high morbidity or mortality without proper treatment regardless of the relationship of animal transmission to humans.
- **Antimicrobials used to treat enteric pathogens in non-foodborne disease:** Enteric pathogens may cause disease other than foodborne illness.
- **No cross-resistance within the drug class and absence of linked resistance with other drug classes:**
- Absence of resistance linked to other antimicrobials makes an antimicrobial more valuable.
- Cross-resistance within antimicrobial classes and absence of linked resistance may change over time and will need to be updated periodically.
- In this context, "cross-resistance" refers to the transmission of resistant determinants between bacterial species or genera and does not refer to transmission of resistant organisms between animals and humans.

- **Difficulty in transmitting resistance elements within or across genera and species of organisms:**
- Antimicrobials to which organisms have chromosomal resistance would be more valuable than antimicrobials whose resistance mechanisms are present on plasmids and transposons.
- This does not refer to "ease of transmissibility" from animals to humans of the resistant pathogen because this is addressed elsewhere in the guidance in the release assessment.

Categories of antimicrobials
The annex of the FDA guidance classifies the antimicrobials (Table 4).

Responsible Use
Guidelines for responsible antimicrobial use provide a set of recommendations for antimicrobial prescribers, and users, to optimize the use of antimicrobials in animals and minimize the risk of AMR from the use of antimicrobials in animals spreading to humans; such guidelines may, or may not, be driven and endorsed by national or international competent authorities or organizations. Recommendations are usually provided for animal species or for production groups (e.g., veal calves). Responsible use guidelines have been changing ever since the first findings of acquired AMR. Earlier recommendations such as "broadspectrum, combination of compounds and prolonged (oral) therapy to avoid secondary infections and relapses" are, following new insights, no longer justified. Randomized controlled trials, reviews, and meta-analysis have led to new responsible use recommendations. Currently, a narrow-spectrum, single compound with high loading dose and a minimum of therapy duration is estimated to be appropriate to maintain clinical efficacy while minimizing the selection and spread of antibiotic resis-

Table 4 Categories of antimicrobials according to the annex of the FDA guidance[a]

Category	Criteria	Classes of antimicrobials
Critically important	Antimicrobial drugs which meet both criteria 1 and 2	Third-generation cephalosporins, fluoroquinolones, macrolides, trimethoprim/sufamethoxazol
Highly important	Antimicrobial drugs which meet either criterium 1 or 2	Natural penicillins, penase resistant penicillins, antipseudomonal penicillins, aminopenicillins, fourth-generation cephalosporins, carbapenems, aminoglycosides, clindamycin, tetracyclines, glycopeptides, streptogramins, oxazolidones, pyrazinamide, rifamycins, chloramphenicol, metronidazole and polymyxin B
Important	Antimicrobial drugs which meet criterion 3 and/or 4 and/or 5	First- and second-generation cephalosporins, cephamycins, monobactams, quinolones

[a]Source: reference 33.

tance (52). Curative treatment and (single-dose) surgical prophylaxis should be the standard, whereas purely preventive treatments should be avoided. Metaphylaxis is only appropriate in clearly defined circumstances when there is a potential for high morbidity due to rapidly spreading disease, as e.g., in current aquaculture and poultry production systems. Even in countries where antimicrobial growth promoters are banned, e.g., in the European Union as of 2006, prophylaxis via large oral group treatments remains routine practice in livestock (52). Whenever possible, individual treatment should be preferred to group or mass treatment, and this also applies for metaphylactic purposes (53). In addition, the use of antimicrobials as feed additives, still allowed in many European countries, causes cross-contamination at different levels and should be discouraged as much as possible (54). To justify appropriate off-label use and assess the public health risks involved (26), the mandatory reporting of off-label use in the future is inherent to responsible use of medication. Mandatory recording is already in place in many European Union member states. Oral group treatments are frequently under- and sometimes overdosed (26, 55), and underlying misevaluation of body weight or dosing instructions should be avoided.

Veterinarians require good advisory skills to address farmers' questions, concerns, and needs related to antimicrobials (51). Adequate sampling and antimicrobial susceptibility testing of organisms at the site of infection is encouraged when symptoms are not indicative of a specific pathogen.

A delay in laboratory results has historically led to empiric broad-spectrum approaches, followed by de-escalation or switching agents. Such additional selection pressure might even aggravate the disorder due to unforeseen multiplication of pathogens due to inactivity and will extend the abundance of resistance determinants present. The development of rapid and reliable patient-side tests (56) should be encouraged. Some mild clinical infections, if supported by adequate diagnostic procedures, can even be cured without antimicrobials, as described for *Rhodococcus equi* infections in foals (57). At the herd level, sample size guidelines should be developed and training given, ideally by syndrome or disease complex. Independent and clinical examination of all animals involved remains the cornerstone of good and responsible veterinary practice and, thus, responsible use of antimicrobial drugs. In countries where monitoring and benchmarking of antimicrobial prescribing has been installed, a substantial decrease in consumption has been documented (58). Illegal use of antimicrobial compounds should be penalized.

Monitoring and Surveillance

For as long as patient-side and on-farm diagnostics do not identify pathogens and susceptibilities during clinical examination, antimicrobial therapy will be guided by the experience of the veterinarian and the history of the animals involved. Regular consultation of monitored resistance trends can further justify the administration of certain antimicrobial classes or compounds. This should not be limited to commensal bacteria (*E. coli*, enterococci) due to substantial differences between trends and resistance rates across production systems and organ systems and depending on whether pathogens are tested (55). In countries where antimicrobial consumption has decreased, monitoring programs made it possible to find some significant relationships with decreasing resistance (58, 59).

Reference centers can validate the susceptibility result in the function of the clinical breakpoint (MIC that bridges susceptible versus resistant isolates). Reference centers also should give guidance on the involvement of pathogens that cannot readily be cultured under routine laboratory conditions (e.g., *Lawsonia intracellularis*, *Brachyspira* spp., *Mycoplasma* spp., and *Ornithobacterium rhinotracheale*).

Marketing authorization holders should provide guidance on identification and susceptibility testing. Multiresistance monitoring should also be integrated in programs to adjust for linked resistance genes (plasmids, transposons, integrons) and horizontal gene transfer. These pathways can easily increase the spread resistance, but if the presence of linked genes and horizontal gene transfer is declining, they also can slow down and even lower the AMR reservoir (59). Defined targets for the reduction of antimicrobial use and benchmarking of farms should be aligned with surveillance of AMR at the appropriate level (farm, veterinary practice, production type, region, country). Zoonotic organisms (e.g., livestock-associated methicillin-resistant *S. aureus*) should be included (60–62). The role of the food industry and that of consumer organizations will likely increase with regard to surveillance and monitoring, including off-label use. Surveillance data of all kinds should be readily available for time-series research purposes, ideally in a global context (31).

CONCLUSION

The challenge of combating AMR has increased the already existent complexity of licensing and approval of antimicrobial agents for use in animals. This article has summarized the evolving data requirements and processes necessary to obtain the marketing authorization for a new antimicrobial agent for use in animals. Due to the possible impact of antimicrobial resistance on animal and public health, a risk assessment framework is currently used in the approval of veterinary medicinal products containing antimicrobial substances.

Citation. Pomba C, Catry B, Edo JT, Jukes H. 2018. Licensing and approval of antimicrobial agents for use in animals. Microbiol Spectrum 6(4):ARBA-0016-2017.

References

1. **Randell AW, Whitehead AJ.** 1997. Codex Alimentarius: food quality and safety standards for international trade. *Rev Sci Tech* **16:**313–321.

2. **VICH (International Cooperation on Harmonisation of Technical Requirements for Registration of Veterinary Medicinal Products).** 2003. VICH Harmonized Tripartite Guideline GL27. Guidance on pre-approval information for registration of new veterinary medicinal products for food producing animals with respect to antimicrobial resistance. http://www.vichsec.org/guidelines/pharmaceuticals/pharma-safety/antimicrobial-safety.html.

3. **VICH (International Cooperation on Harmonisation of Technical Requirements for Registration of Veterinary Medicinal Products).** 2008. VICH Harmonized Tripartide GL43. Target animal safety for veterinary pharmaceutical products. http://www.vichsec.org/guidelines/pharmaceuticals/pharma-safety/environmental-safety.html.

4. **U.S. Department of Health and Human Services, Public Health Service, Food and Drug Administration Center For Veterinary Medicine.** 1996. CVM GFI #49. Target animal safety and drug effectiveness studies for anti-microbial bovine mastitis products (lactating and non-lactating cow products). https://www.fda.gov/AnimalVeterinary/GuidanceComplianceEnforcement/GuidanceforIndustry/ucm053411.htm.

5. **European Medicines Agency.** 2017. Guideline on the conduct of efficacy studies for intramammary products for use in cattle. EMA/CVMP/344/1999-Rev.2. http://www.ema.europa.eu/docs/en_GB/document_library/Scientific_guideline/2017/01/WC500220206.pdf.

6. **Storey S.** 2005. Challenges with the development and approval of pharmaceuticals for fish. *AAPS J* **7:**E335–E343.

7. **VICH (International Cooperation on Harmonisation of Technical Requirements for Registration of Veterinary Medicinal Products).** 2001. VICH harmonized tripartide guideline GL6. Environmental impact assessment (EIAS) for veterinary medicinal products (VMPS) - ECOTOXICITY PHASE I. http://www.vichsec.org/guidelines/pharmaceuticals/pharma-safety/environmental-safety.html.

8. **VICH (International Cooperation on Harmonisation of Technical Requirements for Registration of Veterinary Medicinal Products).** 2004. VICH harmonized tripartide GL38. Environmental impact assessment (EIAs) for veterinary medicinal products (VMPs): ecotoxicity phase II. http://www.vichsec.org/guidelines/pharmaceuticals/pharma-safety/environmental-safety.html.

9. **Joint FAO/WHO Expert Committee on Food Additives (JECFA).** 2016. Guidance document for the establishment of acute reference dose (ARfD) for veterinary drug residues in food. http://www.who.int/foodsafety/chem/jecfa/Guidance_ARfD.pdf.

10. **Spaepen KRI, Van Leemput LJJ, Wislocki PG, Verschueren C.** 1997. A uniform procedure to estimate the predicted environmental concentration of the residues of veterinary medicines in soil. *Environ Toxicol Chem* **16:**1977–1982.

11. **Manaia CM.** 2017. Assessing the risk of antibiotic resistance transmission from the environment to humans: non-direct proportionality between abundance and risk. *Trends Microbiol* **25:**173–181.

12. **VICH (International Cooperation on Harmonisation of Technical Requirements for Registration of Veterinary Medicinal Products).** 2009. VICH harmonized tripartide guideline GL33. Studies to evaluate the safety of residues of veterinary drugs in human food: general approach to testing. http://www.vichsec.org/guidelines/pharmaceuticals/pharma-safety/toxicology.html.

13. **VICH (International Cooperation on Harmonisation of Technical Requirements for Registration of Veterinary Medicinal Products).** 2002. VICH harmonized tripartite guideline GL31. Studies to evaluate the safety of residues of veterinary drugs in human food: repeat-dose (90-day) toxicity testing. http://www.vichsec.org/guidelines/pharmaceuticals/pharma-safety/toxicology.html.

14. **VICH (International Cooperation on Harmonisation of Technical Requirements for Registration of Veterinary Medicinal Products).** 2004. VICH harmonized tripartite guideline GL37. Studies to evaluate the safety of residues of veterinary drugs in human food: repeat-dose (chronic) toxicity testing. http://www.vichsec.org/guidelines/pharmaceuticals/pharma-safety/toxicology.html.

15. **VICH (International Cooperation on Harmonisation of Technical Requirements for Registration of Veterinary Medicinal Products).** 2001. VICH harmonized tripartite guideline GL22. Studies to evaluate the safety of residues of veterinary drugs in human food: reproduction testing. http://www.vichsec.org/guidelines/pharmaceuticals/pharma-safety/toxicology.html.

16. **VICH (International Cooperation on Harmonisation of Technical Requirements for Registration of Veterinary Medicinal Products).** 2001. VICH harmonized tripartite guideline GL23. Studies to evaluate the safety of residues of veterinary drugs in human food: genotoxicity testing. http://www.vichsec.org/guidelines/pharmaceuticals/pharma-safety/toxicology.html.

17. **VICH (International Cooperation on Harmonisation of Technical Requirements for Registration of Veterinary Medicinal Products).** 2002. VICH harmonized tripartite guideline GL32. Studies to evaluate the safety of residues of veterinary drugs in human food: developmental toxicity testing. http://www.vichsec.org/guidelines/pharmaceuticals/pharma-safety/toxicology.html.

18. **VICH (International Cooperation on Harmonisation of Technical Requirements for Registration of Veterinary Medicinal Products).** 2012. VICH harmonized tripartite guideline GL36. Studies to evaluate the safety of residues of veterinary drugs in human food: general approach to establish a microbiological ADI. http://www.vichsec.org/

guidelines/pharmaceuticals/pharma-safety/antimicrobial--safety.html.

19. VICH (International Cooperation on Harmonisation of Technical Requirements for Registration of Veterinary Medicinal Products). 2016. VICH harmonized tripartide GL54. Studies to evaluate the safety of residues of veterinary drugs in human food: general approach to establish an acute reference dose (ARfD). http://www.vichsec.org/guidelines/pharmaceuticals/pharma-safety/toxicology.html.

20. VICH (International Cooperation on Harmonisation of Technical Requirements for Registration of Veterinary Medicinal Products). 2011. VICH harmonized tripartite guideline GL46.Studies to evaluate the safety of residues of veterinary drugs in human food: developmental toxicity testing. http://www.vichsec.org/guidelines/pharmaceuticals/pharma-safety/metabolism-and-residue-kinetics.html.

21. European Medicines Agency. 2016. Guideline for the demonstration of efficacy for veterinary medicinal products containing antimicrobial substances. EMA/CVMP/627/2001-Rev.1. http://www.ema.europa.eu/docs/en_GB/document_library/Scientific_guideline/2016/02/WC500200984.pdf.

22. European Medicines Agency. 2010. Guideline on statistical principles for veterinary clinical trials. EMA/CVMP/EWP/81976/2010. http://www.ema.europa.eu/docs/en_GB/document_library/Scientific_guideline/2010/09/WC500097081.pdf.

23. VICH (International Cooperation on Harmonisation of Technical Requirements for Registration of Veterinary Medicinal Products). 2000. VICH harmonized tripartite guideline GL9. Good clinical practice. http://www.vichsec.org/guidelines/pharmaceuticals/pharma-efficacy/good-clinical-practice.html.

24. Australian Pesticides and Veterinary Medicines Authority. 2009. Veterinary Manual of requirements and guidelines. Part 10. Special data: antibiotic resistance.

25. Graveland H, Wagenaar JA, Heesterbeek H, Mevius D, van Duijkeren E, Heederik D. 2010. Methicillin resistant *Staphylococcus aureus* ST398 in veal calf farming: human MRSA carriage related with animal antimicrobial usage and farm hygiene. *PLoS One* 5:e10990.

26. Persoons D, Haesebrouck F, Smet A, Herman L, Heyndrickx M, Martel A, Catry B, Berge AC, Butaye P, Dewulf J. 2011. Risk factors for ceftiofur resistance in *Escherichia coli* from Belgian broilers. *Epidemiol Infect* 139:765–771.

27. Vose D, Acar J, Anthony F, Franklin A, Gupta R, Nicholls T, Tamura Y, Thompson S, Threlfall EJ, van Vuuren M, White DG, Wegener HC, Costarrica ML, Office International des Epizooties ad hoc Group. 2001. Antimicrobial resistance: risk analysis methodology for the potential impact on public health of antimicrobial resistant bacteria of animal origin. *Rev Sci Tech* 20:811–827.

28. World Organisation for Animal Health (OIE). 2011. *Terrestrial Animal Health Code, chapter 6.10.* www.oie.int/doc/ged/D10905.pdf.

29. Codex Alimentarius Commission. 2005. Code of practice to minimize and contain antimicrobial resistance. CAC/RCP 61-2005. http://www.fao.org/input/download/standards/10213/CXP_061e.pdf.

30. Codex Alimentarius Commission. 2011. Guidelines for risk analysis of foodborne antimicrobial resistance. CAC/GL 77-2011. www.fao.org/input/download/standards/11776/CXG_077e.pdf.

31. World Trade Organization. 2018. The WTO agreement on the application of sanitary and phytosanitary measures (SPS agreement). https://www.wto.org/english/tratop_e/sps_e/spsagr_e.htm#fnt1.

32. U.S. Department of Health and Human Services Food and Drug Administration Center for Veterinary Medicine. 2003. Evaluating the safety of antimicrobial new animal drugs with regard to their microbiological effects on bacteria of human health concern. CVM GFI # 152. https://www.fda.gov/downloads/AnimalVeterinary/GuidanceComplianceEnforcement/GuidanceforIndustry/-UCM052519.pdf.

33. European Medicines Agency. 2015. Guideline on the assessment of the risk to public health from antimicrobial resistance due to the use of an antimicrobial veterinary medicinal product in food-producing animals. EMA/CVMP/AWP/706442/2013. http://www.ema.europa.eu/docs/en_GB/document_library/Scientific_guideline/2015/03/WC500183774.pdf.

34. Health Canada, Veterinary Drugs Directorate. 2005. Current thinking on risk management measures to address antimicrobial resistance associated with the use of antimicrobial agents in food-producing animals. http://www.hc-sc.gc.ca/dhp-mps/vet/antimicrob/amr-ram_reprap_06_05-eng.php.

35. Joint Expert Technical Advisory Committee on Antibiotic Resistance (JETACAR). 1999. *The Use of Antibiotics in Food-Producing Animals: Antibiotic-Resistant Bacteria in Animals and Humans.* Appendix 8. Antibiotic imports to Australia, 1992-97. Commonwealth Department of Health and Aged Care and Commonwealth Department of Agriculture, Fisheries and Forestry, Canberra, Australia.

36. EMEA/CVMP. 2006. Reflection paper on the use of fluoroquinolones in food producing animals: precautions for use in the SPC regarding prudent use guidance. EMEA/CVMP/416168/2006-FINAL). http://www.ema.europa.eu/docs/en_GB/document_library/Other/2009/10/WC500005173.pdf.

37. EMEA/CVMP. 2009. Revised reflection paper on the use of 3rd and 4th generation cephalosporins in food producing animals in the European Union: development of resistance and impact on human and animal health. EMEA/CVMP/SAGAM/81730/2006-Rev.1. http://www.ema.europa.eu/docs/en_GB/document_library/Scientific_guideline/2009/10/WC500004307.pdf.

38. EMA/CVMP. 2011. Reflection paper on the use of macrolides, lincosamides and streptogramins (MLS) in food-producing animals in the European Union: development of resistance and impact on human and animal health. http://www.ema.europa.eu/docs/en_GB/document_library/Scientific_guideline/2011/11/WC500118230.pdf.

39. EMA/CVMP. 2010. Opinion following an Article 35 referral for all veterinary medicinal products containing quinolones including fluoroquinolones intended for use in food-producing species. http://www.ema.europa.eu/ema/index.jsp?curl=pages/medicines/veterinary/referrals/

Quinolones_containing_medicinal_products/vet_referral_000039.jsp&mid=WC0b01ac05805c5170.

40. **EMA/CVMP.** 2012. Opinion following an Article 35 referral for all veterinary medicinal products containing systemically administered (parenteral and oral) 3rd and 4th generation cephalosporins intended for use in food producing species. http://www.ema.europa.eu/ema/index.jsp?curl=pages/medicines/veterinary/referrals/Cephalosporins/vet_referral_000056.jsp&mid=WC0b01ac05805c5170.

41. **European Medicines Agency.** 2013. Reflection paper on the risk of antimicrobial resistance transfer from companion animals. EMA/CVMP/AWP/401740/2013. http://www.ema.europa.eu/docs/en_GB/document_library/Scientific_guideline/2015/01/WC500181642.pdf.

42. **Pomba C, Rantala M, Greko C, Baptiste KE, Catry B, van Duijkeren E, Mateus A, Moreno MA, Pyörälä S, Ružauskas M, Sanders P, Teale C, Threlfall EJ, Kunsagi Z, Torren-Edo J, Jukes H, Törneke K.** 2017. Public health risk of antimicrobial resistance transfer from companion animals. *J Antimicrob Chemother* 72:957–968.

43. **World Health Organization, Advisory Group on Integrated Surveillance of Antimicrobial Resistance (AGISAR).** 2016. *Critically Important Antimicrobials for Human Medicine*, 4th rev. 2013. http://apps.who.int/iris/bitstream/10665/251715/1/9789241511469-eng.pdf?ua=1.

44. **WHO.** 2017. WHO guidelines on use of medically important antimicrobials in food-producing animals. World Health Organization, Geneva, Switzerland.

45. **World Organisation for Animal Health.** 2015. OIE list of antimicrobial agents of veterinary importance. http://www.oie.int/fileadmin/Home/eng/Our_scientific_expertise/docs/pdf/Eng_OIE_List_antimicrobials_May2015.pdf.

46. **European Medicines Agency.** 2014. Answers to the requests for scientific advice on the impact on public health and animal health of the use of antibiotics in animals. EMA/381884/2014. http://www.ema.europa.eu/docs/en_GB/document_library/Other/2014/07/WC500170253.pdf.

47. **European Medicines Agency.** 2016. Sales of veterinary antimicrobial agents in 29 European countries in 2014. EMA/61769/2016. http://www.ema.europa.eu/docs/en_GB/document_library/Report/2016/10/WC500214217.pdf.

48. **European Medicines Agency, Committee for Medicinal Products for Veterinary Use (EMA/CVMP).** Opinion following an Article 35 referral for veterinary medicinal formulations containing colistin at 2 000 000 IU per ml and intended for administration in drinking water to food producing species. http://www.ema.europa.eu/docs/en_GB/document_library/Referrals_document/Colistin_35/WC500093733.pdf.

49. **Catry B, Cavaleri M, Baptiste K, Grave K, Grein K, Holm A, Jukes H, Liebana E, Navas AL, Mackay D, Magiorakos A-P, Romo MAM, Moulin G, Madero CM, Pomba MCMF, Powell M, Pyörälä S, Rantala M, Ružauskas M, Sanders P, Teale C, Threlfall EJ, Törneke K, Van Duijkeren E, Torren Edo J.** 2015. Use of colistin-containing products within the European Union and European Economic Area (EU/EEA): development of resistance in animals and possible impact on human and animal health. *Int J Antimicrob Agents* 46:297–306.

50. **Catry B, Threlfall J.** 2009. Critically important antimicrobial–or not? *Clin Infect Dis* 49:1961–1962, author reply 1962–1963.

51. **RONAFA.** 2017. EMA and EFSA Joint Scientific Opinion on measures to reduce the need to use antimicrobial agents in animal husbandry in the European Union, and the resulting impacts on food safety. *EFSA J* 15:e4666.

52. **Pardon B.** 2012. Morbidity, mortality and drug use in white veal calves with emphasis on respiratory disease. PhD thesis, Ghent University, Ghent, Belgium.

53. **Catry B, Duchateau L, Van de Ven J, Laevens H, Opsomer G, Haesebrouck F, De Kruif A.** 2008. Efficacy of metaphylactic florfenicol therapy during natural outbreaks of bovine respiratory disease. *J Vet Pharmacol Ther* 31:479–487.

54. **Filippitzi ME, Sarrazin S, Imberechts H, Smet A, Dewulf J.** 2016. Risk of cross-contamination due to the use of antimicrobial medicated feed throughout the trail of feed from the feed mill to the farm. *Food Addit Contam Part A Chem Anal Control Expo Risk Assess* 33:644–655 10.1080/19440049.2016.1160442.

55. **Catry B, Dewulf J, Maes D, Pardon B, Callens B, Vanrobaeys M, Opsomer G, de Kruif A, Haesebrouck F.** 2016. Effect of antimicrobial consumption and production type on antibacterial resistance in the bovine respiratory and digestive tract. *PLoS One* 11:e0146488.

56. **Barnum DA, Newbould FH.** 1961. The use of the California mastitis test for the detection of bovine mastitis. *Can Vet J* 2:83–90.

57. **Giguère S.** 2017. Treatment of infections caused by *Rhodococcus equi*. *Vet Clin North Am Equine Pract* 33:67–85.

58. **NethMap.** 2016. Consumption of antimicrobial agents and antimicrobial resistance among medically important bacteria in The Netherlands in 2015. http://www.wur.nl/upload_mm/0/b/c/433ca2d5-c97f-4aa1-ad34-a45ad522d-f95_92416_008804_NethmapMaran2016+TG2.pdf.

59. **Hanon J-B, Jaspers S, Butaye P, Wattiau P, Méroc E, Aerts M, Imberechts H, Vermeersch K, Van der Stede Y.** 2015. A trend analysis of antimicrobial resistance in commensal *Escherichia coli* from several livestock species in Belgium (2011–2014). *Prev Vet Med* 122:443–452.

60. **Catry B, Van Duijkeren E, Pomba MC, Greko C, Moreno MA, Pyörälä S, Ruzauskas M, Sanders P, Threlfall EJ, Ungemach F, Törneke K, Munoz-Madero C, Torren-Edo J, Scientific Advisory Group on Antimicrobials (SAGAM).** 2010. Reflection paper on MRSA in food-producing and companion animals: epidemiology and control options for human and animal health. *Epidemiol Infect* 138:626–644.

61. **DANMAP.** 2016. *DANMAP 2015: Use of Antimicrobial Agents and Occurrence of Antimicrobial Resistance in Bacteria from Food Animals, Food and Humans in Denmark.* http://www.danmap.org/~/media/Projekt%20sites/Danmap/DANMAP%20reports/DANMAP%20%202015/DANMAP%202015.ashx.

62. **Norwegian Ministries.** 2015. National Strategy against Antibiotic Resistance 2015–2020. https://www.regjeringen.no/contentassets/5eaf66ac392143b3b2054aed90b85210/antibiotic-resistance-engelsk-lavopploslig-versjon-for-nett-10-09-15.pdf.

Antimicrobial Resistance in Bacteria from Livestock and Companion Animals
Edited by Frank Møller Aarestrup, Stefan Schwarz, Jianzhong Shen, and Lina Cavaco
© 2018 American Society for Microbiology, Washington, DC
doi:10.1128/microbiolspec.ARBA-0015-2017

Monitoring Antimicrobial Drug Usage in Animals: Methods and Applications

27

Nicole Werner[1], Scott McEwen[2], and Lothar Kreienbrock[1]

INTRODUCTION

To show relationships between the use of antimicrobial agents and the selection and spread of bacteria with resistance characteristics, it is necessary to have access to information about prescription and consumption of antimicrobial drugs in the population to be studied. This requires suitable methods, but also the establishment of figures which adequately describe the use of antimicrobial agents on the level of the enterprise, the veterinarian or the farmer individually, as well as in a cumulative form for countries, regions, or special production forms. The overarching goal of this article, therefore, is to describe the way monitoring systems for antimicrobial drug usage in animals are set up.

Each country applies different systems, and therefore, different calculations for the analysis of data on antimicrobial use are available. As a consequence, the results are not always directly comparable. This article provides an overview of the national and international terminology and variables, summarizes definitions, and identifies those variables that are most suitable for particular objectives.

KEY FIGURES AND VARIABLES TO DESCRIBE ANTIMICROBIAL DRUG USAGE IN ANIMALS

The key figures and variables that are used to describe and evaluate antimicrobial consumption in animals can be divided into categories. Here, the terms and definitions describing antimicrobial consumption are divided into two main categories, following van Rennings et al. (1). The first group defines variables based on quantity. These are terms describing the amount of an active substance administered in grams or kilograms per animal or animal group or per kilogram of body weight of the target animal species. The second group includes variables based on application, defining, for example, the frequency of treatment of a single animal or an animal group with an active substance or drug. To give a better overview of these figures, the glossary (see the Appendix) comprises all given terms.

Key Figures and Variables Based on Quantity

As the first step in characterizing antimicrobial use, we describe variables and measures related to quantity in the broadest sense, in which "dose" and "dosage" are the basic terms.

The dose is the amount of an active substance administered to a single animal in a single application, whereas the dosage corresponds to the amount of active substance applied per kilogram of bodyweight. Based on these terms, the following additional values are defined.

Amount

When analyzing antimicrobial consumption, it is reasonable to first calculate the overall amount applied in the target animal population for every active substance. The (overall) amount is the sum of all doses of one active substance administered to all animals in the target population (e.g., herd, population of a defined region or a country) in kilograms or tons.

The amount is the variable used most often to describe consumption (2), but it does not give detailed information regarding the specific treatment (3, 4). In particular, drugs applied in large doses, such as tetracyclines, may be overrated in their importance, while

[1]Department of Biometry, Epidemiology and Information Processing, WHO Collaborating Centre for Research and Training for Health at the Human-Animal-Environment Interface, University of Veterinary Medicine Hannover, Hannover, Federal Republic of Germany; [2]Department of Population Medicine, Ontario Veterinary College, University of Guelph, Guelph, ON, Canada, N1G 2W1.

drugs applied in small doses may be underrated. Because particularly potent substances such as fluoroquinolones are applied in smaller doses, the presentation of the amount alone might lead to an unintended underrating of their importance (5, 6).

However, taking a look at the amount provides a first overview of the consumption of active substances in different farms, regions, or countries (2). The amount does not give any information about the number or category of animals treated or the route or indication for treatment. Therefore, the interpretation of this variable is limited, and a comparison between animal species and categories is not possible.

Defined daily dose animal (DDDA)

This variable is widely used and was first described as "animal daily dose" in the Danish National Monitoring System for Consumption of Veterinary Drugs (VETSTAT) (7). The term DDDA was recommended by the European Medicines Agency (8). The DDDA describes the average recommended daily dose of an active substance per animal and should be defined for every target animal species, age group, and productive livestock group. The definition is established using specialized information (from drugs containing the same active substance) and expert opinions regarding the main indication for administration of the active substance. It should correspond to the daily dose, which is the assumed average maintenance dose per day for a drug used for a certain indication and animal species. The dose is defined for animals with a standardized body weight that differs depending on the literature source. It has to be kept in mind that the DDDA is a theoretical variable representing an equivalent of application.

The definitions for standardizing the dose are borrowed from the defined daily dose (DDD), which is used in human medicine. According to the WHO, the DDD is "the assumed average maintenance dose per day for a drug used for its main indication in adults" (9). In human medicine, the DDD as a technical measure includes the consumption of all drugs independently from formulation and compound of the single drug, its package size, or from sales data. The DDD is used to compare drug consumption between regions and time periods. It can be applied individually or for trans-boundary comparisons (5, 10).

Some authors use a different definition for DDDA, associating it with the overall amount and the population, thus describing the number of applied doses per animal or person. This can cause confusion and lead to misunderstanding. Therefore, to clearly distinguish between the DDDA and the variable describing the

number of applied doses per animal, for the latter, the term "nDDDA$_{population}$" is recommended (see paragraph on key figures and variables based on application).

Given the lack in veterinary medicine of a variable comparable to the DDD in human medicine, VETSTAT defined the DDDA for every active substance, every animal species, and every age group (11). The DDDA can also be used for comparison of drug consumption between animal groups, veterinary practices, or regions, and it allows for division into animal species, production type, method of application, or indication. In Scandinavia, the DDDA is used regularly to describe amounts of drug consumption.

The Dutch and Belgian counterpart of the DDDA is the DDD (12, 13). Here, it is defined as the daily dose of active substance per animal. In the Dutch monitoring system, there are only data available on the overall amount of active substances used, and no information on the number of treated animals. Using the above-mentioned definition of DDD, the daily dose per animal can be estimated as a mean value per year, i.e., how many kilograms of body weight (kilograms of animal) could be treated with the used amount of active substance by applying the DDD (14).

It is important to note that the DDDA is also an equivalent of application and that it has to be adapted in case of use under practical conditions and known indications. Therefore, calculations based on this measure can only yield estimated values, because the actual dose applied does not always correspond to the recommended one. In the glossary, this is expressed by adding "est" for "estimated" to the term in question.

In addition, it has to be noted that in combination preparations, the DDDA always corresponds exclusively with the main active substance (15), and other active substances of the drug are not considered.

Used daily dose (UDD)

Because the DDDA is a recommended or theoretical variable, Timmerman et al. introduced the UDD (15). This variable was first established in Belgium and displays the actually administered daily dose of one active substance per animal. The UDD can be calculated only from an indicated amount if the number of treated animals and the days of treatment are recorded. The UDD can be estimated for a whole livestock population as an average value per animal by dividing the amount of active substance administered per treatment by the product of the animal count and days of treatment. If the same active substance is used several times in different dosages on a farm, an average dose can be calculated for this farm (15). The UDD is particularly useful for evaluating antimicrobial consumption on the farm level.

Because the DDDA is calculated with an average treatment scenario that may not always reflect the actual field situation, deviations from the UDD are expected. The ratio of UDD and DDDA or UDD and DDD, respectively, described by Timmerman et al. (15) and Persoons et al. (13), compares the actually administered amount with the recommended dosage. By definition, this ratio is not an indicator to establish the correctness of the dosage. Nevertheless, the range of this ratio from 0.8 to 1.25 may be assumed as plausible.

Prescribed daily dose (PDD)

In addition to the DDD and the actually administered UDD, the PDD is the third measure of dose adopted from human medicine, where it is used to describe prescription patterns and offers insights into the habits of individual physicians (10). Because compliance is crucial in the administration of drugs, the ratio between PDD and DDD (physician compliance) and between UDD and PDD (patient compliance) are important measures of consumption.

Arnold et al. (5) used the concept of PDD to evaluate the amount of drug consumption in veterinary medicine. They described PDD as the amount of active substance per prescription divided by the product of average weight, number of treated animals, and days of treatment (in combination preparations every active substance is observed separately). This value has a particular importance in veterinary practice, because depending on the diagnosis of the veterinarian, the active substance can also be dosed individually. In contrast to human medicine (practitioner-patient relation), the definition in veterinary medicine has an additional dimension (veterinarian-farmer-animal relation) and therefore may be used in different settings.

Key Figures and Variables Based on the Course of Application

As a second category, variables indicating whether and how often an antimicrobial drug was used are described here.

Treatment and number of treatments

In the following, as the term is used in Europe, a treatment is the handing over of a drug from the veterinarian to the farmer for its application to the population under study for a defined number of days. The treatment does not consider the number of active substances in the preparation or the number of treatment days. The number of treatments within a certain time period

may represent the number of diseases treated in the population within this time period and is therefore an indicator of animal health in the population.

Single application, sum of single applications, and number of UDDs

The single application can be seen as a basic variable to describe antimicrobial use. It defines the treatment of one animal with one active substance on one day and allows for comparison of applications independently from the prescribed dosage (16). If a drug is applied more often than once a day, this is still seen as only a single application. Hence, if the drug is applied by feed or water, the whole daily ration for one animal represents one single application.

The sum of single applications in a population under study for a given time period is the product of the number of animals treated, the number of days of treatment, and the number of active substances applied. Based on expert consultations at the European Medicines Agency (EMA), this is also described as the number of used daily doses (nUDD) (17).

Regarding preparations with a long-lasting effect, the single application is a variable that requires particular interpretation, because the single application (correlated with duration of effect of one day) is small in comparison to the effect (longer than one day). In such cases, the number of days of treatment may be adjusted with the help of a preparation-specific factor. To evaluate drug consumption, it is more suitable to choose the number of single applications than the amount of used drug in kilograms, because the latter depends on the dosage.

Treatment frequency (TF) and nUDD$_{population}$

The TF indicates for how many days, on average, an animal in the study population is treated within the observation period, e.g., how many single applications were administered to one animal on average (6, 18). Formally, it can also be described as the number of administered UDDs per animal in the study population.

The TF corresponds to cumulative incidence in epidemiology (19). It is independent from the applied amounts and considers the days when an active substance is used. Within the calculation, any observation period can be considered. As a classical ratio, the denominator, i.e., the definition of the population at risk, is of basic importance. Here, several definitions can be used, e.g., the number of places in a farm or the average number of animals present, also taking into account the time present (20).

TF is well suited for comparisons of antimicrobial consumption in the sense of a benchmarking. Because it takes into account the number of active substances in the drug and the days of treatment, it is a value to describe the possibilities in the study population to select resistant bacteria.

Treatment incidence/treatment density

The treatment incidence (TI) described by Timmerman et al. (15) also quantifies the frequency of treatments. Following Persoons et al. (13), the TI is calculated by dividing the overall amount of used active substance by the product of UDDs per kilogram, the overall weight of the treated animals, and the length of the production cycle. Thus, the TI corresponds with the quotient of the product of the number of treated animals and days of treatment, on the one hand, and the product of animals on the farm and the duration of the production cycle on the other hand.

This is an equivalent to the time-at-risk approach in epidemiology, which takes the dynamics within a population into account, and may therefore be denoted as treatment density (21). By definition, the TI is a rate; i.e., it measures consumption per time-at-risk. This time-at-risk displays the sum of all times during which animals were really kept on the farm. When calculating the TI, idle times and periods with different occupancy in a population are included completely. Therefore, the TI shows a more precise picture of the situation within a population under study. But it is important to note that to facilitate the calculation of the TI, much more detailed data have to be collected at the farm level.

If all animals in a population are treated, as is commonly the case for poultry, the TI describes the portion of a production cycle when treatment with the observed active substance takes place.

Sales Data

Sales data are available in many countries and have been widely used since their first application in drug utilization studies (22). These data were first used by the pharmaceutical industry and are still in use for economic purposes. Sales data can be easily obtained from wholesalers, pharmacies, and feed mills, but contain only information on the amount of a product sold (e.g., in tons or kilograms or number of packages) and do not say anything about the species and the number of animals treated or the duration of treatment. Sales data therefore are not appropriate for evaluation of veterinary medical aspects or the relation to antimicrobial resistance. Therefore, it is not recommended to use sales data to evaluate antimicrobial consumption if the purpose is to analyze the impact on selection of antimicrobial resistance. However, as a general measure, sales

data give an overview of the consumption within a population under study.

Nevertheless, sales data can also be used for an overall estimation of the amount of antimicrobial agents that have been consumed in livestock husbandry or in the veterinary sector. In this case, data should always be contrasted to the respective animal population. Because animals differ considerably in their weight, it is not useful to take the number of animals as the value for the animal population. Therefore, standard population figures such as livestock units are usually used (see Glossary).

In Europe, the amounts of veterinary antimicrobial agents sold in different countries are, among others, linked to the animal demographics in each country. The annual sales figures in each country are divided by the estimated weight at treatment of livestock and of slaughtered animals in the corresponding year, taking into account the import and export of animals for fattening or slaughter in another member state. The European Surveillance of Veterinary Antimicrobial Consumption (ESVAC) project introduced a population correction unit (PCU) and expresses sales data in milligrams of active substance/PCU. The PCU is used as the term for the estimated weight, and it is purely a technical unit of measurement, used only to estimate sales corrected by the animal population in individual countries and across countries. In the ESVAC report, 1 PCU = 1 kg of different categories of livestock and slaughtered animals. The data sources used and the methodology for the calculation of PCU are described comprehensively in Appendix 2 of the first report of the EMA (23).

To compare antimicrobial consumption in humans and animals, some countries estimate the biomass of the national human population and use the sales data in milligrams of active substance/kilograms of human and animal biomass/PCU, respectively (for example, the United Kingdom [24] and Sweden [25]).

MONITORING OF ANTIMICROBIAL DRUG USAGE IN FOOD-PRODUCING ANIMALS: SELECTED EXAMPLES

Monitoring Systems in the European Union

Since 2006, the use of antimicrobial substances as growth promoters has been prohibited in the European Union by Regulation (EC) No 1831/2003 on additives for use in animal nutrition (26). The consumption of antimicrobial drugs in livestock is monitored in most European countries, and some countries apply certain measures if the usage of antimicrobial drugs seems inappropriate. Unfortunately, monitoring and surveillance of antimicrobial consumption is not harmonized throughout the European region and not even within the European Union, hampering the comparison of data between countries.

The ESVAC project aims at harmonizing the monitoring of antimicrobial consumption in animals on the European Union level (see passages on "Sales data" and "The ESVAC project"). Some European countries, such as Austria (27), Denmark (28), the Netherlands (29), Norway (30), and Sweden (25), established active monitoring programs years ago, which have been continuously carried out and extended to date. Other countries just started recently. At least information on sales of antimicrobial drugs is collected in most countries, but some countries record more data, enabling in-depth analysis, for example, of target animal species. The variables used and calculated differ in the various systems. Results are usually published in annual reports, mostly together with results from antimicrobial resistance monitoring.

In addition to that, there are also private monitoring systems, such as quality assurance systems, which communicate their data only to the participating farmers and/or veterinarians.

Belgium

The Belgian Veterinary Surveillance of Antibacterial Consumption consortium, founded under the wings of the Belgian Antimicrobial Policy Coordinating Committee, set up surveillance of veterinary antimicrobial consumption in Belgium and started to publish the national consumption report for data from the year 2007. Sales data for all products in all pharmaceutical formulations registered on the Belgian market that contain antimicrobial agents are aggregated. These data are collected from all wholesaler-distributors registered for supplying veterinarians and pharmacies in Belgium with veterinary medicines during the observation period. Reporting is done electronically and is consistent with the Anatomical Therapeutic Chemical (ATC) system for classification of veterinary medicines according to the WHO Collaborating Centre for Drug Statistics Methodology (Norwegian Institute of Public Health). In Belgium, antimicrobial agents are only available by prescription or by delivery from a veterinarian. Information on animal feed containing antimicrobial agents sold to Belgian farms is collected from feed mills, using the same Web-based system. All additional product information in accordance with the ESVAC recommendations is added to the reported data in a database, and

this allows the number of packages sold to be converted to the amount of active substance used. Annual consumption figures with biomass as a yearly adjusted denominator are calculated according to the methodology described by Grave et al. (31). The animal species included are based on the vast majority of the biomass present (estimated to be 92% of the total biomass present in Belgium). This does not include other animal species such as horses, rabbits, small ruminants, and companion animals.

Currently in Belgium, both private (AB register) and governmental (SANITEL MED) herd-level data collection systems are set up that allow for reporting of usage data at the animal species level. For antibacterial premixes, data on animal species are known, and only pigs, poultry, and rabbits receive medicated feed.

Animal population data are taken from Eurostat, and biomass (in kilograms) is calculated, according to the method of Grave et al. (31), as the sum of the amount of beef, pork, and poultry meat produced that year in Belgium plus the number of dairy cattle present in Belgium times 500 kg of metabolic weight per head (32). The Center of Expertise on Antimicrobial Consumption and Resistance in Animals was recently founded in Belgium and became operational on January 2012 (http://www.amcra.be).

Denmark

The Danish Integrated Antimicrobial Resistance Monitoring and Research Program (DANMAP) has monitored antimicrobial resistance and consumption of antimicrobial agents in food animals and in humans in Denmark since 1995. At the beginning, DANMAP published trends on the consumption of antimicrobial agents in production animals based on reports from pharmaceutical companies on their annual sales of veterinary antimicrobial agents to wholesalers without any information on target species (33).

In 2000, VETSTAT was implemented as a second-generation monitoring system based on information on antimicrobial agent consumption at the herd level. Data are entered electronically, and monthly reporting is mandatory for pigs, poultry, cattle, sheep, goats, fish, and mink. Information on pets can be provided on a voluntary basis. Reporters are pharmacies, veterinarians, and feed mills. Information is collected on the reporter, receiver of the antimicrobial agents (e.g., Central Husbandry Register number), ID number of the veterinarian, product number according to the ATCvet list, amount used, animal species, age group, and diagnosis. The overall amount of antimicrobial agent is measured in kilograms of active compound. The VETSTAT system was developed and is maintained by a private contractor (33). From 2003, a national system of animal DDDs for each age group and species determined by VETSTAT was used to measure antimicrobial consumption. The usage was further standardized, taking into account the number of animals in the target population (7).

In 2012, DANMAP introduced new metrics to follow trends in antimicrobial consumption, to ensure the robustness of the analyses over time, and to facilitate comparisons between animal species, as well as comparisons between the veterinary and human sectors by using defined or prescribed animal daily doses. In the context of DANMAP, comparison is based on dosages to keep in focus the newer, potent antimicrobial agents such as fluoroquinolones and cephalosporins that are critically important in the treatment of human infections. Furthermore, the biomass of the live population is used as the denominator to allow for comparisons of selection pressure between animal populations. This follows the concept of nDDDA per biomass, which may be converted to the TF (see Glossary).

In 2010, the Danish Veterinary and Food Administration established the so-called Yellow Card Initiative, a benchmarking system for farmers which was designed to target the highest consumers of antimicrobial agents in pig production. Within this system, thresholds for use of antimicrobial agents were formulated for pig and cattle herds. The threshold is given in Animal Daily Dose per 100 animals per day. When the consumption of antimicrobial agents in a herd exceeds the threshold, the number of annual advisory inspections by a veterinary practitioner increases, and the farmer gets a warning, i.e. a yellow card.

In July 2016, the Differentiated Yellow Card was implemented to also promote responsible use of antimicrobial agents. All classes of antimicrobial agents are assigned a factor, resulting into a so-called Weighted Animal Daily Dose (Weighted ADD). Antimicrobial agents critically important for human medicine, e.g. fluoroquinolones, are assigned factor 10, while simple penicillin is assigned factor 1. Thus, the use of antimicrobial agents with a higher factor accelerates exceeding the threshold for the particular herd (https://www.foedevarestyrelsen.dk/english/Animal/AnimalHealth/Pages/The-Yellow-Card-Initiative-on-Antibiotics.aspx).

France

France has been collecting data on the annual sales of veterinary antimicrobial agents since 1999, and the French Agency for Food Environmental and Occupational Health Safety (ANSES) publishes the results in

annual reports. Data are collected in collaboration with the French Union for the Veterinary Medicinal Product and Reagent Industry, based on annual reporting of antimicrobial sales. These companies also provide an estimated breakdown by target species of the drugs sold. The information collected from the companies covers 100% of authorized drugs. Antimicrobial sales data are compared with other sources of information such as reported turnover from the companies marketing veterinary drugs and data from epidemiological surveys of antimicrobial consumption.

To assess animal exposure to antimicrobial agents, ANSES considers the dosage and duration of administration as well as changes in the animal population over time. As usual in sales data systems, DDDAs per PCU are calculated as well as overall sales figures. By relating the estimates of body weight treated to the mass of the animal population potentially treated with antimicrobial agents, ANSES obtains an estimate of the so-called level of exposure (animal level of exposure to antimicrobial agents, ALEA). This indicator is related to the percentage of animals treated relative to the total population. Data are analyzed for livestock animals, domestic carnivores, horses, and rabbits. In the report, additional indicators are calculated (34) (www.anses.fr).

Germany

In Germany, several systems exist to monitor antimicrobial consumption in livestock animals. Two monitoring systems are official and compulsory, and these include sales data on the one hand and use of antimicrobial agents data on the other hand. Reliable data on total antimicrobial sales were collected for the first time in 2011, based on a legal requirement for the pharmaceutical industry and wholesalers to report total sales data to the German Institute for Medical Documentation and Information (35). Reporting includes information on the annual total sales of veterinary drugs (in tons) containing antimicrobial agents as active substances.

In Germany, veterinarians have the right to dispense and are allowed to obtain drugs from wholesalers and pharmaceutical companies, to deliver drugs to animal owners, and to compound and keep drugs. This activity has to be documented formally by means of the German Medicinal Products Act (in German, Arzneimittelgesetz). Obligatory monitoring of antimicrobial usage was adopted by the 16th amendment of the German Medicinal Products Act in 2014, and reporting started in mid-2014 (36). The variable used to describe antimicrobial consumption is TF. Veterinarians are required to report treatments of animals and the delivery of veterinary drugs to animal owners on specific forms (treatment and delivery forms). With these forms, each application and dispensing of medicine to food-producing animals by the veterinarian is documented for farms with a given minimum number of animals. The farmer has to ensure that twice-a-year reporting is done on time and may designate the veterinarian as the reporter. Reporting is done electronically using the central system HI-Tier (www.hi-tier.de), and data are collected at the farm level on fattening animals (poultry, cattle, and pigs).

The aim of this system is to reduce the usage of antimicrobial agents in fattening animals, and thus the system is used to benchmark the farms. Twice a year, the Federal Office of Consumer Protection and Food Safety calculates two index numbers of the entire distribution of individual farm therapy frequencies, namely, the median and the 75% percentile (www.bvl.bund.de). These index numbers are used to benchmark the farms, and certain measures have to be undertaken if index number 1 or 2 is exceeded. Information on antimicrobial consumption is also summarized in the German report on antimicrobial consumption and antimicrobial resistance in human and veterinary medicine in Germany, GERMAP (37).

The private food quality assurance system, QS Qualität und Sicherheit GmbH, covers all trade levels of meat and meat products from farms to retailers (38). Part of this system involves antimicrobial monitoring for QS members following rules similar to those laid down by legislation and by scientific studies, and with which benchmarking of the participating farms is implemented. The antimicrobial monitoring system has been in place since 2012, and the farmer is responsible for the reporting. The system includes fattening pigs and poultry, and the treatment therapy is registered quarterly. Results are communicated to QS members only.

As a scientific project, the Veterinary Consumption of Antimicrobial Agents (VetCAb) program has collected data from the whole of Germany since 2007 (6, 39). Within this system, participating farmers and veterinarians report the antimicrobial classes used, and this information is collected through the treatment and delivery forms as well.

The Netherlands
The Monitoring of Antimicrobial Resistance and Antimicrobial Usage in Animals in the Netherlands (MARAN) covers two systems of data collection. First, the federation of the Dutch veterinary pharmaceutical industry (FIDIN) reports annually the overall sales of antimicrobial agents. Second, the Wageningen Economic Research Institute of the Wageningen University

and Research (formerly the Landbouw-Economisch Institut, LEI Wageningen UR) monitors the antimicrobial use per animal species. This was first conducted on a stratified sample of farms, but then the large animal production sectors implemented centralized registration systems, monitoring the use on all farms.

Monitoring of annual sales data of all antimicrobial veterinary medicinal products at the level of packages sold in the Netherlands started in 1998. FIDIN reports the total amount of antimicrobial agents (active ingredient in kilograms) sold in the Netherlands at the level of pharmacotherapeutic groups. These data are estimated to cover about 98% of all sales in the Netherlands. Actual consumption can differ from the amounts sold, as a result of stockpiling and cross-border use. The figures give information about the total sales for all animals, not per individual animal species, and are supplemented with antimicrobial veterinary medicinal product data of non-FIDIN members. Since 2011, data have been calculated according to the SDa (Netherlands Veterinary Medicines Authority) method for all antimicrobial veterinary medicinal products, which means only the active base substance mass (excluding the mass of salts and esters) is calculated, including topical applications such as ointments, eye drops, and sprays.

Monitoring of purchased antimicrobial agents on farms in the Farm Accountancy Data Network (FADN) by LEI Wageningen UR started in 2004. In the Netherlands, veterinary antimicrobial agents are sold to the end users (farmers) almost exclusively by veterinarians. Antimicrobial veterinary medicinal product consumption data derived from veterinarians' invoices from farms in the FADN and additional veal calf farmers were used for this survey. In the beginning, the FADN contained a stratified sample of around 1,500 agricultural and horticultural farms in the Netherlands that is representative of Dutch livestock farming (40). On these farms, economic data and key technical figures, all animal medicine data and veterinary services are recorded. This provides information about the true exposure of farm animals to antimicrobial agents and gives insight into the underlying factors that could explain changes in antimicrobial use.

Sales data are converted to the number of defined doses per animal year. Applied antimicrobial veterinary medicinal products are converted to treated animal mass × days by national conversion factors (determined by the nationally authorized dosages and pharmacokinetics of the drug to compensate for duration of action) and related to the animal mass present on a farm. Results are calculated for a period of a year and expressed as the number of days an average animal is treated in that year on that particular farm (DDDA$_F$), which is the TF for one year based on DDDA conversion.

The SDa was established to promote responsible use of veterinary prescription drugs in Dutch animal husbandry. Since 2011, the SDa has prepared husbandry-related consumption reports using consumption data from all farms in the largest sectors of food production animals: pigs, veal calves, broilers, cattle (starting in 2012), and turkeys (starting in 2013). As of 2016, antimicrobial use is also monitored in meat rabbits. Another variable, DDDA$_{NAT}$, is calculated, that represents the days of treatment within one year for an average animal of a certain sector of the whole country. While the calculation method for treated body mass (numerator) is the same, totaled for all farms per sector, the denominator is represented by the whole sector nationwide (29, 41).

Since 2012, the DDDAF is also used to benchmark farms. According to the use of antimicrobials, farms are assigned to a Target, Signaling or Action Zone. The threshold for the Action Zone was first defined as the 75. percentile of the antimicrobial use of the year 2011, splitted into type of farm and sector, and farms exceeding this threshold must take measures to reduce the use immediately. The thresholds are re-evaluated annually since then. A benchmarking method for veterinarians was introduced in March of 2014 and was based on prescription data recorded in 2012. The system aims at documenting prescription patterns of veterinary practitioners and works with the same three benchmark zones, using the Veterinary Benchmark Indicator (VBI) (41).

Sweden

In Sweden, statistics on total sales of antimicrobial agents for use in animals have been available since 1980. Data are compiled through the Swedish Veterinary Antimicrobial Resistance Monitoring (SVARM) system by the National Veterinary Institute. To analyze trends by animal species, information from different sources is used to supplement the sales data.

Overall sales are expressed as kilograms of active substance and are analyzed by the animal population. For antimicrobial agents sold for group treatment in pigs, data are expressed in milligrams of active substance/kilograms of slaughtered pig. In poultry, data are analyzed by calculating milligrams of active compound/kilograms of slaughtered chicken. Raw data on sales are obtained from the Swedish eHealth Agency and represent the sales of products containing antimicrobial agents sold by pharmacies. When products are dispensed for animals, the animal species as given on the prescription is recorded and reported to the Swedish eHealth Agency jointly with the sales, unless the product is sold for use in a veterinary practice (on requisition). For the overall statistics, the data include all products with antimicrobial agents as active substances marketed in Sweden and sold for use in terrestrial animals in certain ATCvet classes. Conclusions on antimicrobial consumption in different animal species or different ways of administration are drawn solely from the sold drugs (e.g., drugs for use in certain animal species or certain ways of administration). In dogs, data are recorded as sold packages. Växa Sweden publishes a yearly report related to the livestock organizations' work to improve animal health and welfare in dairy cows (42). For statistics on the incidence of antimicrobial treatments of dairy cows enrolled in the Swedish milk recording scheme, data are retrieved from a database of veterinarian-reported disease events and treatments (43). Here, antimicrobial use is expressed in treatments per 100 completed/interrupted lactations for systemic treatment of mastitis and in absolute numbers of dose applicators sold for drying off (intramammary use). To compare the consumption of antimicrobial agents in humans and in animals, data are expressed in milligrams per estimated kilograms of biomass, where the animal body mass is estimated by applying the method for calculation of PCU (23). This unit roughly corresponds to the total biomass of major animal populations, excluding dogs and cats.

A review of data from 1980 to 2000 is presented in the report "SVARM 2000." SVARM and Swedres-SVARM reports can be found on the website of the Swedish National Veterinary Institute SVA (http://www.sva.se/en/antibiotics/svarm-reports) (25).

United Kingdom

In the United Kingdom, antimicrobial sales data include antimicrobial agents for systemic, intramammary, and oral use by certain ATCvet code groups of antibiotics. Total annual sales of all veterinary medicines are supplied by marketing authorization holders to the Veterinary Medicines Directorate, where they are collated. From these data, the total weight in tonnes of each antimicrobial active substance is calculated. Data on antimicrobial consumption is estimated in relation to the animal population (livestock, companion animals, and horses) using the PCU as described by ESVAC (24) (www.gov.uk).

Monitoring Systems in non-European Countries

Several non-European countries, including Australia, Canada, Japan, New Zealand and the United States, collect and publish overall veterinary antimicrobial sales data (44–48). Holders of marketing authorizations for veterinary antimicrobial agents are required by law to provide annual quantities (kilograms) sold in each of these countries. In Australia, registrants are requested to estimate proportions used in different species, and Canada, New Zealand, and the United States have declared intentions to follow suit (48, 49). Annual quantities of antimicrobial agents sold are typically reported by drug class, route of administration and, where possible, animal species. Australia, Japan, and New Zealand also provide basic information on numbers of major food animal species in their reports (4- to 5-year intervals) (44, 46, 47). Canadian annual antimicrobial consumption data are adjusted by PCU as developed by ESVAC (45).

Canada and the United States also collect and publish selected species-specific data. The Canadian Integrated Program for Antimicrobial Resistance conducts active surveillance of antimicrobial use on sentinel broiler chicken and grower-finisher pig farms in Canada (45). The numbers of farms included are proportional to the production volume in each participating province. Participation is voluntary, and the farms are recruited by practicing veterinarians, who collect the information on antimicrobial use, herd demographics, and animal health via questionnaires administered to the farmers. For broiler chickens, collected antimicrobial information pertains to sampled flocks, including antimicrobial exposure at the hatchery and farm levels through injection, water, and feed administration. For pigs, antimicrobial use information is limited to the grower-finisher stage of production. Antimicrobial use data are presented qualitatively (broiler chickens, pigs) as antimicrobial exposure by route of administration and quantitatively (pigs, feed administration only) as kilograms of active ingredient per 1,000 pig-days at risk to standardize the number of pigs and duration of treatment (45).

The U.S. Department of Agriculture collects farm-level information on antimicrobial use practices through periodic surveys (50). The National Animal Health Monitoring System conducts nationally representative livestock, poultry, and aquaculture commodity studies that involve voluntary administration of questionnaires to farmers. Major commodities are surveyed at 5- to 7-year intervals, and information on farm management and policies related to antimicrobial use is collected, including reasons for use, numbers of animals treated, antimicrobial class, and route of administration. The Agricultural Resource Management Survey is a survey of farmers that focuses on farm finances but also periodically collects some information on antimicrobial use

(2004 and 2009 for pigs and 2006 and 2011 for broilers) (50).

International Monitoring Activities

The ESVAC Project
The ESVAC project has become a worldwide leader collecting data on veterinary antimicrobial consumption at the supra-national level.

Background
In 2008, the European Commission requested the EMA to develop a harmonized approach for the collection and reporting of data on the use of antimicrobial agents in animals from European Union and European Economic Area member states, based on national sales figures in at least major species groups such as poultry, pigs, veal, other ruminants, pets, and fish. This also included the identification of already existing data and surveillance systems on the national level in the member states. To ensure an integrated approach, the EMA was asked to also consult other European Union agencies such as European Food Safety Authority (EFSA) and European Centre for Disease Prevention and Control (ECDC), as well as the European Reference Laboratory on Antimicrobial Resistance. Following this request, the ESVAC project started its first activities in 2009.

Reporting
The number of countries reporting data to the ESVAC project increased from 9 in 2009 to 30 in 2015. These countries account for approximately 95% of the food-producing animal population in the region. Reporting takes place on a voluntary basis so far, but a new regulation is envisaged that will make reporting mandatory (51). Currently, the ESVAC project is in a pilot stage, during which harmonized overall sales data are collected and analyzed. The main indicator used to express sales is milligrams of active substance sold per PCU (mg/PCU).

Since 2015, data have been collected through a Web-based system in accordance with the ESVAC data collection protocol (52). Reporting includes product information, information on the animal species, packages sold, information on the active substance (using the ATCvet codes), and the calculation of tons of active substances sold during the year. Additional information is collected using a questionnaire (e.g., source of information, sales or purchase data, version of ATCvet classification used). The groups of veterinary antimicrobial agents to be included in ESVAC are also defined.

Some data are collected not directly from the member states, but from other European Union agencies.

The data source for numbers and biomass of food-producing animals slaughtered, as well as data on livestock food-producing animals is Eurostat, the Statistical Office of the European Union. In cases for which data are not available in Eurostat (e.g., for rabbits), national statistics are applied. For horses (a food-producing species according to European Union legislation), national statistics provided by the ESVAC national representatives are used.

Animals exported for fattening or slaughter in another member state are likely to have been treated with antimicrobial agents in the country of origin, and therefore it is important to correct this for the major species (cattle, pigs, poultry, and sheep). Such data are therefore obtained from the Trade Control and Expert System (TRACES) of the European Union, because these are based on health certificates, which are obligatory for all animals passing any border. The ESVAC data collection form and protocol as well as annual reports and other ESVAC documents are published on the ESVAC website (www.ema.europa.eu).

ESVAC Strategy 2016 to 2020
The EMA has developed an ESVAC strategy for 2016 to 2020. The strategy aims to enable the analysis of European-level trends in antimicrobial usage per animal species using data that is standardized between countries. To reach this goal, the harmonization of data collection and analysis methodologies is crucial. The EMA will provide guidance to member states on the collection of data per species, with a specific focus on the three major food-producing species: pigs, cattle, and broilers (poultry) (53).

The WHO Advisory Group on Integrated Surveillance of Antimicrobial Resistance (AGISAR)
AGISAR supports implementation of WHO's Global Action Plan on Antimicrobial Resistance. With respect to monitoring antimicrobial usage in animals, AGISAR maintains guidance on integrated surveillance of antimicrobial resistance and developing indicators/metrics to assess antimicrobial usage in the food chain in member countries. AGISAR also provides support to WHO capacity-building activities (e.g., training modules, protocols) on integrated surveillance of antimicrobial resistance, including collection of antimicrobial usage data (54).

AGISAR's guidance document on integrated surveillance of antimicrobial resistance is intended to assist countries to develop and maintain integrated programs for surveillance of antimicrobial resistance among foodborne bacteria and relevant antimicrobial use in hu-

mans and animals (55). These programs are needed to study trends in antimicrobial use and resistance, identify the need for interventions to address antimicrobial resistance, and measure the impact of these interventions in both animal and human health. Chapter 2 of the guidance addresses surveillance of the use of antimicrobial agents in animals and humans and builds on prior work of WHO as well as the World Organization for Animal Health (OIE), ESVAC, and individual countries. Three main activities are identified: (i) measuring quantities of antimicrobial agents sold (antimicrobial consumption), (ii) collecting information on antimicrobial prescribing, and (iii) collecting information on the actual intake of antimicrobial agents by humans or animals. Various options to undertake these activities are presented, along with examples of templates or protocols, and these largely comprise the various methods used by individual countries and the European Union, which have been described previously in this chapter, and proposed by the OIE (see the following section on the OIE). Important elements include methods for collection of national antimicrobial sales data and methods for collection of data to the species level from pharmacies, veterinary clinics, or farms (e.g., continuous data collection from pharmacies, longitudinal or point prevalence studies at the farm level, species stratification studies). Guidance is also provided on standardized reporting (e.g., use of indicators such as kilograms of active ingredient or milligrams of active substance per PCU, DDDAs) and integrated analysis and reporting of antimicrobial use and of antimicrobial resistance data from human and animal sectors, including examples from established integrated programs (e.g., DANMAP, Canadian Integrated Program for Antimicrobial Resistance, The National Antimicrobial Resistance Monitoring System [NARMS], and the Joint Interagency Antimicrobial Consumption and Resistance Analysis [JIACRA] Report). For countries planning to undertake integrated surveillance, AGISAR's guidance recommends beginning with a small-scale pilot project for surveillance of antimicrobial use and antimicrobial resistance to serve as a proof-of-principle and to allow further refinement and development of an integrated program. Several important steps for such a pilot project are described: establishing governance, building a situation analysis, planning, implementation, identification of key success factors, and evolution toward integrated analysis and reporting (55).

The OIE
The OIE is responsible for improving animal health globally. The OIE has made several important contributions

to the monitoring of antimicrobial drug usage in animals, including the development of international standards for monitoring and building a global database on the use of antimicrobial agents in animals.

OIE standards for monitoring the quantities and usage patterns of antimicrobial agents used in food-producing animals and aquatic animals are published in the Terrestrial Animal Health Code and Aquatic Animal Health Code, respectively (56, 57). These standards include recommendations that address the objectives of antimicrobial usage monitoring, various sources of antimicrobial use data (e.g., pharmaceutical manufacturers, importers, veterinarians, farmers), the types of data that should be monitored (e.g., weight of active ingredient, dosage regimens, numbers of food-producing animals by species), and options for reporting antimicrobial usage data (e.g., total usage by antimicrobial class, by animal species, and by route of administration). The OIE determined through a 2017 survey that 73% of 146 countries reported quantitative data between 2013 to 2016 (58).

The OIE, WHO, and the Food and Agriculture Organization of the United Nations (FAO) have formed a tripartite collaboration to address antimicrobial resistance in the food chain. As part of this collaboration, the OIE was tasked with developing a global database on the usage of antimicrobial agents in animals (58). The OIE has also committed, in its 2016 Strategy on Antimicrobial Resistance and the Prudent Use of Antimicrobials, to supporting member countries in developing and implementing antimicrobial usage monitoring systems and to building and maintaining an international database for the collection, analysis, and reporting of antimicrobial usage in animals, taking into account the animal populations in each country (59).

A template for the collection of harmonized data was sent to 180 OIE member countries in 2016, and responses were received from 143 (79%) countries, representing all five OIE regions. Results of the survey showed that 59% of responding member countries authorized antimicrobial agents as growth promoters. OIE reported that many countries face challenges in collection of quatitative data on antimicrobial use in animals (58).

The FAO

As mentioned above, the FAO participates with WHO and the OIE in a tripartite collaboration. One of its roles is to support the development of local capacity for surveillance and monitoring of antimicrobial use in the food and agriculture sectors (60).

OVERVIEW OF ANTIMICROBIAL CONSUMPTION IN LIVESTOCK

Due to the huge variety of monitoring systems, it is challenging to provide a harmonized overview of the use of antimicrobial agents around the world. Nevertheless, data from national reports on monitoring antimicrobial consumption in animals are shown here as selected examples; total annual sales are shown in Figure 1. Total sales of antimicrobial agents in the veterinary sector are described in the text along with, where available, data per animal species (pigs, cattle, and poultry). For comparison, one should keep in mind that sales data per animal species are often generated by assuming that a drug is used for one (main) species, even if it is approved for use in other species as well. In addition, differences in reporting at the national level (see "Monitoring of Antimicrobial Drug Usage in Food-Producing Animals: Selected Examples" above) are frequent. Because of these differences, data have to be interpreted with caution and are not directly comparable between countries. For descriptions and results of each monitoring system, the corresponding national reports should also be read. If not stated otherwise, the amount always corresponds to the amount of active compound. As described above, some countries have additional systems in place to monitor the use of antimicrobial agents in certain animal species, using different measures and definitions. A few results from these systems are also presented in "Other Countries" below, where we compare data from selected countries. Data on animal populations, if available, are shown here for pigs, cattle, and poultry.

In general, at least for the European countries, an overall decrease in the amount of antimicrobial agents sold in the veterinary sector has been observed during the past years. The antimicrobial classes sold most often are tetracyclines, penicillins, and sulfonamides. Sales of antimicrobial agents that are critically important for human medicine are usually low and/or show a decreasing trend, but this is not the case for all countries included here.

European Countries

The overall sales of antimicrobial agents in Belgium in 2015 were 260.27 tons according to the Belgian Veterinary Surveillance of Antibacterial Consumption national consumption report 2015 (32). Belgian livestock numbers included 6.4 million pigs and 2.5 million cattle in 2015 (61), as well as 294.71 million slaughtered animals (poultry) in 2014 (62).

In Denmark, the total consumption of antimicrobial agents in the veterinary sector in 2015, including agents

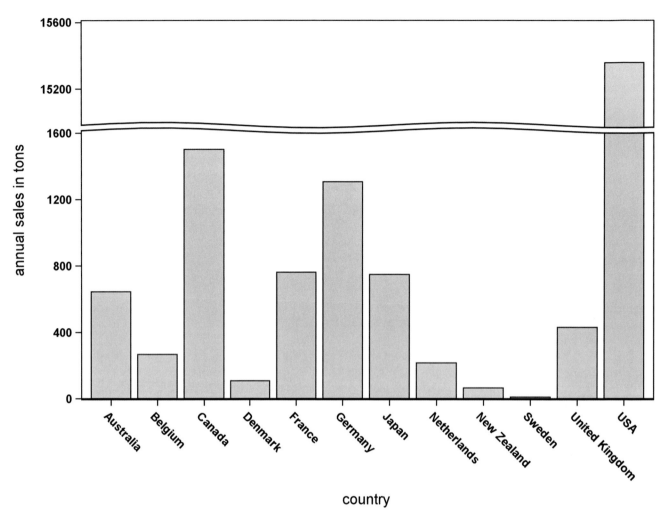

Figure 1 Annual sales of antimicrobial agents in tons (2014; Australian data from 2009/2010). Note that these figures are not adjusted for livestock population sizes and figures for Australia, Canada and the United States include sales of ionophores and/or coccidiostats (see text).

used for companion animals, was 108.6 tons of active compound, showing a 5% decrease from the previous year. The main reason for this was a 5% decrease in antimicrobial usage in the pig industry, which is the main user of antimicrobial agents for animals in Denmark. The total antimicrobial consumption in pigs was 81.5 tons of active compound in 2015, a decrease of 4.5 tons (5%) compared with 2014. The overall consumption of antimicrobial agents in cattle remained at approximately 13 tons, similar to 2014. The total consumption of antimicrobial agents in poultry (all species) was 2.4 tons of active compound, an increase of 58% compared with 2014 due to disease outbreaks in broiler production. This is the highest amount recorded since the DANMAP program began (28). The animal

population in Denmark in 2015 was the following: 12.7 million pigs (63), 522,000 cattle slaughtered, and 561,000 dairy cows, as well as 114.23 million broilers and 598,000 turkeys (28).

In France, a total of 514.26 tons of antimicrobial agents were sold in 2015, of which 185.45 tons were sold for pigs, 124.35 tons for cattle, and 98.98 tons for poultry. This is a 64% decline of sales for pigs compared to 1999, 10.4% for cattle, and 37% for poultry (34). According to Eurostat, the pig population in 2015 consisted of 13.3 million animals—19.4 million cattle (61), 777 million broilers, 49,9 million layers, and 209,9 million other poultry (slaughtered animals) (34).

In Germany, the total sales of antimicrobial agents for usage in animals in 2016 were 742 tons of active compound. Between 2011 and 2016, the amount of sold antimicrobial agents decreased by 56.5%, from 1,706 to 742 tons. From 2015 to 2016, a reduction of 7.8%, or 63 tons of the total sales was recorded. A decrease can also be seen in the sales of antimicrobial agents that are critically important in human medicine (64). The animal population in Germany in 2016 consisted of 12.5 million cattle and 27.4 million pigs; there were 40.2 million layers in 2015 (65).

In the Netherlands, sales of antimicrobial veterinary medicinal products, including topical applications such as ointments, eye drops, and sprays, were 206 tons in 2015. Total sales decreased by 58.4% from 2009 to 2015, while the weight of livestock animals was stable with a small increase during the same period of time. In 2015, the animal population in the Netherlands consisted of 7.59 million pigs, 863,000 turkeys, 49.11 million broilers, 58.64 million other poultry, and 4.27 million cattle (29).

The total sales of antimicrobial agents to the veterinary sector of Sweden were 10.5 tons in 2015. The sales of antimicrobial agents for pigs were 2.13 tons of active substance, compared to 3.37 tons in 2010 (25). The Swedish animal population in 2015 included 1.48 million cattle, 1.36 million pigs, and 9.41 million layers (66).

According to the One Health Report 2015 (24), the total sales of antimicrobial agents for animal use comprised 420 tons in 2013 in the United Kingdom. The livestock population was 4.9 million pigs, 9.8 million cattle, and 163 million poultry in 2013 (67).

Other Countries

In Australia, no distinction is made in data on antimicrobial consumption for therapeutic or prophylactic use. Growth promoters and coccidiostats may be applied without intervention by a veterinarian, and they are listed separately. For the years 2009 to 2010, the total sales of antimicrobial agents for therapeutic and growth promotion purposes (including ionophores and coccidiostats) in food-producing animals were 644.0 tons of active compound in Australia, of which only 288.0 tons were labeled for therapeutic purposes (including prophylactic usage). Of those antimicrobial agents sold for therapeutic purposes, 37.6 tons were sold for cattle and sheep, 160.9 tons for poultry, and 89.4 for pigs. The numbers of livestock in 2013 were 1.74 million pigs, 12.12 million cattle, and 108.4 million chickens according to the inventory of the Australian Bureau of Statistics (68).

In Canada, antimicrobial agents are used in productive animals for the treatment and prevention of disease and to improve feed efficiency/promote growth. In 2014, 1,500 tons of antimicrobial active ingredients (including ionophores and coccidiostats) were sold in the veterinary sector. This number is 5% higher than in 2013 but 12% lower than reported in 2006. From 2010 to 2014, there was a 1% increase. After adjusting for animal populations and weights (PCU), overall sales of antimicrobial agents for use in animals in Canada were relatively stable over the period of 2006 to 2012. (69). The livestock population in 2015 included 8.5 million cattle, 27.9 million pigs, and 630.6 million poultry (70).

In Japan, the overall amount of antimicrobial agents sold for use in animals in 2013 was approximately 780 tons of active compound. Additionally, around 200 tons of feed additives were distributed, including ionophores. The number of slaughtered animals in 2013 was 1.19 million cattle, 16.94 million pigs, 653.99 million broilers, and 86.23 million other poultry (47).

The total sales of antimicrobial agents in 2014 in New Zealand were 64.44 tons. Livestock numbers in this country in 2014 included 8.5 million cattle, 672,108 pigs slaughtered, 118 million broilers, and 3.85 million layers (46).

The total annual domestic sales of antimicrobial agents (including ionophores) to the veterinary sector in 2015 in the United States were 15,577 tons of active compound, including drug applications labeled for both food-producing and non-food-producing animals. From 2009 through 2015, domestic sales and distribution of antimicrobial agents approved for use in food-producing animals increased by 24%, and they increased by 1% from 2014 through 2015. Reporting on estimates of amounts sold per animal species started in 2016. The U.S. population of productive animals comprised 68.3 million pigs (1 December 2015), 91.99 million cattle (1 January 2016), 349.57 million layers during the year, 8.69 billion broilers, and 233.1 million turkeys (1 December 2015) (71).

As shown in "Monitoring of Antimicrobial Drug Usage in Food-Producing Animals: Selected Examples," countries calculate or estimate different variables to describe and analyze antimicrobial consumption in the veterinary sector and/or animal husbandry. Also, there are differences in the legal framework that determines the method of reporting, the responsibilities, and the kind of data collected, even if looking solely at sales data. Additionally, some countries also apply a benchmarking of farms and/or veterinarians, which might influence the choice of antimicrobial classes and number of treatments. All these facts are important to know when interpreting data.

Moreover, sales data have to be seen in relation to the animal population in the country in question. Animal populations can be estimated from different data (slaughtered animals, number of animals at a certain date, average number of animals throughout the year, etc.) and expressed by different measures (e.g., heads, kilograms live weight, kilograms slaughtered animals), and there is no harmonized approach on a global level. Detailed information on how the animal populations are estimated in each country can be found in the respective national reports.

Within the ESVAC project, a harmonized calculation of European data is possible. Figure 2 shows the PCU-corrected overall sales for food-producing animals (including horses) in milligrams per PCU (mg/PCU), by country, for the year 2014 (72). It can be seen that sales data differ significantly between countries. In Scandinavia, sales are very low in comparison to all other countries. The highest sales are reported in Spain, Cyprus, and Italy. However, the data presented here are limited in their informative value, because many factors are not considered in the calculation. For example, the compositions of the animal populations in the countries play an important role, as do the husbandry systems. Thus, any comparison is poor as long as systems for data collection, reporting, and calculation of variables are not harmonized and do not take into account use data by animal species. Until harmonization is reached on an international level, every system has to be looked at separately, especially when interpreting trends over time. All important background information has to be taken into account when analyzing the results of each monitoring system.

FINAL REMARKS

The monitoring of antimicrobial drug usage in animals has now been established in several countries, but there is still a long way to go before most countries around

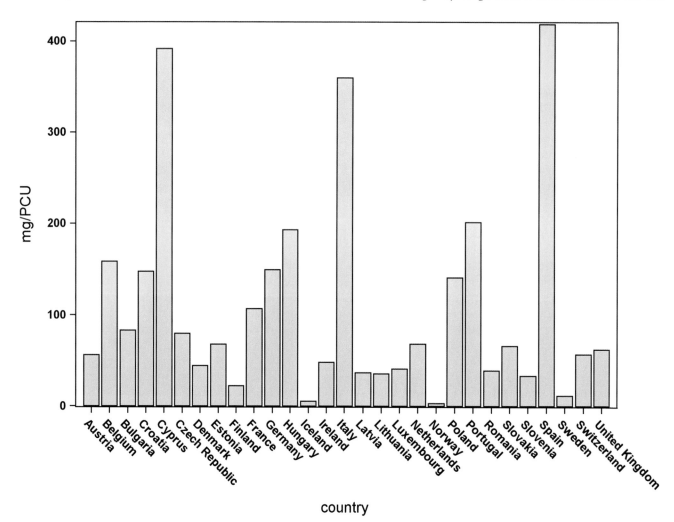

Figure 2   PCU-corrected sales data (mg/PCU) according to the ESVAC report 2016 (72)

the world have systems in place for the collection, analysis, and reporting of comprehensive antimicrobial use data. This is essential so that we have much better information on the types and quantities of antimicrobial agents that are being used in the various animal species around the world. We need this information for improving awareness, identifying opportunities for improved antimicrobial stewardship, assisting in the interpretation of antimicrobial resistance, and assessing the effectiveness of efforts to reduce unnecessary antimicrobial use. Antimicrobial resistance is a global problem, and to effectively address it we need a global program for integrated surveillance of antimicrobial use and resistance in animals and humans. Improved surveillance of this type is a cornerstone of the WHO Global Action Plan on Antimicrobial Resistance, as it is of many other international organizations and individual countries.

A very few countries have sophisticated, centralized, comprehensive antimicrobial use monitoring systems based on high-quality data from one or more of a variety of sources, including pharmaceutical companies, pharmacies, veterinarians, and farmers, covering most if not all animal species and humans. Most other countries, however, currently obtain and report little more than very basic national sales data. As described previously, when coupled with animal population data and stratified to at least the species level, these sales data can provide useful information on overall trends and enable very basic interpretations of antimicrobial resistance data and simple comparisons between countries. However, to accomplish other important functions, such as benchmarking of antimicrobial use at the level of veterinary practices and farms, it is necessary to comprehensively monitor use at those levels. This is much more challenging and requires the cooperation and support of many affected parties so that the necessary high-quality and refined data are collected, shared, analyzed, and utilized in a timely manner. The most progress to date has been made in Europe, where there is longer national-level experience with antimicrobial use monitoring. In addition, directives related to antimicrobial use monitoring have been issued at the European Union level, requiring member states to collect and report use data. Furthermore, the ESVAC project has provided important guidance and support for collection and reporting of use data. In addition, many European countries have capitalized on the prescription-only availability of antimicrobial agents and mandatory treatment record-keeping by veterinarians and farmers in the development of their monitoring systems. Unfortunately, the situation is different in many countries outside of Europe, and they may have to develop other approaches for their monitoring systems. More broadly, there is a need for research and development regarding technologies for collection, sharing, and reporting of antimicrobial use data at the user level. There is also a need for innovation and engagement of veterinary and producer organizations to improve motivation and compliance among end users with regard to data collection and sharing.

Eventually, antimicrobial use monitoring should extend from the major food animal species and humans to include fish, aquaculture, and all other animal and plant species that are treated with antimicrobial agents. This is important from a public health point of view, because companion animals, in particular, have close contact with people, including highly vulnerable populations, but it is also important for animal health, to improve the long-term effectiveness of antimicrobial agents for the treatment of infections in animals.

Acknowledgments. We thank Maria Hartmann for her support in generating Fig. 1. We also express our thanks to Ren Isomura for her assistance with Japanese data.

Citation. Werner N, McEwen SA, Kreienbrock L. 2018. Monitoring antimicrobial drug usage in animals: methods and applications. Microbiol Spectrum 6(4):ARBA-0015-2017.

APPENDIXES Glossary of Terms and Definitions Describing Antimicrobial Drug Usage in Animals (modified from reference 1)

Term	Definitions, interpretation, and Examples
Part I: General terms and definitions	
Animal Unit: number	Definition: animal kept or place. Interpretation: If looking at a period of time, one should consider the overall number of animals kept during this period (e.g., over several production cycles; see below). It is also possible to calculate an average number of animals.

LSU
Livestock unit
Unit: (standardized) number
	Definition: The number of livestock units is calculated based on their live weight by using appropriate conversion keys, taking into account the different groups of productive livestock, age, and usage categories. The reference unit used for the calculation of livestock units (1 LSU) is the grazing equivalent of one adult dairy cow producing 3,000 kg of milk annually, without additional concentrated foodstuffs. One LSU is equivalent to 500 kg live weight. The conversion keys for LSUs indicated in different literature sources are diverse.
	Interpretation: Livestock unit is a measure that can be calculated for every animal species and that allows comparison between different kinds of livestock.
	Example: LSU coefficients according to EUROSTAT [source: http://ec.europa.eu/eurostat/statistics-explained/index.php/Glossary:Livestock_unit_(LSU)]:
	
	Bovine animals
	    Under 1 year old: 0.400
	    Over 1 but less than 2 years old: 0.700
	    Male, 2 years old and over: 1.000
	    Heifers, 2 years old and over: 0.800
	    Dairy cows: 1.000
	    Other cows, 2 years old and over: 0.800
	Sheep and goats: 0.100
	Equidae: 0.800
	Pigs
	    Piglets with a live weight of under 20 kg: 0.027
	    Breeding sows weighing 50 kg and over: 0.500
	    Other pigs: 0.300
	Poultry
	    Broilers: 0.007
	    Laying hens: 0.014
	    Ostriches: 0.350
	    Other poultry: 0.030
	Rabbits, breeding females: 0.020

ESVAC PCU	The PCU is used by ESVAC as a proxy for the size of the animal population of a country. Definition: The PCU for each animal category is calculated by multiplying the number of livestock animals (dairy cows, sheep, sows, and horses) and slaughtered animals (cattle, goat, pigs, sheep, poultry, rabbits, and turkeys) by the theoretical weight at the most likely time for treatment according to Appendix 2 of the ESVAC report for 2005–2009.

Interpretation: The PCU is used as the term for estimated weight. It is purely a technical unit of measurement, used only to estimate sales corrected by the animal population in individual countries and across countries. In the ESVAC report, 1 PCU = 1 kg of different categories of livestock and slaughtered animals.

Example: The PCU is calculated for each species, weight class, and/or production type. Here we take an example for pigs of country X.

PCU domestic:

- Number of pigs slaughtered × estimated weight at treatment: 10,000 × 65 kg = 650,000 kg
- Number of livestock sows × estimated weight at treatment: 240 kg: 3,000 × 240 kg = 720,000 kg

PCU export:

- Number of animals transported to another country for fattening × estimated weight at treatment: 1,000 × 25 kg = 25,000 kg

PCU import:

- Number of animals imported from another country for slaughter × estimated weight at treatment: 500 × 65 kg = 32,500 kg

Total PCU pigs = total PCU$_{Domestic}$ + total PCU$_{Export}$ − total PCU$_{Import}$:

Total PCU pigs = (650,000 kg + 720,000 kg) + 25,000 kg − 32,500 kg = 1,362,500.00 kg

TAR
Time at risk (on a farm)
Unit: (animal) days

Definition: The sum of the lifetime (in days) of all single animals on a farm within a defined period of time.

Interpretation: The duration of stay of an animal on a farm may be shorter than the observation period. The TAR compensates for this problem by recording the duration of stay on a farm in days for every animal.

TAR is a term that originates from human medicine, where it is also called "person time." In Switzerland it is also called "animal years at risk," meaning the time during which an animal could be treated.

Example: 10,000 animals are kept in a broiler farm for 35 days. Afterwards, 2,000 animals are housed out, while the other animals stay another 5 days. For a time period of 40 days this results in

TAR (farm) = (10,000 broilers × 35 days) + (8,000 broilers × 5 days) = 390,000 (animal) days

If, subsequently, the farm is subject to a service period of 10 days, during which no animals are kept, this time at risk is valid also for the time period of 50 days.

Withdrawal time
Unit: days

Definition: The minimum time that has to be followed after a drug has been administered to an animal until this animal can again be used for food production.

Interpretation: The adherence to a defined withdrawal time ensures that maximum residual limits of pharmacologically active substances in food are not exceeded.

Duration of effect
Unit: days

Definition: The period during which a therapeutically effective level of active substance is present at the target site. The duration of effect depends on the drug and the affected organ system (see also one-shot products)

(Production) cycle

Definition: A group of animals (herd) that is at once housed in an empty stable or compartment, fattened, and housed out. Some of the animals may also be housed out earlier than the rest.

Interpretation: In livestock farming, the administration of drugs is often recorded in relation to the production cycle. During evaluations, one should carefully choose the time period and number of housed animals during this period. If data on housing in and out and on the number of animals per production cycle are not available, it is possible to estimate the number of animals by using the number of animal places and overall assumptions on the number of production cycles per year.

(Continued)

APPENDIXES (*Continued*)

Term	Definitions, interpretation, and Examples
	Example: In Germany, the following average numbers are currently valid (source: KTBL, Betriebsplanung Landwirtschaft 2012/2013): Pig: weaner (8.1–28 kg) = 6.89 fattening cycles/stable/year Pig: fattening pig (28–118 kg) = 2.83 fattening cycles/stable/year Poultry: broilers = 7.46 fattening cycles/stable/year Poultry: laying hens = 0.90 cycles/stable/year Poultry: turkey = 2.17 fattening cycles/stable/year
ATC code	Definition: Anatomical therapeutic chemical (ATC) classification system for drugs of the WHO. Interpretation: The classification of active substances is based on the organ system where they are effective (e.g., cardiovascular or gastrointestinal system) and the classes of active substances. Therefore, several ATC codes exist for some substances due to their application in different organ systems (e.g., six for tetracycline). The first letter of the ATC code indicates the anatomic group (1. level); the following double figure, the therapeutic subgroup (2. level); the next letter marks the pharmacological subgroup (3. level); and the last letter, the chemical subgroup (4. level). The 5. level indicates the chemical substance. Example: For tetracycline, the following six ATC codes exist: A01AB13, D06AA04, J01AA07, S01AA09, S02AA08, S03AA02. J01AA07 is the ATC code for systemically applied tetracycline.
ATCvet code	Definition: This system is based on the ATC code from human medicine and has been adapted for veterinary purposes. Interpretation: As a general rule, each ATC code starts with a Q. For veterinary purposes, additional codes are defined if necessary. Example: The following codes exist for oxytetracycline: QD06AA03 (local application), QG01AA07 (gynecological application), QJ01AA06 (systemic application), QS01AA04 (ophthalmologic application).
Combination products	Definition: Combination products contain two or more active substances (e.g., antibiotic substances), that complement each other in their effect. Interpretation: The analysis of such products should be done by active substance. Active substances with a supportive effect to the antibiotic, which have no bactericidal or bacteriostatic effect clinically themselves, are not analyzed separately. Example: Penicillin in combination with streptomycin is analyzed as a combination product of two antibiotics. Amoxicillin in combination with clavulanic acid is not regarded as a combination product, because clavulanic acid has no antibiotic effect.
Products with long-term effects One-shot products	Definition: These are drugs that maintain a constant level of active substance for considerably more than 24 h (up to several days) after one application and that are administered less than once a day. There is no definite labeling of these products. Interpretation: With these drugs, a long duration of effect is reached with a single application or a few applications. When analyzing antibiotic consumption, attention should be paid to these products, because their application should not alter results. The indicated duration of effect should be multiplied by an appropriate factor to adequately display the real duration of effect.

Part II: Terms and definitions based on quantities

Dose
Unit: mg or g per animal

Definition: The amount of active substance administered to a single animal in one application.
Interpretation: The dose depends on the administered active substance, animal species, body weight, and disease to be treated.

Dosage
Unit: mg/kg body weight

$$Dosage = \frac{Dose}{Animal\ weight}$$

Definition: The amount of an active substance administered in one application per kg bodyweight.
Interpretation: The dosage depends on the active substance administered. The dosage of the respective active substance per animal allows calculation of the dose, and it facilitates comparison of the treatment amount independently from the body weight of individual animal.

DDDA (defined daily dose animal)
ESVAC defined daily dose for animals
DDDvet
Unit: mg or g per animal per day

Definition: The DDDA is the average recommended daily maintenance dose of an active substance per animal and is defined for every target animal species, age group, and productive livestock group. The definition is established using specialized information (from drugs containing the same active substance) and expert opinions regarding the main indication the active substance is administered for. The dose is defined for animals with a standardized body weight that differs depending on the literature source.
Interpretation: The principles of standardization of doses comply with the calculation of the DDD in human medicine, where the dose is calculated for a man of 70 kg body weight for every ATC code.
The DDDA was first established in Denmark with the abbreviation ADD (7). In the Netherlands, the concept of DDDA is applied under the term DDD in veterinary medicine. An international procedure was published by the EMA within the ESVAC activity. ESVAC, in 2016, prioritized establishing DDD for animals (DDDvet) values for antimicrobials used in three major food-producing animal species: pigs, cattle, and broilers (poultry). The values are based on average daily dose of active substance according to the manufacturer's instructions. They take account of differences in dosing, pharmaceutical form, and route of administration used in the different species.

DDDA$_{kg}$ (DDDA per kg)
Unit: mg/kg body weight

Definition: The average recommended maintenance dosage of an active substance per kg body weight of a target animal species; it corresponds to the recommended dose.

UDD (used daily dose)
Unit: mg or g per animal and day

Definition: The daily dose of an active substance per animal which is actually administered by the farmer or the veterinarian.

UDD$_{population}$ (used daily dose per population)
Unit: kg

$$UDD = \frac{Overall\ amount\ of\ active\ substance\ administered\ in\ the\ animal\ population}{No.\ of\ animals \times days\ of\ treatment}$$

Amount (of active substance)

Definition: The sum of UDDs of an active substance in the observed population (e.g., in a herd).
Interpretation: The amount of an applied active substance depends on the number of treated animals and on the dose chosen by the veterinarian.
When analyzing the amount, drugs administered in very high doses (e.g., tetracycline) are overestimated in their relevance, but drugs administered in very low doses are underestimated. Because the modern active substances in particular (e.g., fluoroquinolones) are usually administered in low doses, the situation can be misinterpreted when looking at the amounts.
Example 1: Treatment of 100 sucklers at 15 kg over 5 days with tetracycline (recommended reference dose: 85 mg/kg):
Amount = 100 sucklers × 15 kg × 85 mg/kg × 5 days = 640 g
Example 2: Treatment of 100 sucklers at 15 kg over 3 days with enrofloxacin (recommended reference dose: 2.5 mg/kg):
Amount = 100 sucklers × 15 kg × 2.5 mg × 3 days = 11.25 g

UDD$_{kg}$ (UDD per kg)
Unit: mg/kg body weight and day

Definition: The actually administered dosage of an active substance per day and per kg body weight of the treated animal species.

(Continued)

APPENDIXES (Continued)

Term	Definitions, interpretation, and Examples
$UDD_{kg} = \dfrac{\text{Overall amount of active substance administered in the animal population}}{\text{No. of animals} \times \text{body weight} \times \text{days of treatment}}$	Interpretation: The UDD_{kg} animal allows comparison between populations regarding the active substance. It has to be taken into account that these comparisons can only be done for one active substance and that it is not possible to draw overall conclusions regarding antibiotic usage including more than one active substance. If the applied dosage is estimated from overall amounts, this is done usually on the basis of a standardized average animal weight that can differ depending on the source of the literature. In this case UDD_{kg} turns to an estimate due to the unknown body weights in the actual case of treatment. Note, in addition, that standard body weights are not harmonized in the literature.
$UDD_{kg\ est} = \dfrac{\text{Overall amount of active substance administered in the animal population}}{\text{No. of animals} \times \text{standard weight} \times \text{days of treatment}}$	
PDD (prescribed daily dose) Unit: mg or g per animal and day	Definition: The daily dose of an active substance per animal as prescribed by the veterinarian. Interpretation: The PDD originates from human medicine and helps to describe prescribing patterns. In Germany the prescription by the veterinarian and the administration of a drug (on the farm) are recorded simultaneously on the same form. The determination of UDD and PDD therefore usually leads to identical results.
$UDD = \dfrac{\text{Overall amount of active substance prescribed for the animal population}}{\text{No. of animals} \times \text{days of treatment}}$	

Part III: Terms and definitions based on applications

Term	Definitions, interpretation, and Examples
Single application (= application unit) nUDD (number of used daily doses) Unit: number nUDD (sum of single applications) = treated animals × days of treatment × active substance(s)	Definition: The application of one active substance (or sometimes one drug) in one animal on one day. From this, the sum of all single applications in a population under observation over the observation period is calculated. Interpretation: This term quantifies the real application frequency of active substances (or drugs) and days. The number of nUDDs depends on the applied drug, the number of days of treatment, and the number of animals treated. If a drug is applied more often than once a day, this is seen as only a single application. Hence, if the drug is applied by feed or water, the whole daily ration represents one application. The term is usually not related to the active substance and is summarized from all applications. But nUDD for specific active components or even for special drugs under study may be calculated with the same concept. Example 1: Treatment of 100 pigs over 5 days with tetracycline (mono preparation): nUDD = 100 pigs × 5 days × 1 active substance = 500 single applications Example 2: Treatment of 100 pigs over 5 days with sulfadimethoxine and trimethoprim (combination preparation): nUDD = 100 pigs × 5 days × 2 active substances = 1,000 single applications
Adjusted single application (by duration of effect) nUDD_adjust (number of adjusted used daily doses) Unit: number nUDD_adjust = treated animals × factor × active substance	Definition: For drugs with a long-acting effect, the single application should be adjusted by multiplication with a preparation-specific factor. This factor should take into account the time over which an antibiotic effect is expected. Interpretation: This term allows comparison between applications of preparations with long-term effects and other drugs. Currently, there is no official list of long-acting products. Therefore, there is also no access to up-to-date information on preparation-specific factors, and information on levels of effect (in organs) is often absent. So, for the time being, the factor should be chosen so that it corresponds to the average duration of treatment that is expected when using a classic preparation.

TF (treatment frequency)
Unit: single application/animal
$nUDD_{population}$ (number of used daily doses per population)

$$TF = \frac{\text{Sum of single applications}}{\text{Number of animals cared for in population}}$$

Definition: The TF indicates on how many days on average an animal in a population is treated with an active substance (or drug).

Interpretation: The TF is independent from the applied amount and exclusively considers the application of active substances (or drugs). For every treatment, the sum of single applications in a population is divided by the number of animals in that population.

Different time periods can be considered in the calculation by adding all single applications of a period defined in one farm and dividing it by the number of animals kept on the farm during this period.

The TF is a population-based value, which is comparable directly between farms and regions and years. For the application of drugs (without considering the number of active substances included), the TF is sometimes called the animal treatment index.

If applying drugs with a long-acting effect, the number of adjusted single applications may be used in the calculation.

Example 1: Treatment of 100 out of 500 pigs in a farm over 5 days with tetracycline (mono preparation):
TF = (100 pigs × 5 days × 1 active substance)/500 pigs = 1
I.e., on average, every animal in the population was treated for one day with one active substance.

Example 2: Treatment of 100 out of 500 pigs over 5 days with penicillin and streptomycin (combination preparation):
TF = (100 pigs × 5 days × 2 active substances)/500 pigs = 2
I.e., on average, every pig in the population was treated for two days with one active substance.

TI (treatment incidence/treatment density)
Unit: %

$$TI = \frac{\text{Total amount of drugs}}{UDD \times \text{duration of production cycle} \times \text{total weight of animals treated}}$$

$$= \frac{nUDD}{\text{Duration of production cycle} \times \text{number of animals within population}}$$

$$= \frac{\text{Sum of single applications}}{\text{Duration of production cycle} \times \text{number of animals within population}}$$

Definition: The TI is calculated by dividing the overall amount of the applied active substance by the product of the UDD, the overall weight of the treated animals, and the duration of the production cycle.

Interpretation: If the UDD is not known exactly and has to be estimated from the total amount, the TI is calculated as the overall number of UDDs over the duration of the production cycle times the number of animals in the population. For a flock or a farm in which all animals are treated (e.g., an oral treatment for all poultry) the TI again simplifies to the ratio of the number of days treated to the number of days at risk. With this, TI can be interpreted as the percentage treated time at risk.

Example: See above, calculation of treatment density):
TI = (10,000 broilers × 7 days)/390,000 (animal) days = 0.179
I.e., 17.9% of the time at risk, a treatment took place.

Overview of National Monitoring Systems for Antibiotic Consumption

Country	Name of monitoring system or report	Since	Responsible for reporting	Frequency of reporting	Voluntary or mandatory	Type of data	Major metric	Animal species
AU	Quantity of antimicrobial products sold for veterinary use in Australia	Earlier than 2005	Pharmaceutical companies	Annually	Voluntary	Sales data	Total annual sales by species in kg active substances	Food-producing animals, companion animals
BE	BelVet-SAC	2007	Wholesalers, distributors, feed mills	Annually	Mandatory	Sales data	Total sales in mg active substances per kg biomass	Predominantly livestock
BE	AB register (private)	Not yet				Use data		
BE	SANITEL MED (official)	Not yet				Use data		
CA	CIPARS	2006	Pharmaceutical companies	Annually	Voluntary	Sales data	Total annual sales by species in kg active substances	Food-producing animals, companion animals
DE	AMG (official)	2014	Farmers	Half-yearly	Mandatory	Use data	Treatment Frequency (TF)	All fattening animals (cattle, pigs, poultry)
DE	QS (private)	2012	Farmers	Quarterly	Voluntary	Use data	Therapy index (TI)	Fattening animals (pigs, poultry)
DE	DIMDI-AMV (official)	2011	Pharmaceutical companies, wholesalers	Annually	Mandatory	Sales data	Total annual sales in kg active substances	All animals
DK	DANMAP/VETSTAT	1995/2000	Pharmacies, vets, feed mills	Monthly	Mandatory	Sales data/ use data	DADD, DAPD	Food-producing animals and mink; voluntary: pets
FR		1999	Pharmaceutical labs	Annually	Voluntary	Sales data	Total annual sales by species in mg active substances per kg bodyweight; ALEA, number of ACDkg, number of ADDkg	Livestock animals, domestic carnivores, horses, rabbits, fish
JP	JVARM	1999	Pharmaceutical companies	Annually	Mandatory	Sales data	Total annual sales by species in kg active substances	Food-producing animals

Country	Program/Report	Year	Source	Frequency	Type	Data	Description	Animals covered
NL	MARAN	See following rows						
NL	FIDIN	1998	Pharmaceutical companies	Annually	Voluntary	Sales data	Total annual sales in kg active substances	Food-producing animals
NL	FADN (LEI)	2004–2011	Veterinarians	Annually	Voluntary	Use data	Defined doses per animal year on a farm	Pigs, veal calves, broilers, cattle (sentinel farms)
NL	FADN (SDa)	2011	Veterinarians	Annually	Mandatory	Use data	$DDDA_F$, $DDDA_{NAT}$ per sector (species, production group)	Pigs, veal calves, broilers, cattle, turkeys; pets (certain drugs); mink and rabbits from 2016/2017
NZ	2011–2014 Antibiotic sales analysis	2010/2011	Pharmaceutical companies	Annually	Mandatory	Sales data	Total annual sales by species in kg active substances	Food-producing animals, companion animals
SE	SVARM	1980	Pharmacies	Annually	Mandatory	Sales data	Total sales in mg per PCU; sales in mg active substances (or other unit) per species	All terrestrial animals
UK	One Health report	Earlier than 2011	Pharmaceutical companies	Annually?	Mandatory	Sales data	Total sales in mg active substances per PCU	Livestock, horses, companion animals
USA	FDA, Summary Report On Antimicrobials Sold or Distributed for Use in Food-Producing Animals	2009	Pharmaceutical companies	Annually	Mandatory	Sales data	Total sales in kg active substances	Food-producing animals

References

1. van Rennings L, Merle R, von Münchhausen C, Stahl J, Honscha W, Käsbohrer A, Kreienbrock L. 2013. Variablen zur Beschreibung des Antibiotikaeinsatzes beim Lebensmittel liefernden Tier. *Berl Munch Tierarztl Wochenschr* **126**:297–309.

2. Chauvin C, Querrec M, Perot A, Guillemot D, Sanders P. 2008. Impact of antimicrobial drug usage measures on the identification of heavy users, patterns of usage of the different antimicrobial classes and time-trends evolution. *J Vet Pharmacol Ther* **31**:301–311.

3. Chauvin C, Madec F, Guillemot D, Sanders P. 2001. The crucial question of standardisation when measuring drug consumption. *Vet Res* **32**:533–543.

4. Grave K, Kaldhusdal MC, Kruse H, Harr LMF, Flatlandsmo K. 2004. What has happened in Norway after the ban of avoparcin? Consumption of antimicrobials by poultry. *Prev Vet Med* **62**:59–72.

5. Arnold S, Gassner B, Giger T, Zwahlen R. 2004. Banning antimicrobial growth promoters in feedstuffs does not result in increased therapeutic use of antibiotics in medicated feed in pig farming. *Pharmacoepidemiol Drug Saf* **13**:323–331.

6. Merle R, Hajek P, Käsbohrer A, Hegger-Gravenhorst C, Mollenhauer Y, Robanus M, Ungemach F-R, Kreienbrock L. 2012. Monitoring of antibiotic consumption in livestock: a German feasibility study. *Prev Vet Med* **104**:34–43.

7. Jensen VF, Jacobsen E, Bager F. 2004. Veterinary antimicrobial-usage statistics based on standardized measures of dosage. *Prev Vet Med* **64**:201–215.

8. European Medicines Agency. 2013. *Revised ESVAC reflection paper on collecting data on consumption of antimicrobial agents per animal species, on technical units of measurement and indicators for reporting consumption of antimicrobial agents in animals.* European Medicines Agency, London, United Kingdom.

9. WHO Collaborating Centre for Drug Statistics Methodology. 2012. *Guidelines for ATC classification and DDD assignment 2013.* WHO, Oslo, Norway. https://www.whocc.no/filearchive/publications/1_2013guidelines.pdf.

10. Merlo J, Wessling A, Melander A. 1996. Comparison of dose standard units for drug utilisation studies. *Eur J Clin Pharmacol* **50**:27–30.

11. Agersø Y, Hald T, Helwigh B, Borck Høg B, Jensen LB, Jensen VF, Korsgaard H, Larsen LS, Seyfarth AM, Struve T, Hammerum AM, Kuhn KG, Lambertsen LM, Larsen AR, Laursen M, Nielsen EM, Olsen SS, Petersen A, Skjøt-Rasmussen L, Skov RL, Torpdahl M. 2011. *DANMAP 2010: Use of Antimicrobial Agents and Occurrence of Antimicrobial Resistance in Bacteria from Food Animals, Food and Humans in Denmark.* National Food Institute, Søborg, Denmark.

12. MARAN. 2011. *MARAN-2009: Monitoring of Antimicrobial Resistance and Antibiotic Usage in Animals in the Netherlands in 2009.* Central Veterinary Institute of Wageningen University and Research Center, Wageningen, The Netherlands.

13. Persoons D, Dewulf J, Smet A, Herman L, Heyndrickx M, Martel A, Catry B, Butaye P, Haesebrouck F. 2012. Antimicrobial use in Belgian broiler production. *Prev Vet Med* **105**:320–325.

14. Mollenhauer Y. 2010. *Verbrauchsmengenerfassung von Antibiotika bei Lebensmittel liefernden Tieren in landwirtschaftlichen Betrieben im Kreis Kleve.* Dr. med. vet. Stiftung Tierärztliche Hochschule Hannover, Hannover, Germany.

15. Timmerman T, Dewulf J, Catry B, Feyen B, Opsomer G, de Kruif A, Maes D. 2006. Quantification and evaluation of antimicrobial drug use in group treatments for fattening pigs in Belgium. *Prev Vet Med* **74**:251–263.

16. Hajek P, Merle R, Käsbohrer A, Kreienbrock L, Ungemach FR. 2010. Antibiotikaeinsatz in der Nutztierhaltung. Ergebnisse der Machbarkeitsstudie "VetCAb". *Dt Tierärzteblatt* **4**:476–480.

17. European Medicines Agency (EMA). 2013. *Overview of comments received on draft ESVAC reflection paper on collecting data on consumption of antimicrobial agents per animal species, on technical units of measurement and indicators for reporting consumption of antimicrobial agents in animals (EMA/286416/2012).* Division VM, European Medicines Agency, London, United Kingdom. http://www.ema.europa.eu/docs/en_GB/document_library/Other/2013/10/WC500152313.pdf.

18. Anonymous. 2011. *Bericht über den Antibiotikaeinsatz in der Landwirtschaftlichen Nutztierhaltung in Niedersachsen.* Niedersächsisches Miniterium für Ernährung, Landwirtschaft, Verbraucherschutz und Landesentwicklung und Niedersächsisches Landesamt für Verbraucherschutz und Lebensmittelsicherheit, Hannover, Germany.

19. Dohoo I, Martin W, Stryhn H. 2009. *Veterinary Epidemiologic Research*, 2nd ed, **vol 2.** VER Inc., Charlottetown, Canada.

20. EMA. 2013. *Revised ESVAC reflection paper on collecting data on consumption of antimicrobial agents per animal species, on technical units of measurement and indicators for reporting consumption of antimicrobial agents in animals.* European Medicines Agency, London, United Kingdom. http://www.ema.europa.eu/docs/en_GB/document_library/Scientific_guideline/2012/12/WC500136456.pdf.

21. Porta MS, Greenland S, Hernán M, dos Santos Silva I, Last JM. 2014. *A Dictionary of Epidemiology.* Oxford University Press.

22. Dukes MNG. 1993. *Drug Utilization Studies, Methods and Uses.* WHO Regional Office Europe, Copenhagen, Denmark.

23. European Medicines Agency. 2011. *Trends in the Sales of Veterinary Antimicrobial Agents in Nine European Countries (2005–2009).* European Medicines Agency, London, United Kingdom.

24. Public Health England. 2015. *UK One Health Report. Joint Report on Human and Animal Antibiotic Use, Sales and Resistance, 2013.* Public Health England, London, United Kingdom.

25. SVARM. 2015. *SWEDRES/SVARM 2015: Consumption of Antibiotics and Occurrence of Antibiotic Resistance in Sweden.* Public Health Agency of Sweden and National Veterinary Institute, Solna/Uppsala, Sweden.

26. **Anonymous.** Regulation (EC) No. 1831/2003 of the European Parliament and of the Council on Additives for Use in Animal Nutrition. Official Journal L 268, 18 October 2003.29-43.

27. **Bundesministerium für Gesundheit und Frauen (BMGF).** 2016. *Resistenzbericht Österreich, AURES 2015. Antibiotikaresistenz und Verbrauch antimikrobieller Substanzen in Österreich.* Bundesministerium für Gesundheit und Frauen. BMGF, Vienna, Austria.

28. **DANMAP.** 2016. *DANMAP 2015: Use of Antimicrobial Agents and Occurrence of Antimicrobial Resistance in Bacteria from Food Animals, Food and Humans in Denmark.* Microbiology and Infection Control, Statens Serum Institute; National Food Institute, Technical University of Denmark, Søborg/Coopenhagen, Denmark.

29. **MARAN.** 2015. *MARAN: Monitoring of Antimicrobial Resistance and Antibiotic Usage in Animals in The Netherlands in 2014.* Central Veterinary Institute, Wageningen University and Research Center (CVI), Lelystad, The Netherlands.

30. **NORM/NORM-VET.** 2016. *NORM/NORM-VET 2015. Usage of Antimicrobial Agents and Occurrence of Antimicrobial Resistance in Norway.* Norwegian Food Safety Authority, Norwegian Veterinary Institute, Tromsø/Oslo, Norway.

31. **Grave K, Torren-Edo J, Mackay D.** 2010. Comparison of the sales of veterinary antibacterial agents between 10 European countries. *J Antimicrob Chemother* 65: 2037–2040.

32. **BelVetSAC.** 2016. *Belgian Veterinary Surveillance of Antibacterial Consumption National Consumption Report 2015.* Veterinary Epidemiology Unit, Faculty of Veterinary Medicine, Ghent University; Federal Agency for Medicines and Health Products, Merelbeke/Brussels, Belgium.

33. **Stege H, Bager F, Jacobsen E, Thougaard A.** 2003. VETSTAT: the Danish system for surveillance of the veterinary use of drugs for production animals. *Prev Vet Med* 57:105–115.

34. **Moulin G, Chevance A.** 2016. *Sales survey of veterinary medicinal products containing antimicrobial agents in France in 2015.* French Agency for Food, Environmental and Occupational Health & Safety (ANSES) and French Agency for Veterinary Medicinal Products (ANMV), Paris, France.

35. **DIMDI-AMV.** 2010. *Verordnung über das datenbankgestützte Informationssystem über Arzneimittel des Deutschen Instituts für Medizinische Dokumentation und Information (DIMDI-Arzneimittelverordnung - DIMDI-AMV).* BGBl. I S. 140. Bundesministerium für Gesundheit, Bundesministerium für Ernährung, Landwirtschaft und Verbraucherschutz, Bonn, Germany. http://bundesrecht.juris.de/dimdiamv/index.html.

36. **Anonymous.** 2013. *Sechzehntes Gesetz zur Änderung des Arzneimittelgesetzes,* Bundesgesetzblatt *Teil I Nr. 62.*

37. **GERMAP.** 2016. *GERMAP 2015: Bericht über den Antibiotikaverbrauch und die Verbreitung von Antibiotikaresistenzen in der Human- und Veterinärmedizin in Deutschland.* Bundesamt für Verbraucherschutz und Lebensmittelsicherheit (BVL), Paul-Ehrlich-Gesellschaft für Chemotherapie, Rheinbach, Germany.

38. **Anonymous.** 2015. *QS Antibiotikamonitoring bei Schweinen, Mastgeflügel und Mastkälbern.* https://www.q-s.de/tieraerzte/antibiotikamonitoring-tieraerzte.html.

39. **van Rennings L, von Münchhausen C, Ottilie H, Hartmann M, Merle R, Honscha W, Käsbohrer A, Kreienbrock L.** 2015. Cross-sectional study on antibiotic usage in pigs in Germany. *PLoS One* 10:e0119114.

40. **Vrolijk HCJ, van der Veen HB, van Dijk JPM.** 2010. *Sample of Dutch FADN 2008: Design principles and quality of the sample of agricultural and horticultural holdings.* LEI Wageningen UR, The Hague, The Netherlands.

41. **SDa Autoriteit Diergeneesmiddelen.** 2016. *Usage of Antibiotics in Agricultural Livestock in the Netherlands in 2015: Trends, Benchmarking of Livestock Farms and Veterinarians, and a Revision of the Benchmarking Method.* The Netherlands Veterinary Medicines Authority, Utrecht, The Netherlands.

42. **Växa Sverige.** 2016. Account of the Livestock Organisation's Animal Health Services 2014/2015. (In Swedish.)

43. **Mörk MJ, Wolff C, Lindberg A, Vågsholm I, Egenvall A.** 2010. Validation of a national disease recording system for dairy cattle against veterinary practice records. *Prev Vet Med* 93:183–192.

44. **APVMA.** 2014. *Quantities of antimicrobial products sold for veterinary use in Australia.* Australian Pesticides and Veterinary Medicines Authority, Canberra, Australia.

45. **Canada Government.** 2015. *Canadian Integrated Program for Antimicrobial Resistance Surveillance (CIPARS) 2013 Annual Report,* Chapter 1. Design and methods. Public Health Agency of Canada, Guelph, Ontario, Canada.

46. **Ministry for Primary Industries.** 2016. *2011–2014 Antimicrobial sales analysis.* Ministry for Primary Industries, Wellington, New Zealand.

47. **JVARM.** 2016. *Report on the Japanese veterinary antimicrobial resistance monitoring system 2012 to 2013.* National Veterinary Assay Laboratory (NVAL). Ministry of Agriculture, Forestry and Fisheries, Tokyo, Japan.

48. **FDA.** 2016. *Summary report on antimicrobial agents sold or distributed for use in food-producing animals.* Food and Drug Administration, Department of Health and Human Services, Washington, DC.

49. **Mehrotra M, Li X-Z, Ireland MJ.** 2017. Enhancing antimicrobial stewardship by strengthening the veterinary drug regulatory framework. *Can Commun Dis Rep* 43(11): 220–223 https://www.canada.ca/en/public-health/services/reports-publications/canada-communicable-disease-report-ccdr/monthly-issue/2017-43/ccdr-volume-43-11-november-2-2017/enhancing-antimicrobial-stewardship-strengthening-veterinary-drug-regulatory-framework.html.

50. **USDA.** 2014. *Antimicrobial resistance action plan.* United States Department of Agriculture, Washington, DC. https://www.usda.gov/documents/usda-antimicrobial-resistance-action-plan.pdf.

51. **European Commission.** 2014. *Proposal for a regulation of the European Parliament and of the Council on Veterinary Medicinal Products.* European Commission, Brussels, Belgium. http://ec.europa.eu/transparency/regdoc/rep/1/2014/EN/1-2014-558-EN-F1-1.pdf.

52. **European Medicines Agency (EMA).** 2016. *Web based sales data and animal population data collection protocol (version 2).* ESVAC, European Medicines Agency (EMA), London, United Kingdom. http://www.ema.europa.eu/docs/en_GB/document_library/Other/2015/06/WC500188365.pdf.

53. **European Medicines Agency (EMA).** 2016. *ESVAC: Vision, Strategy and Objectives 2016–2020.* ESVAC, London, United Kingdom. http://www.ema.europa.eu/docs/en_GB/document_library/Other/2015/06/WC500188365.pdf.

54. **WHO.** 2015. *Report of the 6th meeting: WHO advisory group on integrated surveillance of antimicrobial resistance with AGISAR 5-year strategic framework to support implementation of the global action plan on antimicrobial resistance (2015–2019).* World Health Organization, Geneva, Switzerland.

55. **WHO.** 2017. *Integrated surveillance of antimicrobial resistance in foodborne bacteria. Application of a One Health approach.* World Health Organization, Advisory Group on Integrated Surveillance of Antimicrobial Resistance, Geneva, Switzerland.

56. **OIE.** 2016. *Terrestrial Animal Health Code,* 25th ed. World Organization for Animal Health, Paris, France.

57. **OIE.** 2016. *Aquatic Animal Health Code,* 19th ed. Paris, France.

58. **OIE.** 2017. *OIE annual report on the use of antimicrobial agents in animals. Second repot.* World Organization for Animal Health, Paris, France. http://www.oie.int/fileadmin/Home/eng/Our_scientific_expertise/docs/pdf/A-MR/Annual_Report_AMR_2.pdf

59. **OIE.** 2016. *The OIE Strategy on Antimicrobial Resistance and the Prudent Use of Antimicrobial Agents.* World Organization for Animal Health, Paris, France. http://www.oie.int/fileadmin/Home/eng/Media_Center/docs/pdf/PortailAMR/EN_OIE-AMRstrategy.pdf.

60. **FAO.** 2016. *The FAO Action Plan on Antimicrobial Resistance 2016–2020.* Food and Agriculture Organization of the United Nations, Rome, Italy. http://www.fao.org/3/a-i5996e.pdf.

61. **Eurostat.** 2016. Livestock population, 2015 (million head), T1. http://ec.europa.eu/eurostat/statistics-explained/index.php/File:Livestock_population,_2015_%28million_head%29_T1.png.

62. **Eurostat.** 2015. Statistics on slaughtering, all species, by country, 2014. http://ec.europa.eu/eurostat/statistics-explained/index.php/File:Statistics_on_slaughtering,_all_species,_by_country,_2014.png.

63. **Danish Agriculture and Food Council.** 2016. *STATISTICS 2015, pigmeat.* Danish Agriculture and Food Council, Copenhagen, Denmark.

64. **Wallmann J, Bender A, Bode C, Köper L, Heberer T.** 2017. Abgabemengenerfassung antimikrobiell wirksamer Stoffe in Deutschland 2016. *Dtsch Tierarzteblatt* **65:** 1650–1659.

65. **Statistisches Bundesamt.** https://www.destatis.de/EN/FactsFigures/EconomicSectors/AgricultureForestryFisheries/AnimalsAnimalProduction/AnimalsAnimalProduction.html. Accessed 16.03.2017.

66. **Swedish Board of Agriculture.** http://www.jordbruksverket.se/swedishboardofagriculture/engelskasidor/statistics/statsec/livestock.4.2d224fd51239d5ffbf780003029.html.

67. **U.K. Government.** 2014. *Agriculture in the United Kingdom 2013.* Department for Environment, Food and Rural Affairs, Department for Agriculture and Rural Development (Northern Ireland), Welsh Assembly Government, The Department for Rural Affairs and Heritage, The Scottish Government, Rural and Environment Research and Analysis Directorate.

68. **Australian Bureau of Statistics.** 2016. 5204.0 Australian System of National Accounts, Table 60. Livestock, value and number of fixed assets and inventories. http://www.abs.gov.au/Agriculture.

69. **Public Health Agency of Canada.** 2016. *Canadian Antimicrobial Resistance Surveillance System Report 2016.* Public Health Agency of Canada, Ottawa, Canada.

70. **Public Health Agency of Canada.** 2017. *Canadian Integrated Program for Antimicrobial Resistance Surveillance (CIPARS) 2015 Annual Report.* Public Health Agency of Canada, Guelph, Canada. http://publications.gc.ca/collections/collection_2017/aspc-phac/HP2-4-2015-eng.pdf.

71. **NASS.** 2016. *Overview of U.S. livestock, poultry, and aquaculture production in 2015.* U.S. Department of Agriculture (USDA), Riverdale, MD. https://www.aphis.usda.gov/animal_health/nahms/downloads/Demographics2015.pdf.

72. **European Medicines Agency.** 2016. *Sales of Veterinary Antimicrobial Agents in 29 European Countries in 2014. Trends from 2011 to 2014.* European Medicines Agency, London, United Kingdom.

Antimicrobial Resistance in Bacteria from Livestock and Companion Animals
Edited by Frank Møller Aarestrup, Stefan Schwarz, Jianzhong Shen, and Lina Cavaco
© 2018 American Society for Microbiology, Washington, DC
doi:10.1128/microbiolspec.ARBA-0028-2017

Present and Future Surveillance of Antimicrobial Resistance in Animals: Principles and Practices

S. Simjee,[1] P. McDermott,[2] D.J. Trott,[3] and R. Chuanchuen[4]

28

INTRODUCTION

There is broad consensus internationally that surveillance of the levels of antimicrobial resistance (AMR) occurring in various systems underpins strategies to address the issue. The key reasons for surveillance of resistance are to determine (i) the size of the problem, (ii) whether resistance is increasing, (iii) whether previously unknown types of resistance are emerging, (iv) whether a particular type of resistance is spreading, and (v) whether a particular type of resistance is associated with a particular outbreak. The implications of acquiring and utilizing this information need to be considered in the design of a surveillance system.

HISTORICAL BACKGROUND

Nearly 50 years ago Anderson (1) reported a spike in infections caused by multidrug-resistant *Salmonella enterica* serovar Typhimurium phage type 29 in calves in the United Kingdom. Such infections became prominent following the adoption of intensive farming practices such as profligate antibiotic use in feed without veterinary prescription. Many human infections resulted. Anderson (1) concluded that the *Salmonella* epidemic could be eliminated "not by the massive use of antibiotics but by improvement in conditions of animal husbandry and reduction in the opportunities for the initiation and spread of the disease." In light of the public health implications of this finding, the Swann Report recommended restricting the use of antimicrobials in livestock production and imposing greater veterinary oversight (2). A national AMR monitoring program for *Salmonella* in animals commenced in the

United Kingdom in 1970 (3), and surveys were conducted in other countries (4). Martel and Coudert (5) reported on the national surveillance of AMR in animal (mainly of bovine origin) isolates of *Salmonella* and *Escherichia coli*, which had been in operation in France since 1969. Although there is scant reference in the literature to national AMR surveillance in animals for the next 20 years, reviews by Cohen and Tauxe (6) and DuPont and Steele (7) confirmed that the use of antimicrobials in livestock contributed to increased AMR in foodborne *Salmonella*. DuPont and Steele (7) recommended national monitoring of the use of antimicrobials in food-producing animals. They also recommended molecular epidemiological investigation to determine whether antimicrobial-resistance determinants arising in food animals as a result of antibiotic use, either by direct cross-infection or through horizontal transfer, influences the pool of genetic resistance determinants that are important to human health. Drug resistance in *Salmonella* was once again identified as the most significant public health threat arising from the use of antibiotics in livestock.

In the late 1980s and 1990s, third-generation cephalosporins and fluoroquinolones became widely available for use in food-producing animals. In 1996, following the emergence of multidrug-resistant *Salmonella* Typhimurium DT104, *S. enterica* serovar Newport resistant to third-generation cephalosporins, and fluoroquinolone-resistant *Campylobacter*, the Centers for Disease Control (CDC), the U.S. Department of Agriculture, and the Food and Drug Administration (FDA) established the National Antimicrobial Resistance Monitoring System (NARMS). Its purpose was to

[1]Elanco Animal Health, Basingstoke, UK; [2]Food and Drug Administration, Center for Veterinary Medicine, Rockville MD; [3]University of Adelaide, Roseworthy, Australia; [4]University of Chulalongkorn, Bangkok, Thailand.

monitor changes in antimicrobial susceptibilities of zoonotic pathogens from human and animal clinical specimens and carcasses of food-producing animals at slaughter plants over time to assess the effectiveness of intervention strategies (8). At the same time, in response to the emergence of vancomycin-resistant enterococci in poultry and pigs in Europe related to avoparcin use, The Danish Integrated Antimicrobial Resistance Monitoring Program (DANMAP) was launched and established baseline levels of resistance in pathogenic, zoonotic, and indicator bacteria of pigs, cattle, and broilers (9). The AMR surveillance strategies and recommendations of these foundational programs have since been adopted in many countries throughout the world (e.g., 10; selected case studies indicated below), and in many cases, linked with antimicrobial use monitoring and human AMR surveillance programs.

CODEVELOPMENT WITH AMR SURVEILLANCE IN HUMANS

Antimicrobial susceptibility testing (AST) for surveillance of AMR in animals essentially evolved from existing surveillance programs focused on human pathogens, with several key differentiating characteristics. While both programs utilize the same AST methodology, namely MIC testing utilizing agar dilution or microbroth dilution techniques, there are major differences in breakpoint determination, types of bacteria screened, and interpretation. Within the animal arena, application of different terminologies, techniques, and clinical breakpoints versus epidemiological cutoff values (ECOFFs) has meant that it has been difficult to compare data across national programs, and sometimes within programs over time as breakpoints are reevaluated or created and methodological advances made.

SIMILARITIES AND DIFFERENCES BETWEEN HUMAN AND ANIMAL AMR SURVEILLANCE PROGRAMS

In human AMR surveillance programs, AST is performed on major bacterial pathogens, collected from primary accession clinical microbiology laboratories. As such, these isolates can be considered convenience samples obtained from either hospitalized patients or outpatients in the community for which a culture and susceptibility test has been requested by the referring clinician. The site of infection is important because the breakpoints used to classify the isolate as susceptible or resistant may differ between an isolate from the urinary tract and a skin or soft tissue infection depending on

the pharmacokinetics of the antimicrobial agent. The main focus of programs also changes over time, often in response to international attempts to harmonize and integrate AST data. For example, in Australia, yearly AMR surveillance of human Gram-negative pathogens focused on hospital-acquired infections in odd-numbered years and community-acquired infections in even-numbered years. However, from 2013, surveillance only focused on sepsis or blood isolates, regardless of the source. In many cases, if the primary accession laboratories utilize the same testing methodology and quality assurance, testing indicates excellent agreement between laboratories (such as use of automated MIC determination technology), the AST data can be collected passively from clinical microbiology laboratory records, and surveillance activities can focus largely on the further characterization and molecular epidemiology of isolates, such as resistance mechanism screening and multilocus sequence typing. Many of these epidemiological characteristics can now be obtained through whole-genome sequence analysis (discussed below), with genomic epidemiology rapidly becoming an important feature of many global surveillance programs.

AMR surveillance in animal pathogens closely mirrors human surveillance programs in that it is focused on isolates obtained from clinical infections in animals. This includes both animal-only pathogens (e.g., *Mannheimia haemolytica*) and zooanthroponotic pathogens (e.g., methicillin-resistant *Staphylococcus aureus* [MRSA]). However, there is often much more variability in AST methodology applied to the isolates, with many veterinary diagnostic laboratories still being heavily reliant on disc diffusion methodology because of its rapidity and price. Automated MIC testing is increasingly available in veterinary laboratories but is often an additional cost for the client. Therefore, AMR surveillance focused on animal pathogens still often relies on centralized collection of isolates by an independent reference laboratory, which then conducts "gold standard" AST (MIC testing), making this a very expensive option for regular ongoing surveillance programs. Where veterinary diagnostic laboratory testing is well coordinated and methodologically similar, such as in France's RESAPATH program, passive collection of animal pathogen AST data is possible and has generated some useful information for antimicrobial stewardship policy and procedures (see example below). Surveillance of animal pathogens directly relates to antimicrobial use in companion animals (defined here as cats and dogs), performance animals (mainly horses, though in some countries horses are food-producing animals), livestock predominantly raised for food and fiber production and, potentially, exotic animals in zoological collections.

AMR surveillance of animals diverges from human surveillance in the development of programs aimed at AMR monitoring of zoonotic foodborne and commensal bacteria that are present in the gastrointestinal tract of food-producing animals at slaughter. In these cases, an epidemiological sampling strategy is used to obtain representative samples postslaughter and isolate key bacteria that are either directly associated with foodborne illness or are indicators or potential reservoirs of AMR determinants. The direct emphasis is monitoring resistance in bacteria from a public health and food safety perspective rather than having a direct benefit to animal health and production. To be included in a targeted livestock surveillance program, the microorganism must either be a commensal of animals that has the potential to provide sentinel information on trends and emergence of AMR, or it is a pathogen of animals and/or humans that has the potential to develop or is known to have developed AMR that is of concern to human health, and its primary route of infection is foodborne.

PRESENT MONITORING OF AMR IN ANIMALS: PRINCIPLES AND PRACTICES

Recommendations for implementation of national surveillance of AMR in animals have been developed by the World Organization for Animal Health, the World Health Organization Advisory Group on Integrated Surveillance of Antimicrobial Resistance, and the EFSA Working Group on Developing Harmonised Schemes for Monitoring Antimicrobial Resistance in Zoonotic Agents (11). In summary, these recommendations cover how to design sampling strategies, target animal and bacterial species, determine which antimicrobials to test, conduct AST and interpret results, and present the data. Some of these points will briefly be covered below.

Scope: Animal Species

AMR in animal and zooanthroponotic pathogens

Major animal species targeted for AMR monitoring in animal pathogens are usually divided into companion animals (i.e., dogs and cats), performance animals, (i.e., horses), livestock including aquaculture species produced for food), and exotics and wildlife. Comparison among animal species can be problematic due to the

differences between clinical breakpoints and site of infection (e.g., skin and soft tissue versus urine), the fact that there are no animal-specific breakpoints for some antimicrobial agents (in which case human breakpoints are used by default), and overall relevance to animal health versus public health.

AMR in zoonotic foodborne and commensal indicator bacteria

Cattle, pigs, and poultry provide the top three sources of meat; are critical in the maintenance of supplies of high-quality, low-cost food for human consumption, providing 13% of human calories and 30% of protein consumption; and produce around 40% of global gross domestic product (12). Most livestock-associated AMR surveillance programs focus on these three main sources. Cattle can be further subdivided into grass-fed (extensive) and lot-fed (intensive) beef cattle, cull dairy cattle, and veal (dairy calf) production systems. Antimicrobial use in each beef production sector varies considerably, from virtually no antimicrobial treatments in grass-fed cattle to a high proportion of animals receiving at least one treatment in feedlots. Poultry production includes both domestic broilers and turkeys, but commercial and free-range laying flocks are also of significant interest from an AMR standpoint given that eggs are a primary source of *Salmonella* food poisoning in many countries and there is only a restricted range of antimicrobial agents that can be used in egg-producing birds. The aquaculture industry, while not the largest in terms of food production in many countries, is the fastest-growing sector, with consumption expected to continue to increase in the coming decades (13). High antimicrobial use was a feature of the industry in its infancy, but as the industry has matured, control of endemic bacterial diseases by vaccination has seen antimicrobial use in some countries drop to very low levels (14). Other minor food animal species that are sometimes considered in country-specific AMR monitoring programs in livestock include horses, rabbits, and wild game species.

Scope: Antimicrobials

Inclusion of an antimicrobial drug in an AMR surveillance program depends upon whether it has been used, currently or historically, in animals to such a degree that development of AMR has been demonstrated or is of future concern to human health, particularly when the antimicrobial is within a class that is deemed to be of critical importance (Table 1). The final list of antimicrobials that are screened can vary considerably between countries and programs and can often change

Table 1   Antibacterial classes and agents registered for human and veterinary use that are often screened in antimicrobial resistance surveillance programs[a,b]

Antibacterial class and antibacterial (use in AMR surveillance)	Principal human use	Principal animal use
Narrow-spectrum penicillins		
Benzylpenicillin (pen G) and phenoxymethylpenicillin (pen V) (AP)	Primary agents in pneumococcal and streptococcal infection	N/A
Procaine penicillin	Intramuscular—occasional substitute for benzylpenicillin	Primary agent for predominantly Gram-positive infections in a wide range of animals, mostly horses (often in combination with gentamicin) and livestock (intramuscular administration only)
Benzathine penicillin	Intramuscular—syphilis treatment and rheumatic fever prophylaxis	N/A
Penethamate hydriodide	N/A	Hydrolized to benzylpenicillin following injection for treatment of mastitis and respiratory and uterine infections, mainly in dairy cattle
Moderate-spectrum penicillins		
Amoxycillin and ampicillin (AP, ZFP, AC)	Principal role in respiratory tract infections; widespread i.v. hospital use in combination for a range of moderate and serious infections; surgical and endocarditis prophylaxis	Broad-spectrum primary agent for a large range of infections in dogs and cats, horses, and livestock (oral or injectable)
Antistaphylococcal penicillin		
Cloxacillin, dicloxacillin, and flucloxacillin (methicillin)	Standard treatment for *Staphylococcus aureus* infections (not MRSA)	Cloxacillin only: intramammary treatment of mastitis due to staphylococci and streptococci in dairy cattle
Oxacillin (AP, ZP [MRSA/MRSP only])	Surgical prophylaxis, especially orthopedics	Oxacillin susceptibility used as a surrogate for MRSP identification in VDLs
Beta-lactamase inhibitor combinations		
Amoxycillin-clavulanate (AP, ZP, ZFP, AC)	Second-line agent for respiratory tract infections; role in certain types of skin/soft tissue infections and mixed staphylococcal/Gram-negative infections and aerobic/anaerobic infections	Primary or second-line broad-spectrum agent in dogs and cats only (oral and injectable) for a wide range of infections (skin, soft tissue, and UTI) Intramammary formulation only for mastitis in dairy cattle
Piperacillin-tazobactam (AP)	Valuable agents for a range of severe mixed aerobic-anaerobic infections including intra-abdominal infections, aspiration pneumonia, skin/soft tissue infections. Neutropenic sepsis	N/A
First-generation cephalosporins		
Cephalexin, cephalothin, and cephazolin (AP, ZP, ZFP, AC)	Treatment of minor and staphylococcal infections in penicillin-allergic patients Prophylaxis in orthopedic and other surgery	Primary agent for skin, soft tissue, and UTIs as well as surgical prophylaxis in dogs and cats only
Cephalonium/cephapirin	N/A	Intramammary treatment of mastitis due to staphylococci and streptococci in dairy cattle/intrauterine treatment for metritis in cattle

Drug	Human use	Animal use
Second-generation cephalosporins and cephamycins		
Cefaclor and cefuroxime-axetil	Treatment of respiratory infections in penicillin-allergic patients	Intramammary treatment of mastitis due to staphylococci and streptococci in dairy cattle
Cefoxitin (AP, ZP, ZFP, AC)	Useful antianaerobic activity, major role in surgical prophylaxis	N/A
Third-generation cephalosporins		
Ceftriaxone (AP, ZP, ZFP, AC)	Major agent in severe pneumonia and meningitis. Used in selected cases for treatment of gonorrhea and alternative for prophylaxis of meningococcal infection	N/A
Cefotaxime (AP, ZP, ZFP, AC)	Major agent in severe pneumonia and meningitis	N/A
Ceftazidime (AP, ZP, ZFP, AC)	Restricted role in pseudomonal infection and neutropenic sepsis	N/A
Cefovecin (AP, ZP)	N/A	Reserve agent for skin, soft tissue, periodontal, and UTIs in dogs and cats only where compliance with oral medication is compromised (injection only)
Ceftiofur (AP, ZP, ZFP, AC)	N/A	Reserve agent for respiratory infections in cattle. Off-label use for infections resistant to first-line therapies in individual food-producing animals (injection only)
Cefpodoxime (AP)	Broad-spectrum oral third-generation cephalosporin available in some countries	Reserve oral agent for skin, soft tissue, periodontal, and UTIs in dogs and cats only
Fourth-generation cephalosporins		
Cefepime	Moderate-to-severe pneumonia, skin and soft tissue infections, complicated and uncomplicated UTIs (broad-spectrum)	N/A
Cefquinome (AP)	N/A	Reserve agent for respiratory infections in cattle and pigs, coliform mastitis in cattle
Carbapenems		
Imipenem (AP, ZP, ZFP, AC), meropenem (AP, ZP, ZFP, AC), doripenem, and ertapenem	Very broad-spectrum reserve agents for multiresistant and serious Gram-negative and mixed infections	Use as a last resort option for multi-resistant Gram-negative infections in dogs has been reported
Tetracyclines/glycylcyclines		
Doxycycline (AP), minocycline (AP), and demeclocycline	Major agents for minor respiratory tract infections and acne. Supportive role in pneumonia for treating *Mycoplasma* and *Chlamydia pneumoniae* Malaria prophylaxis (doxycycline)	Doxycycline only: major primary agent for respiratory skin, soft tissue, urinary tract, and periodontal infections in dogs and cats including *Mycoplasma* and *Chlamydia* (oral only); occasional use of minocycline for MRSP
Chlortetracycline, oxytetracycline, and tetracycline (AP, ZP, ZFP, AC)	N/A	Major broad-spectrum primary agent for systemic infections in livestock
Tigecycline (ZFP, AC)	Reserve agent for multiresistant Gram-positive and some multiresistant Gram-negative infections	N/A

(Continued)

Table 1 Antimicrobial classes and agents registered for human and veterinary use that are often screened in antimicrobial resistance surveillance programs [a,b] (Continued)

Antibacterial class and antibacterial (use in AMR surveillance)	Principal human use	Principal animal use
Glycopeptides		
Vancomycin (AP, ZP, AC)	Drug of choice for serious methicillin-resistant staphylococcal infections Reserve agent for enterococcal infection when there is resistance or penicillin allergy	N/A
Teicoplanin (AC)	Substitute for vancomycin if intolerance or outpatient i.v. therapy *vanB* vancomycin-resistant enterococcal infections	N/A
Aminoglycosides/aminocyclitols		
Neomycin (including framycetin) (AP, AC)	Topical agent for skin infection and gut suppression.	Primary agent for enteric infections in livestock (oral form); broad-spectrum primary agent for a range of systemic infections in livestock and horses (parenteral form)
Gentamicin and tobramycin (AP, ZP, ZFP, AC)	Standard agents in combination for serious and pseudomonal infection Gentamicin used in combination for endocarditis	Gentamicin only: primary agent for broad-spectrum infections in horses (with penicillin); primary agent for short-term treatment of serious/life threatening infections in dogs and cats due to nephrotoxicity Cannot be administered to livestock in Australia
Amikacin (AP, ZP, ZFP, AC)	Reserve agents for Gram-negatives resistant to gentamicin and tobramycin	Use as a last-resort option for multiresistant infections in companion animals Use as a reserve agent for gentamicin-resistant infections in horses
Spectinomycin (AP, AC)	Spectinomycin only used for gonorrhea (infrequently)	Primary agent in combination with lincomycin for gastrointestinal and respiratory infections in pigs and broilers including mycoplasma (oral and injectable)
Streptomycin (AP, ZP, ZFP, AC)	Rare use in treatment of TB and enterococcal endocarditis	N/A
Apramycin (AP)	N/A	Primary agent for *E. coli* and *Salmonella* infections in calves, pigs, and broilers
Dihydrostreptomycin	N/A	Banned in livestock (except in oral or intramammary preparations) due to residue issues (apart from treatment of acute leptospirosis in cattle)
Sulfonamides and DHFR inhibitors		
Trimethoprim (AP, ZP, ZFP, AC)	Treatment and prophylaxis of UTI	N/A
Trimethoprim-sulfamethoxazole (co-trimoxazole) (AP, ZP, ZFP, AC)	Minor infections, especially treatment and prophylaxis of UTI Standard for treatment and prophylaxis of *Pneumocystis carinii* infection and nocardiasis Important for community-acquired MRSA infections	Trimethoprim-sulphonamide combinations are used as primary agents for broad-spectrum infections in livestock, horses, and dogs, including enteritis and pneumonia (oral and injectable)
Sulfadiazine, sulfadoxine, and sulfaquinoxaline	N/A	Oral sulfonamides (without trimethoprim) are also used for coccidiosis in poultry

Drug class / agent		
Oxazolidinones		
Linezolid (AP, ZP, AC)	Treatment of multiresistant Gram-positive infections, especially MRSA and VRE.	N/A
Macrolides		
Azithromycin (ZFP)	Treatment of *Chlamydia trachomatis* infections; Major agent for treatment and suppression of atypical mycobacterial infection	Occasional use in dogs and cats for chlamydia/mycoplasma infection and foals for *Rhodococcus* infection (see erythromycin)
Clarithromycin	Treatment of minor Gram-positive infections; Major agent for treatment and suppression of atypical mycobacterial infection	Occasional use in dogs and cats for chlamydia/mycoplasma infection and foals for *Rhodococcus* infection (see erythromycin)
Erythromycin and roxithromycin (AP, ZFP, AC)	Treatment of minor Gram-positive, *Chlamydia* and *Mycoplasma* infections	Erythromycin only: livestock for respiratory infections and other serious systemic infections including mastitis; respiratory disease in broilers; administered to foals in combination with rifampicin for *Rhodococcus* infection
Spiramycin	Treatment of toxoplasmosis in pregnancy	Periodontal and other anaerobic infections in dogs and cats (with metronidazole)
Oleandomycin	N/A	Intramammary formulation in combination with neomycin and tetracycline for mastitis
Tulathromycin, gamithromycin, and tildipirosin (AP)	N/A	Primary agent for respiratory infections in cattle and pigs
Tilmicosin, tylosin, and kitasamycin (AP)	N/A	Primary agent for respiratory infections in cattle; Treatment and prevention of enteritis and respiratory diseases in cattle, poultry, and pigs (especially *Lawsonia* infection); Growth promotion in pigs
Lincosamides		
Clindamycin and lincomycin (AP)	Reserved for Gram-positive and anaerobic infections in penicillin-allergic patients; Clindamycin topical used for acne	Clindamycin: Gram-positive and anaerobic infections in dogs and cats including osteomyelitis; Lincomycin: oral or injectable in livestock for respiratory and enteric infections (often in combination with spectinomycin)
Streptogramins		
Quinupristin with dalfopristin (AC)	Reserve agent for multiresistant Gram-positive infections (MRSA and vancomycin-resistant *Enterococcus faecium*).	N/A
Pristinamycin	As for quinupristin-dalfopristin	N/A
Virginiamycin	N/A	Laminitis prevention in horses, rumen acidosis prevention in cattle, necrotic enteritis prevention in broilers
Quinolones/Fluoroquinolones		

(Continued)

Table 1 Antimicrobial classes and agents registered for human and veterinary use that are often screened in antimicrobial resistance surveillance programs [a,b] (Continued)

Antibacterial class and antibacterial (use in AMR surveillance)	Principal human use	Principal animal use
Naladixic acid (ZFP, AC)	First-generation quinolone no longer used in human medicine	N/A (often included in AMR surveillance as an indicator of reduced susceptibility to the quinolone class)
Ciprofloxacin (AP, ZP, ZFP, AC)	Major oral agent for the treatment of Gram-negative infections resistant to other agents; Minor role in meningococcal prophylaxis	N/A
Moxifloxacin	Restricted role in the management of serious respiratory infections, especially pneumonia in patients with severe penicillin allergy	N/A
Enrofloxacin, marbofloxacin, and pradofloxacin (AP, ZP)	N/A	Reserve agents for treatment of Gram-negative serious, chronic or life-threatening infections in dogs, cats, and occasionally horses and exotics, treatment of complicated pyoderma due to mixed infections; Respiratory infections in feedlot cattle; historic use in poultry; Cannot be administered to food-producing animals in Australia
Ansamycins		
Rifampicin (rifampin) (AP, ZP)	Meningococcal and *H. influenzae* type b prophylaxis; Standard part of TB regimens; Important oral agent in combination for MRSA infections	Used in combination with a macrolide for treatment of *Rhodococcus* infection in foals
Bacitracin and gramicidin	Topical agents with Gram-positive activity	Treatment and prevention of necrotic enteritis in poultry, topical agents for mucocutaneous infections in companion animals (Gram-positive)
Polymyxins		
Colistin (ZFP, AC)	Reserve agent for very multiresistant Gram-negative infection (both inhaled and intravenous)	N/A
Phenicols		
Chloramphenicol (AP, ZP, ZFP, AC)	Usage largely as topical eye preparation; Occasional need for the treatment of bacterial meningitis.	Reserve agent for multiresistant infections in companion animals (dogs and cats only), especially *E. coli* and MRSP
Florfenicol (AP, ZP, ZFP, AC)	N/A	Respiratory infections in cattle and pigs; Off-label use for multiresistant *E. coli* in pigs
Nitrofurans		
Nitrofurantoin (AP)	Treatment and prophylaxis of UTIs only	N/A
Lipopeptides		
Daptomycin (AP, ZP, AC)	Reserve agent for serious MRSA and VRE infections	N/A

[a] The table focusses on animal pathogens (AP), zooanthroponotic pathogens (ZP), zoonotic foodborne pathogens (ZFP), and animal commensal indictor organisms (AC). Adapted from Shaban et al. (11).
[b] N/A, not applicable; i.v., intravenous; MRSP, methicillin-resistant *Staphylococcus pseudintermedius*; VDL, veterinary diagnostic laboratories; DHFR, dihydrofolate reductase; UTI, urinary tract infection; VRE, vancomycin-resistant enterococci; MRSP, methicillin-resistant *Staphylococcus pseudintermedius*.

between annual reports as new resistance mechanisms are identified or more streamlined approaches are adopted. As an example, the DANMAP 2015 (15) report screened *Salmonella* and *Escherichia coli* isolates for susceptibility to the same 14 antimicrobial agents mainly used in human medicine, whereas in DANMAP 2011 (16) the numbers were 16 and 18 antimicrobials, respectively. The main differences were the historical inclusion of several animal-only antimicrobials such as apramycin and florfenicol, which are no longer included in screening programs. Furthermore, the recent identification of plasmid-mediated mechanisms for resistance to critically important antimicrobials in animal commensal isolates (e.g., Mcr-1 mediated transferable colistin resistance [17] and carbapenemases normally associated with human pathogens [18, 19]) has renewed efforts to ensure that livestock AMR surveillance programs include "last-resort" drug classes in their screening panels. This is particularly the case in countries where there has been reported use of colistin in livestock production, where the *mcr-1* gene remained undetected for a number of years until its chance discovery in humans and livestock.

Scope: Microorganisms

There are four distinct categories of bacteria that can be isolated from animals for inclusion in AMR monitoring programs. This includes animal-only pathogens and/or zooanthroponotic pathogens usually isolated from sick companion/performance animals and livestock, as well as zoonotic foodborne and indicator commensal bacteria isolated from healthy livestock at slaughter. The main organisms targeted for AST in each category are described below and summarized in Table 2.

Animal-only pathogens

While these are rarely involved in causing human infections, they are the main drivers of antibiotic use in either companion or production animals, particularly in the face of developing resistance. In companion animals, methicillin-resistant *Staphylococcus pseudintermedius* is the major bacterium requiring ongoing monitoring, due to its propensity to develop multidrug-resistant and extensive drug-resistant profiles. *S. pseudintermedius* is the resident skin microbiota of dogs and often causes secondary bacterial infections in animals with primary allergic skin disease. The organism is increasingly recognized as a cause of otitis externa and surgical site infections, with nosocomial transmission as an important feature. methicillin-resistant *S. pseudintermedius* epidemiology is characterized by widespread dissemination of resistant clones.

In livestock, the main drivers of antimicrobial use are the bacterial pathogens involved in bovine and porcine respiratory disease complexes. In cattle, *M. haemolytica*, *Pasteurella multocida*, and *Histophilus somni* have traditionally been susceptible to most registered antimicrobials (20). However, in 2012, the first integrative-conjugative element (ICE) containing multiple resistance genes was identified in a *P. multocida* isolate from a case of bovine respiratory disease in the United States (21, 22), and similar ICEs have subsequently been identified in *M. haemolytica* and *H. somni*. Some isolates with ICE elements have also become resistant to fluoroquinolones (23). Among the main respiratory pathogens of pigs, *Actinobacillus pleuropneumoniae*, *Haemophilus parasuis*, and *P. multocida*, AMR to traditional drugs of choice is also increasing, with the first ICE identified in 2016 in *A. pleuropneumoniae* (24).

Enterotoxigenic *E. coli* is a major pathogen of sucker and weaner pigs and neonatal calves. While controlled to some extent by vaccination and management, outbreaks—particularly of postweaning diarrhea in pigs—can be explosive and unpredictable. Resistance to multiple antimicrobials is common, including recent development of resistance to third-generation cephalosporins (e.g., 25) and fluoroquinolones (e.g., 26) in some countries. *Salmonella* that are isolated from cases of infection in animals are usually serotyped and archived by national reference laboratories and are often available for inclusion in more active AMR surveillance focused on carriage by healthy livestock at slaughter (see 3 below).

Zooanthroponotic pathogens

Bacteria that are naturally transmissible from vertebrate animals to humans and vice versa (zooanthroponotic transmission) present public health risks at the human-animal-ecosystem interface. The major organisms include MRSA and extraintestinal pathogenic *E coli*. In companion animals, distinct MRSA clones appear to colonize specific animal host species. For example, health care-associated MRSA clone ST22 (EMRSA-15) is most commonly isolated from dogs and cats, while community-associated MRSA CC 8 (ST8, ST612, and ST254) clones are host-adapted to horses (27). Livestock-associated MRSA (LA-MRSA) ST398 is now endemic in many animal production systems throughout the world and is mainly a risk for humans in direct contact with animals, such as farmers and veterinarians. Additional LA-MRSA sequence types have been identified in dairy cattle, pigs, and poultry. A novel hybrid LA-MRSA CC9/CC398 genotype identi-

Table 2 Microorganisms of interest in AMR monitoring programs focused on both zoonotic foodborne pathogens and commensals in healthy livestock and major animal pathogens[a],[b]

Organism	Animal context	Human context
Methicillin-resistant *Staphylococcus pseudintermedius* (primary animal pathogen)	Recently emerged and spread epidemically in companion animals	Infections in humans are rare, can be a reservoir of SCC*mec*-associated resistance genes
Enterotoxigenic *Escherichia coli*, *Mannheimia haemolytica*, *Pasteurella multocida*, *Histophilus somnus*, *Actinobacillus pleuropneumoniae* (primary animal pathogens)	Relevant to pig and veal production, may drive use of third-generation cephalosporins; major reason for antimicrobial use in feedlot cattle and pigs; resistance to first-choice antimicrobials could result in increased use of third-generation cephalosporins and fluoroquinolones	Multidrug-resistant strains coming through the food chain would drive use of broad-spectrum cephalosporins and carbapenems in humans; uncommon to rare human pathogens
MRSA (zooanthroponotic pathogen/commensal in animals)	Livestock-associated MRSA; some human MRSA subtypes now adapted to animal hosts (i.e., horses and dogs)	Major human AMR surveillance organism; veterinarians in clinical practice have a higher rate of MRSA nasal carriage than the general population
ExPEC (zooanthroponotic pathogen/commensal in animals)	Some human-associated multidrug-resistant subtypes (e.g., ST131, ST648, ST354) can colonize and cause infections in dogs	Major human AMR surveillance organism; similarity between canine, avian, and human strains carrying ESBLs suggests potential for cross-transmission
Multidrug-resistant *Salmonella* (e.g., *S. enterica* serovars Newport, Typhimurium) (zoonotic foodborne pathogens)	Propensity to develop AMR under antimicrobial selection pressure in livestock production; in particular, resistance to critically important antimicrobials	Eggs and meat often implicated in outbreaks; invasive disease in humans often treated with fluoroquinolones in adults and third-generation cephalosporins in children
Fluoroquinolone-resistant *Campylobacter* (zoonotic foodborne pathogen)	Major foodborne risk bacteria associated with poultry; fluoroquinolone use a major selection pressure in livestock systems	Undercooked poultry meat and cross-contamination of fresh food often implicated in outbreaks; macrolides (in children) and fluoroquinolones are the treatments of choice for complicated infections
Commensal *Enterococcus* spp. (commensal indicator organism in livestock)	Gram-positive indicator organism in many surveillance programs; vancomycin resistance related to avoparcin use; streptogramin resistance related to virginiamycin use.	Historical use of avoparcin and other Gram-positive spectrum growth promoters linked to *vanA* type vancomycin resistance in human isolates
Commensal *E. coli.* (commensal indicator organism in livestock)	Have been shown to be reservoirs of plasmid-associated resistance of public health significance (e.g., ESBL and plasmid-borne AmpC β-lactamases).	Gram-negative indicator organisms, frequently harbour multidrug resistance on mobile genetic elements with potential for horizontal movement into human ExPEC

[a] Adapted from Shaban et al. (11).
[b] ESBL, Extended spectrum β-lactamase; MRSA, methicillin-resistant *Staphylococcus aureus*; ExPEC, multidrug-resistant extraintestinal pathogenic *E. coli*.

fied as a cause of infection in Danish citizens without direct contact with livestock (and no reported livestock reservoir in Denmark) has implicated retail poultry meat produced in other European countries as a potential source of infection (28).

Highly similar strains of extraintestinal pathogenic *E. coli* cause clinical infections in both humans and companion animals (29). A number of broad-host-range sequence types that are associated with multidrug resistance, including resistance to both third-generation cephalosporins and fluoroquinolones, have been reported in both humans and animals. These include ST131 (30), ST648 (31), and ST354 (32).

Zoonotic foodborne pathogens

The two main foodborne zoonotic pathogens screened in AMR surveillance programs focused on healthy animals at slaughter are *Salmonella* spp. and *Campylobacter* spp. Together, these organisms comprise the most common causes of foodborne disease derived from the consumption or handling of animal products that may require antimicrobial chemotherapy for severe or invasive infections. It is therefore paramount to report trends in resistance to antimicrobial agents that are likely to be used as first-line treatments for these infections. Multidrug-resistant *Salmonella* strains that also possess resistance to third-generation cephalosporins such as *S. enterica* serovars Newport, Typhimurium, and Heidelberg have been associated with ground beef and chicken meat, respectively (33). Emerging resistance to fluoroquinolones has been documented in *Salmonella* isolates derived from pigs (e.g., 34) and poultry meat (35).

Commensals as indicator bacteria

Monitoring of resistance in indicator bacteria is undertaken in healthy livestock because these organisms are ubiquitous in nature, food, animals, and humans and reflect AMR characteristics arising from selective pressure across these environments. It has also been suggested that they represent potential reservoirs of transferrable resistance genes encoded on mobile genetic elements. *Enterococcus* spp. are included as an AMR indicator organism because they can potentially share mobile genetic elements with other Gram-positive organisms (36). Similarly, plasmid-mediated transfer of AMR genes among commensal *E. coli* in the gut of healthy animals is well documented (37). However, it is important to note that the resident gut commensal *E. coli* may also include phylogenetic groups with the right repertoire of virulence genes to cause extraintestinal infection. Avian pathogenic *E. coli* and other virulent

E. coli lineages are carried in the gut of healthy poultry and have been implicated as sources of foodborne infection in humans, either through direct cross-transmission via meat and eggs or through indirect transmission of plasmids and other mobile genetic elements encoding extended-spectrum beta-lactamases and AMR determinants (38, 39). Broad-host-range commensal *E. coli* sequence types that have acquired resistance to third-generation cephalosporins and/or fluoroquinolones such as ST10 (common between humans and animals) have been isolated in distinct global regions (40, 41). However, a whole-genome sequencing (WGS) study suggested that cephalosporin resistance in human and animal isolates from matching STs was disseminated on different *E. coli* plasmids (42). The availability of rapid and inexpensive WGS platforms (discussed below) is therefore a welcome addition to AMR monitoring programs to provide context and risk assessment.

Laboratory Testing Methodologies for AMR Monitoring

AST results have historically been intended primarily to guide physicians and veterinarians regarding appropriate antimicrobial therapy. Results are generally reported as susceptible, intermediate, or resistant after applying relevant clinical breakpoints, and there has been little incentive to report quantitative AMR data. For the purposes of surveillance, quantitative results achieved using different laboratory methods or applying nonstandard breakpoints are of limited value for detecting trends or evaluating levels of resistance on a broader level, and comparison of the data is rarely useful. However, reporting and retaining quantitative MIC data provides a mechanism to detect shifts in MIC over time and facilitate early detection of emerging resistance. This approach supports comparison with surveillance data from other systems and allows data to be reinterpreted.

MIC testing is the gold standard technique for determining an isolate's individual susceptibility to an antimicrobia agent (defined as the lowest concentration inhibiting growth of the organism using a series of 2-fold dilutions). While a number of techniques for determining MIC have been developed, including broth microdilution using 96-well plates, agar dilution, Etest graded strips, and automated systems, broth microdilution is most applicable to AMR surveillance (43). The Kirby-Bauer disk diffusion technique is often employed in veterinary diagnostic laboratories for AST on individual clinical isolates from animals; however, it is not readily amenable to AMR surveillance projects. The availability of broth microdilution methodologies, such as Sensititre, that utilize freeze-dried, predetermined antimicrobial ranges allows for automated or semiautomated testing, individual plate customization, or adoption of standardized plates (such as the NARMS panel). Nevertheless, there are often cases when additional antimicrobials not available in a standardized plate format need to be evaluated, and thorough knowledge and application of the most appropriate standards are therefore required. The Clinical Laboratory Standards Institute (CLSI) has developed clinical breakpoints for human and veterinary pathogens for both MIC broth microdilution and disk diffusion AST techniques. The European Committee on Antimicrobial Susceptibility Testing (EUCAST) has developed clinical breakpoints for human pathogens, but veterinary pathogen clinical breakpoints are still in development.

CLSI and clinical breakpoints

The CLSI (formerly the National Committee for Clinical Laboratory Standards) is a not-for-profit standards development organization formed in 1968. It has established clinical breakpoints for registered veterinary and human antimicrobial agents according to the label dosing regime when a standard method of testing performance is adopted. Clinical breakpoints are determined using a combination of *in vitro* and *in vivo* data to predict the likelihood of clinical cure based on pharmacokinetic-pharmacodynamic parameters. They do not, however, predict the likely presence of resistance mechanisms in isolates, are not available for all antimicrobials and all animal species (the default is to use human clinical breakpoints if veterinary-specific breakpoints are unavailable), and are subject to change as new pharmacokinetic-pharmacodynamic data are obtained. Based on clinical breakpoints, isolates are designated susceptible (bacterial infection may be appropriately treated with the dosage regimen recommended for that type of infection and infecting species), intermediate (bacterial infection may be appropriately treated in body sites where the drugs are physiologically concentrated or when a high dosage of drug can be used), or resistant (bacteria are not inhibited by the usually achievable concentrations of the agent with normal dosage schedules and/or fall in the range where specific microbial resistance mechanisms are likely and clinical outcome has not been predictable in *in vivo*-based studies) (44). Breakpoints are agreed upon by CLSI's veterinary antimicrobial susceptibility subcommittee (first formed in 1982) after reviewing available data, which includes calculation of ECOFFs (note: the acronym favored by CLSI is ECV). An isolate may be described as non-susceptible if its MIC is above the susceptible clinical

breakpoint (i.e., it is in the intermediate or resistant range).

EUCAST and ECOFFs

EUCAST is a standing committee jointly organized in 1997 by ESCMID, ECDC, and European national breakpoint committees. EUCAST is funded by the European Union. EUCAST first developed the term "ECOFF" and publishes ECOFFs for specific antimicrobials and veterinary pathogen combinations based on MIC distributions of a large number of isolates. ECOFFs classify an organism as wild type or non-wild type based on the normal distribution of MICs for fully susceptible isolates that do not contain any resistance determinants that could influence the MIC phenotype (phenotypically detectable acquired resistance mechanisms). For example, a point mutation in the fluoroquinolone resistance-determining region of *gyrA* imparting reduced susceptibility to enrofloxacin could shift the MIC of an *E. coli* isolate from 0.06 µg/ml (within the wild-type range) to 0.25 µg/ml (the ECOFF). This isolate would be described as non-wild type but should not be described as resistant or be included in percentage resistant calculations for isolate collections, because it is still below the clinical resistance breakpoint of ≥4 µg/ml. MIC distributions are often bimodal, with clinically resistant isolates normally distributed around a high MIC and very few isolates falling within the interval range from the non-wild type ECOFF to the clinical resistance breakpoint. This can best be appreciated in an MIC distribution for a hypothetical antimicrobial (Fig. 1). ECOFF phenotypes can now also be more readily justified on the basis of whole-genome sequence data confirming the presence of specific resistance determinants (see below). However, ECOFFs should not be used to classify an isolate as clinically resistant or to calculate the percentage of isolates that are multidrug-resistant (resistant to at least one drug in three antimicrobial classes) or extensively drug resistant (resistant to all but one or two classes), because this cannot be verified from a statistical analysis of MIC distributions without relevant pharmacological data. It is also extremely important to measure the actual MIC; if it falls below a testing threshold, arbitrary "less than" values cannot be used to calculate an ECOFF (45, 46).

The advantage of measuring and reporting ECOFFs is that AST data, when viewed as an MIC distribution, can be more readily compared over time because the proportion of isolates shifting MICs (either higher or lower) can be directly linked to antimicrobial selection pressure or antimicrobial stewardship policies. Report-

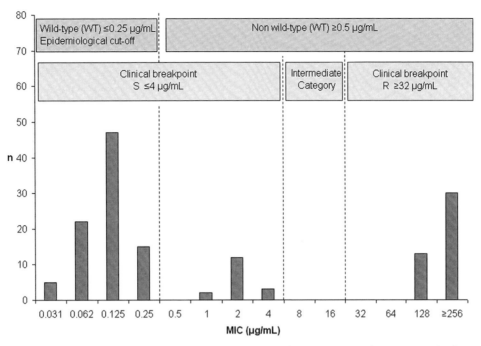

Figure 1 MIC distribution for a hypothetical bacterial species targeted in antimicrobial resistance surveillance programs. Arrows indicate the epidemiological cutoff value (ECOFF) established according to EUCAST recommendations, separating the wild type (no resistance determinants) from the non-wild type (presumed resistance determinants that could be verified by whole-genome sequencing analysis), and the clinical breakpoint. Susceptible, resistant, and intermediate value columns are indicated (45).

ing and retaining quantitative MIC data provides a mechanism to detect shifts in the MIC over time and facilitate early detection of emerging resistance. This approach supports comparison with surveillance data from other systems and allows data to be reinterpreted if breakpoints or cutoff values change—from the perspective of animal clinical breakpoints (if available) versus human clinical breakpoints—if ECOFFs are applied, or if data from different laboratories are compared (47). The current difficulty in interpreting veterinary-specific AST data is where recent changes in clinical breakpoints established for veterinary species have shifted the CLSI clinical breakpoint to below the corresponding ECOFF. This can be seen with current amoxicillin-clavulanate breakpoints for dogs and cats for *E. coli* isolated from skin and soft tissue infections (≥1 µg/ml) and urinary tract infections (≥16 µg/ml) now being below the current ECOFF (≥32 µg/ml), which is also the human clinical breakpoint. Using the veterinary clinical breakpoints, isolates with MICs that do not indicate the presence of resistance mechanisms and are within the wild-type distribution could still be classified as resistant (but the same isolates would be classified as susceptible if they were zooanthroponotic

and had human clinical breakpoints applied). At this time, displaying the MIC data distribution in tabular form with both the ECOFF and clinical breakpoint values clearly marked would appear to be the best way to present the data for interpretation. However, it is disingenuous to present percentage non-wild type as equivalent to percentage resistance if only ECOFFs have been used to define the MIC distribution.

Sampling Strategies for Healthy Livestock at Slaughter Surveys

The relationship between sample numbers and the sensitivity of a surveillance system to detect increases in resistance has been explored (48). For example, if a sample size of 200 yields a resistance rate of 5% to a particular antibiotic, the resistance level measured in a second set of 200 samples would need to rise above 11% before it can be stated that the level of resistance in the population has significantly increased. Sensitivity can be improved by increasing the number of samples. If 1,000 samples were included in each round, an increase from 5 to 7% is indicative of increasing resistance. It is possible that these numbers do not account for the nonrandom distribution (clustering) of resistance isolates, and where clustering occurs, the sample size requirements are much higher. Randomization of sample collection on an abattoir chain represents the best method of avoiding any potential clustering effects. The EFSA Working Group on Developing Harmonised Schemes for Monitoring Antimicrobial Resistance in Zoonotic Agents recommended that European Union member states should collect data on at least 170 isolates each year as the most accurate and achievable number for all possible outcomes (49). This number was determined based on a range of assumptions (95% confidence intervals with 80% power) and to achieve a desired level of accuracy for estimates of resistance. If resistance is already widespread (50% frequency), only a relatively large change in proportion of resistance is considered relevant (15% increase). For the detection of the initial emergence of resistance (such as to critically important human antimicrobials, for example, 0.1 to 5% frequency), an increase of a few percent should be also detectable.

The number of samples per flock or herd is also an important consideration. Current EFSA guidelines suggest that a single animal from a single farm provides enough precision at a national level. However, greater precision (and significant reductions in cost) of sampling for the same estimation of AMR prevalence was achieved in a study of *Campylobacter* isolates by reducing the number of birds per flock (n = 155) sampled from five to two (50). However, if only a single animal was sampled, the flock sample size needed to be increased to 250.

While a wide range of potential samples are listed in the various recommendations, the most appropriate samples (particularly for large countries with long distances between farms) are abattoir specimens in the form of cecal content samples for pigs and beef and carcass rinses or swabs for poultry.

Isolation of Zoonotic and Commensal Bacteria from Gastrointestinal Samples

International or national standardized methods of isolation of each bacterial species need to be employed and applied to each sample (ISO6579:2002 for *Salmonella* and ISO102721:2006 for *Campylobacter*). For *Campylobacter* and *Salmonella* this includes the use of suitable enrichment broth and selective media, preferably employing chromogenic agar. All isolates are required to be confirmed to the species level prior to AST, using appropriate biochemical or genetically based tests. However, matrix-assisted laser desorption ionization–time of flight mass mass spectroscopy is becoming the preferred method in many countries.

Isolates need to be appropriately identified and stored for easy traceability.

Recommendations for Reporting and Database Management

An isolate-level database is at the core of any program for the surveillance of AMR. The database contains relevant details of demographic and microbiological characteristics derived from routine diagnostic samples, convenience samples, or targeted surveillance program samples. Data should be stored in secure databases that facilitate simple entry and retrieval, flexible reporting, and *ad hoc* analysis. Compatibility with similar national and international databases is important. Electronic transfer of data from other systems is highly recommended, rather than manual data entry, which is time- and resource-consuming and error-prone.

SELECTED CASE STUDIES FOR CURRENT AMR SURVEILLANCE IN ANIMALS PROGRAMS

Denmark: DANMAP

DANMAP was established by the Danish Ministry of Food, Agriculture, and Fisheries and the Danish Ministry of Health in 1995 to monitor antimicrobial use in the human and veterinary sectors and to monitor AMR in human and animal pathogens, zoonotic bacteria, and indicator bacteria. DANMAP had its genesis in the 1990s when Danish scientists established the link between avoparcin use in poultry and carriage and contamination of meat with vancomycin-resistant enterococci. It is the first national surveillance program to be initiated by a country and forms a successful blueprint that has been replicated, albeit with modifications, by several other countries. From the outset, DANMAP adopted a coordinated, One Health strategy; they developed a highly integrated, systematic, and continuous program that covered the entire food chain, relating antibiotic consumption with resistance, from "farm to fork to sickbed." Unique methods of integrating data were developed that created outcomes for action through cross-sector collaboration between scientists and authorities. DANMAP has been highly successful due to adequate funding, excellent planning, and collaboration at all sectors, but also because Denmark is a small country with a large economic reliance on high-quality agricultural produce (approximately 80% of antimicrobials used in the animal sector are administered to pigs) and relatively short distances between farms, processing facilities, and laboratories. Susceptibility testing (one isolate per bacterial species per farm, meat sample, or patient) is performed with commercial Sensititre plates according to CLSI guidelines using ECOFFs validated by EUCAST when possible.

Data from DANMAP documenting the increasing prevalence of vancomycin-resistant enterococci in poultry and pig meat was instrumental in the Danish government's decision to ban the use of antimicrobials for growth promotion in the 1990s. Steady increases in the amount of therapeutic use of antimicrobials in animals were recorded following the ban, concomitant with the increased detection of extended-spectrum beta-lactamases in commensal *E. coli* isolates from livestock. Despite the introduction of new guidelines governing the use of antimicrobials, consumption continued to rise. In a further attempt to reduce overall antimicrobial use, the Danish government instituted the "yellow card" system in 2010 for veterinarians and their clients, along with a voluntary withdrawal of the use of cephalosporins in pig production. These efforts resulted in a decrease in detection of extended-spectrum beta-lactamases in indicator *E. coli* from pigs (51).

France: RESAPATH

The French National Observatory for Epidemiology of Bacterial Resistance to Antibiotics (ONERBA) centralizes data from human and animal surveillance covering 17 surveillance networks. Created in 1997, ONERBA is an organization whose scientific and technical activities rely mainly on the networks for surveillance of resistance already established; only one of these networks (RESAPATH) is devoted to isolates obtained from animals. RESAPATH, operated by ANSES, the French Agency for Food, Environmental, and Occupational Health and Safety, coordinates the voluntary contribution of antimicrobial susceptibility data from isolates from diseased food-producing animals and companion animals obtained by 63 public and private diagnostic laboratories distributed throughout the country. It commenced in 1982 and dealt only with bovine isolates; it was expanded to include swine and poultry isolates in 2000, and other animal species including companion animals and horses were added in 2007. RESAPATH is a key component of the EcoAntibio 2017 plan to combat AMR in animals. The EcoAntibio 2017 plan aims to reduce antimicrobial use in the veterinary sector by 25% by 2017 by introducing/refining 40 broad measures. Eco Antibio 2017 supports the mission of EFSA and ESVAC. ANSES manages the *Salmonella* surveillance network and also publishes reports on antimicrobial sales data in the French animal sector (from 1999 onward).

ANSES antimicrobial use data demonstrated a 27.9% increase in the consumption of antimicrobials between 1999 and 2009, though data collected between 2009 and 2010 show a 12.2% decrease. However, during this time there was a concomitant increase in the use of critically important antimicrobials (third- and fourth-generation cephalosporins and fluoroquinolones). RESAPATH confirmed high rates of resistance to critical antimicrobials among *E. coli* isolates from cattle, horses, and companion animals concomitant with increased availability and prescribing of these drugs. However, they were able to demonstrate a drop in resistance frequency in their most recent report when EcoAntibio 2017 energies were focused on education and more appropriate therapeutic guidelines.

Canada: CIPARS

The Canadian Integrated Program for Antimicrobial Resistance Surveillance (CIPARS) was established in 2002. A key feature of CIPARS is that reports are an amalgamation of human data with animal data on AMR and antimicrobial use. CIPARS aims to provide a unified approach for monitoring trends in antimicrobial use and resistance in humans and animals and for facilitating assessment of the public health impact of antimicrobials used in humans and agricultural sectors to enable accurate comparison with data from other countries that use similar surveillance systems.

Surveillance data from CIPARS have been instrumental in strengthening our understanding of how AMR in animals can have an adverse effect on public health. Presentation of human and animal data in an integrated fashion is useful for ensuring that animal surveillance and future interventions both have a focus on human health. Several examples of the impact of CIPARS have been reported, including demonstrating a link between an increasing frequency of detection of multidrug-resistant *Salmonella* Heidelberg in humans and the use of ceftiofur in poultry production in parts of Canada (52).

United States: NARMS

In 1996, collaboration was established between federal, state, and local agencies in the United States for performing surveillance of AMR in enteric bacteria from humans, retail meats, and animals (NARMS). An important feature of NARMS is that methodology in sampling and laboratories has been sufficiently stable since its inception to allow for sound comparison of results between years, thus demonstrating time-based trends in the emergence of resistance. The laboratory methodology is comparable across the three arms of

NARMS (humans, food, and animals) as well, which provides a strong basis for One Health comparisons between these three sources. This provides a powerful mechanism for tracking the evolution of resistance in zoonotic enteric pathogens over time.

Data on the occurrence of fluoroquinolone resistance in *Campylobacter* spp. isolated from poultry have been used in regulatory and legal processes in the United States to reduce the availability of enrofloxacin in animal production. Applications to register new antimicrobial products for use in the animal industries are now evaluated within the context of NARMS findings and through human food safety risk assessments (53). Arguably, one of the most important outcomes of NARMS has been the demonstration of the widespread and increasing level of resistance to third-generation cephalosporins in nontyphoidal *Salmonella* from food animals. These data were clearly very influential in the FDA decision to introduce additional legal constraints on the use of cephalosporin drugs in food-producing animals. The most recent NARMS report (54) is the first to present WGS data in combination with AST. Summarizing the NARMS data, a major finding confirmed that 80% of *Salmonella* isolates from retail meats in the United States have remained susceptible to all antimicrobials tested for the past 10 years, and ceftriaxone resistance has decreased in both human and retail poultry isolates over the same time period (19).

FUTURE MONITORING OF AMR IN ANIMALS

Historically, infectious disease surveillance has been based on a number of laboratory processes that require specialized reagents and dedicated personnel with proficiency in a series of separate methods, each providing a distinct piece of microbiological information to aid the clinician in treating and tracking infectious diseases. These laboratory tests provide species identification based on metabolic byproducts, antibiotic susceptibility patterns derived from the *in vitro* growth response of organisms to different drug concentrations, antigenic structure (e.g., serotype) defined by an algorithm of agglutination reactions, and sometimes virulence properties such as toxin production or the presence of pathognomonic virulence traits (e.g., *stx*) usually revealed by PCR. Phylogenic relationships based on pulsed-field gel electrophoresis (PFGE) patterns, multilocus sequence typing, or other methods were used to investigate and respond to disease outbreaks and to attribute strain types to a source. This daunting assortment of tests is a major impediment to establishing inte-

grated AMR surveillance in many countries. It is also the limiting factor in the design scope of existing surveillance systems, which are necessarily limited in the number and variety of samples and pathogens under surveillance.

In looking toward the future of AMR surveillance, it is clear that the main way in which it will change is through greater use of DNA sequencing technologies. The development of affordable WGS technologies, along with complementary advances in bioinformatics, provides a single, rapid, and comprehensive laboratory procedure by which to characterize bacterial strains. The power of WGS for public health surveillance has already been demonstrated. In a clinical setting, WGS technology is providing solutions to what were once intractable problems in the characterization of pathogens. For zoonotic foodborne infections in particular, WGS now offers a means to more accurately conduct outbreak investigations, to better understand the virulence traits of pathogenic bacteria and the factors that influence their adaptability to food animal environments, and to conduct genetic analysis of surveillance isolates. Moreover, data are growing that show the power of WGS to provide definitive data on AMR determinants regardless of the source of the sample, allowing direct confirmation of the correct ECOFF value separating wild-type strains from those carrying resistance determinants.

Since the array of phenotypic traits provided by traditional microbiology methods can theoretically be deduced from the genotype, and at lower costs, WGS is expected to remove the limitation on surveillance imposed by the need for multiple procedures. For example, DNA sequence analysis has demonstrated the specificity to identify more than 2,300 of the 2,600 *Salmonella* serotypes (SeqSero), to attribute foodborne pathogens to geographic origin (tuna scrape), and to catalogue the array of genes underlying traditional phenotypic testing, including antibiotic resistance genes (see below). For *Listeria* epidemiology, WGS has replaced PFGE for outbreak investigations and will soon replace PFGE and other typing tools for other pathogens. This has started a paradigm shift in the analytical approach to infectious disease by increasing the data that can be quickly extracted from an infectious agent, thereby transforming the laboratory science of pathogen identification, phylogenetic analysis, epidemiology, and surveillance. While the science is still developing, early studies show how WGS data can augment, and in some cases replace, *in vitro* AST for both surveillance and clinical purposes.

The surveillance of AMR is based on *in vitro* AST methods, which measure the growth response of bac teria to different drug concentrations in a defined incubation environment. These methods consist mainly of measuring the MIC of antibiotics arrayed in 2-fold serial dilutions, or the diameter of inhibition zones around disks containing standard amounts of antibiotic. These methods are an uncomplicated and proven way to predict the presence of acquired antibiotic resistance traits and to select appropriate therapy. Despite nearly 100 years of experience with this approach, there are several well-known limitations to methods based on an *in vitro* growth response. There is a lack of harmonization that hinders the interlaboratory comparison of data, an absence of validated methods for many pathogens, practical limitations on the number of agents that can be tested simultaneously, and shifting interpretive standards (55).

THE LIMITATIONS OF PCR FOR RESISTOMICS

In some cases, the results of *in vitro* AST alone are inadequate, and additional genetic information is needed. For example, methicillin resistance in *S. aureus* (MRSA) is conferred by the *mecA* gene. A key characteristic of this gene is its varied expression *in vitro*, which can lead to false-negative results. For this reason, the definition of MRSA includes detection of the *mecA* gene. Similarly, the very slow growth rate of *Mycobacterium tuberculosis* (MTB) in the laboratory causes long delays in the laboratory reporting of susceptibility data. PCR-based testing for rifampin resistance based on mutation in the *rpoB* gene correlates well with phenotypic methods and can be used to provide more timely information for treating infections. Furthermore, in AMR surveillance, phenotype information in the form of MICs or disk diffusion zone sizes usually does not reveal the underlying genetic mechanisms of which there are thousands of known alleles. This information can help attribute pathogens and resistances to different sources, allowing for targeted measures to combat the spread of resistant pathogens.

Since its development in 1983, PCR has been the most common method for detecting the presence of specific genes. Variations on the method have proven indispensable in genotyping bacteria and augmenting the phenotypic susceptibility data in surveillance. Despite the power and ease of PCR, it has several important limitations. In practice, it is limited largely to the detection of known DNA sequences. Even for genes with known sequences, an amplification product usually must be subjected to DNA sequencing to confirm the results, to identify the resistance allele, or to detect structural mutations conferring resistance. False negatives are a problem because amplification can fail due to the presence of a single mutation or to small variations in sample preparation procedures. False positives also can occur, usually through contamination as a result of carryover of DNA template from another specimen.

While it is possible to account for false test results, PCR is limited in the number of genes it can detect in a single assay, and its utility is incomplete without also determining the DNA sequence of the amplicon. DNA microarrays overcome some of the limitations of PCR-based resistance gene detection by enabling the simultaneous detection of thousands of gene alleles. However, microarray methods also rely on known DNA sequences, may give false-positive and -negative results, and are labor-intensive and expensive.

RESISTOME SURVEILLANCE

Since WGS does not depend on known prior sequence information, it circumvents the limitations of PCR and microarray resistance genotyping methods. While WGS reduces the time and resources needed to generate microbiological data, it requires powerful and sophisticated data analysis via bioinformatics to be useful. To facilitate resistome typing from WGS data, several resistance gene databases have been developed that contain all known resistance genes. These include ResFinder (56), CARD (57), Arg-ANNOT (58), and the CVM resistance gene database (59). These databases make analysis easier by reducing the time needed to compile the complement of resistance genes for a given isolate. As with differences in methods and interpretive criteria for *in vitro* susceptibility testing, the variety of resistance gene databases can lead to confusion in the scientific literature without some central reference for harmonized gene naming. The NCBI is attempting to overcome this challenge by resolving discrepancies in the nomenclature of resistance alleles in the GenBank repository, where inaccurate and duplicative annotation is a well-known problem. NCBI recently released the Bacterial Antimicrobial Resistance Reference Gene Database (http://www.ncbi.nlm.nih. gov/bioproject/313047), which is a curated and standardized collection of over 3,440 resistance genes and alleles. NCBI has also taken over curation of the Lahey Clinic's Beta-Lactamase Allele Database, and routinely assigns allele designations for over two dozen beta-lactamase gene families (http://www.ncbi.nlm.nih.gov/ pathogens/submit_beta_lactamase/). In addition, NCBI has developed a tool to automatically catalogue resistance genes in all submitted microbial genome sequences and ultimately will link resistome data automatically with phylogenetic trees and other data produced for the GenomeTrakr Project by NCBI's Pathogen Detection Pipeline. These initiatives will help ensure harmonization of bioinformatics specific to resistome surveillance by providing an index for gene classification.

The effort to develop and curate comprehensive resistance gene databases was motivated to facilitate the use of "resistomics" both to augment AMR surveillance and as a means to guide therapy, related but distinct endeavors. To date, a few studies have examined the correlations between the presence of known resistance determinants and clinical resistance in zoonotic foodborne pathogens. The results show a very high correlation between genotypes and phenotypes for *E. coli*, *Salmonella*, and *Campylobacter* (59–63) for most antimicrobial agents. Some studies have performed similar analyses with *Staphylococcus*, *Klebsiella*, *Pseudomonas*, and *Enterococcus*, although these bacteria do not typically cause serious foodborne infections (60, 61, 64). While there are lower correlations for some antimicrobial agents, overall, these studies show that WGS analysis is very sensitive and specific for identifying acquired resistance determinants. In this way, WGS can provide a corollary to ECVs (ECOFFS) by its ability to identify non-wild-type strains.

In addition to correlating resistance genotypes and phenotypes, WGS-based analysis completes in one step what was unpractical with PCR strategies, namely, identifying new alleles conferring resistance to the same drug class. For example, in one study of gentamicin-resistant *Campylobacter* from human infections and from retail meats, PCR failed to detect aminoglycoside resistance genes in many of the human isolates (65). The use of WGS revealed the presence of six gentamicin-resistance genes that had not previously been found in *Campylobacter*. This included the *aph(2′)-Ig* gene, which has <30% amino acid identity to other *aph(2′)* genes and thus would not have been discovered easily without WGS.

In traditional AMR surveillance, the range of antimicrobial classes that are monitored is determined by various considerations intended to optimize the physical limitations of a 96-well panel format. An important advantage of WGS-based surveillance is the ability to detect resistances that are excluded from phenotypic monitoring for whatever reason. In an early study comparing *Salmonella* genomes, WGS revealed the colocalization of extended-spectrum cephalosporin resistance encoded by the bla_{CMY-2} gene on a plasmid with the *sugE* gene, which confers high-level MICs to cetyl-pyridinium chloride, a chemical used for carcass decontamination. This raises the possibility that chemicals used in processing might influence the resistance profiles of pathogens that reach the food supply. Similarly, WGS has revealed resistance determinants for innate immunity, heavy metals, and less commonly used antibiotics (66). Importantly, WGS supersedes PCR-based methods for plasmid typing by capturing plasmid replicon information, which may signify the animal origin of some resistances.

There is great interest in the potential of WGS to predict the likelihood that a pathogen will respond to anti-infective therapy and thereby serve as a clinical diagnostic test. This is distinct from the utility of WGS in public health surveillance, where a resistance gene is viewed in terms of hazard characterization. The use of WGS to guide clinical treatment options touches on the practice of medicine and standards of care and involves multiple datasets that include clinical outcome information. While DNA tests do serve this purpose for MRSA and MTB as noted above, the parameters for WGS-based susceptibility testing continue to develop for other pathogens. Genomic sequence data have been used to evaluate tentative laboratory breakpoints for streptomycin resistance in *Salmonella* and *E. coli* (67). Similarly, quinolone MICs in *Salmonella* can be distinguished by whether the underlying genetic mechanism for resistance is mutations in *gyrA* (MIC of >16 µg/ml) or *qnr* mutations (MIC of 8 to 16 µg/ml) (63). EUCAST established a subcommittee to explore the role of WGS in AST and released a document for public comment on the topic (http://www.eucast.org/file admin/src/media/PDFs/EUCAST_files/Consultation/ 2016/Aerococcus_and_Kingella_BP_consultation_and_ responses_20161212.pdf.) At the least, WGS can provide information on which antimicrobials are not likely to be effective based on resistance gene content.

RETROSPECTIVE RESISTANCE SURVEILLANCE

In addition to identifying known resistance determinants, WGS allows for rapid retrospective analysis of bacterial genomes as new resistance genes are discovered. An example of this is illustrated by the discovery in 2015 of a mobile colistin resistance (*mcr-1*) gene in *E. coli* from animals, retail meats, and humans in China (17). Colistin is considered a drug of last resort for treating multidrug-resistant Gram-negative infections (68). It has not been part of most routine surveillance, since its use in humans is rare due to toxicity issues. With increasing resistance to front-line drugs, colistin resistance has become more important, and plasmid-mediated resistance adds concern about horizontal spread (17, 69, 70). With WGS, it is now possible to examine historical isolates for the presence of *mcr-1* and other new resistance genes with very little outlay of resources and time. Instead of reviving banked historical isolates and performing traditional susceptibility testing, it is now possible to examine all publicly available genomes to provide a rapid answer. As a result, bacteria with *mcr-1* were detected in over 20 countries within weeks of the original publication (71–73). In the United States, over 55,000 genomes of bacteria from domestic sources were found to be negative for *mcr-1*. This illustrates the unprecedented power of WGS to quickly provide answers to important questions about emerging AMR threats that previously would have been difficult to resolve quickly.

Identifying Resistance Plasmids

One of the drawbacks of Illumina DNA sequencing technologies is the short read length, which results in genomes consisting of many contigs (74). This makes it difficult to localize a given resistance gene to the chromosome or a plasmid. Some databases, such as PlasmidFinder (75), were assembled to help make these determinations, but these databases are far from complete, and while they indicate the presence of plasmid origins of replication, the physical association of resistance genes to particular plasmids is not always obvious.

Technologies that provide longer reads of DNA, and therefore fewer contigs, make it easier to completely close plasmids and chromosomes and to determine the physical linkages of genes with mobile DNA elements (41, 76, 77). This information can be used to assess the phylogenetic relationships of plasmid incompatibility groups and the variations at MDR integration sites where MDR islands are often found. This information sheds light on the likely origins and drivers of resistance and the potential risk associated with the use of antimicrobial drugs where coselection may lead to cross-resistance. Plasmids from food isolates may carry resistance to antimicrobial drugs not used in food animals (76). Furthermore, heavy metals such as copper and zinc used in agriculture and livestock production and aquaculture as antibiotic replacements may coselect for AMR (78). The details of gene arrangements on plasmids and other mobile elements can only be fully understood with closed genomes. Affordable methods to routinely achieve this will significantly enhance surveillance of AMR.

METAGENOMICS AND MOVING BEYOND CULTURE

Although genomic sequencing reveals the panoply of resistance traits in an individual organism, metagenomic methods do not rely on classic cultivation techniques and thus are not limited by which microorganisms can be grown in culture on artificial media. This is due in part to changing laboratory practices and market forces driving the rapid expansion of culture-independent diagnostic tests for foodborne and other illnesses, which do not require or produce a bacterial isolate for analysis. This will impact public health surveillance in a number of ways, including the ability to track trends in antibiotic resistance.

Metagenomics methods provide the total DNA content of a complex biological sample by direct sequencing. They can identify many microorganisms present in a sample and have been used to identify new pathogens. More importantly for resistance surveillance, metagenomic sequencing reveals the overall resistance gene content of a sample, including genes from unknown bacteria, those that are not easy to culture (e.g., anaerobes), and those for which no culture methods exist. This ability to conduct "deep surveillance" into new environments provides a much more complete picture of the microbiome and resistome associated with a given source. It will be important to link resistance genes with their host bacterium in metagenomic assays but more important to understand which genes are traversing ecological bottlenecks to reach human pathogens and compromise treatment. This ability will also enable a more complete One Health approach to combating resistance. This paradigm emphasizes the interconnectedness of animal, human, and environmental systems when addressing sustainability and preventing disease. The cost savings afforded by next-generation sequencing (NGS) technologies will make it possible to expand routine surveillance to more types of environments and enhance our understanding of AMR from a broader ecological perspective.

LIMITATIONS OF GENOME-BASED AMR SURVEILLANCE

There are several limitations to WGS-based AMR surveillance. While the assay does not require a premeditated design based on known sequences, the interpretation of results requires an understanding of structure-function relationships, or at least sufficient sequence similarity to orthologs to allow inferences to be made. For AMR surveillance, this means that some form of phenotypic susceptibility testing will be necessary to detect novel genes, as will a closely curated gene database to add new genes as they are found. The design of phenotypic susceptibility testing may change, however, as certain agents selected especially for epidemiological purposes (e.g., streptomycin, chloramphenicol) in *Salmonella* may be tracked adequately by WGS alone. Beyond the quinolones, WGS has not been adequately vetted for its ability to detect resistance resulting from a combination of mutations, which would require straightforward bioinformatics pipelines to evaluate multiple acquired mechanisms working together. Nor can WGS easily detect changes in susceptibility caused by differential gene expression, such as the combination of loci in the Mar regulon that lead to MIC changes or to silent genes whose expression depends on the genetic background of the host.

Despite these limitations, NGS technologies will make it easier to collect larger data sets at lower costs. With freely available bioinformatics tools, along with efforts to automate informatics at GenBank and other places online, it is anticipated that this technology will become automated in the near future for microbial surveillance while replacing programs and processes that require separate laboratory processes. As data on the relationship between genotype and MIC increase, NGS methods may replace traditional susceptibility testing for more pathogens. WGS has already largely replaced PFGE in strain typing, PCR for speciation, and a number of other traditional microbiological techniques (79, 80). Thus, it can be expected that veterinarians, physicians, and other public health officials who make decisions based on the characteristics of microbial pathogens will come to rely more and more on what can be gleaned from the genome as NGS methods become routine.

SUMMARY AND CONCLUSION

AMR surveillance is the cornerstone to address many of the global aspects of AMR. It provides a foundation for assessing the burden of AMR and for providing the necessary evidence for developing efficient and effective control and prevention strategies. The codevelopment of AMR surveillance programs in humans and animals is essential, but there remain several key elements that make data comparisons between human and animal AMR monitoring programs difficult. Differences in AMR programs between regions and countries also create challenges for data comparison. Currently, AMR surveillance relies on uncomplicated *in vitro* antimicrobial susceptibility methods. However, the lack of harmonization across programs and the limitation of

genetic information of AMR remain the major drawbacks of these phenotypic methods. The future of AMR surveillance is moving toward genotypic detection, and molecular analysis methods are expected to yield a wealth of information. However, the expectation that these molecular techniques will surpass phenotypic susceptibility testing in routine diagnosis and monitoring of AMR remains a distant reality, and phenotypic testing remains necessary in the detection of emerging resistant bacteria, new resistance mechanisms, and trends of AMR.

DISCLAIMER

The views expressed in this article are those of the authors and do not necessarily reflect the official policy of the Department of Health and Human Services, the U.S. Food and Drug Administration, or the U.S. government.

Acknowledgments. The authors thank Ramon Shaban, Geoff Simons, David Jordan, and John Turnidge for critical review and intellectual contributions.

Citation. Simjee S, McDermott P, Trott DJ, Rungtip C. 2018. The present and future surveillance of antimicrobial resistance in animals: principles and practices. Microbiol Spectrum 6(4):ARBA-0028-2017.

References

1. **Anderson ES.** 1968. Drug resistance in *Salmonella typhimurium* and its implications. *BMJ* **3:**333–339.

2. **UK Joint Committee of Houses of Parliament.** 1969. Report on the use of antibiotics in animal husbandry and veterinary medicine ('Swann Report'). Her Majesty's Stationery Office, London.

3. **Wray C, McLaren IM, Beedell YE.** 1993. Bacterial resistance monitoring of salmonellas isolated from animals, national experience of surveillance schemes in the United Kingdom. *Vet Microbiol* **35:**313–319.

4. **Pocurull DW, Gaines SA, Mercer HD.** 1971. Survey of infectious multiple drug resistance among *Salmonella* isolated from animals in the United States. *Appl Microbiol* **21:**358–362.

5. **Martel JL, Coudert M.** 1993. Bacterial resistance monitoring in animals: the French national experiences of surveillance schemes. *Vet Microbiol* **35:**321–338.

6. **Cohen ML, Tauxe RV.** 1986. Drug-resistant *Salmonella* in the United States: an epidemiologic perspective. *Science* **234:**964–969.

7. **DuPont HL, Steele JH.** 1987. Use of antimicrobial agents in animal feeds: implications for human health. *Rev Infect Dis* **9:**447–460.

8. **Tollefson L, Angulo FJ, Fedorka-Cray PJ.** 1998. National surveillance for antibiotic resistance in zoonotic enteric pathogens. *Vet Clin North Am Food Anim Pract* **14:**141–150.

9. Aarestrup FM, Bager F, Jensen NE, Madsen M, Meyling A, Wegener HC. 1998. Resistance to antimicrobial agents used for animal therapy in pathogenic-, zoonotic- and indicator bacteria isolated from different food animals in Denmark: a baseline study for the Danish Integrated Antimicrobial Resistance Monitoring Programme (DANMAP). *APMIS* 106:745–770.

10. Moyaert H, de Jong A, Simjee S, Thomas V. 2014. Antimicrobial resistance monitoring projects for zoonotic and indicator bacteria of animal origin: common aspects and differences between EASSA and EFSA. *Vet Microbiol* 171:279–283.

11. Shaban RZ, Simon GI, Trott DJ, Turnidge J, Jordan D. 2014. Surveillance and reporting of antimicrobial resistance and antibiotic usage in animals and agriculture in Australia. Report to the Department of Agriculture, Griffith University and University of Adelaide, Australia.

12. Pagel SW, Gautier P. 2012. Use of antimicrobial agents in livestock. *Rev Sci Tech* 31:145–188.

13. Weir M, Rajić A, Dutil L, Uhland C, Bruneau N. 2012. Zoonotic bacteria and antimicrobial resistance in aquaculture: opportunities for surveillance in Canada. *Can Vet J* 53:619–622.

14. Brudeseth BE, Wiulsrød R, Fredriksen BN, Lindmo K, Løkling KE, Bordevik M, Steine N, Klevan A, Gravningen K. 2013. Status and future perspectives of vaccines for industrialised fin-fish farming. *Fish Shellfish Immunol* 35:1759–1768.

15. DANMAP. 2016. *DANMAP 2015. Use of Antimicrobial Agents and Occurrence of Antimicrobial Resistance in Bacteria from Food Animals, Food and Humans.* https://www.danmap.org/.

16. DANMAP. 2012. *DANMAP 2011. Use of Antimicrobial Agents and Occurrence of Antimicrobial Resistance in Bacteria from Food Animals, Food and Humans.* https://www.danmap.org/.

17. Liu YY, Wang Y, Walsh TR, Yi LX, Zhang R, Spencer J, Doi Y, Tian G, Dong B, Huang X, Yu LF, Gu D, Ren H, Chen X, Lv L, He D, Zhou H, Liang Z, Liu JH, Shen J. 2016. Emergence of plasmid-mediated colistin resistance mechanism MCR-1 in animals and human beings in China: a microbiological and molecular biological study. *Lancet Infect Dis* 16:161–168.

18. Guerra B, Fischer J, Helmuth R. 2014. An emerging public health problem: acquired carbapenemase-producing microorganisms are present in food-producing animals, their environment, companion animals and wild birds. *Vet Microbiol* 171:290–297.

19. Johnson TJ. 2017. Carbapenemase-producing Enterobacteriaceae in swine production in the United States: impact and opportunities. *Antimicrob Agents Chemother* 61:e02348-16.

20. El Garch F, de Jong A, Simjee S, Moyaert H, Klein U, Ludwig C, Marion H, Haag-Diergarten S, Richard-Mazet A, Thomas V, Siegwart E. 2016. Monitoring of antimicrobial susceptibility of respiratory tract pathogens isolated from diseased cattle and pigs across Europe, 2009–2012: VetPath results. *Vet Microbiol* 194:11–22.

21. Michael GB, Kadlec K, Sweeney MT, Brzuszkiewicz E, Liesegang H, Daniel R, Murray RW, Watts JL, Schwarz S. 2012. ICEPmu1, an integrative conjugative element (ICE) of *Pasteurella multocida*: structure and transfer. *J Antimicrob Chemother* 67:91–100.

22. Michael GB, Kadlec K, Sweeney MT, Brzuszkiewicz E, Liesegang H, Daniel R, Murray RW, Watts JL, Schwarz S. 2012. ICEPmu1, an integrative conjugative element (ICE) of *Pasteurella multocida*: analysis of the regions that comprise 12 antimicrobial resistance genes. *J Antimicrob Chemother* 67:84–90.

23. Lubbers BV, Hanzlicek GA. 2013. Antimicrobial multidrug resistance and coresistance patterns of *Mannheimia haemolytica* isolated from bovine respiratory disease cases: a three-year (2009–2011) retrospective analysis. *J Vet Diagn Invest* 25:413–417.

24. Bossé JT, Li Y, Fernandez Crespo R, Chaudhuri RR, Rogers J, Holden MT, Maskell DJ, Tucker AW, Wren BW, Rycroft AN, Langford PR, the BRaDP1T Consortium. 2016. ICEApl1, an integrative conjugative element related to ICEHin1056, identified in the pig pathogen *Actinobacillus pleuropneumoniae*. *Front Microbiol* 7:810.

25. Jahanbakhsh S, Smith MG, Kohan-Ghadr HR, Letellier A, Abraham S, Trott DJ, Fairbrother JM. 2016. Dynamics of extended-spectrum cephalosporin resistance in pathogenic *Escherichia coli* isolated from diseased pigs in Quebec, Canada. *Int J Antimicrob Agents* 48:194–202.

26. Smith M, Do TN, Gibson JS, Jordan D, Cobbold RN, Trott DJ. 2014. Comparison of antimicrobial resistance phenotypes and genotypes in enterotoxigenic *Escherichia coli* isolated from Australian and Vietnamese pigs. *J Glob Antimicrob Resist* 2:162–167.

27. Walther B, Monecke S, Ruscher C, Friedrich AW, Ehricht R, Slickers P, Soba A, Wleklinski CG, Wieler LH, Lübke-Becker A. 2009. Comparative molecular analysis substantiates zoonotic potential of equine methicillin-resistant *Staphylococcus aureus*. *J Clin Microbiol* 47:704–710.

28. Larsen J, Stegger M, Andersen PS, Petersen A, Larsen AR, Westh H, Agersø Y, Fetsch A, Kraushaar B, Käsbohrer A, Feler AT, Schwarz S, Cuny C, Witte W, Butaye P, Denis O, Haenni M, Madec JY, Jouy E, Laurent F, Battisti A, Franco A, Alba P, Mammina C, Pantosti A, Monaco M, Wagenaar JA, de Boer E, van Duijkeren E, Heck M, Domínguez L, Torres C, Zarazaga M, Price LB, Skov RL. 2016. Evidence for human adaptation and foodborne transmission of livestock-associated methicillin-resistant *Staphylococcus aureus*. *Clin Infect Dis* 63:1349–1352.

29. Platell JL, Johnson JR, Cobbold RN, Trott DJ. 2011. Multidrug-resistant extraintestinal pathogenic *Escherichia coli* of sequence type ST131 in animals and foods. *Vet Microbiol* 153:99–108.

30. Platell JL, Cobbold RN, Johnson JR, Heisig A, Heisig P, Clabots C, Kuskowski MA, Trott DJ. 2011. Commonality among fluoroquinolone-resistant sequence type ST131 extraintestinal *Escherichia coli* isolates from humans and companion animals in Australia. *Antimicrob Agents Chemother* 55:3782–3787.

31. Ewers C, Bethe A, Stamm I, Grobbel M, Kopp PA, Guerra B, Stubbe M, Doi Y, Zong Z, Kola A, Schaufler K, Semmler T, Fruth A, Wieler LH, Guenther S. 2014. CTX-M-15-D-ST648 *Escherichia coli* from companion animals and horses: another pandemic clone combining multiresistance and extraintestinal virulence? *J Antimicrob Chemother* **69**:1224–1230.

32. Vangchhia B, Abraham S, Bell JM, Collignon P, Gibson JS, Ingram PR, Johnson JR, Kennedy K, Trott DJ, Turnidge JD, Gordon DM. 2016. Phylogenetic diversity, antimicrobial susceptibility and virulence characteristics of phylogroup F *Escherichia coli* in Australia. *Microbiology* **162**:1904–1912.

33. Iwamoto M, Reynolds J, Karp BE, Tate H, Fedorka-Cray PJ, Plumblee JR, Hoekstra RM, Whichard JM, Mahon BE. 2017. Ceftriaxone-resistant nontyphoidal *Salmonella* from humans, retail meats, and food animals in the United States, 1996–2013. *Foodborne Pathog Dis* **14**:74–83.

34. Jiu Y, Zhu S, Khan SB, Sun M, Zou G, Meng X, Wu B, Zhou R, Li S. 2016. Phenotypic and genotypic resistance of *Salmonella* isolates from healthy and diseased pigs in China during 2008–2015. *Microb Drug Resist* **23**:651–659.

35. Lin D, Chen K, Wai-Chi Chan E, Chen S. 2015. Increasing prevalence of ciprofloxacin-resistant food-borne *Salmonella* strains harboring multiple PMQR elements but not target gene mutations. *Sci Rep* **5**:14754.

36. Clewell DB, Weaver KE, Dunny GM, Coque TM, Francia MV, Hayes F. 2014. Extrachromosomal and mobile elements in *Enterococci*: transmission, maintenance, and epidemiology. *In* Gilmore MS, Clewell DB, Ike Y, Shankar N (ed), *Enterococci: from Commensals to Leading Causes of Drug Resistant Infection*. [Internet.] Massachusetts Eye and Ear Infirmary, Boston, MA.

37. Al-Tawfiq JA, Laxminarayan R, Mendelson M. 2017. How should we respond to the emergence of plasmid-mediated colistin resistance in humans and animals? *Int J Infect Dis* **54**:77–84.

38. Kluytmans JA, Overdevest IT, Willemsen I, Kluytmans-van den Bergh MF, van der Zwaluw K, Heck M, Rijnsburger M, Vandenbroucke-Grauls CM, Savelkoul PH, Johnston BD, Gordon D, Johnson JR. 2013. Extended-spectrum β-lactamase-producing *Escherichia coli* from retail chicken meat and humans: comparison of strains, plasmids, resistance genes, and virulence factors. *Clin Infect Dis* **56**:478–487.

39. Mitchell NM, Johnson JR, Johnston B, Curtiss R III, Mellata M. 2015. Zoonotic potential of *Escherichia coli* isolates from retail chicken meat products and eggs. *Appl Environ Microbiol* **81**:1177–1187.

40. Abraham S, Jordan D, Wong HS, Johnson JR, Toleman MA, Wakcham DL, Gordon DM, Turnidge JD, Mollinger JL, Gibson JS, Trott DJ. 2015. First detection of extended-spectrum cephalosporin- and fluoroquinolone-resistant *Escherichia coli* in Australian food-producing animals. *J Glob Antimicrob Resist* **3**:273–277.

41. Doi Y, Hazen TH, Boitano M, Tsai YC, Clark TA, Korlach J, Rasko DA, Chattaway MA, DoNascimento V, Wain J, Helmuth R, Guerra B, Schwarz S, Threlfall J, Woodward MJ, Coldham N, Doi Y, Hazen TH, Boitano M, Tsai YC, Clark TA, Korlach J, Rasko DA. 2014. Whole-genome assembly of *Klebsiella pneumoniae* co-producing NDM-1 and OXA-232 carbapenemases using single-molecule, real-time sequencing. *Antimicrob Agents Chemother* **58**:5947–5953.

42. de Been M, Lanza VF, de Toro M, Scharringa J, Dohmen W, Du Y, Hu J, Lei Y, Li N, Tooming-Klunderud A, Heederik DJ, Fluit AC, Bonten MJ, Willems RJ, de la Cruz F, van Schaik W. 2014. Dissemination of cephalosporin resistance genes between *Escherichia coli* strains from farm animals and humans by specific plasmid lineages. *PLoS Genet* **10**:e1004776.

43. Jorgensen JH, Ferraro MJ. 2009. Antimicrobial susceptibility testing: a review of general principles and contemporary practices. *Clin Infect Dis* **49**:1749–1755.

44. Lubbers BV, Turnidge J. 2015. Antimicrobial susceptibility testing for bovine respiratory disease: getting more from diagnostic results. *Vet J* **203**:149–154.

45. CLSI. 2011. Generation, presentation and application of antimicrobial susceptibility test data for bacteria of animal origin. https://clsi.org/standards/products/veterinary-medicine/documents/vet05/.

46. Silley P. 2012. Susceptibility testing methods, resistance and breakpoints: what do these terms really mean? *Rev Sci Tech* **31**:33–41.

47. European Food Safety Authority. 2012. Technical specifications for the analysis and reporting of data on antimicrobial resistance (AMR) in the European Union Summary Report. Parma, Italy.

48. World Health Organization. 2002. *Surveillance Standards for Antimicrobial Resistance*. WHO, Geneva, Switzerland.

49. European Food Safety Authority–Working Group on Developing Harmonised Schemes for Monitoring Antimicrobial Resistance in Zoonotic Agents. 2008. Harmonised monitoring of antimicrobial resistance in *Salmonella* and *Campylobacter* isolates from food animals in the European Union. *Clin Microbiol Infect* **14**:522–533.

50. Regula G, Lo Fo Wong DMA, Ledergerber U, Stephan R, Danuser J, Bissig-Choisat B, Stärk KDC. 2005. Evaluation of an antimicrobial resistance monitoring program for *Campylobacter* in poultry by simulation. *Prev Vet Med* **70**:29–43.

51. Agersø Y, Aarestrup FM. 2013. Voluntary ban on cephalosporin use in Danish pig production has effectively reduced extended-spectrum cephalosporinase-producing *Escherichia coli* in slaughter pigs. *J Antimicrob Chemother* **68**:569–572.

52. Parmley EJ, Pintar K, Majowicz S, Avery B, Cook A, Jokinen C, Gannon V, Lapen DR, Topp E, Edge TA, Gilmour M, Pollari F, Reid-Smith R, Irwin R. 2013. A Canadian application of One Health: integration of *Salmonella* data from various Canadian surveillance programs (2005–2010). *Foodborne Pathog Dis* **10**:747–756.

53. Gilbert JM, White DG, McDermott PF. 2007. The US national antimicrobial resistance monitoring system. *Future Microbiol* **2**:493–500.

54. FDA. 2016. National Antimicrobial Resistance Monitoring System - Enteric Bacteria (NARMS): NARMS Integrated Report 2014. Rockville, Maryland: U.S. Department of Health and Human Services, Food & Drug Administration. Available at: http://www.fda.gov/AnimalVeterinary/SafetyHealth/AntimicrobialResistance/NationalAntimicrobialResistanceMonitoringSystem/default.htm.

55. Kahlmeter G. 2014. Defining antibiotic resistance-towards international harmonization. *Ups J Med Sci* **119**:78–86.

56. Zankari E, Hasman H, Cosentino S, Vestergaard M, Rasmussen S, Lund O, Aarestrup FM, Larsen MV. 2012. Identification of acquired antimicrobial resistance genes. *J Antimicrob Chemother* **67**:2640–2644.

57. McArthur AG, Waglechner N, Nizam F, Yan A, Azad MA, Baylay AJ, Bhullar K, Canova MJ, De Pascale G, Ejim L, Kalan L, King AM, Koteva K, Morar M, Mulvey MR, O'Brien JS, Pawlowski AC, Piddock LJV, Spanogiannopoulos P, Sutherland AD, Tang I, Taylor PL, Thaker M, Wang W, Yan M, Yu T, Wright GD. 2013. The comprehensive antibiotic resistance database. *Anti microb Agents Chemother* **57**:3348–3357.

58. Gupta SK, Padmanabhan BR, Diene SM, Lopez-Rojas R, Kempf M, Landraud L, Rolain JM. 2014. ARG-ANNOT, a new bioinformatic tool to discover antibiotic resistance genes in bacterial genomes. *Antimicrob Agents Chemother* **58**:212–220.

59. Tyson GH, McDermott PF, Li C, Chen Y, Tadesse DA, Mukherjee S, Bodeis-Jones S, Kabera C, Gaines SA, Loneragan GH, Edrington TS, Torrence M, Harhay DM, Zhao S. 2015. WGS accurately predicts antimicrobial resistance in *Escherichia coli*. *J Antimicrob Chemother* **70**:2763–2769.

60. Stoesser N, Batty EM, Eyre DW, Morgan M, Wyllie DH, Del Ojo Elias C, Johnson JR, Walker AS, Peto TE, Crook DW. 2013. Predicting antimicrobial susceptibilities for *Escherichia coli* and *Klebsiella pneumoniae* isolates using whole genomic sequence data. *J Antimicrob Chemother* **68**:2234–2244.

61. Zankari E, Hasman H, Kaas RS, Seyfarth AM, Agersø Y, Lund O, Larsen MV, Aarestrup FM. 2013. Genotyping using whole-genome sequencing is a realistic alternative to surveillance based on phenotypic antimicrobial susceptibility testing. *J Antimicrob Chemother* **68**:771–777.

62. Zhao S, Tyson GH, Chen Y, Li C, Mukherjee S, Young S, Lam C, Folster JP, Whichard JM, McDermott PF. 2015. Whole-genome sequencing analysis accurately predicts antimicrobial resistance phenotypes in *Campylobacter* spp. *Appl Environ Microbiol* **82**:459–466.

63. Mcdermott PF, Tyson GH, Kabera C, Chen Y, Li C, Folster JP, Ayers SL, Lam C, Tate HP, Zhao S. 2016. The use of whole genome sequencing for detecting antimicrobial resistance in nontyphoidal *Salmonella*. *Antimicrob Agents Chemother*. **60**:5515–5520.

64. Gordon NC, Price JR, Cole K, Everitt R, Morgan M, Finney J, Kearns AM, Pichon B, Young B, Wilson DJ, Llewelyn MJ, Paul J, Peto TE, Crook DW, Walker AS, Golubchik T. 2014. Prediction of *Staphylococcus aureus* antimicrobial resistance by whole-genome sequencing. *J Clin Microbiol* **52**:1182–1191.

65. Zhao S, Mukherjee S, Chen Y, Li C, Young S, Warren M, Abbott J, Friedman S, Kabera C, Karlsson M, McDermott PF. 2015. Novel gentamicin resistance genes in *Campylobacter* isolated from humans and retail meats in the USA. *J Antimicrob Chemother* **70**:1314–1321.

66. Pal C, Bengtsson-Palme J, Rensing C, Kristiansson E, Larsson DG. 2014. BacMet: antibacterial biocide and metal resistance genes database. *Nucleic Acids Res* **42** (D1):D737–D743.

67. Tyson GH, Li C, Ayers S, McDermott PF, Zhao S. 2016. Using whole-genome sequencing to determine appropriate streptomycin epidemiological cutoffs for *Salmonella* and *Escherichia coli*. *FEMS Microbiol Lett* **363**:363.

68. Kaye KS, Pogue JM, Tran TB, Nation RL, Li J. 2016. Agents of last resort: polymyxin resistance. *Infect Dis Clin North Am* **30**:391–414.

69. Hu Y, Liu F, Lin IY, Gao GF, Zhu B. 2016. Dissemination of the *mcr-1* colistin resistance gene. *Lancet Infect Dis* **16**:146–147.

70. Stoesser N, Mathers AJ, Moore CE, Day NP, Crook DW. 2016. Colistin resistance gene *mcr-1* and pHNSHP45 plasmid in human isolates of *Escherichia coli* and *Klebsiella pneumoniae*. *Lancet Infect Dis* **16**:285–286.

71. Hasman H, Hammerum AM, Hansen F, Hendriksen RS, Olesen B, Agersø Y, Zankari E, Leekitcharoenphon P, Stegger M, Kaas RS, Cavaco LM, Hansen DS, Aarestrup FM, Skov RL. 2015. Detection of *mcr-1* encoding plasmid-mediated colistin-resistant *Escherichia coli* isolates from human bloodstream infection and imported chicken meat, Denmark 2015. *Euro Surveill* **20**:20.

72. McGann P, Snesrud E, Maybank R, Corey B, Ong AC, Clifford R, Hinkle M, Whitman T, Lesho E, Schaecher KE. 2016. *Escherichia coli* harboring *mcr-1* and *blaCTX-M* on a novel IncF plasmid: first report of *mcr-1* in the United States. *Antimicrob Agents Chemother* **60**:4420–4421.

73. Suzuki S, Ohnishi M, Kawanishi M, Akiba M, Kuroda M. 2016. Investigation of a plasmid genome database for colistin-resistance gene *mcr-1*. *Lancet Infect Dis* **16**:284–285.

74. Lesho E, Clifford R, Onmus-Leone F, Appalla L, Snesrud E, Kwak Y, Ong A, Maybank R, Waterman P, Rohrbeck P, Julius M, Roth A, Martinez J, Nielsen L, Steele E, McGann P, Hinkle M. 2016. The challenges of implementing next generation sequencing across a large healthcare system, and the molecular epidemiology and antibiotic susceptibilities of carbapenemase-producing bacteria in the healthcare system of the U.S. Department of Defense. *PLoS One* **11**:e0155770.

75. Carattoli A, Zankari E, García-Fernández A, Voldby Larsen M, Lund O, Villa L, Møller Aarestrup F, Hasman H. 2014. *In silico* detection and typing of plasmids using PlasmidFinder and plasmid multilocus sequence typing. *Antimicrob Agents Chemother* **58**:3895–3903.

76. Chen Y, Mukherjee S, Hoffmann M, Kotewicz ML, Young S, Abbott J, Luo Y, Davidson MK, Allard M, McDermott P, Zhao S. 2013. Whole-genome sequencing of gentamicin-resistant *Campylobacter coli* isolated from U.S. retail meats reveals novel plasmid-mediated amino-

glycoside resistance genes. *Antimicrob Agents Chemother* 57:5398–5405.

77. Wang J, Stephan R, Power K, Yan Q, Hächler H, Fanning S. 2014. Nucleotide sequences of 16 transmissible plasmids identified in nine multidrug-resistant *Escherichia coli* isolates expressing an ESBL phenotype isolated from food-producing animals and healthy humans. *J Antimicrob Chemother* 69:2658–2668.

78. Seiler C, Berendonk TU. 2012. Heavy metal driven co-selection of antibiotic resistance in soil and water bodies impacted by agriculture and aquaculture. *Front Microbiol* 3:399.

79. Larsen MV, Cosentino S, Lukjancenko O, Saputra D, Rasmussen S, Hasman H, Sicheritz-Pontén T, Aarestrup FM, Ussery DW, Lund O. 2014. Benchmarking of methods for genomic taxonomy. *J Clin Microbiol* 52:1529–1539.

80. Salipante SJ, SenGupta DJ, Cummings LA, Land TA, Hoogestraat DR, Cookson BT. 2015. Application of whole-genome sequencing for bacterial strain typing in molecular epidemiology. *J Clin Microbiol* 53:1072–1079.

Antimicrobial Resistance in Bacteria from Livestock and Companion Animals
Edited by Frank Møller Aarestrup, Stefan Schwarz, Jianzhong Shen, and Lina Cavaco
© 2018 American Society for Microbiology, Washington, DC
doi:10.1128/microbiolspec.ARBA-0027-2017

Source Attribution and Risk Assessment of Antimicrobial Resistance

29

Sara M. Pires[1], Ana Sofia Duarte[2], and Tine Hald[2]

INTRODUCTION

Antimicrobial use in humans and animals has been identified as a main driver of antimicrobial resistance (AMR), and bacteria harboring resistance to antimicrobials can be found in humans, animals, foods, and the environment. As a consequence, humans can be exposed to antimicrobial-resistant bacteria through a wide range of sources and transmission pathways. To inform policies aimed at reducing the burden of AMR in animals and foods, risk managers need evidence about the most important sources and transmission routes and the critical points throughout the production chain for the prevention and control of AMR. While this process is complex and deeply reliant on the integration of surveillance data from humans, animals, and foods, it is supported by scientific disciplines that have evolved rapidly in the past decades, including source attribution and quantitative risk assessment.

Source attribution is a relatively new discipline that has been developed to assist risk managers to identify and prioritize effective food safety intervention measures. It is defined as the *partitioning of the human disease burden of one or more foodborne illnesses to specific sources, where the term source includes reservoirs and vehicles* (1). A variety of source attribution methods is available to estimate the relative contribution of different reservoirs or vehicles of foodborne pathogens, including methods relying on data on the occurrence of the pathogen in sources and humans, epidemiological studies, intervention studies, and expert elicitations. These methods have been applied to inform food safety policy-making at the national or international level, particularly regarding *Salmonella* and *Campylobacter* intervention strategies (see, e.g., 2–6). Source attribution methods differ in their approaches and data requirements, and as a consequence, they attribute disease at different points along the food chain (points of attribution), i.e., at the point of reservoir (e.g., animal production stage, environment emissions) or the point of exposure (end of the transmission chain) (Fig. 1). The application and utility of each method, therefore, depends on the risk management question being addressed and on the availability of data.

Microbial risk assessment is a systematic and science-based approach to estimating the risk of microbial hazards in the production-to-consumption chain (8, 9). Microbial risk assessment can be used to detect critical control points along the food chain and for the assessment of control and intervention strategies. It is a well-established discipline that has been widely applied to estimate the risk of an extensive variety of pathogen-food commodity pairs, and it is also systematically applied to inform food safety risk management in many countries and international bodies such as the European Food Safety Authority (e.g., 10–12). In coordination with source attribution studies, it is particularly useful to focus on the production chain of the most important source(s) of the hazard of interest (as identified in the source attribution step), identify the steps in the food chain that are critical for hazard control, and identify and suggest strategies for reduction of the risk to humans.

While source attribution and risk assessment have been widely used to provide evidence that can support strategies to reduce the burden of a number of food-

[1]Risk Benefit Research Group, Division of Diet, Disease Prevention and Toxicology, National Food Institute, Technical University of Denmark, 2800 Kgs. Lyngby; [2]Unit for Genomic Epidemiology, National Food Institute, Technical University of Denmark, 2800 Kgs. Lyngby, Denmark.

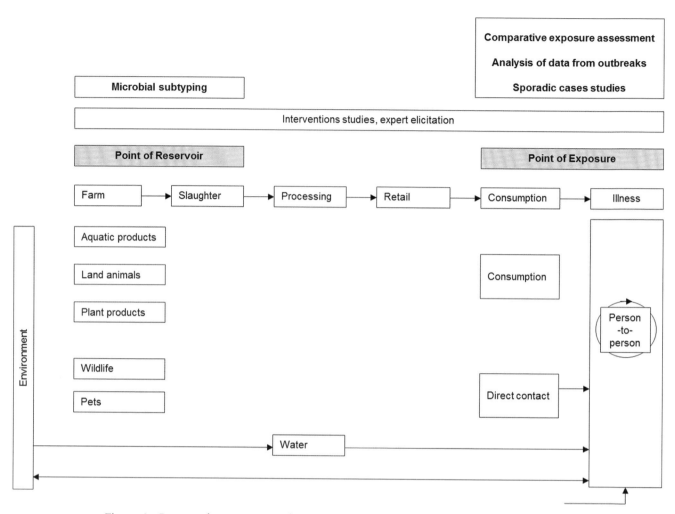

Figure 1   Routes of transmission of zoonotic pathogens and points of source attribution. Adapted from reference 7.

borne pathogens, the transmission and spread of pathogens carrying resistance to antimicrobials adds an extra layer of complexity to this integrated food safety paradigm. On one hand, virtually any foodborne pathogen can acquire resistance to antimicrobials, which may lead to prolonged and more severe disease and even be life-threatening, when antimicrobial therapy is required but fails to succeed due to resistance to the prescribed drug(s). On the other hand, the potential transfer of AMR genes (i.e., the gene[s] carrying the resistance trait) between pathogenic and commensal bacteria in the human gut can amplify the public health impact of foodborne AMR (13). As a consequence, it is not only challenging to estimate the direct risk posed by resistant foodborne pathogens, but also to quantify the relative contribution to risk of the transfer of AMR genes, e.g., from commensals originating from animal reservoirs to human pathogens.

This article describes the overall concepts and methods in source attribution and microbial risk assessment, describes the state of the art of their application in the area of AMR, and discusses current challenges and future perspectives for the development of methods to inform policies to reduce the disease burden of AMR in human populations.

SOURCE ATTRIBUTION

Source Attribution of AMR

The purpose of applying source attribution methods to antimicrobial-resistant pathogens (i.e., a pathogen that has acquired resistance to at least one antimicrobial drug) or AMR genes is to identify the most important sources and transmission routes for human exposure to AMR. It is widely recognized that one of the main drivers of resistance in zoonotic bacteria is antimicrobial use in livestock production (i.e., in the reservoirs) (14). Identifying the most important reservoirs for human exposure to AMR is hence critical to direct policy-making aimed at reducing antimicrobial use at the primary production level. In addition, knowledge of the transmission routes from reservoirs to humans is crucial for the prioritization of risk management along the food chain.

While a range of source attribution methods attributing disease to the original reservoirs or to exposure routes of foodborne pathogens exists, only a few studies have applied these in the context of AMR, and the relative importance of transmission pathways of resistance remains a critical knowledge gap.

The challenges of applying source attribution methods for AMR include the fact that virtually any pathogen can become resistant to antimicrobials and that most zoonotic pathogens can be transmitted to humans via a variety of foodborne and nonfoodborne routes. Thus far, source attribution has typically focused on a single pathogen (e.g., *Salmonella* or *Escherichia coli*) and on resistance profiles found among that pathogen in different sources (15–17). In addition, AMR genes are often located on plasmids, which can be transferred between bacterial species (plasmid-mediated horizontal gene transfer) and therefore also from commensal bacteria to human pathogens (e.g., *Klebsiella* spp.). Focusing on a single bacterial species is therefore likely to underestimate the overall exposure and thus the risk posed by AMR.

To address this challenge, source attribution of the AMR determinant may be more efficient. Such studies require knowledge of and data on the prevalence, abundance, and transmission of genes and on horizontal gene transfer rates, which is still being gathered (e.g., in the European Union project EFFORT—Ecology from Farm to Fork of Microbial Drug Resistance and Transmission; http://www.effort-against-amr.eu/).

Existing Source Attribution Approaches

Microbial subtyping

The microbial subtyping approach involves characterization of the hazard by subtyping methods (e.g., phenotypic or genotypic subtyping of bacterial strains), and the principle is to compare the subtypes of isolates from different sources (e.g., animals, food) with the subtypes isolated from humans. The subtyping approach attributes illness at the point of reservoir and is enabled by the identification of strong associations between some of the dominant subtypes and a specific

reservoir or source, providing a heterogeneous distribution of subtypes among the sources (1).

Microbial subtyping methods for source attribution include frequency-matched models and population genetic models. While the frequency-matched methods are based on the comparison of human strain types and the distribution of those types in the sources, the population genetic models are based on modeling the organism's evolutionary history (18). In the frequency-matched models, subtypes exclusively or almost exclusively isolated from one source are regarded as indicators for the human health impact of that particular source, assuming that all human cases caused by these subtypes originate only from that source. Human cases of disease caused by subtypes found in several reservoirs are then distributed relative to the prevalence of the indicator types (2, 3, 19). Population genetics approaches use genotyping data to infer evolutionary and clonal relationships among different strains, including the occurrence of novel (combinations of) alleles in strains from humans that are unobserved in source populations (20).

All microbial subtyping models require a collection of temporally and spatially related isolates from various sources and thus are facilitated by an integrated foodborne disease surveillance program providing a collection of isolates from the major animal reservoirs of foodborne diseases. These models do not require prevalence data and can rely on the distribution of the isolates' subtypes in the different sources and in humans.

Both types of models have been applied to attribute foodborne pathogens to sources in a variety of countries. Microbial subtyping approaches have been particularly successful to attribute *Salmonella* and *Campylobacter* infections (see e.g., 3, 21–24). This method has also been applied to other pathogens (namely, *Listeria monocytogenes* and Shiga toxin-producing *E. coli* [25, 26]), even though less frequently due to a lack of available surveillance data in most countries.

The microbial subtyping approach has seldom been used to estimate the relative contribution of sources of antimicrobial-resistant pathogens to AMR in humans. To our knowledge, two frequency-matched studies have been conducted, both using antimicrobial susceptibility patterns as a typing method for *Salmonella* (15, 16). Both studies demonstrate that AMR data can be used to characterize pathogen subtypes in a microbial subtyping source-attribution model and discuss its utility in terms of discriminatory power but do not focus on the source origin of specific AMR genes.

Microbial subtyping methods are recognized as one of the most robust types of data-driven methods for source attribution. They have the advantage of attributing illness to the reservoirs of the pathogens, thus informing risk-management strategies that are the closest possible to the original sources and preventing further spread to other routes or sources of transmission (1). Another advantage of this approach is that it does not require data on the prevalence and concentration of the pathogen in the different sources (which is often difficult to obtain) or on the exposure frequency in the population. Still, these methods are often limited by the requirement of comparable subtyping data originating from an operative integrated surveillance of human cases and food/animals. In addition, the methods cannot distinguish between different transmission routes from a specific animal reservoir to humans.

Comparative exposure assessment

Comparative exposure assessments determine the relative importance of the known transmission routes by estimating the human exposure to the hazard (e.g., pathogen) via each route. For each known transmission route, this approach requires information on the prevalence and/or dose/concentration of the pathogen in the source, the changes of the prevalence and quantity of the pathogen throughout the transmission chain, and the frequency at which humans are exposed by that route (e.g., consumption data). Exposure doses are then compared, and the relative contribution of each of the various transmission routes to human exposure in the population is estimated, proportionally to the size of each exposure dose.

The data requirements of the comparative exposure assessment approach depend on the overall transmission groups considered in the model (i.e., foodborne, environmental, and/or contact with animals), as well as on the point in the transmission chain where the "origin" of the pathogen is set. In general, contamination data for each source, information on the main steps in the transmission chain and data on the effects of these on contamination, and exposure data are needed. If transmission via contact with live animals is considered, the exposure model needs to be expanded to consider different possibilities for direct and indirect contact with a contaminated animal.

Exposure assessments have been used with different degrees of success to source-attribute disease by several microbial agents (namely, *Listeria*, *Campylobacter*, Verocytotoxigenic *Escherichia coli* (VTEC), and *Toxoplasma gondii*) and by chemical hazards (aflatoxins, cadmium, and lead) (27–34).

In the context of AMR, this approach is particularly useful to address a widely recognized knowledge gap, which is understanding the relative contribution of the exposure routes of AMR from animals to humans. Specifically, it can be used to estimate the relative importance of the food chain, companion animals, and the environment for exposure of the general population to antimicrobial-resistant bacteria or AMR genes. Thus far (and to our knowledge), two comparative exposure assessments have been applied to estimate the relative contribution of different types of meat to the exposure of consumers to extended-spectrum beta-lactamase-producing and AmpC beta-lactamase-producing *E. coli* in the Netherlands (17) and in Denmark (35).

An important drawback of this approach is that, due to data limitations and gaps (e.g., in food preparation habits and the effect of these on the contamination of foods), exposure estimates for microbial pathogens are likely to present wide uncertainty intervals. Furthermore, in the context of AMR, these studies focus on specific antimicrobial-resistant pathogens and do not address all concomitant transmission routes contributing to overall transmission of resistance to humans (e.g., the same AMR determinant present in other members of the meat bacterial community), which adds to the uncertainty of the relative exposure estimates.

Epidemiological approaches

Epidemiological approaches for source attribution include analyses of data from outbreak investigations and studies of sporadic infections; both approaches attribute illness at the point of exposure. An outbreak is here defined as (i) the occurrence of two or more cases of a similar illness resulting from the exposure to a common source (36) or (ii) a situation in which the observed number of cases exceeds the expected number and where the cases are linked to the same food source. Sporadic cases are those that have not been associated with known outbreaks (37). Even though outbreak-associated cases are more likely to be captured by public health surveillance systems, an unknown proportion of cases classified as sporadic may be part of undetected outbreaks.

Many outbreak investigations are successful in identifying the specific contaminated source or ingredient causing human infections. A simple descriptive analysis or summary of outbreak investigations is useful for quantifying the relative contribution of different foods to outbreak illnesses. However, these implicated foods may be composed of multiple ingredients, and thus outbreak data do not always allow pinpointing of the actual source of infection. Probabilistic models using outbreak data to estimate the total number of illnesses in the population attributable to different foods provide a useful way to generalize outbreak data to a broader population of foodborne illnesses. These models are used not only to generalize the results of outbreak investigations, but also to estimate the contaminated sources in composite or "complex" foods.

Analyses of data from outbreak investigations benefit from detailed data on each reported outbreak and require the adoption of a food categorization scheme for classification of implicated foods (see, e.g., 38). Composite foods are assigned to two or more food categories depending on the number and nature of their ingredients. By assigning a probability to each ingredient, corresponding to the likelihood that it was the source of the outbreak, outbreak data, including data about both simple and complex foods, can be used to attribute foodborne illnesses to sources.

Several analyses of outbreak data for source attribution have been published in recent years, most of them modeling (39–41) or summarizing (42, 43) data from multiple pathogens. The strength of this method is that it uses data that is readily available in many countries worldwide, and thus its use is not restricted to countries with integrated foodborne disease surveillance programs. Also, it attributes foodborne illnesses at the point of exposure, which means that it is particularly useful to identify which foods (including processed foods) most frequently cause disease, as well as which risk factors contribute more to contamination of foods at the end of the food chain (e.g., cross-contamination). This type of information is valuable to define interventions at the processing and consumption level but does not provide evidence to inform risk management strategies at the origin of the pathogen (reservoirs).

Several outbreaks caused by antimicrobial-resistant pathogens have been reported and investigated in the past decades (see, e.g., 44, 45). A review of outbreak data has also been used for source attribution of antimicrobial-resistant *Salmonella* in the United States, suggesting that antimicrobial susceptibility data on isolates from foodborne outbreaks can help determine which foods are associated with resistant infections (46). Even though few countries or regions are likely to have sufficient data for a robust source attribution analysis using AMR-related outbreaks, summarizing available information may provide evidence on the relative contribution of different foods to infection with antimicrobial-resistant pathogens.

Another epidemiological approach that can be used for source attribution of foodborne disease is the case control study of sporadic cases. Case-control studies are a valuable tool to identify potential risk factors for human illness, including sources and predisposing, behavioral, or seasonal factors (47). In addition to individual case-control studies, a systematic review of published case-control studies of sporadic infections of a given pathogen can provide an overview of the relevant exposures and risk factors for that disease and a summary of the estimated population-attributable fractions for each exposure (48). A systematic review follows a rigorous search strategy to identify all potentially relevant peer-reviewed case-control studies for a hazard, studies being conducted in a variety of countries and time periods, designed with different settings, and potentially focused on specific age groups within the population. A meta-analysis is then performed to compare and combine information from different studies. To do this, risk factors may be stratified according to source-categorization schemes, location of exposures, and if appropriate, frequency of exposure. An overall population-attributable fraction derived from a meta-analysis or weighted summary of several case-control studies of a certain hazard can be combined with estimates of the burden of disease caused by that hazard to estimate the burden of disease attributed to each exposure.

This method is particularly useful for hazards that do not frequently cause outbreaks but that have been extensively studied (49). In addition, it is valuable to attribute illness at a regional or global level when data are scarce in most countries. A number of case-control studies have been conducted to investigate risk factors for infection with foodborne pathogens resistant to antimicrobials (see, e.g., 50, 51). However, the utility of a meta-analysis of case-control studies to investigate the relative contribution of different sources and risk factors to infection with antimicrobial-resistant pathogens may be limited if a low number of case-control studies focused on specific antimicrobial-resistant pathogens or AMR genes have been conducted.

Other approaches

Other approaches for source attribution of foodborne pathogens include intervention studies and expert elicitations. Intervention studies are large-scale, well-structured prospective studies that are specifically tailored to evaluate direct impacts of a specific intervention on the risk of disease in a population. While they would be the "gold standard" of attribution studies, they have the disadvantages of being resource-demanding, expensive, and difficult to implement because other concurrent factors may affect occurrence of disease.

Expert elicitations can be designed as structured methods to gather and analyze knowledge from experts, which is communicated with a measure of uncertainty. They are particularly useful to attribute the burden of foodborne diseases to the main transmission pathways (i.e., foodborne, environmental, direct contact), for which data-driven methods are typically insufficient (49). There are numerous methods used for expert elicitation, including methods that are based on iteration and finding consensus among a small group of experts (e.g., the Delphi method). Expert judgments are subjective by nature and may be biased by the specific background and scientific expertise of the respondents, and several methods to evaluate the experts' performance have been described. Several expert elicitation studies have been conducted for source attribution of foodborne disease (e.g., 52, 53). The World Health Organization's Initiative to Estimate the Global Burden of Foodborne Diseases (WHO-FERG) has undertaken a large-scale and successful expert elicitation to attribute disease due to 19 foodborne hazards to main transmission groups at global, regional, and subregional levels (54). The study applied structured expert judgment using Cooke's classical model (55) to obtain estimates for the relative contributions of different transmission pathways for several foodborne hazards.

Applications and Results

Despite the increased recognition of the importance of source attribution of foodborne pathogens to direct risk management strategies, and the growing use of these approaches in several countries and research groups, source attribution of AMR is still in its infancy. There are few published examples of the methods described here, and the identified challenges are still being addressed. The two microbial subtyping studies that have been published are both frequency-matched studies that used antimicrobial susceptibility patterns as a typing method for *Salmonella* (15, 16). These studies use AMR profiles as a typing method (i.e., to characterize pathogen subtypes) but do not focus on the source origin of specific AMR genes. Still, they are able to estimate the distribution of AMR in human cases attributed to different sources, as is done routinely in the *Salmonella* source attribution activities in Denmark (56). Similarly, the two comparative exposure assessments that have been applied to estimate the relative contribution of different types of meat to the exposure of consumers to AMR have focused on the same causative agent, extended spectrum beta-lactamase-producing and AmpC beta-lactamase-producing *E. coli* (17, 35). These studies demonstrate that the method

could be extended to other countries and agents. The recent review of outbreak data for source attribution of antimicrobial-resistant *Salmonella* in the United States suggests that antimicrobial susceptibility data on isolates from foodborne outbreaks can help determine which foods are associated with resistant infections (46). This method could be applied in countries that have sufficient data or to regional data in an attempt to gather information from multiple countries. Numerous epidemiological studies of sporadic infections (case-control or cohort studies) investigating risk factors for antimicrobial-resistant infections in humans demonstrate these methods' usefulness to identify routes of AMR (e.g., 57–59). While their use focusing on foodborne or direct or indirect contact to animals' transmission has been limited, available studies still provide information that is useful for food safety risk management (50, 51).

Strengths and Weaknesses

Source attribution of AMR genes and of antimicrobial-resistant pathogens is a research area under active development. The application of the methods described here remains a challenge, for reasons that depend on each method considered.

For the application of subtyping frequency-matched studies, two of the main challenges are the limited availability of animal, food, and human AMR data from established surveillance systems and the difficulty of defining the number of AMR profiles highly specific to a particular source/transmission route, a cornerstone of this method. Furthermore, the fact that the method does not determine the actual transmission route from each specific reservoir to humans is another limitation for the use of frequency-matched models. Due to the public health need for understanding the transmission of AMR, population genetics approaches may eventually be a good complement to frequency-matched models, especially considering the increasing availability of whole-genome sequencing and metagenomics data, which describe the occurrence of AMR genes in populations. For instance, population genetics can help in identifying reservoir-specific AMR genes' patterns that can then be used in frequency-matched models. New-generation sequencing data may also contribute to unraveling details that contribute to a more accurate source attribution, such as the evolution of AMR patterns over time in different sources and resistance in humans that is not transmitted from animals or foods.

While single genomics and metagenomics studies may support the development of novel subtyping source-attribution methods, they may hinder the application of comparative exposure assessment. Information on the prevalence and quantity of AMR genes or antimicrobial-resistant pathogens in each source, as well as their changes throughout the transmission chain, are difficult to assess from those data and are impaired by a high degree of uncertainty.

Epidemiological methods of source attribution, e.g., those based on outbreak investigation, have the advantage of not relying on a sophisticated, data-abundant, and integrated surveillance system encompassing animal reservoirs, foods, and humans. However, they require consistent AMR investigation on food sources and human cases, based at least on bacterial isolation and phenotypic susceptibility testing. Eventually, new-generation sequencing may overtake traditional diagnostic methods in outbreak investigation (14, 60), which will also require modification of the current epidemiological approaches.

Intervention studies have, in the context of AMR, the same limitations as when applied to bacterial pathogens. It is difficult to evaluate the exact impact of a specific intervention (e.g., reducing antimicrobial use at the farm level) on the population where disease is attributed (e.g., AMR occurrence in humans). Control measures that reduced antimicrobial use in primary production have been successfully implemented with the aim of reducing AMR in animals (e.g., the antimicrobial growth promoter intervention, the voluntary ban on the use of cephalosporins, and the yellow card antimicrobial scheme in swine herds in Denmark [61–63]). However, to assess the real success of such measures in terms of public health impact, it is necessary to collect data prior to and following the intervention (14), at all dimensions of AMR transmission to humans, i.e., also including other transmission routes such as the environment and antimicrobial use in humans.

RISK ASSESSMENT

Microbial risk assessment of AMR

Risk assessment is the process of estimating the likelihood that exposure to a biological, chemical, or physical hazard will result in an adverse health effect in exposed individuals. Microbial risk assessment has been established as a part of the food safety risk analysis paradigm by international and national bodies in recent decades, with harmonized guidelines being proposed and widely adopted worldwide (8, 64). In the context of AMR, risk assessments are useful to inform regulatory decision-making for the mitigation of poten-

tial health consequences in both humans and animals (65). While the importance and need for AMR risk assessments have been recognized for decades (66), their application has been complicated by several knowledge gaps. Challenges of the development of AMR risk assessment include the following:

- The nature of the hazard is difficult to identify and will determine the nature of the adverse consequence of the exposure. In the context of AMR risk assessment, different hazards can be considered (67, 68). For example, Salisbury et al. (67) discussed three interrelated hazards that can be assessed separately: the antimicrobial drug, the antimicrobial-resistant bacteria, and the AMR determinant, leading to three different health consequences, respectively—development of resistance, infection and treatment failure, and transference of resistance. Similarly, Manaia (68) describes that resistome-associated risks have been discussed considering the microbial community, the genome, and transmission of resistance.

- The nature of the risk posed by antimicrobial use and AMR to human health is inherently complex and logically linked to the nature of the hazard, as mentioned above. In other words, while the likelihood that humans will be infected by pathogens that are resistant to one or several antimicrobials can be estimated, the resulting adverse health consequences can be one or several of the following: development of disease due to infection with the pathogen, failure of treatment of the infection due to resistance to the drug(s) used, and spread of AMR genes to commensal bacteria in the human host (which can amplify the risk and extend the impact of an isolated exposure in time).

- Numerous factors are involved in the process of selection and spread of resistance in bacterial populations, between and within animal species, humans, and the environment and within different bacterial populations in those same reservoirs. These factors include the several drivers of the emergence and spread of AMR in food production, specifically at the farm. At this level, antimicrobial use is recognized as the most important driver but is not always necessary (if, for example, coresistance and co-selection occur) and not always sufficient; additional drivers are, e.g., poor prevention and control of infectious diseases leading to increased antimicrobial use and the spread of clones that have established themselves in the herd/environment and keep selective pressure, even if antimicrobial use is interrupted. These factors, among many others, influence the development of exposure assessment in microbial risk assessment.

- In addition to the challenges described above, estimating the likelihood of adverse health effects, given exposure to an antimicrobial-resistant pathogen or determinant, is difficult due to the absence of a well-defined dose-response effect for AMR and the existence of various possibilities of adverse effects.

Recognizing the need for AMR risk assessments to identify strategies aimed at preventing and reducing the disease burden of AMR transmitted through foods, a number of reviews and scientific articles proposed frameworks for such risk assessments in the late 1990s and early 2000s (66, 67, 69). Even though such proposals were comprehensive and structured to address the challenges identified at that time, they were not widely adopted, mostly due to remaining knowledge and data gaps regarding AMR transmission and impact. More recent frameworks apply current available data and are either mostly qualitative or semiquantitative (see, e.g., 70, 71), take a linear approach (e.g., 72), and/or focus on marketing authorization applications for antimicrobial veterinary medicinal products for use in food-producing species (73).

The Four Steps of Microbial Risk Assessment Focusing on AMR

The microbial risk assessment process is, as described by the *Codex Alimentarius* guidelines (8), constituted by four main components: hazard identification, hazard characterization, exposure assessment, and risk characterization.

In an AMR risk assessment, the hazard can be the antimicrobial drug, the antimicrobial-resistant pathogen, or the AMR determinant. Ultimately, the identification of the hazard of interest depends on the risk-assessment question to be addressed. In a traditional microbial risk assessment (i.e., focused on a pathogen-food pair, without considering resistance to antimicrobial drugs), the hazard identification step consists of the qualitative description of the hazard, including the evaluation of the presence of the pathogen in a food product available for consumption in a population and the host interface (types of disease caused, susceptible populations). In the context of AMR, this step is complicated by a number of factors: (i) selection of resistance in a pathogen can occur by multiple mechanisms (namely, mutation and horizontal gene transfer of mobile genetic elements containing AMR genes) (74); (ii) one or more genes may be necessary for the development of AMR; (iii) AMR genes can be located in

chromosomal or extra-chromosomal DNA, such as plasmids (74); and (iv) several bacterial species or strains can harbor and serve as a reservoir for resistance.

The hazard characterization step of a risk assessment consists of the review and collection of information on the relationship between the dose of the hazard and the onset of disease in the exposed individuals (i.e., infectious dose) and the relationship between different doses and the probability of occurrence of disease (i.e., dose-response). The response of a human population to exposure to a foodborne pathogen is highly variable, reflecting the fact that the incidence of disease is dependent on a variety of factors such as the virulence characteristics of the pathogen, the numbers of cells ingested, the general health and immune status of the hosts, and the attributes of the food that alter microbial-host interactions (75). Thus, the likelihood that any individual becomes ill due to an exposure to a foodborne pathogen is dependent on the integration of host, pathogen, and food matrix effects. Again, in AMR risk assessment, the required data to assess a dose-response relationship depend on the hazard considered; it can be one of the three: the dose level of the antimicrobial for observing resistance usually expressed by the MIC breakpoint (74), or any other factor that can affect the development or amplification of resistance, the dose of the pathogen needed to cause disease, or any factor related to the stability and transfer potential of the AMR gene in a bacterial population (67).

In the exposure assessment step, the likelihood that an individual or a population will be exposed to a hazard and the numbers of the microorganism that are likely to be ingested are estimated (76). The exposure assessment requires data on the prevalence and concentration of the hazard in the food source(s), as well as information on the potential changes of the pathogen load throughout the food-processing chain (e.g., growth, reduction) (77); in addition, it requires data on the frequency and amount of food consumed by individuals of the population. As mentioned above, numerous factors influence the process of selection and spread of resistance, consequently influencing the final exposure of the consumer to AMR genes or antimicrobial-resistant pathogens. These factors are either still unknown or there are limited data reporting their influence on AMR transmission throughout the food chain.

In the last component of a risk assessment, risk characterization, the final risk to the consumer is estimated by integrating the previous three components. Specifically, the measure of exposure (i.e., the likely dose an individual is exposed to in a given food consumption/

exposure event) is integrated with the dose-response relationship to estimate the likelihood of an adverse health effect. In the context of AMR microbial risk assessment, even after an appropriate definition of the risk question and the targeted hazard identification (which determine the adverse effect to be assessed) and the estimation of the likelihood of exposure to the hazard of interest, characterizing the risk in the absence of an appropriate and comprehensive hazard characterization step remains a challenge. A "dose-response" step becomes particularly demanding when the "dose" at exposure is expressed in genotypic terms (by use of genomics or metagenomics AMR data) and the "response" must be expressed in phenotypic terms (e.g., expression of resistance in a pathogen or horizontal transfer of an AMR gene between commensal and pathogenic bacteria).

Applications and Results

A number of risk assessments focused on specific antimicrobial-resistant pathogen-food/animal pairs have been conducted since the publication of the various proposed guidelines. These include qualitative, semiquantitative, and quantitative risk assessments performed by food authorities, academia, or industry. Here, we provide examples of the three types of risk assessment that have been important to highlight the challenges and limitations they still face, the applications of their results, and the need for further studies.

Qualitative risk assessments

One of the first studies published assessed the health impact of residues of antibacterial and antiparasitic drugs in foods of animal origin and was published over 2 decades ago (78). It was a qualitative and comprehensive review that focused on residues of a variety of drugs in multiple foods, and it was an important step for the recognition of several of the challenges described in this chapter. More drug- and pathogen-focused qualitative assessments have been conducted since then, including in recent years, such as the qualitative risk assessment focused on methicillin-resistant *Staphylococcus aureus* (MRSA) conducted by a multisectorial and interdisciplinary expert group in Denmark (79). This study is a good example of an applied risk assessment, conducted upon request from the food and veterinary authorities with the aims of (i) assessing the risk of livestock MRSA based on the existing knowledge and the results of veterinary screening studies conducted in herds and (ii) providing a recommendation for control measures to reduce the spread of MRSA from the affected herds to the

surrounding environment and community. The method consisted of a comprehensive evaluation of all available data on the prevalence of MRSA in animals and humans, as well as on the risk factors for infection by livestock MRSA from the environment, from meat, from occupational activities (e.g., risk for slaughterhouse or farm workers), and from the community. The risk assessment consisted of a descriptive evaluation of the risk of these types of transmission in the Danish population.

Another recent study has applied the risk assessment framework developed by the European Medicines Agency (73) to assess the AMR risk to public health due to use of antimicrobials in pigs, using pleuromutilins as an example (80). Livestock-associated MRSA of clonal complex 398 (MRSA CC398) and enterococci were identified as relevant hazards. This framework followed the International Organization for Animal Health's approach to risk assessment and consisted of four steps describing the risk pathway, combined into a risk estimate. The study applied a qualitative approach, where the output of each step was defined on a scale. Likewise, the level of uncertainty was described qualitatively in the different steps and the output (as high, medium, or low). The authors discuss the value of mathematical modeling as a tool to simulate pathways and identify ways of reducing resistance. Still, they stress that the relationship between reducing consumption of antibiotics and reducing resistance is not necessarily linear and defend that this relationship needs to be better established for modeling to have full value (80). Despite the fact that this study is recent at the time of writing of this chapter and thus could build on all newly available evidence on AMR mechanisms, it still dealt with substantial data and knowledge gaps that enhanced uncertainty around outputs (80).

Another example of a qualitative assessment is the WHO's list of critically important antimicrobials (70). The list applies criteria to rank antimicrobials according to their relative importance in human medicine. The purpose of this assessment is to provide clinicians, regulatory agencies, policy-makers, and other stakeholders' with information to develop risk management strategies for the use of antimicrobials in food-production animals globally. The first WHO list of critically important antimicrobials was developed in a WHO expert meeting in 2005, where participants considered the list of all antimicrobial classes used in human medicine and categorized them into the three groups "critically important," "highly important," and "important" based on two criteria that describe, first, the availability or lack of availability of alternatives to the antimicrobial for treatment of serious bacterial infections in people, and second, if the antimicrobial is used to treat infections by (i) bacteria that may be transmitted to humans from nonhuman sources or (ii) bacteria that may acquire resistance genes from nonhuman sources. The output of the qualitative assessment is a list of classes of drugs that meet all three of a set of defined priorities. Since its original publication, the assessment has been revised several times and is now in its fifth edition.

Semiquantitative risk assessments

One example of a semiquantitative assessment is the study integrating a probabilistic quantitative risk assessment conducted in Denmark to assess the human health risk of macrolide-resistant *Campylobacter* infection associated with the use of macrolides in Danish pig production (81). This model was able to account for exposure through imported and domestic meat (i.e., that could be a vehicle for antimicrobial-resistant bacteria as a consequence of antimicrobial drug use in animal production in that country) and used evidence available at the time. One important feature of this study is that, while it measured exposure probabilistically and thus reflected model and data uncertainty, the final step of the risk assessment—risk characterization—used an ordinal scale, and thus risk was described in a qualitative scale.

Quantitative risk assessments

Several quantitative risk assessments have been published since the early 2000s. These include the high-profile assessment of fluoroquinolone-resistant *Campylobacter* from chicken in the United States (82), which ultimately prompted the Food and Drug Administration to propose withdrawal of the approval of new animal drug applications for fluoroquinolone use in poultry, an action that would prohibit fluoroquinolone use in chickens and turkeys in that country (83).

Another early study employed probabilistic methodology to analyze the potential public health risk from *Campylobacter jejuni* and fluoroquinolone-resistant *C. jejuni* due to fresh beef and ground beef consumption (84). The model focused on the beef product at retail and modelled consumer handling in the kitchen, processing, and consumption. The model estimated, first, the risk of *Campylobacter* infection through consumption of beef and then the risk of treatment failure given infection, concluding an increased health impact due to resistance.

In another study, a risk assessment followed the Food and Drug Administration's Center for Veterinary Medicine Guidance (85) and was commissioned by a pharmaceutical company to estimate the risk of human infection treatment failure associated with the use of an antimicrobial drug in food animals (86). The deterministic model included all uses of two macrolides in poultry, swine, and beef cattle. The hazard was defined as illness (i) caused by foodborne bacteria with a resistance determinant, (ii) attributed to a specified animal-derived meat commodity, and (iii) treated with a human use drug of the same class. Risk was defined as the probability of this hazard combined with the consequence of treatment failure due to resistant *Campylobacter* spp. or *Enterococcus faecium*. At the time, this microbial risk assessment had the advantage of being quantitative and thus more transparent when compared to previous assessments focusing on AMR. Thus, the authors highlighted several limitations, particularly with regard to data gaps on the probability of treatment failure due to the antimicrobial-resistant bacteria and the probability of resistant determinant development. In contrast to many evidence and risk assessments conducted elsewhere, the results of this study led the authors to conclude that the current use of macrolides in cattle, poultry, and swine created a risk much lower than the potential benefit to food safety, animal welfare, and public health (86).

The same author published another risk assessment a few years later, applying a similar approach to estimate the risk of a different combination of antimicrobial-pathogen-fluoroquinolone-resistant *Salmonella* and *Campylobacter* in beef in the United States (87). This approach was able to provide a better measure of uncertainty but was similar in its findings, concluding that the risk of health consequences in humans was minimal.

The most recent quantitative risk assessment study published is also the more novel and promising of the AMR studies reviewed here (88). It considered the existence of environmental compartments resulting from sewage-treatment plants, agriculture production, and manufacturing industries and assessed their roles in the maintenance, emergence, and possible dissemination of antibiotic resistance. This study used probabilistic methods to assess the risks of antibiotic resistance development and neutralizing antibiotic pressures in hotspot environments. Importantly, this study presents a modeling approach to assess the selective pressure exerted by antibiotics in bacterial communities and to calculate antibiotic resistance development risks. While the described approach was exemplarily when used to model antibiotic resistance risks in an intensive aquaculture production scenario of Southeast Asia, it has the potential to be applied to other cases, including other types of animal production, settings, and drugs.

Strengths and Weaknesses

Microbial risk assessment is a science-based tool with proven benefits in supporting food safety authorities in policy-making. It is hence commended to continue its use in assessing the consequences for the consumer of the transmission of AMR genes/pathogens through the food chain. The fact that it is a well-defined, stepwise-structured method facilitates its adaptation to the food safety challenge of AMR. However, several limitations have already been identified and require the joint focus of the scientific community, risk assessors, and authorities. Examples of a few critical challenges are the following:

- The definition of AMR is critical for the four steps of microbial risk assessment and needs, therefore, to be well established at the start of a risk assessment study. Martínez et al. (74) explains the existence of several possible definitions of resistance (namely, clinical, epidemiological, and operational) and two definitions of resistance gene (ecological and operational). The adoption of standard concepts and terminology is a requirement for the transparency of microbial risk assessment and an important part of its development. Although transmission of AMR genes and antimicrobial-resistant bacteria may be perceived and have been defined as two separate hazards, it has also been recently suggested that the risk of AMR transmission to humans cannot be estimated unless the AMR gene pool and the presence and quantity of antimicrobial-resistant bacteria that are able to colonize and multiply in the human body are both taken into consideration (68).
- Exposure assessment often relies on available knowledge of the changes in the microbial hazard levels throughout the food chain, due to, e.g., growth or inactivation. In the context of microbiomes and resistomes, it is difficult to model these changes, because the very composition of the microbial population (and corresponding AMR genes) may significantly change between "farm" and "fork" (89, 90). Consequently, microbial risk assessment for AMR is highly dependent on data collected at several points of the transmission pathway, both from the source(s) of AMR and from exposed human subjects.
- While new-generation sequencing attractively provides a broad characterization of the presence and abundance of AMR genes in a particular pathogen or in the microbiome from a particular reservoir, it remains a challenge to determine variability of the resistome and of the potential to exchange AMR genes (i.e., presence of phage recombination sites, plasmids, integrons, or transposons) between different pathogen strains (68). This knowledge is crucial to assign the AMR genes detected with metagenomics to the corresponding bacterial hosts and to account for the occurrence of horizontal gene transfer between commensal and pathogenic bacteria in a population.
- An important challenge for the integration of metagenomics data in microbial risk assessment is the harmonization of languages between the "omics" and the food microbiology communities (91).
- Risk characterization requires knowledge of the relationship between a "dose," resulting from the exposure assessment, and a "response," i.e., the adverse health effect of exposure. However, the infective dose and the modes of transmission of most of the antimicrobial-resistant bacteria of relevance are still unknown (68), which represents an important knowledge gap for the development of microbial risk assessment for AMR.
- Finally, a major limitation of the current microbial risk assessment frameworks is that they do not allow estimation of the long-term impact of exposure to AMR. Particularly serious public health consequences of AMR arise when multiresistant bacteria emerge and become widespread. There is therefore the need to develop microbial risk assessment methods that include a different characterization of the risk of AMR. In addition to immediate consequences to human health due to a single exposure to an antimicrobial-resistant pathogen, it is necessary to estimate the likelihood that such exposure (eventually together with past and subsequent ones, to the same or other types of AMR) will lead to the development of antimicrobial multiresistance in the future. Also, it is necessary to assess the potential of multiresistance spread, to characterize the severity of the consequences of exposure to multiresistance, and to estimate the time from initial exposure to those consequences.

DISCUSSION AND FUTURE PERSPECTIVES

Several position and stakeholder papers have stressed the need for improved quality and an increased amount of data for risk assessment of AMR (see, e.g., 92). These include, e.g., data on antimicrobial use in animal production; AMR surveillance data in animals, foods, and humans; and gene transfer and spread of AMR genes. All data requirements apply for most source attribution studies, and thus are transversal to the methods described in this article. Likewise, many of the challenges to the application of these methods in the context of AMR are common to source attribution and risk assessment approaches (Table 1).

The studies described here all show the importance of knowledge of (i) the most important sources and routes of transmission of antimicrobial-resistant bacteria or AMR genes, (ii) the actual risk for human health, and (iii) the points in the transmission chain where interventions could be effective to reduce this risk. While all findings so far have been crucial to direct policies and raise awareness to the public health impact of AMR in animals and foods, they are insufficient for a complete understanding of the underlying transmission mechanisms and the real impact of AMR. Several challenges have been addressed, including the fact that emergence and spread of AMR is complex. From an epidemiological point of view, the risk of AMR probably follows the "sufficient-component causes" principle (93). The sufficient-component causes principle is an epidemiological causal modeling approach that can be used to explain diseases, or conditions like AMR, characterized by many causes, none of which alone is necessary or sufficient. The relations among the causes are described such that a "sufficient cause" is a set of minimal conditions that will definitely lead to the outcome (e.g., antimicrobial-resistant infection), and a "component cause" is one of the minimal conditions included in a sufficient cause (93). For example, a

particular resistance gene can be a component cause of an antimicrobial-resistant infection, but the sufficient cause of the latter includes other conditions, such as the bacterial strain carrying that particular gene, that pathogen causing infection, treatment of the infection with antimicrobial(s) for which resistance is encoded in the gene, and the actual expression of that resistance gene. The future of microbial risk assessment for AMR may therefore include defining the components sufficient to cause AMR transmission from animals/foods/the environment to humans followed by treatment failure of infections by antimicrobial-resistant pathogens.

Recent developments in omics technologies (whole-genome sequencing and metagenomics, transcriptomics, proteomics, metabolomics, fluxomics) provide unique opportunities to fill in some of our knowledge gaps. It is now widely recognized that these omics technologies have advantages compared to traditional phenotypic culture-based methods for characterizing microorganisms (91, 94).

Brul et al. (91) described in detail how omics can be integrated in each step of microbial risk assessment, contributing to a mechanistic insight into the interaction between microorganisms and their hosts, new perspectives on strain diversity and variability and physiological uncertainty, and overall more robust risk assessments. den Besten et al. (94) discussed the utility of omics technologies applied by the food industry, to help identify the influence of different bacterial ecosystems on both patho-

Table 1   Definition, overview of methods and main challenges of source attribution and microbial risk assessment approaches

	Source attribution	Microbial risk assessment
Definition	Partitioning of human cases of illness to the responsible sources (e.g., foods, animal reservoirs)	Systematic and science-based approach to estimate the risk of microbial hazards in the production-to-consumption chain
Methods	Microbial subtyping	Qualitative RA[a]
	Comparative exposure assessment	Semiquantitative RA
	Outbreak-data analysis	Quantitative RA
	Case-control studies	Deterministic
	Expert elicitations	Probabilistic
	Intervention studies	
Main challenges in the context of AMR	Hazard identification, e.g., the antimicrobial drug, the antimicrobial-resistant pathogen, or the AMR determinant	
	Lack of occurrence/prevalence data	
	Definition of the health outcome, i.e., infection with antimicrobial-resistant agent, treatment failure (in case treatment is needed), or spread of resistance determinant between commensal and pathogenic organisms	
	Lack of epidemiological data	Establishment of dose-response relationship
		Determining variability of the resistome and of the potential to exchange AMR genes between different pathogen strains

[a]RA. risk assessment.

gen survival and growth—information that can eventually contribute to the future definition of food safety objectives.

A particular advantage of metagenomics is that it provides a picture of the whole microbial community and its resistome, which is key to understanding AMR emergence and spread in a population. Importantly, these new "typing" techniques have been rapidly followed by new bioinformatics and new statistics/modeling tools that allow for the analysis and sense-making of such (big) data (91, 95). For example, machine learning has the potential to be applied on the analysis of omics data. Combining machine learning approaches with metagenomics and farm-specific data could allow for describing, e.g., health, production efficiency, and the relative abundance of AMR genes, based on the identification of (clusters of) genetic factors in the farm microbiome. In addition, such techniques could be used to examine the predictive importance of (clusters of) genetic factors to characterize (i) a "healthy farm microbiome" or (ii) AMR genes in a specific animal reservoir. They can also be used to identify (combinations of) specific husbandry practices that are associated with, e.g., a particular resistome or a healthy farm microbiome. The latter could lead to recommendations on how to shift the farm microbiome to improve the overall health of the farm and consequently, in the long term, to reduce the level of antimicrobial use and antimicrobial-resistant bacteria. It is possible that promoting a healthy farm microbiome will have a more long-term impact on the overall reduction of AMR than focusing exclusively on the farm resistome. Metagenomics and other omics technologies hence have enormous potential for the future development of source attribution and microbial risk assessment of AMR through foods. To explore their full potential, different technologies will be combined. For example, genomics studies should be coupled with proteomics, because gene-expression studies do not always reflect the actual protein levels (91). Also, genomic similarities may not imply similarities in behavior, because the surrounding environment (food matrix, bacterial ecosystem, etc.) also plays a role (94). Furthermore, omics data are not sufficient without accompanying epidemiological data that allow for the identification of risk factors for AMR.

CONCLUDING REMARKS

Recent developments in source-attribution and microbial risk assessment of AMR are promising and have significantly contributed to the evolution of each of these methods. However, the adaptation to the omics big data era is happening at a much slower pace than the speed at which these data are becoming available. This is due to the many challenges encountered when interpreting those data.

AMR at the animal reservoir, food, environment, and human levels is increasingly described by the characterization of the resistomes of single bacteria isolates (by whole-genome sequencing) or the bacterial whole community (by metagenomics) representing each of those populations. Gradually, AMR surveillance will convert from phenotypic to genotypic (e.g., PulseNet International is already on its way to standardizing whole-genome sequencing-based subtyping of foodborne disease [95]). For a successful transition, it is crucial to pair genomic data with phenotypic data and relevant explanatory epidemiological data.

This transition will require a parallel adaptation of the existing analysis methods, which will include the development of new source-attribution and microbial risk assessment modeling approaches. It is therefore with great expectation that we foresee in the near future a surge of influencing and inspiring scientific output in both fields.

Citation. Pires SM, Duarte AS, Hald T. 2018. Source attribution and risk assessment of antimicrobial resistance. *Microbiol Spectrum* 6(3):ARBA-0027-2017.

References

1. **Pires SM, Evers EG, van Pelt W, Ayers T, Scallan E, Angulo FJ, Havelaar A, Hald T, Schroeter A, Brisabois A, Thebault A, Käsbohrer A, Schroeder C, Frank C, Guo C, Wong DLF, Döpfer D, Snary E, Nichols G, Spitznagel H, Wahlström H, David J, Pancer K, Stark K, Forshell LP, Nally P, Sanders P, Hiller P, Med-Vet-Net Workpackage 28 Working Group.** 2009. Attributing the human disease burden of foodborne infections to specific sources. *Foodborne Pathog Dis* 6:417–424.

2. **Mullner P, Jones G, Noble A, Spencer SEF, Hathaway S, French NP.** 2009. Source attribution of food-borne zoonoses in New Zealand: a modified Hald model. *Risk Anal* 29:970–984.

3. **Hald T, Vose D, Wegener HC, Koupeev T.** 2004. A Bayesian approach to quantify the contribution of animal-food sources to human salmonellosis. *Risk Anal* 24:255–269.

4. **de Knegt LV, Pires SM, Hald T.** 2015. Using surveillance and monitoring data of different origins in a *Salmonella* source attribution model: a European Union example with challenges and proposed solutions. *Epidemiol Infect* 143:1148–1165.

5. **Pires SM, Vigre H, Makela P, Hald T.** 2010. Using outbreak data for source attribution of human salmonellosis and campylobacteriosis in Europe. *Foodborne Pathog Dis* 7:1351–1361.

6. Guo C, Hoekstra RM, Schroeder CM, Pires SM, Ong KL, Hartnett E, Naugle A, Harman J, Bennett P, Cieslak P, Scallan E, Rose B, Holt KG, Kissler B, Mbandi E, Roodsari R, Angulo FJ, Cole D. 2011. Application of Bayesian techniques to model the burden of human salmonellosis attributable to U.S. food commodities at the point of processing: adaptation of a Danish model. *Foodborne Pathog Dis* 8:509–516.

7. Pires SM, Evers EG, van Pelt W, Ayers T, Scallan E, Angulo FJ, Havelaar A, Hald T, Med-Vet-Net Workpackage 28 Working Group. 2009. Attributing the human disease burden of foodborne infections to specific sources. *Foodborne Pathog Dis* 6:417–424.

8. FAO. 1999. *Principles and Guidelines for the Conduct of Microbiological Risk Assessment*. FAO, Rome, Italy.

9. Office International des Epizooties. 2002. International Animal Health Code, eleventh edition. Rue de Prony 12, 75017 Paris, France.

10. USDA. 2012. *Microbial Risk Assessment Guideline: Pathogenic Microorganisms with Focus on Food and Water*. Prepared by the Interagency Microbiological Risk Assessment Guideline Workgroup Microbial Risk Assessment Guideline. US Department of Agriculture, Washington, DC.

11. Wegener HC. 2010. Danish initiatives to improve the safety of meat products. *Meat Sci* 84:276–283.

12. Snary EL, Swart AN, Hald T. 2016. Quantitative microbiological risk assessment and source attribution for *Salmonella*: taking it further. *Risk Anal* 36:433–436.

13. Lester CH, Frimodt-Møller N, Sørensen TL, Monnet DL, Hammerum AM. 2006. *In vivo* transfer of the vanA resistance gene from an *Enterococcus faecium* isolate of animal origin to an *E. faecium* isolate of human origin in the intestines of human volunteers. *Antimicrob Agents Chemother* 50:596–599.

14. Aarestrup FM. 2015. The livestock reservoir for antimicrobial resistance: a personal view on changing patterns of risks, effects of interventions and the way forward. *Philos Trans R Soc Lond B Biol Sci* 370:20140085.

15. Hald T, Lo Fo Wong DM, Aarestrup FM. 2007. The attribution of human infections with antimicrobial resistant *Salmonella* bacteria in Denmark to sources of animal origin. *Foodborne Pathog Dis* 4:313–326.

16. Vieira AR, Grass J, Fedorka-Cray PJ, Plumblee JR, Tate H, Cole DJ. 2016. Attribution of *Salmonella enterica* serotype Hadar infections using antimicrobial resistance data from two points in the food supply system. *Epidemiol Infect* 144:1983–1990.

17. Evers EG, Pielaat A, Smid JH, van Duijkeren E, Vennemann FBC, Wijnands LM, Chardon JE. 2017. Comparative exposure assessment of ESBL-producing *Escherichia coli* through meat consumption. *PLoS One* 12:e0169589.

18. Barco L, Barrucci F, Olsen JE, Ricci A. 2013. *Salmonella* source attribution based on microbial subtyping. *Int J Food Microbiol* 163:193–203.

19. Mughini-Gras L, Barrucci F, Smid JH, Graziani C, Luzzi I, Ricci A, Barco L, Rosmini R, Havelaar AH, Van Pelt W, Busani L. 2014. Attribution of human *Salmonella* infections to animal and food sources in Italy (2002–2010): adaptations of the Dutch and modified Hald source attribution models. *Epidemiol Infect* 142:1070–1082.

20. Wilson DJ, Gabriel E, Leatherbarrow AJH, Cheesbrough J, Gee S, Bolton E, Fox A, Fearnhead P, Hart CA, Diggle PJ. 2008. Tracing the source of campylobacteriosis. *PLoS Genet* 4:e1000203.

21. Pires SM, Vieira AR, Hald T, Cole D. 2014. Source attribution of human salmonellosis: an overview of methods and estimates. *Foodborne Pathog Dis* 11:667–676.

22. de Knegt LV, Pires SM, Löfström C, Sørensen G, Pedersen K, Torpdahl M, Nielsen EM, Hald T. 2016. Application of molecular typing results in source attribution models: the case of multiple locus variable number tandem repeat analysis (MLVA) of *Salmonella* isolates obtained from integrated surveillance in Denmark. *Risk Anal* 36:571–588.

23. Boysen L, Rosenquist H, Larsson JT, Nielsen EM, Sørensen G, Nordentoft S, Hald T. 2014. Source attribution of human campylobacteriosis in Denmark. *Epidemiol Infect* 142:1599–1608.

24. Mullner P, Spencer SEF, Wilson DJ, Jones G, Noble AD, Midwinter AC, Collins-Emerson JM, Carter P, Hathaway S, French NP. 2009. Assigning the source of human campylobacteriosis in New Zealand: a comparative genetic and epidemiological approach. *Infect Genet Evol* 9:1311–1319.

25. Little CL, Pires SM, Gillespie IA, Grant K, Nichols GL. 2010. Attribution of human *Listeria monocytogenes* infections in England and Wales to ready-to-eat food sources placed on the market: adaptation of the Hald *Salmonella* source attribution model. *Foodborne Pathog Dis* 7:749–756.

26. Mughini-Gras L, van Pelt W, van der Voort M, Heck M, Friesema I, Franz E. 2018. Attribution of human infections with Shiga toxin-producing *Escherichia coli* (STEC) to livestock sources and identification of source-specific risk factors, The Netherlands (2010–2014). *Zoonoses Public Health* 65:e8–e22.

27. Evers EG, Van Der Fels-Klerx HJ, Nauta MJ, Schijven JF, Havelaar AH. 2008. Campylobacter source attribution by exposure assessment. *Int J Risk Assess Manag* 8:174.

28. Kosmider RD, Nally P, Simons RRL, Brouwer A, Cheung S, Snary EL, Wooldridge M. 2010. Attribution of human VTEC O157 infection from meat products: a quantitative risk assessment approach. *Risk Anal* 30: 753–765.

29. Opsteegh M, Prickaerts S, Frankena K, Evers EG. 2011. A quantitative microbial risk assessment for meatborne *Toxoplasma gondii* infection in The Netherlands. *Int J Food Microbiol* 150:103–114.

30. FDA. 2003. Quantitative assessment of relative risk to public health from foodborne *Listeria monocytogenes* among selected categories of ready-to-eat foods. Summary of public comments and FDA/FSIS revisions to risk assessment. https://www.fda.gov/Food/FoodScience Research/RiskSafetyAssessment/ucm183966.htm.

31. EFSA. 2009. Scientific opinion: cadmium in food. Scientific opinion of the Panel on Contaminants in the Food Chain. *EFSA J* **980:**1–139.

32. EFSA. 2010. Scientific opinion on lead in food. *EFSA J* **8:**1570.

33. Cassini A, Hathaway S, Havelaar A, Koopmans M, Koutsoumanis K, Messens W, Müller-Seitz G, Nørrung B, Rizzi V, Scheutz F. 2016. Microbiological risk assessment. *EFSA J* **14:**1–10.

34. EFSA. 2007. Opinion of the scientific panel on contaminants in the food chain [CONTAM] related to the potential increase of consumer health risk by a possible increase of the existing maximum levels for aflatoxins in almonds, hazelnuts and pistachios and derived products. *EFSA J* **5:**446.

35. Carmo LP, Nielsen LR, da Costa PM, Alban L. 2014. Exposure assessment of extended-spectrum beta-lactamases/AmpC beta-lactamases-producing *Escherichia coli* in meat in Denmark. *Infect Ecol Epidemiol* **4:**1–10.

36. Olsen SJ, MacKinnon LC, Goulding JS, Bean NH, Slutsker L. 2000. Surveillance for foodborne-disease outbreaks: United States, 1993–1997. *MMWR CDC Surveill Summ* **49:**1–62.

37. Neimann J, Engberg J, Mølbak K, Wegener HC. 2003. A case-control study of risk factors for sporadic campylobacter infections in Denmark. *Epidemiol Infect* **130:**353–366.

38. Painter JA, Ayers T, Woodruff R, Blanton E, Perez N, Hoekstra RM, Griffin PM, Braden C. 2009. Recipes for foodborne outbreaks: a scheme for categorizing and grouping implicated foods. *Foodborne Pathog Dis* **6:**1259–1264.

39. Pires SM, Vigre H, Makela P, Hald T. 2010. Using outbreak data for source attribution of human salmonellosis and campylobacteriosis in Europe. *Foodborne Pathog Dis* **7:**1351–1361.

40. Painter JA, Hoekstra RM, Ayers T, Tauxe RV, Braden CR, Angulo FJ, Griffin PM. 2013. Attribution of foodborne illnesses, hospitalizations, and deaths to food commodities by using outbreak data, United States, 1998–2008. *Emerg Infect Dis* **19:**407–415.

41. Pires SM, Vieira AR, Perez E, Lo Fo Wong D, Hald T. 2012. Attributing human foodborne illness to food sources and water in Latin America and the Caribbean using data from outbreak investigations. *Int J Food Microbiol* **152:**129–138.

42. Ravel A, Greig J, Tinga C, Todd E, Campbell G, Cassidy M, Marshall B, Pollari F. 2009. Exploring historical Canadian foodborne outbreak data sets for human illness attribution. *J Food Prot* **72:**1963–1976.

43. King N, Lake R, Campbell D. 2011. Source attribution of nontyphoid salmonellosis in New Zealand using outbreak surveillance data. *J Food Prot* **74:**438–445.

44. Jones TF, Kellum ME, Porter SS, Bell M, Schaffner W. 2002. An outbreak of community-acquired foodborne illness caused by methicillin-resistant *Staphylococcus aureus*. *Emerg Infect Dis* **8:**82–84.

45. Mølbak K, Baggesen DL, Aarestrup FM, Ebbesen JM, Engberg J, Frydendahl K, Gerner-Smidt P, Petersen AM, Wegener HC. 1999. An outbreak of multidrug-resistant, quinolone-resistant *Salmonella enterica* serotype typhimurium DT104. *N Engl J Med* **341:**1420–1425.

46. Brown AC, Grass JE, Richardson LC, Nisler AL, Bicknese AS, Gould LH. 2017. Antimicrobial resistance in *Salmonella* that caused foodborne disease outbreaks: United States, 2003–2012. *Epidemiol Infect* **145:**766–774.

47. Engberg J. 2006. Contributions to the epidemiology of *Campylobacter* infections: a review of clinical and microbiological studies. *Dan Med Bull* **53:**361–389.

48. Domingues AR, Pires SM, Halasa T, Hald T. 2012. Source attribution of human campylobacteriosis using a meta-analysis of case-control studies of sporadic infections. *Epidemiol Infect* **140:**970–981.

49. Pires SM. 2013. Assessing the applicability of currently available methods for attributing foodborne disease to sources, including food and food commodities. *Foodborne Pathog Dis* **10:**206–213.

50. Varma JK, Marcus R, Stenzel SA, Hanna SS, Gettner S, Anderson BJ, Hayes T, Shiferaw B, Crume TL, Joyce K, Fullerton KE, Voetsch AC, Angulo FJ. 2006. Highly resistant *Salmonella* Newport-MDRAmpC transmitted through the domestic US food supply: a FoodNet case-control study of sporadic *Salmonella* Newport infections, 2002–2003. *J Infect Dis* **194:**222–230.

51. Kassenborg HD, Smith KE, Vugia DJ, Rabatsky-Ehr T, Bates MR, Carter MA, Dumas NB, Cassidy MP, Marano N, Tauxe RV, Angulo FJ, Emerging Infections Program FoodNet Working Group. 2004. Fluoroquinolone-resistant *Campylobacter* infections: eating poultry outside of the home and foreign travel are risk factors. *Clin Infect Dis* **38**(Suppl 3):S279–S284.

52. Havelaar AH, Galindo AV, Kurowicka D, Cooke RM. 2008. Attribution of foodborne pathogens using structured expert elicitation. *Foodborne Pathog Dis* **5:**649–659.

53. Ravel A, Davidson VJ, Ruzante JM, Fazil A. 2010. Foodborne proportion of gastrointestinal illness: estimates from a Canadian expert elicitation survey. *Foodborne Pathog Dis* **7:**1463–1472.

54. Hald T, Aspinall W, Devleesschauwer B, Cooke R, Corrigan T, Havelaar AH, Gibb HJ, Torgerson PR, Kirk MD, Angulo FJ, Lake RJ, Speybroeck N, Hoffmann S. 2016. World Health Organization estimates of the relative contributions of food to the burden of disease due to selected foodborne hazards: a structured expert elicitation. *PLoS One* **11:**e0145839.

55. Cooke R. 1991. *Experts in Uncertainty: Opinion and Subjective Probability in Science.* Oxford University Press, Oxford, UK.

56. Anonymous. 2017. *Annual Report on Zoonoses in Denmark 2016.* National Food Institute, Technical University of Denmark, Kgs. Lyngby, Denmark.

57. Kim H, Kim YA, Park YS, Choi MH, Lee GI, Lee K. 2017. Risk factors and molecular features of sequence type (ST) 131 extended-spectrum β-lactamase-producing *Escherichia coli* in community-onset bacteremia. *Sci Rep* **7:**14640.

58. Vos T, Barber RM, Bell B, Bertozzi-Villa A, Biryukov S, Bolliger I, Charlson F, Davis A, Degenhardt L, Dicker D, Duan L, Erskine H, Feigin VL, Ferrari AJ, Fitzmaurice C, Fleming T, Graetz N, Guinovart C, Haagsma J, Hansen GM, Hanson SW, Heuton KR, Higashi H, Kassebaum N, Kyu H, Laurie E, Liang X, Lofgren K, Lozano R, MacIntyre MF, Moradi-Lakeh M, Naghavi M, Nguyen G, Odell S, Ortblad K, Roberts DA, Roth GA, Sandar L, Serina PT, Stanaway JD, Steiner C, Thomas B, Vollset SE, Whiteford H, Wolock TM, Ye P, Zhou M, Ávila MA, Aasvang GM, Abbafati C, et al. 2015. Global, regional, and national incidence, prevalence, and years lived with disability for 301 acute and chronic diseases and injuries in 188 countries, 1990–2013: a systematic analysis for the Global Burden of Disease Study 2013. *Lancet* **386**:743–800.

59. Harb A, O'Dea M, Hanan ZK, Abraham S, Habib I. 2017. Prevalence, risk factors and antimicrobial resistance of *Salmonella* diarrhoeal infection among children in Thi-Qar Governorate, Iraq. *Epidemiol Infect* **145**:3486–3496.

60. Loman NJ, Constantinidou C, Christner M, Rohde H, Chan JZ-M, Quick J, Weir JC, Quince C, Smith GP, Betley JR, Aepfelbacher M, Pallen MJ. 2013. A culture-independent sequence-based metagenomics approach to the investigation of an outbreak of Shiga-toxigenic *Escherichia coli* O104:H4. *JAMA* **309**:1502–1510.

61. Aarestrup FM, Seyfarth AM, Emborg HD, Pedersen K, Hendriksen RS, Bager F. 2001. Effect of abolishment of the use of antimicrobial agents for growth promotion on occurrence of antimicrobial resistance in fecal enterococci from food animals in Denmark. *Antimicrob Agents Chemother* **45**:2054–2059.

62. Jensen VF, de Knegt LV, Andersen VDWA, Wingstrand A. 2014. Temporal relationship between decrease in antimicrobial prescription for Danish pigs and the "Yellow Card" legal intervention directed at reduction of antimicrobial use. *Prev Vet Med* **117**:554–564.

63. Agersø Y, Aarestrup FM. 2013. Voluntary ban on cephalosporin use in Danish pig production has effectively reduced extended-spectrum cephalosporinase-producing *Escherichia coli* in slaughter pigs. *J Antimicrob Chemother* **68**:569–572.

64. Alban L, Olsen AM, Nielsen B, Sørensen R, Jessen B, OIE. 2002. Qualitative and quantitative risk assessment for human salmonellosis due to multi-resistant *Salmonella* Typhimurium DT104 from consumption of Danish dry-cured pork sausages. *Prev Vet Med* **52**:251–265.

65. Claycamp HG, Hooberman BH. 2004. Antimicrobial resistance risk assessment in food safety. *J Food Prot* **67**:2063–2071.

66. Snary EL, Kelly LA, Davison HC, Teale CJ, Wooldridge M. 2004. Antimicrobial resistance: a microbial risk assessment perspective. *J Antimicrob Chemother* **53**:906–917.

67. Salisbury JG, Nicholls TJ, Lammerding AM, Turnidge J, Nunn MJ. 2002. A risk analysis framework for the long-term management of antibiotic resistance in food-producing animals. *Int J Antimicrob Agents* **20**:153–164.

68. Manaia CM. 2017. Assessing the risk of antibiotic resistance transmission from the environment to humans: non-direct proportionality between abundance and risk. *Trends Microbiol* **25**:173–181.

69. Bezoen A, Van Haren W, Hanekamp JC. 1999. *Emergence of a Debate: AGPs and Public Health*. HAN, Amsterdam, The Netherlands.

70. WHO. 2016. *Critically Important Antimicrobials for Human Medicine*, 5th revision. WHO, Geneva, Switzerland.

71. Collineau L, Carmo LP, Endimiani A, Magouras I, Müntener C, Schüpbach-Regula G, Stärk KDC. 2017. Risk ranking of antimicrobial-resistant hazards found in meat in Switzerland. *Risk Anal*.

72. Bartholomew MJ, Vose DJ, Tollefson LR, Travis CC. 2005. A linear model for managing the risk of antimicrobial resistance originating in food animals. *Risk Anal* **25**:99–108.

73. CVMP. 2013. Guideline on the assessment of the risk to public health from antimicrobial resistance due to the use of an antimicrobial VMPs in food-producing animals. Available at http://www.ema.europa.eu/docs/en_GB/document_library/Scientific_guideline/2015/03/WC500183774.pdf.

74. Martínez JL, Coque TM, Baquero F. 2015. What is a resistance gene? Ranking risk in resistomes. *Nat Rev Microbiol* **13**:116–123.

75. Buchanan RL, Smith JL, Long W. 2000. Microbial risk assessment: dose-response relations and risk characterization. *Int J Food Microbiol* **58**:159–172.

76. Lammerding AM, Fazil A. 2000. Hazard identification and exposure assessment for microbial food safety risk assessment. *Int J Food Microbiol* **58**:147–157.

77. Nauta MJ. 2008. The modular process risk model (MPRM): a structured approach to food chain exposure assessment, p 99–136. *In* Schaffner DW (ed), *Microbial Risk Analysis of Foods*. ASM Press, Washington, DC.

78. Waltner-Toews D, McEwen SA. 1994. Residues of antibacterial and antiparasitic drugs in foods of animal origin: a risk assessment. *Prev Vet Med* **20**:219–234.

79. Anonymous. 2014. MRSA risk assessment. Prepared by the MRSA expert group. Available at https://www.foedevarestyrelsen.dk/english/SiteCollectionDocuments/Dyresundhed/Rapport_fra_MRSA-ekspertgruppe%20EN.pdf.

80. Alban L, Ellis-Iversen J, Andreasen M, Dahl J, Sönksen UW. 2017. Assessment of the risk to public health due to use of antimicrobials in pigs: an example of pleuromutilins in Denmark. *Front Vet Sci* **4**:74.

81. Alban L, Nielsen EO, Dahl J. 2008. A human health risk assessment for macrolide-resistant *Campylobacter* associated with the use of macrolides in Danish pig production. *Prev Vet Med* **83**:115–129.

82. FDA. 2000. *Human health impact of fluoroquinolone resistant campylobacter attributed to the consumption of chicken*. Food and Drug Administration Center for Veterinary Medicine, Rockville, MD.

83. Nelson JM, Chiller TM, Powers JH, Angulo FJ. 2007. Fluoroquinolone-resistant *Campylobacter* species and the

withdrawal of fluoroquinolones from use in poultry: a public health success story. *Clin Infect Dis* **44:**977–980.

84. **Anderson SA, Woo RWY, Crawford LM.** 2001. Risk assessment of the impact on human health of resistant *Campylobacter jejuni* from fluoroquinolone use in beef cattle. *Food Control* **12:**13–25.

85. **FDA.** 2003. *Guidance for industry #152: evaluating the safety of antimicrobial new animal drugs with regard to their microbiological effects on bacteria of human health concern.* Food and Drug Administration Center for Veterinary Medicine, Rockville, MD.

86. **Hurd HS, Doores S, Hayes D, Mathew A, Maurer J, Silley P, Singer RS, Jones RN.** 2004. Public health consequences of macrolide use in food animals: a deterministic risk assessment. *J Food Prot* **67:**980–992.

87. **Hurd HS, Vaughn MB, Holtkamp D, Dickson J, Warnick L.** 2010. Quantitative risk from fluoroquinolone-resistant *Salmonella* and *Campylobacter* due to treatment of dairy heifers with enrofloxacin for bovine respiratory disease. *Foodborne Pathog Dis* **7:**1305–1322.

88. **Rico A, Jacobs R, Van den Brink PJ, Tello A.** 2017. A probabilistic approach to assess antibiotic resistance development risks in environmental compartments and its application to an intensive aquaculture production scenario. *Environ Pollut* **231:**918–928.

89. **Chaillou S, Chaulot-Talmon A, Caekebeke H, Cardinal M, Christieans S, Denis C, Desmonts MH, Dousset X, Feurer C, Hamon E, Joffraud J-J, La Carbona S, Leroi F, Leroy S, Lorre S, Macé S, Pilet M-F, Prévost H, Rivollier M, Roux D, Talon R, Zagorec M, Champomier-Vergès M-C.** 2015. Origin and ecological selection of core and food-specific bacterial communities associated with meat and seafood spoilage. *ISME J* **9:**1105–1118.

90. **De Filippis F, La Storia A, Villani F, Ercolini D.** 2013. Exploring the sources of bacterial spoilers in beefsteaks by culture-independent high-throughput sequencing. *PLoS One* **8:**e70222.

91. **Brul S, Bassettb J, Cookc P.** 2012. "Omics" technologies in quantitative microbial risk assessment. *Trends Food Sci Technol* **27:**12–24.

92. **McEwen SA, Singer RS.** 2006. Stakeholder position paper: the need for antimicrobial use data for risk assessment. *Prev Vet Med* **73:**169–176.

93. **Madsen AM, Hodge SE, Ottman R.** 2011. Causal models for investigating complex disease. I. A primer. *Hum Hered* **72:**54–62.

94. **den Besten HMW, Amézquita A, Bover-Cid S, Dagnas S, Ellouze M, Guillou S, Nychas G, O'Mahony C, Pérez-Rodriguez F, Membré J-M.** 2017. Next generation of microbiological risk assessment: potential of omics data for exposure assessment. *Int J Food Microbiol.* [Epub ahead of print.]

95. **Nadon C, Van Walle I, Gerner-Smidt P, Campos J, Chinen I, Concepcion-Acevedo J, Gilpin B, Smith AM, Man Kam K, Perez E, Trees E, Kubota K, Takkinen J, Nielsen EM, Carleton H, FWD-NEXT Expert Panel.** 2017. PulseNet International: vision for the implementation of whole genome sequencing (WGS) for global food-borne disease surveillance. *Euro Surveill* **22:**30544.

Antimicrobial Resistance in Bacteria from Livestock and Companion Animals
Edited by Frank Møller Aarestrup, Stefan Schwarz, Jianzhong Shen, and Lina Cavaco
© 2018 American Society for Microbiology, Washington, DC
doi:10.1128/microbiolspec.ARBA-0018-2017

Optimization of Antimicrobial Treatment to Minimize Resistance Selection

30

Luca Guardabassi,[1] Mike Apley,[2] John Elmerdahl Olsen,[1]
Pierre-Louis Toutain,[3] and Scott Weese[4]

INTRODUCTION

Optimization of antimicrobial use is a cornerstone in the fight against antimicrobial resistance (AMR) and one of the five objectives of the WHO global action plan on AMR (1). The growing evidence that antimicrobial use in animals may contribute to some multidrug-resistant (MDR) bacterial infections in humans has increased consumer demand and governmental pressure to optimize antimicrobial use in the veterinary sector (2). Promoting appropriate use of antimicrobials in veterinary medicine and strengthening of the regulatory framework on veterinary medicines and medicated feed are key actions in the European Union One Health action plan against AMR (3). Following a request from the EU Commission, the European Food Safety Authority and the European Medicines Agency (EMA) published a joint scientific opinion on how to reduce the need for antimicrobial use in food-producing animals (4). In 2015, the EU Commission provided the member states with a set of guidelines for prudent antimicrobial use in veterinary medicine (5), which covers the main animal production types (pigs, cattle, poultry, aquaculture, and rabbits) as well as other species (pets, fur animals, and other non-food-producing species). In the same year, the USA government released a national action plan for combating antimicrobial-resistant bacteria, which includes a plan to eliminate the use of medically important antimicrobials for growth promotion and to foster antimicrobial stewardship in animals (6).

Antimicrobials are essential for both human and animal health. Any use of antimicrobials, in humans or in animals, can select for AMR. However, selective pressure is amplified by unnecessary use, overuse of broad-spectrum antimicrobials, subinhibitory dosage, or inappropriate duration of treatment. In our opinion, optimal antimicrobial treatment should balance clinical efficacy with minimal risk of AMR selection in the strain causing infection as well as in the patient's/herd's commensal microbiota. This concept is, however, not easy to implement because it requires that veterinarians are guided to choose the most appropriate drug, administration form, dosage regimen, and treatment duration for every disease condition, taking into consideration both clinical efficacy and AMR prevention. Various international authorities, professional veterinary associations, and farming associations have released generic veterinary guidelines on prudent antimicrobial use (5, 7, 8). However, international animal species- and disease-specific guidelines, which are essential for implementing rational antimicrobial use in veterinary practice, are lacking for many species and disease conditions, and national practice guidelines are only available in a few countries. Scientific guidance about optimal drug selection and dosing regimens is also sparse, particularly in terms of their influence on AMR. Thus, while it is easy to agree that antimicrobials should be used rationally, actually doing so can be a challenge, even to the most motivated veterinarians.

This article provides an overview of the general principles of optimal antimicrobial treatment, including species-specific recommendations for improving antimicrobial use in pig, cattle, small animal, and equine

[1]Department of Veterinary and Animal Sciences, Faculty of Health and Medical Sciences, University of Copenhagen, 1870 Frederiksberg C, Denmark; [2]Kansas State University College of Veterinary Medicine, Manhattan, Kansas, 66506; [3]INTHERES, Université de Toulouse, INRA, ENVT, Toulouse, France; [4]Department of Pathobiology, Ontario Veterinary College, University of Guelph, Guelph, Canada.

veterinary practices. The focus of the article is on the food-producing and companion animal species that account for the most antimicrobials used in the veterinary sector, even though we recognize the importance of optimizing antimicrobial treatment in all animals, including poultry, small ruminants, rabbits, and fish. Due to the great variety of disease conditions that may be treated with antimicrobial drugs, we concentrated our attention on the most common conditions that are responsible for antimicrobial use in each animal species, highlighting key situations where the current antimicrobial drug products, treatment recommendations, and practices, which were developed to ensure clinical efficacy, contain costs, and/or enhance compliance, may be insufficient to minimize the impact on AMR selection.

GENERAL PRINCIPLES FOR OPTIMAL ANTIMICROBIAL TREATMENT

Optimal antimicrobial treatment implies selection of the most appropriate drug, the right time of administration, the appropriate administration route, and an optimal dosage regimen and treatment duration based on a variety of factors, such as intrinsic and local patterns of

antimicrobial susceptibility of the target pathogen, infection site, drug pharmacokinetics (PK) and pharmacodynamics (PD), and host factors that affect drug efficacy or toxicity (e.g., species, age, size, pregnancy, comorbidities, immunocompetence, and drug interactions), as well as a concern related to the economic and noneconomic value of the individual animal, the cost of treatment, withdrawal times, and herd productivity. The striking differences between animal species make a one-size-fits-all approach to antimicrobial stewardship difficult. However, there is a basic logical thought process which can enable antimicrobial stewardship across all animal species and therapeutic challenges. This logical process requires (i) veterinary guidance in constructing case definitions and validating the definitions through caretaker training and diagnostics; (ii) consideration of possible alternatives to prevent, control, or treat the bacterial disease; (iii) choice of a first-line agent for empiric treatment if there are no alternatives to antimicrobials; and (iv) safe and effective usage of the selected agent (Fig. 1). Moreover, treatment outcome should be adequately monitored to allow the necessary adjustments if the health conditions of the patient or herd do not improve after initial treat-

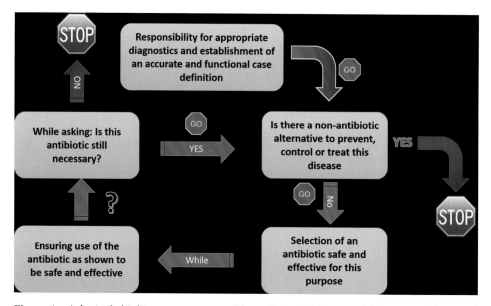

Figure 1 A logical thinking process to enable antimicrobial stewardship across all animal species and therapeutic challenges. This logical process requires (1) veterinary guidance in constructing case definitions and validating the definitions through caretaker training and diagnostics, (2) consideration of possible alternatives to prevent, control, or treat the bacterial disease, (3) choice of a first-line agent for empiric treatment if there are no alternatives to antimicrobials, and (4) safe and effective usage of the selected agent. During the time of antimicrobial use, it is appropriate to constantly evaluate if the disease challenge is still present according to the definitions established in step 1 above. If not, stop the antimicrobial use and monitor according to these definitions and diagnostics. If the challenge is still present, constantly evaluate step 2.

ment or if clinical cure is achieved before the end of the prescribed course of treatment. The goal in this process is to avoid the ultimate antimicrobial transgression, that of antimicrobial exposure with no beneficial effect on disease outcome.

There is evidence that AMR is at least in part driven by the overall volume of antimicrobials used (9–11) as well as by drug type (12), mode of administration (13), dosage regimen (14), and treatment duration (15). Based on this, we have identified four key targets for implementing the concept of optimal antimicrobial treatment in veterinary medicine and livestock production: (i) reduction of overall antimicrobial consumption, (ii) improved use of diagnostic testing, (iii) prudent use of second-line, critically important antimicrobials, and (iv) optimization of dosage regimens.

Reduction of Antimicrobial Consumption

Since the use of antimicrobials is considered the main driving force for the selection of resistant bacteria and any use (not only overuse or misuse) of antimicrobial drugs can promote AMR, it is reasonable to assume that AMR can be at least in part mitigated by reducing overall antimicrobial consumption. There is a good correlation between antimicrobial use and levels of resistant bacteria isolated from the exposed animal population (9–11), even though this is not a straight correlation (16). Exceptions to the general rule exist for specific pathogens, which have remained sensitive for decades despite antimicrobial selection pressure, such as group C streptococci in animals (17). Moreover, resistance may also spread in the absence of any apparent selective pressure because of vertical spread of resistant bacteria in the production pyramid (18) or as a consequence of coselection by other substances, such as feed supplements containing zinc and copper in pig farming (8, 19).

Regulating antimicrobial dispensation and consumption

In many countries, any sort of antimicrobial products, including medically important antimicrobials, can be purchased over the counter without the need for veterinary prescription. These conditions are not compatible with optimal antimicrobial treatment, because they facilitate indiscriminate consumption of antimicrobials. In the European Union countries, any veterinary drug for systemic use can only be obtained with a written prescription from a veterinarian. In the United States, as of 1 January 2017, the use of medically important antimicrobials in the feed or water of food animals requires authorization through either a veterinary feed directive or prescription, respectively (20). Other regulatory measures that can be used to reduce antimicrobial consumption include bans or restriction of the use of specific drugs, taxation of antimicrobial products, and benchmarking approaches to attain specific reduction targets in antimicrobial consumption (21) or to penalize farmers using high amounts of antimicrobials (22). The two latter interventions require sophisticated surveillance programs for monitoring prescription patterns at the farm level.

Banning or restricting growth promotion use

An effective way of drastically reducing the overall consumption of antimicrobials in livestock without directly impacting animal health is the ban or restriction of antimicrobial use for growth promotion, i.e., exposure of healthy animals to low (subtherapeutic) concentrations in feed to improve growth rate, efficiency of feed utilization, and reproductive performance. In Denmark, the ban on growth promotion decreased overall consumption from more than 200 tons in 1994 to around 120 tons in 2015, even though the number of pigs increased during this period (23, 24). The ban demanded management changes, especially in poorly managed herds, but on average, it did not result in significant production drops in either pig (25) or poultry production (26), even though an increase in the use of antimicrobials for treatment of diarrheal diseases was observed immediately after the ban (23).

The use of antimicrobials for growth promotion was officially banned in the European Union in 2006 (27). As of 1 January 2017, the use of medically important antimicrobials for growth promotion is prohibited in the United States, with the use of non-medically important antimicrobials, such as the ionophores, still allowed (28). In 2014, the Canadian government launched a voluntary phase-out of the use of medically important antibiotics as growth promoters (29). To date, antimicrobial growth promoters have been banned in three non-European Union members of the Organisation for Economic Co-operation and Development (Mexico, South Korea, and New Zealand) but are still authorized in most other countries, including major meat-producing countries such as Argentina, Brazil, China, India, Indonesia, Japan, Philippines, Russian Federation, and South Africa (30). We agree that growth promotion use should be banned, especially for medically important antimicrobials, since their use at subtherapeutic doses in healthy animals is likely to have negative effects on both drug efficacy and AMR prevention. The positive and negative consequences deriving from the use of specific antimicrobial growth promoters that are not classified as medically important antimicrobials are less clear since some of these products (e.g., Flavomycin) do not seem to have an impact on the efficacy of medically important antimicrobials. Use of these substances for growth promotion is less critical, but ideally their short- and long-term effects on animal health and AMR selection and coselection, including their environmental impact, should be carefully assessed in a drug-specific fashion.

Avoiding unnecessary prophylaxis

Antimicrobial prophylaxis refers to the administration of an antimicrobial drug to a healthy animal in the presence of a specific risk factor (e.g., weaning for piglets, transportation for calves, drying off for dairy cows, contaminated surgery for companion animals, etc.). The question of whether prophylactic treatment is optimal is more difficult to address and has multifaceted answers. According to the WHO (31), antimicrobial prophylaxis should not be used as a substitute for good animal health management but should be restricted to situations where there is a veterinary patient or a group of animals at high risk for developing infections that significantly impact animal health and herd productivity. This requires veterinary oversight and continuous risk assessment to evaluate clinical outcome and possible treatment discontinuation and relies on subjective assessment of what constitutes "high risk" and "significant impact." In the recent European Union guidelines (5), it is recommended to reserve prophylactic treatment for exceptional case-specific indications. In line with this recommendation, the authors believe that prophylactic use is only justified in cases where other control measures are not available or effective, and only while other means of controlling the disease are being pursued. Any form of routine prophylaxis to prevent neonatal diseases should be avoided since there are efficient production systems where neonatal diseases are prevented by appropriate sanitation measures.

Rationalizing the use of metaphylaxis

Herd or group medication, also referred to as metaphylaxis, refers to the administration of an antimicrobial product to both diseased and clinically healthy (but presumably infected) in-contact animals, to prevent them from developing clinical signs and to prevent further spread of the disease (32). Metaphylaxis should be avoided whenever it is possible and sustainable to isolate sick animals and treat them individually (e.g., by parenteral drugs). However, there are times and certain situations where metaphylaxis may be appropriate, not only for animal welfare but also to avoid thera-

peutic use and minimize AMR development. Indeed, it has been shown in rodent models and in calves that the efficacious dose of an antimicrobial can be much lower when treatment is initiated at very early stages of infection, most likely because of the lower bacterial inoculum at the infection site (33–35). Interestingly, simple mathematical modelling suggests that treatment of infected human patients at early stages of an infection favors treatment success and hinders selection of AMR (36). No experimental validation for this observation has been performed, and the model used in this study does not capture the large variability in the gut microbiota that exists between individual animals in real life, even within the same herd (37). Nevertheless, these data suggest that there may be a trade-off between early treatment and limited AMR development. Altogether, we believe that metaphylactic treatment is justified for the control of disease outbreaks, provided that clear diagnostic cutoff values are used to initiate treatment.

Avoiding unnecessary antimicrobial therapy

Antimicrobial consumption can also be reduced by avoiding unnecessary therapy. For example, antimicrobials are not required for management of viral infections, self-limiting bacterial infections, and diseases that have a noninfectious cause or can be treated with surgery or topical therapy. Some countries where antimicrobial growth promoters are banned and prophylaxis is strictly regulated, such as The Netherlands and Denmark, have achieved further significant reductions in the sales of veterinary antimicrobials through benchmarking of antimicrobial use per herd and per veterinarian, improvement of herd health, and definition of reduction targets for antimicrobial consumption as a whole (22, 23). Other countries are planning to follow this approach in the near future. Notably, this and other approaches aimed at reducing antimicrobial consumption imply clear responsibilities for veterinarians, which in turn require access to species-specific practice guidelines for antimicrobial use and evidence-based diagnostic protocols to accomplish the reduction targets adopted by national authorities without negatively impacting animal health and welfare. The most common disease conditions for which the authors perceive room for improved stewardship are listed for each animal species in the section "Optimization of Antimicrobial Treatment in Veterinary Practice."

Preventing and controlling infection

Any measures aimed at preventing and controlling infection contribute to decreased antimicrobial consumption by reducing the need for antimicrobials. Effective measures include internal and external biosecurity, good management practices, disease control and vaccination programs in livestock production, and hospital infection control programs in companion animal medicine. As an example, a 52% reduction in antimicrobial consumption, including an important reduction in the use of critically important antimicrobials, was achieved in Belgian pig farms undergoing guided interventions based on optimization of herd management, improvement of the biosecurity level, and guidance on prudent antimicrobial use, with beneficial effects on production parameters such as the number of weaned piglets per sow per year, daily weight gain, and mortality in the finisher period (38). Indeed, another study in Belgium demonstrated that there may even be an economic advantage to the farmers to changing from antimicrobial-based health management systems to systems based on improved use of vaccines, optimal feeding, and higher internal and external biosecurity (39). The efficacy of vaccination alone was shown in a Danish pig farm, where antimicrobial use was reduced by 79% by vaccinating against *Lawsonia intracellularis*, with highly significant improvements of average daily weight gain and carcass weight, as well as a shortened fattening period (40). It is up to the veterinarian to constantly seek new information related to vaccines, biosecurity, and animal husbandry practices, as well as alternative measures such as antibodies to specific pathogens, immunomodulatory agents, bacteriophages, antimicrobial peptides, and feed supplements based on pro- and prebiotics or symbiotic mixtures of the two (41).

Improved Use of Diagnostic Testing
Whenever possible and relevant, diagnosis of bacterial infection and drug choice should be guided by cytology and culture. The information provided by cytology has generally limited value to guide drug choice, but it may be useful to diagnose bacterial infection as opposed to viral infection and consequently to decide whether antimicrobial treatment is needed. For some disease conditions (e.g., otitis externa in dogs), it can also be used to select drugs active against specific groups of bacteria based on the morphology of the infecting strain (Gram-positive cocci versus Gram-negative rods) and to identify nonbacterial pathogens (e.g., fungi, ectoparasites). Culture and antimicrobial susceptibility testing (AST) are almost never contraindicated and are particularly indicated if the infection is severe or requires long treatment or if the patient/herd has not responded to therapy or has a history of relapse, reinfection, or infection with MDR bacteria, is immunosuppressed, or suffers

from comorbidities. Notably, clinical specimens can be submitted to the diagnostic laboratory even when empiric treatment is prescribed. This approach can be usefully employed to correct therapy if the clinical conditions of the patient/herd have not improved after initial treatment and the cultured strain is reported as resistant to the first-line agent used for empiric treatment.

It is the responsibility of the veterinarian to decide whether empiric therapy and laboratory diagnosis are needed based on the clinical conditions of the individual patient or herd. Unfortunately, it is generally recognized that the use of laboratory microbiology is too infrequent in veterinary practice, in both companion animals and livestock. According to a recent survey conducted on a large sample of European veterinarians (42), rapid results and cheaper testing were the two main factors that could increase use of AST according to the majority of the respondents (71% and 68%, respectively); however, other factors such as lack of confidence in testing, assumptions of what the results will be based on clinical experience, and poor understanding of how to use the results of susceptibility tests likely also play a role. Use of diagnostic testing can be increased through educational approaches, which have the dual function of promoting use and training veterinarians for correct interpretation of the results. Notably, diagnostic tests are not beneficial if they are inaccurate or biologically irrelevant. Diagnostic laboratories typically have complete freedom to offer any test, regardless of how well (or even if) it has been scrutinized. The quality of diagnostic testing, particularly molecular testing, is variable, and inaccurate test results can lead to errors in patient care and antimicrobial use. Accordingly, veterinarians should give attention to selecting diagnostic laboratories that have the resources and expertise necessary to perform up-to-date microbiological analyses. The European Society for Clinical Microbiology and Infectious Diseases Study Group for Veterinary Microbiology has recently recommended the use of laboratories that employ mass spectrometry for bacterial identification and MIC determination for susceptibility testing and that offer assistance from expert microbiologists on pre- and postanalytical issues (43).

Increasing use of broad-range diagnostic testing such as PCR panels can provide abundant information, but sometimes at the expense of clinical specificity. In many ways, the ability to test has outpaced the ability to properly interpret test results in a clinical context, and the default approach to identification of a pathogen of unknown clinical relevance is often to try to eliminate it with antimicrobials. Molecular assays for bacterial pathogens are also associated with another important limitation: they cannot provide antimicrobial susceptibility data. Therefore, while identification of a pathogen can be helpful, antimicrobial selection must be done empirically, something that might result in the use of broader-spectrum antimicrobials. Improvement in antimicrobial use through diagnostic testing involves greater use of testing, provided tests are properly validated and performed and the clinical relevance of results is understood. Optimally, in-clinic and in-stable point-of-care tests that provide information on the causative agent(s) and their antimicrobial susceptibility within minutes should be the goal, but such tests are generally not yet available on the market.

Prudent Use of Second-Line, Critically Important Agents

If empiric treatment is required, drugs listed as first-line agents in antimicrobial guidelines should be preferred over second-line agents with broader spectrums of activity and critical importance for managing "difficult-to-treat" infections. In principle, the broader is the spectrum of a drug, the wider is the impact on the commensal flora and on selection of AMR. Even though the definition of spectrum is quite arbitrary and AMR selection is complicated by complex mechanisms of coselection, it is generally recognized that certain antimicrobial drugs have great clinical importance, and their efficacy should be preserved by using them as second-line or reserve agents. This is the case for cephalosporins, macrolides, and fluoroquinolones, which have been classified as the most critically important agents in human and veterinary medicine by the WHO and the World Organization for Animal Health, respectively (44, 45). The biggest public health concerns are associated with veterinary use of extended-spectrum third- and fourth-generation cephalosporins and fluoroquinolones. A multitude of studies indicate that these two antimicrobial classes promote selection of MDR bacteria of veterinary importance and zoonotic potential that have emerged in animal populations over the past decade, namely, methicillin-resistant *Staphylococcus aureus* in livestock, methicillin-resistant *Staphylococcus pseudintermedius* in companion animals, and extended-spectrum β-lactamase (ESBL)-producing *Enterobacteriaceae* in all animal species; these MDR bacteria are, by definition, resistant to (and therefore selected by) extended-spectrum cephalosporins and display relatively high rates of fluoroquinolone resistance compared to their cephalosporin-susceptible counter-

parts (8–10, 20). Use of these critically important drugs should be reserved for management of difficult-to-treat infections, and empiric use should be avoided except for specific disease conditions where they are recommended as first-line agents by expert guidelines. Their use in livestock is regulated or banned in some countries, where it is only indicated if susceptibility data demonstrate that the pathogen involved is resistant to other veterinary drugs with proven clinical efficacy for the disease condition to be treated.

Macrolides have also been classified as high-priority, critically important agents for both human and animal health. There is, however, little evidence that their use in animals favors the spread of macrolide-resistant bacterial infections and impacts the efficacy of macrolides in human medicine. The only significant exception is *Campylobacter*, for which macrolides are regarded as first-line agents for managing severe infections in humans. Even though severe infections that require antimicrobial treatment represent a minority of the infections caused by this zoonotic pathogen and the prevalence of macrolide resistance is very low in animal, food, and human clinical isolates (46), macrolides should be used prudently in livestock, strictly according to guidelines. There are public health concerns also regarding veterinary use of polypeptides (colistin) and glycopeptides, which are ranked as "high priority critically important" in the most recent revision of the WHO classification (44) but not in the World Organization for Animal Health classification (45). Recently, concerns have also been raised regarding the use of several other antimicrobial drugs that are not ranked as critically important in the WHO classification, namely zinc oxide and tetracyclines (see species-specific sections).

The ranking of antimicrobials by importance to human medicine provides one context, but this cannot be the only method of selecting the most appropriate antimicrobial. To simply pick the appropriate antimicrobial by its ranking on this list would ignore the important considerations of efficacy, local AMR patterns, route of administration, duration of exposure, and relative efficacy for possible pathogens. Also, there are welfare and economic concerns related to using a less effective antimicrobial with a lower human importance ranking when a higher-ranked antimicrobial may actually treat the disease with a shorter period of treatment. A prioritization based strictly on ranking of medical importance may also be misleading when consideration is given to the frequent association of multiple resistance genes in the same bacterial strain or mobile genetic element, including genes conferring resistance to drugs that are not used or have low importance in human medicine. As a consequence of this phenomenon (i.e., coresistance), use of one of these drugs may result in coselection for resistance to medically important drugs.

Dose Regimen Optimization

Dose regimen optimization consists of choosing an appropriate dose, dosage interval, time of initiation, and duration of treatment. The risks of selecting AMR in the target pathogen and in the commensal and environmental microbiota can be minimized by using different strategies to optimize antimicrobial PD and PK.

Optimizing the PK/PD Relationship to Minimize AMR Selection in the Target Pathogen

The delimiting range of drug concentrations (and thus of doses) favoring selection of resistant mutants has been termed for the fluoroquinolones the "mutant selective window" and is delimited by two critical plasma concentrations: the MIC in the initial (wild-type) population of the infecting strain and the MIC of the first-mutant subpopulation, also termed the mutant prevention concentration (MPC) (Fig. 2) (47). An optimal dosage regimen should limit the overall time during which the drug concentration at the infection site is within the mutant selective window. This goal can be achieved by using a specific PK/PD index (fT > MPC [time for free plasma concentration above the MPC] or fAUC [area under the free concentration-time curve]/ MPC). This approach has been shown to be useful for preventing the emergence of fluoroquinolone resistance during treatment since these drugs have a stepwise mechanism of resistance development based on mutation of the drug target. For example, the *in vitro* predicted "antimutant" AUC/MPC ratio for ciprofloxacin has been estimated to be 58 h for *Escherichia coli* and 60 to 69 h for *S. aureus* (48). Although MIC/MPC ratios have been proposed for a variety of veterinary antimicrobials (e.g., macrolides, cephalosporins, and florfenicol) (49), the usefulness of this approach is unclear for other antimicrobial classes for which resistance is acquired in one step by horizontal gene transfer. MPC should be measured *in vitro* using a larger inoculum size than the one used for MIC determination (approximately 10^{10} instead 10^5 cells per ml) (49). This value would need to be known to optimize dosage

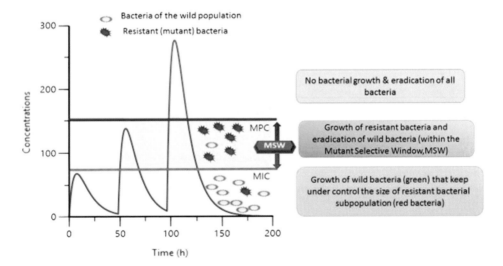

Figure 2 Mutant selection window and mutant prevention concentration (MPC). Optimal dosage regimens should maintain as long as possible the drug concentration at or above the MPC (blue area), which reflects the highest possible MIC of the resistant mutants (red bacteria). The minimum amount of time required to prevent selection of the resistant mutants can be estimated for each species by using a specific PK/PD index (fT > MPC or fAUC/MPC). The mutant selective window delimitates the range of antimicrobial concentrations selecting for the resistant mutants, which range from the MPC (upper horizontal red line) to the MIC (lower horizontal green line) of the initial (wild-type) bacterial population (green bacteria). Drug concentrations below the MIC inhibit neither the mutants nor the wild-type population. Abbreviations: T, drug concentration time; AUC, area under the concentration-time curve, C max, maximum drug concentration; C min, minimum drug concentration.

regimens based on AUC/MPC ratios. However, at present, methods for MPC measurement are not standardized, and microbiological laboratories do not routinely provide MPC testing.

Optimizing PK to minimize AMR selection in the commensal microbiota

A high priority of optimal antimicrobial treatment is to have minimal or no impact on the commensal microbiota, especially in the large intestine, where the largest fraction of the commensal microbiota resides, including important zoonotic and veterinary opportunistic pathogens. Unfortunately, nearly all the currently available veterinary antimicrobial products are eliminated into the gastrointestinal (GI) tract (50). For the oral route, this is mainly due to very low bioavailability. For example, tetracyclines have very low oral bioavailability in pigs and poultry, with values typically between 5 and 15% (51–53). The situation is not better for antimicrobials that are administered parenterally, because most products available for veterinary use are extensively eliminated by the digestive tract, either by the bile or by intestinal clearance, and can attain intestinal concentrations capable of selecting resistant organisms (14, 54). A recent study of ciprofloxacin in piglets has shown that the emergence of AMR in the GI tract is indeed related to the local drug exposure levels (55). Using a rodent model, low efficacious doses of marbofloxacin (33), amoxicillin, or cefquinome (34, 56) were shown to have minimal impact on the gut microbiota when administered in the early stages of lung infection. These data suggest that the lowest clinically effective dose might be the best to prevent AMR selection in the gut microbiota.

Doses are currently determined preclinically by dose-titration trials, which lead to the selection of an effective dose but not to an optimal dosage regimen for minimizing selection of AMR in the target pathogen and in the commensal gut microbiota (57, 58). In addition, this approach does not consider variables related to pathogen susceptibility or host factors influencing PK parameters such as plasma clearance and bioavailability. Plasma clearance, which together with bioavailability is the main factor controlling antimicrobial exposure, can be extremely variable within a given species because it depends on certain physiological or pathological factors. For example, the plasma clearance of marbofloxacin was reported to be nearly 3-fold lower in experimentally infected calves (1.3 ± 0.16 ml/kg/min) than in healthy calves (3.0 ± 0.36 ml/kg/min) (59), meaning that a 3-fold lower dose in infected calves would ensure exactly the same overall marbo-

floxacin exposure as the full dose between preruminant animals (half-life of 12 h) and ruminant animals (half-life of 4 h), but the same dosage regimen is recommended (60). These data clearly indicate that a standard dose covering all types of treatment (e.g., therapy versus metaphylaxis) or all individuals within a given species need to be questioned to be consistent with optimal antimicrobial use. It should be noted that current dosage regimens are determined by PK studies conducted preclinically in healthy animals. To determine the most appropriate dosage regimens, the variability of plasma clearance needs to be more extensively documented by population PK studies conducted on infected animals during clinical trials. Similarly, differences in bioavailability can be huge between routes of administration and for a given route (especially the oral route) between species or between animals of different ages within the same species. Just as an example, amoxicillin has an oral bioavailability of about 5% in adult horses (61), 36% in 1-week-old foals (62), 28 to 33% in pigs (63), 64 to 77% in dogs (64), and 93% in humans (65).

An optimal dosage should ensure coverage of most animals in a population (e.g., 90%), taking into account all the different variables, including pathogen susceptibility (MIC) and key drug properties such as plasma clearance, protein binding, and bioavailability. Such a dose can be computed with an equation using the actual population distribution for each variable; then using Monte Carlo simulations, a population distribution of doses can be established instead of a single "average" dose, and an optimal dose can be defined as the 90th percentile of this distribution. The principles of this stochastic approach have been described for various antimicrobials in human medicine (66–68). A veterinary example is given by a study of tulathromycin for respiratory infections in calves (69). For this drug-animal species combination, it was concluded that the main source of variability was the pathogen's MIC (77%), whereas the variability associated with serum clearance was significantly lower (23.0%), and that of protein binding was negligible. Similar results have been obtained for many antimicrobials and fully justify use of the actual MIC of the pathogen involved to eliminate this source of uncertainty. Adjusting (reducing) the dose, especially if the MIC of the infecting strain is low, is a promising approach that can be used to optimize antimicrobial dosage regimens in the future (see the "Future Perspectives" section).

Optimizing duration of treatment

Generally, the duration of treatment should be as indicated on the label. Insufficient duration of administration can lead to recrudescence of the infection and increase the likelihood of selecting organisms with reduced sensitivity. On the other hand, treatment should be stopped as soon as the animal's own host defense system can control the infection to avoid an unnecessary extension of the antimicrobial selective pressure on the commensal microbiota. The challenge is determining when this pivotal decision point has been reached. The duration of antimicrobial treatment can play a major role in the development of bacterial resistance, and both clinical studies and *in vitro* models have demonstrated that longer treatments are associated with higher rates of AMR (47, 70). Higher prevalence of AMR is observed in pig and poultry farms that use longer antimicrobial treatments (15, 71). The latest trend in human medicine is that unnecessary treatment should be avoided after clinical resolution of symptoms (36). This has led to alterations in educational campaigns from "take all the antimicrobial that was prescribed" to "take the antimicrobial for as long as your physician says to," since stopping prior to the initially prescribed course may be indicated in some patients. Such an approach is potentially confusing and requires more communication between patient and prescriber but ultimately can result in more appropriate treatment.

OPTIMIZATION OF ANTIMICROBIAL TREATMENT IN VETERINARY PRACTICE

General principles for optimal antimicrobial treatment need to be translated into veterinary practice. This requires knowledge of the species and AMR properties of the infecting organisms (microbiology), the pharmacological properties, dosage and label instructions of the available antimicrobial products (pharmacology), and the practical consequences of the use and nonuse of antimicrobials on patient care (veterinary medicine) and livestock productivity (animal husbandry). In the following paragraphs, we outline practice recommendations to achieve the four targets defined above in "General Principles for Optimal Antimicrobial Treatment" for optimizing antimicrobial treatment, with particular reference to specific disease conditions that account for the most antimicrobial use in pigs, cattle, dogs and cats, and horses. Whenever possible, our recommendations are based on the current international veterinary guidelines. National veterinary guidelines, human guidelines, or expert opinion were used for those disease conditions that are not covered by internationally recognized veterinary guidelines.

Optimal Antimicrobial Treatment in Pig Veterinary Practice

Practice guidelines providing recommendations on first- and second-line drug choices have been developed for pig veterinarians in several countries (72–74), and some key measures for prudent antimicrobial use in pigs are recommended in the European Union guidelines (5) and in textbooks (75). While veterinarians can guide farmers in best practices to prudent antimicrobial use, often the responsibility for implementation lies with the farmer. In recognition of the important role of the farmer in reducing antimicrobial consumption, the Danish Pig Farmer Association has developed antimicrobial use guidelines (in English) specifically targeting the farmers, with emphasis on infection prevention (76). These examples may serve as models for other countries where guidelines have not yet been developed.

The highest incidence of antimicrobial treatment in pigs is seen in the postweaning period. Data from Denmark in 2015 showed that 43% of antimicrobials were used in weaners, 29% in sows and piglets, and 28% in finisher pigs (24). Diarrhea in weaner pigs and respiratory diseases in weaners and finisher pigs were the main indications for antimicrobial use (24, 77). In general, GI and respiratory diseases account for a high proportion of antimicrobial use in modern pork production, ranking either number one or number two in countries with detailed reporting of antimicrobial use (24, 77–79). Thus, optimization of treatment of these two disease conditions is likely to have the biggest impact on reducing antimicrobial consumption and preventing AMR development.

Reducing overall antimicrobial consumption
A long list of possible means to reduce the need for antimicrobial agents in animal husbandry has recently been published as a joint EMA/European Food Safety Authority scientific opinion (4). Many of these tools are highly relevant to pig production. The following paragraphs focus on prevention and metaphylaxis for GI and respiratory disease.

GI disease prevention
The safest way to reduce antimicrobial consumption is to avoid infection. Transport, mixing of pigs originating from different pens/farms, unsuitable feeding methods, improper colostrum management, and insufficient biosecurity measures are the main risk factors for the development of GI disease in pigs. As such, optimal management of these risk factors is the best way to prevent disease and reduce antimicrobial use at the farm level. The need for pig production systems that avoid

the stress associated with mixing animals and long-distance transport (e.g., closed farrow-to-finishing farms and an integrated approach between breeding and fattening farms) is underlined by the European Union guidelines for prudent antimicrobial use (5). Important tools to prevent the most treatment-costly GI infections in nursery pigs are improved feeding regimens (80) and vaccination against some of the most important pathogens (40, 81). Similarly, sow vaccination can be used to minimize bacterial diarrhea caused by *E. coli* and *Clostridium perfringens* in neonatal pigs (82, 83). Unfortunately, effective vaccines against postweaning diarrhea and swine dysentery are currently not available. Many substrates have been tested as feed additives for the prevention of diarrhea in pigs. Generally, these aim at either stabilizing the intestinal flora (84), downregulating the expression of virulence factors of intestinal pathogens (85), or enhancing the immune responses (86). This efficacy of nonantimicrobial alternatives has recently been reviewed (87). The most well-documented effects are seen with administration of short-chain fatty acids to weaner pigs as a feed supplement (84). However, contradictory results have been published regarding the efficacy of this approach (88), suggesting that it is likely influenced by management factors.

Respiratory disease prevention

Management and housing factors play a critical role in the outcome of respiratory disease in pigs. Factors that increase the risk and severity of respiratory disease include the lack of all-in all-out production, mixing pigs of different ages, moving pigs between areas, and suboptimal air flow (89, 90). Thus, any attempt to reduce antimicrobial use starts with optimizing these factors. Vaccination plays an important role in the prevention of disease in herds where the disease is endemic, and strategic use of vaccines should be preferred to antimicrobial-based control. The use of vaccination often reduces clinical symptoms, production losses, and medication (91), but it cannot prevent colonization and eliminate the disease. Systematic efforts to reduce disease prevalence, in particular, the two most treatment-demanding respiratory disease conditions, enzootic pneumonia caused by *Mycoplasma hyopneumoniae* and porcine pleuropneumonia caused by *Actinobacillus pleuropneumoniae*, are cost-effective but rely on depopulation and require strict measures afterward to prevent reintroduction of disease (92). Like antimicrobial treatment, vaccination is complicated by the fact that infections may be caused by combinations of pathogens; for example, the presence of porcine reproductive and respiratory syn-

drome virus and porcine circovirus type 2 significantly affects the efficacy of *M. hyopneumoniae* vaccination (93).

Rational metaphylaxis

A vast proportion of group treatments in pigs can be considered metaphylaxis. There is no doubt that minimizing flock treatment can significantly reduce the amount of antimicrobials used in pig production. For example, unselective metaphylactic treatment of herds with tulathromycin for control of the porcine respiratory disease complex has been shown to be unjustified (94). A large proportion of the significant drop in antimicrobial consumption observed in the pig industry in The Netherlands in recent years has been due to reduced use of group treatment (95). However, in certain situations, where clinical signs or laboratory methods cannot detect sick animals in the early stages of disease, it may be advantageous to use a metaphylactic approach. For example, single-animal treatment may not be efficient with diarrheal diseases. It has been shown that group treatment (full batch treatment) was superior to pen-wise and single-animal treatment in reducing levels of *L. intracellularis* in pigs; the single-animal treatment performed the poorest and did not result in a significant reduction of disease-positive pigs compared to the before-treatment situation, probably because of the poor sensitivity of currently available diagnostic tests and hence undertreatment (96). Moreover, and perhaps more surprisingly, group treatment with oxytetracycline did not increase the numbers of tetracycline-resistant coliform bacteria in the intestine compared to the group of individually treated pigs, even though only 55% of pigs were treated in the latter group. A possible explanation of this result is that untreated pigs shared the pen with treated pigs, thereby facilitating transmission of resistant bacteria within the group (97). It is unknown whether this result can be extended to diarrheal diseases caused by other pathogenic bacteria. However, until improved diagnostic procedures are available, metaphylaxis should be regarded as a valuable tool for the control of diseases with high in-herd prevalence. The diagnostic criteria that justify initiation of metaphylaxis for disease control should always be clear, as described for GI infections in the next section.

Improving diagnostic testing

Prudent use of antimicrobials for pigs starts with defining treatment plans and treatment options for each herd based on a thorough diagnostic investigation and using the knowledge of the underlying etiology for the important disease complexes in the herd. Where available, sampling and diagnostic procedures should take into account national guidelines provided by either health authorities or professional organizations. To justify metaphylaxis, it is important to ensure proper knowledge of the pathogen involved and its local susceptibility patterns.

GI disease

The major pathogens of relevance for diarrhea in the nursery period in most countries are *E. coli*, *L. intracellularis*, and *Brachyspira pilosicoli*. In addition, classical swine dysentery, caused by *Brachyspira hyodysenteriae*, has reappeared in some countries. Salmonellosis may cause postweaning diarrhea too. The importance of viral agents differs substantially between countries. Where porcine endemic diarrheal virus and transmissible GI virus are present, they may cause widespread disease. In such areas, microbiological diagnosis to rule out viral disease is an important step in optimizing antimicrobial treatment. The choice of drug for the treatment of diarrhea in pigs is complicated by the fact that a high proportion of cases are mixed infections (98). Ideally, the choice should be guided by frequent susceptibility testing of isolates, but in practice, only testing of *E. coli* and *Salmonella* can be performed in nonspecialized laboratories. For *E. coli* and *Salmonella*, MDR isolates are not uncommon (99, 100), underlining the need to guide drug choice based on susceptibility patterns of isolates originating from the case herd. Recent studies of antimicrobial susceptibility of *Brachyspira* species paint a picture of increasing AMR problems for these organisms (101, 102), again underlining the importance of updated information on strains circulating locally. *Brachyspira* species have been reported to display high *in vitro* susceptibility to tiamulin, valnemulin, and carbadox; medium susceptibility to doxycycline; and low susceptibility to lincomycin and tylosin (103). However, in the absence of approved breakpoints for these bacteria, we do not recommend trusting *in vitro* susceptibility data for predicting *in vivo* treatment outcome. Due to the inability to culture *L. intracellularis*, only two investigations of antimicrobial susceptibility are available, both based on very few strains. One report from Korea (two strains) found tylosin and tilmicosin to be the most efficacious antimicrobials (104). The other one, which was based on 10 strains from North America, the United Kingdom, and Denmark, found carbadox, tiamulin, and valnemulin to be the most efficacious drugs. In particular, valnemulin had an effect on both intracellular and extracellular organisms (105). In addition to

the technical difficulties of culturing *L. intracellularis*, *B. hyodyseteriae*, and *B. pilosicoli*, there are no internationally recognized species- or disease-specific breakpoints for some of these organisms. This makes clinical susceptibility testing cumbersome for this disease condition. For example, the percentage of porcine *B. pilosicoli* isolates with reduced susceptibility or resistance to lincomycin was reported as ranging from 4 to 92%, depending on the interpretative criteria used (101). Consequently, diarrhea is often treated empirically. As far as *Lawsonia* and *Brachyspira* are concerned, pleuromutilins are generally regarded as first choice drugs for these pathogens. However, they are not effective against *E. coli*. For this pathogen, resistance patterns are extremely variable, even between farms in the same geographic area, and knowledge of the susceptibility profile of the causative strain is needed. In cases where infection is caused by *E. coli* in combination with one of the two other organisms, combination treatment may be justified.

Respiratory disease

A fairly high number of pathogens are commonly found associated with respiratory disease in pigs. The most common are (i) viruses such as porcine reproductive and respiratory syndrome virus, swine influenza virus, and porcine circovirus type 2; (ii) mycoplasmas such as *M. hyopneumoniae*; and (iii) bacteria such as *A. pleuropneumoniae* and *Pasteurella multocida*. While testing for the latter bacterial species is straightforward according to the standard Clinical and Laboratory Standards Institute (CLSI) guidelines (106), testing for *M. hyopneumoniae* is uncommonly performed outside specialized laboratories. The few available reports show that *M. hyopneumoniae* has acquired resistance to macrolides and lincosamides (107, 108). In common with GI disease, porcine respiratory disease is commonly the result of infection with combinations of pathogens, which changes benign mono-infections into severe treatment-requiring conditions (109). The fact that polymicrobial infections are so widely observed makes diagnosis difficult and sets a high demand for optimal diagnostic procedures to guide decision making by the veterinarian. To our knowledge, no systematic investigation to support such decision making has yet been published.

For both GI and respiratory diseases in pigs, diagnosis is further complicated by the fact that the major bacterial causative agents may occur in healthy animals (110, 111). Multiplex quantitative PCR (qPCR) tests have been developed and are extensively used for porcine diarrheal disease (112). Based partly on clinical observations and partly on validation studies, cutoff values for the important bacterial pathogens for the presence of enteritis have been established (113–115). To obtain representative samples, so-called sock samples can be used, in which the farmer or veterinarian walks through several pens wearing a (to begin with) sterile sock over his or her boots (116). To our knowledge, multiplex qPCR methods are not available for the full set of relevant respiratory pathogens. Single-pathogen qPCR methods have been developed for *M. hyopneumoniae* (117), *A. pleuropneumoniae* (118), and toxigenic *P. multocida* (119); these could be used to assess pathogen load in infected herds. However, so far, nobody has validated these methods for use as a decision tool for herds where the disease is endemic and the causative pathogen(s) is present in both sick and healthy animals. Multiplex traditional PCR exists for all relevant viral agents (120), but also in this case, no validation has been performed in endemic situations.

For metaphylactic treatment of diarrhea, Pedersen et al. (121) proposed a cutoff at 15% of pigs affected before antimicrobial treatment is indicated. qPCR based on pooled fecal samples was the best method to determine this cutoff; alternatively, the cutoff could be determined by observation of diarrheal stools, with approximately 1.5 diarrheal stools per pen (20 to 25 pigs) as a cutoff value (121). While qPCR methods ensure that decisions on metaphylactic treatment are based on a correct microbiological diagnosis, they have the drawback that no colonies are available for susceptibility testing. qPCR methods for quantification of relevant AMR genes directly in fecal samples have been developed and validated, and it has been determined how to sample to obtain a good representation of the AMR level in a herd (113). A recent study has shown promising results to quantify resistance genes in fecal samples by metagenomics (122). However, it is not yet possible to link these results to the actual detection of relevant pathogens. In some cases, no pathogens can be found in relation to outbreaks of GI disease in pigs (123). Antimicrobial treatment of such cases is not indicated, and treatment may be terminated when microbiological analysis shows negative results.

Limiting empiric use of second-line, critically important agents

Generally, drugs that are categorized as highest-priority critically important for human health, especially fluoroquinolones, third- and fourth-generation cephalosporins, and colistin (44), are prescribed more commonly for GI than for respiratory diseases in pigs (42). Multidrug resistance is rare in most porcine pathogens ex-

cept *Enterobacteriaceae*, suggesting that replacement of these critically important drugs with less critical drugs would not have any major consequence on treatment outcome and animal health. Even though significant differences exist between geographical regions, it is not easy to encounter porcine strains that require therapy with these agents. This is confirmed by the example provided by one of the largest pig-producing countries, Denmark, where the pig industry has restricted the use of these two antimicrobial classes to rare circumstances where their use is justified by multidrug resistance. A study across Europe with representative strain collections found that less than 1% of isolates of *A. pleuropneumoniae*, *P. multocida*, and *Streptococcus suis* were resistant to any of 16 antimicrobials, except tetracycline (124). In contrast, resistance was more common in *A. pleuropneumoniae* and *P. multocida* isolates from pigs in Australia, and resistance to macrolides was on the level of resistance to tetracycline (125). In Italy, a large study comparing the susceptibility of *A. pleuropneumoniae* isolates from 1994 to 2009 revealed a temporal increase in resistance to penicillins and aminopenicillins and a decrease in resistance to aminoglycosides and quinolones (126). Such reports emphasize the importance of knowing local resistance trends based on recent data. One of the most challenging respiratory pathogens is *A. pleuropneumoniae*, but here the true challenge is to achieve sufficient antimicrobial concentrations at the infection site rather that multidrug resistance. This may promote the use of second-line agents, especially the fluoroquinolones for their excellent penetration and activity against this important respiratory pathogen (127), even with a single-dose regimen (128). However, uncertainty with regard to transfer of resistant zoonotic bacteria in the pork chain, most importantly *Salmonellae* and *Campylobacter* (4), makes it unwise to advocate the use of fluroquinolones unless all other treatment options have been ruled out.

With regard to colistin, the EMA Committee for Medicinal Products for Veterinary Use has recommended restricting the use of this polymyxin due to its widespread use in livestock production, especially for management of GI disease in pigs, and due to the recent discovery of plasmid-mediated transferrable colistin resistance in pathogenic *E. coli* of animal origin (129, 130). The Committee for Medicinal Products for Veterinary Use recommendations include restriction of the use of colistin for treatment of enteric infections caused by susceptible noninvasive *E. coli* only, removal of any indications for prophylactic use, restriction of the duration of treatment to a maximum of 7 days, and withdrawal of any marketing authorizations for veterinary medicinal products containing colistin in combination with other antimicrobial substances (129). Recently, a penalty factor of 10 was added to the use of colistin in the Danish yellow card system, in essence banning the use of this drug for herd treatment. Among the possible alternatives to colistin for treatment of *E. coli* GI infections are tetracyclines and zinc oxide, and even though these agents are not categorized as critically important antimicrobials, in some parts of the world there are increasing concerns about their widespread use in pig production since they have been identified as likely drivers for the selection of methicillin-resistant *S. aureus* in livestock (131, 132). As a consequence, the use of tetracycline is associated with an extra penalty in the Danish yellow card system (22), which regulates the use of antimicrobials in pig farms, and the EMA has recommended stopping granting new marketing authorizations for zinc and withdrawing the existing ones (133).

Optimizing dosage regimens

Both modelling and experimental studies on a herd level show that the selection of antimicrobial-resistant bacteria varies significantly between pigs receiving the same treatment (134–136). Probably for that reason, studies show very little effect of antimicrobial dosage on AMR development (137). The same appears to be the case for dosage intervals (135, 136). As a general recommendation, one should aim at the lowest dose and shortest treatment duration that ensure clinical efficacy. In support of this recommendation, a recent randomized trial investigating three different doses (5 to 20 mg/kg) of oxytetracyline for treatment of diarrhea induced by *L. intracellularis* in nursery pigs did not show any significant differences in the microbiological and clinical outcomes or in average weight gain (138). Using an experimental model of porcine *A. pleuropneumoniae* infection, it was shown that the efficacy of a single dose of amoxicillin (20 mg/kg) did not differ from that achieved when the same dose was split into four daily administrations (128). Similarly, no significant differences were reported in a study comparing two florfenicol dosage regimens (15 mg/kg daily versus 15 mg twice, 48 h apart) (139). An *in silico* study evaluating clinical efficacy and AMR development following treatment with three dose levels (2, 4, and 8 mg/kg) of marbofloxacin showed that a single shot at the highest dose was the best method to ensure clinical outcome and to reduce the risk of resistance development in *A. pleuropneumoniae* and *Haemophilus parasuis* (140).

Optimal Antimicrobial Treatment in Cattle Veterinary Practice

Veterinary practitioners should be well acquainted with relevant guidelines. The European Union Guidelines for the Prudent Use of Antimicrobials in Veterinary Medicine list several key components of antimicrobial stewardship in cattle (5). Guidelines for the appropriate use of antimicrobials in seven common diseases of cattle were published in 2008 (141). The most recent guidelines for cattle in the United States are from the American Association of Bovine Practitioners (142). These guidelines emphasize the veterinarian's responsibility in implementing all measures that aid in reducing the incidence of disease and, thereby, the need for antimicrobials (e.g., design management, immunization, housing, and nutritional programs). The veterinarian should base actions and recommendations on strong clinical evidence of the identity of the pathogen causing the disease using clinical signs, history, necropsy examination, laboratory data, and experience. They also remark that the use of antimicrobials for prevention or control of disease should be based on a group, source, or production unit evaluation by the herd veterinarians rather than being utilized as a standard practice and that the veterinarian should regularly monitor antimicrobial use on the farm by reviewing treatment records, inventory, and drug purchase history. The final component of antimicrobial stewardship is to constantly monitor for protocol drift away from prescribed practices and protocols, as well as constant vigilance to evaluate if the need for the antimicrobial interventions are still present. The veterinarian is ultimately responsible for constructing clinical and laboratory diagnostic protocols for themselves and for their clients. Training on these protocols on a periodic basis is essential to minimize protocol drift and to enable timely updates.

According to a survey of veterinarians in Europe (42), mastitis (42%) and respiratory disease (20%) are the main indications for antimicrobial use in cattle (42). The examples of bovine respiratory disease complex (BRDC) and mastitis highlight the opportunities offered by advancing antimicrobial stewardship. Both diseases have multiple avenues of animal, environment, and pathogen management, which should be pursued to minimize the need for antimicrobial intervention. When intervention is necessary, the application of well-constructed clinical detection and diagnostic protocols are also essential. In selecting antimicrobial management tools, such as treatment to control BRDC or dry cow therapy for mastitis, stewardship is only present when rational selection protocols are implemented, and then only when all other possible efforts are made to reduce the need for these antimicrobial-based management practices.

Reducing overall antimicrobial consumption

The benefits of managing the environment, nutrition, colostrum transfer, and overall stress of cattle should first be recognized as the foundation of proper animal husbandry. The following paragraphs focus on the prevention of BRDC and mastitis and the optimal use of metaphylaxis.

BRDC prevention

Good husbandry practices such as low-stress weaning practices, intermediate steps between weaning and the feedlot (backgrounding), and stress control at all stages of production are advocated to control BRDC (143). The relationship of even the earliest management practices to BRDC morbidity has been demonstrated by research showing that the status of passive immune transfer immediately after birth can have an influence on preweaning and feedlot BRDC morbidity (144). Immunization should be a foundation of infectious disease prevention. Vaccines against BRDC viral pathogens such as infectious bovine rhinotracheitis virus, bovine viral diarrhea virus, and bovine respiratory syncytial virus are essential components of most BRDC prevention protocols. A 2015 meta-analysis of the literature related to the efficacy of these vaccines found a decreased BRDC morbidity risk with various antigen combinations in natural exposure trials (145). Results were more variable in experimental challenge models, with concerns about the external validity of these studies. A 2016 review of the efficacy of bovine respiratory syncytial virus vaccines pointed out the complexity of evaluating vaccine efficacy based on clinical morbidity alone and that disease-sparing attributes should also be considered (146). The concept that the timing of vaccination and the conditions in which vaccines are applied are critical to the difference between vaccination and immunization is supported by a recent review of these interventions (147). The literature evaluating vaccination against the primary bacterial pathogens of BRDC has also been evaluated in a meta-analysis (148). The authors reported that BRDC bacterial pathogen vaccines in feedlot cattle demonstrated no consistent efficacy; the available data showed a central tendency of no effect when administered on arrival in feedlots. This review does not rule out the effect of these vaccines in other husbandry systems but does again support the concept of variable effects. Alternative options for the prevention and control BRDC include agents that interact with the immune system. As for vaccines, realistic

expectations must be determined. A DNA-liposome immunostimulant acting on the innate immune system, labeled for BRDC, has recently been released in the United States (149). Currently, the peer-reviewed literature is minimal for this product, with sponsor-conducted studies serving as the main source of information on efficacy. Nonantimicrobial alternatives for BRDC control have varying efficacy depending on the type of production environment, when they are applied, and animal husbandry practices. While every effort should be made to include alternatives as a component of preventive and therapeutic programs, it is also important to have a realistic viewpoint related to their efficacy.

Mastitis prevention

Different strategies are implemented in relation to contagious and environmental pathogens, although basic practices often address both types of mastitis. For the contagious pathogens, there is a primary focus on preventing transfer and exposure in quantities that overwhelm the host defenses of the cow. Control measures of the two main contagious pathogens, *Streptococcus agalactiae* and *S. aureus*, have been emphasized as management during the milking procedure to include basic sanitation as well as pre- and postmilking teat disinfection (150). Additional factors correlated with the control of contagious mastitis pathogens are attention to the function of the milking equipment, strategic culling, biosecurity procedures for new herd additions, as well as dry cow antimicrobial therapy, which is discussed below. For environmental mastitis pathogens, critical prevention practices include frequent manure removal, avoiding standing water in the environment, and avoiding overcrowding (151). Washed sand bedding was reported to have 100-fold less pathogen load than alternative organic beddings. The greatest period of environmental mastitis occurs in the dry period and early lactation, with contributing factors of higher ambient temperature and greater moisture in the environment; this information informs decisions on when prevention intensity should be maximal. Premilking teat dipping was cited as decreasing mastitis by 50% in herds with low mastitis incidence. However, this also likely includes a substantial decrease in contagious mastitis as well. Mastitis vaccine development has ranged from the more successful *E. coli* J-5 vaccine to the more challenging *S. aureus* vaccines (152). The search for therapeutic and immunologic alternatives to antimicrobials for the prevention and control of mastitis is alive and well. Vaccines, bacteriophages, nanoparticles, cytokines, and animal- and plant-derived antibacterial compounds have all been evaluated, with varying results to date (152). Similarly, for BRDC, the struggle is to find nonantimicrobial alternatives that are as effective as antimicrobials in the control or prevention of mastitis.

Rational metaphylaxis

When environmental and immunological prevention strategies have not been successful in preventing infectious disease, the use of antimicrobials to control BRDC and mastitis are an alternative practice. Obviously, all efforts should be made to minimize the need for and the use of this practice. There is a substantial body of data in which the efficacy of antimicrobials in the control of BRDC has been compared in high-risk calves both against untreated controls and between antimicrobials. An analysis of available trials involving negative controls found that the number needed to treat (NNT) for preventing one acute BRDC case by treating for control of BRDC at feedlot arrival is 5 (153), which means that 5 animals must be treated to create a difference in clinical outcome in 1 animal. For high-risk cattle, the median NNT for creating a positive effect on BRDC case outcome with individual animal therapy was 2. The median NNT for preventing a mortality through individual animal therapy was estimated to be 6. These values would be expected to change depending on the many factors contributing to disease severity and outcome. Other authors took a meta-analysis approach to the effects of BRDC control treatment in high-risk calves, finding the mean morbidity of untreated calves to be 55% (95% confidence interval, 44.5 to 65.1%), while calves treated for control of BRDC had observed morbidities of 29% (95% confidence interval, 21.2 to 38.6%) (154). This fits with a common concept of treatment for control of BRDC resulting in a decrease in morbidity of approximately 50%.

Another component of using antimicrobials to control BRDC is what proportion of the population to treat. It has been shown in a randomly designed clinical experiment that selective metaphylaxis with florfenicol in calves (carried out only in animals with a body temperature $\geq 39.7°C$) was not significantly different from metaphylaxis of the entire group when considering clinical, pathological, and productivity outcomes (155). This kind of observation highlights the potential of "precision medicine" (see the "Future Perspectives" section), aiming to benefit from the biological advantage of an early metaphylactic treatment while dissociating it from mass medication. This kind of approach may be combined with increasingly sensitive and spe-

cific diagnostic methods to further reduce the number of animals in a population which must be treated to achieve the desired clinical outcome at the herd level.

When considering using antimicrobials to control mastitis, strategies range from blanket therapy (all cows at dry off) to different selection criteria, often focusing on somatic cell count. A simulation analysis of different selection criteria related to udder health, overall antimicrobial usage, and economics illustrated that the criteria have a significant effect on outcomes of the program (156). An entire book could be written on the benefits and concerns of dry cow therapy; a recent editorial by veterinarians captures the necessity of reappraisal of this practice with a focus on identifying cows for which this antimicrobial exposure provides a benefit (157).

Improving the use of diagnostic testing

When preventive efforts have failed, the next step in reducing antimicrobial consumption is to ensure that only animals requiring intervention receive an antimicrobial and that the antimicrobial is appropriately matched to the bacterial target.

BRDC

A recognized challenge is accurate and timely identification of animals that require antimicrobial intervention through diagnosis of BRDC. A 2016 meta-analysis of the literature pertaining to the use of visual clinical illness evaluation in beef feedlots provided an estimate of test sensitivity and specificity of 0.27 (0.12 to 0.65) and 0.92 (0.72 to 0.98) expressed as pooled estimates (95% Bayesian credible interval) (158). The authors reported high heterogeneity between studies, highlighting the variability of clinical score application for BRDC detection in different clinical settings. Different scoring systems have also been evaluated in preweaned dairy calves (159). The diagnostic sensitivity for the California and Wisconsin screening systems were 72.6% and 71.1%, respectively, while the specificity values were 87.4% and 91.2%, respectively. The "gold standard" diagnostics were thoracic ultrasound and auscultation. Additional clinical diagnostic criteria such as rectal temperature, remote temperature sensing, lung auscultation, ultrasonography, and behavioral patterns have been investigated to improve sensitivity and specificity, based on the concept that early detection provides the best chance of treatment success (160–163). The ultimate clinical diagnostic approach remains to be found, but these continued efforts are encouraging.

Laboratory diagnostics is an important part of the confirmation of bacterial pathogens and their antimicrobial susceptibility. The identification, and resulting control efforts, of viral components of this multifactorial disease is also critically important. A review of AMR in bovine respiratory disease pathogens found some troubling trends in *Mannheimia haemolytica* isolated from diagnostic isolates in the United States (164). While the applicability of diagnostic isolate AMR trends, and even the applicability of AST, remains contested, it is clear that in the reviewed literature there is a trend toward increasing levels of multidrug resistance for *M. haemolytica* in these regions. The use of AST for BRDC should be done within the context of understanding approved breakpoints and limitations of conclusions from the results. A recent review highlighted the importance of knowing whether the testing adhered to CLSI guidelines and also recognizing the source of the tested isolates (165).

Mastitis

In the treatment of bovine mastitis, it is important not only to diagnose that mastitis is present, but also to understand the factors of the disease which contribute to the likelihood of a positive impact of antimicrobials on case outcome. The focus should be on both the cow and the pathogen. This section primarily addresses clinical mastitis, although consideration of subclinical mastitis is also very important in dairy herd health, especially for contagious pathogens. A study with multiple pathogens in naturally occurring mastitis cases found that strategic mastitis treatment decisions were well informed by considering the pathogen, parity, and history of clinical and subclinical mastitis for that cow (166). These cow factors, along with the pathogen characteristics described below, should have a great influence on the decision to treat or to cull the cow from the herd. There is well-established documentation that for some pathogens antimicrobial treatment is not warranted. Reinforcing the concept that treatment protocols to support antimicrobial stewardship in mastitis therapy should be based on evaluation of disease severity and culture, a review by Roberson established that antimicrobial therapy is not warranted for mild to moderate severity Gram-negative clinical mastitis, nor for yeast, fungal, and no-growth culture result cases (167). A decision tree analysis of treatment strategies for mild and moderate cases of mastitis in early lactation also concluded that optimal approaches were to avoid antimicrobials when Gram-negative pathogens were identified or when no culture growth was detected (168). The optimal strategy as identified by economic analysis was to treat Gram-positive pathogens for 2 days, while the use of extended intra-

mammary antimicrobial therapy resulted in the least economic return.

Knowing the mastitis pathogens in an individual case or in a population is critical to the rational use of antimicrobials. Antimicrobial treatment has little chance to have a positive impact on clinical outcome if the species of microorganisms isolated from a mastitis sample are not primary pathogens. These include *Arcanobacterium pyogenes*, *Bacillus* spp., *Mycobacterium* spp., *Mycoplasma bovis*, *Nocardia* spp., *Pasteurella* spp., *Proteus* spp., *Pseudomonas* spp., *Serratia* spp., algae such as *Prototheca* spp., and yeasts (166). In contrast, the contagious mastitis pathogen *S. agalactiae* typically responds well to antimicrobial therapy, depending on accompanying case parameters of the cow as described above. *S. aureus* mastitis therapy varies greatly based on the cow factors described above and on whether the strain involved produces β-lactamase. Cow factors affecting treatment outcome for *S. aureus* mastitis include increasing age, somatic cell count, colony counts in milk, duration of infection, and number of quarters affected (169). Culturing of mastitis cases is not a common practice in USA dairies. A survey of 600 eastern USA dairy farms published in 2016 revealed that only 17% of milk samples from cows with high somatic cell counts and 18% of samples from cows with clinical mastitis were cultured (170). Although culturing mastitis cases results in added costs and labor, this practice has been demonstrated to dramatically reduce the number of cows that are treated with an antimicrobial. A 2011 multistate study in the United States demonstrated that the use of an on-farm culture system reduced intramammary antimicrobial administration by half (171). This reduction was accomplished with no significant effects on days to clinical cure, bacteriological cure rate, new intramammary infection risk, or treatment failure risk within the 21 days following the initial mastitis event. In contrast to AST for BRDC, testing for mastitis pathogens is more controversial and has been questioned by some authors (172, 173). There are few CLSI-approved breakpoints for mastitis, and clinical outcomes related to susceptibility testing results may vary (174).

Based on the fact that the vast majority of mastitis cases in cows are caused by just a few agents, veterinarians in Denmark have used a simplified microbiological approach for several decades. In this approach, milk samples are cultured on blood esculin agar and blood agar supplemented with benzylpenicillin. Combined analysis of colony morphology, hemolysis, Gram reaction, cell morphology, and catalase reaction allows for quick identification. The penicillin concentration in the blood agar is calibrated to detect penicillin-resistant *S. aureus* but is commonly used as an indication of whether simple penicillin would be a suitable treatment option in acute mastitis. The system has been quality controlled by a number of ring tests (175). Recently, real-time PCR tests have been introduced as an alternative and shown to perform well for diagnosis of the common mastitis pathogens. Primers for amplification of the *blaZ* gene, which encodes penicillin resistance in *S. aureus*, are included in some of these tests, maintaining the ability to evaluate for penicillin resistance in *S. aureus* (176). Low-quality samples are a problem when qPCR is used to diagnose mastitis pathogens. Even low-grade contamination of milk samples from the environment can result in false-positive results, and there is concern about whether samples drawn from milking robots in herds with automated milking systems can be considered cow-specific.

Prudent use of second-line, critically important agents

Comparison of the expected efficacy of different antimicrobials is critical in decision making. The effectiveness of approved antimicrobials for respiratory disease in the United States has been evaluated in a mixed treatment meta-analysis (177). Tulathromycin and enrofloxacin were ranked the highest (most efficacious), while oxytetracycline was just above the bottom ranking of the nonactive controls in the studies. Of the 12 antimicrobials evaluated, macrolides and fluoroquinolones made up the top six in the ranking of efficacy. The WHO considers both of these antimicrobial classes highest priority within critically important antimicrobials, while oxytetracycline ranks as highly important (44). These reviews focused on the use of these antimicrobials in high-risk calves entering feedlots. This high-risk category results from extensive comingling and handling immediately prior to feedlot entry. There are substantially fewer prospective, randomized, masked, negative-control datasets available for dairy cows or very young calves. Great caution must be used in extrapolating these comparative results to respiratory disease in lower-risk cattle, such as yearlings or calves directly from a ranch. In cases of BRDC in lower-risk cattle, this is the most likely situation where an antimicrobial such as oxytetracycline could be considered for first-line treatment.

As for BRDC, the primary basis of antimicrobial selection for mastitis therapy should begin with clinical efficacy studies. Clinical evidence for efficacy of antimicrobials against appropriate mastitis pathogens has been reviewed, with detailed reporting of case definitions for study entry and outcomes, reported as both clinical and microbiological cure rate (178). These outcomes should be evaluated when selecting an appropriate therapeutic intervention, with careful attention being paid to the external validity of the trials related to the specific clinical situation(s) being considered. It is interesting to note that NNT values for intramammary mastitis therapy tended to range from 3 to 4, compared to the median NNT of 2 for BRDC therapy reported above. The primary route to restricting the use of critically important antimicrobials for therapy of mastitis lies in instituting routine culturing procedures with defined protocols for which pathogens are treated or not treated. Blanket treatment of all acute mastitis cases with an empirically selected antimicrobial is clearly not consistent with stewardship principles. Guidelines for prudent treatment have been issued that emphasize the importance of an etiological diagnosis and following evidence-based, best practices. For empiric treatment, the drug of choice must be based on herd data and the veterinarian's personal experience. In general, however, antimicrobials with a primary Gram-positive aerobic spectrum among mastitis pathogens, such as penicillin-G, can be used except when Gram-negative bacteria are suspected as the cause of the infection. This is because streptococci and penicillin-susceptible staphylococci are the most common causes of mastitis. Third- and fourth-generation cephalosporins should be avoided as first-line drugs against these common pathogens (179). For these reasons, penicillin is recommended as a first-line drug for mastitis in Scandinavian countries (180).

Optimizing dosage regimens

Many of the antimicrobials used to treat BRDC are single-injection formulations with a predefined duration of antimicrobial exposure that is controlled by their more or less prolonged terminal half-life due to prolonged release from the injection site, characteristics of the antimicrobial itself, or a combination of both. Therefore, after cattle have been treated for BRDC, the next key decision is when to evaluate them for the need for further treatment (success/failure). A review of evidence for when to conduct this evaluation noted that data are lacking to support defining the optimal antimicrobial exposure period for BRDC therapy (181). Data cited in the review were used to suggest that, lacking other specific data for a single-injection antimicrobial used in the therapy of BRDC, a posttreatment interval of 7 days is likely appropriate. Application of success-failure criteria after daily-administered antimicrobials for BRDC has typically been the day after the last dose.

Guidance on duration of therapy prior to application of success-failure criteria for daily-administered antimicrobials in BRDC is lacking; the approval process has focused on evaluating different doses at the same duration and frequency. This lack of clear guidance highlights the need for research to focus on optimal duration of administration and timing of success/failure determination. The impact of doses of marbofloxacin (2 versus 10 mg/kg) on the microbiological, pathological, and clinical outcomes of calves challenged with *M. haemolytica* has been reported for early (2 to 4 h) versus late (35 to 39 h) treatment (35). It was shown that an early 2-mg/kg-dose treatment was more efficacious to prevent pulmonary lesions and led to a rapid and total microbiological cure, supporting the hypothesis that a reduced antibiotic regimen given at an early stage of the disease is efficacious in the management of BRDC. The clinical application of this finding is unknown at present due to the imprecision of clinical diagnosis and subsequently the inability to stage naturally occurring disease in the field. For concentration-dependent antimicrobials such as the fluoroquinolones, it is recommended to minimize treatment duration to decrease the likelihood of AMR emergence in the target respiratory pathogen. For example, a single high dose (10 mg/kg) is preferable to multiple-dose administration of 2 mg/kg (182). The goal in single high-dose therapy is to kill the target pathogens as rapidly as possible or at least a sufficient fraction of the initial load to allow eradication of the remnant bacterial population by the host's natural defenses.

The need for additional research on optimal duration of treatment for mastitis pathogens was supported by a study of dairy farmers in The Netherlands and Germany; extending therapy beyond the label duration was primarily based on the social norm that discontinuing treatment while there were still clinical symptoms was inconsistent with "being a good farmer" (183). A clinical trial evaluating extended therapy of cefquinome for *S. aureus* mastitis in the United Kingdom, France, Hungary, Italy, and The Netherlands found that extending the therapy beyond label indications resulted in improved clinical, but not bacteriological, cures and should not be recommended (184). More studies like these are needed to further define the optimal duration of therapy.

Optimal Antimicrobial Treatment in Small Animal Veterinary Practice

The International Society for Companion Animal Infectious Diseases (ISCAID) has published international disease-specific guidelines for urinary tract infections (185), superficial folliculitis (186), and respiratory infections (187) in small animals. Guidelines for systemic treatment of bacterial skin infections have been proposed by Beco et al. (188). Recommendations on prudent antimicrobial choice covering all disease conditions are available in textbooks (189) and national guidelines (190, 191). It is generally recognized that antimicrobial use in small animal veterinary practice should be optimized by implementing dedicated antimicrobial stewardship programs (ASPs), which are typically multimodal (involving a variety of measures at once) and multidisciplinary (e.g., involving clinicians, pharmacists, microbiologists, and administrators) (192). ASPs have been proven to be useful to reduce total or targeted antimicrobial use, reduce AMR, and improve patient care in human health care facilities. Unfortunately, the use of ASPs in small animal medicine is in its infancy but will likely increase, through either formal programs or less formal measures directed at controlling antimicrobial use at the clinic or facility level. It has been demonstrated that the introduction of antimicrobial policies at the clinic level has a positive impact on prescribing patterns, with a general reduction in antimicrobial use and a relative reduction in the use of second-line agents (193). Unfortunately, the practice of developing and updating antimicrobial policies is uncommon in veterinary practice, and people with expertise to help develop and implement ASPs in veterinary medicine are limited. According to a cross-sectional survey conducted in small animal veterinary practices in the United Kingdom, an antimicrobial policy was established in only 3.5% of the clinics (194). Data are not available on a global scale, but our perception is that the overall frequency of clinics that have an antimicrobial policy in place is similar or even lower in other countries.

Reducing overall antimicrobial consumption

As for other animal species, the most important generic approach for reducing antimicrobial consumption in small animal medicine is the prevention of infections so that there is no need to consider antimicrobials. This can take various forms, including measures directed at patients as well as infection control measures in veterinary facilities and other group situations (195). A survey of small animal practitioners in Europe indicated skin (52%), genitourinary (11%), respiratory, and GI (10%) diseases as the most frequent indications for antimicrobial prescription in dogs (42). The indications for which antimicrobials are prescribed in cats were similar, with the notable exception of periodontal and GI disease, which accounted for 14% and less than 3%, respectively, of the prescriptions claimed by veterinarians for this animal species. Studies conducted in veterinary teaching hospitals (196, 197) have confirmed the perception that most antimicrobials are prescribed for skin (23 to 30%), GI (11 to 19%), genitourinary (12 to 14%), and respiratory (6 to 14%) diseases. Accordingly, significant reductions in antimicrobial consumption can mainly be attained by optimizing the prevention and treatment of these diseases.

Skin disease

Superficial pyoderma accounts for a major proportion of antimicrobial consumption in dogs. Antimicrobial use can be reduced by preventing recurrent infections and controlling predisposing factors (e.g., atopic dermatitis). Moreover, there is an increasing amount of scientific evidence supporting the notion that superficial pyoderma can effectively be managed by biocide-containing shampoos and other topical products as an alternative to systemic therapy (198, 199). National and international guidelines recommend topical therapy alone (without coadministration of systemic antimicrobial drugs) unless precluded by owner and/or patient factors (186, 190, 191). The topical approach is particularly encouraged for management of (i) localized lesions, (ii) early stages of generalized superficial pyoderma, and (iii) to prevent recurrence. However, most veterinarians continue to use topical therapy as an adjunctive therapy in combination with systemic antimicrobials, if they use it at all. A recent UK study based on electronic patient records revealed that 92% of dogs with a diagnosis of pyoderma were prescribed systemic therapy, whereas only 5% of dogs were prescribed topical therapy alone (200). These data suggest that the overall antimicrobial consumption could significantly be reduced if the international guidelines were implemented in veterinary dermatology. Other common skin conditions for which systemic antimicrobial therapy is often unnecessary include abscesses and wound infections. These conditions can usually be managed by mechanical cleansing, debridement of necrotic tissue, drainage, and suturing. According to the Swedish and Danish guidelines (190, 191), systemic antimicrobial treatment is only indicated if (i) there is evidence of systemic infection, (ii) surgical procedures alone are not sufficient to achieve wound healing, (iii) the tissue damage is extensive, or (iv) the injury affects a structure particularly susceptible to infection (e.g., a joint). For abscesses, it should be noted that penetration of certain systemic antimicrobials may be compromised and their efficacy hampered by the presence of pus (e.g., penicillin) and various local factors such as low pH (e.g., aminoglycosides and macrolides) and protein binding, and that incision and drainage is an effective sole measure for discrete abscesses.

GI disease

Although unspecified acute gastroenteritis (i.e., acute diarrhea and vomiting without evidence of hemorrhage and systemic disease) is usually self-limiting and can be managed by supportive therapy, antimicrobial use is widespread for this disease condition. According to a questionnaire survey in the United Kingdom in 2009 (194), 23% of the respondents reported that they prescribed antimicrobial therapy for cases of unspecified gastroenteritis. A similar response was given by approximately 70% of the respondents in an older survey in Australia (201). According to a qualitative study of factors associated with antimicrobial usage in small animal veterinary practices in the United Kingdom (202), antimicrobial drugs are more likely to be prescribed for therapy of unspecified gastroenteritis in the presence of an elderly animal or if the owners are "particularly worried," suggesting a likely conflict between rational antimicrobial use and the perception of veterinary practice as a "business" that should satisfy the client's expectations. However, antimicrobial treatment is normally not indicated since bacterial gastroenteritis (or at least bacterial enteritis that is effectively controlled through administration of an antimicrobial) is relatively infrequent in small animals. The occurrence of acute diarrhea with the presence of blood in the feces is common, but this clinical sign alone is not an indication for antimicrobial treatment, which is only indicated for patients displaying poor general conditions and fever.

There is no evidence that antimicrobial therapy may be beneficial for dogs affected by acute hemorrhagic diarrhea syndrome (previously known as hemorrhagic gastroenteritis) without signs of sepsis. A placebo-controlled study showed no significant effect of antimicrobial therapy with amoxicillin clavulanate on mortality rate, dropout rate, duration of hospitalization, or severity of clinical signs (203). Anecdotally, the incidence of systemic complications (e.g., meningitis, arthritis, sepsis) following GI disease, even acute hemorrhagic disease, appears to be low. However, some patient populations are likely at increased risk of complications of bacterial translocation, and while inadequately studied, antimicrobials may be justifiable. For example, puppies with parvovirus infection may be at higher risk because of their young age and degree of intestinal mucosal compromise, and short parenteral antimicrobial treatment is commonly used to prevent bacterial translocation. Adverse drug reactions associated with disruption of the gut microbiota should be carefully considered in adult patients. As studies of this microbiota and GI disease increase, it is becoming more apparent that diarrhea, particularly chronic diarrhea, is often associated with broad effects on the microbiota, not overgrowth of single pathogens, and that the drugs that are commonly used to empirically treat GI disease (e.g., tylosin, metronidazole) would impact bacteria that are increasingly recognized as critical for gut health (e.g., members of the *Clostridiales*).

Genitourinary disease

Overall antimicrobial use can be reduced by avoiding antimicrobial treatment of subclinical bacteriuria or pyuria and feline lower urinary tract disease (FLUTD). Treatment of subclinical bacteriuria, pyuria, or other cytological abnormalities is generally not recommended in the absence of clinical abnormalities. While the bladder is often considered a sterile environment, studies of various patient populations make it clear that the presence of bacteria in the absence of disease (subclinical bacteriuria) is a common event. There is no evidence that subclinical bacteriuria progresses to disease or that treatment is protective. In fact, a recent study of humans has noted a detrimental impact of treatment of subclinical bacteriuria (204), with an increased risk of recurrence compared to untreated controls. Even though previous guidelines supported the treatment of animals with no clinical signs but cytological evidence of inflammation (185), there is no evidence supporting a different approach in veterinary medicine, and recent guideline revisions have discouraged treatment in the absence of clinical evidence of disease (205). As for FLUTD, this is a relatively common noninfectious condition associated with environmental stressors and rarely involving bacterial infection. However, according to a study conducted on primary care veterinary practices in Canada (206), 74% of cases associated with FLUTD were treated with antimicrobials. In a UK interview study (202), nearly half of veterinarians interviewed in first opinion practices believed that FLUTD was an infectious condition that should be treated with antimicrobials. Altogether, these data suggest antimicrobial overuse for the treatment of FLUTD.

Respiratory disease

Other conditions that require attention in antimicrobial prescription include feline upper respiratory tract disease and canine infectious respiratory disease complex (previously known as canine infectious tracheobronchitis, or kennel cough complex). A Canadian study revealed that 70% of cats affected by feline upper respiratory tract disease and 67% dogs affected by canine

infectious respiratory disease complex were treated with antimicrobials (206). It is plausible that overall antimicrobial use could be reduced for these disease conditions, which are often caused by viral agents. In particular, most feline upper respiratory tract disease cases are associated with feline herpesvirus or calicivirus, and a considerable proportion of canine infectious respiratory disease complex cases are associated with either canine adenovirus 2, canine distemper virus, canine respiratory coronavirus, canine influenza viruses, canine herpesvirus, canine pneumovirus, or canine parainfluenza virus, which may or may not develop secondary bacterial infections. Moreover, even if bacteria are involved, infection can be self-limiting, especially if the causative agents are *Bordetella bronchiseptica* in dogs and *Chlamydophila felis* in cats. Based on these considerations, the recent guidelines for treatment of respiratory tract disease published by the ISCAID Antimicrobial Working Group recommend a 10-day observation period before prescribing antimicrobials. Antimicrobial therapy should only be considered within the 10-day observation period if fever, lethargy, or inappetence is present together with mucopurulent discharges (187). While requiring more owner monitoring and veterinary follow-up, this type of approach is likely to be effective at limiting the impact of disease, reducing AMR pressures, and reducing costs and potential adverse effects of antimicrobial administration.

Improving the use of diagnostic testing

Unfortunately, definitive diagnoses are rarely made during first-opinion small animal consultations. For the common disease conditions requiring antimicrobial prescription, definitive diagnoses have been estimated to be as low as 21% for skin, 10% for GI cases, 4% for urinary tract, and 3% for respiratory cases (207). The use of culture and AST is low despite the recommendations by many national and international veterinary organizations. The frequency of bacterial culture and AST has been estimated by different studies to be approximately 2 to 8% of all cases where antimicrobials are prescribed (197, 207). According to a recent survey on veterinarian prescription practices in Europe (42), the frequency of AST in small animal practice is higher than in livestock practice but lower than in equine practice. Poor response to therapy was the main reason for performing AST according to 90% of small animal veterinarians. The diffusion of pet insurance covering microbiology diagnostics would be an important contribution to promote the use of AST by reducing the costs for pet owners. However, pet insurance is not well established in most countries.

Bacterial culture is always advisable but is of particular importance in the following situations: (i) complicated or life-threatening infection, (ii) treatment failure, (iii) recurrent infection, (iv) immunosuppressed patients, and (v) patients at risk of infection with MDR bacteria. The latter situation is increasingly difficult to define, given the rapid spread of resistant bacteria such as methicillin-resistant *S. pseudintermedius* and ESBL-producing *Enterobacteriaceae* in the companion animal population, but factors such as previous hospital exposure, contact with a person harboring an MDR bacterium, and previous antimicrobial exposure all increase the risk. In Denmark, because of the need to increase microbiological surveillance of AMR, culture and AST are recommended for all cases of pyoderma where systemic antimicrobial therapy is to be used and for urinary tract infections (190). These infections are the commonest reasons for antimicrobial prescription in companion animal and are frequently associated with bacterial species that may display multidrug resistance. Moreover, pyoderma requires prolonged treatment, and treatment failure from ineffective empirical antimicrobial selection can have consequences on both the patient's welfare and the owner's finances. Routine culture is recommended in veterinary referral hospitals situated in geographical areas with high prevalence of methicillin-resistant *S. pseudintermedius* and ESBL-producing *E. coli*.

Limiting the empiric use of second-line, critically important agents

Among the drugs ranked as high-priority critically important by the WHO (44), macrolides are rarely used in small animals due to poor efficacy and adverse side effects. Various studies have documented overuse of fluoroquinolones (e.g., enrofloxacin, ciprofloxacin, marbofloxacin, and pradofloxacin) and extended-spectrum cephalosporins (e.g., cefovecin and cefpodoxime). In a Canadian study, these two antimicrobial classes accounted for 12% and 29% of all antimicrobial prescriptions in dogs and cats, respectively (206). In an Italian study, fluoroquinolones exceeded 20% of the total prescriptions and 60% of the prescriptions for urinary tract infections (197). A recent study in the United Kingdom identified skin infections (48.2%), urinary tract infections (13.7%), and respiratory infections (9.8%) as the most common cat disease conditions for which cefovecin is prescribed in first-opinion practices. Another study in the United Kingdom reported that this cephalosporin accounted for 13% of antimicrobial prescriptions for respiratory disease (194). Cefovecin is a long-acting third-generation cephalosporin that re-quires a single subcutaneous administration for covering a course treatment of 14 to 21 days. This atypical pharmacological feature makes this drug very attractive in patients where oral administration can be difficult, particularly cats. However, both fluoroquinolones and extended-spectrum cephalosporins are high-priority, critically important drugs in both human and veterinary medicine and have a considerable impact on the gut microbiota of dogs (208–211). For these reasons, these drugs are generally classified by international guidelines as second- or third-line agents for use in companion animals, except for severe life-threatening infections (e.g., sepsis, peritonitis, and lower respiratory tract infections) or rare situations (e.g., prostatitis and pyelonephritis) in which fluoroquinolones outcompete other antimicrobial classes in terms of both clinical efficacy and safety (189). For other disease conditions, fluoroquinolones and extended-spectrum cephalosporins should only be used with the support of culture and susceptibility data indicating a lack of appropriate first-line options.

The European Union guidelines for prudent antimicrobial use in veterinary medicine recommend that off-label (cascade) use of antimicrobials not authorized in veterinary medicine should be avoided, especially for last-resort drugs that are of high critical importance for human health, namely, the carbapenems and vancomycin (5). The use of these "reserve" drugs should only be considered in very exceptional cases, e.g., when laboratory susceptibility testing has confirmed that no other antimicrobials will be effective and where there are ethical reasons to justify such a course of treatment. The British Small Animal Veterinary Association guideline on companion animals (212) considers there to be a strong argument that "last resort" antimicrobials, such as carbapenems and vancomycin, should not be used for veterinary patients. In Sweden, the use of these drugs in veterinary medicine has been banned by law, and other countries may follow this example in the near future. The emergence of ESBL-producing *Enterobacteriaceae* has created increasing challenges in this area, because carbapenems are a drug of choice for these infections from a clinical standpoint. As resistance becomes more common, the potential need for last resort antimicrobials correspondingly increases, emphasizing the need for infection control and a proactive approach to if, how, when, and where to use these antimicrobials.

Optimizing dosage regimens

Unfortunately, evidence of how to optimize dosage regimens, particularly treatment duration, is often lacking in small animal veterinary medicine, where antimicrobial mis-dosing seems not to be uncommon. Summers et al. (200) reported that prescribed doses were below the minimum recommended daily dose for approximately 26% of the dogs diagnosed with pyoderma in primary care veterinary practice in the United Kingdom. According to another study in the United Kingdom, amoxicillin, amoxicillin clavulanate, and fluoroquinolones were underdosed in approximately 8%, 4% and 3% of the cases and overdosed in 16%, 26% and 12% of the cases, respectively (194). The most frequently underdosed drugs were metronidazole (25.64%) and trimethoprim-sulfadiazine (15.63%).

In theory, antimicrobial dosage regimens should follow the label instructions even if some historical dosage regimens are likely not optimal because they were established prior the current PK/PD era. For certain drugs (e.g., doxycycline), different dosage regimens (e.g., 10 mg/kg per day or twice a day) are indicated for the same product in different countries. In human medicine this question of antimicrobial dosage regimen obsolescence led to the suggestion to re-evaluate regular dosing regimens and to recommend that market authorization should be awarded for a limited time period (e.g., 5 years) instead of granting unlimited duration (213). When the label instructions indicate a range of possible drug doses, the highest dose is recommended for concentration-dependent drugs such as the fluoroquinolones to enhance therapeutic efficacy as well as to prevent selection of resistant mutants ("shoot high") (214, 215), except in situations where toxicity is of particular concern (e.g., enrofloxacin in cats, aminoglycosides in animals with renal compromise). It has been suggested, as a general rule, that the average levels of concentration-dependent drugs should exceed at least 8 to 10 times the MIC in the target pathogen to prevent selection of resistant subpopulations at the infection site (216). This recommendation is often expressed in the veterinary literature by saying that the value of the corresponding PK/PD index predictive of clinical and bacteriological efficacy, AUC/MIC, should be equal to 125 to 250 h, which is equivalent to saying that the average plasma concentration should be equal to 5- to 10-fold the MIC in steady-state conditions (217). However, a recent investigation on MPC in *S. pseudintermedius* has shown that the lowest doses within the clinically recommended dose ranges of all veterinary fluoroquinolones are too low to prevent selection of resistant mutants with AUC/MIC$_{90}$ ≤ 26 (218). Actually, there is no straightforward relationship between MIC and MPC for fluoroquinolones (219), rendering it difficult to express a general recommendation

on the dose preventing the emergence of resistant mutant. For marbofloxacin, a similar ratio was reported for *E. coli* and *S. aureus* (9.2 and 9.0), but this ratio was 9 and 17 for orbifloxacin and 7.8 and 35 for enrofloxacin (220). The same situation exists for β-lactams (221). Notably, although laboratory data indicate a benefit from using high doses of fluoroquinolones, the actual impact on prevention of emergence of AMR in clinical practice is still questioned by some authors (222). However, while principles of antimicrobial use based on factors such as time above MIC and AUC/MIC are well founded, the lack of MIC data for clinical isolates hampers clear application of these principles.

Maintaining a regular administration interval is particularly important for time-dependent antimicrobials such as all β-lactams since their clinical efficacy is affected if *f*T > MIC [Time for free plasma concentration above the MIC] for less than 40 to 50% of the dosing interval ("shoot regular") (223). From here, it is important to communicate to the animal owners the critical role that compliance plays in the treatment outcome. In theory, the administration interval could also influence the prevention of resistance to fluoroquinolones, since delayed administration may increase the time below the MPC, with the consequent risk that resistant mutants may be selected during therapy. However, a single daily administration is recommended for all veterinary fluoroquinolones. It should be noted that in veterinary medicine, the doses and dosing interval can significantly differ from those recommended for the same drug in human medicine. The latter situation may at least in part reflect differences in species-specific PK properties of the selected antimicrobial drug. For example, clindamycin is recommended at a dosage of 5 to 10 mg/kg every 12 h in small animals and at 3 to 400 mg (20 mg/kg/day) every 8 h in children for the treatment of skin staphylococcal infections (224). This can simply reflect that the half-life of clindamycin is of 2.0 h in 6- to 12-year-old children (225), in contrast to 4.4 h in dogs (226). Similarly, cephalexin is recommended at 15 to 30 mg/kg every 12 h in small animals and at 250 mg (25 mg/kg/day) every 6 h in children for the same indication (225). This may simply reflect that the typical half-life of cephalexin in humans (oral route) is about 1.4 h (226), in contrast to 4.74 h in dogs (227). On one hand, there is evidence to discourage easy translation of human recommendations on dosage regimens to veterinary medicine. On the other hand, the current veterinary dosage regimens were defined in the pre-PK/PD era and might have been influenced by marketing considerations.

Small animals are generally treated for significantly longer periods than humans. For example, courses of treatment as short as 3 days have proven to be sufficient to treat uncomplicated bacterial cystitis in dogs (227). Accordingly, the joint IDSA/European Society for Clinical Microbiology and Infectious Diseases guidelines recommend treatment for 3 to 5 days depending on the specific drug (228). However, uncomplicated urinary tract infections are traditionally treated for 7 to 14 days in small animal practice. A 7-day treatment has been regarded as "reasonable" by the ISCAID Antimicrobial Working Group in the absence of objective data and encouraged clinical trials supporting shorter treatment durations in dogs and cats (185), with revised guidelines suggesting that 3 to 5 days of treatment should be considered, similar to humans (205). A similar discrepancy is evident between human and veterinary guidelines for treatment of superficial skin infections. Veterinary guidelines recommend at least 3 weeks of treatment and 1 week beyond clinical cure (186, 189), whereas human guidelines recommend treating staphylococcal skin infections for approximately 7 days depending on clinical response (229).

Optimal Antimicrobial Treatment in Equine Veterinary Practice

Education regarding indications for antimicrobial use, dosing regimens, and potential adverse consequences is an important aspect of antimicrobial stewardship and may be particularly important in horses, where multiple levels of decision making (e.g., veterinarian, trainer, owner) are involved. While various commentaries have been published directed at equine veterinarians (230–232), antimicrobial stewardship efforts directed at lay personnel have been lacking. There is also limited availability of international treatment guidelines (233), especially in comparison to small animals, for which guidelines are now available for selected conditions (185–188). Antimicrobials are commonly used in equine veterinary practice for the treatment and prevention of bacterial infections, as well as in situations where bacterial infections are unlikely (234). Despite the commonness of antimicrobial use in horses, clear data regarding how antimicrobials are used in this species are very limited. Yet available data raise concerns about how and when antimicrobials are used. A study of Swiss, German, and Austrian equine veterinarians evaluated responses to specific scenarios, with a majority of respondents indicating that they would prescribe an antimicrobial for situations most consistent with viral infections (235). The use of unapproved antimicrobials was common, as was the use of inadequate doses.

Reducing overall antimicrobial consumption

The incidence of antimicrobial use in situations where bacterial infections are unlikely provides much opportunity for reducing antimicrobial use, yet achieving such reductions can be challenging and requires consideration of the forces that drive antimicrobial decisions. These can include economic factors in performance horses (e.g., decreased performance or missing competitions because of infections), concerns about fear of complications developing in expensive animals, and defaulting to the use of antimicrobials when bacterial infections are not definitely excluded because of the risk aversion of owners, trainers, and clinicians, often with less consideration of the potential adverse effects of antimicrobial use. For example, some antimicrobials (e.g., doxycycline) have some nonantimicrobial properties (236) that might have therapeutic or performance-enhancing effects. It has been recommended that antimicrobials not be used for nonantimicrobial properties (8), but the demand for such uses will likely remain in the competitive equine world. Examples of situations where antimicrobials are often used (and potentially misused) in equine practice are discussed below.

Use of local treatment

The overall use of systemic antimicrobial drugs can be reduced by increasing the use of local antimicrobial delivery. Local approaches such as the use of antimicrobial-impregnated materials, topical therapy, regional limb perfusion, and intra-articular and intra-osseous administration are well studied in horses (237–239) and are potentially effective for certain types of infections. These approaches can result in high drug levels at the site of infection and minimize systemic antimicrobial exposure, reducing the corresponding toxicity and adverse effects (e.g., colitis), as well as cost. The large size of horses makes some of these approaches both more practical and more cost-effective, and they are widely used in some situations.

Upper respiratory tract disease

Upper respiratory tract disease is a leading cause of morbidity and poor performance in horses. A variety of etiologies may be encountered, including bacterial infections caused by pathogens such as *Streptococcus equi* subsp. *equi*, *S. equi* subsp. *zooepidemicus*, and *Actinobacillus* spp. However, inflammatory airway disease (a noninfectious condition) is common, particularly among performance horses, where subtle impacts on respiratory function can lead to significant impacts on performance. Antimicrobial use for poor performance believed to be associated with the respiratory tract is not uncommon, despite little indication that bacterial infections are a common or important cause. A study of racing standardbreds and thoroughbreds identified treatment of 69% of horses diagnosed with nonseptic inflammatory airway disease, a noninfectious condition (240). Horses had received up to three antimicrobials and 20 days of treatment prior to pursuing diagnostic testing and identification of a noninfectious cause.

Neonatal foal care

Antimicrobial treatment is common in both healthy and sick neonatal foals. Prophylactic administration of antimicrobials such as gentamicin to all foals has been recommended, yet data have indicated that this is not effective (241). While routine treatment of all newborn foals is perhaps less common now than in the past, anecdotal information indicates that it is still performed on some farms. Although there is little argument for the need for antimicrobials to treat foals with evidence of (or at high risk of) sepsis, routine treatment is likely both ineffective and potentially detrimental. Regular use of a standard foal antimicrobial regimen on a farm would reasonably be suspected of increasing the likelihood of emergence of AMR, potentially impacting treatment efficacy when antimicrobials are used on ill foals. Further, with increasing evidence of the importance of the microbiota (the body's vast microbial population) and the potentially long-term health impacts of early antimicrobial exposure in other species (242, 243), more consideration of the potential adverse effects of routine antimicrobial use in foals is warranted.

Surgical prophylaxis

Antimicrobials are widely used for peri-operative prophylaxis. In some situations, antimicrobials are probably critical for prevention of surgical site infections; however, many low-risk procedures are performed in horses. Limited studies that have been conducted have highlighted potential issues with the use of antimicrobials for surgical prophylaxis. A study of elective arthroscopies, a clean procedure where antimicrobials are not recommended in humans (244, 245), identified peri-operative antimicrobial administration to 98% of horses (246). Whether antimicrobials are truly needed in equine arthroscopy is not established, with proponents of prophylaxis often citing the potentially devastating impacts of (rare) postoperative septic arthritis. The predominant use of sodium penicillin raises additional questions about the necessity and appropriateness of use, considering the expected high prevalence of β-lactamase production among staphylococci, the main

causes of septic arthritis in horses (247). There are also concerns about the use of peri-operative antimicrobials based on the timing of administration (see the section below on improving the use of diagnostic testing). Large-scale, multicenter studies using clear study criteria and infection definitions are needed to properly assess optimal peri-operative antimicrobial practices, balancing preventing infections and avoiding adverse effects (e.g., antimicrobial-associated colitis, AMR).

Improving the use of diagnostic testing

Inadequate, inaccurate, or improperly interpreted diagnostic testing can foster imprudent antimicrobial use, while prompt and accurate diagnostic testing can limit unnecessary use of antimicrobials and help optimize drug choices. Surprisingly, in a survey on prescribing habits among veterinarians in Europe (42), equine practitioners claimed to perform susceptibility testing more frequently compared to other types of veterinary practice. Because antimicrobials are often used empirically and in situations where viral infections (e.g., upper respiratory viruses) or noninfectious conditions (e.g., inflammatory airway disease) are common, rapid (and ideally horse-side) diagnostic tests could have a significant impact on antimicrobial use. However, there is currently limited availability of such tests.

Limiting empiric use of second-line, critically important agents

Drugs within the WHO's definition of "highest priority critically important antimicrobials" (45) are all used in horses, to variable extents ranging from relatively common (third-generation cephalosporins and macrolides) to infrequent (fluoroquinolones) or rare (glycopeptides). The evaluation of drugs within this category and their use in horses highlights many issues and challenges in terms of minimizing and optimizing their use. Third-generation cephalosporins are desirable in some situations because of their broad spectrum. Use of this class has presumably increased with the licensing of ceftiofur crystalline-free acid in some countries, a long-acting drug that requires infrequent administration. While dosing convenience can be beneficial by facilitating compliance (which would have positive impacts on outcome and proper antimicrobial use), concerns exist about the use of broad-spectrum, long-acting agents when the spectrum or duration is excessive but chosen because of convenience. This becomes evident in situations where ceftiofur is used instead of narrower-spectrum antimicrobials that would be effective anyway, such as penicillins or potentiated sulfonamides, for treatment of *S. equi* infections. Similarly, while not particularly frequent (42,

235), the use of third-generation cephalosporins or fluoroquinolones for peri-operative prophylaxis is still high since their use is often not indicated.

Macrolides have a unique and important niche in equine medicine, being used primarily for *Rhodococcus equi* infection in foals, a common and important disease. Macrolides are the main recommendation (typically in combination with rifampin) (248, 249), and their use is easy to justify from a medical standpoint. The potential contribution of this rather widespread use in horses to resistance in horses or humans is poorly understood; however, given the limited other good options for treatment of this infection, macrolide use will likely remain high in foals. A variety of macrolides have been recommended or used for treatment of *R. equi* infection, including erythromycin, azithromycin, and clarithromycin (249). Whether there is any benefit or risk of using newer macrolides versus older drugs, from an AMR standpoint, is unclear.

While fluoroquinolones are used frequently in companion animals, their use is relatively low in horses (42, 235, 250). Whether limited use of fluoroquinolones in most regions reflects concern about the use of this antimicrobial class, cost, or other factors is unknown. Use of glycopeptides (vancomycin) has been reported in horses (251) but is exceedingly rare in clinical practice, with some facilities having restriction policies and some countries having regulatory bans. At the population level, use of this drug has minimal impact on horse health, being reserved for very rare situations in certain areas.

Compared to some animal species, a relatively limited number of antimicrobials are commonly used in horses. The unavailability or high risk of adverse effects of some antimicrobials that are commonly used as first-line agents in other species, particularly oral options (e.g., amoxicillin/clavulanic acid, cephalexin, clindamycin), and the availability of fluoroquinolones and third-generation cephalosporins inherently increases the likelihood of these critically important agents being used as first-line agents. Dosing interval and route can play an important role in treatment decisions (235), which can drive the use of some second-line options (e.g., enrofloxacin and ceftiofur crystalline-free acid). However, first-line drugs such as trimethoprim-sulfonamide combinations and penicillins are practical, cost effective, and useful for many infections. Information about how to more broadly restrict the use of second-line agents is lacking but needed.

Optimizing dosing regimens

Dosing accuracy is a key aspect of dosage regimen optimization in equine veterinary medicine. The need to es-

timate body weight is a potential barrier to proper antimicrobial dosing, because access to a scale is very limited in field situations. While various methods for assessing weight are available, underestimation is common (252), which can lead to underdosing. This is a challenge that is difficult to address in the field, since increasing availability of scales is unrealistic. Veterinarians need to take the time and effort to attempt accurate weight estimation to try to optimize drug administration. Various calculations can be used to improve on completely empirical estimation, with varying accuracy (252, 253). Although the estimate can be inaccurate and contribute to mis-dosing, no better alternatives are available.

Compared to food-producing animals, PK studies in horses are limited. Limited objective information about dosing is available for many antimicrobials that are used in an extra-label manner, something that accounts for a large percentage of antimicrobial use in many areas. While often reasonable, empirical dosing regimens can pose risks of poor treatment efficacy and increased likelihood of adverse effects, particularly GI effects. There are specific concerns about the timing of antimicrobial administration in peri-operative prophylaxis. A study based on the medical records of 192 horses with septic arthritis/tenosynovitis revealed that only 6.3% of the horses received their peri-operative antimicrobials within 60 minutes prior to the first incision, and in 91% of cases, more than 2 half-lives (the standard duration time at which redosing is indicated during surgical prophylaxis) had passed prior to the end of surgery, with no intra-operative redosing (247). Thus, there would be expected to be minimal to no impact of antimicrobials on infection prevention. Similar concerns exist for peri-operative prophylaxis in colic surgery. A study of antimicrobial administration for colic surgery identified appropriate intra-operative redosing in only 1.8% of situations where it was indicated (254). Underdosing was also common, with 41% of horses that received gentamicin being underdosed. This occurred in a teaching facility where there is access to scales. Dosing errors are a particular concern in the field when estimation of weight is almost always required and where underestimation is common (252). While these studies involved single surgical facilities, there is little reason to think that similar issues are not present elsewhere. Further, these studies were all based at referral centers, and information about peri-operative practices associated with primary care equine medicine is lacking. More PK data, along with clinical efficacy studies, are needed to optimize antimicrobial dosing in horses.

FUTURE PERSPECTIVES

While the previous sections describe how antimicrobial treatment in animals can be optimized using the presently available knowledge and tools, this final section addresses future perspectives for improving antimicrobial use in the years to come. Both education and research efforts are needed to achieve this goal. As extensively emphasized by the recent European Food Safety Authority/EMA Joint Scientific Opinion (4), education for veterinarians and users of antimicrobials is a key area for optimization of antimicrobial use. Resources should be allocated to educate both antimicrobial prescribers and users. Veterinary and agricultural schools should provide students with up-to-date teaching on pharmacology and use of antimicrobial agents and on public and animal health consequences related to AMR and, especially, should expose them to the general principles of antimicrobial stewardship, infection control, and prevention, which probably have the biggest impact on reducing antimicrobial use and on preventing the spread of certain MDR clones such as methicillin-resistant *S. aureus* in livestock. Education regarding indications for antimicrobial use, dosing regimens, and potential adverse consequences is an important aspect of antimicrobial stewardship and requires continuing education courses specialized for each type of veterinary practice. While generic guidelines and various commentaries have been published, directed at different types of veterinary practices, antimicrobial stewardship efforts directed at lay personnel have been lacking, and sustained and comprehensive stewardship programs are largely lacking for veterinary equine clinics too. International and national veterinary organizations should ensure that these educational needs are met. They should also support and coordinate efforts for developing and implementing international and national guidelines, respectively. International species- and disease-specific practice guidelines are presently limited to selected conditions in small animals, and national guidelines are missing in most countries. International clinical treatment guidelines are essential to set the basis for the development and harmonization of national guidelines since the expertise and resources necessary for their development are not available in all countries. National guidelines complement international guidelines because they consider national patterns of antimicrobial use and AMR, drug availability in the market, specificities of national livestock production systems, and cultural and regulatory differences between countries. Guideline development alone does not ensure translation of expert recommendations into veterinary practice and should be followed by an adequate implementation plan using national and regional meetings with veterinarians and farmers.

A lack of scientific evidence and clinical data is in many instances the main limitation to making informed decisions. Accordingly, sustained research is required to fill knowledge gaps that hamper optimization of dosage regimens and development of evidence-based guidelines, including comparative analysis of the *in vivo* effects of different drugs, drug formulations, doses, administration forms, and treatment durations on AMR selection and clinical efficacy. In the diagnostic field, research is needed for development of evidence-based diagnostic protocols, as are cheap and reliable point-of-care tests that facilitate discrimination between viral and bacterial disease or that rapidly detect bacterial resistance to first-line antimicrobials. Finally, research on new and innovative pharmaceuticals, including vaccines, new antimicrobials, and alternative treatments, is urgently needed to prevent the occurrence of key bacterial diseases that impact antimicrobial consumption, to replace antimicrobials that are being restricted or phased out because of public health concerns related to their use in livestock, and to meet the demand for effective systemic antimicrobials that can be used to manage MDR infections in companion animals, avoiding the use of high-priority critically important drugs in human medicine. Ideally, new veterinary antimicrobials should not be chemically related to medically important antimicrobials for human use and should have a minimal ecological impact on the animal commensal microbiota as well as on the environmental microbiota. Drugs with these ideal features have been termed "green antimicrobials" (50). This new generation of antimicrobials should possess appropriate PK/PD selectivity, i.e., they should be pathogen-targeted and have narrow spectrums of activity and be restricted to the infection site or at least excluded from the large intestine to minimize impact on the gut microbiota of the treated animal and on the environmental microbiota. For orally administered drugs, this goal can be achieved by substances with high bioavailability and minimal affinity for feed constituents such as cellulose. For nonoral routes of administration, the ideal drug should be water soluble to concentrate in the extracellular space and have low plasma clearance to allow a long half-life and single-dose administration. Preferential elimination via the kidneys would be highly desirable because this route of elimination is not associated with unwanted direct exposure of the gut commensal microbiota. Accordingly, screening funnels for discovery of veterinary-specific green antimicrobials should be targeted to drugs with no affinity for the biliary and GI tract efflux pumps.

A future cutting-edge therapeutic option for food-producing animals is so-called precision medicine; its goal is to treat animals selectively but at the herd level, and for a given animal, to tailor the most appropriate dosage regimen (right time of administration, right dose, right duration of treatment). In the framework of metaphylaxis, precision medicine is the opposite of what is currently mass medication, which is imprecision medicine. Metaphylaxis (or control) should be biologically understood as being only an early treatment during the incubation of the disease, i.e., before the full clinical expression of symptoms while the pathogen load to eradicate is still relatively low. The current difficulty is how to selectively initiate such early metaphylactic treatment; the main bottleneck is the lack of validated diagnostic signal(s) to ensure real-time individual monitoring of all animals at the herd level and allow early detection of disease with an appropriate specificity and sensitivity. Radio frequency identification feeding systems (255), monitoring of drinking behavior (256), and other precision livestock farming technologies for early detection of disease (257) are under investigation and hopefully will soon be translated into precision livestock medicine.

Acknowledgments. Luca Guardabassi and Pierre-Louis Toutain contributed to this chapter on behalf of the European Society of Clinical Microbiology and Infectious Diseases Study Group for Veterinary Microbiology (ESGVM), which endorsed the content of the chapter.

Citation. Guardabassi L, Apley M, Olsen JE, Toutain P-L, and Weese JS. 2018. Optimization of antimicrobial treatment to minimize resistance selection. Microbiol Spectrum 6(3): ARBA-0018-2017.

References

1. **World Health Organization (WHO).** 2015. AMR: draft global action plan on antimicrobial resistance. http://www.who.int/antimicrobial-resistance/global-action-plan/en/.
2. **Review on Antimicrobial Resistance.** 2015. Antimicrobials in agriculture and the environment: reducing unnecessary use and waste. https://amr-review.org/sites/default/files/Antimicrobials%20in%20agriculture%20and%20the%20environment%20-%20Reducing%20unnecessary%20use%20and%20waste.pdf.
3. **European Commission.** 2017. EU One Health action plan against AMR. https://ec.europa.eu/health/amr/.
4. **European Medicines Agency (EMA) Committee for Medicinal Products for Veterinary Use (CVMP) and EFSA Panel on Biological Hazards (BIOHAZ).** 2017. EMA and EFSA Joint Scientific Opinion on measures to reduce the need to use antimicrobial agents in animal husbandry in the European Union, and the resulting impacts on food safety (RONAFA). *EFSA J* 15:4666.
5. **European Commission.** 2015. Commission notice. Guidelines for the prudent use of antimicrobials in veterinary medicine. Commission notice 2015/C 299/04. http://ec.europa.eu/health//sites/health/files/antimicrobial_resistance/docs/2015_prudent_use_guidelines_en.pdf.
6. **The White House.** 2015. National action plan for combating antibiotic-resistant bacteria. https://obamawhitehouse.archives.gov/sites/default/files/docs/national_action_plan_for_combating_antibotic-resistant_bacteria.pdf.
7. **Teale CJ, Moulin G.** 2012. Prudent use guidelines: a review of existing veterinary guidelines. *Rev Sci Tech* 31:343–354.
8. **Weese JS, Giguère S, Guardabassi L, Morley PS, Papich M, Ricciuto DR, Sykes JE.** 2015. ACVIM consensus statement on therapeutic antimicrobial use in animls and antimicrobial resistance. *J Vet Intern Med* 29:487–498.
9. **Chantziaras I, Boyen F, Callens B, Dewulf J.** 2014. Correlation between veterinary antimicrobial use and antimicrobial resistance in food-producing animals: a report on seven countries. *J Antimicrob Chemother* 69:827–834.
10. **Dorado-García A, Dohmen W, Bos ME, Verstappen KM, Houben M, Wagenaar JA, Heederik DJ.** 2015. Dose-response relationship between antimicrobial drugs and livestock-associated MRSA in pig farming. *Emerg Infect Dis* 21:950–959.
11. **Catry B, Dewulf J, Maes D, Pardon B, Callens B, Vanrobaeys M, Opsomer G, de Kruif A, Haesebrouck F.** 2016. Effect of antimicrobial consumption and production type on antibacterial resistance in the bovine respiratory and digestive tract. *PLoS One* 11:e0146488.
12. **Cavaco LM, Abatih E, Aarestrup FM, Guardabassi L.** 2008. Selection and persistence of CTX-M-producing *Escherichia coli* in the intestinal flora of pigs treated with amoxicillin, ceftiofur, or cefquinome. *Antimicrob Agents Chemother* 52:3612–3616.
13. **Zhang L, Huang Y, Zhou Y, Buckley T, Wang HH.** 2013. Antibiotic administration routes significantly influence the levels of antibiotic resistance in gut microbiota. *Antimicrob Agents Chemother* 57:3659–3666.
14. **Bibbal D, Dupouy V, Ferré JP, Toutain PL, Fayet O, Prère MF, Bousquet-Mélou A.** 2007. Impact of three ampicillin dosage regimens on selection of ampicillin resistance in *Enterobacteriaceae* and excretion of blaTEM genes in swine feces. *Appl Environ Microbiol* 73:4785–4790.
15. **Gibbons JF, Boland F, Egan J, Fanning S, Markey BK, Leonard FC.** 2016. Antimicrobial resistance of faecal *Escherichia coli* isolates from pig farms with different durations of in-feed antimicrobial use. *Zoonoses Public Health* 63:241–250.
16. **Garcia-Migura L, Hendriksen RS, Fraile L, Aarestrup FM.** 2014. Antimicrobial resistance of zoonotic and commensal bacteria in Europe: the missing link between consumption and resistance in veterinary medicine. *Vet Microbiol* 170:1–9.
17. **Erol E, Locke SJ, Donahoe JK, Mackin MA, Carter CN.** 2012. Beta-hemolytic *Streptococcus* spp. from horses: a

retrospective study (2000–2010). *J Vet Diagn Invest* **24**: 142–147.

18. **Petersen A, Christensen JP, Kuhnert P, Bisgaard M, Olsen JE.** 2006. Vertical transmission of a fluoroquinolone-resistant *Escherichia coli* within an integrated broiler operation. *Vet Microbiol* **116**:120–128.

19. **Bednorz C, Oelgeschläger K, Kinnemann B, Hartmann S, Neumann K, Pieper R, Bethe A, Semmler T, Tedin K, Schierack P, Wieler LH, Guenther S.** 2013. The broader context of antibiotic resistance: zinc feed supplementation of piglets increases the proportion of multi-resistant *Escherichia coli in vivo*. *Int J Med Microbiol* **303**: 396–403.

20. **Food and Drug Administration.** 2015. Department of Human Health and Services. Veterinary Feed Directive. *Fed Regist* **80**:31708–31735. ••• https://www.gpo.gov/fdsys/pkg/FR-2015-06-03/pdf/2015-13393.pdf.

21. **Dorado-García A, Mevius DJ, Jacobs JJ, Van Geijlswijk IM, Mouton JW, Wagenaar JA, Heederik DJ.** 2016. Quantitative assessment of antimicrobial resistance in livestock during the course of a nationwide antimicrobial use reduction in the Netherlands. *J Antimicrob Chemother* **71**:3607–3619.

22. **Jensen VF, de Knegt LV, Andersen VD, Wingstrand A.** 2014. Temporal relationship between decrease in antimicrobial prescription for Danish pigs and the "Yellow Card" legal intervention directed at reduction of antimicrobial use. *Prev Vet Med* **117**:554–564.

23. **National Food Institute, Statens Serum Institut.** 2012. DANMAP 2011. Use of antimicrobial agents and occurrence of antimicrobial resistance in bacteria from food animals, food and humans in Denmark. https://danmap.org/~/media/Projekt%20sites/Danmap/DANMAP%20reports/Danmap_2011.ashx.

24. **National Food Institute, Statens Serum Institut.** 2016. DANMAP 2015. Use of antimicrobial agents and occurrence of antimicrobial resistance in bacteria from food animals, food and humans in Denmark. https://danmap.org/~/media/Projekt%20sites/Danmap/DANMAP%20%202015/DANMAP%202015.ashx.

25. **Aarestrup FM, Jensen VF, Emborg HD, Jacobsen E, Wegener HC.** 2010. Changes in the use of antimicrobials and the effects on productivity of swine farms in Denmark. *Am J Vet Res* **71**:726–733.

26. **Emborg H, Ersbøll AK, Heuer OE, Wegener HC.** 2001. The effect of discontinuing the use of antimicrobial growth promoters on the productivity in the Danish broiler production. *Prev Vet Med* **50**:53–70.

27. **EU Commission.** 2003. Regulation (EC) No 1831/2003 of the European Parliament and of the Council of 22 September 2003 on additives for use in animal nutrition. http://eur-lex.europa.eu/legal-content/EN/TXT/?uri=CELEX%3A32003R1831.

28. **Food and Drug Administration Center for Veterinary Medicine.** 2017. FDA announces implementation of GFI#213, outlines continuing efforts to address antimicrobial resistance. CVM update 3 January 2017. Accessed 28 March 2017. https://www.fda.gov/Animal Veterinary/NewsEvents/CVMUpdates/ucm535154.htm.

29. **Government of Canada.** 2014. Notice to stakeholders: collaborative efforts to promote the judicious use of medically-important antimicrobial drugs in food animal production. http://www.hc-sc.gc.ca/dhp-mps/vet/antimicrob/amr-notice-ram-avis-20140410-eng.php.

30. **Center for Disease Dynamics, Economics & Policy (CDDEP).** 2015. State of the World's Antibiotics, 2015. CDDEP, Washington, DC. http://cddep.org/publications/state_worlds_antibiotics_2015#sthash.u0R3NX7U.dpbs.

31. **World Health Organization (WHO).** 2000. WHO global principles for the containment of antimicrobial resistance in animals intended for food. *In* Report of a WHO consultation with the participation of the Food and Agriculture of the United Nations and the Office International des Epizooties, 5–9 June, Geneva, Switzerland. WHO/CDS/CSR/APH/2000.4. http://apps.who.int/iris/bitstream/10665/68931/1/WHO_CDS_CSR_APH_2000.4.pdfE/.

32. **European Medicines Agency (EMA).** 2016. Question and answer on the CVMP guideline on the SPC for antimicrobial products (EMEA/CVMP/SAGAM/383441/2005). EMA/CVMP/414812/2011-Rev.2. Veterinary Medicines Division. http://www.ema.europa.eu/docs/en_GB/document_library/Other/2011/07/WC500109155.pdf.

33. **Ferran AA, Toutain PL, Bousquet-Mélou A.** 2011. Impact of early versus later fluoroquinolone treatment on the clinical; microbiological and resistance outcomes in a mouse-lung model of *Pasteurella multocida* infection. *Vet Microbiol* **148**:292–297.

34. **Vasseur MV, Laurentie M, Rolland JG, Perrin-Guyomard A, Henri J, Ferran AA, Toutain PL, Bousquet-Mélou A.** 2014. Low or high doses of cefquinome targeting low or high bacterial inocula cure *Klebsiella pneumoniae* lung infections but differentially impact the levels of antibiotic resistance in fecal flora. *Antimicrob Agents Chemother* **58**:1744–1748.

35. **Lhermie G, Ferran AA, Assié S, Cassard H, El Garch F, Schneider M, Woerhlé F, Pacalin D, Delverdier M, Bousquet-Mélou A, Meyer G.** 2016. Impact of timing and dosage of a fluoroquinolone treatment on the microbiological, pathological, and clinical outcomes of calves challenged with *Mannheimia haemolytica*. *Front Microbiol* **7**:237.

36. **D'Agata EM, Dupont-Rouzeyrol M, Magal P, Olivier D, Ruan S.** 2008. The impact of different antibiotic regimens on the emergence of antimicrobial-resistant bacteria. *PLoS One* **3**:e4036.

37. **Herrero-Fresno A, Larsen I, Olsen JE.** 2015. Genetic relatedness of commensal *Escherichia coli* from nursery pigs in intensive pig production in Denmark and molecular characterization of genetically different strains. *J Appl Microbiol* **119**:342–353.

38. **Postma M, Vanderhaeghen W, Sarrazin S, Maes D, Dewulf J.** 2017. Reducing antimicrobial usage in pig production without jeopardizing production parameters. *Zoonoses Public Health* **64**:63–74.

39. **Rojo-Gimeno C, Postma M, Dewulf J, Hogeveen H, Lauwers L, Wauters E.** 2016. Farm-economic analysis of reducing antimicrobial use whilst adopting improved

management strategies on farrow-to-finish pigfarms. *Prev Vet Med* **129**:74–87.

40. Bak H, Rathkjen PH. 2009. Reduced use of antimicrobials after vaccination of pigs against porcine proliferative enteropathy in a Danish SPF herd. *Acta Vet Scand* **51**:1.

41. Cheng G, Hao H, Xie S, Wang X, Dai M, Huang L, Yuan Z. 2014. Antibiotic alternatives: the substitution of antibiotics in animal husbandry? *Front Microbiol* **5**:217.

42. De Briyne N, Atkinson J, Pokludová L, Borriello SP, Price S. 2013. Factors influencing antibiotic prescribing habits and use of sensitivity testing amongst veterinarians in Europe. *Vet Rec* **173**:475.

43. Guardabassi L, Damborg P, Stamm I, Kopp PA, Broens EM, Toutain PL, ESCMID Study Group for Veterinary Microbiology. 2017. Diagnostic microbiology in veterinary dermatology: present and future. *Vet Dermatol* **28**: 146-e30.

44. World Health Organization (WHO). 2016. *Critically Important Antimicrobials for Human Medicine*, 5th rev. http://www.who.int/foodsafety/publications/antimicrobials-fifth/en/.

45. World Organization for Animal Health (OIE). 2007. OIE list of antimicrobials of veterinary importance. http://www.oie.int/doc/ged/D9840.PDF.

46. European Food Safety Authority (EFSA). 2016. The European Union summary report on antimicrobial resistance in zoonotic and indicator bacteria from humans, animals and food in 2014. *EFSA J* **14**:4380. https://www.efsa.europa.eu/en/efsajournal/pub/4380

47. Tam VH, Louie A, Deziel MR, Liu W, Drusano GL. 2007. The relationship between quinolone exposures and resistance amplification is characterized by an inverted U: a new paradigm for optimizing pharmacodynamics to counterselect resistance. *Antimicrob Agents Chemother* **51**:744–747.

48. Firsov AA, Strukova EN, Shlykova DS, Portnoy YA, Kozyreva VK, Edelstein MV, Dovzhenko SA, Kobrin MB, Zinner SH. 2013. Bacterial resistance studies using *in vitro* dynamic models: the predictive power of the mutant prevention and minimum inhibitory antibiotic concentrations. *Antimicrob Agents Chemother* **57**: 4956–4962.

49. Blondeau JM, Borsos S, Blondeau LD, Blondeau BJ, Hesje CE. 2012. Comparative minimum inhibitory and mutant prevention drug concentrations of enrofloxacin, ceftiofur, florfenicol, tilmicosin and tulathromycin against bovine clinical isolates of *Mannheimia haemolytica*. *Vet Microbiol* **160**:85–90.

50. Toutain PL, Ferran AA, Bousquet-Melou A, Pelligand L, Lees P. 2016. Veterinary medicine needs new and innovative green antimicrobial drugs. *Front Microbiol* **7**:1196.

51. Pollet RA, Glatz CE, Dyer DC, Barnes HJ. 1983. Pharmacokinetics of chlortetracycline potentiation with citric acid in the chicken. *Am J Vet Res* **44**:1718–1721.

52. Pijpers A, Schoevers EJ, van Gogh H, van Leengoed LA, Visser IJ, van Miert AS, Verheijden JH. 1991. The influ-

ence of disease on feed and water consumption and on pharmacokinetics of orally administered oxytetracycline in pigs. *J Anim Sci* **69**:2947–2954.

53. Nielsen P, Gyrd-Hansen N. 1996. Bioavailability of oxytetracycline, tetracycline and chlortetracycline after oral administration to fed and fasted pigs. *J Vet Pharmacol Ther* **19**:305–311.

54. Lindecrona RH, Friis C, Nielsen JP. 2000. Pharmacokinetics and penetration of danofloxacin into the gastrointestinal tract in healthy and in *Salmonella typhimurium* infected pigs. *Res Vet Sci* **68**:211–216.

55. Nguyen TT, Chachaty E, Huy C, Cambier C, de Gunzburg J, Mentré F, Andremont A. 2012. Correlation between fecal concentrations of ciprofloxacin and fecal counts of resistant *Enterobacteriaceae* in piglets treated with ciprofloxacin: toward new means to control the spread of resistance? *Antimicrob Agents Chemother* **56**:4973–4975.

56. Vasseur M, Ferran A, Bousquet-Mélou A, Toutain PL. 2012. Impact of early versus later beta-lactam treatments on clinical and microbiological outcomes in an original mouse model of airborne *Pasteurella multocida* lung infection, p 124. *In* EAVPT (ed), 12th International Congress of the European Association for Veterinary Pharmacology and Toxicology, Noordwijkerhout, The Netherlands.

57. Toutain PL, del Castillo JRE, Bousquet-Mélou A. 2002. The pharmacokinetic-pharmacodynamic approach to a rational dosage regimen for antibiotics. *Res Vet Sci* **73**: 105–114.

58. Toutain PL, Lees P. 2004. Integration and modelling of pharmacokinetic and pharmacodynamic data to optimize dosage regimens in veterinary medicine. *J Vet Pharmacol Ther* **27**:467–477.

59. Ismail M, El-Kattan YA. 2007. Comparative pharmacokinetics of marbofloxacin in healthy and *Mannheimia haemolytica* infected calves. *Res Vet Sci* **82**:398–404.

60. Mzyk DA, Baynes RE, Messenger KM, Martinez M, Smith GW. 2017. Pharmacokinetics and distribution in interstitial and pulmonary epithelial lining fluid of danofloxacin in ruminant and preruminant calves. *J Vet Pharmacol Ther* **40**:179–191.

61. Ensink JM, Klein WR, Mevius DJ, Klarenbeek A, Vulto AG. 1992. Bioavailability of oral penicillins in the horse: a comparison of pivampicillin and amoxicillin. *J Vet Pharmacol Ther* **15**:221–230.

62. Baggot JD, Love DN, Stewart J, Raus J. 1988. Bioavailability and disposition kinetics of amoxicillin in neonatal foals. *Equine Vet J* **20**:125–127.

63. Agersø H, Friis C. 1998. Bioavailability of amoxycillin in pigs. *J Vet Pharmacol Ther* **21**:41–46.

64. Küng K, Wanner M. 1994. Bioavailability of different forms of amoxycillin administered orally to dogs. *Vet Rec* **135**:552–554.

65. Sánchez Navarro A. 2005. New formulations of amoxicillin/clavulanic acid: a pharmacokinetic and pharmacodynamic review. *Clin Pharmacokinet* **44**:1097–1115.

66. Ambrose PG, Grasela DM. 2000. The use of Monte Carlo simulation to examine pharmacodynamic variance

of drugs: fluoroquinolone pharmacodynamics against *Streptococcus pneumoniae*. *Diagn Microbiol Infect Dis* **38**:151–157.

67. Drusano GL, Preston SL, Hardalo C, Hare R, Banfield C, Andes D, Vesga O, Craig WA. 2001. Use of preclinical data for selection of a phase II/III dose for evernimicin and identification of a preclinical MIC breakpoint. *Antimicrob Agents Chemother* **45**:13–22.

68. Dudley MN, Ambrose PG. 2000. See comment in PubMed Commons below Pharmacodynamics in the study of drug resistance and establishing *in vitro* susceptibility breakpoints: ready for prime time. *Curr Opin Microbiol* **3**:515–21.

69. Toutain PL, Potter T, Pelligand L, Lacroix M, Illambas J, Lees P. 2017. Standard PK/PD concepts can be applied to determine a dosage regimen for a macrolide: the case of tulathromycin in the calf. *J Vet Pharmacol Ther* **40**:16–27.

70. Guillemot D, Carbon C, Vauzelle-Kervroëdan F, Balkau B, Maison P, Bouvenot G, Eschwège E. 1998. Inappropriateness and variability of antibiotic prescription among French office-based physicians. *J Clin Epidemiol* **51**:61–68.

71. Randall LP, Cooles SW, Coldham NC, Stapleton KS, Piddock LJ, Woodward MJ. 2006. Modification of enrofloxacin treatment regimens for poultry experimentally infected with *Salmonella enterica* serovar Typhimurium DT104 to minimize selection of resistance. *Antimicrob Agents Chemother* **50**:4030–4037.

72. Ungemach FR, Müller-Bahrdt D, Abraham G. 2006. Guidelines for prudent use of antimicrobials and their implications on antibiotic usage in veterinary medicine. *Int J Med Microbiol* **296**(Suppl 41):33–38.

73. Anonymous. 2015. Pig Veterinary Society: prescribing principles for antimicrobials. http://www.pigvetsoc.org.uk/files/document/92/1401%20PIG%20VETERINARY%20SOCIETY-PP%20final.pdf.

74. Anonymous. 2016. Guidelines for the use of antimicrobials in the South African pig industry. http://www.sava.co.za/2017/05/26/antibiotic-guidelines-pig-industry/.

75. Burch DGS, Duran OC, Aarestrup FM. 2009. Guidelines for antimicrobial use in swine, p 102–125. *In* Guardabassi L, Jensen LB, Kruse H (ed), *Guide to Antimicrobial Use in Animals*. Blackwell Publishing, Oxford, United Kingdom.

76. Anonymous. 2013. Guidelines on Good Antibiotic Practice: As Little As Possible, but As Often As Possible. Videncenter for Svineproduktion, Landbrug og Fødevarer. http://svineproduktion.dk/viden/i-stalden/management/manualer/antibiotika.

77. Jensen VF, Emborg HD, Aarestrup FM. 2012. Indications and patterns of therapeutic use of antimicrobial agents in the Danish pig production from 2002 to 2008. *J Vet Pharmacol Ther* **35**:33–46.

78. Callens B, Persoons D, Maes D, Laanen M, Postma M, Boyen F, Haesebrouck F, Butaye P, Catry B, Dewulf J. 2012. Prophylactic and metaphylactic antimicrobial use in Belgian fattening pig herds. *Prev Vet Med* **106**:53–62.

79. van Rennings L, von Münchhausen C, Ottilie H, Hartmann M, Merle R, Honscha W, Käsbohrer A, Kreienbrock L. 2015. Cross-sectional study on antibiotic usage in pigs in Germany. *PLoS One* **10**:e0119114.

80. Heo JM, Opapeju FO, Pluske JR, Kim JC, Hampson DJ, Nyachoti CM. 2013. Gastrointestinal health and function in weaned pigs: a review of feeding strategies to control post-weaning diarrhoea without using in-feed antimicrobial compounds. *J Anim Physiol Anim Nutr (Berl)* **97**:207–237.

81. Melkebeek V, Goddeeris BM, Cox E. 2013. ETEC vaccination in pigs. *Vet Immunol Immunopathol* **152**:37–42.

82. Taylor D. 1999. Clostridial infections, p 395–412. *In* Straw BE, D'Allaire S, Mengeling WL, Taylor D (ed), *Diseases of Swine*. Iowa State University Press, Ames, IA.

83. Riising HJ, Murmans M, Witvliet M. 2005. Protection against neonatal *Escherichia coli* diarrhoea in pigs by vaccination of sows with a new vaccine that contains purified enterotoxic *E. coli* virulence factors F4ac, F4ab, F5 and F6 fimbrial antigens and heat-labile *E. coli* enterotoxin (LT) toxoid. *J Vet Med B Infect Dis Vet Public Health* **52**:296–300.

84. Suiryanrayna MVAN, Ramana JV. 2015. A review of the effects of dietary organic acids fed to swine. *J Anim Sci Biotechnol* **6**:45.

85. Gantois I, Ducatelle R, Pasmans F, Haesebrouck F, Hautefort I, Thompson A, Hinton JC, Van Immerseel F. 2006. Butyrate specifically down-regulates *Salmonella* pathogenicity island 1 gene expression. *Appl Environ Microbiol* **72**:946–949.

86. Hu Q, Zhao Z, Fang S, Zhang Y, Feng J. 2017. Phytosterols improve immunity and exert anti-inflammatory activiey in weaned piglets. *J Sci Food Agric* **97**:4103–4109.

87. Den Hartog LA, Smits CHM, Henridks WH. 2016. Feed additive strategies for replacement of antimicrobial growth promoters and a responsible use of antimicrobials. Feedipedia www.feedipedia.org No 34, October 2016.

88. Thacker PA. 2013. Alternatives to antibiotics as growth promoters for use in swine production: a review. *J Anim Sci Biotechnol* **4**:35.

89. Jäger HC, McKinley TJ, Wood JL, Pearce GP, Williamson S, Strugnell B, Done S, Habernoll H, Palzer A, Tucker AW. 2012. Factors associated with pleurisy in pigs: a case-control analysis of slaughter pig data for England and Wales. *PLoS One* **7**:e29655.

90. Fablet C, Dorenlor V, Eono F, Eveno E, Jolly JP, Portier F, Bidan F, Madec F, Rose N. 2012. Noninfectious factors associated with pneumonia and pleuritis in slaughtered pigs from 143 farrow-to-finish pig farms. *Prev Vet Med* **104**:271–280.

91. Maes D, Segales J, Meyns T, Sibila M, Pieters M, Haesebrouck F. 2008. Control of *Mycoplasma hyopneumoniae* infections in pigs. *Vet Microbiol* **126**:297–309.

92. Stärk KD, Miserez R, Siegmann S, Ochs H, Infanger P, Schmidt J. 2007. A successful national control prog-

ramme for enzootic respiratory diseases in pigs in Switzerland. *Rev Sci Tech* 26:595–606.

93. Chae C. 2016. Porcine respiratory disease complex: interaction of vaccination and porcine circovirus type 2, porcine reproductive and respiratory syndrome virus, and *Mycoplasma hyopneumoniae*. *Vet J* 212:1–6.

94. Ramirez CR, Harding AL, Forteguerri EB, Aldridge BM, Lowe JF. 2015. Limited efficacy of antimicrobial metaphylaxis in finishing pigs: a randomized clinical trial. *Prev Vet Med* 121:176–178.

95. Bos ME, Taverne FJ, van Geijlswijk IM, Mouton JW, Mevius DJ, Heederik DJ, Netherlands Veterinary Medicines Authority (SDa). 2013. Consumption of antimicrobials in pigs, veal calves, and broilers in the Netherlands: quantitative results of nationwide collection of data in 2011. *PLoS One* 8:e77525.

96. Larsen I, Nielsen SS, Olsen JE, Nielsen JP. 2016. The efficacy of oxytetracycline treatment at batch, pen and individual level on *Lawsonia intracellularis* infection in nursery pigs in a randomised clinical trial. *Prev Vet Med* 124:25–33.

97. Græsbøll K, Damborg P, Mellerup A, Herrero-Fresno A, Larsen I, Holm A, Nielsen JP, Christiansen LE, Angen Ø, Ahmed S, Folkesson A, Olsen JE. 2017. Effect of tetracycline dose and treatment mode on selection of resistant coliform bacteria in nursery pigs. *Appl Environ Microbiol* 83:e00538–e17.

98. Weber N, Nielsen JP, Jakobsen AS, Pedersen LL, Hansen CF, Pedersen KS. 2015. Occurrence of diarrhoea and intestinal pathogens in non-medicated nursery pigs. *Acta Vet Scand* 57:64.

99. Alali WQ, Scott HM, Harvey RB, Norby B, Lawhorn DB, Pillai SD. 2008. Longitudinal study of antimicrobial resistance among *Escherichia coli* isolates from integrated multisite cohorts of humans and swine. *Appl Environ Microbiol* 74:3672–3681.

100. Liu Z, Zhang Z, Yan H, Li J, Shi L. 2015. Isolation and molecular characterization of multidrug-resistant *Enterobacteriaceae* strains from pork and environmental samples in Xiamen, China. *J Food Prot* 78:78–88.

101. Mirajkar NS, Davies PR, Gebhart CJ. 2016. Antimicrobial susceptibility patterns of *Brachyspira* species isolated from swine herds in the United States. *J Clin Microbiol* 54:2109–2119.

102. Pringle M, Landén A, Unnerstad HE, Molander B, Bengtsson B. 2012. Antimicrobial susceptibility of porcine *Brachyspira hyodysenteriae* and *Brachyspira pilosicoli* isolated in Sweden between 1990 and 2010. *Acta Vet Scand* 54:54.

103. Kirchgässner C, Schmitt S, Borgström A, Wittenbrink MM. 2016. Antimicrobial susceptibility of *Brachyspira hyodysenteriae* in Switzerland. *Schweiz Arch Tierheilkd* 158:405–410.

104. Yeh JY, Lee JH, Yeh HR, Kim A, Lee JY, Hwang JM, Kang BK, Kim JM, Choi IS, Lee JB. 2011. Antimicrobial susceptibility testing of two *Lawsonia intracellularis* isolates associated with proliferative hemorrhagic enteropathy and porcine intestinal adenomatosis in South Korea. *Antimicrob Agents Chemother* 55:4451–4453.

105. Wattanaphansak S, Singer RS, Gebhart CJ. 2009. *In vitro* antimicrobial activity against 10 North American and European *Lawsonia intracellularis* isolates. *Vet Microbiol* 134:305–310.

106. Clinical and Laboratory Standards Institute (CLSI). 2013. Performance standards for antimicrobial disk and dilution susceptibility tests for bacteria isolated from animals. Approved standard VET01-A4. CLSI, Wayne, PA.

107. Vicca J, Stakenborg T, Maes D, Butaye P, Peeters J, de Kruif A, Haesebrouck F. 2004. *In vitro* susceptibilities of *Mycoplasma hyopneumoniae* field isolates. *Antimicrob Agents Chemother* 48:4470–4472.

108. Stakenborg T, Vicca J, Butaye P, Maes D, Minion FC, Peeters J, De Kruif A, Haesebrouck F. 2005. Characterization of *in vivo* acquired resistance of *Mycoplasma hyopneumoniae* to macrolides and lincosamides. *Microb Drug Resist* 11:290–294.

109. Opriessnig T, Giménez-Lirola LG, Halbur PG. 2011. Polymicrobial respiratory disease in pigs. *Anim Health Res Rev* 12:133–148.

110. Ruiz VL, Bersano JG, Carvalho AF, Catroxo MH, Chiebao DP, Gregori F, Miyashiro S, Nassar AF, Oliveira TM, Ogata RA, Scarcelli EP, Tonietti PO. 2016. Case-control study of pathogens involved in piglet diarrhea. *BMC Res Notes* 9:22.

111. Palzer A, Ritzmann M, Wolf G, Heinritzi K. 2008. Associations between pathogens in healthy pigs and pigs with pneumonia. *Vet Rec* 162:267–271.

112. Ståhl M, Kokotovic B, Hjulsager CK, Breum SO, Angen Ø. 2011. The use of quantitative PCR for identification and quantification of *Brachyspira pilosicoli*, *Lawsonia intracellularis* and *Escherichia coli* fimbrial types F4 and F18 in pig feces. *Vet Microbiol* 151:307–314.

113. Clasen J, Mellerup A, Olsen JE, Angen Ø, Folkesson A, Halasa T, Toft N, Birkegård AC. 2016. Determining the optimal number of individual samples to pool for quantification of average herd levels of antimicrobial resistance genes in Danish pig herds using high-throughput qPCR. *Vet Microbiol* 189:46–51.

114. Pedersen KS, Ståhl M, Guedes RM, Angen Ø, Nielsen JP, Jensen TK. 2012. Association between faecal load of *Lawsonia intracellularis* and pathological findings of proliferative enteropathy in pigs with diarrhoea. *BMC Vet Res* 8:198.

115. Pedersen KS, Stege H, Jensen TK, Guedes R, Ståhl M, Nielsen JP, Hjulsager C, Larsen LE, Angen Ø. 2013. Diagnostic performance of fecal quantitative real-time polymerase chain reaction for detection of *Lawsonia intracellularis*-associated proliferative enteropathy in nursery pigs. *J Vet Diagn Invest* 25:336–340.

116. Pedersen KS, Okholm E, Johansen M, Angen Ø, Jorsal SE, Nielsen JP, Bækbo P. 2015. Clinical utility and performance of sock sampling in weaner pig diarrhoea. *Prev Vet Med* 120:313–320.

117. Vangroenweghe F, Karriker L, Main R, Christianson E, Marsteller T, Hammen K, Bates J, Thomas P, Ellingson J, Harmon K, Abate S, Crawford K. 2015. Assessment of litter prevalence of *Mycoplasma hyopneumoniae* in preweaned piglets utilizing an antemortem tracheobron-

chial mucus collection technique and a real-time polymerase chain reaction assay. *J Vet Diagn Invest* 27: 606–610.

118. **Tobias TJ, Bouma A, Klinkenberg D, Daemen AJ, Stegeman JA, Wagenaar JA, Duim B.** 2012. Detection of *Actinobacillus pleuropneumoniae* in pigs by rcal-time quantitative PCR for the apxIVA gene. *Vet J* 193: 557–560.

119. **Scherrer S, Frei D, Wittenbrink MM.** 2016. A novel quantitative real-time polymerase chain reaction method for detecting toxigenic *Pasteurella multocida* in nasal swabs from swine. *Acta Vet Scand* 58:83.

120. **Zhang M, Xie Z, Xie L, Deng X, Xie Z, Luo S, Liu J, Pang Y, Khan MI.** 2015. Simultaneous detection of eight swine reproductive and respiratory pathogens using a novel GeXP analyser-based multiplex PCR assay. *J Virol Methods* 224:9–15.

121. **Pedersen KS, Johansen M, Angen O, Jorsal SE, Nielsen JP, Jensen TK, Guedes R, Ståhl M, Bækbo P.** 2014. Herd diagnosis of low pathogen diarrhoea in growing pigs: a pilot study. *Ir Vet J* 67:24.

122. **Munk P, Andersen VD, de Knegt L, Jensen MS, Knudsen BE, Lukjancenko O, Mordhorst H, Clasen J, Agersø Y, Folkesson A, Pamp SJ, Vigre H, Aarestrup FM.** 2017. A sampling and metagenomic sequencing-based methodology for monitoring antimicrobial resistance in swine herds. *J Antimicrob Chemother* 72:385–392.

123. **Pedersen KS, Kristensen CS, Nielsen JP.** 2012. Demonstration of non-specific colitis and increased crypt depth in colon of weaned pigs with diarrhea. *Vet Q* 32: 45–49.

124. **de Jong A, Thomas V, Simjee S, Moyaert H, El Garch F, Maher K, Morrissey I, Butty P, Klein U, Marion H, Rigaut D, Vallé M.** 2014. Antimicrobial susceptibility monitoring of respiratory tract pathogens isolated from diseased cattle and pigs across Europe: the VetPath study. *Vet Microbiol* 172:202–215.

125. **Dayao DA, Gibson JS, Blackall PJ, Turni C.** 2014. Antimicrobial resistance in bacteria associated with porcine respiratory disease in Australia. *Vet Microbiol* 171:232–235.

126. **Vanni M, Merenda M, Barigazzi G, Garbarino C, Luppi A, Tognetti R, Intorre L.** 2012. Antimicrobial resistance of *Actinobacillus pleuropneumoniae* isolated from swine. *Vet Microbiol* 156:172–177.

127. **Sweeney MT, Quesnell R, Tiwari R, Lemay M, Watts JL.** 2013. *In vitro* activity and rodent efficacy of clinafloxacin for bovine and swine respiratory disease. *Front Microbiol* 4:154.

128. **Lauritzen B, Lykkesfeldt J, Friis C.** 2003. Evaluation of a single dose versus a divided dose regimen of danofloxacin in treatment of *Actinobacillus pleuropneumoniae* infection in pigs. *Res Vet Sci* 74:271–277.

129. **European Medicines Agency (EMA).** 2016. Updated advice on the use of colistin products in animals within the European Union: development of resistance and possible impact on human and animal health EMA/231573/2016. http://www.ema.europa.eu/docs/en_GB/ document_library/Scientific_guideline/2016/05/W-C500207233.pdf.

130. **Kempf I, Jouy E, Chauvin C.** 2016. Colistin use and colistin resistance in bacteria from animals. *Int J Antimicrob Agents* 48:598–606.

131. **Moodley A, Nielsen SS, Guardabassi L.** 2011. Effects of tetracycline and zinc on selection of methicillin-resistant *Staphylococcus aureus* (MRSA) sequence type 398 in pigs. *Vet Microbiol* 152:420–423.

132. **Slifierz MJ, Friendship R, Weese JS.** 2015. Zinc oxide therapy increases prevalence and persistence of methicillin-resistant *Staphylococcus aureus* in pigs: a randomized controlled trial. *Zoonoses Public Health* 62:301–308.

133. **European Medicines Agency (EMA).** 2016. Committee for Medicinal Products for Veterinary Use (CVMP) Meeting of 06-08 December 2016 EMA/CVMP/794393/2016. http://www.ema.europa.eu/docs/en_GB/document_library/Press_release/2016/12/WC500217843.pdf.

134. **Madson DM, Magstadt DR, Arruda PH, Hoang H, Sun D, Bower LP, Bhandari M, Burrough ER, Gauger PC, Pillatzki AE, Stevenson GW, Wilberts BL, Brodie J, Harmon KM, Wang C, Main RG, Zhang J, Yoon KJ.** 2014. Pathogenesis of porcine epidemic diarrhea virus isolate (US/Iowa/18984/2013) in 3-week-old weaned pigs. *Vet Microbiol* 174:60–68.

135. **Ahmad A, Zachariasen C, Christiansen LE, Græsbøll K, Toft N, Matthews L, Nielsen SS, Olsen JE.** 2016. Modeling the growth dynamics of multiple *Escherichia coli* strains in the pig intestine following intramuscular ampicillin treatment. *BMC Microbiol* 16:205.

136. **Herrero-Fresno A, Zachariasen C, Nørholm N, Holm A, Christiansen LE, Olsen JE.** 2017. Effect of different oral oxytetracycline treatment regimes on selection of antimicrobial resistant coliforms in nursery pigs. *Vet Microbiol* 208:1–7.

137. **Burow E, Simoneit C, Tenhagen BA, Käsbohrer A.** 2014. Oral antimicrobials increase antimicrobial resistance in porcine *E. coli*: a systematic review. *Prev Vet Med* 113:364–375.

138. **Larsen I, Hjulsager CK, Holm A, Olsen JE, Nielsen SS, Nielsen JP.** 2016. A randomised clinical trial on the efficacy of oxytetracycline dose through water medication of nursery pigs on diarrhoea, faecal shedding of *Lawsonia intracellularis* and average daily weight gain. *Prev Vet Med* 123:52–59.

139. **Zolynas R, Cao J, Simmons R.** 2003. Evaluation of the efficacy and safety of Nuflor injectable solution (15mg/kg twice 48hours apart) in the treatment of swine respiratory disease (SRD). Proceedings of the AASV meeting, Orlando, FL, p 211–214.

140. **Vilalta C, Giboin H, Schneider M, El Garch F, Fraile L.** 2014. Pharmacokinetic/pharmacodynamic evaluation of marbofloxacin in the treatment of *Haemophilus parasuis* and *Actinobacillus pleuropneumoniae* infections in nursery and fattener pigs using Monte Carlo simulations. *J Vet Pharmacol Ther* 37:542–549.

141. **Constable PD, Pyörälä S, Smith GW.** 2008. Guidelines for antimicrobial use in cattle, p 143–160. *In* Guardabassi L, Jensen LB, Kruse H (ed), *Guide to*

Antimicrobial Use in Animals. Blackwell Publishing, Oxford, United Kingdom.

142. **American Association of Bovine Practitioners (AABP).** 2013. Prudent antimicrobial use guidelines. http://www.aabp.org/about/AABP_Guidelines.asp.

143. **Edwards TA.** 2010. Control methods for bovine respiratory disease for feedlot cattle. *Vet Clin North Am Food Anim Pract* 26:273–284.

144. **Wittum TE, Perino LJ.** 1995. Passive immune status at postpartum hour 24 and long-term health and performance of calves. *Am J Vet Res* 56:1149–1154.

145. **Theurer ME, Larson RL, White BJ.** 2015. Systematic review and meta-analysis of the effectiveness of commercially available vaccines against bovine herpesvirus, bovine viral diarrhea virus, bovine respiratory syncytial virus, and parainfluenza type 3 virus for mitigation of bovine respiratory disease complex in cattle. *J Am Vet Med Assoc* 246:126–142.

146. **Ellis JA.** 2017. How efficacious are vaccines against bovine respiratory syncytial virus in cattle? *Vet Microbiol* 206:59–68.

147. **Murray GM, O'Neill RG, More SJ, McElroy MC, Earley B, Cassidy JP.** 2016. Evolving views on bovine respiratory disease: an appraisal of selected control measures. Part 2. *Vet J* 217:78–82.

148. **Larson RL, Step DL.** 2012. Evidence-based effectiveness of vaccination against *Mannheimia haemolytica, Pasteurella multocida,* and *Histophilus somni* in feedlot cattle for mitigating the incidence and effect of bovine respiratory disease complex. *Vet Clin North Am Food Anim Pract* 28:97–106.

149. **Health BA.** 2017. *Zelnate 2016 1-4-2017.* https://academic.oup.com/jas/article/87/10/3418/4563405

150. **Keefe G.** 2012. Update on control of *Staphylococcus aureus* and *Streptococcus agalactiae* for management of mastitis. *Vet Clin North Am Food Anim Pract* 28:203–216.

151. **Hogan J, Smith KL.** 2012. Managing environmental mastitis. *Vet Clin North Am Food Anim Pract* 28:217–224.

152. **Gomes F, Henriques M.** 2016. Control of bovine mastitis: old and recent therapeutic approaches. *Curr Microbiol* 72:377–382.

153. **DeDonder KD, Apley MD.** 2015. A review of the expected effects of antimicrobials in bovine respiratory disease treatment and control using outcomes from published randomized clinical trials with negative controls. *Vet Clin North Am Food Anim Pract* 31:97–111, vi.

154. **Wileman BW, Thomson DU, Reinhardt CD, Renter DG.** 2009. Analysis of modern technologies commonly used in beef cattle production: conventional beef production versus nonconventional production using meta-analysis. *J Anim Sci* 87:3418–3426.

155. **González-Martín JV, Elvira L, Cerviño López M, Pérez Villalobos N, Calvo López-Guerrero E, Astiz S.** 2011. Reducing antibiotic use: selective metaphylaxis with florfenicol in commercial feedlots. *Livest Sci* 141:173–181.

156. **Scherpenzeel CG, den Uijl IE, van Schaik G, Riekerink RG, Hogeveen H, Lam TJ.** 2016. Effect of different scenarios for selective dry-cow therapy on udder health, antimicrobial usage, and economics. *J Dairy Sci* 99:3753–3764.

157. **Biggs A, Barrett D, Bradley A, Green M, Reyher K, Zadoks R.** 2016. Antibiotic dry cow therapy: where next? *Vet Rec* 178:93–94.

158. **Love WJ, Lehenbauer TW, Van Eenennaam AL, Drake CM, Kass PH, Farver TB, Aly SS.** 2016. Sensitivity and specificity of on-farm scoring systems and nasal culture to detect bovine respiratory disease complex in preweaned dairy calves. *J Vet Diagn Invest* 28:119–128.

159. **DeDonder K, Thomson DU, Loneragan GH, Noffsinger T, Taylor W, Apley MD.** 2010. Lung auscultation and rectal temperature as a predictor of lung lesions and bovine respiratory disease treatment outcome in feedyard cattle. *Bov Pract* 44:146–153.

160. **Rose-Dye TK, Burciaga-Robles LO, Krehbiel CR, Step DL, Fulton RW, Confer AW, Richards CJ.** 2011. Rumen temperature change monitored with remote rumen temperature boluses after challenges with bovine viral diarrhea virus and *Mannheimia haemolytica. J Anim Sci* 89:1193–1200.

161. **Ollivett TL, Buczinski S.** 2016. On-farm use of ultrasonography for bovine respiratory disease. *Vet Clin North Am Food Anim Pract* 32:19–35.

162. **White BJ, Goehl DR, Amrine DE, Booker C, Wildman B, Perrett T.** 2016. Bayesian evaluation of clinical diagnostic test characteristics of visual observations and remote monitoring to diagnose bovine respiratory disease in beef calves. *Prev Vet Med* 126:74–80.

163. **Wolfger B, Timsit E, White BJ, Orsel K.** 2015. A systematic review of bovine respiratory disease diagnosis focused on diagnostic confirmation, early detection, and prediction of unfavorable outcomes in feedlot cattle. *Vet Clin North Am Food Anim Pract* 31:351–365.

164. **DeDonder KD, Apley MD.** 2015. A literature review of antimicrobial resistance in pathogens associated with bovine respiratory disease. *Anim Health Res Rev* 16:125–134.

165. **Lubbers BV, Turnidge J.** 2015. Antimicrobial susceptibility testing for bovine respiratory disease: getting more from diagnostic results. *Vet J* 203:149–154.

166. **Wagner SA, Erskine RJ.** 2013. Antimicrobial drug use in mastitis, p 519–528. *In* Giguère S, Prescott JF, Dowling PM, (ed), *Antimicrobial Therapy in Veterinary Medicine.* Wiley Blackwell, Ames, IA.

167. **Roberson JR.** 2012. Treatment of clinical mastitis. *Vet Clin North Am Food Anim Pract* 28:271–288.

168. **Pinzón-Sánchez C, Ruegg PL.** 2011. Risk factors associated with short-term post-treatment outcomes of clinical mastitis. *J Dairy Sci* 94:3397–3410.

169. **Barkema HW, Schukken YH, Zadoks RN.** 2006. Invited review: the role of cow, pathogen, and treatment regimen in the therapeutic success of bovine *Staphylococcus aureus* mastitis. *J Dairy Sci* 89:1877–1895.

170. **Kayitsinga J, Schewe RL, Contreras GA, Erskine RJ.** 2016. Antimicrobial treatment of clinical mastitis in the eastern United States: the influence of dairy farmers'

mastitis management and treatment behavior and attitudes. *J Dairy Sci* 100(2):1388–1407.

171. Lago A, Godden SM, Bey R, Ruegg PL, Leslie K. 2011. The selective treatment of clinical mastitis based on on-farm culture results. I. Effects on antibiotic use, milk withholding time, and short-term clinical and bacteriological outcomes. *J Dairy Sci* 94:4441–4456.

172. Constable PD, Morin DE. 2003. Treatment of clinical mastitis. Using antimicrobial susceptibility profiles for treatment decisions. *Vet Clin North Am Food Anim Pract* 19:139–155.

173. Barlow J. 2011. Mastitis therapy and antimicrobial susceptibility: a multispecies review with a focus on antibiotic treatment of mastitis in dairy cattle. *J Mammary Gland Biol Neoplasia* 16:383–407.

174. Hoe FG, Ruegg PL. 2005. Relationship between antimicrobial susceptibility of clinical mastitis pathogens and treatment outcome in cows. *J Am Vet Med Assoc* 227:1461–1468.

175. Hendriksen RS, Karlsmose S, Aarestrup FM, Krogh K, Voss H. 2009. Fra gram positiv til negativ og fra kokker til stave – Sammendrag af resultaterne af årets ringtest for identifikation og resistensbestemmelse af mastitispatogener. *Dansk Vettidsskr* 92:28–33.

176. Koskinen MT, Holopainen J, Pyörälä S, Bredbacka P, Pitkälä A, Barkema HW, Bexiga R, Roberson J, Sølverød L, Piccinini R, Kelton D, Lehmusto H, Niskala S, Salmikivi L. 2009. Analytical specificity and sensitivity of a real-time polymerase chain reaction assay for identification of bovine mastitis pathogens. *J Dairy Sci* 92:952–959.

177. O'Connor AM, Yuan C, Cullen JN, Coetzee JF, da Silva N, Wang C. 2016. A mixed treatment meta-analysis of antibiotic treatment options for bovine respiratory disease: an update. *Prev Vet Med* 132:130–139.

178. Royster E, Wagner S. 2015. Treatment of mastitis in cattle. *Vet Clin North Am Food Anim Pract* 31:17–46.

179. Pyörälä S. 2009. Treatment of mastitis during lactation. *Ir Vet J* 62(Suppl 4):S40–S44.

180. Nordiske Meieriorganisasjoners Samarbeidsutvalg for Mjolkekvalitetsarbeid (NMSM). 2009. Nordic guidelines for mastitis therapy. http://www.sva.se/globalassets/redesign2011/pdf/antibiotika/antibiotikaresistens/nordic-guidelines-for-mastitis-therapy.pdf.

181. Apley MD. 2015. Treatment of calves with bovine respiratory disease: duration of therapy and post-treatment intervals. *Vet Clin North Am Food Anim Pract* 31:441–453, vii.

182. Vallé M, Schneider M, Galland D, Giboin H, Woehrlé F. 2012. Pharmacokinetic and pharmacodynamic testing of marbofloxacin administered as a single injection for the treatment of bovine respiratory disease. *J Vet Pharmacol Ther* 35:519–528.

183. Swinkels JM, Hilkens A, Zoche-Golob V, Krömker V, Buddiger M, Jansen J, Lam TJ. 2015. Social influences on the duration of antibiotic treatment of clinical mastitis in dairy cows. *J Dairy Sci* 98:2369–2380.

184. Swinkels JM, Cox P, Schukken YH, Lam TJ. 2013. Efficacy of extended cefquinome treatment of clinical

Staphylococcus aureus mastitis. *J Dairy Sci* 96:4983–4992.

185. Weese JS, Blondeau JM, Boothe D, Breitschwerdt EB, Guardabassi L, Hillier A, Lloyd DH, Papich MG, Rankin SC, Turnidge JD, Sykes JE. 2011. Antimicrobial use guidelines for treatment of urinary tract disease in dogs and cats: antimicrobial guidelines working group of the international society for companion animal infectious diseases. *Vet Med Int* 2011:263768.

186. Hillier A, Lloyd DH, Weese JS, Blondeau JM, Boothe D, Breitschwerdt E, Guardabassi L, Papich MG, Rankin S, Turnidge JD, Sykes JE. 2014. Guidelines for the diagnosis and antimicrobial therapy of canine superficial bacterial folliculitis (Antimicrobial Guidelines Working Group of the International Society for Companion Animal Infectious Diseases). *Vet Dermatol* 25:163–175, e42-3.

187. Lappin MR, Blondeau J, Boothe D, Breitschwerdt EB, Guardabassi L, Lloyd DH, Papich MG, Rankin SC, Sykes JE, Turnidge J, Weese JS. 2017. Antimicrobial use guidelines for treatment of respiratory tract disease in dogs and cats: Antimicrobial Guidelines Working Group of the International Society for Companion Animal Infectious Diseases. *J Vet Intern Med* 31:279–294.

188. Beco L, Guaguère E, Lorente Méndez C, Noli C, Nuttall T, Vroom M. 2013. Suggested guidelines for using systemic antimicrobials in bacterial skin infections (1): diagnosis based on clinical presentation, cytology and culture. *Vet Rec* 172:72–78.

189. Guardabassi L, Frank L, Houser G, Papich M. 2008. Guidelines for antimicrobial use in dogs and cats, p 183–206. *In* Guardabassi L, Jensen LB, Kruse H (ed), *Guide to Antimicrobial use in Animals.* Blackwell Publishing, Oxford, United Kingdom.

190. Danish Small Animal Veterinary Association (SvHKS). 2013. Antibiotic use guidelines for companion animal practice. https://www.ddd.dk/sektioner/hundkatsmaedyr/antibiotikavejledning/Documents/AntibioticGuidelines.pdf.

191. Swedish Veterinary Association. 2009. Guidelines for the clinical use of antibiotics in the treatment of dogs and cats. http://www.svf.se/Documents/S%C3%A4llskapet/Sm%C3%A5djurssektionen/Policy%20ab%20english%2010b.pdf.

192. Guardabassi L, Prescott JF. 2015. Antimicrobial stewardship in small animal veterinary practice: from theory to practice. *Vet Clin North Am Small Anim Pract* 45:361–376, vii.

193. Weese JS. 2006. Investigation of antimicrobial use and the impact of antimicrobial use guidelines in a small animal veterinary teaching hospital: 1995–2004. *J Am Vet Med Assoc* 228:553–558.

194. Hughes LA, Williams N, Clegg P, Callaby R, Nuttall T, Coyne K, Pinchbeck G, Dawson S. 2012. Cross-sectional survey of antimicrobial prescribing patterns in UK small animal veterinary practice. *Prev Vet Med* 104:309–316.

195. Stull JW, Weese JS. 2015. Infection control in veterinary small animal practice. *Vet Clin North Am Small Anim Pract* 45:xi–xii.

196. Rantala M, Hölsö K, Lillas A, Huovinen P, Kaartinen L. 2004. Survey of condition-based prescribing of anti-

microbial drugs for dogs at a veterinary teaching hospital. *Vet Rec* **155**:259–262.

197. Escher M, Vanni M, Intorre L, Caprioli A, Tognetti R, Scavia G. 2011. Use of antimicrobials in companion animal practice: a retrospective study in a veterinary teaching hospital in Italy. *J Antimicrob Chemother* **66**: 920–927.

198. Mueller RS, Bergvall K, Bensignor E, Bond R. 2012. A review of topical therapy for skin infections with bacteria and yeast. *Vet Dermatol* **23**:330–341.

199. Borio S, Colombo S, La Rosa G, De Lucia M, Damborg P, Guardabassi L. 2015. Effectiveness of a combined (4% chlorhexidine digluconate shampoo and solution) protocol in MRS and non-MRS canine superficial pyoderma: a randomized, blinded, antibiotic-controlled study. *Vet Dermatol* **26**:339–344, e72.

200. Summers JF, Hendricks A, Brodbelt DC. 2014. Prescribing practices of primary-care veterinary practitioners in dogs diagnosed with bacterial pyoderma. *BMC Vet Res* **10**:240.

201. Watson AD, Maddison JE. 2001. Systemic antibacterial drug use in dogs in Australia. *Aust Vet J* **79**:740–746.

202. Mateus AL, Brodbelt DC, Barber N, Stärk KD. 2014. Qualitative study of factors associated with antimicrobial usage in seven small animal veterinary practices in the UK. *Prev Vet Med* **117**:68–78.

203. Unterer S, Strohmeyer K, Kruse BD, Sauter-Louis C, Hartmann K. 2011. Treatment of aseptic dogs with hemorrhagic gastroenteritis with amoxicillin/clavulanic acid: a prospective blinded study. *J Vet Intern Med* **25**: 973–979.

204. Cai T, Nesi G, Mazzoli S, Meacci F, Lanzafame P, Caciagli P, Mereu L, Tateo S, Malossini G, Selli C, Bartoletti R. 2015. Asymptomatic bacteriuria treatment is associated with a higher prevalence of antibiotic resistant strains in women with urinary tract infections. *Clin Infect Dis* **61**:1655–1661.

205. Weese JS, Blondeau J, Boothe D, Guardabassi L, Gumley N, Lappin M, Papich M, Rankin S, Sykes J, Westropp J. 2016. Guidelines for management of urinary tract infections in dogs and cats. American College of Veterinary Internal Medicine Forum, Denver, CO, 10 June 2016.

206. Murphy CP, Reid-Smith RJ, Boerlin P, Weese JS, Prescott JF, Janecko N, McEwen SA. 2012. Out-patient antimicrobial drug use in dogs and cats for new disease events from community companion animal practices in Ontario. *Can Vet J* **53**:291–298.

207. Robinson NJ, Dean RS, Cobb M, Brennan ML. 2016. Factors influencing common diagnoses made during first-opinion small-animal consultations in the United Kingdom. *Prev Vet Med* **131**:87–94.

208. Trott DJ, Filippich LJ, Bensink JC, Downs MT, McKenzie SE, Townsend KM, Moss SM, Chin JJ. 2004. Canine model for investigating the impact of oral enrofloxacin on commensal coliforms and colonization with multidrug-resistant *Escherichia coli. J Med Microbiol* **53**:439–443.

209. Lawrence M, Kukanich K, Kukanich B, Heinrich E, Coetzee JF, Grauer G, Narayanan S. 2013. Effect of

cefovecin on the fecal flora of healthy dogs. *Vet J* **198**: 259–266.

210. Ding Y, Jia YY, Li F, Liu WX, Lu CT, Zhu YR, Yang J, Ding LK, Yang L, Wen AD. 2012. The effect of staggered administration of zinc sulfate on the pharmacokinetics of oral cephalexin. *Br J Clin Pharmacol* **73**:422–427.

211. Papich MG, Davis JL, Floerchinger AM. 2010. Pharmacokinetics, protein binding, and tissue distribution of orally administered cefpodoxime proxetil and cephalexin in dogs. *Am J Vet Res* **71**:1484–1491.

212. British Small Animal Veterinary Association (BSAVA). 2015. British Small Animal Veterinary Association (BSAVA) Guideline on Companion Animals. https://www.bsava.com/Resources/Veterinary-resources/Medicines-Guide.

213. Mouton JW, Ambrose PG, Canton R, Drusano GL, Harbarth S, MacGowan A, Theuretzbacher U, Turnidge J. 2011. Conserving antibiotics for the future: new ways to use old and new drugs from a pharmacokinetic and pharmacodynamic perspective. *Drug Resist Updat* **14**:107–117.

214. Stein GE, Schooley SL, Nicolau DP. 2008. Urinary bactericidal activity of single doses (250, 500, 750 and 1000 mg) of levofloxacin against fluoroquinolone-resistant strains of *Escherichia coli. Int J Antimicrob Agents* **32**:320–325.

215. Katz DE, Lindfield KC, Steenbergen JN, Benziger DP, Blackerby KJ, Knapp AG, Martone WJ. 2008. A pilot study of high-dose short duration daptomycin for the treatment of patients with complicated skin and skin structure infections caused by Gram-positive bacteria. *Int J Clin Pract* **62**:1455–1464.

216. Levison ME, Levison JH. 2009. Pharmacokinetics and pharmacodynamics of antibacterial agents. *Infect Dis Clin North Am* **23**:791–815, vii.

217. Toutain PL, Bousquet-Mélou A, Martinez M. 2007. AUC/MIC: a PK/PD index for antibiotics with a time dimension or simply a dimensionless scoring factor? *J Antimicrob Chemother* **60**:1185–1188.

218. Awji EG, Tassew DD, Lee JS, Lee SJ, Choi MJ, Reza MA, Rhee MH, Kim TH, Park SC. 2012. Comparative mutant prevention concentration and mechanism of resistance to veterinary fluoroquinolones in *Staphylococcus pseudintermedius. Vet Dermatol* **23**:376–380, e68-9.

219. Drlica K, Zhao X, Blondeau JM, Hesje C. 2006. Low correlation between MIC and mutant prevention concentration. *Antimicrob Agents Chemother* **50**:403–404.

220. Wetzstein HG. 2005. Comparative mutant prevention concentrations of pradofloxacin and other veterinary fluoroquinolones indicate differing potentials in preventing selection of resistance. *Antimicrob Agents Chemother* **49**:4166–4173.

221. Gugel J, Dos Santos Pereira A, Pignatari AC, Gales AC. 2006. beta-Lactam MICs correlate poorly with mutant prevention concentrations for clinical isolates of *Acinetobacter* spp. and *Pseudomonas aeruginosa. Antimicrob Agents Chemother* **50**:2276–2277.

222. Falagas ME, Bliziotis IA, Rafailidis PI. 2007. Do high doses of quinolones decrease the emergence of antibac-

terial resistance? A systematic review of data from comparative clinical trials. *J Infect* **55**:97–105.

223. Craig WA. 2007. Pharmacodynamics of antimicrobials: general concepts and applications, p 1–19. *In* Nightingale CH, Ambrose PG, Drusano GL, Murakawa K (ed), *Antimicrobials Pharmacodynamics in Theory and in Clinical Practices*, 2nd ed. Informa Healthcare, New York, NY.

224. Stevens DL, Bisno AL, Chambers HF, Dellinger EP, Goldstein EJ, Gorbach SL, Hirschmann JV, Kaplan SL, Montoya JG, Wade JC. 2014. Practice guidelines for the diagnosis and management of skin and soft tissue infections: 2014 update by the infectious diseases society of America. *Clin Infect Dis* **59**:147–159.

225. Gonzalez D, Delmore P, Bloom BT, Cotten CM, Poindexter BB, McGowan E, Shattuck K, Bradford KK, Smith PB, Cohen-Wolkowiez M, Morris M, Yin W, Benjamin DK Jr, Laughon MM. 2016. Clindamycin pharmacokinetics and safety in preterm and term infants. *Antimicrob Agents Chemother* **60**:2888–2894.

226. Batzias GC, Delis GA, Athanasiou LV. 2005. Clindamycin bioavailability and pharmacokinetics following oral administration of clindamycin hydrochloride capsules in dogs. *Vet J* **170**:339–345.

227. Clare S, Hartmann FA, Jooss M, Bachar E, Wong YY, Trepanier LA, Viviano KR. 2014. Short- and long-term cure rates of short-duration trimethoprim-sulfamethoxazole treatment in female dogs with uncomplicated bacterial cystitis. *J Vet Intern Med* **28**:818–826.

228. Gupta K, Hooton TM, Naber KG, Wullt B, Colgan R, Miller LG, Moran GJ, Nicolle LE, Raz R, Schaeffer AJ, Soper DE. 2011. Infectious Diseases Society of America.; European Society for Microbiology and Infectious Diseases. International clinical practice guidelines for the treatment of acute uncomplicated cystitis and pyelonephritis in women: a 2010 update by the Infectious Diseases Society of America and the European Society for Microbiology and Infectious Diseases. *Clin Infect Dis* **52**:e103-20.

229. Stevens DL, Bisno AL, Chambers HF, Dellinger EP, Goldstein EJ, Gorbach SL, Hirschmann JV, Kaplan SL, Montoya JG, Wade JC; Infectious Diseases Society of America. 2014. Practice guidelines for the diagnosis and management of skin and soft tissue infections: 2014 update by the Infectious Diseases Society of America. *Clin Infect Dis.* **59**:e10-52.

230. Bowen M. 2013. Antimicrobial stewardship: time for change. *Equine Vet J* **45**:127–129.

231. Haggett EF. 2014. Antimicrobial use in foals: do we need to change how we think? *Equine Vet J* **46**:137–138.

232. Weese JS. 2015. Antimicrobial use and antimicrobial resistance in horses. *Equine Vet J* **47**:747–749.

233. Weese SJ, Baptiste KE, Baverud V, Toutain PL. 2008. Guidelines for antimicrobial use in horses, p 161–182. *In* Guardabassi L, Jensen LB, Kruse H (ed), *Guide to Antimicrobial use in Animals*. Blackwell Publishing, Oxford, United Kingdom.

234. Hughes LA, Pinchbeck G, Callaby R, Dawson S, Clegg P, Williams N. 2013. Antimicrobial prescribing practice in UK equine veterinary practice. *Equine Vet J* **45**:141–147.

235. Schwechler J, van den Hoven R, Schoster A. 2016. Antimicrobial prescribing practices by Swiss, German and Austrian equine practitioners. *Vet Rec* **178**:216.

236. Maher MC, Schnabel LV, Cross JA, Papich MG, Divers TJ, Fortier LA. 2014. Plasma and synovial fluid concentration of doxycycline following low-dose, low-frequency administration, and resultant inhibition of matrix metalloproteinase-13 from interleukin-stimulated equine synoviocytes. *Equine Vet J* **46**:198–202.

237. Cribb NC, Bouré LP, Hanna WJ, Akens MK, Mattson SE, Monteith GJ, Weese JS. 2009. *In vitro* and *in vivo* evaluation of ferric-hyaluronate implants for delivery of amikacin sulfate to the tarsocrural joint of horses. *Vet Surg* **38**:498–505.

238. Harvey A, Kilcoyne I, Byrne BA, Nieto J. 2016. Effect of dose on intra-articular amikacin sulfate concentrations following intravenous regional limb perfusion in horses. *Vet Surg* **45**:1077–1082.

239. Newman JC, Prange T, Jennings S, Barlow BM, Davis JL. 2013. Pharmacokinetics of tobramycin following intravenous, intramuscular, and intra-articular administration in healthy horses. *J Vet Pharmacol Ther* **36**:532–541.

240. Weese JS, Sabino C. 2005. Scrutiny of antimicrobial use in racing horses with allergic small airway inflammatory disease. *Can Vet J* **46**:438–439.

241. Wohlfender FD, Barrelet FE, Doherr MG, Straub R, Meier HP. 2009. Diseases in neonatal foals. Part 1: the 30 day incidence of disease and the effect of prophylactic antimicrobial drug treatment during the first three days post partum. *Equine Vet J* **41**:179–185.

242. Arboleya S, Sánchez B, Milani C, Duranti S, Solís G, Fernández N, de los Reyes-Gavilán CG, Ventura M, Margolles A, Gueimonde M. 2015. Intestinal microbiota development in preterm neonates and effect of perinatal antibiotics. *J Pediatr* **166**:538–544.

243. Greenwood C, Morrow AL, Lagomarcino AJ, Altaye M, Taft DH, Yu Z, Newburg DS, Ward DV, Schibler KR. 2014. Early empiric antibiotic use in preterm infants is associated with lower bacterial diversity and higher relative abundance of *Enterobacter*. *J Pediatr* **165**:23–29.

244. Bert JM, Giannini D, Nace L. 2007. Antibiotic prophylaxis for arthroscopy of the knee: is it necessary? *Arthroscopy* **23**:4–6.

245. Wieck JA, Jackson JK, O'Brien TJ, Lurate RB, Russell JM, Dorchak JD. 1997. Efficacy of prophylactic antibiotics in arthroscopic surgery. *Orthopedics* **20**:133–134.

246. Weese JS, Cruz A. 2009. Retrospective study of perioperative antimicrobial use practices in horses undergoing elective arthroscopic surgery at a veterinary teaching hospital. *Can Vet J* **50**:185–188.

247. Schneider RK, Bramlage LR, Moore RM, Mecklenburg LM, Kohn CW, Gabel AA. 1992. A retrospective study of 192 horses affected with septic arthritis/tenosynovitis. *Equine Vet J* **24**:436–442.

248. Giguère S, Prescott JF. 1997. Clinical manifestations, diagnosis, treatment, and prevention of *Rhodococcus equi* infections in foals. *Vet Microbiol* **56**:313–334.

249. Giguère S, Cohen ND, Chaffin MK, Slovis NM, Hondalus MK, Hines SA, Prescott JF. 2011. Diagnosis, treatment, control, and prevention of infections caused by *Rhodococcus equi* in foals. *J Vet Intern Med* **25**: 1209–1220.

250. Ross SE, Duz M, Rendle DI. 2016. Antimicrobial selection and dosing in the treatment of wounds in the United Kingdom. *Equine Vet J* **48**:676–680.

251. Orsini JA, Snooks-Parsons C, Stine L, Haddock M, Ramberg CF, Benson CE, Nunamaker DM. 2005. Vancomycin for the treatment of methicillin-resistant staphylococcal and enterococcal infections in 15 horses. *Can J Vet Res* **69**:278–286.

252. Wagner EL, Tyler PJ. 2011. A comparison of weight estimation methods in adult horses. *J Equine Vet Sci* **31**: 706–710.

253. Carroll CL, Huntington PJ. 1988. Body condition scoring and weight estimation of horses. *Equine Vet J* **20**: 41–45.

254. Dallap Schaer BL, Linton JK, Aceto H. 2012. Antimicrobial use in horses undergoing colic surgery. *J Vet Intern Med* **26**:1449–1456.

255. Wolfger B, Manns B, Barkema HW, Schwartzkopf-Genswein KSG, Dorin C, Orsel K. 2015. Evaluating the cost implications of radio frequency identification feeding system for early detection of bovine respiratory disease in feedlot cattle. *Prev Vet Med* **118**:285–292.

256. Maselyne J, Adriaens I, Huybrechts T, De Ketelaere B, Millet S, Vangeyte J, Van Nuffel A, Saeys W. 2016. Measuring the drinking behaviour of individual pigs housed in group using radio frequency identification (RFID). *Animal* **10**:1557–1566.

257. Berckmans D. 2014. Precision livestock farming technologies for welfare management in intensive livestock systems. *Rev Sci Tech* **33**:189–196.

Antimicrobial Resistance in Bacteria from Livestock and Companion Animals
Edited by Frank Møller Aarestrup, Stefan Schwarz, Jianzhong Shen, and Lina Cavaco
© 2018 American Society for Microbiology, Washington, DC
doi:10.1128/microbiolspec.ARBA-0023-2017

Antimicrobial Stewardship in Veterinary Medicine

31

David H. Lloyd[1] and Stephen W. Page[2]

STEWARDSHIP AND THE USE OF ANTIMICROBIAL DRUGS

Stewardship implies a process of caring and responsible management (1), and as we face the progressive extension of multiresistance amongst bacteria in veterinary and human medicine, and in agriculture, there is a need to apply stewardship efficiently to the use of antimicrobial drugs so that we can preserve and extend their efficacy.

The relationship between the use of antimicrobial drugs and the development of resistant bacteria is now well established (2). The problem of antimicrobial resistance has been extensively reviewed by the O'Neill committee in the United Kingdom, which published its final report and recommendations in May 2016 (3). The committee examined the problem in all fields of antimicrobial use and on a worldwide basis. It concluded that human deaths as a consequence of antimicrobial resistance and inability to treat and control microbial infections were already of the order of 700,000 per year and estimated to rise to 10 million per annum (a figure that includes infections with resistant HIV and malaria, as well as tuberculosis and other bacterial infections), with a cumulative cost to global productivity of $100 trillion to the year 2050, unless appropriate actions are taken to deal with this problem.

An important driver of resistance in bacteria is the use of antimicrobials in agriculture and veterinary medicine. This is rising rapidly, driven by the unprecedented rate of increase in global demand for animal protein for human consumption, particularly in middle-income countries where extensive farming is being replaced by large-scale intensive production systems that routinely use large quantities of antimicrobials, often

with no veterinary intervention (4). The O'Neill committee concluded that the total amount of antimicrobial agents being used in agriculture was at least as great as that used in human medicine. Furthermore, using data from the U.S. Food and Drug Administration (FDA), it calculated that, in 2012 in the United States, 70% of the total weight of antibiotics defined by the FDA as medically important in humans was sold for use in animals (5). This situation may no longer apply, because new guidelines for antimicrobial use, including expanded need for veterinary prescription, were introduced by the Center for Veterinary Medicine in the United States on 1 January 2017.

It is recognized that resistant bacteria emerging in farm animals can pose a risk not only to the animals but also to farmers, veterinarians and their families, to workers in meat and milk production and sales, and to consumers; such bacteria include commensal organisms which may not necessarily cause significant disease among farm animals but can pose a significant risk through direct or indirect transfer to members of the public (6). Although antimicrobial use in companion animal practice is much lower than that in farm animals, the close relationship between treated animals, veterinary staff, owners and their families, and the public has increased the risk of transfer and infection among them (7). It is noteworthy that transfer occurs not only from animals to humans but also in the other direction, as evidenced by the occurrence of hospital-associated methicillin-resistant *Staphylococcus aureus* (MRSA) colonization and infection in dogs and cats (8–10). Furthermore, the greatly increased international movement of companion animals (11), including both pets and horses, and international trade and illegal transportation of foodstuffs (12), coupled with their

[1]Department of Clinical Sciences and Services, Royal Veterinary College (University of London), Hawkshead Campus North Mymms, Hatfield AL9 7TA, United Kingdom; [2]Advanced Veterinary Therapeutics, Newtown, NSW 2042, Australia.

ability to carry resistant bacteria, increase the risk of global dissemination. Better surveillance of the impact of international trade and movement of these animals and animal products is required so that their impact on the development of antimicrobial resistance can be more accurately assessed, facilitating the establishment of appropriate control measures (13).

We have now reached a situation where bacteria involved in colonization and infection of both farm and companion animals include organisms that can be resistant to all registered veterinary drugs. These include organisms such as MRSA and methicillin-resistant *Staphylococcus pseudintermedius*, extended-spectrum β-lactamase-producing *Escherichia coli*, carbapenemase-producing *E. coli* and *Klebsiella pneumoniae*, and multidrug-resistant enterococci and *Acinetobacter baumannii*. These organisms, their resistance factors, and their local and global dissemination have been covered elsewhere and will not be considered here.

The generation of antimicrobial agents and the development of resistance mechanisms is part of the normal biology of bacteria and other microorganisms, a process that has been involved in bacterial evolution over a long period, as demonstrated by the identification of genes encoding resistance to a wide range of modern antibiotics in ancient DNA from 30,000-year-old Beringian permafrost sediments and from the Lechuguilla Cave, New Mexico, which has been isolated for more than 4 million years (14, 15). Indeed, predictions of the time of origin of the B3 subclass of metallo-β-lactamases, based on dating of biosynthetic gene clusters, has been estimated at 2.2 billion years ago (16). Thus, bacteria are very capable of evolving resistance to antimicrobials, and prospects for the development of new agents which will not generate resistance are very low. Implementation of effective antimicrobial stewardship (AMS) strategies is now an urgent necessity if we are to preserve the efficacy of our existing drugs and ensure optimal longevity of any new agents that are developed.

This article focuses on the processes involved in effective AMS, reviewing what has been achieved in the human medicine field, the tools and mechanisms for implementation that are becoming available for veterinary use, evidence for success, and the need for incentives or legislation in promoting compliance.

AMS in Human Medicine

The need for AMS in human medicine is now well recognized, and it is being applied in a variety of ways in human hospitals in an increasing number of countries. Systematic reviews of the effects of stewardship have

been carried out by Davey et al., who reported an initial study in 2005 and followed this up in 2017 (17, 18), work corroborated by Schuts et al. (19). Each of these studies demonstrated overall beneficial effects. Davey et al. (17, 18) studied the impact of interventions designed to influence the prescription of antimicrobials to hospital inpatients and reduce antimicrobial resistance or *Clostridium difficile* associated diarrhea (CDAD) and their effects on clinical outcomes in a total of 155 studies. They found that interventions aiming to reduce excessive prescription were associated with reduction in *C. difficile* infections and colonization or infection with aminoglycoside- or cephalosporin-resistant Gram-negative bacteria, MRSA, and vancomycin-resistant *Enterococcus*. Interventions designed to increase effective prescribing were also able to improve clinical outcome. Meta-analysis showed that restrictive interventions such as form filling and the need to obtain approval from an infection specialist prior to antimicrobial prescription were more effective than persuasive interventions (advice on how to prescribe or feedback after prescriptions were made) for up to 6 months, but the two approaches were equally effective after that. Disturbingly, they concluded that prescribing was often suboptimal, and up to 50% of use could be inappropriate. On a positive note, Davey et al. (18) demonstrated that enablement (increasing means or reducing barriers to increase capability or opportunity) consistently increased the effect of interventions and that feedback further increased the positive impact. Schuts et al. (19) focused on four outcomes in 145 studies: clinical responses, adverse events, costs, and rates of bacterial resistance. They found that for the objectives of empirical therapy according to guidelines, de-escalation of therapy, switching from intravenous to oral treatment, therapeutic drug monitoring, use of a list of restricted antimicrobials, and bedside consultation, there were overall significant benefits for one or more of the four outcomes.

These studies show the benefits that can be obtained by the application of AMS in human hospitals. However, implementation of antimicrobial use guidelines has been problematic even in countries with vigorous policies aimed at the control of antimicrobial resistance. An example is the introduction of consensus-based guidelines developed by a multidisciplinary expert group for antimicrobial use in the treatment of meningitis in the Netherlands in 1997, which were disseminated in booklet form. A year later, a prospective study (20) showed that only one-third of patients had been treated in accordance with the guidelines. For the study, patients were divided into four groups according to risk factor status. The largest group was composed of patients with no risk factors, and 39% of these were treated empirically with third-generation cephalosporins, whereas the guidelines, which reflected the very low incidence of local resistance among likely pathogens, recommended penicillin. In a leading article referring to this study, Brown (21) speculated on the reasons why so few clinicians in The Netherlands had adopted the guidelines. These included mistrust, a feeling that the guidelines were too narrow, preference for locally developed guidelines, poor dissemination, and lack of incentives for implementation. He pointed out that such failure to adopt guidelines was far from unique and went on to review the principles underlying the generation of effective guidelines, with a particular emphasis on the need for planning and the allocation of sufficient resources for effective dissemination and implementation.

Although there is broad recognition of the need for AMS in the human field, there continues to be a lack of appropriate guidelines and effective implementation in many medical institutions and disciplines. A notable example is pediatrics, where the need for formal AMS programs has only recently been recognized and there are continuing problems relating to implementation, most importantly, the need for financial resources and for administrative consensus enabling the education of pediatricians and the creation of multidisciplinary interprofessional teams able to prepare guidelines and administer AMS programs (22). The need for AMS to be adapted to different settings is important if it is to be accepted by those involved, and it has become apparent that the impact of behavioral determinants and social norms is not being given sufficient attention (23). Clinicians often emulate the incorrect prescribing behavior of fellow clinicians, and junior doctors are likely to be influenced by their seniors (24, 25). Senior doctors like to have autonomy in decision-making and may be reluctant to interfere with their peers' prescribing decisions (23). Thus, senior clinicians and consultants need to be involved in the development of tailored guidelines in their disciplines, aligning the guidelines with the evidence base and consultants' preferences and ensuring that the teaching of junior doctors focuses on adherence while also indicating when deviation is justified (26).

There is particular concern regarding the excessive and indiscriminate use of agents that are regarded as being of special importance in human medicine. These have been listed by the World Health Organization (WHO) (27) under the title "critically important antimicrobials" in a document intended for public health and animal health authorities, physicians, veterinarians, and others involved in managing antimicrobial resistance. The document categorizes a wide range of agents and places them into three categories on the basis of their importance in human medicine: critically important, highly important, and important. These lists are designed to help formulate and prioritize risk assessment and management strategies for containing antimicrobial resistance due to human and nonhuman antimicrobial use when designing guidelines. Fluoroquinolones; third-, fourth-, and fifth-generation cephalosporins; macrolides and ketolides; glycopeptides; and polymyxins have been categorized as being of the highest priority for risk management. The document recommends that carbapenems, glycopeptides, oxazolidinones, and any new classes of antimicrobials developed for human therapy should not be used in animals, plants, or aquaculture. Classes of antimicrobials used in animals but not in humans are also identified and include aminocoumarins, orthosomycins, phosphoglycolipids, polyether ionophores, and quinoxalines. Antimicrobials used in food-producing animals have also been listed and categorized by the World Organisation for Animal Health as critically important, highly important, and important together with the animal species to which they are applied, the indications for their use, and whether they are essential or have few alternatives (28).

While the adoption and implementation of AMS in the human medicine field has moved forward and is being developed in the wealthier countries of the world, this is not the case in low- and middle-income countries where insufficient political commitment, scarcity of funding, and a lack of expertise create major difficulties (29). In such countries, this lack of AMS programs is compounded by high levels of inappropriate antimicrobial drug use, particularly in emerging economies where increasing funds are available for their purchase and where dispensing of antimicrobials without prescription and self-medication are common practices. This problem is exacerbated by the sale of poorly formulated and counterfeit antimicrobials (30, 31) and by the increasing availability of antimicrobials through illicit online pharmacies (32). Such inappropriate antimicrobial use drives resistance and can lead to rapid transfer of resistant microorganisms and resistance genes on a global basis.

Emergence of resistance among livestock and companion animals and the risk of its transfer to humans is an issue that is causing increasing concern. This is a true One Health issue because transfer may occur in either direction, a situation that is exemplified by the occurrence of human hospital-associated MRSA infections in animals, particularly in domestic pets (33). The emerging problem of MRSA CC398 colonization of pigs and other farm animals illustrates the complexity of the situation. CC398 has become established with high rates of carriage in pig farms in Denmark and, while typically causing little pathology in the pigs, it has now become the dominant MRSA clone found in humans in Denmark (34) and a cause of infection in those having no direct contact with the pigs (35). Although CC398 is believed to have originated as a human strain of *S. aureus* which became adapted to pigs (36), it is now evolving to produce distinct animal-adapted and human-adapted strains, as well as strains with increased invasive capacity for both humans and animals (37). This has led to the recommendation that human hospitals with MRSA exclusion policies should screen farmers and veterinarians with livestock contacts for carriage of CC398 prior to admission. Recognition of this problem in Norway has led to a search and destroy policy on pig farms aimed at keeping pig populations MRSA free and preventing them from becoming reservoirs for transmission of CC398 to humans (38), but this approach will be more difficult to establish in countries with larger pig populations. Public health risks posed by enterobacterial species producing extended-spectrum and AmpC β-lactamases in food and food-producing animals have also been highlighted by the European Food Safety Authority, with the identification of cephalosporin use and international trade in animals as risk factors (39).

More recently, the identification of the plasmid-mediated colistin resistance gene, *mcr-1*, from *E. coli* from pigs, poultry, and hospital patients in China (40) and the subsequent recognition that it is present worldwide with more frequent isolation from animals, coupled with the much greater use of colistin in livestock, has caused the European Medicines Agency to issue new advice on its use in animals on the basis that this gene has probably arisen in animals and transferred to humans (41, 42). European Union member states are recommended to minimize sales of colistin for use in animals to achieve a 65% reduction, and colistin is to be added to the critical category of medicines reserved for treating clinical conditions for which there are no effective alternative treatments for the respective target species and indication (42), while WHO has added colistin (a polymyxin) to the list of highest-priority critically important antimicrobials (27).

AMS in the human medicine field has been principally focused on reduction of antimicrobial use and more critical choice of appropriate antimicrobial therapy. However, there is increasing attention on the unintended consequences which may occur following the use of antimicrobial drugs (43), and particularly the effects of intestinal dysbiosis (44). The effect of antimicrobial therapy on the occurrence of *C. difficile*-associated diarrhea is well recognized, but there is now increasing evidence associating antimicrobial exposure with inflammatory bowel disease and childhood obesity (45–47) and with juvenile idiopathic arthritis occurring in children aged 1–15 years (48). Disturbance of the microbial ecology of the gut has also been associated with neurodevelopmental disorders (49). More study is required in these areas, and it seems likely that other diseases associated with disturbance of the microbiome by antimicrobial drugs will emerge.

AMS in Veterinary Medicine

The development of AMS in veterinary medicine has lagged behind that in the human medicine field but has gained impetus with increasing evidence of the worldwide multiple-resistance crisis in human medicine and the possible contributions from antimicrobial use and resistance selection in animals. Recommendations on the establishment of AMS programs and guidelines on prudent antimicrobial use and disease prevention have been published by a number of authors and by international and national organizations, and there is an accumulating literature providing a framework for their implementation in the companion animal and farming sectors.

At the international governmental level, the European Union moved to control the use of antimicrobial drugs in food production at an early stage. Chloramphenicol use for therapeutic purposes was banned in food production animals in the European Community in 1994 because of public health toxicological concerns. Owing to concerns about antimicrobial resistance selection, antimicrobial drugs were progressively withdrawn from use as growth promoters in animal feed in Europe beginning in 1972, with a complete ban in 2006 (50). The WHO adopted a global action plan on antimicrobial resistance in 2015 with the principal goal of ensuring treatment and prevention of infectious diseases with quality-assured, safe, and effective medicines. The plan outlines five strategic objectives (Table 1), all of which relate to the development and implementation of effective AMS (51). These objectives are being implemented in collaboration with the United Nations Food and Agriculture Organization (FAO) and World Organisation for Animal Health in a coordinated "One Health" approach involving a wide range of sectors including human and veterinary medicine,

Table 1 Objectives of the WHO Global Action Plan on Antimicrobial Resistance[a]

1 To improve awareness and understanding of antimicrobial resistance through effective communication, education, and training
2 To strengthen the knowledge and evidence base through surveillance and research
3 To reduce the incidence of infection through effective sanitation, hygiene, and infection prevention measures
4 To optimize the use of antimicrobial medicines in human and animal health
5 To develop the economic case for sustainable investment that takes account of the needs of all countries and to increase investment in new medicines, diagnostic tools, vaccines, and other interventions

[a]Source: reference 51.

agriculture, finance, environment, and consumers. The aim was to have multisectorial national plans in place in 2017. In February 2016, WHO, the FAO, and the World Organisation for Animal Health jointly released a manual and toolkit for developing national action plans (52), and the FAO released its action plan, which deals with the food and agricultural sectors, including terrestrial and aquatic animal health and production, crop production, food safety standard-setting, and legal aspects, in September 2016 (53). The FAO plan focuses on four components: (i) awareness of antimicrobial resistance and related threats, (ii) surveillance and monitoring of antimicrobial resistance and antimicrobial use, (iii) strengthening governance related to antimicrobial use and antimicrobial resistance, including implementation of international guidelines/standards on antimicrobial resistance such as the Codex Alimentarius (54), and (iv) promoting good practice in food and agricultural systems and prudent antimicrobial use at the country level, including the capacity for implementation of international standards and guidelines relating to antimicrobial resistance and use, and consideration of antimicrobial resistance issues in the development of voluntary guidelines for sustainable agricultural production.

The European Union has also been active in working with WHO to develop plans dealing with antimicrobial resistance and covering both human and veterinary medicine and agriculture. WHO Europe published the European strategic action plan on antibiotic resistance in 2011, which aimed to promote coordination and development of European national action plans. These are listed by the European Centre for Disease Prevention and Control (55), which shows 13 countries with programs initiated between 2011 and 2016. Other

countries have also published strategies which aim to support development of the WHO One Health global plan including the Public Health Agency of Canada, the Australian Government (Departments of Health and of Agriculture) and the U.S. government (56–58). Although the United States has relied on guidance documents and voluntary action to regulate antimicrobial use in farm animals (59), it is now increasingly restricting the use of antimicrobials in feed and water for food animals (60).

The development of effective AMS programs in both human and veterinary medicine in low-income and medium-income countries continues to be problematic owing to insufficient political commitment and the lack of funding and expertise (29, 61–63), as discussed earlier.

At the institutional level, veterinary AMS and responsible antimicrobial use guidelines have been developed by a wide range of national and international organizations. In the United Kingdom, the Responsible Use of Medicines in Agriculture Alliance (RUMA, http://www.ruma.org.uk/) brings together organizations involved in all stages of the food chain with the objective of promoting food safety, animal health, and animal welfare. Established in 1997, it publishes guidelines on antimicrobial use and vaccination in poultry, pigs, cattle, sheep, and fish while also promoting and providing links to AMS and disease control schemes by producers' organizations. The European Platform for the Responsible Use of Medicines in Animals (EPRUMA, http://www.epruma.eu/) has similar objectives and broad international membership. Established in 2005, it works at the European Union level facilitating and promoting coordinated and integrated action, including the production of framework documents providing guidance on responsible antimicrobial use in food-producing animals.

While the focus on AMS among international and national governmental organizations has principally been directed at farming and food production, recommendations and guidelines for companion animals have been chiefly developed by veterinary societies and associations. In North America, the American Veterinary Medical Association and its constituent allied organizations, the American College of Veterinary Internal Medicine, and the Canadian Veterinary Medical Association have been particularly active (64–66). Within Europe, national veterinary organizations have also produced guidelines and posters on AMS and responsible use of antimicrobials, and the Federation of European Companion Animal Veterinary Associations, which brings together European national associations, has produced a series of posters for veterinary surgeons and owners.

More specific guidelines for responsible antimicrobial use in particular diseases are also being increasingly made available. The International Society for Companion Animal Infectious Disease (ISCAID) Antimicrobial Working Group is working to produce a range of guidelines and has already published on the treatment of urinary tract infections, respiratory diseases, and superficial bacterial folliculitis (67–69). The ISCAID website (http://www.iscaid.org/guidelines) also lists a range of guidelines produced by other organizations.

In Europe, The Netherlands has been particularly successful in promoting AMS and reducing antimicrobial use. It recorded a 58.4% decrease in sales between 2009 and 2015, and this has been associated with a clear reduction in levels of antimicrobial resistance in broilers, veal calves, and pigs. Its policy has been proposed by the European Union as a model of good practice for other European community states (70). The prudent use policies were set up as a public-private partnership which took responsibility for the institution of effective measures based on expert scientific advice. The partnership involved stakeholders in the major livestock production sectors together with the Royal Netherlands Veterinary Association, facilitated and supervised by the national government, and led to the establishment of the independent Netherlands Veterinary Medicine Authority, which analyzed data on antimicrobial use at the farm level and set benchmarks. Veterinarians that are found to be noncompliant with specified prudent use policies may be subject to a range of sanctions including official warnings, application of administrative or criminal law, and reference to the veterinary disciplinary board, leading to suspension or the application of fines.

DEVELOPING AND IMPLEMENTING GOOD STEWARDSHIP PRACTICE

Good stewardship practice (GSP) describes the active, dynamic, and motivated approach to antimicrobial use reinforced by a mindset for continuous improvement (71). However, despite the many calls for prudent antimicrobial use and the wide range of guidelines that is now available, the benefits of effective implementation of GSP both in human and in animal medicine are only just starting to be recognized. A review of key AMS literature (72–81) that continues to evolve and influence the development and implementation of AMS plans in human medicine has revealed a number of

important messages to guide the establishment of a more effective veterinary AMS framework, the core elements of which—goals, key strategies, and success factors—are presented in Table 2.

The 5R Antimicrobial Framework

There is a growing experience with a collaborative and participatory approach to antimicrobial use that sets out to bring about change by recognizing the importance of sociology and using practical knowledge that is useful in local practice (82–84). The participatory approach works particularly well at the farm level, where changes in antimicrobial use can be discussed by the veterinarian and the farmer, and a jointly owned plan can be prepared and implemented (85–89).

Related to the participatory approach is that of handshake stewardship (90, 91), which is defined by the lack of a restriction and preauthorization but includes a collaborative review of all prescribed antimicrobials and an in-person approach to feedback. Handshake stewardship is ironically named, because handshakes are associated with pathogen transmission and may be replaced with alternative greetings (92).

This less intrusive approach to modifying antimicrobial use is likely to be more acceptable to veterinarians who may be similar to family physicians who have been reported to oppose any measure aimed at restricting freedom of prescription (93). Fortunately, several authoritative studies have demonstrated that postprescription review with feedback can have a greater impact on modifying antimicrobial prescribing than restrictive approaches (18, 94).

The value of feedback in improving antimicrobial use is the subject of many studies (18, 95–98). Dunn and Dunn (99) described the most striking effects of clinical audit and feedback in small animal practice: "with a modicum of work, the standards within practice have been improved, and a plan to improve them further demonstrates that a simple audit process works."

From this background, a veterinary framework of AMS has evolved (100, 101), with each core element mapping to the major features of currently described AMS programs. The framework is customized to meet the varying requirements across the veterinary profession, which encompasses everything from single animal treatment to herd and flock health management. The framework is summarized in Fig. 1, which describes GSP and the application of five core elements (the 5Rs: responsibility, reduce, replace, refine, review). Responsibility is the fundamentally important and essential starting point; AMS programs will not succeed without senior management commitment. Under the aegis of

Table 2 Principal elements in the establishment of an effective veterinary AMS framework

Core elements	1. Generate enthusiasm, commitment, and support among senior management
	2. Identify resistance patterns and antimicrobial use in treated animals
	3. Select priority areas and devise intervention plans
	4. Determine how progress and success will be measured
	5. Implement at least one readily achievable policy or practice of improved antimicrobial use to allow the group to experience early success
	6. Implement quantitative and qualitative measurement of prescribing practice, including self-audit, if appropriate
	7. Customize the AMS plan to serve the special needs of each practice or other operation
	8. Provide educational resources and access to expertise on optimizing antimicrobial prescribing
AMS goals	1. Ensure that each patient receives the most appropriate treatment: the right drug, at the right time, at the right dose for the right duration by the right route of delivery (5 rights)
	2. Eliminate antimicrobial overuse and misuse
	3. Minimize the selection, maintenance, and dissemination of antimicrobial resistance
Key strategies	1. Implement clinical guidelines that take into account local microbiology and susceptibility patterns
	2. Establish formulary restriction and approval systems that restrict later generation and critically important antimicrobials to patients where clinical need is justified
	3. Review antimicrobial prescribing with intervention and direct feedback to the prescriber
	4. Ensure that the clinical microbiology laboratory uses selective reporting of susceptibility results that is consistent with clinical guidelines
Success factors	1. Presence of a motivated team leader
	2. Motivated team sharing responsibility for GSP

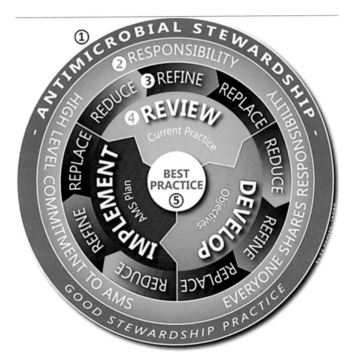

Figure 1 Key elements of antimicrobial stewardship. 1. GSP requires embedded thinking and action to improve antimicrobial use and minimize resistance selection and impact. 2. Responsibility implies high-level commitment, with everybody taking and sharing responsibility 3. The 3Rs of responsible use—reduce, refine, and replace—should be applied wherever possible. 4. Review antimicrobial use and infection control and develop objectives to improve current practice and implementation of the stewardship plan. 5. Every cycle of 5R stewardship reflects continuous improvement (*kaizen*) and leads to best practices in infection prevention and control and antimicrobial use. (Figure graphics by Ed Hewson.)

corporate support, GSP requires that all uses of antimicrobials are examined under the multiple lenses of the potential to reduce, replace, or refine each use. The final element, review, involves the measurement and assessment of use, antimicrobial resistance, and resources needed, which may often include continuing professional development. The process is self-motivating and a continuous form of improvement.

Two important features distinguish this model from that of current human AMS programs. First, the GSP 5R model includes consideration of both improved antimicrobial use and infection prevention and control, which necessarily work in tandem and cannot be naturally separated. Second, a fundamental objective of the framework is to consider ways not to use antimicrobials. It is only when antimicrobials are necessary that optimal use is considered.

Responsibility

It is widely acknowledged that a fundamental requirement for a successful and sustained AMS program is to have executive or senior management support (102–105). This element of the 5R framework maps to the first core element of AMS programs (106), outpatient AMS (81) and hospital AMS (107), described as 'leadership commitment" and requiring dedication to and accountability for optimizing antimicrobial prescribing and patient safety. There are many enabling mechanisms to ensure that a collaborative and participatory

team approach is taken with effective communication with all stakeholders. A particularly powerful positive influence is associated with skilled leadership and social cohesion (108), which has been observed to transform even conservative clinicians into early adopters.

Reduction

A common theme of veterinary science for more than 100 years that remains pivotal to the reduction of antimicrobial resistance is the implementation of improved infection prevention and control measures (109, 110), a process described by the concept of biosecurity, which includes the set of preventive measures designed to reduce the risk of introduction, development, and spread of infectious disease within an animal population (111). An excellent review of how biosecurity can reduce antimicrobial use and antimicrobial resistance selection has been published (112), and pivotal features and examples of biosecurity actions are summarized in Table 3.

Modern precision farming could not take place in the absence of high levels of biosecurity, and it underpins production practices in poultry (113, 114), dairy cattle (115), feedlot cattle (116), pigs (117), and aquaculture (118). A quantitative tool to measure biosecurity on broiler farms has been developed (119), making self-assessment much easier. There can be competing interests that have to be balanced. The increasing growth of outdoor livestock production systems

Table 3 Biosecurity and disease prevention

Biosecurity phase	Examples of effective actions
Primary prevention: external biosecurity (bioexclusion)	Minimize the introduction of animals
	Minimize the number of sources of introduced animals
	Clean and disinfect transport vehicles and containers
	Isolate sick animals before introduction
	Provide clean water, feed, air
	Exclude pests from and control human access to housing, filter exhaust to reduce pathogen load
Secondary prevention: internal biosecurity (biocontainment)	All-in-all-out production system
	Hygiene, infection control protocols
	Housing design: ventilation, drainage
	Litter/bedding materials
	Early diagnosis of disease
	Once pathogen is present, introduce measures to eliminate or reduce transmission—guided by on-farm microbiological risk assessment
	Reduce stocking density, segregation, sick pens
Tertiary prevention: individual animal resilience (adaptive capacity to changing environment)	Genetic selection
	Vaccination
	Management (handling, low stress, enrichment)
	Nutrition
	Housing (ventilation, temperature, stocking rate, hygiene)

can be incompatible with the maintenance of biosecurity, as well illustrated by the introduction of a requirement to enhance biosecurity in United Kingdom bird enterprises to help reduce the risk of avian influenza introduction (120).

Biosecurity is equally important in small animal (121) and equine practices and hospitals (122), and practice-specific infection control plans have been widely advocated (123), with model plans available for adaptation (124–126).

GSP requires consideration of the entire spectrum of possible reduction approaches, which also include genetic selection for disease resistance (127–132), use of vaccines (which have repeatedly been shown to reduce antimicrobial use in a variety of food animal species, including fish [133], calves [134], pigs [135–138], and poultry [139]), identifying modifiable risk factors (140–143), and of course, measuring current practice. The importance of this has been demonstrated by Elbers et al. (144, 145), who identified otherwise inapparent opportunities to reduce antimicrobial use, and by Greko (146), who demonstrated that feedback on personal or practice antimicrobial use can lead to reductions.

Replacement

Replacement of the use of antimicrobials with alternative, nonantimicrobial measures, wherever possible and appropriate, is another critical AMS tenet. Key considerations include whether or not the alternative approach will select for antimicrobial resistance and the quality and strength of the evidence supporting the use of the selected approach. The most comprehensive recent review of the use of alternative products in livestock (112) concluded that "due to limitation in data availability, the potential impact of the alternative measures on the occurrence of antimicrobial resistance in bacteria from food-producing animals and food cannot be established." High-quality research is needed to overcome this critical information gap.

While the impact on antimicrobial resistance may not be clear, the subject is attracting substantial interest (147–150); several alternatives have been demonstrated to have positive impacts on animal health in particular circumstances, and their use is increasing in livestock production. These alternatives include the use of dietary acidifiers or organic acids in broilers (151) and pigs (152); the use of probiotic yeasts (153–155) and probiotic bacteria (156–158) in fish, monogastric, and ruminant species; and the use of prebiotics (nondigestible food ingredients that beneficially affect the host by selectively stimulating the growth and/or activity of one or a limited number of bacteria in the colon) and their

combination with probiotics (known as synbiotics) (159–162) in livestock and companion animal species.

The literature is also providing support for a number of other options that include antimicrobial peptides (163, 164), bacteriophages (165–171), essential oils (172, 173), honey (174), nitric oxide (175), predatory bacteria (176, 177), and immunoglobulins, both IgY from hyperimmune chicken egg yolk (178–180) and spray dried immune plasma (181, 182).

Two alternative products that replace antimicrobials have already received regulatory approval in major markets worldwide and are having a significant impact in replacing antimicrobial use in dairy cattle, where mastitis is a major indication for antimicrobial treatment. Teat-sealing pastes containing an inert heavy metal, such a bismuth subnitrate, are available for use in suitably selected dairy cattle at the end of each lactation, where they provide a physical barrier that prevents new infections from ascending the teat canal during the dry period (183). More recently, pegbovigrastim (184), a modified form of the naturally occurring immunoregulatory cytokine bovine granulocyte colony-stimulating factor, which restores normal neutrophil function to cattle during the periparturient period, thereby reducing susceptibility to clinical mastitis infections, has become available and also has the potential to replace the need for later antimicrobial use.

Although the movement away from the use of antimicrobial growth promoters has been a strong driver for research and development of antimicrobial replacement approaches in livestock, there is also keen interest in companion animal and equine practice to identify and use replacements (185). However, experience with probiotic use in horses suggests that the beneficial effects seen in livestock species cannot always be expected in foals and horses (186, 187) and highlights the need for careful selection and testing of probiotic strains.

Where infections can be reached with topical therapy, this can be a very effective way of replacing systemic antimicrobial drugs (68, 188–190). Topical antimicrobials are commonly active in the face of resistance to systemically administered agents because they can be used at much higher concentrations. It should be noted that antimicrobial susceptibility tests are normally based on the expectation of systemic therapy and their results cannot therefore be applied to the assessment of resistance when topical therapy is being considered.

The potential benefits of antimicrobial replacements are increasingly being studied and reported, but it cannot be assumed that their use is innocuous. A growing list of unintended consequences, some extremely serious, is being reported. Examples relating to animal feed supplementation in pigs include apparent coselection of MRSA, and of tetracycline and sulfonamide resistance in Gram-negative bacteria, by high concentrations of dietary ZnO (191–193) and apparent coselection of macrolide and glycopeptide resistance by diets with high concentrations of copper (194, 195). In cattle, selection of tetracycline-resistant *E. coli* by dietary menthol has been reported (196). Clays routinely added to animal feed to improve growth and animal product quality appear to facilitate horizontal transfer of resistance determinants in the digestive tracts of farm animals (197). Worryingly, *in vitro* serial passage studies of MRSA and host-derived antimicrobial peptides have demonstrated evolution of stable virulent mutants with cross-resistance to human innate immunity as well as antimicrobial therapy (198).

Refinement

Opportunities for refinement of antimicrobial use are identified in Fig. 2, which summarizes the steps in initi-

ating and implementing an antimicrobial therapeutic plan. The process begins with diagnosis, often the most tenuous link in the chain as identified by O'Neill (199), who further noted that uncertainty of diagnosis of bacterial infection is a major driver of antimicrobial overuse and antimicrobial resistance selection in humans. It is likely that in many situations this is the same in veterinary practice. For example, it is notoriously difficult to establish an accurate diagnosis of bovine respiratory disease in feedlot cattle, especially early in the pathogenesis (200). These issues have been reviewed by Griffin (201), who concludes that a major factor that is seldom considered in the treatment response in bovine respiratory disease is correctness of the clinical diagnosis; misdiagnosis as a cause of treatment failure is a common necropsy finding.

The pivotal role that diagnosis plays in ensuring appropriate antimicrobial use has led to a massive investment in research to find better diagnostic tests. Substantial rewards are available to those that can meet the diagnostic needs. The European Commission (202)

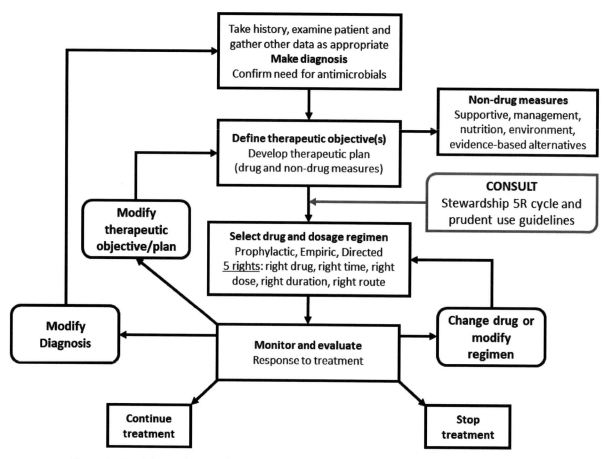

Figure 2   Decision-making and application of GSP in suspected bacterial infection.

awarded the €1 million Horizon Prize to the innovators of a breakthrough test which distinguishes between viral and bacterial infections in humans. The United Kingdom Longitude Prize (203) is a challenge with a £10 million prize fund to reward a diagnostic test that helps solve the problem of global antimicrobial resistance by identifying when antimicrobials are needed and, if they are, which ones to use. Criteria that the test must satisfy are that it is needed, accurate, affordable, rapid, easy to use, scalable, safe, connected, and available to anyone, anywhere in the world. These criteria are very similar to those enunciated by WHO as the ASSURED (affordable, sensitive, specific, user-friendly, rapid and robust, equipment-free, and deliverable) criteria (204) for novel diagnostic tests suitable for global use.

While it is expected that any technological breakthroughs in diagnostic tests for medical use will find ready application in the animal health world, in the meantime there has been substantial research into improved methods of disease diagnosis in livestock, driven by the desire to detect infections early in individual animals to allow more targeted treatment with more rapid responses. Examples of new approaches that are actively being investigated include remote automatic sensing of animal behavior, including feeding and drinking, in chickens (205–207), pigs (208), calves (209), and cattle (210–212), with evidence of the possibility of earlier detection of clinical illness from 1 day to 14 days in advance of observed disease. Remote detection of cough sounds in pigs (208, 213) and cattle (214) also presents opportunities for earlier diagnosis and intervention. A variety of other promising approaches have also been reported, including computer-aided lung auscultation in cattle for bovine respiratory disease diagnosis (215), infrared thermography of cattle (216) and pigs (217), and a diversity of acute phase protein (218–220), bacteriological (221, 222), genomic (223–226), proteomic (227), and immunological (228, 229) tests.

Already, improved culture-based diagnostic tests are allowing selective treatment of dairy cattle with purulent vaginal discharge (222) or clinical mastitis (230–232), and improved use of somatic cell count data is guiding selective dry cow treatment of dairy cattle (233, 234), each decreasing antimicrobial use.

Depending on the strength of the diagnosis, prophylactic (risk factors for infection present), empiric (bacterial infection suspected), or directed (bacterial infection and site of infection known) treatment can be planned. It is then important to be guided by local treatment guidelines incorporating the judicious use principles set out in Table 4, which have been derived from an analysis of existing guidelines and present a taxonomy divided into stage of treatment.

While the therapeutic objective of local antimicrobial prescribing guidelines is frequently stated as attaining optimal use where effectiveness is maximized and adverse effects, including antimicrobial resistance, are minimized, the recommended dosage regimens of existing antimicrobial products have been developed to demonstrate efficacy, not to minimize resistance.

A dosage regimen for a particular route of systemic administration consists of a dose (mg/kg), a dosing interval (either continuous via feed, water or infusion, or one or more administrations each day) and a duration (days). These are the only parameters that can be changed, though it is a reasonable expectation that in the majority of cases it is likely that the label dose recommendation will lead to satisfactory therapeutic efficacy. However, it seems unlikely that a single dosage regimen could apply to all situations all the time (especially when pathogen MICs are forever increasing), and even optimal use of systemic drugs will delay but not prevent the spread of resistance (235). The father of antimicrobial chemotherapy, Nobel laureate Paul Ehrlich, famously advocated antimicrobial use regimens characterized by *"frapper fort et frapper vite"*—hit hard and hit quickly (236). Interestingly, this approach is again finding favor as it is realized that appropriate doses early in the course of a bacterial infection have greater efficacy and lower propensity to select for antimicrobial resistance (237, 238). In addition, the possibility of using topical or anatomically targeted therapy should always be considered. This is likely to be applicable most often for surface wounds and infections involving mucosae and skin and for accessible sites of infection such as the mammary gland, uterus, and eye. Topical and targeted therapy has the advantage that the antimicrobial agents can be administered at much higher concentrations than those used systemically. This can overcome existing resistance to systemic drugs and is less likely to facilitate development of resistance among susceptible organisms. It is being increasingly used and recommended in small-animal dermatology, particularly in the face of methicillin-resistant staphylococcal infection (68, 239).

Review: the basis of continuous improvement
Review of the AMS program is a fundamental core principle. At the outset, stock-taking or audit of current antimicrobial use practice, infection prevention and control measures, and the antimicrobial resistance status defines the starting point and allows an examination of those areas where improvements can inform

Table 4 Core principles of judicious use of antimicrobial agents

Category	Principles
Pretreatment principles	Disease prevention
	Apply appropriate biosecurity, husbandry, hygiene, health monitoring, vaccination, nutrition, housing, and environmental controls.
	Use codes of practice, quality assurance programs, flock or herd health surveillance programs, and education programs that promote responsible and prudent use of antimicrobial agents.
	Professional intervention
	Ensure that use (labelled and extra-label) of antimicrobials meets all the requirements of a valid veterinarian-client-patient relationship.
	Alternatives to antimicrobial agents
	Efficacious, scientific, evidence-based alternatives to antimicrobial agents can be an important adjunct to good husbandry practices.
Diagnosis	Accurate diagnosis
	Make clinical diagnosis of bacterial infection with appropriate point of care and laboratory tests and epidemiological information.
Therapeutic objective and plan	Develop outcome objectives (for example, clinical or microbiological cure) and implementation plan (including consideration of therapeutic choices, supportive therapy, host, environment, infectious agent, and other factors).
Drug selection	Justification of antimicrobial use
	Consider other options first; antimicrobials should not be used to compensate for or mask poor farm or veterinary practices.
	Use informed professional judgment balancing the risks (especially the risk of antimicrobial resistance selection and dissemination) and benefits to humans, animals, and the environment.
	Guidelines for antimicrobial use
	Consult disease- and species-specific guidelines to inform antimicrobial selection and use.
	Critically important antimicrobial agents
	Use all antimicrobial agents, including those considered important in treating refractory infections in human or veterinary medicine, only after careful review and reasonable justification.
	Culture and sensitivity testing
	Utilize culture and susceptibility (or equivalent) testing when clinically relevant to aid selection of antimicrobials, especially if initial treatment has failed.
	Spectrum of activity
	Use narrow-spectrum in preference to broad-spectrum antimicrobials whenever appropriate.
	Extra-label (off-label) antimicrobial therapy
	Must be prescribed only in accordance with prevailing laws and regulations.
	Confine use to situations where medications used according to label instructions have been ineffective or are unavailable and where there is scientific evidence, including residue data if appropriate, supporting the off-label use pattern.
Drug use	Dosage regimens
	Where possible, optimize regimens for therapeutic antimicrobial use following current pharmacokinetic and pharmacodynamic guidance.
	Duration of treatment
	Minimize therapeutic exposure to antimicrobials by treating for only as long as needed to meet the therapeutic objective.
	Labelling and instructions
	Ensure that the veterinarian gives the end user written instructions on drug use, with clear details for method of administration, dose rate, frequency and duration of treatment, precautions, and withholding period.
	Target animals
	Limit therapeutic antimicrobial treatment to ill or at-risk animals, treating the fewest animals possible.
	Record keeping
	Keep accurate records of diagnosis (indication), treatment, and outcome to allow therapeutic regimens to be evaluated by the prescriber and permit benchmarking as a guide for continuous improvement.

(Continued)

Table 4   *(Continued)*

Category	Principles
	Compliance
	Encourage and ensure that instructions for drug use are implemented appropriately
	Monitor response to treatment
	Report to appropriate authorities any reasonable suspicion of an adverse reaction to the medicine in either treated animals or farm staff having contact with the medicine, including any unexpected failure to respond to the medication.
	Thoroughly investigate every treated case that fails to respond as expected.
Posttreatment activities	Environmental contamination
	Minimize environmental contamination with antimicrobials whenever possible.
	Surveillance of antimicrobial resistance
	Undertake susceptibility surveillance periodically and provide the results to the prescriber, supervising veterinarians, and other relevant parties.
	Continuous evaluation
	Evaluate veterinarians' prescribing practices continually, based on such information as the main indications and types of antimicrobials used in different animal species and their relation to available data on antimicrobial resistance and current use guidelines.

AMS objectives and lead to early gains (99). Review remains an essential element of AMS as each cycle of continuous improvement is achieved. Review includes the measurement of progress toward each objective. Information on the use of antimicrobials can be obtained from both quantitative and qualitative assessments. There are many indices describing the quantity of antimicrobial agents used (240), each related to the objective, whether to assess trends in use over time, to compare use in different populations of animals (for example, in different countries), to benchmark, or to assess the relationship of antimicrobial use and AMS. Unfortunately, there is no consensus on the most appropriate index. However, all indices rely on limited data (see Fig. 3), which include species of animal treated, number of animals, bodyweight, daily dose, and duration of use. If this information is captured, then any of the many indices of quantitative use can be derived. When quantities of antimicrobial use are reduced, there is much to learn from an assessment of the quality of antimicrobial use.

While it is generally not difficult to measure the quantity of antimicrobials used, the ability to measure the quality of use can be challenging. However, it can be argued that achieving a high level of quality use of antimicrobials is an important AMS goal.

One approach that facilitates measuring quality of use is the development of antimicrobial prescribing survey tools (241), an example of which is provided in Table 5. The basic principle of assessment of quality is whether or not the prescription or use of antimicrobials was compliant with the most appropriate local or national antimicrobial use guideline. To be able to assess quality of use, it is necessary that the indication or

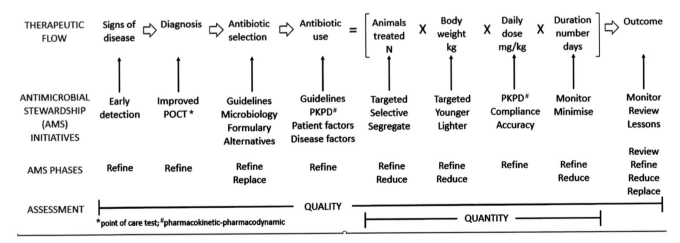

Figure 3   Interventions that can guide enhanced AMS.

Table 5 Assessment of quality of use

Appropriate		
1	Optimal	Antimicrobial prescription optimally follows a national or endorsed local guideline, including indication, antimicrobial choice, dosage, route, and duration (including for surgical prophylaxis).
2	Adequate	Antimicrobial prescription does not optimally follow the national or endorsed local guideline, including antimicrobial choice, dosage, route, or duration, but is a reasonable alternative choice for the likely causative or cultured pathogens; or for surgical prophylaxis, as above and duration is less than 24 hours.
Inappropriate		
3	Suboptimal	Antimicrobial prescription including antimicrobial choice, dosage, route, and duration, is an unreasonable choice for the likely causative or cultured pathogens, including spectrum excessively broad or an unnecessary overlap in spectrum of activity; and/or failure to appropriately de-escalate when microbiological results are available.
4	Inadequate	Antimicrobial prescription including indication, antimicrobial choice, dosage, route, or duration is unlikely to treat the likely causative or cultured pathogens; or an antimicrobial is not indicated for the documented or presumed indication; or there may be the potential risk of toxicity due to drug interaction; or for surgical prophylaxis, the duration is greater than 24 hours (except where guidelines endorse this).
Unknown		
5	Not assessable	The indication is not documented and cannot be determined from the clinical case notes; or the case notes are not comprehensive enough to assess appropriateness; or the patient is too complex, due to multiple comorbidities, microbiology results, etc.

reason for antimicrobial use is recorded, and there must be an antimicrobial use guideline available as the reference standard for quality determination. There is a growing literature focused on how best to determine quality of use (242–245) which cautions against the dogmatic use of guidelines because clinical factors may mean that deviations are warranted (246) and emphasizes the need to validate quality indicators based on quality of use (247).

Review also includes the assessment of educational needs, review of the literature and other sources of information on antimicrobial resistance and AMS, use of benchmarking and infection prevention and control measures, seeking external assessments to broaden the basis of decision making, determination of risk factors for infectious disease to identify risk management interventions, and setting of new objectives for the next cycle of improvement.

A summary of interventions that can guide enhanced AMS is presented in Fig. 3, which identifies the steps from diagnosis to clinical outcomes, highlighting opportunities for improvement.

MAINTAINING GSP

Maintaining and extending GSP implies continual revision and improvement. This needs to take into account not only development of new therapeutic agents and methods of treating and preventing infections but also increasing demand for antimicrobials created by the extension of infectious disease and changes in the livestock industry as global population growth drives increasing intensification. Allied to this are the threats posed by the increasing availability of counterfeit products and substandard generic drugs, rising demand for antimicrobials for human medicine and both livestock and companion animal medicine in emerging countries with increasingly wealthy populations, and the lack of effective legislation and enforcement of regulations controlling the prescription of antimicrobial drugs in much of the world. These threats will exacerbate the problem of inappropriate antimicrobial use and continue to drive the development of antimicrobial resistance. Global travel, migration, and the international market in animals and animal products will transport resistant organisms and continue to threaten stewardship even in countries with effective antimicrobial usage policies.

It is very unlikely that the situation will be resolved by the development of new and powerful antimicrobial agents. However, increased biosecurity and a focus on the development of disease prevention and control methods are likely to be highly effective and will need to be increasingly prominent components of GSP in the future.

Citation. Lloyd DH, Page SW. 2018. Antimicrobial stewardship in veterinary medicine. Microbiol Spectrum 6(3):ARBA-0023-2017.

References

1. **Rollin BE.** 2005. Reflections on stewardship. Proceedings of the North American Veterinary Conference, January 8–12, 2005, Orlando, FL. http://www.ivis.org/proceedings/navc/2005/SAE/180.pdf?LA=1.
2. **Bell BG, Schellevis F, Stobberingh E, Goossens H, Pringle M.** 2014. A systematic review and meta-analysis

of the effects of antibiotic consumption on antibiotic resistance. *BMC Infect Dis* 14:13.

3. O'Neill J (chair). 2016. The review on antimicrobial resistance. Tackling drug resistant infections globally: final report and recommendations. https://amr-review.org/sites/default/files/160525_Final%20paper_with%20cover.pdf.

4. Van Boeckel TP, Brower C, Gilbert M, Grenfell BT, Levin SA, Robinson TP, Teillant A, Laxminarayan R. 2015. Global trends in antimicrobial use in food animals. *Proc Natl Acad Sci USA* 112:5649–5654.

5. O'Neill J (chair). 2015. The review on antimicrobial resistance. Antimicrobials in agriculture and the environment: reducing unnecessary use and waste. https://amr-review.org/sites/default/files/Antimicrobials%20in%20agriculture%20and%20the%20environment%20-%20Reducing%20unnecessary%20use%20and%20waste.pdf.

6. Landers TF, Cohen B, Wittum TE, Larson EL. 2012. A review of antibiotic use in food animals: perspective, policy, and potential. *Public Health Rep* 127:4–22.

7. Damborg P, Broens EM, Chomel BB, Guenther S, Pasmans F, Wagenaar JA, Weese JS, Wieler LH, Windahl U, Vanrompay D, Guardabassi L. 2016. Bacterial zoonoses transmitted by household pets: state-of-the-art and future perspectives for targeted research and policy actions. *J Comp Pathol* 155(Suppl 1):S27–S40.

8. Soares Magalhães RJ, Loeffler A, Lindsay J, Rich M, Roberts L, Smith H, Lloyd DH, Pfeiffer DU. 2010. Risk factors for methicillin-resistant *Staphylococcus aureus* (MRSA) infection in dogs and cats: a case-control study. *Vet Res* 41:55.

9. Loeffler A, Pfeiffer DU, Lindsay JA, Soares Magalhães RJ, Lloyd DH. 2011. Prevalence of and risk factors for MRSA carriage in companion animals: a survey of dogs, cats and horses. *Epidemiol Infect* 139:1019–1028.

10. Fritz SA, Hogan PG, Singh LN, Thompson RM, Wallace MA, Whitney K, Al-Zubeidi D, Burnham CA, Fraser VJ. 2014. Contamination of environmental surfaces with *Staphylococcus aureus* in households with children infected with methicillin-resistant *S aureus*. *JAMA Pediatr* 168:1030–1038.

11. Sluyter FJ. 2001. Traceability of *Equidae*: a population in motion. *Rev Sci Tech* 20:500–509.

12. Müller A, Seinige D, Jansen W, Klein G, Ehricht R, Monecke S, Kehrenberg C. 2016. Variety of antimicrobial resistances and virulence factors in *Staphylococcus aureus* isolates from meat products legally and illegally introduced to Germany. *PLoS One* 11:e0167864.

13. Queenan K, Häsler B, Rushton J. 2016. A One Health approach to antimicrobial resistance surveillance: is there a business case for it? *Int J Antimicrob Agents* 48:422–427.

14. D'Costa VM, King CE, Kalan L, Morar M, Sung WW, Schwarz C, Froese D, Zazula G, Calmels F, Debruyne R, Golding GB, Poinar HN, Wright GD. 2011. Antibiotic resistance is ancient. *Nature* 477:457–461.

15. Bhullar K, Waglechner N, Pawlowski A, Koteva K, Banks ED, Johnston MD, Barton HA, Wright GD. 2012. Antibiotic resistance is prevalent in an isolated cave microbiome. *PLoS One* 7:e34953.

16. Hall BG, Barlow M. 2004. Evolution of the serine β-lactamases: past, present and future. *Drug Resist Updat* 7:111–123.

17. Davey P, Brown E, Fenelon L, Finch R, Gould I, Hartman G, Holmes A, Ramsay C, Taylor E, Wilcox M, Wiffen P. 2005. Interventions to improve antibiotic prescribing practices for hospital inpatients. *Cochrane Database Syst Rev* Oct 19;(4):CD003543.

18. Davey P, Marwick CA, Scott CL, Charani E, McNeil K, Brown E, Gould IM, Ramsay CR, Michie S. 2017. Interventions to improve antibiotic prescribing practices for hospital inpatients. *Cochrane Database Syst Rev* Feb 9;2:CD003543.

19. Schuts EC, Hulscher MEJL, Mouton JW, Verduin CM, Stuart JWTC, Overdiek HWPM, van der Linden PD, Natsch S, Hertogh CMPM, Wolfs TFW, Schouten JA, Kullberg BJ, Prins JM. 2016. Current evidence on hospital antimicrobial stewardship objectives: a systematic review and meta-analysis. *Lancet Infect Dis* 16:847–856.

20. van de Beek D, de Gans J, Spanjaard L, Vermeulen M, Dankert J. 2002. Antibiotic guidelines and antibiotic use in adult bacterial meningitis in The Netherlands. *J Antimicrob Chemother* 49:661–666.

21. Brown EM. 2002. Guidelines for antibiotic usage in hospitals. *J Antimicrob Chemother* 49:587–592.

22. Principi N, Esposito S. 2016. Antimicrobial stewardship in paediatrics. *BMC Infect Dis* 16:424.

23. Charani E, Edwards R, Sevdalis N, Alexandrou B, Sibley E, Mullett D, Franklin BD, Holmes A. 2011. Behavior change strategies to influence antimicrobial prescribing in acute care: a systematic review. *Clin Infect Dis* 53:651–662.

24. Charani E, Castro-Sánchez E, Sevdalis N, Kyratsis Y, Drumright L, Shah N, Holmes A. 2013. Understanding the determinants of antimicrobial prescribing within hospitals: the role of "prescribing etiquette". *Clin Infect Dis* 57:188–196.

25. Mattick K, Kelly N, Rees C. 2014. A window into the lives of junior doctors: narrative interviews exploring antimicrobial prescribing experiences. *J Antimicrob Chemother* 69:2274–2283.

26. Parker HM, Mattick K. 2016. The determinants of antimicrobial prescribing among hospital doctors in England: a framework to inform tailored stewardship interventions. *Br J Clin Pharmacol* 82:431–440.

27. World Health Organization. 2017. *Critically Important Antimicrobials for Human Medicine*, 5th revision. World Health Organization, Geneva. http://www.who.int/foodsafety/publications/antimicrobials-fifth/en/.

28. World Organisation for Animal Health (OIE). 2015. OIE list of antimicrobials of veterinary importance. 2015. Available at http://www.oie.int/fileadmin/Home/eng/Our_scientific_expertise/docs/pdf/Eng_OIE_List_antimicrobials_May2015.pdf.

29. Tiong JJ, Loo JS, Mai CW. 2016. Global antimicrobial stewardship: a closer look at the formidable implementation challenges. *Front Microbiol* 7:1860.

30. Hajjou M, Krech L, Lane-Barlow C, Roth L, Pribluda VS, Phanouvong S, El-Hadri L, Evans L III, Raymond C, Yuan E, Siv L, Vuong TA, Boateng KP, Okafor R, Chibwe KM, Lukulay PH. 2015. Monitoring the quality of medicines: results from Africa, Asia, and South America. *Am J Trop Med Hyg* **92**(Suppl):68–74.

31. Kelesidis T, Falagas ME. 2015. Substandard/counterfeit antimicrobial drugs. *Clin Microbiol Rev* **28**:443–464.

32. Mackey TK, Nayyar G. 2016. Digital danger: a review of the global public health, patient safety and cybersecurity threats posed by illicit online pharmacies. *Br Med Bull* **118**:110–126.

33. Loeffler A, McCarthy A, Lloyd DH, Musilová E, Pfeiffer DU, Lindsay JA. 2013. Whole-genome comparison of meticillin-resistant *Staphylococcus aureus* CC22 SCC*mec*IV from people and their in-contact pets. *Vet Dermatol* **24**:538–e128.

34. DANMAP. 2014. *Use of Antimicrobial Agents and Occurrence of Antimicrobial Resistance in Bacteria from Food Animals, Food and Humans in Denmark.* http://www.danmap.org/~/media/Projekt%20sites/Danmap/DANMAP%20reports/DANMAP%202014/Danmap_2014.ashx.

35. Larsen J, Petersen A, Sørum M, Stegger M, van Alphen L, Valentiner-Branth P, Knudsen LK, Larsen LS, Feingold B, Price LB, Andersen PS, Larsen AR, Skov RL. 2015. Meticillin-resistant *Staphylococcus aureus* CC398 is an increasing cause of disease in people with no livestock contact in Denmark, 1999 to 2011. *Euro Surveill* **20**:30021.

36. Cuny C, Wieler LH, Witte W. 2015. Livestock-associated MRSA: the impact on humans. *Antibiotics (Basel)* **4**:521–543.

37. van der Mee-Marquet NL, Corvaglia A, Haenni M, Bertrand X, Franck JB, Kluytmans J, Girard M, Quentin R, François P. 2014. Emergence of a novel subpopulation of CC398 *Staphylococcus aureus* infecting animals is a serious hazard for humans. *Front Microbiol* **5**:652.

38. Grøntvedt CA, Elstrøm P, Stegger M, Skov RL, Skytt Andersen P, Larssen KW, Urdahl AM, Angen Ø, Larsen J, Åmdal S, Løtvedt SM, Sunde M, Bjørnholt JV. 2016. Methicillin-resistant *Staphylococcus aureus* CC398 in humans and pigs in Norway: a "One Health" perspective on introduction and transmission. *Clin Infect Dis* **63**:1431–1438.

39. Liebana E, Carattoli A, Coque TM, Hasman H, Magiorakos AP, Mevius D, Peixe L, Poirel L, Schuepbach-Regula G, Torneke K, Torren-Edo J, Torres C, Threlfall J. 2013. Public health risks of enterobacterial isolates producing extended-spectrum β-lactamases or AmpC β-lactamases in food and food-producing animals: an EU perspective of epidemiology, analytical methods, risk factors, and control options. *Clin Infect Dis* **56**:1030–1037.

40. Liu YY, Wang Y, Walsh TR, Yi LX, Zhang R, Spencer J, Doi Y, Tian G, Dong B, Huang X, Yu LF, Gu D, Ren H, Chen X, Lv L, He D, Zhou H, Liang Z, Liu JH, Shen J. 2016. Emergence of plasmid-mediated colistin resistance mechanism MCR-1 in animals and human beings in China: a microbiological and molecular biological study. *Lancet Infect Dis* **16**:161–168.

41. Skov RL, Monnet DL. 2016. Plasmid-mediated colistin resistance (*mcr-1* gene): three months later, the story unfolds. *Euro Surveill* **21**:30155.

42. European Medicines Agency. 2016. Updated advice on the use of colistin products in animals within the European Union: development of resistance and possible impact on human and animal health. http://www.ema.europa.eu/docs/en_GB/document_library/Scientific_guideline/2016/07/WC500211080.pdf.

43. Goldman JL, Jackson MA. 2015. Tip of the iceberg: understanding the unintended consequences of antibiotics. *Pediatrics* **136**:e492–e493.

44. Dethlefsen L, Huse S, Sogin ML, Relman DA. 2008. The pervasive effects of an antibiotic on the human gut microbiota, as revealed by deep 16S rRNA sequencing. *PLoS Biol* **6**:e280.

45. Bailey LC, Forrest CB, Zhang P, Richards TM, Livshits A, DeRusso PA. 2014. Association of antibiotics in infancy with early childhood obesity. *JAMA Pediatr* **168**:1063–1069.

46. Saari A, Virta LJ, Sankilampi U, Dunkel L, Saxen H. 2015. Antibiotic exposure in infancy and risk of being overweight in the first 24 months of life. *Pediatrics* **135**:617–626.

47. Scott FI, Horton DB, Mamtani R, Haynes K, Goldberg DS, Lee DY, Lewis JD. 2016. Administration of antibiotics to children before age 2 years increases risk for childhood obesity. *Gastroenterology* **151**:120–129.e5.

48. Horton DB, Scott FI, Haynes K, Putt ME, Rose CD, Lewis JD, Strom BL. 2015. Antibiotic exposure and juvenile idiopathic arthritis: a case–control study. *Pediatrics* **136**:e333–e343.

49. Buffington SA, Di Prisco GV, Auchtung TA, Ajami NJ, Petrosino JF, Costa-Mattioli M. 2016. Microbial reconstitution reverses maternal diet-induced social and synaptic deficits in offspring. *Cell* **165**:1762–1775.

50. Cogliani C, Goossens H, Greko C. 2011. Restricting antimicrobial use in food animals: lessons from Europe. *Microbe* **6**:274–279.

51. World Health Organization. 2015. *Global Action Plan on Antimicrobial Resistance.* http://www.wpro.who.int/entity/drug_resistance/resources/global_action_plan_eng.pdf.

52. Food and Agriculture Organisation of the United Nations. 2016. The FAO action plan on antimicrobial resistance 2016–2020. FAO Rome, September 2016. http://www.fao.org/3/a-i5996e.pdf.

53. World Health Organization, Food and Agriculture Organization, World Organisation for Animal Health. 2016. *Antimicrobial Resistance. A Manual for Developing National Action Plans, version 1.* http://apps.who.int/iris/bitstream/10665/204470/1/9789241549530_eng.pdf?ua=1.

54. FAO/WHO Codex Alimentarius. 2015. Codex texts on foodborne antimicrobial resistance. ftp://ftp.fao.org/codex/Publications/Booklets/Antimicrobial/Antimicrobial_2015Tri.pdf.

55. European Centre for Disease Prevention and Control. 2016. Antibiotic resistance strategies and action plans. http://

ecdc.europa.eu/en/healthtopics/Healthcare-associated_infections/guidance-infection-prevention-control/Pages/antimicrobial-resistance-strategies-action-plans.aspx. Accessed 20 December 2016.

56. **Commonwealth of Australia.** 2015. *Responding to the Threat of Antimicrobial Resistance. Australia's first National Antimicrobial Resistance Strategy 2015–2019.* Commonwealth of Australia, Canberra, Australia. https://www.amr.gov.au/australias-response/national-amr-strategy.

57. **Public Health Agency of Canada.** 2015. *Federal Action Plan on Antimicrobial Resistance and Use in Canada. Building on the Federal Framework for Action.* Public Health Agency of Canada, Ottawa, Canada. http://healthycanadians.gc.ca/alt/pdf/publications/drugs-products-medicaments-produits/antibiotic-resistance-antibiotique/action-plan-daction-eng.pdf. Accessed December 20 2016.

58. **The White House.** 2014. National strategy for combating antibiotic-resistant bacteria, September 2014. Available at http://obamawhitehouse.archives.gov/sites/default/files/docs/carb_national_strategy.pdf. Accessed December 20 2016.

59. **Elliott K.** 2015. Antibiotics on the farm: agriculture's role in drug resistance. CGD Policy Paper 59. Center for Global Development, Washington, DC. http://www.cgdev.org/publication/antibiotics-farm-agricultures-role-drug-resistance.

60. **Center for Veterinary Medicine (CVM).** 2017. FDA announces implementation of GFI #213, outlines continuing efforts to address antimicrobial resistance. http://www.fda.gov/AnimalVeterinary/NewsEvents/CVMUpdates/ucm535154.htm. Accessed 9 June 2017.

61. **Kimang'a AN.** 2012. A situational analysis of antimicrobial drug resistance in Africa: are we losing the battle? *Ethiop J Health Sci* 22:135–143.

62. **Nguyen KV, Thi Do NT, Chandna A, Nguyen TV, Pham CV, Doan PM, Nguyen AQ, Thi Nguyen CK, Larsson M, Escalante S, Olowokure B, Laxminarayan R, Gelband H, Horby P, Thi Ngo HB, Hoang MT, Farrar J, Hien TT, Wertheim HF.** 2013. Antibiotic use and resistance in emerging economies: a situation analysis for Viet Nam. *BMC Public Health* 13:1158.

63. **Huttner B, Harbarth S, Nathwani D, ESCMID Study Group for Antibiotic Policies (ESGAP).** 2014. Success stories of implementation of antimicrobial stewardship: a narrative review. *Clin Microbiol Infect* 20:954–962.

64. **Bender JB, Barlam TF, Glore RP, Gumley N, Grayzel SE, Hoang C, Murphy MJ, Papich MG, Sykes JE, Watts JL, Whichard JM, AVMA Task Force for Antimicrobial Stewardship in Companion Animal Practice.** 2015. Antimicrobial stewardship in companion animal practice. *J Am Vet Med Assoc* 246:287–288.

65. **Weese JS, Giguère S, Guardabassi L, Morley PS, Papich M, Ricciuto DR, Sykes JE.** 2015. ACVIM consensus statement on therapeutic antimicrobial use in animals and antimicrobial resistance. *J Vet Intern Med* 29:487–498.

66. **Prescott JF, Szkotnicki J, McClure JT, Reid-Smith RJ, Léger DF.** 2012. Conference report: antimicrobial stewardship in Canadian agriculture and veterinary medi-cine. How is Canada doing and what still needs to be done? *Can Vet J* 53:402–407.

67. **Weese JS, Blondeau JM, Boothe D, Breitschwerdt EB, Guardabassi L, Hillier A, Lloyd DH, Papich MG, Rankin SC, Turnidge JD, Sykes JE.** 2011. Antimicrobial use guidelines for treatment of urinary tract disease in dogs and cats: antimicrobial guidelines working group of the international society for companion animal infectious diseases. *Vet Med Int* 2011:263768.

68. **Hillier A, Lloyd DH, Weese JS, Blondeau JM, Boothe D, Breitschwerdt E, Guardabassi L, Papich MG, Rankin S, Turnidge JD, Sykes JE.** 2014. Guidelines for the diagnosis and antimicrobial therapy of canine superficial bacterial folliculitis (Antimicrobial Guidelines Working Group of the International Society for Companion Animal Infectious Diseases). *Vet Dermatol* 25:163–175, e42–e43.

69. **Lappin MR, Blondeau J, Boothe D, Breitschwerdt EB, Guardabassi L, Lloyd DH, Papich MG, Rankin SC, Sykes JE, Turnidge J, Weese JS.** 2017. Antimicrobial use guidelines for treatment of respiratory tract disease in dogs and cats: Antimicrobial Guidelines Working Group of the International Society for Companion Animal Infectious Diseases. *J Vet Intern Med* 31:279–294.

70. **European Commission Directorate-General for Health and Food Safety.** 2017. Final report of a fact-finding mission carried out in The Netherlands from 13 September 2016 to 20 September 2016 in order to gather information on the prudent use of antimicrobials in animals. Audit number 2016-8889, March 1 2017. http://ec.europa.eu/food/audits-analysis/audit_reports/details.cfm?rep_id=3753.

71. **Prescott JF, Boerlin P.** 2016. Antimicrobial use in companion animals and Good Stewardship Practice. *Vet Rec* 179:486–488.

72. **Barlam TF, Cosgrove SE, Abbo LM, MacDougall C, Schuetz AN, Septimus EJ, Srinivasan A, Dellit TH, Falck-Ytter YT, Fishman NO, Hamilton CW, Jenkins TC, Lipsett PA, Malani PN, May LS, Moran GJ, Neuhauser MM, Newland JG, Ohl CA, Samore MH, Seo SK, Trivedi KK.** 2016. Implementing an Antibiotic Stewardship Program: Guidelines by the Infectious Diseases Society of America and the Society for Healthcare Epidemiology of America. *Clin Infect Dis* 62:e51–e77.

73. **de With K, Allerberger F, Amann S, Apfalter P, Brodt H-R, Eckmanns T, Fellhauer M, Geiss HK, Janata O, Krause R, Lemmen S, Meyer E, Mittermayer H, Porsche U, Presterl E, Reuter S, Sinha B, Strauß R, Wechsler-Fördös A, Wenisch C, Kern WV.** 2016. Strategies to enhance rational use of antibiotics in hospital: a guideline by the German Society for Infectious Diseases. *Infection* 44:395–439.

74. **Doron S, Davidson LE.** 2011. Antimicrobial stewardship. *Mayo Clin Proc* 86:1113–1123.

75. **Duguid M, Cruickshank M (ed).** 2011. *Antimicrobial Stewardship in Australian Hospitals.* Australian Commission on Safety and Quality in Health Care, Sydney, Australia.

76. **Hanson A, Crank CW.** 2017. Development and execution of stewardship interventions, p 290–301. *In* LaPlante

KL, Cunha CB, Morrill HJ, Rice LB, Mylonakis E (ed), *Antimicrobial Stewardship: Principles and Practice.* CAB International, Wallingford, Oxfordshire, United Kingdom.

77. Jeffs L, Thampi N, Maione M, Steinberg M, Morris AM, Bell CM. 2015. A qualitative analysis of implementation of antimicrobial stewardship at 3 academic hospitals: understanding the key influences on success. *Can J Hosp Pharm* **68:**395–400.

78. LaPlante KL, Cunha CB, Morrill HJ, Rice LB, Mylonakis E. 2017. *Antimicrobial Stewardship: Principles and Practice.* CAB International, Wallingford, Oxfordshire, United Kingdom.

79. Laundy M, Gilchrist M, Whitney L. 2016. *Antimicrobial Stewardship.* Oxford University Press, Oxford, United Kingdom.

80. Pulcini C, Ergonul O, Can F, Beovic B. 2017. *Antimicrobial Stewardship.* Elsevier Science Publishing Co., Inc., San Diego, CA.

81. Sanchez GV, Fleming-Dutra KE, Roberts RM, Hicks LA. 2016. Core elements of outpatient antibiotic stewardship. *MMWR Recomm Rep* **65:**1–12.

82. Sedrak A, Anpalahan M, Luetsch K. 2017. Enablers and barriers to the use of antibiotic guidelines in the assessment and treatment of community-acquired pneumonia: a qualitative study of clinicians' perspectives. *Int J Clin Pract* **71:**e12959.

83. Sikkens JJ, van Agtmael MA, Peters EJG, Lettinga KD, van der Kuip M, Vandenbroucke-Grauls CMJE, Wagner C, Kramer MHH. 2017. Behavioral approach to appropriate antimicrobial prescribing in hospitals: The Dutch Unique Method for Antimicrobial Stewardship (DUMAS) participatory intervention study. *JAMA Intern Med* **177:**1130–1138.

84. van Buul LW, Sikkens JJ, van Agtmael MA, Kramer MHH, van der Steen JT, Hertogh CMPM. 2014. Participatory action research in antimicrobial stewardship: a novel approach to improving antimicrobial prescribing in hospitals and long-term care facilities. *J Antimicrob Chemother* **69:**1734–1741.

85. McDougall S, Compton C. 2015. Effect of infusing an internal teat sealant into a gland infected with a major pathogen. *Livestock (Lond)* **20:**194–200.

86. Postma M, Vanderhaeghen W, Sarrazin S, Maes D, Dewulf J. 2017. Reducing antimicrobial usage in pig production without jeopardizing production parameters. *Zoonoses Public Health* **64:**63–74.

87. Reyher KK, Barrett DC, Tisdall DA. 2017. Achieving responsible antimicrobial use: communicating with farmers. *In Pract* **39:**63–71.

88. Tisdall DA, Reyher KK, Barrett DC. 2017. Achieving responsible medicines use at practice and farm level. *In Pract* **39:**119–127.

89. van Dijk L, Hayton A, Main DCJ, Booth A, King A, Barrett DC, Buller HJ, Reyher KK. 2017. Participatory policy making by dairy producers to reduce anti-microbial use on farms. *Zoonoses Public Health* **64:**476–484.

90. Hurst AL, Child J, Pearce K, Palmer C, Todd JK, Parker SK. 2016. Handshake stewardship: a highly effective rounding-based antimicrobial optimization service. *Pediatr Infect Dis J* **35:**1104–1110.

91. Messacar K, Campbell K, Pearce K, Pyle L, Hurst AL, Child J, Parker SK. 2017. A handshake from antimicrobial stewardship opens doors for infectious disease consultations. *Clin Infect Dis* **64:**1449–1452.

92. Gorman A. 2017. Handshake-free zone: stopping the spread of germs in the hospital. *Medscape.* http://www.medscape.com/viewarticle/880856. Accessed 30 May 2017.

93. Giry M, Pulcini C, Rabaud C, Boivin JM, Mauffrey V, Birgé J. 2016. Acceptability of antibiotic stewardship measures in primary care. *Med Mal Infect* **46:**276–284.

94. Tamma PD, Avdic E, Keenan JF, Zhao Y, Anand G, Cooper J, Dezube R, Hsu S, Cosgrove SE. 2017. What is the more effective antibiotic stewardship intervention: pre-prescription authorization or post-prescription review with feedback? *Clin Infect Dis* **64:**537–543.

95. Hallsworth M, Chadborn T, Sallis A, Sanders M, Berry D, Greaves F, Clements L, Davies SC. 2016. Provision of social norm feedback to high prescribers of antibiotics in general practice: a pragmatic national randomised controlled trial. *Lancet* **387:**1743–1752.

96. Meeker D, Linder JA, Fox CR, Friedberg MW, Persell SD, Goldstein NJ, Knight TK, Hay JW, Doctor JN. 2016. Effect of behavioral interventions on inappropriate antibiotic prescribing among primary care practices: a randomized clinical trial. *JAMA* **315:**562–570.

97. Mitchell MW, Fowkes FG. 1985. Audit reviewed: does feedback on performance change clinical behaviour? *J R Coll Physicians Lond* **19:**251–254.

98. van Buul LW, van der Steen JT, Achterberg WP, Schellevis FG, Essink RTGM, de Greeff SC, Natsch S, Sloane PD, Zimmerman S, Twisk JWR, Veenhuizen RB, Hertogh CMPM. 2015. Effect of tailored antibiotic stewardship programmes on the appropriateness of antibiotic prescribing in nursing homes. *J Antimicrob Chemother* **70:**2153–2162.

99. Dunn F, Dunn J. 2012. Clinical audit: application in small animal practice. *In Pract* **34:**243–245.

100. Page S, Prescott J, Weese S. 2014. The 5Rs approach to antimicrobial stewardship. *Vet Rec* **175:**207–208.

101. Weese JS, Page SW, Prescott JF. 2013. Antimicrobial stewardship in animals, p 117–132. *In* Giguère S, Prescott JF, Dowling PM (ed), *Antimicrobial Therapy in Veterinary Medicine,* 5th ed. John Wiley & Sons, Inc., Ames, IA.

102. Guardabassi L, Prescott JF. 2015. Antimicrobial stewardship in small animal veterinary practice: from theory to practice. *Vet Clin North Am Small Anim Pract* **45:**361–376, vii.

103. Morris AM, Stewart TE, Shandling M, McIntaggart S, Liles WC. 2010. Establishing an antimicrobial stewardship program. *Healthc Q* **13:**64–70.

104. Traynor K. 2016. Smaller size no barrier to effective antimicrobial stewardship. *Am J Health Syst Pharm* **73:**1116–1120.

105. Turnidge J. 2015. Antimicrobial stewardship: what is it, and how does it work? *Anim Prod Sci* **55:**1432–1436.

106. Robb F, Seaton A. 2016. What are the principles and goals of antimicrobial stewardship? p 12–19. *In* Laundy M, Gilchrist M, Whitney L (ed), *Antimicrobial Stewardship.* Oxford University Press, Oxford, United Kingdom.

107. CDC. 2017. Core elements of hospital antibiotic stewardship programs. https://www.cdc.gov/getsmart/health care/implementation/core-elements.html. Accessed 1 March 2017.

108. Kwok YLA, Harris P, McLaws M-L. 2017. Social cohesion: the missing factor required for a successful hand hygiene program. *Am J Infect Control* 45:222–227.

109. Bonansea SJ. 1906. Veterinary hygiene: applied to the protection of man against zoonosis. *Public Health Pap Rep* 32:320–324.

110. Jones LM. 1955. Suggestions for antibiotic therapy. *Cornell Vet* 45:316–326.

111. Koblentz GD. 2010. Biosecurity reconsidered: calibrating biological threats and responses. *Int Secur* 34:96–132.

112. EMA (European Medicines Agency), EFSA (European Food Safety Authority). 2017. EMA and EFSA Joint Scientific Opinion on measures to reduce the need to use antimicrobial agents in animal husbandry in the European Union, and the resulting impacts on food safety (RONAFA). *EFSA J* 15(1).

113. Aviagen. 2014. *Ross Broiler Management Manual.* Aviagen, Newbridge, Midlothian, Scotland.

114. Cobb. 2013. *Cobb Broiler Management Guide.* Cobb-Vantress Inc, Siloam Springs, AK.

115. Green M, Bradley A, Breen J, Higgins H, Hudson C, Huxley J, Statham J, Green L, Hayton A. 2012. *Dairy Herd Health.* CABI, Wallingford, Oxfordshire, United Kingdom.

116. Sanderson M. 2009. Biosecurity for feedlot enterprises, p 633–636. *In* Anderson DE, Rings DM (ed), *Food Animal Practice,* 5th ed. W.B. Saunders, Saint Louis, MO.

117. Laanen M, Persoons D, Ribbens S, de Jong E, Callens B, Strubbe M, Maes D, Dewulf J. 2013. Relationship between biosecurity and production/antimicrobial treatment characteristics in pig herds. *Vet J* 198:508–512.

118. Palić D, Scarfe AD, Walster CI. 2015. A standardized approach for meeting national and international aquaculture biosecurity requirements for preventing, controlling, and eradicating infectious diseases. *J Appl Aquacult* 27:185–219.

119. Gelaude P, Schlepers M, Verlinden M, Laanen M, Dewulf J. 2014. Biocheck.UGent: a quantitative tool to measure biosecurity at broiler farms and the relationship with technical performances and antimicrobial use. *Poult Sci* 93:2740–2751.

120. DEFRA. 2017. *Biosecurity and Preventing Disease in Captive Birds within a Prevention Zone.* Department for Environment, Food & Rural Affairs, London, United Kingdom.

121. Burgess BA, Morley PS. 2015. Veterinary hospital surveillance systems. *Vet Clin North Am Small Anim Pract* 45:235–242, v.

122. Burgess BA, Morley PS. 2014. Infection control in equine critical care settings. *Vet Clin North Am Equine Pract* 30:467–474, ix–x.

123. Stull JW, Weese JS. 2015. Hospital-associated infections in small animal practice. *Vet Clin North Am Small Anim Pract* 45:217–233, v.

124. AVA. 2017. *Guidelines for Veterinary Personal Biosecurity,* 3rd ed. Australian Veterinary Association, St. Leonards, NSW, Australia.

125. Canadian Committee on Antibiotic Resistance. 2008. *Infection Prevention and Control Best Practices for Small Animal Veterinary Clinics.* Department of Pathobiology, University of Guelph, Guelph, Ontario, Canada.

126. Williams CJ, Scheftel JM, Elchos BL, Hopkins SG, Levine JF. 2015. Compendium of veterinary standard precautions for zoonotic disease prevention in veterinary personnel: National Association of State Public Health Veterinarians: Veterinary Infection Control Committee 2015. *J Am Vet Med Assoc* 247:1252–1277.

127. Bishop SC, Axford RFE, Nicholas FW, Owen JB. 2010. *Breeding for Disease Resistance in Farm Animals,* 3rd ed. CABI, Wallingford, Oxfordshire, United Kingdom.

128. Burkard C, Lillico SG, Reid E, Jackson B, Mileham AJ, Ait-Ali T, Whitelaw CBA, Archibald AL. 2017. Precision engineering for PRRSV resistance in pigs: macrophages from genome edited pigs lacking CD163 SRCR5 domain are fully resistant to both PRRSV genotypes while maintaining biological function. *PLoS Pathog* 13:e1006206.

129. Gadde U, Kim WH, Oh ST, Lillehoj HS. 2017. Alternatives to antibiotics for maximizing growth performance and feed efficiency in poultry: a review. *Anim Health Res Rev* 18:26–45.

130. Reiner G. 2016. Genetic resistance: an alternative for controlling PRRS? *Porcine Health Manag* 2:27.

131. Swaggerty CL, Pevzner IY, He H, Genovese KJ, Kogut MH. 2017. Selection for pro-inflammatory mediators produces chickens more resistant to *Campylobacter jejuni. Poult Sci* 96:1623–1627.

132. Whyte J, Blesbois E, McGrew MJ. 2016. Increased sustainability in poultry production: new tools and resources for genetic management. *In* Burton E, Gatcliffe J, O'Neill HM, Scholey D (ed), *Sustainable Poultry Production in Europe,* vol. 31. CABI, Wallingford, Oxfordshire, United Kingdom.

133. NORM/NORM-VET. 2016. *Usage of Antimicrobial Agents and Occurrence of Antimicrobial Resistance in Norway. 2015.* Tromsø/Oslo, Norway.

134. Fertner M, Toft N, Martin HL, Boklund A. 2016. A register-based study of the antimicrobial usage in Danish veal calves and young bulls. *Prev Vet Med* 131:41–47.

135. Bak H, Rathkjen PH. 2009. Reduced use of antimicrobials after vaccination of pigs against porcine proliferative enteropathy in a Danish SPF herd. *Acta Vet Scand* 51:1.

136. Beskow P, Söderlind O, Thafvelin B. 1989. *Actinobacillus (Haemophilus) pleuropneumoniae* infections in swine: serological investigations and vaccination trials in combination with environmental improvements. *Zentralbl Veterinarmed B* 36:487–494.

137. Kyriakis SC, Alexopoulos C, Vlemmas J, Sarris K, Lekkas S, Koutsoviti-Papadopoulou M, Saoulidis K.

2001. Field study on the efficacy of two different vaccination schedules with HYORESP in a *Mycoplasma hyopneumoniae*-infected commercial pig unit. *J Vet Med B Infect Dis Vet Public Health* **48:**675–684.

138. Maass P. 2016. Ileitis vaccine: an alternative to antibiotics? *Pig Prog (Doetinchem)* **32:**13–15.

139. Kleven SH. 2008. Control of avian mycoplasma infections in commercial poultry. *Avian Dis* **52:**367–374.

140. Hay KE, Barnes TS, Morton JM, Gravel JL, Commins MA, Horwood PF, Ambrose RC, Clements ACA, Mahony TJ. 2016. Associations between exposure to viruses and bovine respiratory disease in Australian feedlot cattle. *Prev Vet Med* **127:**121–133.

141. Hay KE, Morton JM, Clements ACA, Mahony TJ, Barnes TS. 2016. Associations between feedlot management practices and bovine respiratory disease in Australian feedlot cattle. *Prev Vet Med* **128:**23–32.

142. Hay KE, Morton JM, Mahony TJ, Clements ACA, Barnes TS. 2016. Associations between animal characteristic and environmental risk factors and bovine respiratory disease in Australian feedlot cattle. *Prev Vet Med* **125:**66–74.

143. Hay KE, Morton JM, Schibrowski ML, Clements ACA, Mahony TJ, Barnes TS. 2016. Associations between prior management of cattle and risk of bovine respiratory disease in feedlot cattle. *Prev Vet Med* **127:**37–43.

144. Elbers AR, Cromwijk WA, Hunneman WA, Tielen MJ. 1990. Log book registration of farms for slaughtering pigs in the Integrated Quality Control Project. I. Use of drugs and vaccines. *Tijdschr Diergeneeskd* (In Dutch.) **115:**249–261.

145. Elbers AR, Tielen MJ, Cromwijk WA, vd Voorst PH, Bais JT, Verhaegh G, de Bruyn AA. 1992. Logbook registration in slaughtering pig farms within the project Integrated Quality Control. II. Drug utilization in relation to clinical observation, farm conditions and prevalence of pathological findings. *Tijdschr Diergeneeskd* (In Dutch.) **117:**41–48.

146. Greko C. 2013. Reduction of sales of antimicrobials for dogs: Swedish experiences. *Eur J Companion Anim Pract* **23:**55–60.

147. Allen HK, Trachsel J, Looft T, Casey TA. 2014. Finding alternatives to antibiotics. *Ann N Y Acad Sci* **1323:**91–100.

148. Cheng G, Hao H, Xie S, Wang X, Dai M, Huang L, Yuan Z. 2014. Antibiotic alternatives: the substitution of antibiotics in animal husbandry? *Front Microbiol* **5:**217.

149. Gao Y, Wu H, Wang Y, Liu X, Chen L, Li Q, Cui C, Liu X, Zhang J, Zhang Y. 2017. Single Cas9 nickase induced generation of *NRAMP1* knockin cattle with reduced off-target effects. *Genome Biol* **18:**13.

150. United States Department of Agriculture and World Organisation for Animal Health. 2016. 2nd International Symposium on Alternatives to Antibiotics (ATA). *Challenges and Solutions in Animal Production.* https://www.ars.usda.gov/alternativestoantibiotics/Symposium2016/ATA%20Abstracts%202016.pdf.

151. Palamidi I, Paraskeuas V, Theodorou G, Breitsma R, Schatzmayr G, Theodoropoulos G, Fegeros K,

152. Mountzouris KC. 2017. Effects of dietary acidifier supplementation on broiler growth performance, digestive and immune function indices. *Anim Prod Sci* **57:**271–281.

152. Lynch H, Leonard FC, Walia K, Lawlor PG, Duffy G, Fanning S, Markey BK, Brady C, Gardiner GE, Argüello H. 2017. Investigation of in-feed organic acids as a low cost strategy to combat *Salmonella* in grower pigs. *Prev Vet Med* **139(Pt A):**50–57.

153. Finck DN, Ribeiro FRBP, Burdick NC, Parr SL, Carroll JA, Young TR, Bernhard BC, Corley JR, Estefan AG, Rathmann RJ, Johnson BJ. 2014. Yeast supplementation alters the performance and health status of receiving cattle. *Prof Anim Sci* **30:**333–341.

154. Mountzouris KC, Dalaka E, Palamidi I, Paraskeuas V, Demey V, Theodoropoulos G, Fegeros K. 2015. Evaluation of yeast dietary supplementation in broilers challenged or not with *Salmonella* on growth performance, cecal microbiota composition and *Salmonella* in ceca, cloacae and carcass skin. *Poult Sci* **94:**2445–2455.

155. Vohra A, Syal P, Madan A. 2016. Probiotic yeasts in livestock sector. *Anim Feed Sci Technol* **219:**31–47.

156. Banerjee G, Ray AK. 2017. The advancement of probiotics research and its application in fish farming industries. *Res Vet Sci* **115:**66–77.

157. Callaway TR, Edrington TS, Byrd JA, Nisbet DJ, Ricke SC. 2017. Use of direct-fed microbials in layer hen production: performance response and salmonella control, p 301–322. *In* Ricke S, Gast R (ed), *Producing Safe Eggs.* Academic Press, San Diego, CA.

158. Wisener LV, Sargeant JM, O'Connor AM, Faires MC, Glass-Kaastra SK. 2015. The use of direct-fed microbials to reduce shedding of *Escherichia coli* O157 in beef cattle: a systematic review and meta-analysis. *Zoonoses Public Health* **62:**75–89.

159. Ducatelle R, Eeckhaut V, Haesebrouck F, Van Immerseel F. 2015. A review on prebiotics and probiotics for the control of dysbiosis: present status and future perspectives. *Animal* **9:**43–48.

160. Hoseinifar SH, Esteban MA, Cuesta A, Sun Y. 2015. Prebiotics and fish immune response: a review of current knowledge and future perspectives. *Rev Fish Sci Aquacult* **23:**315–328.

161. Rose L, Rose J, Gosling S, Holmes M. 2017. Efficacy of a probiotic-prebiotic supplement on incidence of diarrhea in a dog shelter: a randomized, double-blind, placebo-controlled trial. *J Vet Intern Med* **31:**377–382.

162. Stover MG, Watson RR, Collier RJ. 2016. Pre- and probiotic supplementation in ruminant livestock production, p 25–36. *In* Preedy VR, Watson RR (ed), *Probiotics, Prebiotics, and Synbiotics: Bioactive Foods in Health Promotion.* Academic Press, San Diego, CA.

163. Ben Lagha A, Haas B, Gottschalk M, Grenier D. 2017. Antimicrobial potential of bacteriocins in poultry and swine production. *Vet Res (Faisalabad)* **48:**22.

164. Wang S, Zeng X, Yang Q, Qiao S. 2016. Antimicrobial peptides as potential alternatives to antibiotics in food animal industry. *Int J Mol Sci* **17:**E603.

165. Carvalho C, Costa AR, Silva F, Oliveira A. 2017. Bacteriophages and their derivatives for the treatment and control of food-producing animal infections. *Crit Rev Microbiol* 43:583–601.

166. Doss J, Culbertson K, Hahn D, Camacho J, Barekzi N. 2017. A review of phage therapy against bacterial pathogens of aquatic and terrestrial organisms. *Viruses* 9:E50.

167. Oechslin F, Piccardi P, Mancini S, Gabard J, Moreillon P, Entenza JM, Resch G, Que YA. 2017. Synergistic interaction between phage therapy and antibiotics clears *Pseudomonas aeruginosa* infection in endocarditis and reduces virulence. *J Infect Dis* 215:703–712.

168. Porter J, Anderson J, Carter L, Donjacour E, Paros M. 2016. *In vitro* evaluation of a novel bacteriophage cocktail as a preventative for bovine coliform mastitis. *J Dairy Sci* 99:2053–2062.

169. Richards GP. 2014. Bacteriophage remediation of bacterial pathogens in aquaculture: a review of the technology. *Bacteriophage* 4:e975540.

170. Verstappen KM, Tulinski P, Duim B, Fluit AC, Carney J, van Nes A, Wagenaar JA. 2016. The effectiveness of bacteriophages against methicillin-resistant *Staphylococcus aureus* ST398 nasal colonization in pigs. *PLoS One* 11:e0160242.

171. Wagenaar JA, Van Bergen MA, Mueller MA, Wassenaar TM, Carlton RM. 2005. Phage therapy reduces *Campylobacter jejuni* colonization in broilers. *Vet Microbiol* 109:275–283.

172. Hammer KA, Carson CF. 2011. Antibacterial and antifungal activities of essential oils, p 255–306. *In* Thormar H (ed), *Lipids and Essential Oils as Antimicrobial Agents*. John Wiley & Sons, Ltd., Chichester, United Kingdom.

173. Chávez-González ML, Rodríguez-Herrera R, Aguilar CN. 2016. Essential oils: a natural alternative to combat antibiotics resistance, p 227–237. *In* Kon K, Rai M (ed), *Antibiotic Resistance. Mechanisms and New Antimicrobial Approaches*. Academic Press, San Diego CA.

174. Maruhashi E, Braz BS, Nunes T, Pomba C, Belas A, Duarte-Correia JH, Lourenço AM. 2016. Efficacy of medical grade honey in the management of canine otitis externa: a pilot study. *Vet Dermatol* 27:93-8e27.

175. Timsit E, Workentine M, Crepieux T, Miller C, Regev-Shoshani G, Schaefer A, Alexander T. 2017. Effects of nasal instillation of a nitric oxide-releasing solution or parenteral administration of tilmicosin on the nasopharyngeal microbiota of beef feedlot cattle at high-risk of developing respiratory tract disease. *Res Vet Sci* 115:117–124.

176. Shatzkes K, Connell ND, Kadouri DE. 2017. Predatory bacteria: a new therapeutic approach for a post-antibiotic era. *Future Microbiol* 12:469–472.

177. Tyson J, Sockett RE. 2017. Predatory bacteria: moving from curiosity towards curative. *Trends Microbiol* 25:90–91.

178. Gadde U, Rathinam T, Lillehoj HS. 2015. Passive immunization with hyperimmune egg-yolk IgY as prophylaxis and therapy for poultry diseases: a review. *Anim Health Res Rev* 16:163–176.

179. Li X, Wang L, Zhen Y, Li S, Xu Y. 2015. Chicken egg yolk antibodies (IgY) as non-antibiotic production enhancers for use in swine production: a review. *J Anim Sci Biotechnol* 6:40.

180. Xu Y, Li X, Jin L, Zhen Y, Lu Y, Li S, You J, Wang L. 2011. Application of chicken egg yolk immunoglobulins in the control of terrestrial and aquatic animal diseases: a review. *Biotechnol Adv* 29:860–868.

181. Niewold TA, van Dijk AJ, Geenen PL, Roodink H, Margry R, van der Meulen J. 2007. Dietary specific antibodies in spray-dried immune plasma prevent enterotoxigenic *Escherichia coli* F4 (ETEC) post weaning diarrhoea in piglets. *Vet Microbiol* 124:362–369.

182. Torrallardona D. 2010. Spray dried animal plasma as an alternative to antibiotics in weanling pigs: a review. *Asian-Australas J Anim Sci* 23:131–148.

183. McDougall S, Compton C, Botha N. 2017. Factors influencing antimicrobial prescribing by veterinarians and usage by dairy farmers in New Zealand. *N Z Vet J* 65:84–92.

184. Ruiz R, Tedeschi LO, Sepúlveda A. 2017. Investigation of the effect of pegbovigrastim on some periparturient immune disorders and performance in Mexican dairy herds. *J Dairy Sci* 100:3305–3317.

185. Lloyd DH. 2012. Alternatives to conventional antimicrobial drugs: a review of future prospects. *Vet Dermatol* 23:299–304, e259–260.

186. Schoster A, Guardabassi L, Staempfli HR, Abrahams M, Jalali M, Weese JS. 2016. The longitudinal effect of a multi-strain probiotic on the intestinal bacterial microbiota of neonatal foals. *Equine Vet J* 48:689–696.

187. Schoster A, Weese JS, Guardabassi L. 2014. Probiotic use in horses: what is the evidence for their clinical efficacy? *J Vet Intern Med* 28:1640–1652.

188. Frank LA, Loeffler A. 2012. Meticillin-resistant *Staphylococcus pseudintermedius*: clinical challenge and treatment options. *Vet Dermatol* 23:283–291, e256.

189. Karki S, Cheng AC. 2012. Impact of non-rinse skin cleansing with chlorhexidine gluconate on prevention of healthcare-associated infections and colonization with multi-resistant organisms: a systematic review. *J Hosp Infect* 82:71–84.

190. Jeffers JG. 2013. Topical therapy for drug-resistant pyoderma in small animals. *Vet Clin North Am Small Anim Pract* 43:41–50.

191. Poole K. 2017. At the nexus of antibiotics and metals: the impact of Cu and Zn on antibiotic activity and resistance. *Trends Microbiol* 25:820–832.

192. Slifierz MJ, Friendship RM, Weese JS. 2015. Methicillin-resistant *Staphylococcus aureus* in commercial swine herds is associated with disinfectant and zinc usage. *Appl Environ Microbiol* 81:2690–2695.

193. Vahjen W, Pietruszyńska D, Starke IC, Zentek J. 2015. High dietary zinc supplementation increases the occurrence of tetracycline and sulfonamide resistance genes in the intestine of weaned pigs. *Gut Pathog* 7:23.

194. Amachawadi RG, Scott HM, Alvarado CA, Mainini TR, Vinasco J, Drouillard JS, Nagaraja TG. 2013. Occurrence of the transferable copper resistance gene *tcrB*

among fecal enterococci of U.S. feedlot cattle fed copper-supplemented diets. *Appl Environ Microbiol* 79: 4369–4375.

195. Hasman H, Kempf I, Chidaine B, Cariolet R, Ersbøll AK, Houe H, Bruun Hansen HC, Aarestrup FM. 2006. Copper resistance in *Enterococcus faecium*, mediated by the *tcrB* gene, is selected by supplementation of pig feed with copper sulfate. *Appl Environ Microbiol* 72: 5784–5789.

196. Aperce CC, Amachawadi R, Van Bibber-Krueger CL, Nagaraja TG, Scott HM, Vinasco-Torre J, Drouillard JS. 2016. Effects of menthol supplementation in feedlot cattle diets on the fecal prevalence of antimicrobial-resistant *Escherichia coli*. *PLoS One* 11:e0168983.

197. Rodríguez-Rojas A, Rodríguez-Beltrán J, Valverde J, Blázquez J. 2015. Can clays in livestock feed promote antibiotic resistance and virulence in pathogenic bacteria? *Antibiotics (Basel)* 4:299–308.

198. Kubicek-Sutherland JZ, Lofton H, Vestergaard M, Hjort K, Ingmer H, Andersson DI. 2017. Antimicrobial peptide exposure selects for *Staphylococcus aureus* resistance to human defence peptides. *J Antimicrob Chemother* 72:115–127.

199. O'Neill J (chair). 2015. Review on antimicrobial resistance. Rapid diagnostics: stopping unnecessary use of antibiotics. https://amr-review.org/sites/default/files/Rapid%20Diagnostics%20-%20Stopping%20Unnecessary%20use%20of%20Antibiotics.pdf.

200. Timsit E, Dendukuri N, Schiller I, Buczinski S. 2016. Diagnostic accuracy of clinical illness for bovine respiratory disease (BRD) diagnosis in beef cattle placed in feedlots: a systematic literature review and hierarchical Bayesian latent-class meta-analysis. *Prev Vet Med* 135: 67–73.

201. Griffin D. 2009. Respiratory disease treatment considerations in feedyards, p 509–519. *In* Anderson DE, Rings DM (ed), *Food Animal Practice*, 5th ed. W.B. Saunders, Saint Louis, MO.

202. European Commission. 2017. Commission awards €1 million to breakthrough test which distinguishes between viral or bacterial infections. http://europa.eu/rapid/press-release_IP-17-205_en.htm.

203. Nesta. 2017. Longitude prize. https://longitudeprize.org/. Accessed 1 March 2017.

204. Okeke IN, Peeling RW, Goossens H, Auckenthaler R, Olmsted SS, de Lavison JF, Zimmer BL, Perkins MD, Nordqvist K. 2011. Diagnostics as essential tools for containing antibacterial resistance. *Drug Resist Updat* 14:95–106.

205. Colles FM, Cain RJ, Nickson T, Smith AL, Roberts SJ, Maiden MCJ, Lunn D, Dawkins MS. 2016. Monitoring chicken flock behaviour provides early warning of infection by human pathogen *Campylobacter*. *Proc Biol Sci* 283:283.

206. Dawkins MS, Roberts SJ, Cain RJ, Nickson T, Donnelly CA. 2017. Early warning of footpad dermatitis and hockburn in broiler chicken flocks using optical flow, bodyweight and water consumption. *Vet Rec* 180:499.

207. De Montis A, Pinna A, Barra M, Vranken E. 2013. Analysis of poultry eating and drinking behavior by software eYeNamic. *J Agric Eng Res* 44:166–173.

208. Matthews SG, Miller AL, Clapp J, Plötz T, Kyriazakis I. 2016. Early detection of health and welfare compromises through automated detection of behavioural changes in pigs. *Vet J* 217:43–51.

209. Johnston D, Kenny DA, McGee M, Waters SM, Kelly AK, Earley B. 2016. Electronic feeding behavioural data as indicators of health status in dairy calves. *Ir J Agric Food Res* 55:159.

210. Jackson KS, Carstens GE, Tedeschi LO, Pinchak WE. 2016. Changes in feeding behavior patterns and dry matter intake before clinical symptoms associated with bovine respiratory disease in growing bulls. *J Anim Sci* 94:1644–1652.

211. White BJ, Goehl DR, Amrine DE, Booker C, Wildman B, Perrett T. 2016. Bayesian evaluation of clinical diagnostic test characteristics of visual observations and remote monitoring to diagnose bovine respiratory disease in beef calves. *Prev Vet Med* 126:74–80.

212. Wolfger B, Schwartzkopf-Genswein KS, Barkema HW, Pajor EA, Levy M, Orsel K. 2015. Feeding behavior as an early predictor of bovine respiratory disease in North American feedlot systems. *J Anim Sci* 93:377–385.

213. Ferrari S, Silva M, Guarino M, Aerts JM, Berckmans D. 2008. Cough sound analysis to identify respiratory infection in pigs. *Comput Electron Agric* 64:318–325.

214. Vandermeulen J, Bahr C, Johnston D, Earley B, Tullo E, Fontana I, Guarino M, Exadaktylos V, Berckmans D. 2016. Early recognition of bovine respiratory disease in calves using automated continuous monitoring of cough sounds. *Comput Electron Agric* 129:15–26.

215. Mang AV, Buczinski S, Booker CW, Timsit E. 2015. Evaluation of a computer-aided lung auscultation system for diagnosis of bovine respiratory disease in feedlot cattle. *J Vet Intern Med* 29:1112–1116.

216. Schaefer AL, Cook NJ, Bench C, Chabot JB, Colyn J, Liu T, Okine EK, Stewart M, Webster JR. 2012. The non-invasive and automated detection of bovine respiratory disease onset in receiver calves using infrared thermography. *Res Vet Sci* 93:928–935.

217. Martínez-Avilés M, Fernández-Carrión E, López García-Baones JM, Sánchez-Vizcaíno JM. 2017. Early detection of infection in pigs through an online monitoring system. *Transbound Emerg Dis* 64:364–373.

218. Abdallah A, Hewson J, Francoz D, Selim H, Buczinski S. 2016. Systematic review of the diagnostic accuracy of haptoglobin, serum amyloid A, and fibrinogen versus clinical reference standards for the diagnosis of bovine respiratory disease. *J Vet Intern Med* 30:1356–1368.

219. Cray C. 2012. Acute phase proteins in animals. *Prog Mol Biol Transl Sci* 105:113–150.

220. Schneider A. 2015. Acute phase proteins for diagnosis of diseases in dairy cattle. *Vet J* 205:333–334.

221. Guardabassi L, Hedberg S, Jessen LR, Damborg P. 2015. Optimization and evaluation of Flexicult Vet for detection, identification and antimicrobial susceptibility

testing of bacterial uropathogens in small animal veterinary practice. *Acta Vet Scand* 57:72.

222. Madoz LV, Prunner I, Jaureguiberry M, Gelfert CC, de la Sota RL, Giuliodori MJ, Drillich M. 2017. Application of a bacteriological on-farm test to reduce antimicrobial usage in dairy cows with purulent vaginal discharge. *J Dairy Sci* 100:3875–3882.

223. Bosward KL, House JK, Deveridge A, Mathews K, Sheehy PA. 2016. Development of a loop-mediated isothermal amplification assay for the detection of *Streptococcus agalactiae* in bovine milk. *J Dairy Sci* 99:2142–2150.

224. Hasman H, Saputra D, Sicheritz-Ponten T, Lund O, Svendsen CA, Frimodt-Møller N, Aarestrup FM. 2014. Rapid whole-genome sequencing for detection and characterization of microorganisms directly from clinical samples. *J Clin Microbiol* 52:139–146.

225. Kinoshita Y, Niwa H, Katayama Y. 2015. Use of loop-mediated isothermal amplification to detect six groups of pathogens causing secondary lower respiratory bacterial infections in horses. *Microbiol Immunol* 59:365–370.

226. Li Y, Fan P, Zhou S, Zhang L. 2017. Loop-mediated isothermal amplification (LAMP): a novel rapid detection platform for pathogens. *Microb Pathog* 107:54–61.

227. Oved K, Cohen A, Boico O, Navon R, Friedman T, Etshtein L, Kriger O, Bamberger E, Fonar Y, Yacobov R, Wolchinsky R, Denkberg G, Dotan Y, Hochberg A, Reiter Y, Grupper M, Srugo I, Feigin P, Gorfine M, Chistyakov I, Dagan R, Klein A, Potasman I, Eden E. 2015. A novel host-proteome signature for distinguishing between acute bacterial and viral infections. *PLoS One* 10:e0120012.

228. Jacob ME, Crowell MD, Fauls MB, Griffith EH, Ferris KK. 2016. Diagnostic accuracy of a rapid immunoassay for point of-care detection of urinary tract infection in dogs. *Am J Vet Res* 77:162–166.

229. Seidel C, Peters S, Eschbach E, Feßler AT, Oberheitmann B, Schwarz S. 2017. Development of a nucleic acid lateral flow immunoassay (NALFIA) for reliable, simple and rapid detection of the methicillin resistance genes *mecA* and *mecC*. *Vet Microbiol* 200:101–106.

230. Lago A, Godden SM, Bey R, Ruegg PL, Leslie K. 2011. The selective treatment of clinical mastitis based on on-farm culture results. I. Effects on antibiotic use, milk withholding time, and short-term clinical and bacteriological outcomes. *J Dairy Sci* 94:4441–4456.

231. Lago A, Godden SM, Bey R, Ruegg PL, Leslie K. 2011. The selective treatment of clinical mastitis based on on-farm culture results. II. Effects on lactation performance, including clinical mastitis recurrence, somatic cell count, milk production, and cow survival. *J Dairy Sci* 94:4457–4467.

232. Vasquez AK, Nydam DV, Capel MB, Eicker S, Virkler PD. 2017. Clinical outcome comparison of immediate blanket treatment versus a delayed pathogen-based treatment protocol for clinical mastitis in a New York dairy herd. *J Dairy Sci* 100:2992–3003.

233. Higgins HM, Golding SE, Mouncey J, Nanjiani I, Cook AJ. 2017. Understanding veterinarians' prescribing decisions on antibiotic dry cow therapy. *J Dairy Sci* 100:2909–2916.

234. Scherpenzeel CGM, den Uijl IEM, van Schaik G, Riekerink RGMO, Hogeveen H, Lam TJGM. 2016. Effect of different scenarios for selective dry-cow therapy on udder health, antimicrobial usage, and economics. *J Dairy Sci* 99:3753–3764.

235. Courvalin P. 2008. Can pharmacokinetic-pharmacodynamic parameters provide dosing regimens that are less vulnerable to resistance? *Clin Microbiol Infect* 14:989–994.

236. Ehrlich P. 1913. Address in pathology on chemotherapeutics. Scientific principles, methods, and results. *Lancet* 182:445–451.

237. Lhermie G, Gröhn YT, Raboisson D. 2017. Addressing antimicrobial resistance: an overview of priority actions to prevent suboptimal antimicrobial use in food-animal production. *Front Microbiol* 7:2114.

238. Martinez MN, Papich MG, Drusano GL. 2012. Dosing regimen matters: the importance of early intervention and rapid attainment of the pharmacokinetic/pharmacodynamic target. *Antimicrob Agents Chemother* 56:2795–2805.

239. Bajwa J. 2016. Canine superficial pyoderma and therapeutic considerations. *Can Vet J* 57:204–206.

240. Collineau L, Belloc C, Stärk KDC, Hémonic A, Postma M, Dewulf J, Chauvin C. 2017. Guidance on the selection of appropriate indicators for quantification of antimicrobial usage in humans and animals. *Zoonoses Public Health* 64:165–184.

241. James R, Upjohn L, Cotta M, Luu S, Marshall C, Buising K, Thursky K. 2015. Measuring antimicrobial prescribing quality in Australian hospitals: development and evaluation of a national antimicrobial prescribing survey tool. *J Antimicrob Chemother* 70:1912–1918.

242. Kallen MC, Prins JM. 2017. A systematic review of quality indicators for appropriate antibiotic use in hospitalized adult patients. *Infect Dis Rep* 9:6821.

243. Retamar P, Martín ML, Molina J, del Arco A. 2013. Evaluating the quality of antimicrobial prescribing: is standardisation possible? *Enferm Infecc Microbiol Clin* 31(Suppl 4):25–30.

244. Schouten JA, Berrevoets MAH, Hulscher ME. 2017. Quality indicators to measure appropriate antibiotic use: some thoughts on the black box. *Clin Infect Dis* 64:1295.

245. Spivak ES, Cosgrove SE, Srinivasan A. 2016. Measuring appropriate antimicrobial use: attempts at opening the black box. *Clin Infect Dis* 63:1639–1644.

246. Schwartz DN, Wu US, Lyles RD, Xiang Y, Kieszkowski P, Hota B, Weinstein RA. 2009. Lost in translation? Reliability of assessing inpatient antimicrobial appropriateness with use of computerized case vignettes. *Infect Control Hosp Epidemiol* 30:163–171.

247. van den Bosch CM, Hulscher ME, Natsch S, Wille J, Prins JM, Geerlings SE. 2016. Applicability of generic quality indicators for appropriate antibiotic use in daily hospital practice: a cross-sectional point-prevalence multicenter study. *Clin Microbiol Infect* 22:888.e1–888.e9.

Index

A

Abortion, listeriosis in food-producing animals, 241–242

Acinetobacter spp.
acquired carbapenem resistance mechanisms, 381
acquired resistance, 378
antimicrobial resistance in, 378–379
antimicrobial resistance in, from companion animals, 380–381
antimicrobial resistance in, from food-producing animals, 379–380
infections in animal hosts, 377–381
intrinsic resistance, 378
lethality of infections, 377
overview of, 381
sequence types, 381

Acinetobacter baumannii, 296, 387
acquired resistance, 378
aminoglycosides resistance in, 378–379
common mobile genetic elements in, 379
fluoroquinolones resistance, 379
intrinsic resistance, 378
β-lactam resistance in, 378
overview of, 381
public health concern, 378
resistance mechanism, 113
resistance to antibiotics in, 379

Acquired resistance
Acinetobacter spp., 378
Clostridium difficile, 454–455
Pseudomonas aeruginosa, 383

Actinobacillus spp., 331–332
antimicrobial resistance genes and mutations, 336–337
antimicrobial susceptibility, 332–335
dissemination, coselection and persistence of resistance genes in, 354–356
macrolides resistance, 350
streptomycin and/or spectinomycin resistance, 343
subset of resistance plasmids in, 344–345
sulfonamide resistance, 348–349
tetracyclines resistance, 335, 338–339, 341

Actinobacillus pleuropneumoniae, 17
fluoroquinolones resistance, 354
gentamicin resistance, 347
β-lactam resistance, 341, 343
lincosamides resistance, 350
macrolide resistance, 350
percentages of resistance against antimicrobial agents, 334
phenicols resistance, 351–352
structure and organization of genes in plasmids from, 338, 339
structure and organization of plasmids from, 340, 342, 346, 353
subset of resistance plasmids in, 344, 345
tetracyclines resistance, 335, 339, 341
trimethoprim resistance, 349

Actinobacillus porcitonsillarum
gentamicin resistance, 347
macrolide resistance, 350
structure and organization of plasmids from, 342, 346
trimethoprim resistance, 349

Actionobacillus pleuropneumoniae, macrolides resistance, 350

Aeromonas spp., heavy metal resistance, 89

Aeromonas salmonicida, 502, 503–504, 512, 513

Agar dilution
for anaerobic bacteria, 448
heavy metal method, 89
method and test conditions, 397

Agar disk diffusion, method and test conditions, 397

AGISAR (Advisory Group on Integrated Surveillance of Antimicrobial Resistance), World Health Organization, 578

Alcaligenaceae family, *Bordetella bronchiseptica*, 365

Aluvibrio salmonicida, 502, 509

American Association of Bovine Practitioners, 649

American College of Veterinary Internal Medicine, 679

American Veterinary Medical Association, 679

Amikacin, 2

Aminocyclitols
animal staphylococci resistance to, 137–138
Bordetella bronchiseptica resistance, 371
human and animal use, 600
origins of, 52
resistance of *Pasturellaceae* family, 343, 347–348
resistance to, 60–61

699